MW00989346

Master Techniques in Orthopaedic Surgery®

Reconstructive Knee Surgery

FOURTH EDITION

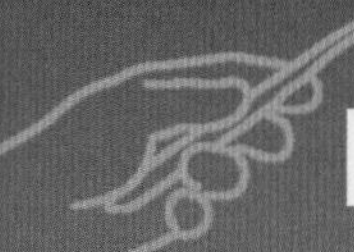

Master Techniques in Orthopaedic Surgery®

Reconstructive Knee Surgery

FOURTH EDITION

Darren L. Johnson, MD
Professor and Chairman
Department of Orthopaedic Surgery
Director of Sports Medicine
University of Kentucky School of Medicine
Lexington, Kentucky

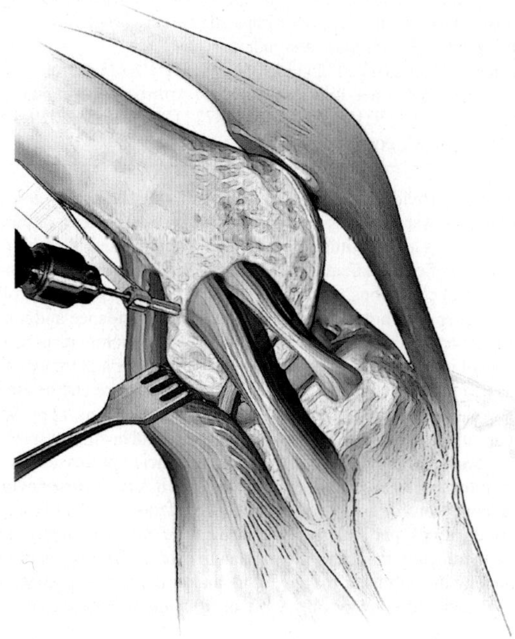

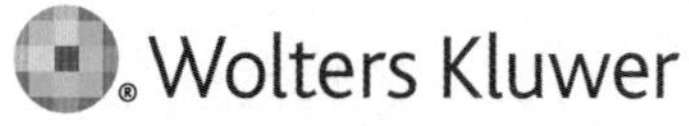
Wolters Kluwer

Philadelphia • Baltimore • New York • London
Buenos Aires • Hong Kong • Sydney • Tokyo

Acquisitions Editor: Brian Brown
Editorial Coordinator: Dave Murphy
Marketing Manager: Daniel Dressler
Production Project Manager: David Saltzberg
Design Coordinator: Stephen Druding
Manufacturing Coordinator: Beth Welsh
Prepress Vendor: SPi Global

4th edition

9 8 7 6 5 4 3 2 1

Printed in China

Library of Congress Cataloging-in-Publication Data
Names: Johnson, Darren L., editor.
Title: Reconstructive knee surgery / [edited by] Darren L. Johnson.
Other titles: Master techniques in orthopaedic surgery.
Description: Fourth edition. | Philadelphia : Wolters Kluwer, [2017] | Series: Master techniques in orthopaedic surgery | Includes bibliographical references and index.
Identifiers: LCCN 2017007255 | ISBN 9781496318275 (hardback)
Subjects: | MESH: Knee Injuries—surgery | Arthroscopy—methods | Knee Joint—surgery
Classification: LCC RD561 | NLM WE 872 | DDC 617.5/82059—dc23 LC record available at https://lccn.loc.gov/2017007255

LWW.com

Contributors

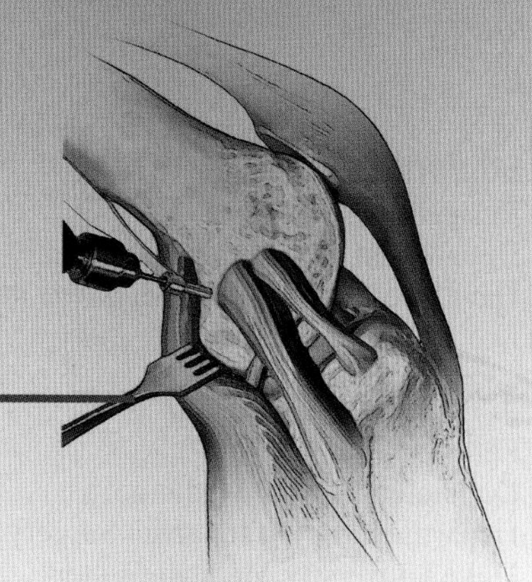

Christopher S. Ahmad, MD
Head Team Physician New York Yankees
Vice Chair of Clinical Research
Chief, Sports Medicine Service
Co-Director, Center for Shoulder, Elbow, and Sports Medicine
Director, Pediatric and Adolescent Sports Medicine, Biomechanics Research
Professor of Orthopaedic Surgery
Columbia University Medical Center
New York, New York

Eduard Alentorn-Geli, MD, PhD, MSc, FEBOT
Fellow
Division of Sports Medicine
Department of Orthopaedic Surgery
Duke University Medical Center
Durham, North Carolina

Annunziato Amendola, MD
Professor and Vice Chair
Department of Orthopaedic Surgery
Chief, Division of Sports Medicine
Duke University
Durham, North Carolina

Allen F. Anderson, MD
Physician
Department of Orthopaedics
Tennessee Orthopaedic Alliance
St. Thomas Hospital
Nashville, Tennessee

Christian N. Anderson, MD
Tennessee Orthopaedic Alliance
Nashville, Tennessee

Robert A. Arciero, MD
Professor, Orthopaedics
University of Connecticut Health Center
Director, Orthopaedic Sports Medicine Fellowship
Orthopaedic Team Physician
University of Connecticut
Farmington, Connecticut

Davide E. Bonasia, MD
Department of Orthopaedics and Traumatology
University of Torino
Torino, Italy

Craig R. Bottoni, MD
Chief, Sports Medicine
Director, Residency Research
Orthopaedic Surgery Service
Tripler Army Medical Center
Honolulu, Hawaii

Charles H. Brown Jr, MD
International Knee & Joint Centre
Abu Dhabi, United Arab Emirates

William Bugbee, MD
Orthopaedic Surgeon
Joint Replacement/Lower Extremity Reconstruction
Cartilage Transplantation/Restoration
Division of Orthopaedic Surgery
Scripps Clinic
La Jolla, California

Kirk A. Campbell, MD
Sports Medicine Fellow
Department of Orthopaedic Surgery
Rush University Medical Center
Chicago, Illinois

Jourdan M. Cancienne, MD
Orthopaedic Surgery Resident
University of Virginia
Charlottesville, Virginia

James L. Carey, MD, MPH
Director, Penn Center for Advanced Cartilage Repair and Osteochondritis Dissecans Treatment
Penn Sports Medicine Center
Philadelphia, Pennsylvania

Edward S. Chang, MD
Fellow of Orthopaedic Sports Medicine
Department of Orthopaedic Surgery
University of Pittsburgh
Pittsburgh, Pennsylvania

Edward C. Cheung, MD
Resident
Department of Orthopaedic Surgery
David Geffen School of Medicine at UCLA
Los Angeles, California

J. H. James Choi, MD
Fellow
Division of Sports Medicine
Department of Orthopaedic Surgery
Duke University Medical Center
Durham, North Carolina

Randy M. Cohn, MD
Assistant Professor
Hofstra North Shore-LIJ School of Medicine
North Shore-LIJ Orthopaedic Institute at Garden City
Garden City, New York

Brian J. Cole, MD, MBA
Professor
Department of Orthopaedic Surgery and Anatomy and Cell Biology
Rush University Medical Center
Chicago, Illinois

Tyler R. Cram, MA, ATC, OTC
The Steadman Clinic
Vail, Colorado

David Dejour, MD
Orthopaedic Surgeon
Lyon-Ortho-Clinic
Lyon, France

David R. Diduch, MD
Vice Chair, Orthopaedic Surgery
A. R. Shands Professor
Head Orthopaedic Team Physician
University of Virginia
UVA Sports Medicine Clinic
Charlottesville, Virginia

Zachary B. Domont, MD
Orthopaedic Surgeon
AMG-Lincolnshire Orthopaedics
Village Green, Illinois

John B. Doyle, BA
Department of Orthopedic Surgery
Hospital for Special Surgery
New York, New York

Michael P. Elliott, DO
Orthopaedic Sports Fellow
Department of Orthopaedics
University of Kentucky
Lexington, Kentucky

Peter D. Fabricant, MD, MPH
Assistant Attending Orthopedic Surgeon
Hospital for Special Surgery
New York, New York

Gregory C. Fanelli, MD, FAAOS
Associate, Department of Orthopaedics
Geisinger Health System
Danville, Pennsylvania

German Jose Filippi, MD
Hospital Universitario CEMIC
Buenos Aires, Argentina

Freddie H. Fu, MD
Chair, Department of Orthopaedic Surgery
Distinguished Service Professor
David Silver Professor, Division of Sports Medicine
Head Team Physician, Department of Athletics
Professor, Physical Therapy, School of Health and Rehabilitation Sciences
Professor, Health and Physical Activity, School of Education
Professor, Mechanical Engineering & Materials Science
Swanson School of Engineering
University of Pittsburgh
Pittsburgh, Pennsylvania

John P. Fulkerson, MD
Orthopedic Associates of Hartford, PC
Hartford, Connecticut

Theodore J. Ganley, MD
Director, Sports Medicine
Children's Hospital of Philadelphia
Philadelphia, Pennsylvania

G. Keith Gill, MD
Chief Resident
UNM Orthopaedics
University of New Mexico hospital
Albuquerque, New Mexico

Megan Gleason, MD
Fellow, Sports Medicine
Department of Orthopaedic Surgery
University of Virginia Health System
Charlottesville, Virginia

Simon Görtz, MD
Fellow
Department of Orthopedic Surgery
Washington University
St. Louis, Missouri

Chad Griffith, MD
Orthopaedic Sports Medicine Fellow
Department of Orthopaedic Surgery
University of Pittsburgh
Pittsburgh, Pennsylvania

Daniel Guenther, MD
Research Fellow
Department of Orthopaedic Surgery
University of Pittsburgh
Pittsburgh, Pennsylvania

Arielle J. Hall, MD
Research Assistant
Tissue Engineering, Regeneration and Repair Program
Hospital for Special Surgery
New York, New York

Christopher D. Harner, MD
Professor
Vice Chair of Academic Affairs, Director of the Sports Medicine Fellowship
Department of Orthopaedic Surgery
The University of Texas Health Science Center at Houston – UT Health
Houston, Texas

Benjamin V. Herman, MD, FRCSC
Orthopaedic Sport Medicine Fellow
Fowler Kennedy Sport Medicine Centre
Department of Surgery
Western University
London, Ontario

K. J. Hippensteel, MD
Lieutenant Medical Corps United States Naval Reserves
Orthopaedic Surgery Resident
Washington University in Saint Louis
St. Louis, Missouri

Ian D. Hutchinson, MD
Research Fellow
Tissue Engineering, Regeneration and Repair Program
Hospital for Special Surgery
New York, New York

John Jasko, MD
Marshall Sports Medicine Institute
Huntington, West Virginia

Darren L. Johnson, MD
Professor and Chairman
Department of Orthopaedic Surgery
Director of Sports Medicine
University of Kentucky School of Medicine
Lexington, Kentucky

Nirav B. Joshi, MD
Orthopaedic Research Fellow
Department of Orthopaedic Surgery
David Geffen School of Medicine at UCLA
Los Angeles, California

Jay V. Kalawadia, MD
Fellow of Orthopaedic Sports Medicine
Department of Orthopaedic Surgery
University of Pittsburgh
Pittsburgh, Pennsylvania

Nicholas I. Kennedy, BA
The Steadman Philippon Research Institute
Vail, Colorado

Vinícius Canello Kuhn, MD
Instituto de Ortopedia e Traumatologia de Passo Fundo (IOT)
Passo Fundo, Brazil

Robert F. LaPrade, MD, PhD
Complex Knee and Sports Medicine Surgeon
The Steadman Clinic
Chief Medical Officer, Steadman Philippon Research Institute
Co-Director, Sports Medicine Fellowship Program
Director, International Scholar Program
Adjunct Professor, Orthopaedic Surgery
University of Minnesota
Affiliate Faculty, College of Veterinary Medicine and Biomedical Sciences
Colorado State University
Vail, Colorado

Christian Lattermann, MD
Director, Center for Cartilage Repair and Restoration
Associate Professor
Department of Orthopaedic Surgery and Sports Medicine
University of Kentucky
Lexington, Kentucky

Bruce A. Levy, MD
Professor of Orthopedic Surgery
Department of Orthopedic Surgery
Mayo Clinic
Rochester, Minnesota

Joshua Lindsey, MD
Orthopaedic Sports Fellow
University of Rochester
Rochester, New York

Robert Litchfield, MD, FRCS
Medical Director
Fowler Kennedy Sport Medicine Clinic
Associate Professor
Schulich School of Medicine & Dentistry
London, Ontario

David P. Lustenberger, MD
Orthopaedic Surgery Resident
University of Virginia
Charlottesville, Virginia

T. Sean Lynch, MD
Assistant Attending Physician
New York Presbyterian Hospital
Assistant Professor of Orthopedic Surgery
Department of Orthopaedic Surgery
Columbia University Medical Center
New York, New York

Michael Maloney, MD
Professor
Orthopaedic Sports Department
University of Rochester
Rochester, New York

Robert G. Marx, MD, MSc
Professor of Orthopedic Surgery
Weill Cornell Medical College
Attending Orthopedic Surgeon
Hospital for Special Surgery
New York, New York

Matthew J. Matava, MD
Professor, Orthopedic Surgery
Professor, Physical Therapy
Chief, Sports Medicine Service
Department of Orthopedic Surgery
Washington University
St. Louis, Missouri

Cristin J. Mathew, DO
Chief Resident
Department of Orthopaedic Surgery
North Shore-LIJ Health System
New York, New York

David R. McAllister, MD
Professor and Chief of Sports Medicine
Department of Orthopaedic Surgery
David Geffen School of Medicine at UCLA
Los Angeles, California

Eric McCarty, MD
Associate Professor
Chief of Sports Medicine and Shoulder Surgery
University of Colorado Hospital
CU Sports Medicine
Boulder, Colorado

Heather Menzer, MD
Resident
Orthopaedics & Rehabilitation
University of New Mexico
Albuquerque, New Mexico

Adam V. Metzler, MD
Commonwealth Orthopaedic Centers
Edgewood, Kentucky

Mark D. Miller, MD
S. Ward Casscells Professor
Head, Division of Sports Medicine
Department of Orthopaedic Surgery
University of Virginia
Team Physician, James Madison University Director, Miller Review Course
Charlottesville, Virginia

Andrew A. Millis, MD
Fellow
Department of Orthopaedic Surgery, Sports Medicine
Cleveland Clinic Foundation
Cleveland, Ohio

Claude T. Moorman III, MD
Executive Director
Sports Sciences Institute
Professor of Orthopaedic Surgery
Vice-Chairman, Department of Orthopaedic Surgery
Duke University Medical Center
Durham, North Carolina

Samuel G. Moulton, BA
The Steadman Philippon Research Institute
Vail, Colordo

Philippe Neyret, MD
Department of Orthopaedic Surgery
Centre Albert Trillat
Hôpital de la Croix-Rousse
Lyon, France

Richard D. Parker, MD
President of Marymount Hospital
Department of Orthopaedic Surgery, Sports Medicine
Cleveland Clinic Foundation
Garfield Heights, Ohio

Kushal V. Patel, MD
Fellow
Orthopaedic Sports Medicine and Shoulder Surgery
University of Colorado
Denver, Colorado

Matthew R. Prince, MD
Resident
Department of Orthopedic Surgery
Mayo Clinic
Rochester, Minnesota

Lauren H. Redler, MD
Fellow
Hospital for Special Surgery
New York, New York

James Robinson, FRCS (Orth), MS
International Knee & Joint Centre
Abu Dhabi, United Arab Emirates

Scott A. Rodeo, MD
Co-Chief Emeritus
Sports Medicine and Shoulder Service
Co-Director of the Tissue Engineering, Regeneration and Repair Program
Hospital for Special Surgery
New York, New York

Olivier Reynaud, MD
Department of Orthopaedic Surgery
Centre Albert Trillat
Hôpital de la Croix-Rousse
Lyon, France

Marcus A. Rothermich, MD
Orthopaedic Sports Medicine Fellow
American Sports Medicine Institute
Birmingham, Alabama

Paulo Renato Fernandes Saggin, MD
Orthopedist—Traumatologist
Instituto de Ortopedia e Traumatologia de Passo Fundo (IOT)
Passo Fundo, Brazil

Robert C. Schenck Jr, MD
Professor and Chair
Department of Orthopaedics & Rehabilitation
University of New Mexico
Albuquerque, New Mexico

Nicholas A. Sgaglione, MD
Chairman of Orthopaedic Surgery, Long Island Jewish Medical Center
Chairman of Orthopaedic Surgery—Research & Education
North Shore University Hospital
Professor, Hofstra North Shore-LIJ School of Medicine
University Orthopaedic Associates at Great Neck
Great Neck, New York

Harris S. Slone, MD
Assistant Professor
Department of Orthopaedics
Medical University of South Carolina
Charleston, South Carolina

Elad Spitzer, MD
Research Fellow
Department of Orthopaedic Surgery
Hospital for Special Surgery
New York, New York

Beth E. Shubin Stein, MD
Associate Attending Physician
Sports Medicine and Shoulder Service
Hospital for Special Surgery
Associate Professor of Orthopaedic Surgery
Weill Cornell Medical College
New York, New York

Sabrina M. Strickland, MD
Associate Attending
Sports Medicine and Shoulder Service
Hospital for Special Surgery
Associate Professor of Orthopaedic Surgery
Weill Cornell Medical College
New York, New York

Joseph J. Stuart, MD
Fellow
Division of Sports Medicine
Department of Orthopaedic Surgery
Duke University Medical Center
Durham, North Carolina

Michael J. Stuart, MD
Professor of Orthopedic Surgery
Department of Orthopedic Surgery
Mayo Clinic
Rochester, Minnesota

Annemarie K. Tilton, BS
Sports Medicine Research Fellow
Department of Orthopaedic Surgery
Rush University Medical Center
Chicago, Illinois

Gehron Treme, MD
Assistant Professor
Department of Orthopaedics
University of New Mexico
Albuquerque, New Mexico

Robert Van Gorder, MD
Orthopaedic Sports Fellow
University of Rochester
Rochester, New York

Garth Nyambi Walker, MD
Orthopaedic Research Fellow
Department of Orthopaedic Surgery
University of Pittsburgh
Pittsburgh, Pennsylvania

Dean Wang, MD
Professor and Chief of Sports Medicine
Department of Orthopaedic Surgery
David Geffen School of Medicine at UCLA
Los Angeles, California

Daniel C. Wascher, MD
Professor
Department of Orthopaedics
University of New Mexico
Albuquerque, New Mexico

Rick W. Wright, MD
Jerome J. Gilden Distinguished Professor of Orthopaedic Surgery
Executive Vice Chairman
Washington University School of Medicine
St. Louis, Missouri

John W. Xerogeanes, MD
Professor of Orthopaedic Surgery
Department of Orthopaedic Surgery
Emory University
Atlanta, Georgia

Justin Shu Yang, MD
Orthopaedic Sports Medicine Fellow
Department of Orthopaedics
University of Connecticut
Storrs, Connecticut

Foreword

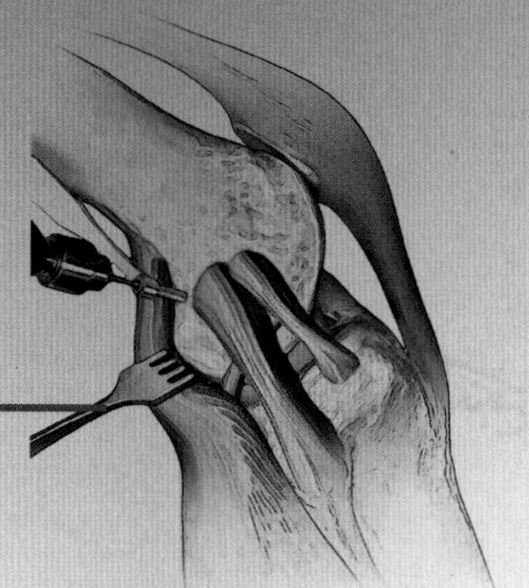

It is my distinct pleasure to introduce the fourth edition of the "*Master Techniques in Orthopaedic Surgery, Reconstructive Knee Surgery*," edited by Darren Johnson, MD. This edition represents a continuum of improved knowledge, science, and surgical techniques in the management of common and complex knee disorders. This volume is in keeping with the established reputation of this work as one of the foremost treatise on instruction in the surgical care of these knee disorders.

The highlights of this particular work is the format of providing tips and pearls from some of the leading surgeons in the world. It is refreshing to observe the generosity of these leading surgeons in sharing their clinical and surgical expertise on so many different topics. This is a true reflection that the patient comes first, so that many other treating surgeons can learn and apply the principles demonstrated in this book and apply them in their individual clinical practice.

A review of the offerings in this new book will show in Part I the latest techniques and indications for extensor mechanism disorders to include not only medial patellofemoral ligament reconstruction and tibial tubercle osteotomy but also the newer and perhaps controversial topics of trochleoplasty and patellofemoral replacement. Part II will feature meniscal repair surgery to include inside-out, and all-inside techniques as well as meniscal transplantation. Part III will feature "everything you wanted to know about knee ligament surgery." The topics of ACL reconstruction, extra-articular augmentation, three different types of PCL reconstruction, posterolateral corner reconstruction, MCL, and the role of osteotomy in managing chronic knee ligament deficient knees are outstanding chapters. Finally, Part IV is devoted to articular cartilage injuries and potential surgical solutions and options. The topics range from microfracture to bulk allograft and autograft and include cell-based techniques.

In short, this is simply an outstanding textbook that will serve as up-to-date education on current effective techniques and demonstrated by leaders in the field. The book will serve as instruction and a ready reference for the practicing surgeon as he or she prepares for any of these types of cases. The constellation of topics, illustration, and authorship by experts in these areas make the *Master Techniques in Orthopaedic Surgery, Reconstructive Knee Surgery* an important resource for the practicing orthopaedist.

Robert A. Arciero, MD
Professor, Orthopaedics
University of Connecticut

Preface

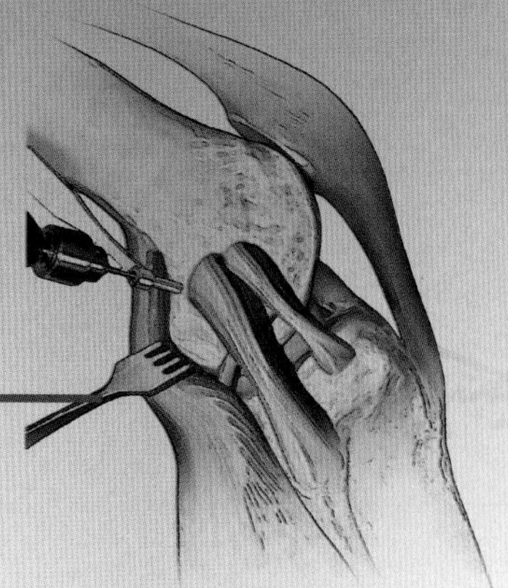

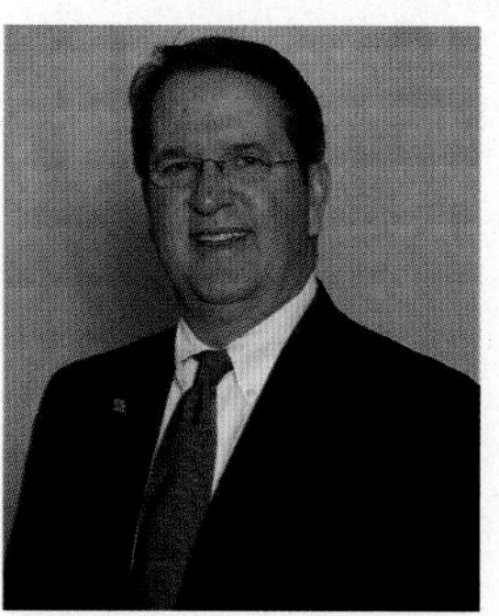

It is my distinct pleasure to serve as the editor of the fourth edition of the *Master Techniques in Orthopaedic Surgery, Reconstructive Knee Surgery*. I am personally humbled and honored to serve as your guest editor. This is a fully updated version of the *Reconstructive Knee Surgery* volume edited by Douglas W. Jackson, MD, in 2008. Much has changed in our field over the last 9 years. This fourth edition represents a continuum of knowledge, science, and latest surgical techniques in the management of common and complex knee disorders. I want to personally thank each of the authors who have contributed valuable time and expertise to this outstanding volume. They have worked tirelessly over the last year to make this a truly exceptional knee surgical textbook/atlas on surgical techniques. I firmly believe that this volume will be a great addition to any master knee surgeon.

Since the publication of the first edition of the series/textbook in 1995, much has changed in the field of surgical treatment about the knee. This edition represents the most important, time-tested operations over the last 20-plus years. You will see that we have added new chapters, new topics, with improved surgical technical experience outlined by master technique knee surgeons who are the authors. I want to congratulate each of the authors on a job well-done making this a corner stone of any knee surgeon's library when learning or reviewing about surgical techniques around the knee.

The surgeon masters contributing to this volume were carefully chosen for their expertise and experience in the clinical application and the latest techniques and technologies of specific knee disorders. They present surgical innovations, clinical judgment expertise, operation room methodology, and decision making. They share their indications and contraindications, as well as the pitfalls they may occur during surgery. Each chapter includes specific details that lead to success in the operating room but more importantly improved patient outcomes. Each chapter represents a selected individual author's approach to a specific knee problem; the references at the end of each chapter are limited. These authors have given us the specific surgical technical pearls that lead to outstanding patient outcomes. My personal involvement in selecting the authors, reviewing, and editing these chapters has drastically improved the surgical care that I am personally able to offer my patients. I am forever in debt to them for their expertise knowledge they have shared. I am thoroughly convinced that this fourth edition of *Master Techniques in Orthopaedic Surgery, Reconstructive Knee Surgery* will be a tremendous benefit and will help all of those who desire to be master knee surgeon. It has been a pleasure and lifelong learning experience to serve as your editor.

Darren L. Johnson, MD

Series Preface

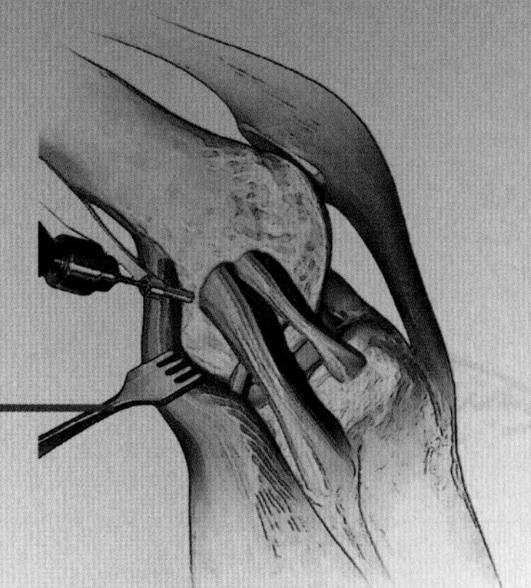

Since its inception in 1994, the *Master Techniques in Orthopaedic Surgery* series has become the gold standard for both physicians in training and experienced surgeons. Its exceptional success may be traced to the leadership of the original series editor, Roby Thompson, whose clarity of thought and focused vision sought "to provide direct, detailed access to techniques preferred by orthopedic surgeons who are recognized by their colleagues as 'masters' in their specialty," as he stated in his series preface. It is personally very rewarding to hear testimonials from both residents and practicing orthopedic surgeons on the value of these volumes to their training and practice.

A key element of the success of the series is its format. The effectiveness of the format is reflected by the fact that it is now being replicated by others. An essential feature is the standardized presentation of information replete with tips and pearls shared by experts with years of experience. Abundant color photographs and drawings guide the reader through the procedures step by step.

The second key to the success of the *Master Techniques* series rests in the reputation and experience of our volume editors. The editors are truly dedicated "masters" with a commitment to share their rich experience through these texts. We feel a great debt of gratitude to them and a real responsibility to maintain and enhance the reputation of the *Master Techniques* series that has developed over the years. We are proud of the progress made in formulating the third edition volumes and are particularly pleased with the expanded content of this series. Six new volumes will soon be available covering topics that are exciting and relevant to a broad cross section of our profession. While we are in the process of carefully expanding *Master Techniques* topics and editors, we are committed to the now-classic format.

The first of the new volumes is—*Relevant Surgical Exposures*—which I have had the honor of editing. The second new volume is *Pediatrics*. Subsequent new topics to be introduced are *Soft Tissue Reconstruction*, *Management of Peripheral Nerve Dysfunction*, *Advanced Reconstructive Techniques in the Joint*, and finally *Essential Procedures in Sports Medicine*. The full library thus will consist of 16 useful and relevant titles. I am pleased to have accepted the position of series editor, feeling so strongly about the value of this series to educate the orthopedic surgeon in the full array of expert surgical procedures. The true worth of this endeavor will continue to be measured by the ever-increasing success and critical acceptance of the series. I remain indebted to Dr. Thompson for his inaugural vision and leadership, as well as to the *Master Techniques* volume editors and numerous contributors who have been true to the series style and vision. As I indicated in the preface to the second edition of The Hip volume, the words of William Mayo are especially relevant to characterize the ultimate goal of this endeavor: "The best interest of the patient is the only interest to be considered." We are confident that the information in the expanded *Master Techniques* offers the surgeon an opportunity to realize the patient-centric view of our surgical practice.

Bernard F. Morrey, MD

Contents

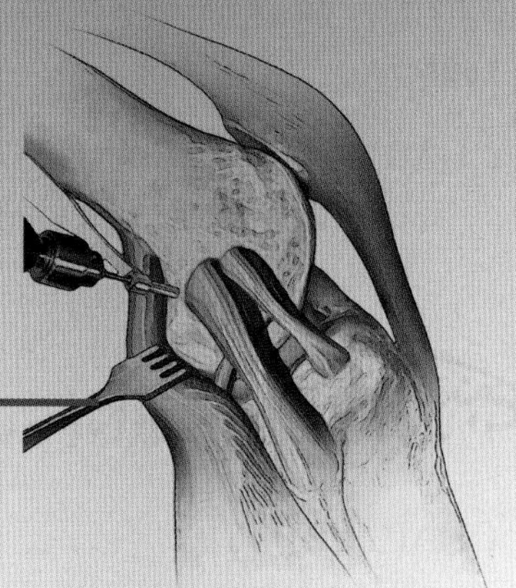

PART IV Articular Cartilage and Synovium 436

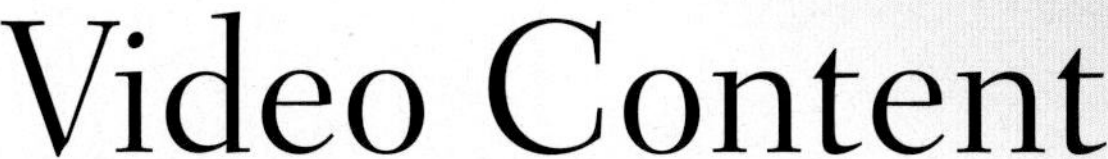

Video Content

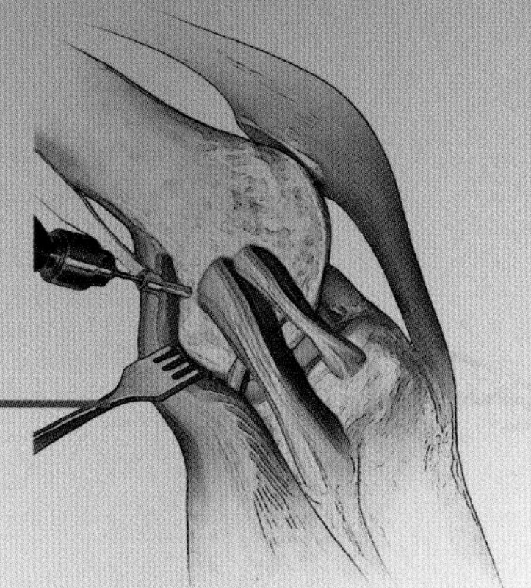

VIDEO 1-1	After passage of locking sutures, the quadriceps tendon is easily mobilized to the proximal patella.
VIDEO 1-2	Preparation of proximal patellar pole with burr.
VIDEO 1-3	Extensor lag associated with chronic failed quad tendon repair.
VIDEO 6-1	Patellofemoral joint replacement.
VIDEO 9-1	All-inside meniscus repair FasT-Fix.
VIDEO 10-1	Inside-out meniscus repair technique of the medial meniscus using zone specific instrumentation.
VIDEO 14-1	How I do a BCB ACL reconstruction.
VIDEO 28-1	Lachman exam under anesthesia.
VIDEO 28-2	Arthroscopic exam under anesthesia.
VIDEO 30-1	Chondroplasty and synovectomy.
VIDEO 36-1	Proximal tibial osteotomy for management of unicompartmental arthritis.

PART I EXTENSOR MECHANISM-PATELLOFEMORAL PROBLEMS

1 Quadriceps and Patellar Tendon Repair

Michael Maloney, Joshua Lindsey, and Robert Van Gorder

ACUTE QUADRICEPS TENDON REPAIR

Introduction and Diagnosis

An acute quadriceps tendon rupture (QTR) is a rare injury in the United States, with a reported incidence of about 1.37/100,000. Those affected are generally males over 40 years of age, and rupture occurs by direct or indirect trauma (1,2). Older patients often present after a low-energy fall (61%), while younger patients may incur rupture during sporting activity (1). Eccentric contraction of the quadriceps mechanism is the predominant mechanism of injury and is heightened in the setting of age-related degenerative tendinopathy. Predisposing factors to rupture include chronic renal disease, diabetes, gout, hyperparathyroidism, lupus, morbid obesity, and rheumatoid arthritis (1–4). Pharmacologic risk factors include long-term corticosteroid use and fluoroquinolone antibiotics (2,3,5). In addition, these systemic factors can result in bilateral ruptures in up to 12% of affected individuals (6).

Prompt diagnosis is critical to guiding treatment. Predominantly a clinical diagnosis, acute QTR can be missed in up to 50% of patients (3). The classic triad of acute pain, absence of active knee extension, and a palpable soft tissue defect 1 to 2 cm proximal to the patella (an avascular region) is usually sufficient to make an accurate diagnosis of QTR (1–3,7). Radiographic findings may include suprapatellar effusion, a soft tissue mass representing the retracted tendon, avulsion of the superior pole of the patella, or patellar baja. We generally obtain AP and lateral x-rays to rule out patella fracture. Routine use of advanced imaging is not necessary but provides additional information if the diagnosis is unclear. Ultrasound is less expensive, is time consuming, and can be performed in an outpatient clinic setting, yet is plagued by a specificity of 67% as noted in two recent studies (8,9). On the contrary, MRI has a sensitivity and specificity approaching 100% and can characterize the location and precise nature of a tear (3,8–10). We reserve the use of MRI in rare cases when our clinical suspicion for rupture is elevated but confounded by physical exam findings, such as weak active knee extension in the setting of an intact extensor retinaculum. However, surgery should not be delayed to obtain an MRI.

The literature is consistent and unequivocal in support of acute quadriceps tendon repair to avoid unsatisfactory patient outcomes. A recent systematic review of 12 studies involving early repair demonstrated near-unanimous good to excellent patient outcomes, while those of delayed repair had poor results (1). Two common techniques, simple sutures and transosseous patellar drill holes, had no significant impact on patient function or satisfaction despite the presence of quadriceps atrophy and decreased strength (1,7). Up to 97% of patients are able to return to their preinjury level of activity (2,4). Delayed surgery, however, consistently led to worse outcomes independent of injury mechanism, patient risk factors, and technique. Chronic tears generally show improvement with surgery but not to the degree as acute repairs. Moreover, delayed surgical intervention is more extensive including repair with augmentation (Scuderi technique), V-Y tendon lengthening (Codvilla method), or allograft reconstruction.

Indications and Patient Selection

We have a low threshold for prompt surgical intervention in complete QTR in most patients. Ideally, repair should occur within 2 weeks to mitigate tendon retraction, muscle contraction, and scar formation. Significant retraction can occur in just 72 hours, thus emphasizing the need for urgent repair. Contraindications include patients who are medically unstable or nonambulatory, have open wounds with gross contamination or infection, or have limb-threatening vasculopathy.

Surgery

Patient Positioning

Patients undergo a preoperative screening by anesthesia. Critical health problems are addressed and optimized. Most QTRs are repaired at an outpatient surgery center. A femoral nerve block is administered for postoperative pain management.

The patient is positioned supine after anesthesia induction, and a well-padded thigh tourniquet and ipsilateral hip bump are placed, followed by a ramp of towels or Bone-Foam. The leg is prepped with ChloraPrep and draped free from mid-thigh to mid-calf. Prophylactic antibiotics are administered prior to incision.

Surgical Technique

The leg is exsanguinated with an Esmarch and the tourniquet inflated. A midline incision centered over the suprapatellar defect is made approximately 15 to 20 cm in length (Fig. 1-1). Sharp dissection is carried down to the quadriceps fascia, deep to which is often a tense hematoma. After hematoma evacuation and irrigation, the quadriceps mechanism is inspected. The medial and lateral retinacula are often torn to the mid-coronal plane (Fig. 1-2A,B). As a critical component of the extensor mechanism, it is imperative to inspect and later repair the retinacula.

The quadriceps tendon stump is isolated and sharply debrided to remove hematoma, clot, and avascular scar tissue (Fig. 1-3A,B). In parallel fashion, two no. 2 FiberWire sutures (Arthrex, Naples, FL) are whipstitched with a locking Krackow suture from the stump to the musculotendinous junction (Fig. 1-4). The four strands should exit distally from the terminal stump, making sure there is adequate length for passage through the patella. Ease of tendon excursion is noted (Video 1-1).

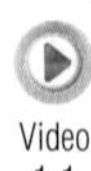
Video 1-1

The proximal pole of the patella is prepared next. Generally, the tendon is completely avulsed from the osseous-tendinous insertion. Residual fibers are sharply debrided until all borders of the proximal pole, including the articular surface, are adequately visualized. The proximal pole is decorticated with a 3-mm bur to create a bleeding base for tendon healing

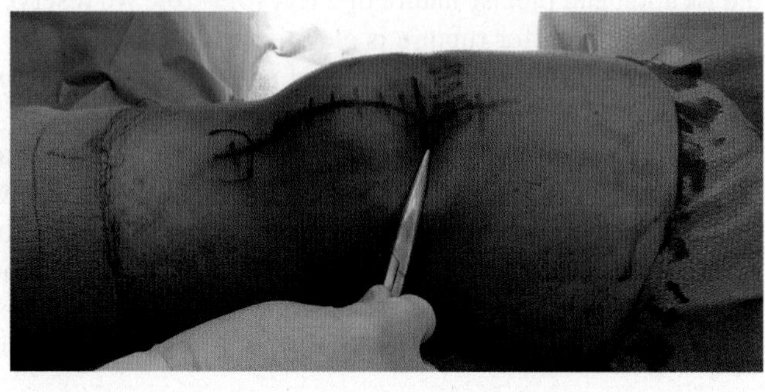

FIGURE 1-1

Preparation of knee for surgery. Disruption of the quadriceps tendon is clearly palpated.

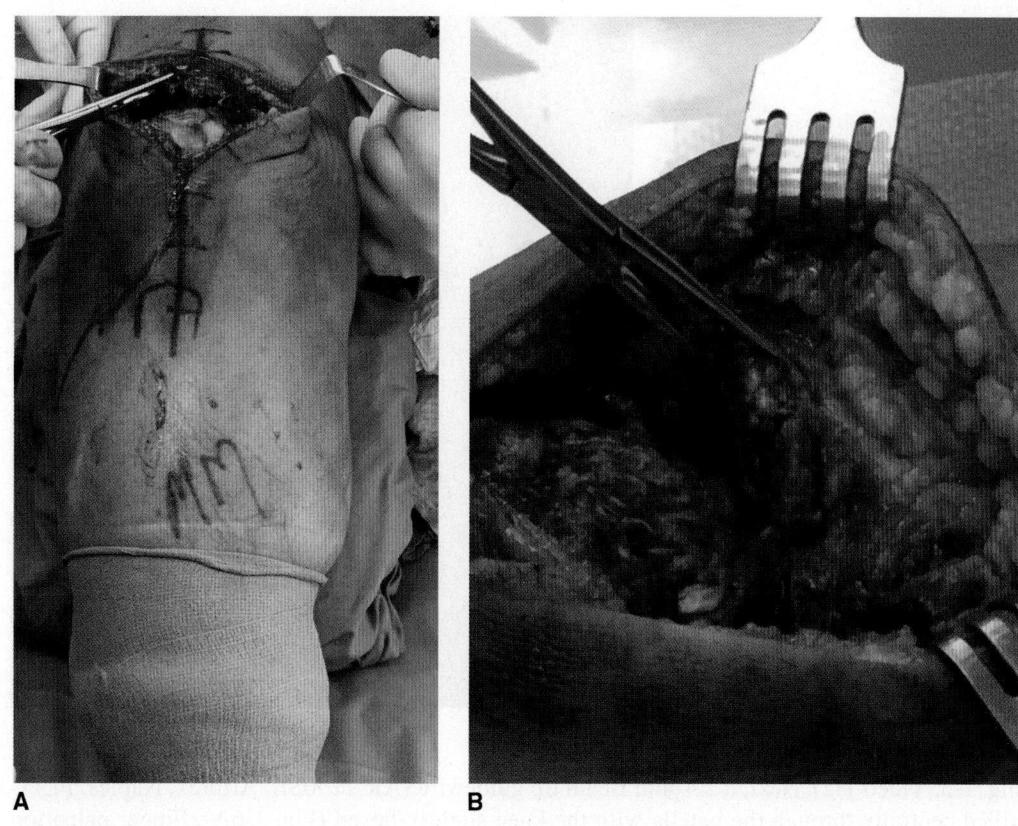

FIGURE 1-2

A, B: Full-thickness QTR with disruption of extensor retinacula.

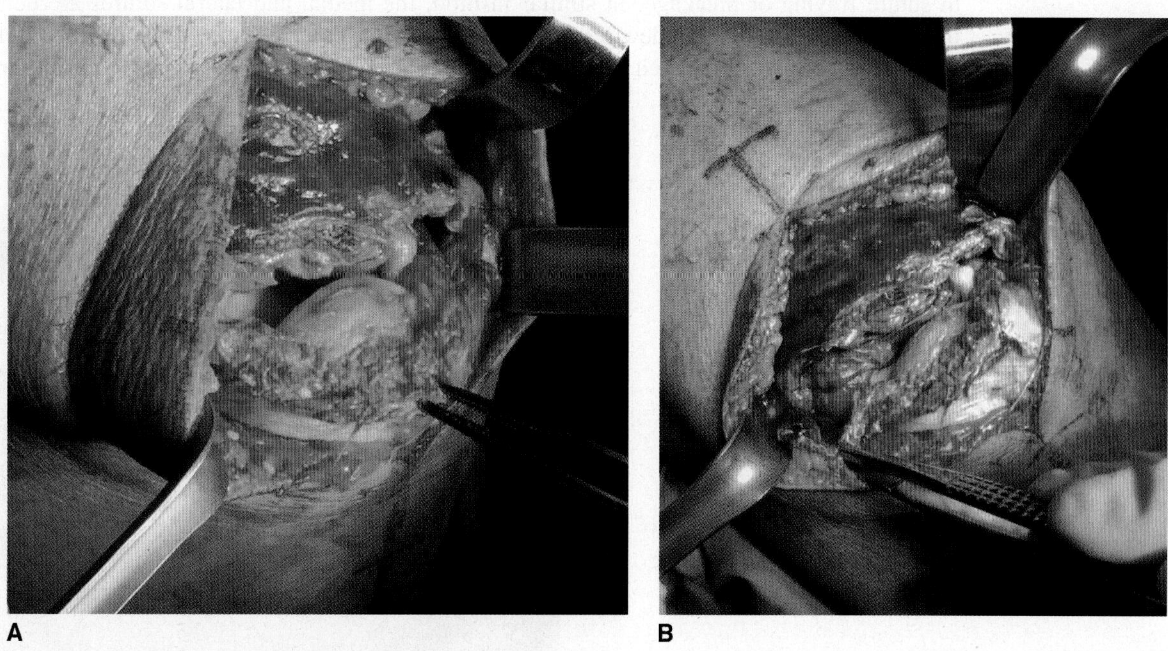

FIGURE 1-3

A, B: After preparation of the tendon stump (superior), the extent of the extensor retinacula injury is seen. The articular margin of the proximal patella is also identified.

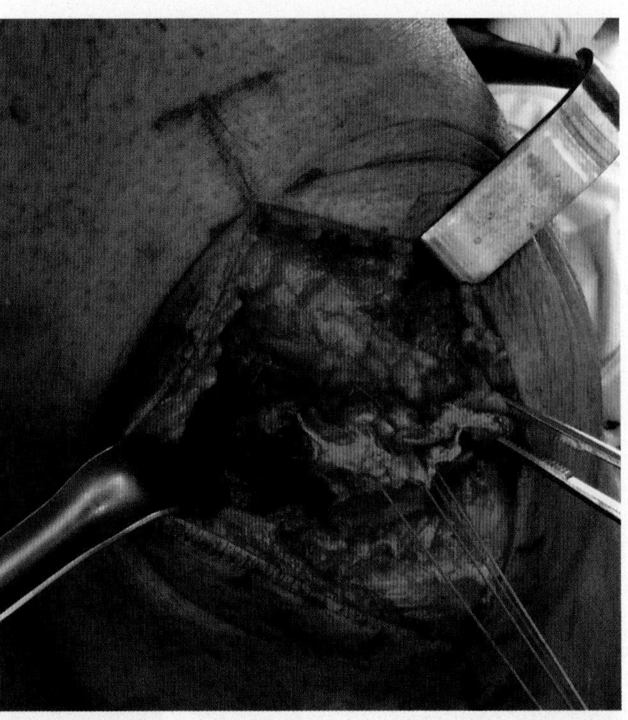

FIGURE 1-4

No. 2 FiberWire (Arthrex) running sutures in a locking Krackow fashion with four strands exiting distally.

Video 1-2

(Fig. 1-5, Video 1-2). Next, a 2.4-mm Beath tip guidewire (AR-1250SB, Arthrex, Naples, FL) is drilled centrally through the patella with the knee slightly flexed (Fig. 1-6A). Finger palpation of the articular surface helps prevent its violation from the guidewire. Two additional 2.4-mm guidewires are drilled in parallel fashion, one medial and one lateral (Fig. 1-6B). An adequate amount of each wire must be exposed distally to allow each to each to be pulled through the patella once the sutures are loaded. The two middle sutures are loaded through the central guidewire. The guidewire is then pulled distally through the patella with a locking chuck handle or heavy pliers (Fig. 1-7) with the aid of a mallet. We avoid rotating the guidewire as this may lead to suture fraying or breakage. In similar fashion, the medial and lateral sutures are delivered through their respective guidewires to the distal patellar pole. With the knee in full extension, firm tension is placed on each suture, the tendon is reduced to its anatomic footprint, and the

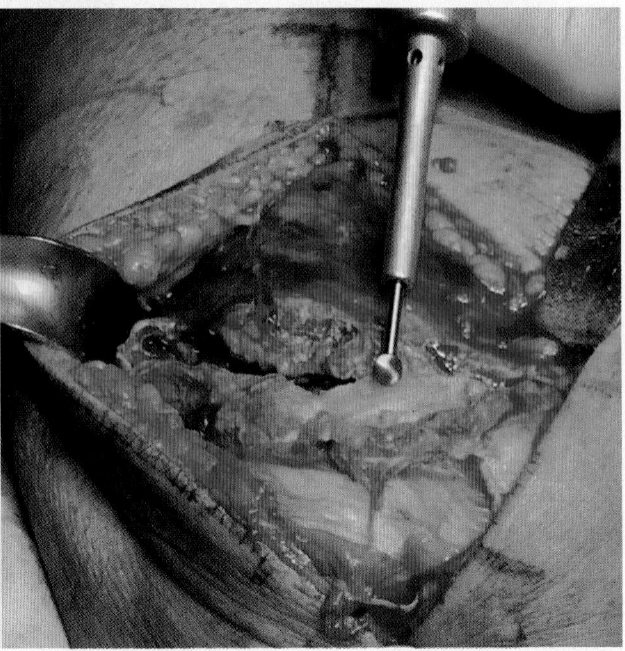

FIGURE 1-5

Preparation of the proximal patellar pole with a high-speed 3-mm bur.

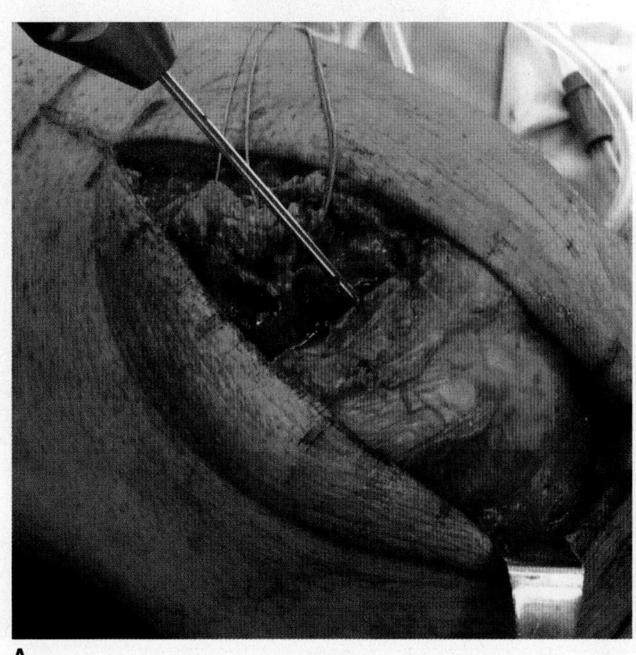
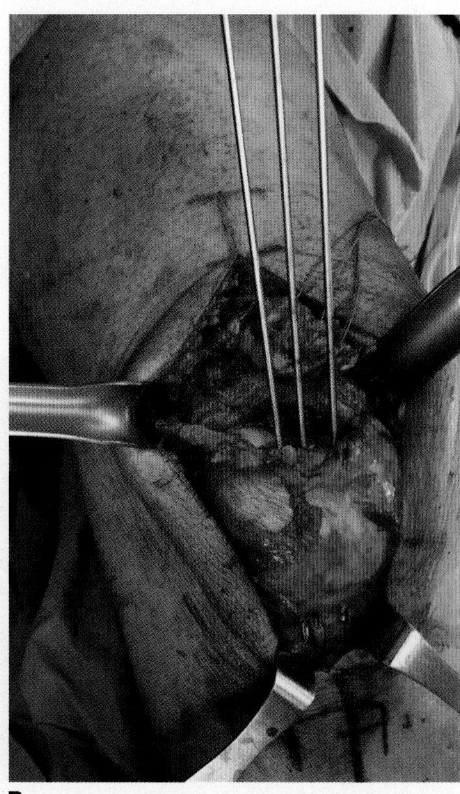

A B

FIGURE 1-6

A, B: Placement of three parallel 2.4-mm Beath tip guidewires, starting with the central wire. Army/Navy retractors help protect the skin as the wires exit distally.

sutures are tied down securely over the patellar bone bridge (Fig. 1-8A,B). If difficulty in tendon mobility or reduction is encountered, the tourniquet is deflated, relaxing the quadriceps and improving tendon excursion.

The wound is then copiously irrigated and the retinacula repaired with no. 1 Vicryl suture in interrupted fashion to create a watertight closure (Fig. 1-9). Meticulous repair of this layer is crucial to well-functioning extensor mechanism postoperatively. Gentle flexion is performed to assess the integrity of the repair and is a reference for post-op range of motion (ROM) parameters. Soft tissues are closed in layers, and a compressive dressing and locked extension brace are placed prior to cessation of anesthesia.

Pearls and Pitfalls

While acute QTR is generally straightforward, several critical steps ensure a good outcome. First, tension across the suture line must be minimized and is accomplished by complete release of adhesions, deflating the tourniquet, and keeping the knee in full extension during final suture tying. A robust repair of the retinaculum not only restores the extensor mechanism but also augments and protects the main tendon repair. Second, reestablishing the anatomic tendon insertion is vital to prevent patellar maltracking or patellofemoral malalignment. Lastly, careful guidewire advancement prevents suture failure and minimizes patellar torque, safeguarding against a devastating patella fracture.

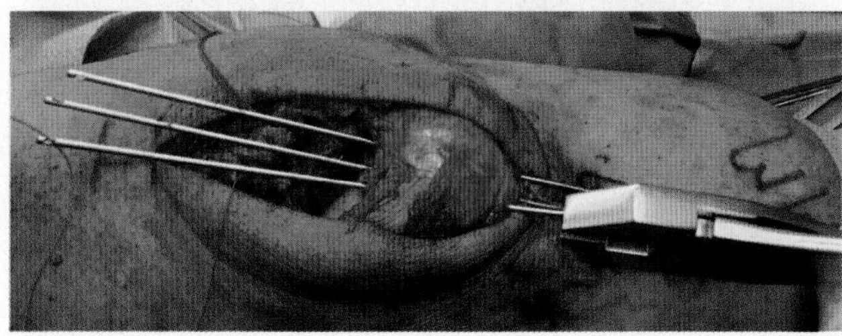

FIGURE 1-7

Advancing the guidewires and sutures through patellar bone tunnels with pliers. It is imperative to pull in-line traction, often assisted by a mallet on the proximal end of the wires.

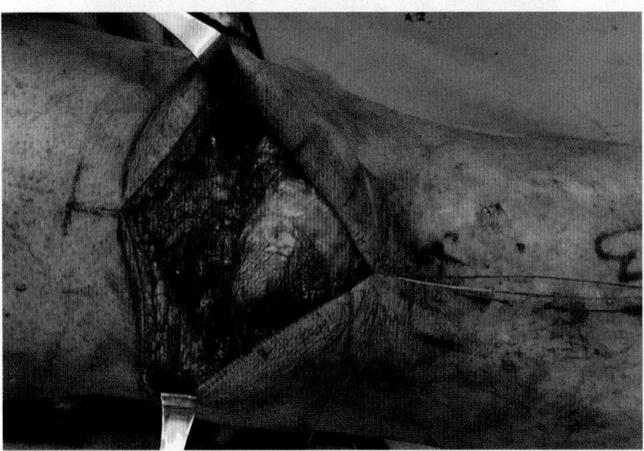

A

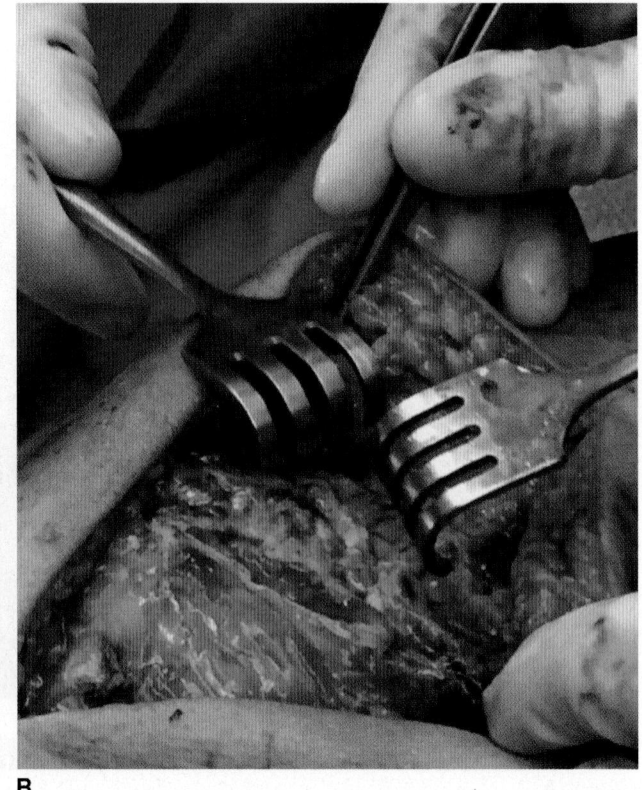

B

FIGURE 1-8

A, B: The sutures are tied down securely over the distal patella, achieving good fixation of the quadriceps tendon.

Postoperative Management

The first phase of rehab consists of immobilization in an extension brace for 2 weeks. Patients are touch-down weight bearing on crutches with progression to full weight bearing by 6 weeks. Isometrics and modalities to reduce swelling are begun immediately. Phase two occurs from 3 to 6 weeks postoperatively, with a focus on restoration of motion. The goal is for full active flexion by 6 weeks. During this time, only passive extension is allowed. Strengthening occurs from 7 to 12 weeks. The brace and crutches are discontinued once the patient can perform a straight leg raise without an extensor lag and has normal gait, respectively. Weeks 9 to 12 focus on open- and closed-chain quadriceps exercises. Sport-specific functional rehab begins 4 months after surgery, with the goal of return to sport by 6 months.

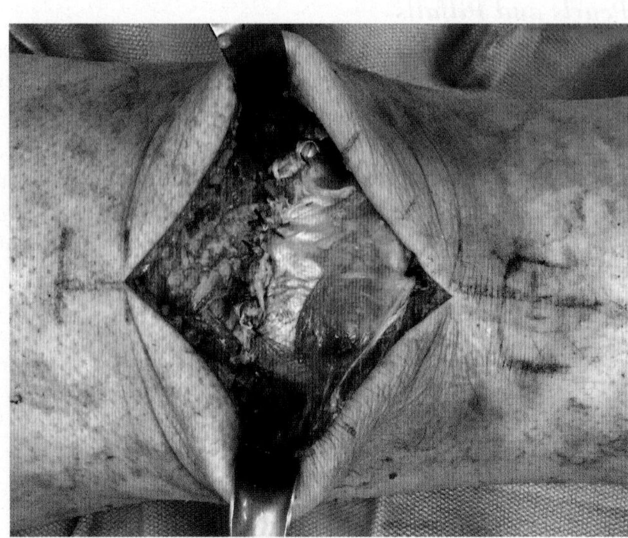

FIGURE 1-9

The medial and lateral retinacula are repaired with interrupted sutures, completing the extensor mechanism repair.

Complications

Early repair, good surgical technique, and a good physical therapy program are important factors in minimizing complications. Overall complications (3%) are rare (2). Lost motion and extensor weakness are the most commonly cited; both are unaffected by type of repair or length of immobilization up to 6 weeks (11–13). Rerupture rate is very low (2%). Early postoperative motion has not been shown to increase the risk of rerupture and may improve functional ROM (12). Other reported complications include DVT, infection, radiographic evidence of patellofemoral arthritis, patella fracture, and complex regional pain syndrome.

RESULTS

Acute QTRs are relatively uncommon but disproportionately affect males 8:1 versus females (4). Prompt surgical management is necessary to restore knee extensor strength, ROM, and gait in an otherwise debilitating injury. Good to excellent outcomes including return to preinjury activity level and patient satisfaction are significantly improved in acute versus delayed repair. While atrophy and strength reduction of the quadriceps do occur despite surgical management (20% to 30%), overall outcomes are significantly improved over nonoperative repair (1).

CHRONIC QUADRICEPS TENDON REPAIR AND RECONSTRUCTION

Introduction

Orthopaedic literature demonstrates that chronic tears repaired in a delayed fashion have poorer outcomes. Chronic tears often have poor tissue quality, are significantly retracted, and are difficult to mobilize and repair in a tension-free fashion. Atrophy and weakness of the quadriceps are more pronounced. Dissatisfaction among patients treated in a delayed fashion can be upward of 50%. Despite this, however, delayed repair or reconstruction and revision of failed repairs confer significant improvement in patient outcomes over nonoperative treatment. We promote repair of the quadriceps tendon, even in a delayed fashion: a testament to the truly debilitating nature of knee extensor mechanism disruption.

Surgery

Technique

Our initial approach to treating chronic or failed QTR begins with the same goal as acute injuries: reapproximation of the quadriceps tendon to its anatomic patellar attachment with a tension-free repair. If the tendon can be advanced to the patella with the knee in full extension, we proceed with the same repair technique as acute QTR (Figs. 1-10 to 1-12; Video 1-3).

Video 1-3

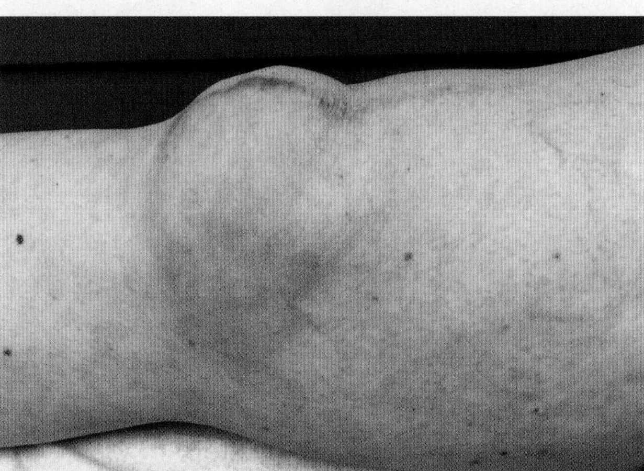

FIGURE 1-10

Chronic failed quadriceps repair. Defect in quad tendon is demonstrated.

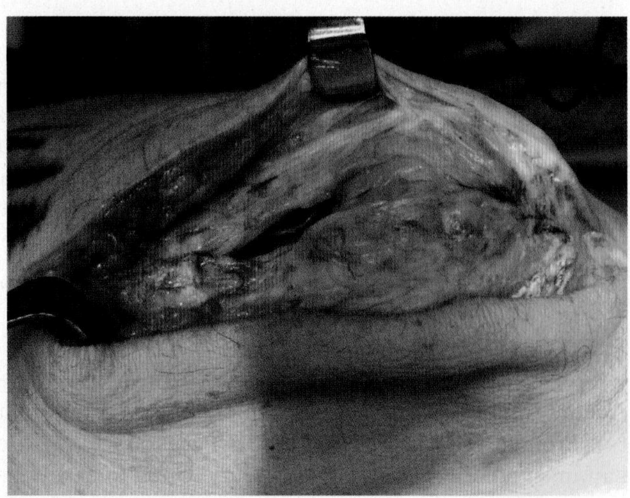

FIGURE 1-11

Failure of prior quad tendon repair. Notice the gapping between retracted quadriceps tendon on the left, patella on the right.

In these settings, the environment for healing is less hospitable, and additional measures to promote tendon healing are required. We have begun placing platelet-rich plasma (PRP) using the Arthrex ACP (Autologous Conditioned Plasma) system within the repair site of chronic QTR repairs. A systematic review of PRP in the treatment of patellar tendinopathy demonstrated improved clinical outcomes (14), but evidence for the use of PRP in chronic QTR repair is currently lacking. However, a case report of a patient with bilateral QTR demonstrated greater vascularity and more robust reparative process in the PRP injected tendon repair, yet did not reach clinical significance (15).

Reconstruction with an Achilles allograft is performed if the tendon cannot be mobilized or significant tendon deficiency exists. The distal end of the graft is whipstitched with two no. 2 FiberWire (Arthrex, Naples, FL) locking Krackow sutures with the tails exiting distally (Fig. 1-13). The sutures are passed through patellar bone tunnels using 2.4-mm Beath tip guidewires and tied down over the distal patellar pole similar to an acute quad tendon repair (Fig. 1-14). The graft is tensioned to the required length and then sutured to the distal extent of the native quadriceps tendon with no. 2 FiberWire (Fig. 1-15). The broad proximal portion of the Achilles graft is then reflected distally and sutured to the anterior patella (Fig. 1-16) and extensor retinacula with no. 1 Vicryl sutures (Fig. 1-17). Augmentation with the proximal graft provides additional structural support to the extensor mechanism and protection to the reconstructed quadriceps tendon. We feel this will facilitate a reduction in the rate of failure and lead to improved patient outcomes. The postoperative rehab protocol is the same as with an acute quadriceps tendon repair.

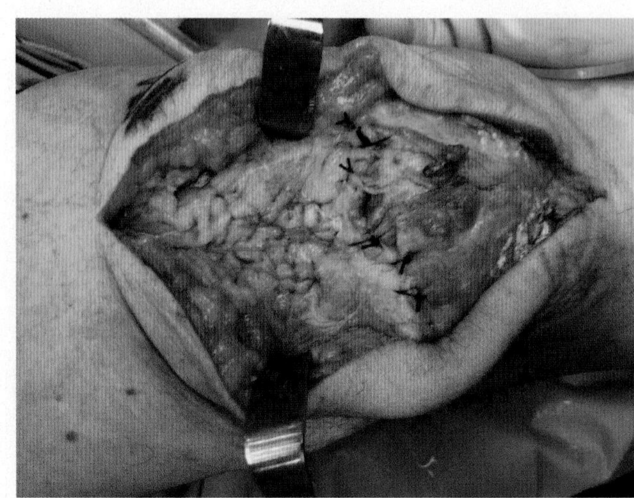

FIGURE 1-12

Revision quad tendon repaired primarily. Tendon easily mobilized to proximal patella. Extensor retinacula repaired. PRP (Arthrex ACP system) was added to the repair site prior to closure.

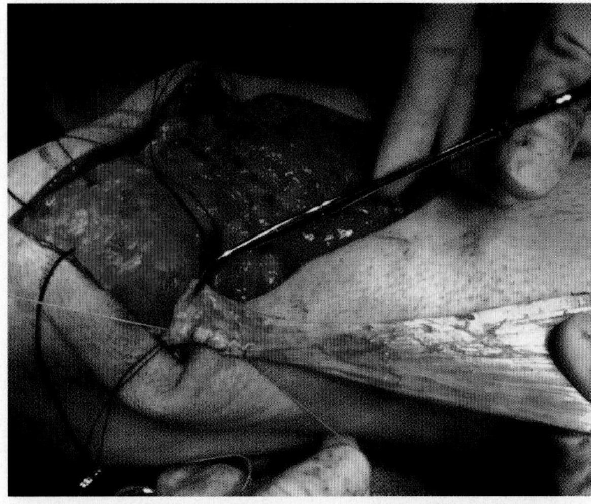

FIGURE 1-13

Achilles allograft reconstruction of a chronic QTR. No. 2 FiberWire (Arthrex, Naples, FL) sutures are placed in the distal allograft in a running Krackow fashion.

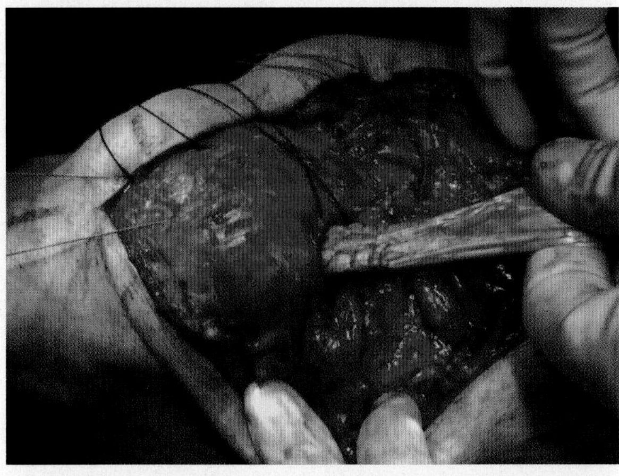

FIGURE 1-14

The graft sutures are passed through patellar bone tunnels and tied over the distal patella.

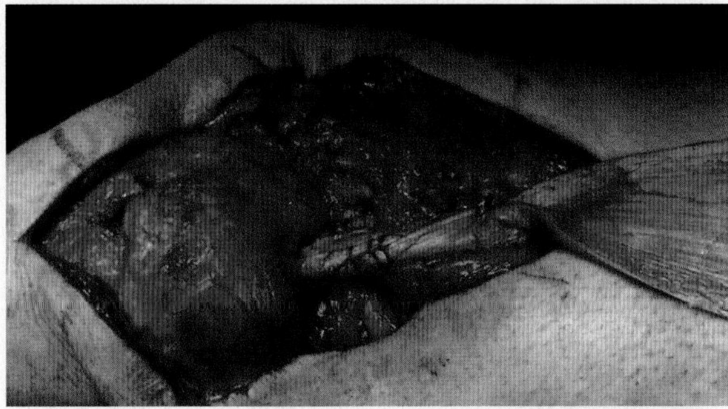

FIGURE 1-15

Achilles allograft is fixed securely to proximal patella in chronic quad tendon rupture. The graft Is tensloned to the required length and then sutured to the distal extent of the native quadriceps tendon.

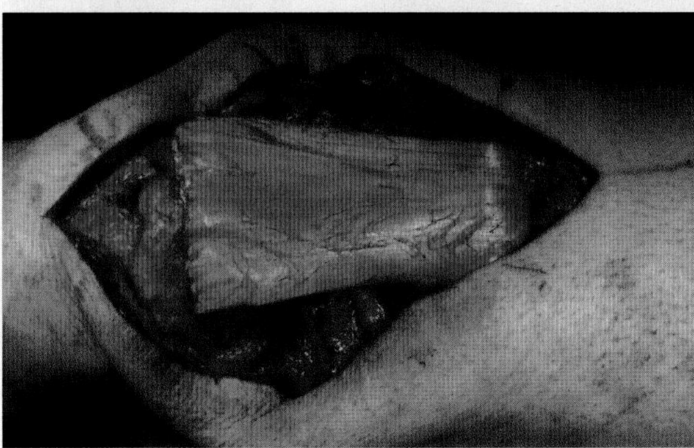

FIGURE 1-16

The proximal portion of the allograft is reflected and sutured to the anterior patella to augment the quadriceps tendon reconstruction.

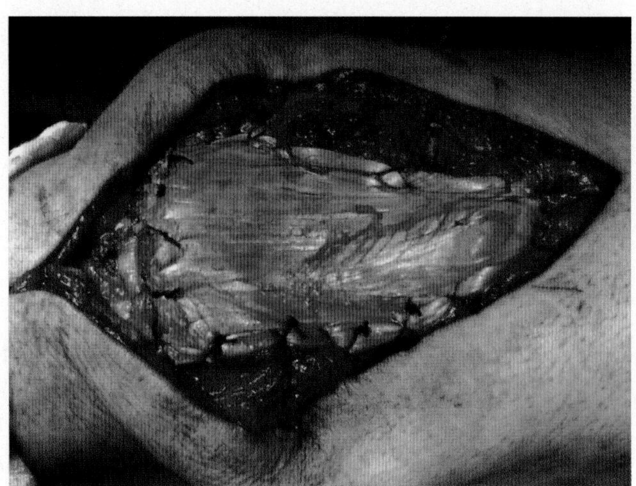

FIGURE 1-17

The reflected portion of the graft is repaired to the extensor retinacula, providing further augmentation to the quadriceps extensor mechanism. Reconstruction of the chronic quad tendon rupture is complete.

PATELLAR TENDON DISRUPTION

Introduction and Diagnosis

The mechanism of injury is typically an eccentric load to the tendon or secondary to trauma. Patellar disruption can occur in the setting of prior surgery or after mid-patellar tendon harvest for an anterior cruciate ligament (ACL) reconstruction.

The diagnosis of an acute patellar tendon disruption is usually obvious as the tendon is very superficial. There is usually a visible defect in the tendon upon palpation (Fig. 1-18). The patient either will not be able to perform a straight leg raise or will have an extensor lag with attempted straight leg raise. In obese patients or patient with a history of prior surgery, it can be more difficult to assess on physical exam. The location of the disruption is key to surgical planning as various repair or reconstruction techniques should be planned based upon the tear location.

Preoperative Planning

Radiographs of the knee should be obtained in the setting of trauma to assess for fractures. A lateral radiograph will demonstrate patella alta, or a superior position of the patella relative to the knee joint. An MRI should be obtained if the diagnosis is in question (Fig. 1-19). The surgeon should have all tools available in case a midsubstance or tibial tubercle avulsion is encountered.

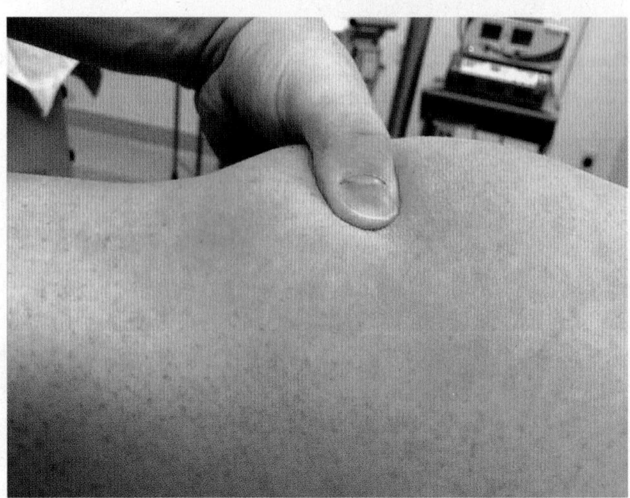

FIGURE 1-18

A palpable defect is usually present on physical exam.

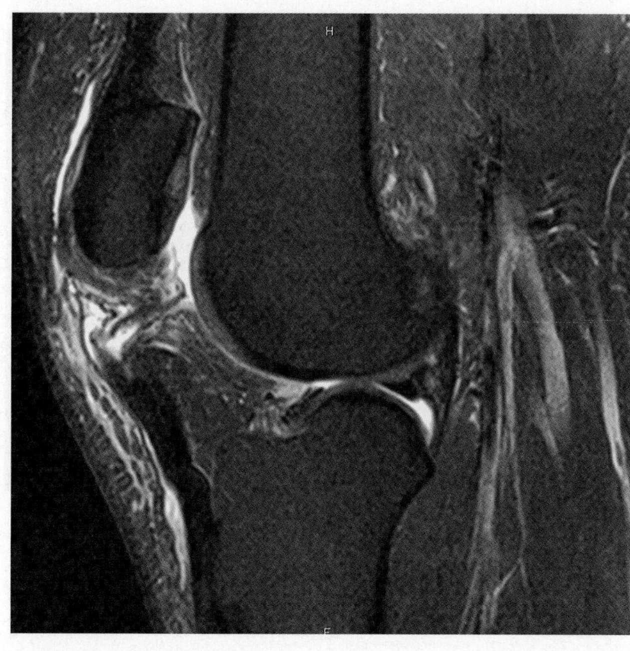

FIGURE 1-19

MRI of a patellar tendon disruption from the inferior pole of the patella.

Surgery

Patient Position

The patient should be positioned supine on the operating room table. To keep the knee in neutral position, we advocate for a towel or wedge bump (Bone Foam—Lateral Wedge) placed under the patient's ipsilateral pelvis and torso. A bump can then be used to elevate the operative leg (Fig. 1-20). A tourniquet can be used but is not required. If a tourniquet is used, it should be placed as far proximal as possible to prevent interference with the extensor mechanism excursion during the repair. Flexing the knee at the time of tourniquet inflation will also help prevent shortening of the extensor mechanism during surgery.

Technique

A midline incision should be made, and if possible, the surgeon should err on the side of making the incision medial for the potential of future surgery on the knee joint. Depending upon the tear location, the exposure should allow access superior to the patella and to the level of the tibial tubercle. Once the incision has been made, wide full-thickness skin flaps should be created to allow for adequate exposure to the paratenon covering the patellar tendon (Fig. 1-21). Gelpi retractors can be used for retraction. The paratenon is then incised in line with the tendon fibers, and this layer will be later closed over the future repair.

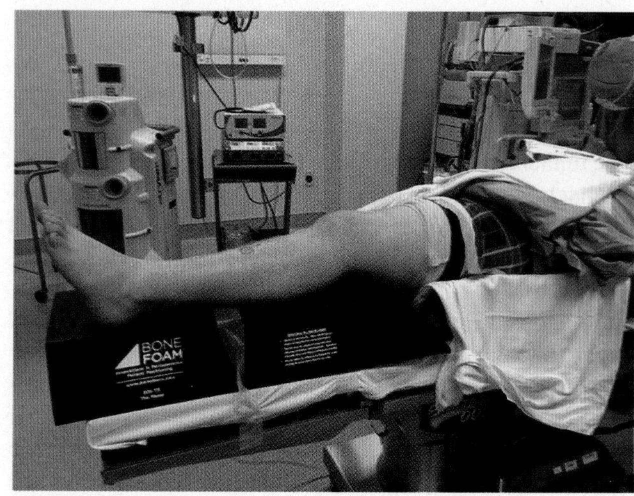

FIGURE 1-20

The patient is positioned supine with a wedge under the ipsilateral torso and pelvis. A nonsterile tourniquet is placed as far proximal as possible. The leg can be elevated on a ramp with the nonoperative leg secured to the table with the use of tape.

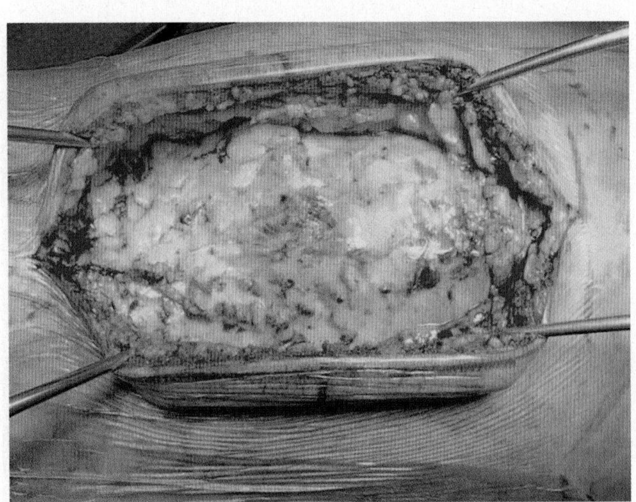

FIGURE 1-21

After a midline incision, generous skin flaps are created to allow for separation of the paratenon from the superficial layers. Large Gelpi retractors are helpful for exposure.

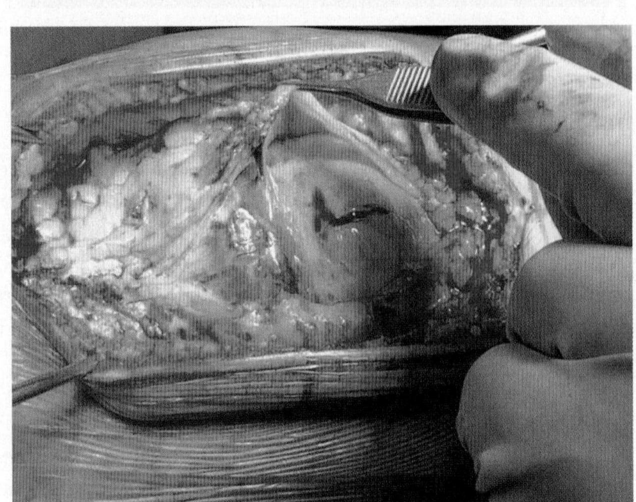

FIGURE 1-22

The paratenon is incised in line with the tendon. The thickened layer should be separated from the tendon surface to allow for later closure.

Upon entering the paratenon, the tendon is visible with an associated hematoma (Fig. 1-22). The Gelpi retractors can then be replaced inside the paratenon for exposure. The tendon ends can have a soupy, unhealthy appearance to them. The nonviable ends are debrided and cleaned for the planned repair.

REPAIR OF A PROXIMAL PATELLAR TENDON AVULSION INJURY

Proximal rupture is repaired utilizing bone tunnels through the patella or suture anchors.

Our preference is to utilize osseous tunnels for fixation. The inferior aspect of the patella is cleared of soft tissue, and a bone trough is created for the tendon. The bone trough can be created with the use of a rongeur or a high-speed bur. Once created, the tendon is then prepared using a polyethylene suture such as an Arthrex no. 2 FiberWire. Two sutures are then passed through the tendon, one on the medial side and the other on the lateral side in a Krackow stitch configuration (Fig. 1-23). The interlocking stitches add excellent strength to the repair.

Once the tendon has been prepared, we prefer to use three 2.4-mm ACL short guide pins (AR-1250SB) with eyelets to make tunnels in the patella. A rolled towel bump is then placed under the knee, flexing the knee approximately 30 degrees. The index finger of the free hand is placed on the chondral surface of the patella to obtain the appropriate trajectory of the guide pins, preventing

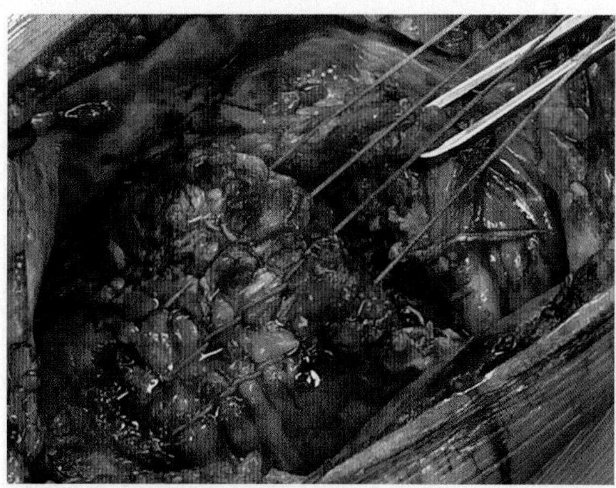

FIGURE 1-23

Two no. 2 FiberWire stitches are passed using a Krackow stitch configuration from the tear site distally and then returning proximally to the midportion of the tendon. The sutures should be evenly spaced, and care must be taken to not inadvertently puncture a previously placed stitch, which would weaken the construct.

a breach of the articular surface (Fig. 1-24). The first pin should be placed in the middle of the patella in the medial to lateral direction and midway in the anterior to posterior direction. If the guide pins are placed too superficial in the patella, this will create inferior tilt of the patella with the final repair.

The three pins are placed parallel to one another in the patella. We feel it is critical to use three individual guide pins as the patella is very dense bone and using dull guide pins can result in thermal necrosis. After breaching the superior cortex of the patella, an Army/Navy retractor is then used to guide the pin out of the quadriceps tendon and over the skin. Each of the guide pins is then advanced until just the eyelets are visible. The FiberWire sutures are then passed through the eyelets. The central guide pin will have two suture limbs, one from each FiberWire suture strand passed through the tendon. We then advocate that the end of the drill bit is held with a vise grips or pliers, and a mallet is used to advance the guide pins with sutures out of the patella (Fig. 1-25). It is tempting to grab the drill bit with a wire driver; however, this will potentially split the suture as they become bound up during passage through the patella. The rolled bump is then removed from behind the knee and placed behind the ankle. This will hold the leg in hyperextension, allowing for reduction of the tendon.

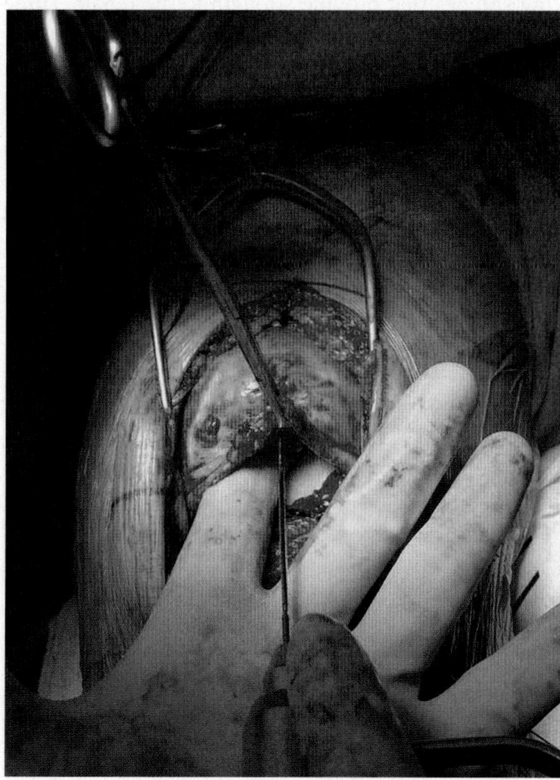

FIGURE 1-24

The free hand index finger is placed along the chondral surface of the patella. This serves as a guide to prevent chondral injury with the guide pin placement.

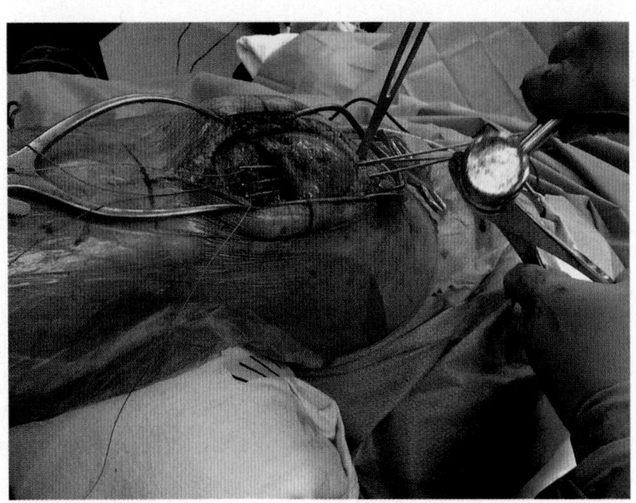

FIGURE 1-25

The guide pins are grasped with pliers, and a mallet is used to shuttle the stitches through the patellar tendon.

The sutures are then tied to one another above the patella (Fig. 1-26). One suture limb from the central drill tunnel is tied to each of the suture limbs from the peripheral tunnels.

Once the FiberWire sutures have been tied, the medial and lateral retinacula are then closed side to side with an interrupted cruciate stitch pattern using an 0 or 1 Vicryl stitch. At this point in time, the repair should be stressed to help guide the postoperative therapy protocol. The knee is then bent until there is visible tension on the repair. The patient should be allowed passive range of motion from neutral to this degree of flexion in the postoperative period (Fig. 1-27). The paratenon is then closed using no. 2 Vicryl in an interrupted fashion along its length.

Midsubstance Repair

A midsubstance repair is completed primarily with suture in an end-to-end fashion. We favor the use of a polyethylene-based suture material such as an Arthrex no. 2 FiberWire with tapered needles. The tendon is prepared in the manner described by Krackow. The suture is placed starting at the ruptured end and traveling away from the tear. The suture is then brought back down the tendon and through the rupture end. The sutures are locking stitches that provide strength to the repair. Three locking loops are sufficient for strength; however, we typically recommend multiple passes along the length of the remaining tendon. We try to have four suture limbs to tie at the end of the case. The same tendon preparation is done on the other side of the tear. At the time of tying the suture ends together, we recommend that the assistant hold the neighboring sutures under tension to allow for a tight end-to-end repair. The leg should also be held in full extension with a bump under the operative ankle.

If there is concern that a primary repair would fail, the repair can be augmented by the use of either hamstring tendon or suture material. Mersilene tape or FiberWire suture can be used for

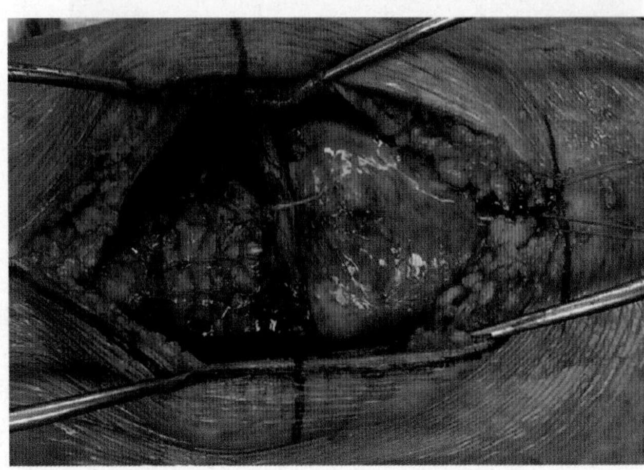

FIGURE 1-26

The repair after the sutures have been passed through the osseous tunnels.

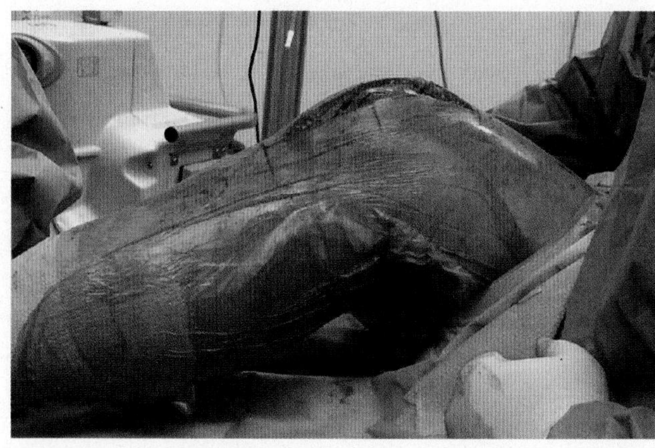

FIGURE 1-27
The knee is gently flexed to determine the point at which the repair is stressed. This will help determine where the patient can begin with the active range of motion in the repair protocol.

augmentation. A drill hole is made transversely through the patella, and suture is passed through this hole. An additional hole is then made in the tibial tubercle for passage of the suture. The suture is then tightened to offload the repair on the patellar tendon.

The semitendinosus has been used for augmentation in the literature. The tendon can be harvested from its distal insertion. Once harvested, it can be passed through a transverse hole in the patella and then attached to the tubercle with a suture anchor or side-to-side stitch configuration.

Inferior Patellar Tendon Disruptions

Although less common, inferior patellar tendon disruptions provide a technical challenge to repair. In general, these are treated with suture anchors for fixation. It is important for the surgeon to remember that the cortical bone in this region of the tibia will split when a suture anchor is forced. A drill or tap may be necessary depending upon the material and size of the anchor used. Two anchors are placed. Once the anchor has been placed, the tails of the anchor are made such that one is longer than the other. The longer limb is then used as a running Krackow stitch along the length of the tendon and back. The same occurs with the other anchor sutures. The sutures are then tied to one another with the knee in extension securing the patellar tendon to its insertion. The capsule and retinacular tissue should also be closed to enhance the repair.

Chronic Repairs

Chronic repairs can be augmented with the use of Achilles allograft with the associated calcaneal bone block. A trough is created in the tibia to allow for an inset of the bone block. The bone block is then secured using two 4.5-mm screws, which are placed bicortically for fixation. We advocate the use of fluoroscopy during the drilling of these screws as the neurovascular bundle is directly posterior to the path of the drill.

Any available tissue for repair of the native patellar tendon should be used to perform a repair similar to a primary repair prior to augmentation. Once secured distally, the Achilles tendon graft is laid over the top of the native patellar tendon to the quadriceps if the length allows. The graft is then sewn into the native patellar tendon reenforcing the native tissue. The rehab protocol should be adjusted for these repairs.

REFERENCES

1. Ciriello V, Gudipati S, Tosounidis T, et al. Clinical outcomes after repair of quadriceps tendon rupture: a systematic review. *Injury*. 2012;43:1931–1938.
2. Boudissa M, Roudet A, Rubens-Duval B, et al. Acute quadriceps tendon ruptures: a series of 50 knees with an average follow-up of more than 6 years. *Orthop Traumatol Surg Res*. 2014;100:217–220.
3. Saragaglia D, Pison A, Rubens-Duval B. Acute and old ruptures of the extensor apparatus of the knee in adults (excluding knee replacement). *Orthop Traumatol Surg Res*. 2013;99(suppl 1):S67–S76.
4. O'Shea K, Kenny P, Donovan J, et al. Outcomes following quadriceps tendon ruptures. *Injury*. 2002;33:257–260.
5. Khalid Y, Zhanel GG. Musculoskeletal injury associated with fluoroquinolones antibiotics. *Clin Plast Surg*. 2005;32:495–502.
6. Vidil A, Ouaknine M, Anract P, et al. Trauma-induced tears of the quadriceps tendon: 47 cases. *Rev Chir Orthop Reparatrice Apar Mot*. 2004;90:40–48.
7. Ramseier L, Werner C, Heinzelmann M. Quadriceps and patellar tendon rupture. *Injury*. 2006;37:516–519.

8. Swamy GN Nanjayan SK, Yallappa S, et al. Is ultrasound diagnosis reliable in acute extensor tendon injuries of the knee? *Acta Orthop Belg*. 2012;78(6):764–770.
9. Perfitt JS, Petrie MJ, Blundell CM, et al. Acute quadriceps rupture: a pragmatic approach to diagnostic imaging. *Eur J Orthop Surg Traumatol*. 2014;24(7):1237–1241.
10. Ilan DI, Tejwani N, Keschner M, et al. Quadriceps tendon rupture. *J Am Acad Orthop Surg*. 2003;11(3):192–200.
11. Rougraff BT, Reeck CC, Essenmacher J. Complete quadriceps tendon ruptures. *Orthopedics*. 1996;19:509–514.
12. West JL, Keene JS, Kaplan LD. Early motion after quadriceps and patellar tendon repairs: outcomes with single-suture augmentation. *Am J Sports Med*. 2008;36:316–323.
13. Wenzl ME, Kirchner R, Seide K, et al. Quadriceps tendon ruptures—is there a complete functional restitution? *Injury*. 2004;35:922–926.
14. Jeong DU, Lee CR, Lee JH, et al. Clinical applications of platelet-rich plasma in patellar tendonopathy. *BioMed Res Intern*. 2014;2014:1–15.
15. Lanzetti RM, Vadala A, Morelli F, et al. Bilateral Quadriceps rupture: results with and without platelet-rich plasma. *Orthopedics*. 2013;36(11):e1474–e1478.

2 Medial Patellofemoral Ligament Reconstruction Superficial Quadriceps Technique in the Young Athlete

Theodore J. Ganley, Zachary B. Domont, Peter D. Fabricant, and James L. Carey

Patellar instability in the skeletally immature patient may result from a primary, traumatic, laterally directed blow to the affected knee, but more often is the result of a low-energy or noncontact mechanism with knee twisting on a planted foot in patients at increased risk. Risk factors that predispose patients to patellar dislocation include a high Q-angle, trochlear dysplasia, excessive femoral anteversion, and collagen hyperlaxity.

Medial patellofemoral ligament (MPFL) reconstruction is a mainstay of patellar stabilization procedures, and due to the relationship of the distal femoral physis to the MPFL femoral origin, close attention must be paid to femoral tunnel placement. The goal of surgery is anatomic restoration of the patella medial check reign to properly restore the articulation of the patella within the femoral trochlea during early flexion.

It is understood that all patellofemoral dislocation patients will have underlying medical conditions, bone deformity, and soft tissue contractures addressed in concert with any patellofemoral ligament reconstruction. Patients with a lateralized tibial tubercle may have a pathologically elevated lateral tibial tubercle to trochlea groove (TT-TG) distance causing undue stress to any medial soft tissue procedure. In those circumstances, the most common surgeries performed in concert with an MPFL reconstruction are tibial tubercle medialization in patients with closed physes and the Roux-Goldthwait procedure, which lateralizes the patellar tendon insertion site without compromising the tibial tubercle growth center.

This chapter will address MPFL reconstruction in patients with appropriate alignment and insufficient medial patellofemoral restraint, specifically focusing on the clinical and radiographic evaluation, surgical technique, and rehabilitation for the superficial quadriceps technique. This chapter will not address osteotomies, skeletal dysplasia, and soft tissue contracture release following congenital patella dislocation.

Nonoperative treatment remains a viable form of treatment for a patient sustaining a patellar dislocation that has not sustained concurrent osteochondral avulsion fractures. Nonoperative treatment typically consists of postinjury activity restriction but early motion and brace treatment including lateral patellar support when swelling resolves. This treatment also entails rehabilitation involving core, hip, and isometric and closed chain kinetic quadriceps strengthening as well as early passive motion. Risk factors that diminish the success of nonoperative treatment include trochlear dysplasia, valgus deformity, a markedly lateralized tibial tubercle, and habitual subluxation or dislocation of the patella.

INDICATIONS FOR SURGERY

- Recurrent patella dislocation in those with appropriate alignment who have failed appropriate conservative treatment
- Primary or recurrent patella dislocation in patients with disrupted medial soft tissue restraints and chondral or osteochondral avulsions from the medial facet of the patella and/or the distal lateral trochlea
- MPFL rupture in a high-risk collision sport athlete

CONTRAINDICATIONS

- Active infection
- Inability to participate fully with postoperative restrictions
- Patients with medial patellofemoral instability following a prior excessive lateral release

PREOPERATIVE PLANNING

- **History:** Patients with patellofemoral instability commonly report a history of a distinct patellar dislocation event. It is helpful to gauge whether the instability episode required a reduction maneuver such as an extension of the knee on the sidelines or in the emergency room. The discreet history of the injury such as a direct blow to the lateral aspect of the knee or a twisting on a planted foot is additionally important as is the number of dislocation events. Further inquiry should be made regarding the development of an effusion, the activity or activities that elicit apprehension or dislocation, and mechanical symptoms such as locking or clicking. It is also important to note any family history of collagen or connective tissue disorders.
- **Physical Examination:** Physical examination of the patient with patellar instability begins with assessing for overall alignment and rotational mechanics. Particularly, genu valgum and excessive femoral anteversion (measured as excessive femoral internal rotation) should be recorded. Any knee effusion should be noted, and the patella should be translated laterally to assess for apprehension and quadrant mobility and endpoint firmness. A complete knee exam is performed to ensure that no additional injuries exist, and if there is concern for hypermobility, a Beighton score is calculated by evaluating palms to the floor and joint hypermobility of the fingers, wrists, elbows, and knees.
- **Radiographic Imaging:** Standard, weight-bearing knee radiographs including anteroposterior, 45 degrees of flexed posteroanterior, lateral in 30 degrees of flexion, and patellar views such as Merchant views are obtained. The patellar view is most helpful to show trochlear dysplasia, patellar tilt, and osteochondral fragments or loose bodies. Hyperflexion patellofemoral views should be avoided as they falsely depict anatomic patellar tracking by forcing the patella into the trochlear groove.
- **Magnetic Resonance Imaging:** In patients who have generalized laxity and experience a patellar dislocation without significant trauma or knee effusion, magnetic resonance imaging is not routinely used. For patients experiencing a traumatic patellar dislocation episode, magnetic resonance imaging is more commonly obtained along with plain radiographs to further delineate the integrity and location of injury of the MPFL, the degree of trochlear dysplasia, the presence of osteochondral fragments or loose bodies, the TT-TG distance, and the presence of concomitant injuries. Classically, there is bony edema within the medial patellar facet and the lateral aspect of the lateral femoral condyle due to impaction during reduction after a dislocation event.

TECHNIQUE

- **Preparation:** The patient is positioned in the supine position with lateral side post, and a tourniquet may be inflated based on surgeon preference.
- **Surgical Arthroscopy:** Routine surgical diagnostic arthroscopy is performed through standard anterolateral and anteromedial portals. The knee is then brought into extension and the arthroscope is positioned to evaluate the patellofemoral joint. Examination of the trochlea for dysplasia or osteochondral injuries is performed followed by evaluation of the distal lateral aspect of the lateral femoral condyle for impaction injury. If loose bodies are suspected based on MRI, these are commonly found in the lateral gutter or suprapatellar pouch. The patella is then evaluated with careful attention paid to the medial patellar facet and patellar tracking is dynamically evaluated by flexing and extending the knee.

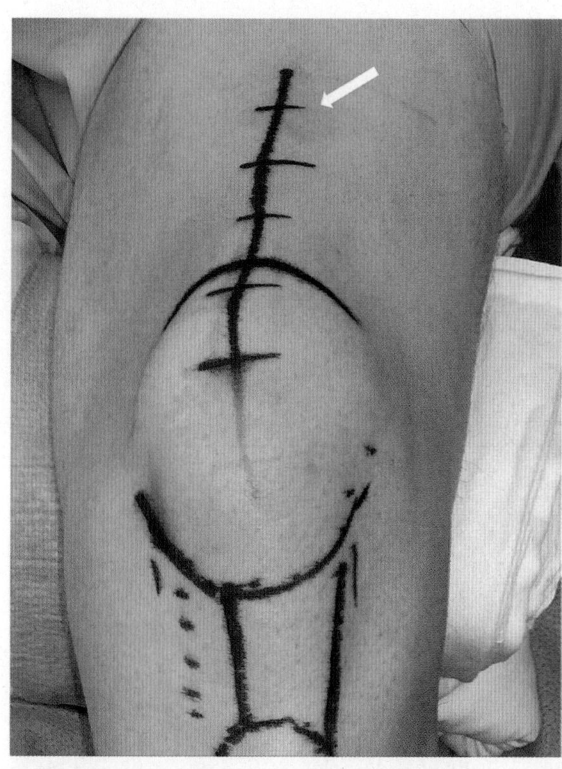

FIGURE 2-1

The *arrow* shows the location of the midline incision for the quadriceps turndown medial patellofemoral ligament reconstruction procedure.

Quadriceps Tendon Harvest

An incision is made midline from the superior third of the patella proximally for a distance of 10 cm (Fig. 2-1) through the dermis, and hemostasis is achieved using electrocautery. Metzenbaum scissors are used to release and develop the plane superficial to the retinaculum and quadriceps tendon. The proper location of the graft harvest (Fig. 2-2) 7 to 10 mm in width and 10 cm proximal to the patella is outlined using a marking pen. A longitudinal incision is made at least 2 to 3 cm proximal to the proximal pole of the patella to dissect (Fig. 2-3) beneath the superficial slip of the quadriceps tendon (rectus femoris portion) while leaving the deep slip (vastus intermedius) intact (Fig. 2-4). Dissection is carried through the superficial quadriceps tendon and the width of the desired graft is typically 7 to 10 mm. (Figs. 2-4 and 2-5). Dissection is developed proximally

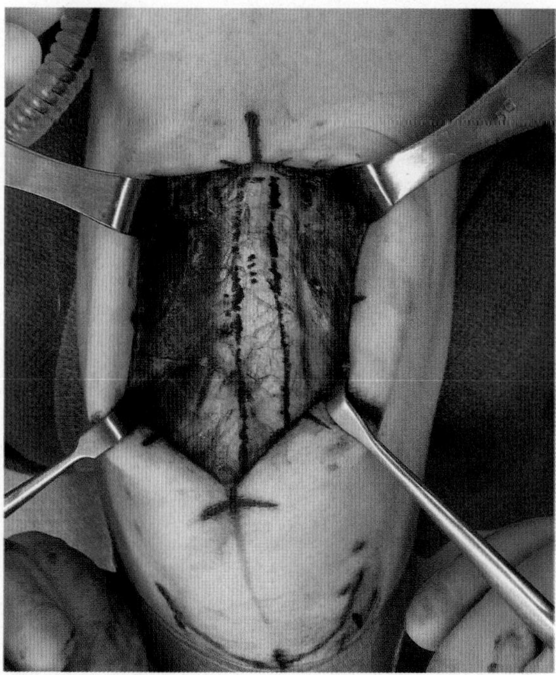

FIGURE 2-2

The proper location for the superficial quadriceps graft harvest is outlined using a sterile marking pen.

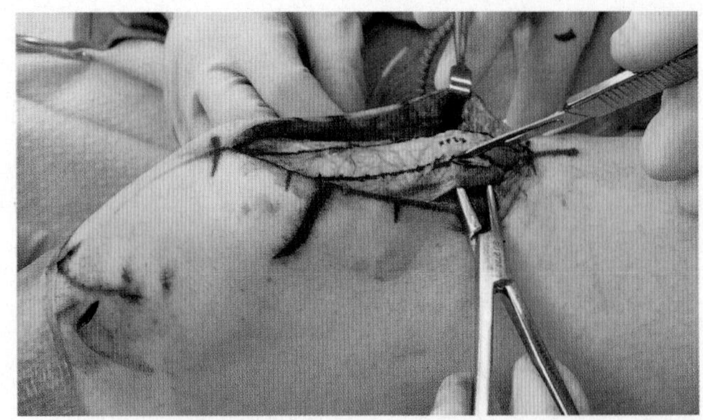

FIGURE 2-3

A longitudinal incision is made through to the superficial slip of the quadriceps tendon at least 2 to 3 cm proximal to the proximal pole of the patella.

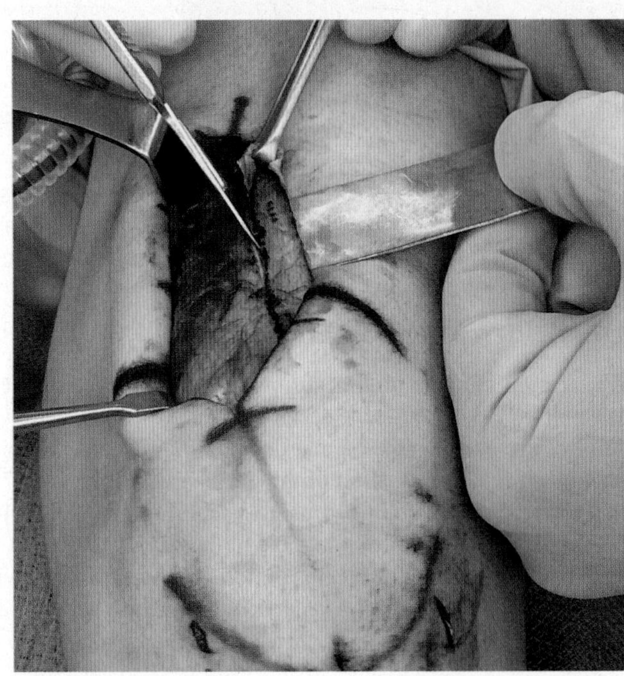

FIGURE 2-4

A longitudinal incision is made through the superficial slip of the quadriceps, and a metal ribbon is shown protecting deeper structures including the deep slip of the quadriceps.

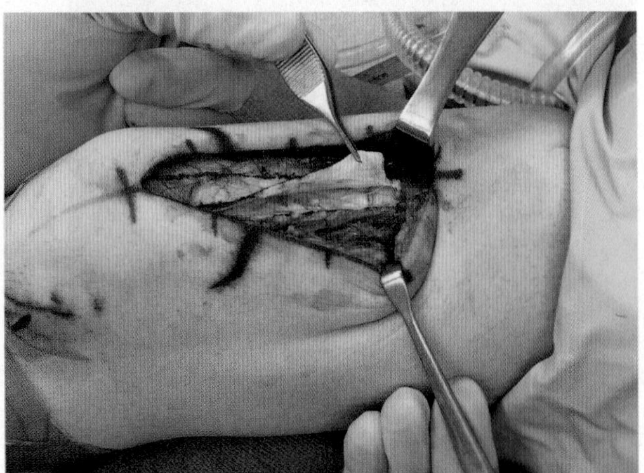

FIGURE 2-5

The forceps is shown on the proximal aspect of the superficial slip of the quadriceps tendon.

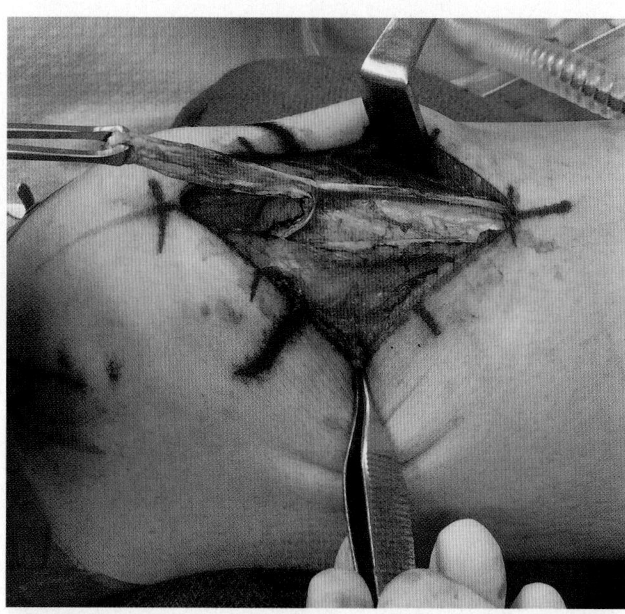

FIGURE 2-6

An Allis clamp is placed on the superficial quadriceps graft, which has been detached proximally.

toward the muscle-tendon junction to a point roughly 10 cm proximal to the proximal pole of the patella. Metzenbaum scissors are then used to connect the longitudinal incisions and create a free graft end proximally (Fig. 2-6). A no. 15 blade is then used to carry the intratendinous dissection distally and to skeletonize the quadriceps tendon from the proximal third of the patella. Slightly more tendon is released distally on the lateral limb overlying the patella than on the medial limb such that the graft is reflected medially with minimal prominence anteriorly (Figs. 2-7 and 2-8). When the graft is reflected toward the femur, high-strength "rip stop" sutures are to be placed at the distal most point of dissection on the patella (Figs. 2-8 and 2-9).

Medial Dissection

Medial to the patella, sharp dissection is performed to enter the potential space between layers two and three, which lies superficial to the joint capsule (Fig. 2-10). Blunt dissection is performed without resistance toward the adductor tubercle, opening this area widely to avoid graft impingement.

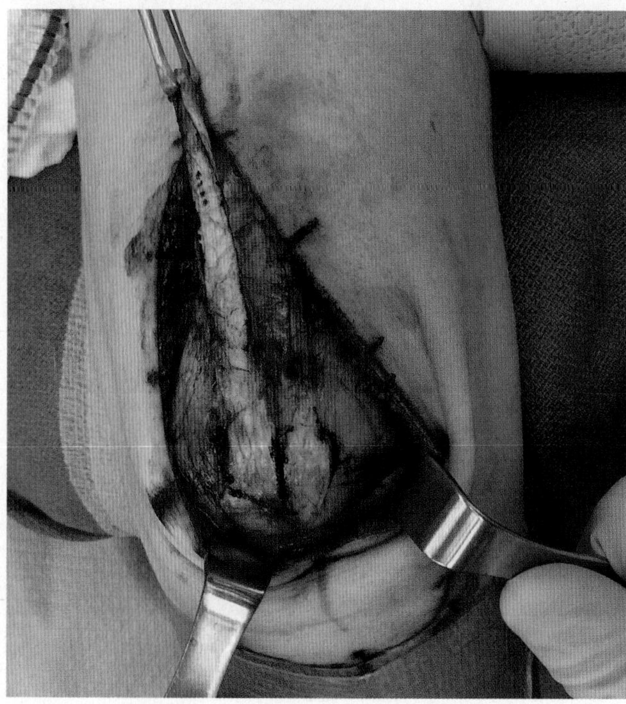

FIGURE 2-7

Dissection is performed to the midpatella and is carried slightly more distally and laterally than medially.

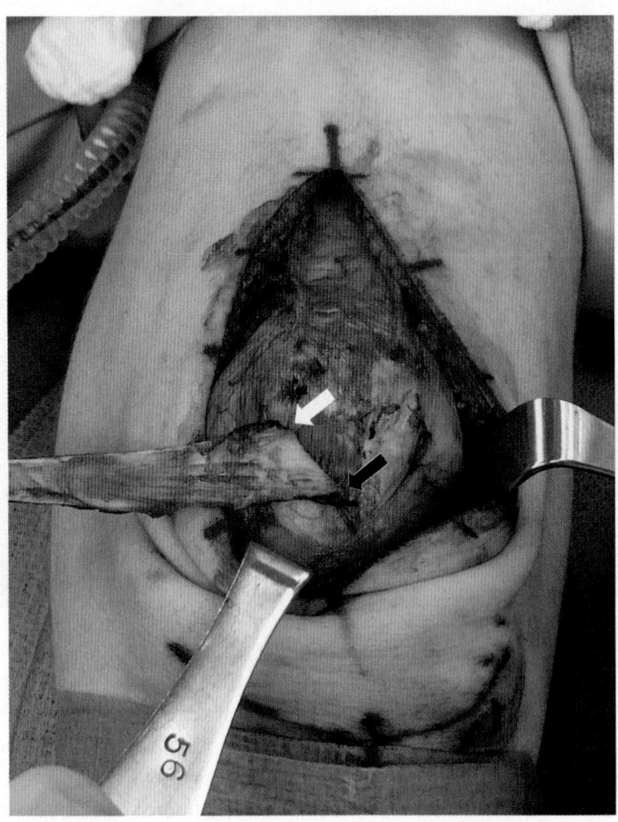

FIGURE 2-8

The graft is reflected medially, and the lateral limb (*black arrow*) is carried more distal than the medial limb (*white arrow*).

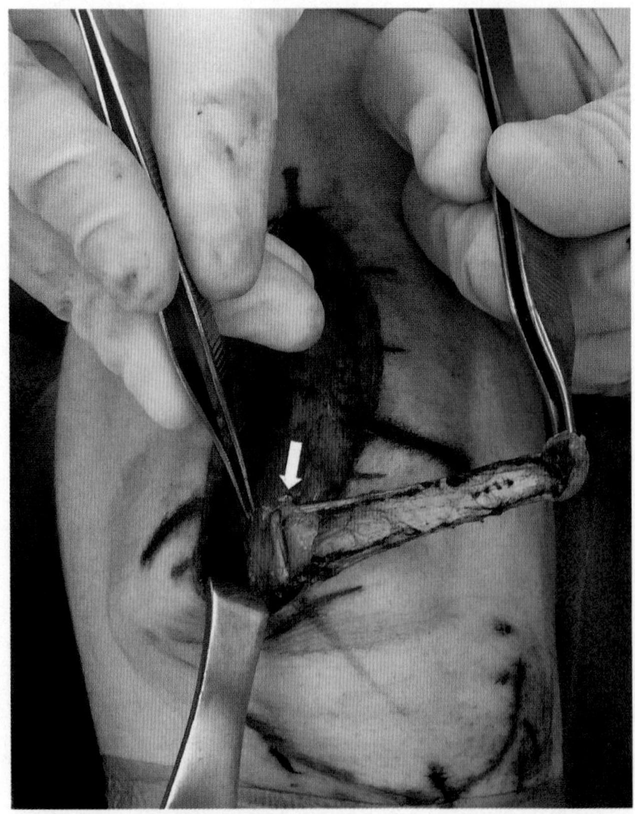

FIGURE 2-9

A high-strength suture (*white arrow*) is placed at the points where the graft is reflected.

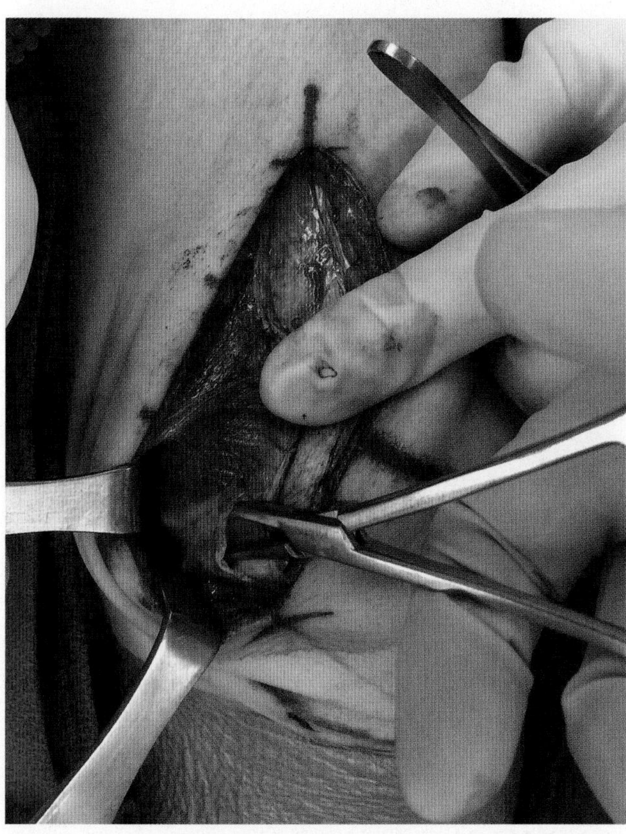

FIGURE 2-10
Dissection is carried distal to the vastus medialis between layers two and three.

A 2-cm incision is made directly overlying the saddle between the adductor tubercle and the medial epicondyle through which the graft will be secured (Fig. 2-11).

Femoral Tunnel

Attention is then turned to the creation of the femoral tunnel. Palpation of the medial side of the knee is performed to the medial epicondyle, which is slightly anterior and distal to the adductor tubercle (which is in turn slightly proximal and posterior to the medial epicondyle). Between these two structures is the saddle-shaped origin of the MPFL. A 2.4-mm guide wire is passed through the medial femoral skin incision. Under fluoroscopic guidance, the pin is advanced. If a physeal-avoiding technique is preferred, the guide pin is aimed just distal to the medial physeal flare, which is typically 6 mm distal to the distal femoral physis. When the patient is skeletally immature with open physes, locate the footprint by palpating between the medial epicondyle and adductor tubercle, confirm with C-arm, and place the tunnel just distal to the physis. When using the all-epiphyseal

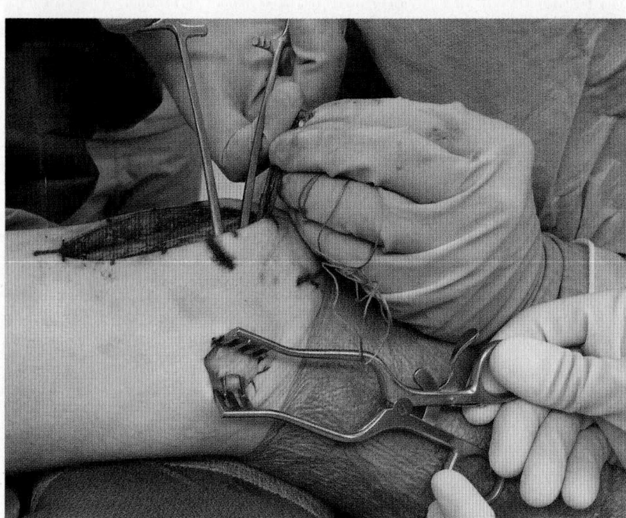

FIGURE 2-11
A curved clamp is placed between layers two and three and is spread widely to prevent graft impingement.

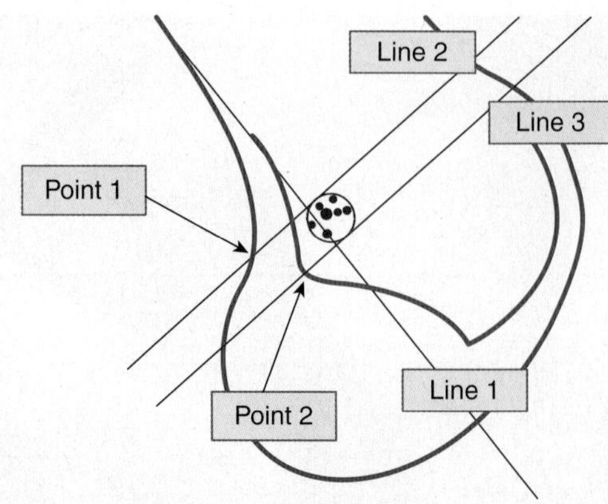

FIGURE 2-12

The *circle* represents the optimal guide pin position for femoral tunnel drilling, as described by Schöttle et al.

technique, place the tunnel in the epiphysis. If the optimal position for the tunnel is at the physis, then use two limbs and secure just above and below the physis via tunnels or sutures only, as described by Noyes and Albright. If the patient is approaching skeletal maturity and in valgus, then the surgeon may intentionally drill and place the tunnel across the physis to get some slight correction to neutral prior to skeletal maturity. A perfect lateral radiograph is then obtained such that the medial and lateral femoral condyles completely overlap. The optimal position for the guide pin is, as described by Schöttle et al., 1.3 mm anterior to a line drawn along the posterior cortex, 2.5 mm distal to a perpendicular that crosses at the posterior origin of the medial femoral condyle, and 3 mm proximal to a perpendicular that intersects the most proximal point of the Blumensaat line (Fig. 2-12). Once the guide pin has been placed into the anatomic footprint of the MPFL, an 18-gauge needle or a hemostat is placed to allow for accurate identification of the starting point on the plain radiograph (Fig. 2-13). Once this is confirmed, the guide pin is advanced into the femur. The guide pin is then overdrilled with a 6-mm drill to 25 to 30 mm.

Graft Preparation

The distance from the medial border of the proximal half of the patella to the anatomic footprint on the femur for the MPFL is measured by placing a suture within the soft tissue plane native to the MPFL between those two points. Once harvested proximally, the quadriceps tendon graft is folded medially to note the length of tendon that will be to the anatomic footprint and the length that will be in the femoral tunnel. A mark is made on the graft with a marking pen at the level of the MPFL

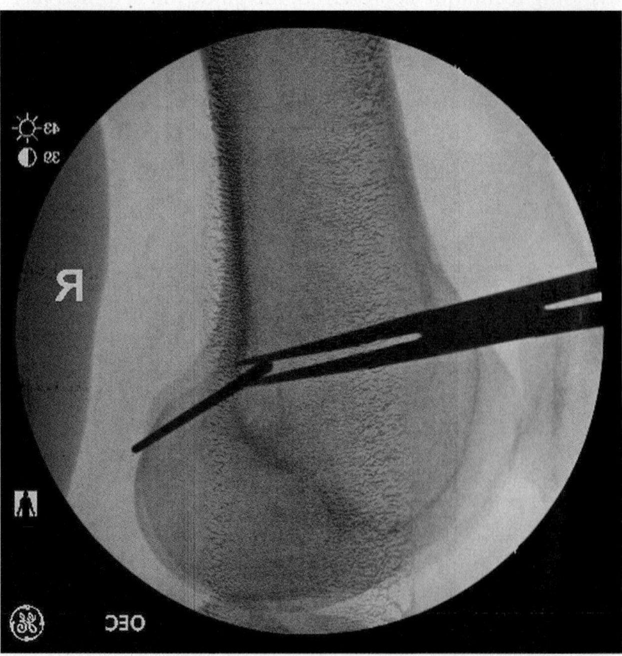

FIGURE 2-13

A hemostat is placed over the guide pin to show the pin entry point on the radiograph.

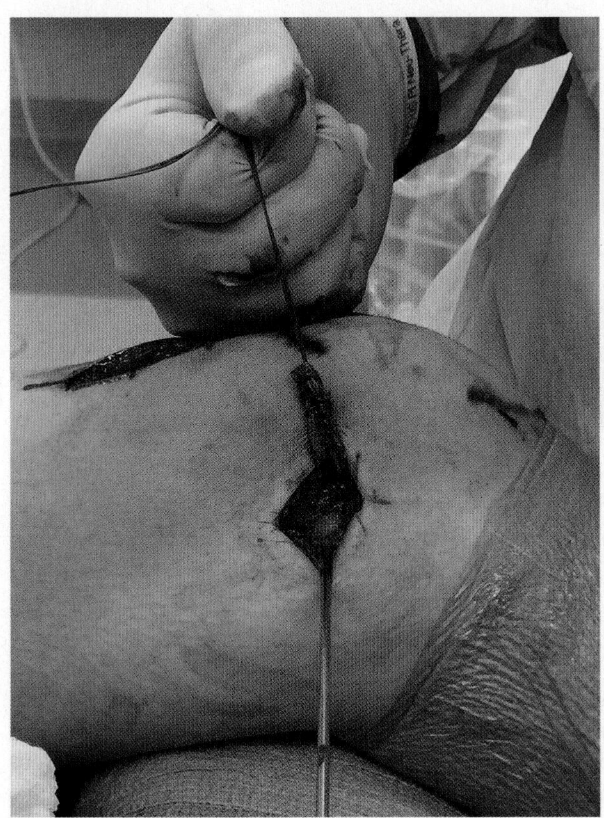

FIGURE 2-14

The graft is shown traversing the distal medial incision.

footprint on the femur, and the graft is whipstitched from that point 20 mm to the end of the graft using a no. 2 nonresorbable suture to create a Krakow or locking whipstitch (Fig. 2-14).

Graft Passage and Fixation

A pull suture is placed between layers two and three to allow for smooth passage of the graft from the anterior incision to and out of the medial incision (Fig. 2-15). The authors prefer to tubularize and size the graft to 6 mm and use a 6 × 23 mm interference screw for femoral fixation (Figs. 2-16 and 2-17). The knee is taken through a range of motion and stopped at the flexion angle that creates the greatest degree of tension, which is typically between 45 and 60 degrees of flexion. The screw is docked into the femoral tunnel and tightened until the head of the screw is flush with the cortical bone at the medial distal femur. The knee is then taken

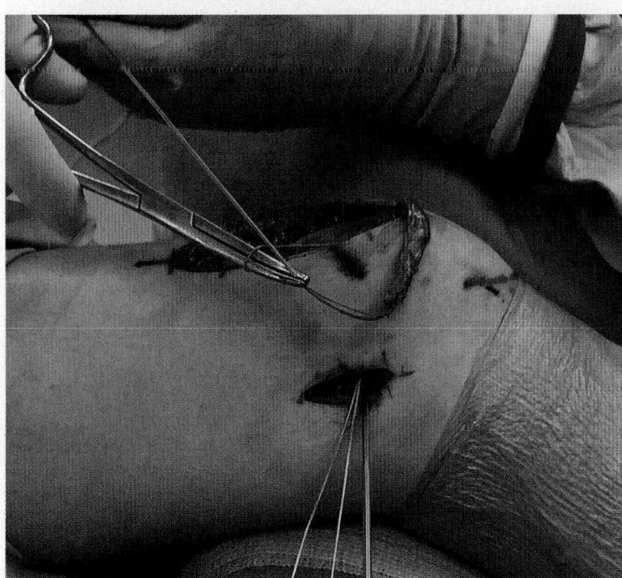

FIGURE 2-15

A pull suture, which can facilitate graft passage, is shown traversing layers two and three.

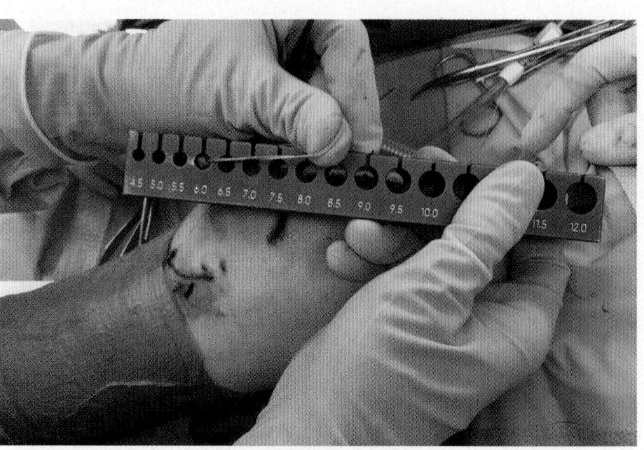

FIGURE 2-16

The tubularized graft is shown in a graft sizer.

through a full range of motion with particular attention paid to full extension and full flexion (ensuring the heel can touch the ipsilateral buttock). The MPFL that has been placed is palpated, and the patella is checked to ensure that appropriate medial to lateral translation is noted in all degrees of flexion and extension.

Closure

The wounds are copiously irrigated and the deep retinacular layer on the femoral side is closed with 0 resorbable braided suture as are the remaining superficial quadriceps tendon slip and paratenon. Subcutaneous tissue is closed with 2-0 resorbable braided suture, and a running subcuticular running suture is placed using 4-0 monofilament resorbable suture.

PEARLS/PITFALLS

- It is best to define the plane between the superficial and deep slips of the quadriceps tendon 2 to 3 cm above the superior pole of the patella, as distal to this point they are confluent.
- Use caution when dissecting the quadriceps tendon from the anterior patella. Excessive distal dissection traction can cause the tendon to begin to detach from the patella.
- When placing the guide pin for the medial femoral tunnel, use a second metal instrument (such as a large-bore needle or hemostat) at the medial femoral cortex to allow for accurate identification of the entry point of the pin into the distal medial femur.

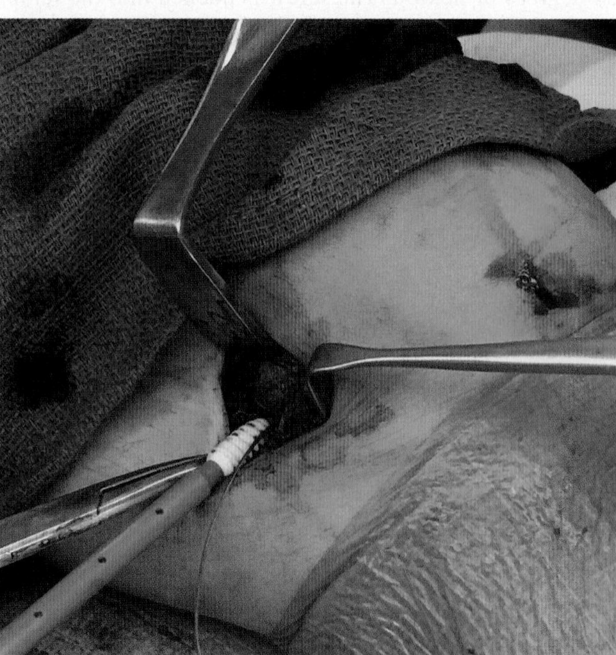

FIGURE 2-17

An interference screw, which is the same size as the graft and the tunnel, is placed.

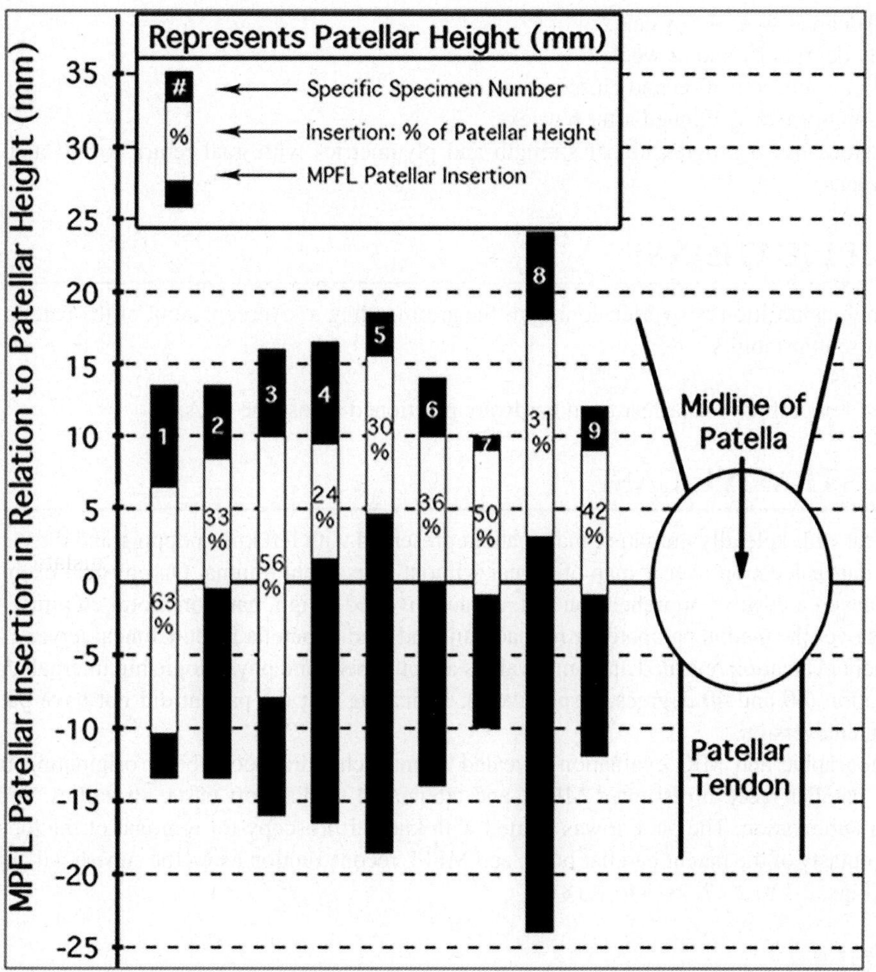

FIGURE 2-18
An anatomic study conducted by Shea et al. demonstrates the location of the MPFL patellar insertion. (From Shea KG, Polousky JD, Jacobs JC Jr, et al. The patellar insertion of the medial patellofemoral ligament in children: a cadaveric study. *J Pediatr Orthop.* 2015;35(4):e31–e35.)

- Use stay sutures on the medial aspect of the patella as a "rip-stop" to secure the graft to the anatomic footprint on the patella.
- Dissect the quadriceps tendon from the anterior patella slightly more distal laterally then medially to allow the quadriceps tendon graft to be appropriately folded and avoid excessive tendon graft prominence. Dissecting more distal laterally and in the proximal half of the patella medially allows for a broad expanse of tissue at the medial patella to mimic the native origin of the MPFL that has been noted in anatomic study (Fig. 2-18).
- Ensure that the knee is at roughly 45 degrees of knee flexion when the graft is secured into the femur.
- When the graft has been secured, take the knee through a full range of motion, and confirm that there is appropriate medial to lateral patella excursion and full flexion.
- Do not overtension the graft, as the MPFL functions not to constrain as a physiologic check rein against lateral patellar translation during early flexion.

POSTOPERATIVE MANAGEMENT

- Toe-touch weight bearing with crutches, continuous passive motion machine 0 to 30 degrees and advance to 10 degrees per day as tolerated.
- Wean crutches between weeks 2 and 4 and progress to full weight bearing at 4 weeks.
- Promote knee flexion.

- 90 degrees by end of week 2
- 130 degrees by end of week 4
- Begin muscle activation and closed-chain exercises.
- Post-op brace discontinued after 6 weeks.
- Milestone-based progression of strength and plyometrics with goal return to full activities at 24 weeks.

COMPLICATIONS

- Tunnel malposition or overtensioning of the graft leading to overconstraint of the patella
- Recurrent instability
- Stiffness
- Distal femoral physeal arrest from hardware positioned across the physis

ILLUSTRATIVE CASE

A 14-year-old skeletally immature male patient presented with left knee popping and three episodes of patellar dislocation over a span of 1 year without antecedent trauma. On physical examination, he displayed a positive apprehension test, a trace inverted J-sign, patellofemoral crepitus, and tenderness over the medial parapatellar retinaculum and medial patella facet. Clinical lower extremity alignment evaluation revealed anatomic valgus at both knees and physiologic hip internal and external rotation (60 and 40 degrees, respectively), indicating that the patient did not have pathologic femoral anteversion.

Radiographic and MRI evaluation revealed a small chondral loose body originating from the medial patellar facet, a disrupted MPFL and attenuated medial soft tissue structures, and lateral patellar subluxation. The patient was treated with knee arthroscopy for removal of the loose body, chondroplasty of the parent patellar bone, and MPFL reconstruction using the superficial quad technique (Figs. 2-1 to 2-12, 2-15 to 2-18).

RESULTS

Steensen et al. described the superficial quadriceps technique for MPFL reconstruction reporting on the results of 14 knees in 13 patients, none of whom experienced recurrent dislocation at an average of 37 months. They did not comment on the presence of any complications or report on patient-reported outcomes. The superficial quad technique for reconstruction of the MPFL was first described by Noyes et al. and further reported upon by Goyal in 32 patients with no patella complications and Kujala score improvements similar to other techniques using hamstring grafts.

RECOMMENDED READINGS

Beighton PH, Horan F. Orthopedic aspects of the Ehlers-Danlos syndrome. *J Bone Joint Surg Br.* 1969;51:444–453.

Goyal D. Medial patellofemoral ligament reconstruction: the superficial quad technique. *Am J Sports Med.* 2013;41(5):1022–1029.

Noyes FR, Albright JC. Reconstruction of the medial patellofemoral ligament with autologous quadriceps tendon. *Arthroscopy.* 2006;22(8):904.e1–904.e7.

Palmu S, Kallio PE, Donell ST, et al. Acute patellar dislocation in children and adolescents: a randomized clinical trial. *J Bone Joint Surg Am.* 2008;90:463–470.

Schöttle PB, Schmeling A, Rosenstiel N, et al. Radiographic landmarks for femoral tunnel placement in medial patellofemoral ligament reconstruction. *Am J Sports Med.* 2007;35(5):801–804.

Shea KG, Polousky JD, Jacobs JC, et al. The patellar insertion of the medial patellofemoral ligament in children: a cadaveric study. *J Pediatr Orthop.* 2015;35(4):e31–e35.

Steensen RN, Dopirak RN, Maurus PB. A simple technique for reconstruction of the medial patellofemoral ligament using a quadriceps tendon graft. *Arthroscopy.* 2005;21:365–370.

Warren LF, Marshall JL. The supporting structures and layers on the medial side of the knee: an anatomical analysis. *J Bone Joint Surg Am.* 1979;61(1):56–62.

3 Medial Patellofemoral Ligament Reconstruction

T. Sean Lynch and Christopher S. Ahmad

MPFL BASICS

The medial patellofemoral ligament (MPFL) is the primary static restraint to lateral translation of the patella. The MPFL is most important for the first 30 to 50 degrees of knee flexion as the patella engages into the trochlea when the articular geometry subsequently increases its contribution to stability as knee flexion increases. The MPFL originates between the medial epicondyle and the adductor tubercle on the femur and attaches to the proximal medial edge of the patella.

MPFL injury has been termed "the essential lesion." First time dislocators have a 50% chance of recurrent episodes of patellar dislocations or subluxations. Causes of patellofemoral instability are multifactorial with bony and soft tissues contributors that can include the following:

- Abnormal mechanical alignment
  - Increased quadriceps angle
  - External tibial torsion
  - Patella alta
  - Increased femoral anteversion
  - Pes planus
  - Genu valgum
- Deficient static and dynamic soft tissue stabilizers
  - Generalized ligamentous laxity
  - Vastus medialis obliquus atrophy
  - MPFL insufficiency
- Abnormal cartilage and osseous abnormalities of the patella and trochlea

PATIENT PRESENTATION

Patellar instability represents a continuum ranging from minor incidental subluxation episodes to traumatic fixed dislocations that require reductions.

- Indirect: patellar dislocations can occur from an indirect twisting mechanism as the upper body rotates while the foot remains planted on the ground. During athletic motions, this at-risk knee position is termed functional valgus. With the knee in flexion, the femur is relatively internally rotated and adducted, while the tibia is externally rotated and abducted.
- Direct: traumatic blow to the medial aspect of the patella forcing it laterally during a sporting event or motor vehicle accident is a less common mechanism.

Regardless of mechanism, patients with patellar instability are at risk of chondral injuries. Franzone et al. showed that the increasing chronicity of a patient's patellar instability may have a higher likelihood of and higher grade of patellofemoral chondral injuries, specifically for trochlear lesions. The patella may spontaneously reduce as the knee is extended or may require a formal reduction maneuver.

With a first dislocation, the patient will usually experience significant pain and swelling that is caused by soft tissue and intra-articular damage. The resulting hematoma/hemarthrosis and residual quadriceps weakness may take several weeks to resolve.

The patient will usually describe an episode of "giving way" when going into a flexed position while pivoting. Sometimes, the event is associated with an audible pop and a rapid onset of an effusion; therefore, the history can resemble an anterior cruciate ligament (ACL) tear (in fact, patella instability event is often confused for an ACL injury).

Patients with multiple episodes of instability tend to experience less severe symptoms and often describe a sense that their knee may "give out."

Physical Exam

- Inspection:
  - Tibiofemoral alignment with patient standing or walking
  - Assess for effusion and extra-articular swelling
  - J sign: during active knee extension, observe patellar tracking for the tendency of the patellar to slip laterally as the knee approaches the last 20 degrees of extension when the patella is no longer constrained by the lateral trochlear ridge
- Palpation:
  - Along the course of the MPFL, identify the area of greatest tenderness as this usually identifies the location of the tear.
    - Acute dislocators typically exhibit tenderness along the adductor tubercle, suggesting an injury at the insertion.
    - Direct compression of the patella into the trochlea at various degrees of knee flexion may elicit pain and/or crepitance to help localize potential articular cartilage injuries.
- Ligamentous assessment:
  - It is necessary to rule out concomitant cruciate or collateral ligament tears.
    - Medial collateral ligament (MCL) injuries commonly occur at the time of patellar dislocation.
- Provocative testing:
  - Patellar translation: estimate in quadrants by applying laterally directed force to the medial aspect of the patella with the knee in extension.
    - Normal is two quadrants of displacement in either direction.
    - Soft end point suggests MPFL incompetence.
  - Apprehension sign: with laterally directed pressure on medial aspect of patella at 30 degrees of knee flexion, a sense of apprehension or an indistinct end point supports the diagnosis of instability.
  - Moving patellar apprehension test (MPAT): patient lies supine and relaxed with ankle held off the examination table by the physician. The first part of the test includes translation of the patella laterally with the examiners thumb as far as possible with the knee in full extension. The lateral force on the patella is maintained while the knee is flexed to 90 degrees and brought back to full extension (Fig. 3-1A). The second part of the test consists of a medially directed force placed on the patella by the examiners index finger attempting to translate the patella medially with the knee in full extension to 90 degrees of flexion and back to full extension (Fig. 3-1B).

Imaging

Plain radiographs: weight-bearing anteroposterior (AP), lateral with the knee flexed to 30 degrees, and Merchant views can help to confirm patellar location, presence of osteochondral fracture, and patellofemoral relationships.

- The presence of an osteochondral fracture on x-ray is likely a significant lesion that should be followed by a magnetic resonance imaging (MRI) and possible surgical excision or fixation.
- Lateral view with the knee flexed 30 degrees can indicate patella height. A Caton-Deschamps index of more than 1.3 implies patella alta, which predisposes the patella to lateral instability as the medial patellar facet is not captured by the lateral femoral condyle in early flexion (Fig. 3-2).
- The lateral view with the posterior condyles aligned can evaluate trochlear dysplasia with the "crossing sign," where the curve of the trochlear floor crosses the anterior contour of the lateral femoral condyle. This represents flattening of the trochlear groove and an absence of trochlear constraint against patellar displacement.

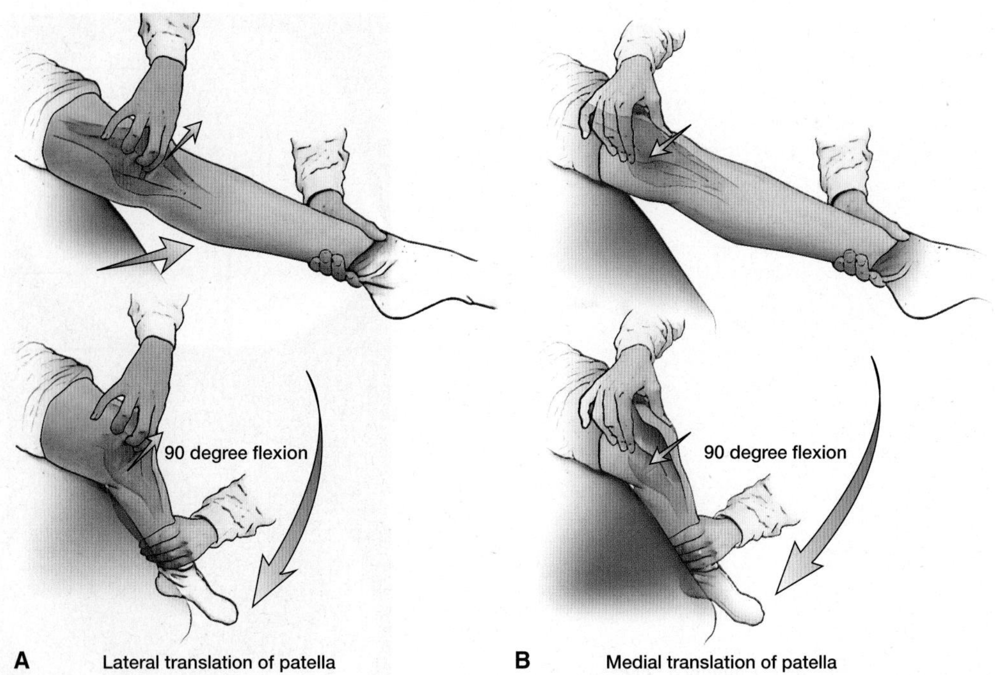

FIGURE 3-1

Moving patellar apprehension test. Part 1 of the test is considered positive if the patient expresses apprehension and may activate his/her quadriceps to stop flexion. Part 2 is considered positive if free flexion and extension are completed with no sign of apprehension. MPAT is considered positive if both parts 1 and 2 are positive.

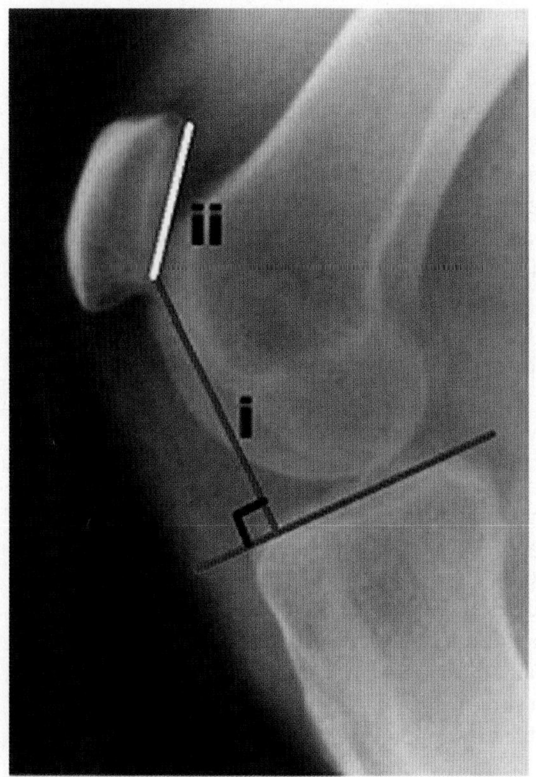

FIGURE 3-2

The Caton-Deschamps index is a ratio between the length of (a) the tibial plateau to the lower end of the patellar articular surface and (b) patellar articular surface length. If the quotient is greater than 1.3, the patient has patella alta.

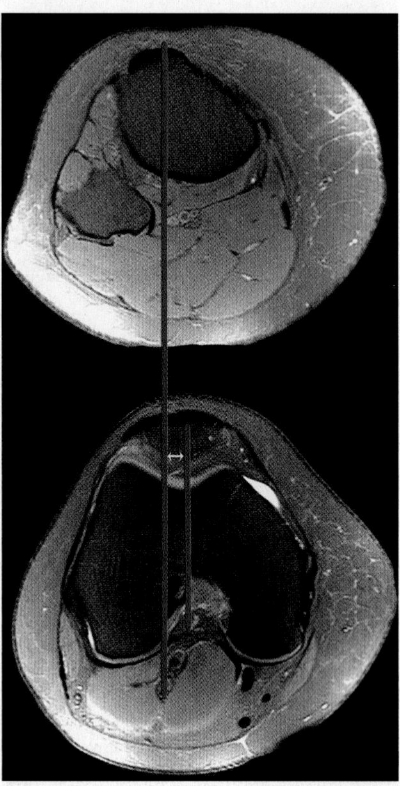

FIGURE 3-3

TT-TG distance measures the distance between two perpendicular lines from the posterior cortex to the tibial tubercle and the trochlear groove. Distance greater than 20 mm usually considered abnormal.

- Although MPFL reconstruction does not directly address trochlear dysplasia, it is helpful to understand the forces contributing to patellar instability as a severely hypoplastic femoral condyle can allow for continued lateral instability and place stress on the reconstructed MPFL and potentially put it at risk for reinjury.
- Merchant view demonstrates patellar tilt or subluxation and allows visualization of trochlear morphology as well as joint space (indicating possible cartilage wear).
- MRI evaluates osteochondral injuries and soft tissue structures.
- The secondary objective of the MRI is to identify the location of the MPFL lesion, which has prognostic value.
  - An MPFL avulsion at the femoral attachment in primary traumatic patellar dislocations predicts subsequent patellar instability.
- It should be noted that MRI detection of chronic laxity of the MPFL in the absence of bleeding or edema is poor; therefore, this places an even greater emphasis on physical examination with maneuvers such as the MPAT that mimics the actual dislocation or instability event.
- Typical bone bruise pattern on the medial patella and lateral trochlea can indicate diagnosis of patellar dislocation independent of the MPFL imaging.
- Axial MR images are also used to determine tibial tubercle-trochlear groove (TT-TG) distance, which drives the decision on whether to perform a tibial tubercle osteotomy in addition to the MPFL reconstruction (Fig. 3-3).

SURGICAL INDICATIONS

Symptomatic recurrent lateral patellar instability without bony malalignment that has failed nonoperative management that includes activity modification, physical therapy, and knee bracing. The ideal candidate has minimal pain between these instability episodes. Acute patellar dislocation with concomitant intra-articular abnormality (osteochondral fracture, loose body, or meniscal injury) as these additional injuries will frequently need repair.

Patients with chondral lesions to the medial facet of the patella are not universally excluded from reconstruction as many of these patients are disabled by continued dislocations and still experience improvement with this procedure.

SURGICAL CONTRAINDICATIONS

- Medial instability
- Isolated anterior knee pain
- Patellofemoral osteoarthritis
- Extreme malalignment or trochlea hypoplasia

PREOPERATIVE PLANNING

- Equipment:
  - Standard arthroscopy tower and instruments
  - Hamstring stripper for graft harvest
  - Drill set (usually 3.2-mm drills are sufficient)
  - Curved suture passing device and suture
  - No. 5 braided nonabsorbable suture to be used as pullout suture
  - No. 2 nonabsorbable suture to secure the graft to the patella
  - Multiple no. 0 absorbable sutures on a taper needle to whipstitch the free and looped graft ends
  - BioTenodesis interference screw

SURGICAL PROCEDURE

There are two surgical goals of this operation:

- To restore a checkrein against lateral patellar motion
- To maintain normal limits of passive lateral motion

Numerous surgical techniques have been described; however, the author's preference is a technique that minimizes risk of complications such as patellar fracture, overconstraining the patella, and hardware complications. The authors prefer the **docking technique** as this procedure allows for precise tunnel placement that maximizes native ligament isometry and simplifies graft tensioning and fixation.

The procedure can be performed on an outpatient basis with general or regional anesthesia.

Patient preparation

Patient is placed supine on a standard operating room table. Examination under anesthesia (EUA) should be performed after successful induction of anesthesia. Patellar stability, translation, and tilt are usually easier to characterize when the patient is anesthetized.

A vertical thigh post is used to facilitate arthroscopic evaluation and can be removed prior to proceeding with reconstruction. A tourniquet is place around the proximal thigh of the operative leg with an Esmarch used to exsanguinate the extremity, and the tourniquet is inflated to 300 mm Hg prior to incision.

Hamstring Harvest

A vertical incision is made along the anteromedial aspect of the proximal tibia (Fig. 3-4). Once skin flaps have been raised, sartorial fascia is then divided horizontally between the gracilis and semitendinosus (Fig. 3-5). A tendon stripper is then used to harvest the semitendinosus proximally (Fig. 3-6).

In some patients, we have elected to use semitendinosus allograft, to minimize postoperative discomfort and improve immediate postoperative function.

Graft Preparation

- The tendon is cleared of any remaining muscular tissue and folded in half (Fig. 3-7).
- The diameter of the folded graft is checked with a sizing guide with the goal of approximately 5 to 6 mm.

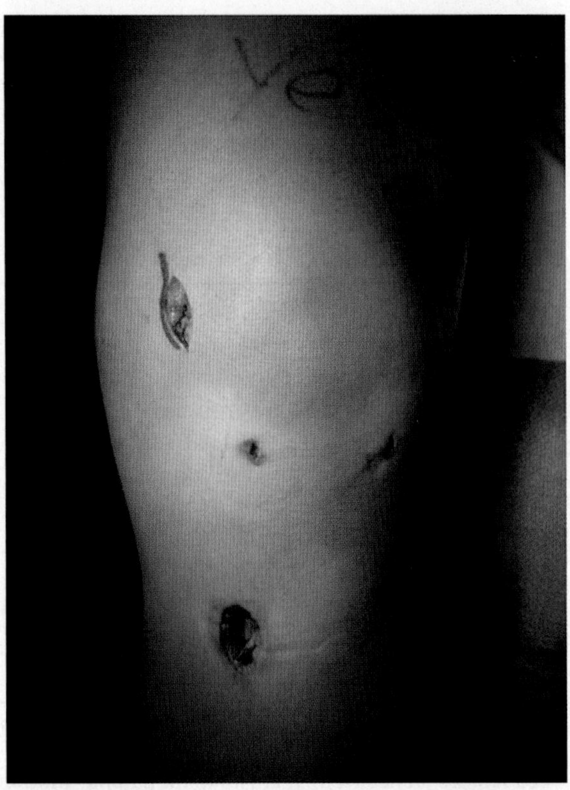

FIGURE 3-4

Hamstring harvest: approximately three to four fingerbreadths below the joint line and midway between the anterior tibial crest and posteromedial border of the tibia.

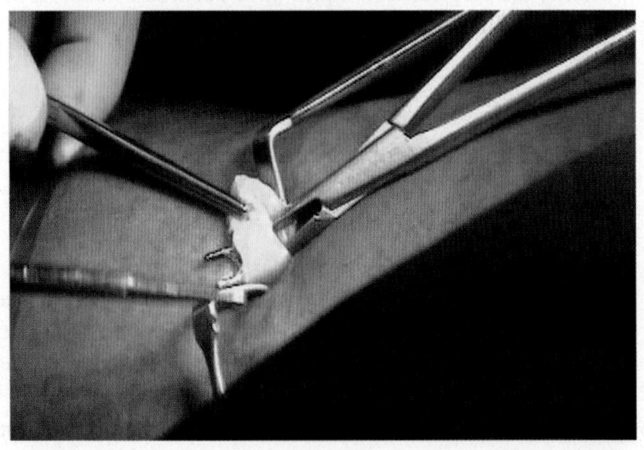

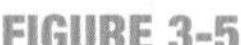

FIGURE 3-5

The semitendinosus is freed from the sartorial fascia and incised at its distal insertion and a no. 2 nonabsorbable whipstitch suture is placed into the free tendon stump. All attachments between the semitendinosus and the medial head of the gastrocnemius are released.

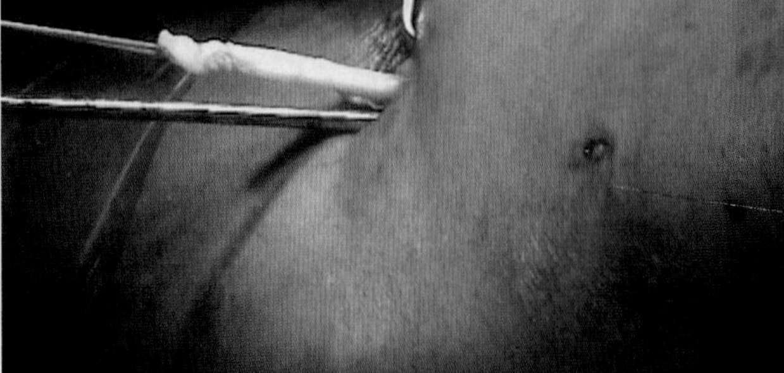

FIGURE 3-6

Hamstring harvest.

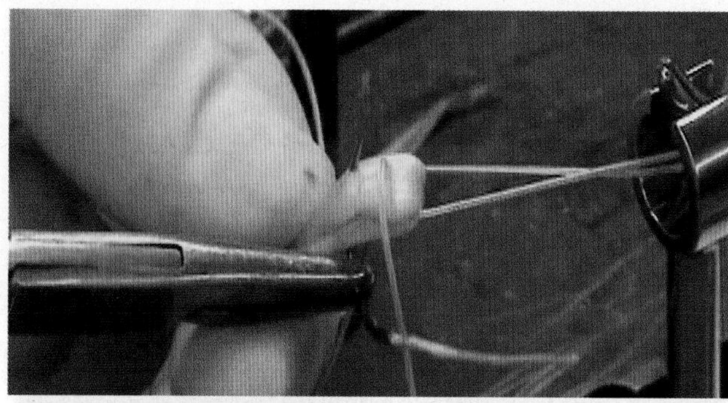

FIGURE 3-7

The folded graft is whipstitched together with a no. 2 suture for a distance of approximately 15 mm from the folded end, leaving two free suture limbs for later graft passage.

Diagnostic Arthroscopy

- Facilitates assessment of chondral injuries at the patellofemoral joint or loose bodies.
  - Chondroplasty is performed when indicated to remove any unstable cartilage flaps.
  - Loose bodies are removed and large osteochondral fragments can be reduced and fixed if technically feasible.
- Hemorrhage may be noted in the soft tissue adjacent to the medial edge of the patella in patients with recent MPFL avulsions.
- If the preoperative examination demonstrated negative patellar tilt suggestive of tight lateral structures, then a lateral release can be performed.
  - Lateral release is not routinely necessary in patients with generalized ligamentous laxity.

Creation of "Moving Window"

Approximately halfway between the adductor tubercle and the medial border of the patella, a 3-cm longitudinal incision is made at the medial aspect of the knee (Fig. 3-8). With the knee in full extension, skin flaps are raised and dissection is carried laterally into the prepatellar space.

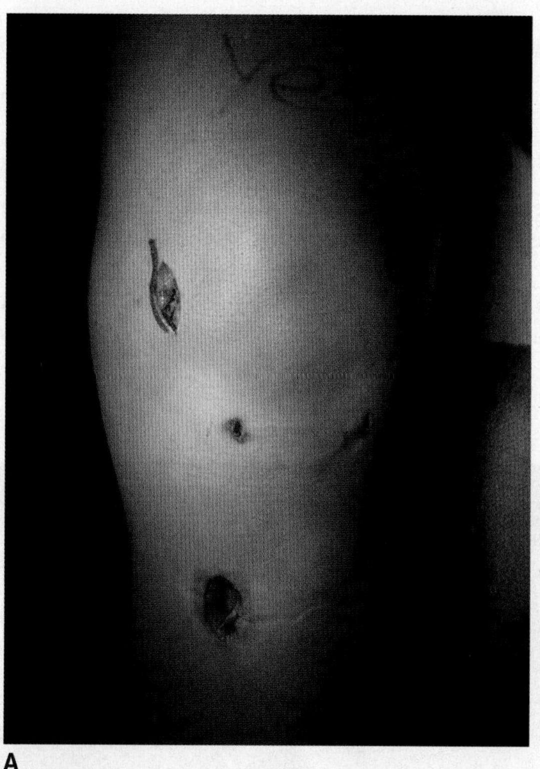

A

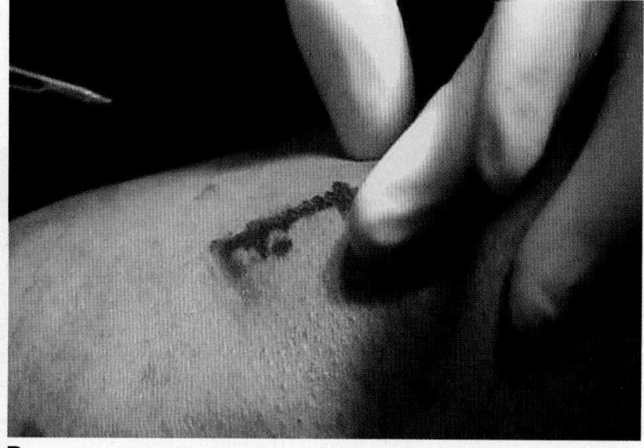

B

FIGURE 3-8

Medial incision: this "moving window" incision allows for lateral exposure of the patella with the knee in full extension and medial exposure of the femoral MPFL attachment with the knee in flexion.

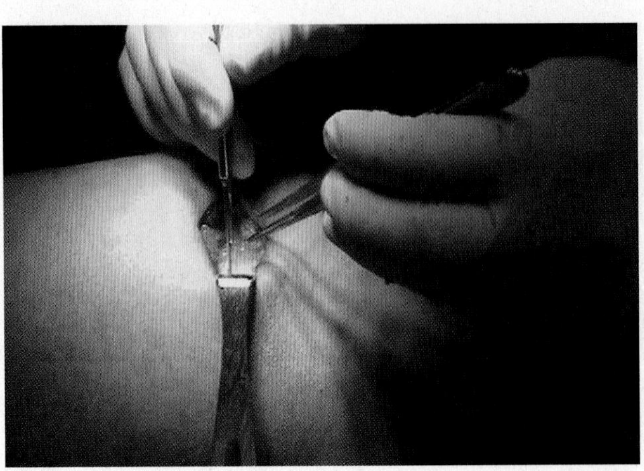

FIGURE 3-9

The retinacular split facilitates patellar exposure as well as allows for later imbrication of the VMO and medial soft tissues over the reconstructed MPFL graft.

For the medial exposure, the knee is flexed to approximately 60 degrees and the medial epicondyle is identified. The medial retinaculum is incised horizontally just distal to the vastus medialis obliquus (VMO) attachment onto the patella (proximal one-third of the patella) being mindful to not violate the capsule (Fig. 3-9). The plane between the retinaculum and the capsule is developed medially to the level of the medial epicondyle.

Patellar Tunnel Preparation

Soft tissue on the medial patella is debrided with a rongeur. Place a 2.4-mm guide pin into the medial patella at the insertion site of the native MPFL. Insert slightly anterior to avoid penetration into the deep subchondral bone to a depth of 20 mm (Fig. 3-10).

- In the setting of small-sized patella, the depth of the tunnel may be decreased.
- If the graft diameter is too large, the graft can be trimmed to a smaller size to accommodate the smaller tunnel.
- Once the docking tunnel has been created, two divergent holes are drilled from the base of the tunnel using a 2.4-mm (or 1.5 mm) pin with an eyelet (Fig. 3-11).

Patellar Tunnel Graft Docking

After each hole is drilled, the eyelet in the pin is used to pass a shuttle suture loop through the drill hole. Then, one free end of nonabsorbable suture from the midportion of the folded graft is loaded into each shuttle loop and pulled through the drill holes to exit laterally (Fig. 3-12). The free ends are tensioned at the lateral patella to dock the graft within the patellar tunnel until it is fully seated (Fig. 3-13). Through the medial incision and the prepatellar space, the sutures are tied over the lateral bone bridge (Fig. 3-14).

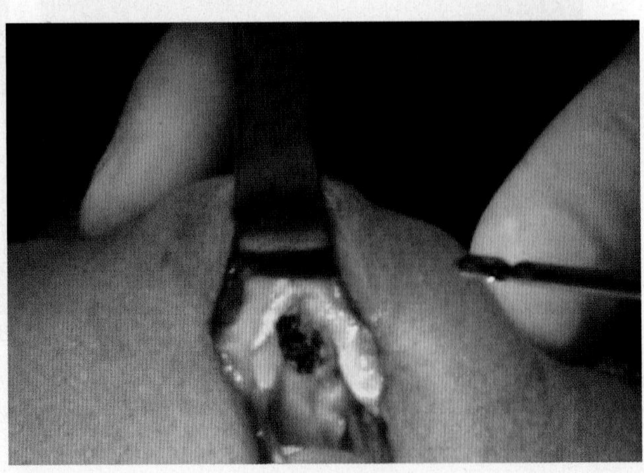

FIGURE 3-10

Patellar tunnel location should be drilled at the intersection of the proximal one-third and distal two-thirds of the patella. The patellar docking tunnel is then drilled over the guide pin to a depth of 15 to 20 mm with a diameter equal to that of the graft (5 to 6 mm).

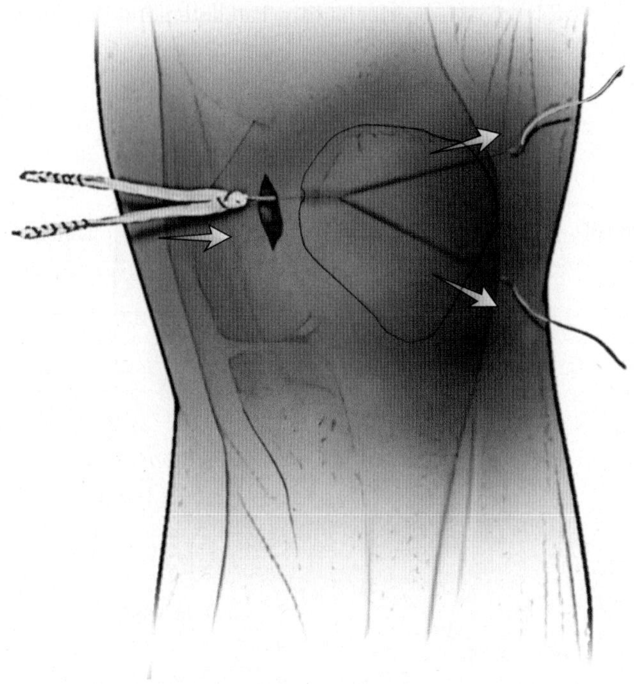

FIGURE 3-11

One pin should be directed proximally and the other distally, maintaining a minimum 1-cm bone bridge between the pins at the lateral aspect of the patella and exit laterally by piercing the skin.

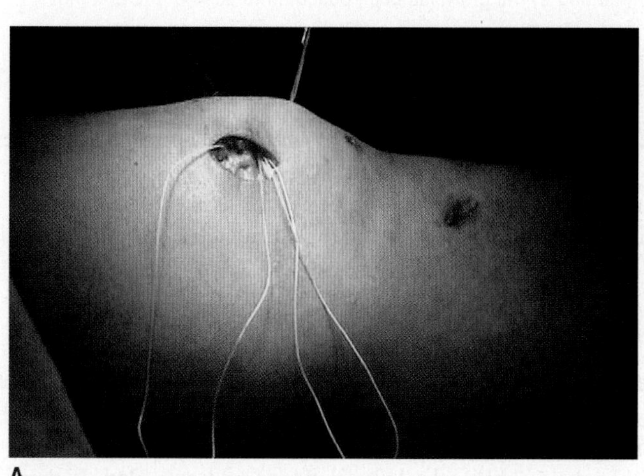

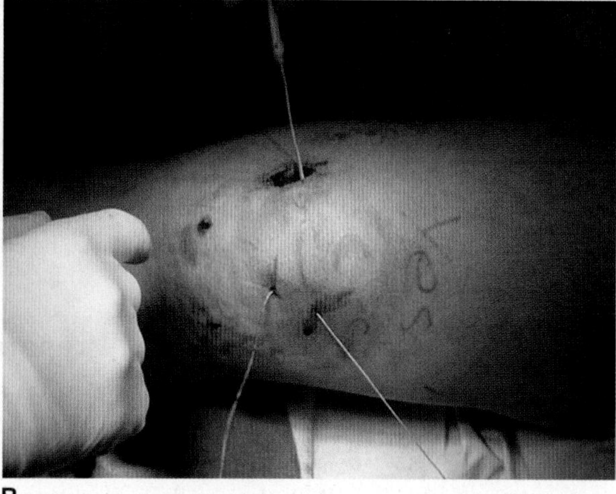

A B

FIGURE 3-12

A: Suture shuttling using the eyelet of the pin. **B:** Docking of the graft into the patellar tunnel. One limb of the whipstitch at the folded end of the graft has been passed into each of the 2.4 mm divergent holes.

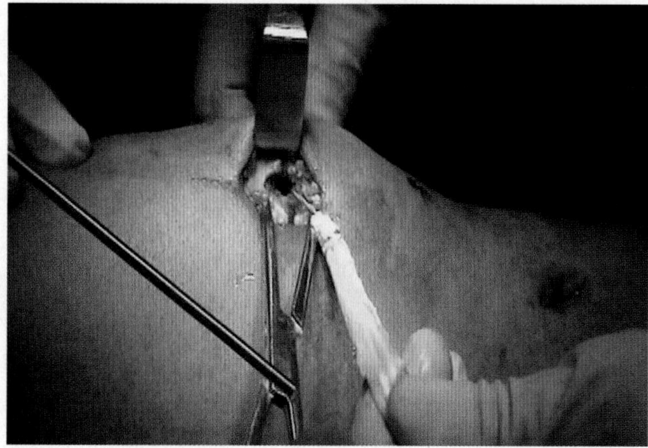

FIGURE 3-13

Pulling sutures from the lateral aspect of the knee will allow for docking of the graft.

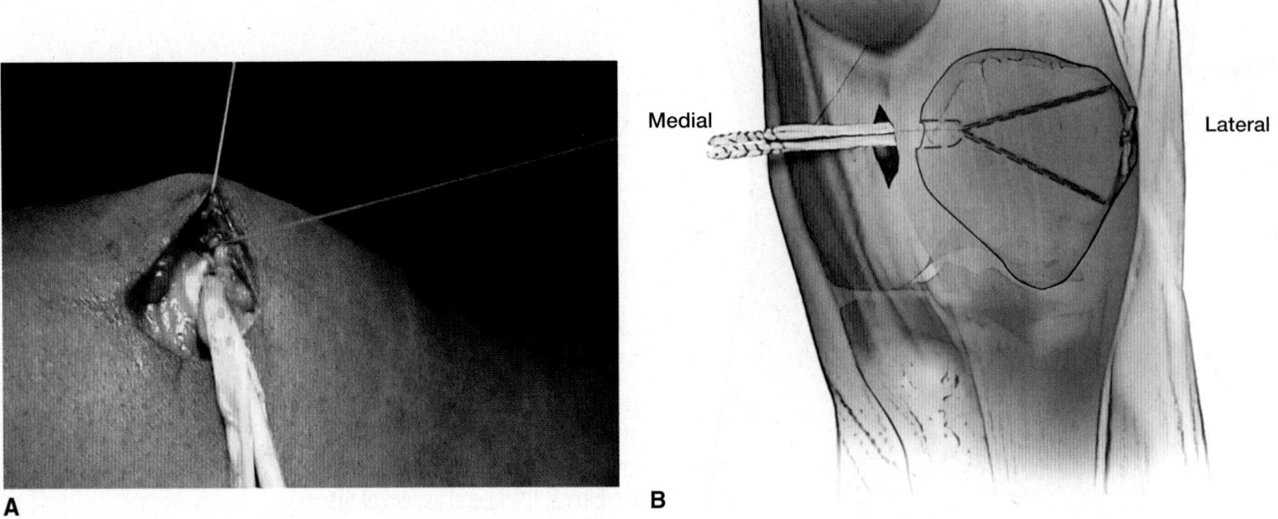

FIGURE 3-14

A: The sutures exiting the lateral skin can then be retrieved into the skin incision with an arthroscopic probe placed in the prepatellar space. This step is facilitated by developing the prepatellar bursa all the way to the lateral patella before tunnel creation. **B:** Docking of the graft into the patellar tunnel. One limb of the whipstitch at the folded end of the graft has been passed into each of the 2.4-mm divergent holes.

- During this step, the patella can be displaced medially to simplify knot tying, and the tying fingers can be placed into the prepatellar space to appropriately tension the knot.
- Sutures should be cut short to minimize any knot prominence below the skin.
- Graft security should also be confirmed by pulling medially on the semitendinosus graft as it exits the docking tunnel.

Femoral Tunnel Preparation

With the knee is flexed to 60 degrees, a guide pin is inserted at the exact site of the MPFL attachment to the medial epicondyle (Fig. 3-15A). Once the pin has been placed, isometry is inspected by wrapping the graft around the pin with gentle tension (Fig. 3-15B).

With the patella held reduced within the trochlea, the knee is flexed and extended. If there is excursion of the graft more than 3 mm relative to the pin, the femoral pin site should be considered nonisometric. The pin often needs to be repositioned in a slightly more inferior and posterior position. Once the femoral isometric point has been confirmed, a 7-mm tunnel is drilled to a depth of 25 mm over the guide pin (Fig. 3-16).

Femoral Tunnel Graft Fixation

The graft tension is established with the knee flexed to 60 degrees so that the patella is fully engaged within the trochlea. This anatomic position of the patella is therefore not influenced by the medially directed force placed on the patella during tensioning the graft.

The graft is provisionally positioned over the femoral tunnel and marked with a pen at the tunnel entrance (Fig. 3-17). The BioTenodesis driver should be prepared with a 7 × 23 mm BioTenodesis screw and a free looped no. 2 suture within the cannulation of the driver. The looped suture is placed around the graft at its distal extent. Using the tip of the driver, the graft is delivered under tension into the femoral tunnel. The screw is then advanced, keeping the tip of the driver in place to maintain appropriate graft tension and position (Fig. 3-18).

Tension and isometry should again be evaluated by ranging the knee from 0 to 110 degrees, confirming proper tracking of the patella and ensuring that the reconstruction has not constrained motion (Fig. 3-19).

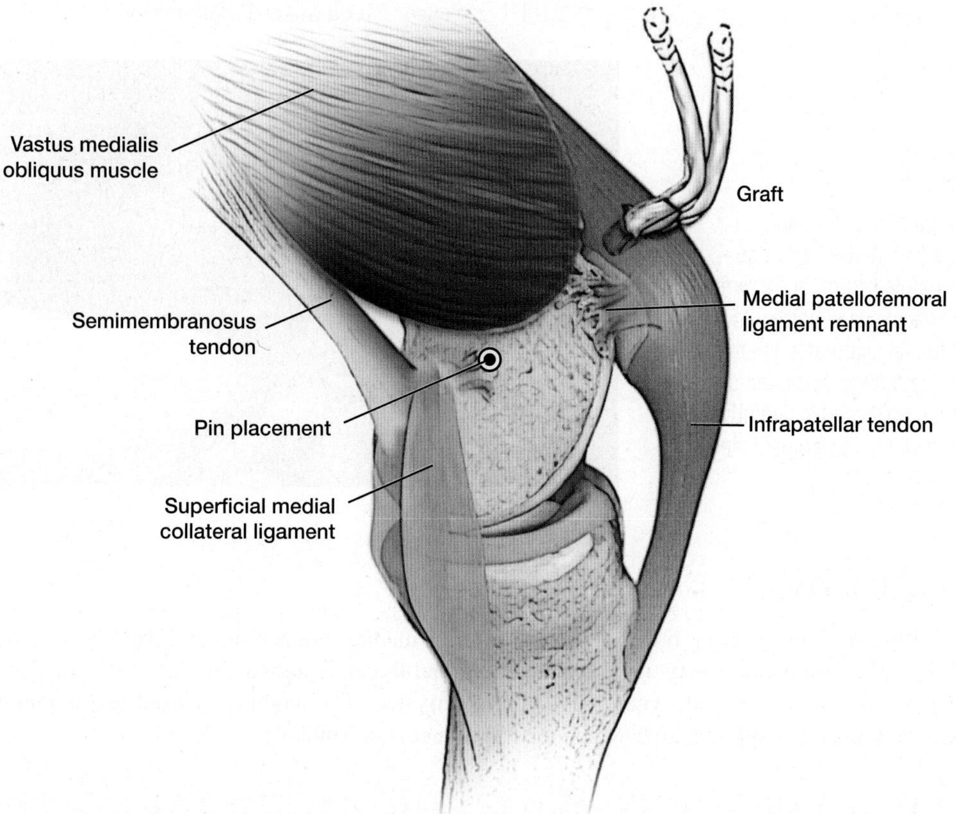

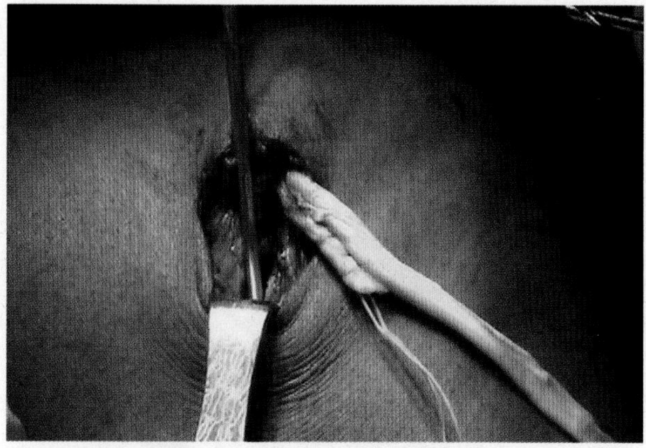

FIGURE 3-15

The pin is placed just proximal to origin of the superficial MCL and is directed slightly anterior and superior to avoid penetration of the posterior aspect of the medial femoral condyle during reaming.

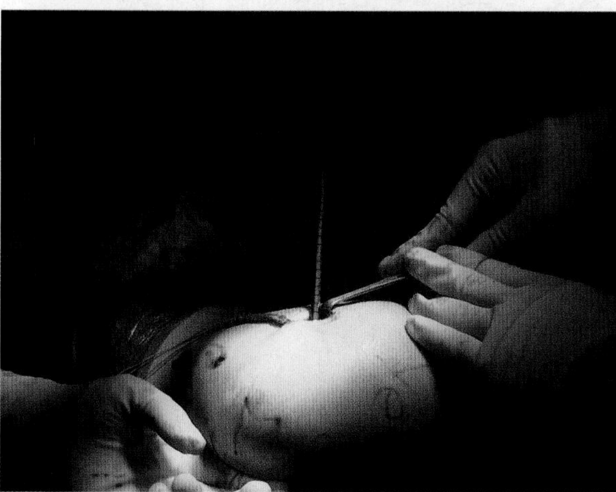

FIGURE 3-16

Femoral drilling over the guide pin. The tunnel should be directed slightly anterior and superior to avoid penetration of the medial femoral condyle.

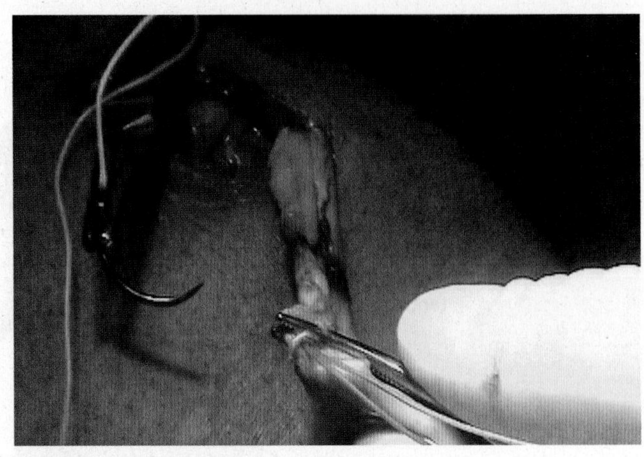

FIGURE 3-17

The two graft limbs are then whipstitched together with a no. 2 nonabsorbable suture for 20 mm from the anticipated site of entry into the femoral tunnel, starting at the marked point on the graft and working distally. Any excess graft can be carefully trimmed distal to the whipstitched suture.

VMO Imbrication

VMO is imbricated by suturing it distally to the inferior medial retinaculum and the MPFL graft (Fig. 3-20). This imbrication may also provide additional dynamic support to the reconstruction, theoretically tensioning the graft when the VMO is activated. The wound is closed and a gentle compressive dressing is applied, after which the tourniquet is deflated.

SURGICAL VARIATIONS

- Patella fixation with screws or button
  - Avoid drilling large tunnels across patella
- The use of two incisions for the reconstruction
- The use of allograft to reconstruct the ligament
- Fluoroscopy to confirm location of femoral tunnel prior to drilling

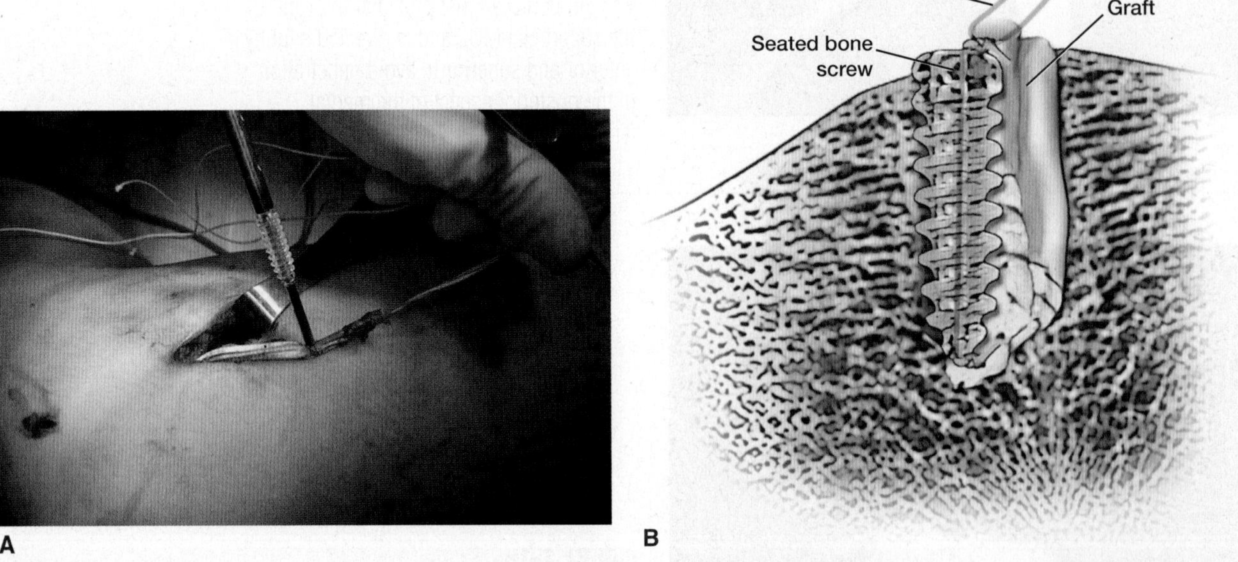

FIGURE 3-18

After the screw is seated, the driver is removed, leaving the looped suture exiting from the cannulation of the screw. The central sutures are tied to the sutures previously whipstitched into the graft, resulting in a combined suture anchor and interference screw construct.

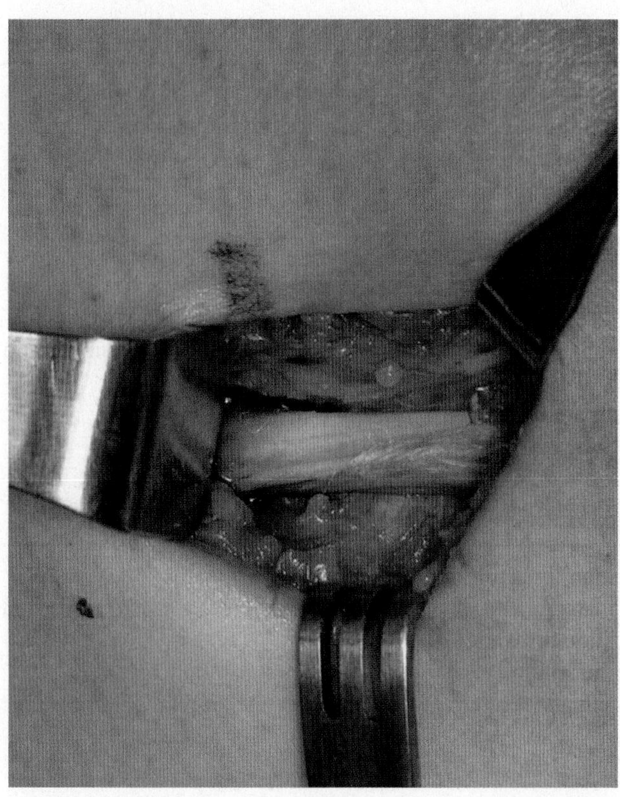

FIGURE 3-19

Appropriately tensioned and securely fixed MPFL reconstruction with semitendinosus autograft.

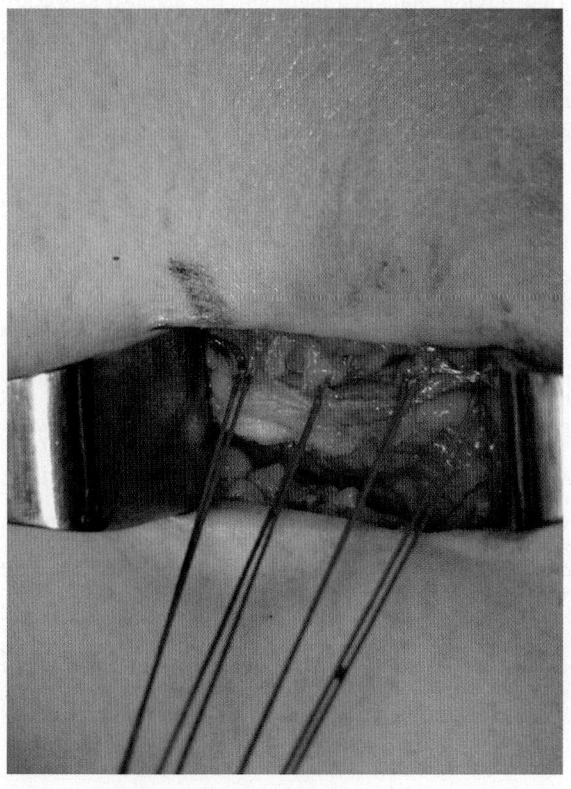

FIGURE 3-20

The previous horizontal incision in the medial retinacular tissue allows for inferior advancement of the VMO, restoring the intimate anatomic relationship between the MPFL and inferior quadriceps mechanism.

POSTOPERATIVE MANAGEMENT

- The operative knee is immobilized in full extension allowing for full weight bearing without activation of the quadriceps for 4 weeks or until adequate quadriceps control is obtained.
- Range of motion is started immediately with using a continuous passive motion (CPM) and progressed to achieve a minimum of 90 degrees of flexion by 6 weeks.
- Therapy protocol
  - Weeks 0 to 2: home program for quadriceps strengthening.
  - Week 2: formal physical therapy is initiated with emphasis on passive and active range of motion.
  - Week 6: more aggressive strengthening of the quadriceps and hamstrings with inclusion of hip and core muscles.
  - Week 12: running and agility training are permitted.
  - Week 16: return to full sporting activities.

COMPLICATIONS TO AVOID

- Most common postoperative complication is stiffness.
  - Flexion deficits may also be secondary to intraoperative technical errors (graft malposition from inaccurate femoral tunnel location or overtensioning).
- Other complications include recurrent instability, painful hardware, and patellar fracture.
- Patellar chondrosis at time of surgery can also lead to post-op pain despite alleviation of instability symptoms.

PEARLS AND PITFALLS

- An incision over the midportion of the MPFL allows exposure of both the medial border of the patella and the medial femoral epicondyle.
- The femoral tunnel should be referenced from the MCL: proximal to the origin of the superficial MCL and is directed slightly anterior and superior to avoid penetration of the posterior aspect of the medial femoral condyle during reaming.
- Final femoral fixation should occur at the knee flexion angle that facilitates the greatest necessary graft length with the goal of reproducing the same amount of lateral patellar translation as was appreciated on the contralateral normal side with the knee extended during the EUA.
- Great care should be taken to not to overtighten the MPFL or malposition the graft.
  - This can result in excessive medial patellofemoral joint pressures and could exacerbate patellofemoral pain.

RECOMMENDED READINGS

Ahmad CS, Brown GD, Stein BS. The docking technique for medial patellofemoral ligament reconstruction: surgical technique and clinical outcome. *Am J Sports Med.* 2009;37:2021–2027.

Ahmad CS, McCarthy M, Gomez JA, et al. The moving patellar apprehension test for lateral patellar instability. *Am J Sports Med.* 2009;37:791–796.

Elias JJ, Cosgarea AJ. Technical errors during medial patellofemoral ligament reconstruction could overload medial patellofemoral cartilage: a computational analysis. *Am J Sports Med.* 2006;34:1478–1485.

Farrow LD, Alentado VJ, Abdulnabi Z, et al. The relationship of the medial patellofemoral ligament attachment to the distal femoral physis. *Am J Sports Med.* 2014;42:2214–2218.

Franzone JM, Vitale MA, Shubin Stein BE, et al. Is there an association between chronicity of patellar instability and patellofemoral cartilage lesions? An arthroscopic assessment of chondral injury. *J Knee Surg.* 2012;25:411–416.

Kohn LM, Meidinger G, Beitzel K, et al. Isolated and combined medial patellofemoral ligament reconstruction in revision surgery for patellofemoral instability: a prospective study. *Am J Sports Med.* 2013;41:2128–2135.

Lippacher S, Dreyhaupt J, Williams SR, et al. Reconstruction of the medial patellofemoral ligament: clinical outcomes and return to sports. *Am J Sports Med.* 2014;42:1661–1668.

Shah JN, Howard JS, Flanigan DC, et al. A systematic review of complications and failures associated with medial patellofemoral ligament reconstruction for recurrent patellar dislocation. *Am J Sports Med.* 2012;40:1916–1923.

Trentacosta NE, Vitale MA, Ahmad CS. The effects of timing of pediatric knee ligament surgery on short-term academic performance in school-aged athletes. *Am J Sports Med.* 2009;37:1684–1691.

4 Anteromedial Tibial Tubercle Transfer

John P. Fulkerson

INDICATIONS/CONTRAINDICATIONS

The best candidate for anteromedial tibial tubercle transfer (1–3) (Fig. 4-1) is a patient with lateral patellar tilt (and/or subluxation) associated with grade III or IV articular degeneration localized on the lateral and/or distal medial patellar facets following the failure of nonsurgical therapy. If there is no articular degeneration or pain, there is no need to anteriorize the TT, and a straight medial transfer of the TT as described by Trillat (4) and reviewed by Carney, Mologne, Muldoon, and Cox (5) is more appropriate for correcting subluxation. However, some patients have distal and/or lateral patella articular softening (grade I) or cartilage breakdown (grade II to IV).

In such patients, the surgeon may wish to anteriorize the extensor mechanism to some extent at the time of realignment. An oblique osteotomy will transfer load off an area of articular degeneration, particularly when damage is noted on the distal aspect of the patella (anteriorization "tips" up the distal patella, thereby unloading it). Anteromedial tibial tubercle transfer is appropriate whenever the surgeon wishes to shift contact stress on the patella from the lateral and distal aspects of the patella to the more proximal and medial patellar articular cartilage. Most important is to recognize that TT anteriorization at the time of medialization gives the added benefit of removing articulation with the distal patella, which is often a fragmented or softened source of pain.

Before considering anteromedial tibial tubercle transfer, alternative nonsurgical treatment methods must fail. In particular, a well-structured program of rehabilitation should be tried involving mobilization of a lateralized and tight extensor mechanism supplemented by patellar bracing (6). I use the Tru-Pull braces (DJ Ortho, Vista, CA). A tight extensor mechanism and hamstrings should be mobilized through stretching and strengthening. Prone quadriceps stretching has been very helpful and is easy for patients to do at home. Lower extremity core stability including hip stabilization exercises is important in these patients. Nonsteroidal anti-inflammatory medication is often helpful for symptomatic treatment during the period of nonsurgical therapy.

Failed lateral release is another potential indication for anteromedial tibial tubercle transfer. If a patient is left with residual articular pain or symptomatic lateral malalignment of the patella following lateral release, anteromedial tibial tubercle transfer may be helpful.

Contraindications to anteromedial tibial tubercle transfer include the following:

- Diffuse patella articular breakdown. Particularly, if the cartilage loss involves the proximal medial patella (dashboard or crush injury), patients are less likely to benefit from anteromedial tibial tubercle transfer.
- Tilt alone and no significant subluxation or lateral facet collapse. Such patients may benefit from simple lateral retinacular release; therefore, anteromedial tibial tubercle transfer is not recommended as a first procedure.
- Reflex sympathetic dystrophy and complex regional pain syndrome (CRPS).
- Patients with a bleeding tendency, clotting disorder, or history of deep venous thrombosis are less desirable candidates for this type of surgery.
- Poor healing capacity, diabetes, gross obesity, and smoking are relative contraindications for tibial tubercle transfer.

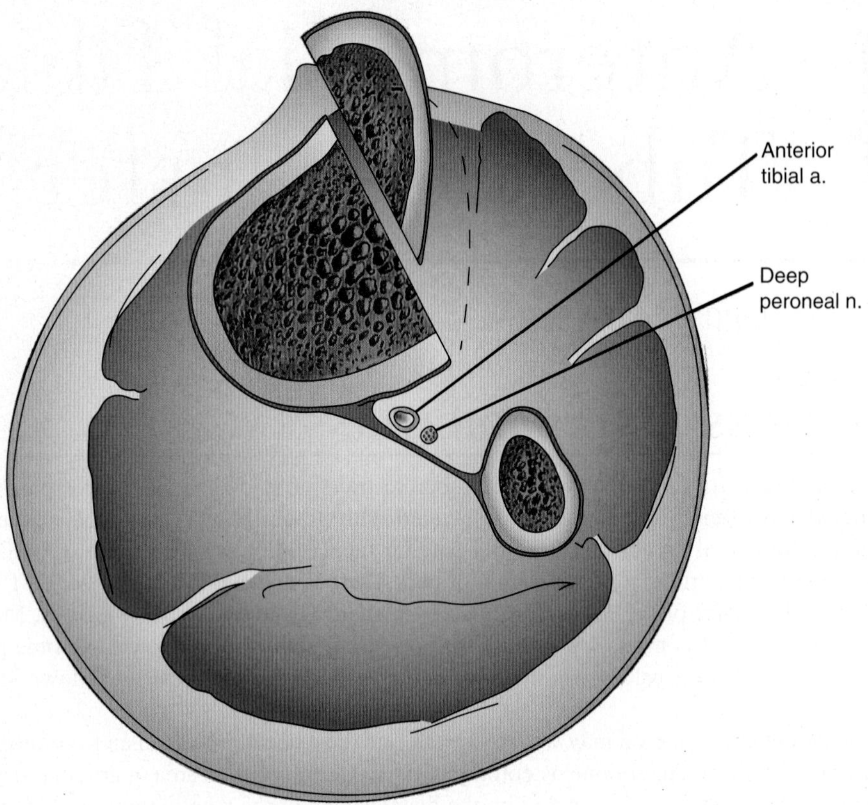

FIGURE 4-1
Anteromedial tibial tubercle transfer.

PREOPERATIVE PLANNING

Clinical examination is important in preoperative planning for anteromedial tibial tubercle transfer. The examination should include compression of the patella while flexing and extending the knee to see if articular pain can be elicited (Fig. 4-2). The examining surgeon should also rule out other nonarticular causes of pain such as neuroma, isolated retinacular pain, patellar tendonitis, referred pain, plica, meniscus derangement, synovitis, and osteochondritis dissecans. The physical examination should be done with the patient in both standing and supine positions. The examiner should look for evidence of lateralization of the extensor mechanism and tilt. Presence or absence of passive patellar tilt and/or tightness of the lateral retinaculum should be noted (1). Pain on compression of the patella with flexion and extension of the knee suggests an articular source. A positive step-down test further confirms a distal patella articular pain source and therefore the importance of anteromedial versus medial tibial tubercle. If lateralization and lateral tilt of the patella are prominent, the patient may be a candidate for anteromedial tibial tubercle transfer, particularly if the step-down test suggests a painful distal patella articular lesion that will be completely unloaded on anteriorization of the tibial tubercle. It is important to be certain that pain is not due to a retinacular neuroma, painful scar, or intra-articular cause that might be corrected by a smaller surgical procedure or injection.

Standard anteroposterior and lateral radiographs should be taken on all surgical candidates and supplemented with an axial (tangential) view. A standard axial (7) view (knee flexed 45 degrees and x-ray beam 30 degrees from the horizontal plane) provides a good idea of patella orientation in the trochlea and is our view of choice. If a specific malalignment pattern is identifiable on the axial radiograph, no further radiographic evaluation is necessary, particularly if the lateral patellofemoral joint is narrow. On the other hand, some patients with significant malalignment of the extensor mechanism will demonstrate a normal axial radiograph yet have significant lateral subluxation and/or tilt on computed tomography (CT) of the patellofemoral joint. In such cases, I recommend a more steep, anteriorizing osteotomy, with less medialization.

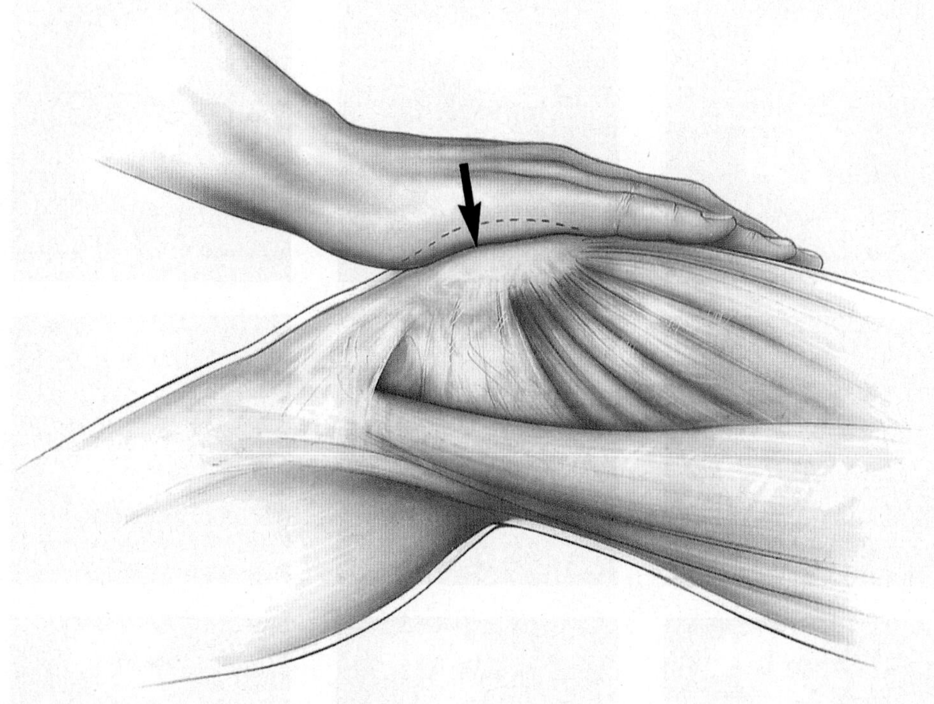

FIGURE 4-2

Compression of the patella while passing the knee through a range of motion will give an impression of the extent of articular damage and pain emanating from the articular surfaces of the patellofemoral joint.

A true lateral radiograph of the knee (posterior condyles superimposed) at 0 and 30 degrees knee flexion will help greatly in understanding trochlea morphology from top to bottom. Despite trochlear dysplasia, trochleoplasty is contraindicated in patients with lateral patellofemoral arthritis.

CT of the patellofemoral joint may be done with normal standing alignment of the patient reproduced in the scanner gantry. Midpatellar transverse tomographic images should be made with the CT cut directed to include the posterior condyles of the femur (Fig. 4-3). These tomographic slices should be taken with the knees flexed 15, 30, and 45 degrees (2). The patella is significantly tilted if the patellar tilt angle (the angle created by lines drawn along the lateral facet of the patella and the posterior femoral condyles) is less than 12 degrees on the tomographic image with the knee flexed 15 degrees. The patella should be centered in the trochlea on the tomographic image in which the knee is flexed at 15 degrees. (In other words, the congruence angle (7) should be 0 or slightly negative). Furthermore, CT provides an ideal opportunity to understand the relationship of the tibial tubercle to the central trochlea (TT-TG index as described by Goutallier (8)). As the TT-TG index rises, TT transfer becomes increasingly desirable, particularly when it exceeds 20 mm.

Following full clinical evaluation and radiographic study, the surgeon will know whether the patella is malaligned and will have some idea of the degree of lateral and distal articular degeneration, particularly as demonstrated by pain and crepitation on flexion/extension of the knee while compressing the patella and by a positive step-down test. If appropriate nonsurgical treatment has failed, the patient may be a candidate for anteromedial tibial tubercle transfer, given significant malalignment (tilt and/or subluxation) and evidence of pain coming from the patellar articular surface (particularly if articular degeneration is distal and/or lateral) (9).

WHEN AMZ VERSUS PATELLOFEMORAL ALLOGRAFT OR ARTHROPLASTY?

Anteromedial tibial tubercle transfer (AMZ or AMTTT) is a joint preservation procedure versus allograft or metal/plastic arthroplasty joint replacement procedures. I usually recommend AMZ for active patients under 50 years old who have painful lateral and distal patella arthrosis with intact medial patellofemoral cartilage. A lateralized tibial tubercle makes tibial tubercle medialization particularly desirable (10).

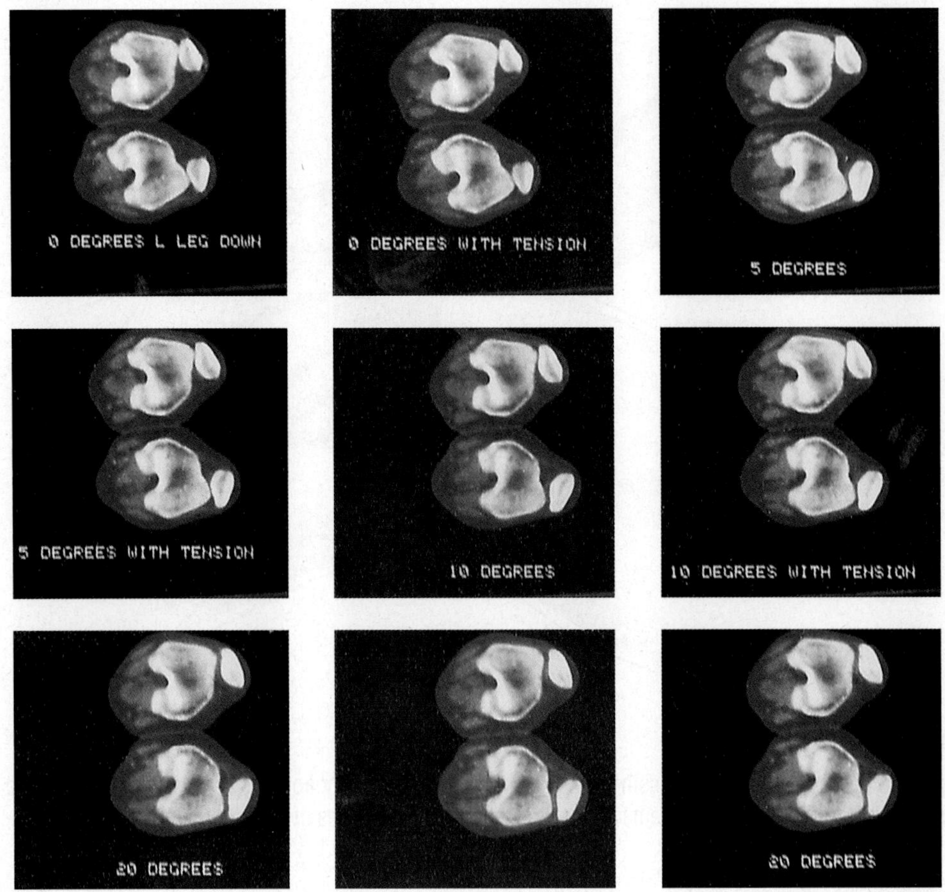

FIGURE 4-3

CT imaging of the patellofemoral joint should include precise midpatellar transverse cuts directed through the posterior femoral condyles.

Patellofemoral replacement is more appropriate for patients with diffuse patellofemoral arthrosis, particularly involving the medial patella. I lean toward recommending allograft in patients under 40 with diffuse patella degeneration and metal/plastic unicompartmental PF replacement over 40 in patients who are not candidates for joint preservation, as long as the medial and lateral compartments are intact and pain free.

Recently, patellofemoral arthroplasty has become more popular as more alternative prostheses have become available. Nonetheless, it is important to remember the inevitable wear of polyethylene and risk of loosening, particularly in younger, more active patients.

AMZ, in my practice, is a 45-minute same-day surgery joint preservation procedure versus a more extensive knee arthrotomy, usually inpatient, joint replacement procedure. I believe AMZ is preferable in younger patients.

SURGERY

The patient is positioned supine on the operating room table, and the anesthesiologist may apply a percutaneous nerve stimulator over the femoral nerve at the groin level. A tourniquet is applied on the proximal thigh and the patient is prepped from the tourniquet level down to and including the toes. Impermeable drapes are used.

Technique

An arthroscopy is routine at the outset of anteromedial tibial tubercle transfer. A superomedial portal, two finger-breadths above the medial proximal pole of the patella, allows an excellent view of the patellar articular surfaces (Fig. 4-4), but standard arthroscopic evaluation using medial and

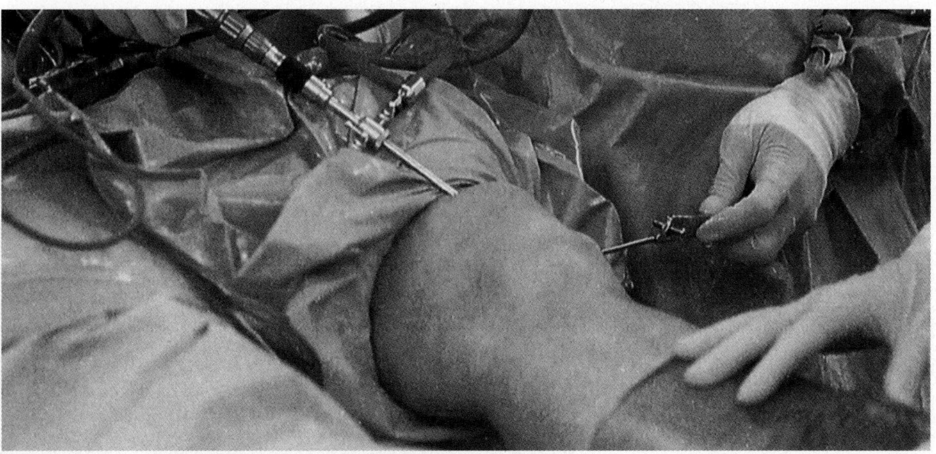

FIGURE 4-4

Arthroscopy of the patellofemoral joint using the superomedial approach gives an excellent view of the entire patellar articular surface as well as the medial and lateral recesses.

lateral infrapatellar portals is often sufficient. By distending the knee to 60 mm Hg pressure, the surgeon can determine the extent of articular damage as well as the extent and location of articular breakdown. Reducing the fluid inflow pressure gives an idea of the extent of patellar subluxation and/or tilt with flexion and extension of the knee. The femoral nerve may be stimulated (to brief tetany) with the knee in progressive flexion to help determine the dynamic alignment/malalignment. The arthroscopy is completed through an infrapatellar portal to evaluate the rest of the knee and to confirm the patellar findings noted if a proximal approach was used.

The surgeon must first characterize and document (by print or video) the nature and location of any articular lesion. A precise description of all articular lesions and their location should be dictated later in the operation report.

Loose flaps of articular cartilage or fibrillated cartilage can be removed most easily at the time of arthroscopy. Abrasion or resection of exposed sclerotic bone can also be done at the time of arthroscopy or with the knee open at the time of anteromedial tibial tubercle transfer. Drilling of the patella is best accomplished after lateral release. Debridement of inflamed synovium, preferably using cautery, and removal of loose bodies are best accomplished arthroscopically.

Most important at the time of arthroscopy is a critical assessment of whether anteromedial tibial tubercle transfer will remove the loading from soft or fragmented articular surfaces and transfer it to better cartilage. Experience has shown that patients in whom the proximal medial facet is preserved are those most likely to benefit from anteromedial tibial tubercle transfer. The operation effectively transfers load from the more lateral and distal aspects of the patella onto proximal medial articular cartilage. Since most patients with chronic patellar malalignment have breakdown of the lateral facet or distal patella, anteromedial tibial tubercle transfer is helpful to many if not most patients with patellar articular degeneration related to chronic malalignment. Patients with dashboard injuries, which occur with the knee flexed, often have destruction of proximal patellar cartilage and may be less amenable to anteromedial tibial tubercle transfer, since this operation transfers load onto proximal and medial patellar cartilage. Failure of straight medial tibial tubercle transfer may result from a failure to unload a distal patella articular pain source.

In performing an anteromedial tibial tubercle transfer, a longitudinal incision is made immediately along the patellar tendon and extended to a point 6 cm distal to the tibial tubercle at the anterior midline (Fig. 4-5). The patellar tendon is identified by sharp dissection (Fig. 4-6) and a lateral retinacular release is accomplished, taking care to dissect away the subcutaneous tissues (Fig. 4-7) bluntly and to release all components of the lateral retinaculum (3) and distal vastus lateralis obliquus (6), but *not the main vastus lateralis tendon*. In fact, it is best to do a limited lateral release, only to the level of the top of the patella, in most patients, to minimize the risk of creating a medial subluxation problem. At this time also release any indurated fat pad that might tether the distal patella and limit free movement of the patella anteriorly after the osteotomy is completed. Inspect the patellar surface and debride carefully to remove loose cartilage flaps while abrading

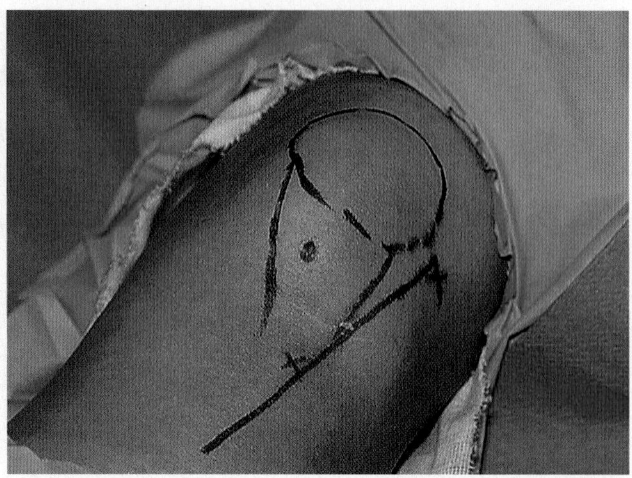

FIGURE 4-5

The incision for anteromedial tibial tubercle transfer should extend from the lateral patella to a point 6 cm distal to the tibial tubercle at the midline.

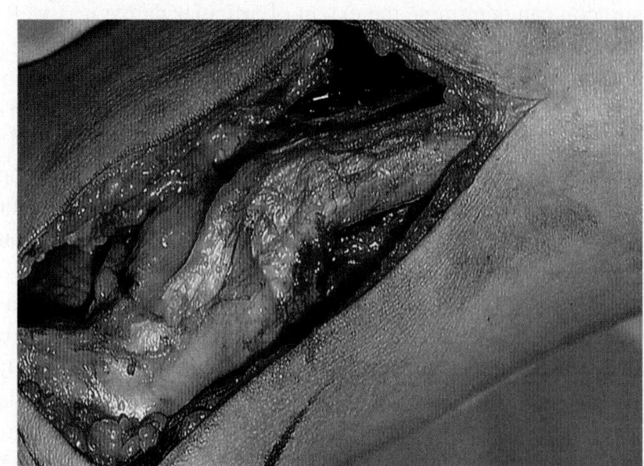

FIGURE 4-6

The patellar tendon is identified by sharp dissection.

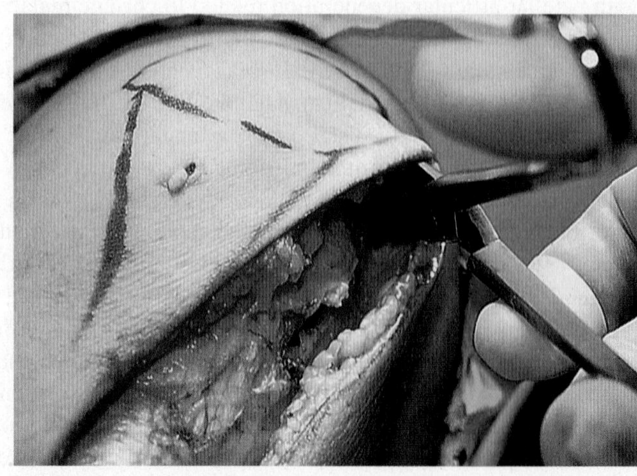

FIGURE 4-7

The lateral retinacular release should extend through the entire retinaculum, with care taken to release any tight fibrous bands in the retropatellar fat-pad area. The lateral release should extend only to the superior pole of the patella, avoiding the main tendon of the vastus lateralis. Do not overrelease. Leaving some of the proximal muscle/vastus lateralis obliquus attached to the main vastus lateralis tendon is a good idea in most cases.

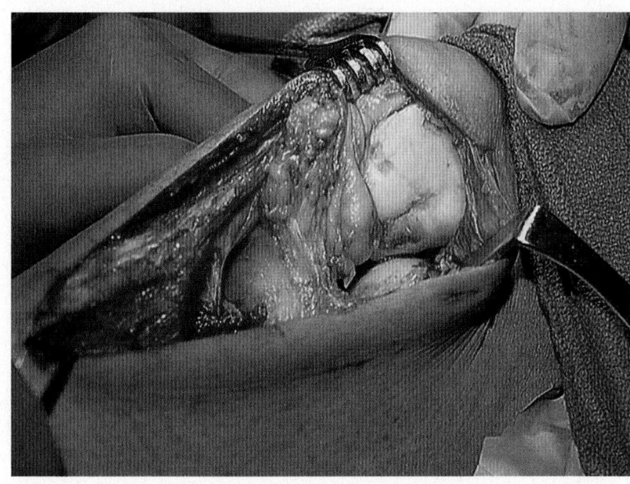

FIGURE 4-8
The patella can be inspected thoroughly following lateral release.

or drilling eburnated bone (Fig. 4-8). Also at this time, determine the need for any autologous, allogeneic, or synthetic osteochondral allograft resurfacing. Place Kelly clamp behind the patellar tendon (Fig. 4-9) and incise longitudinally into the periosteum parallel to the anterior crest of the tibia, just medial to the crest and lateral at the muscle origin of the anterior compartment, reflecting the periosteum and muscle belly to expose the entire lateral tibia for 8 to 10 cm. Periosteum is elevated carefully, and a drill guide is used to define the osteotomy plane, allowing a cut close to the anterior tibial crest medially (Fig. 4-10). A special drill guide with a cutting slot, such as the Tracker guide (Mitek), can make this process easier. The drill bits are pointed posterolaterally, with the most proximal drill bit penetrating the lateral tibial cortex under direct visualization and with careful retraction of the tibialis anterior (Fig. 4-11). Multiple parallel drill holes are made (Figs. 4-12 and 4-13). The angle can be modified according to the desired degree of anteriorization and medialization of the tibial tuberosity. The drill bits should be aligned to limit the depth of the distal tibial pedicle tip to 2 mm, so that fracture of the distal pedicle will be possible. Great care must be taken to avoid drill penetration too far posteriorly into the posterior neurovascular structures. Although the pedicle of bone deep to the tibial tubercle is fairly thick, it tapers anteriorly to the tip of the pedicle distally.

An oscillating saw or osteotomes are used to carefully fashion a cut connecting the drill holes (Figs. 4-14 and 4-15), adding an oblique cut from the most proximal drill hole to a spot just proximal to the insertion of the lateral patellar tendon (Fig. 4-16). This avoids cutting into the broad metaphyseal region of the tibia. The osteotomy must be made in the defined plane only, and care should be taken to work at all times in the osteotomy plane. The cut is completed at about 5 to 8 cm from the tibial tuberosity. The length of this bone pedicle should provide good surface contact and avoid tilting the fragment medially. With great care, the bone fragment is carefully mobilized (Fig. 4-16) and

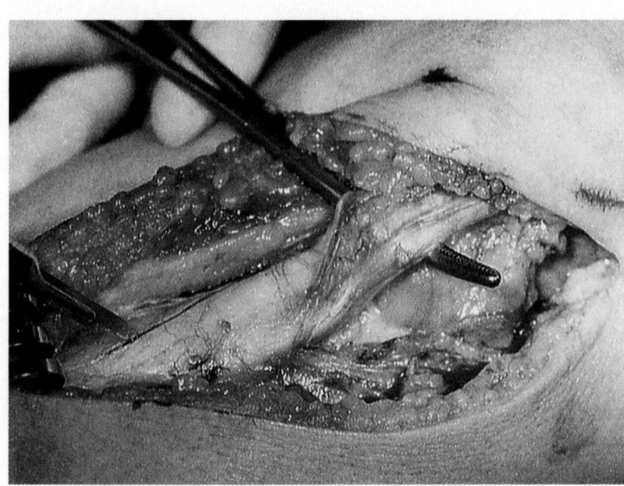

FIGURE 4-9
The patellar tendon insertion is carefully identified and elevated with a Kelly clamp.

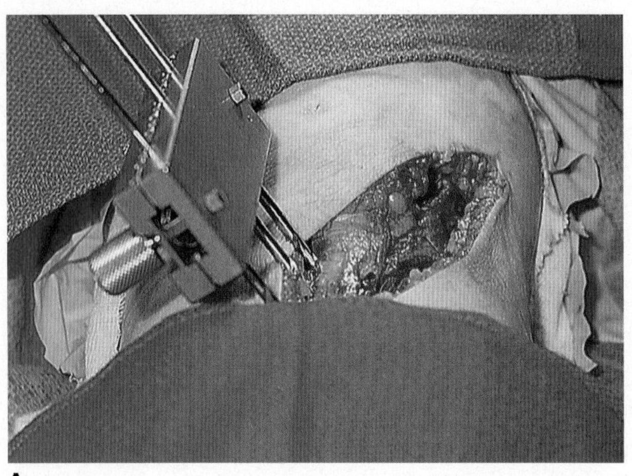

A

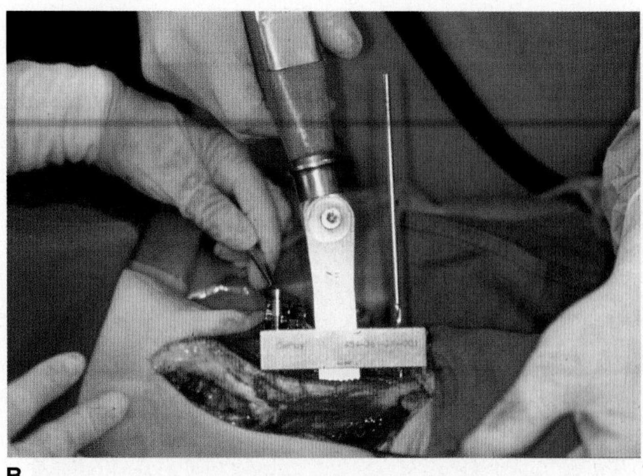

B

FIGURE 4-10

A: A drill guide allowing parallel drill placement along the osteotomy plane allows for precise definition of the osteotomy plane. It is most important to taper the osteotomy distally toward the anterior cortex, leaving only 1 to 2 mm of cortical bone at the distal anterior aspect of the bone pedicle. **B:** The Mitek Tracker guide is ideal for this purpose.

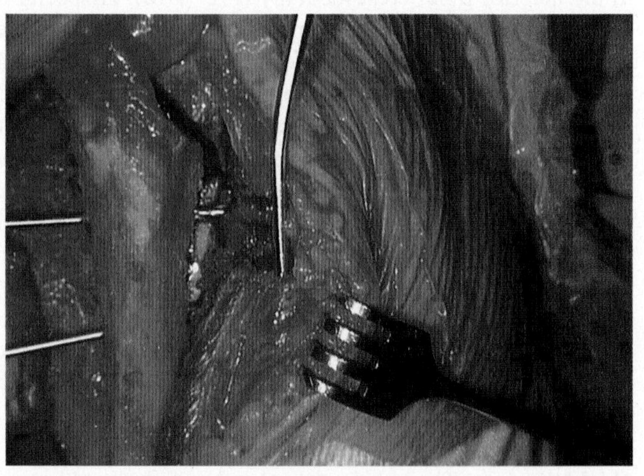

FIGURE 4-11

Exiting of the drill bits at the lateral tibial cortex must be directly visualized by carefully retracting the tibialis anterior muscle from the lateral tibia. The deep peroneal nerve and anterior tibial artery are just behind the posterolateral corner of the tibia.

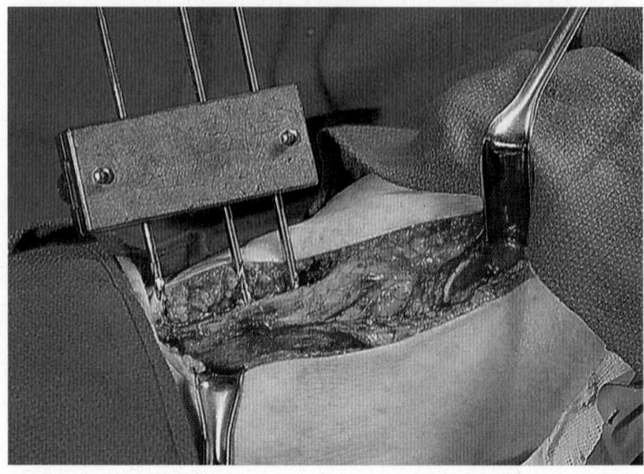

FIGURE 4-12

The obliquity of the osteotomy plane is demonstrated.

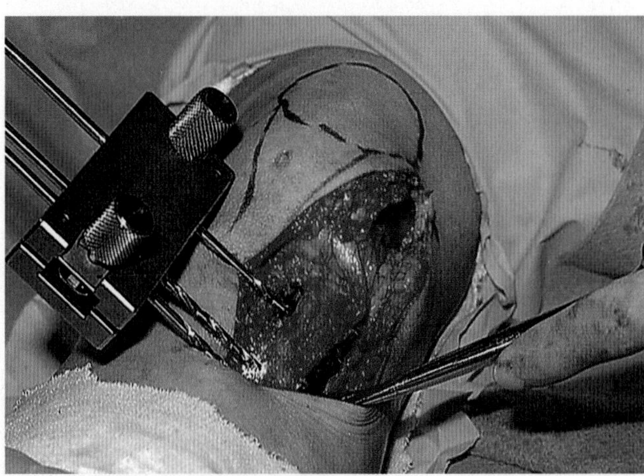

FIGURE 4-13

Great care must be taken to place the drill bits parallel to each other so that an accurate osteotomy will be defined before cutting the anterior tibial bone pedicle. The Mitek Tracker guide works very well for this purpose and has a cutting slot for an oscillating saw.

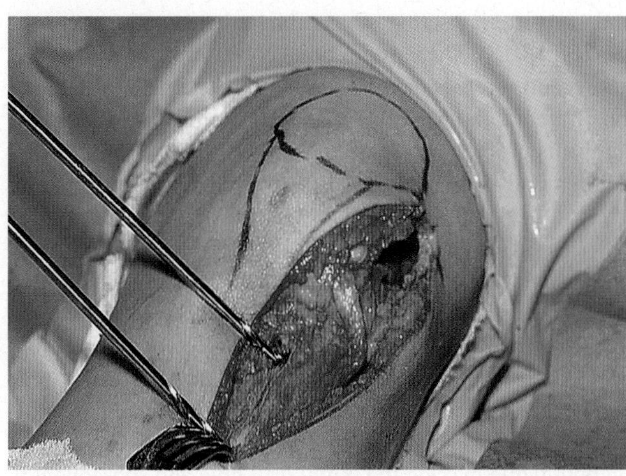

FIGURE 4-14

The proximal and distal drill bits are left in place to help define the plane while cutting the bone pedicle.

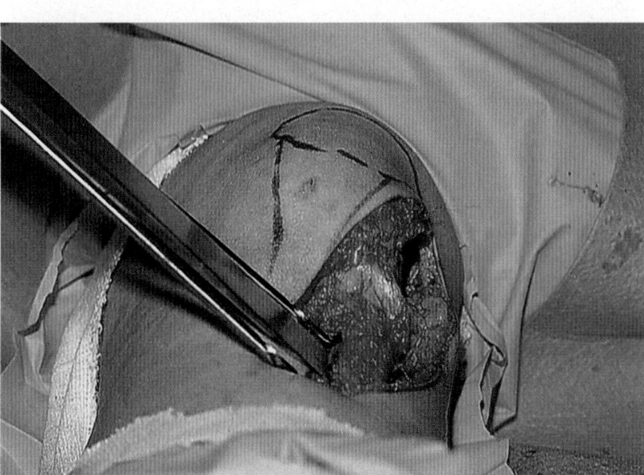

FIGURE 4-15

A sharp, broad osteotome works well for fashioning the osteotomy. The surgeon may wish to use an oscillating saw.

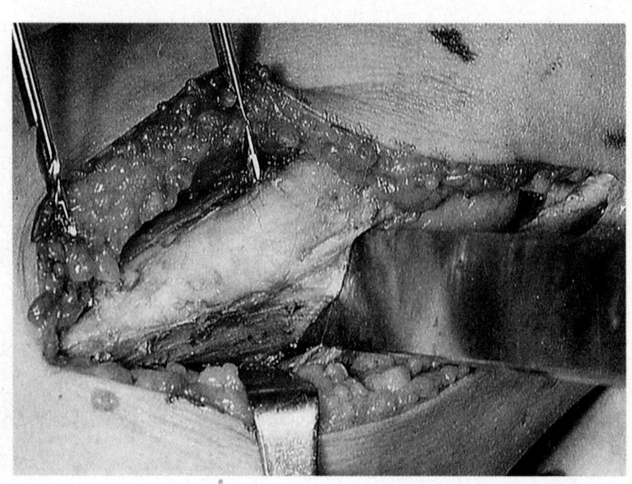

FIGURE 4-16

An osteotome or oscillating saw is used to connect the proximal drill bit tip with the tibial bone posterior and proximal to the patellar tendon insertion. Full visualization of the cutting tool as it exits the lateral tibia is mandatory. Note taper of the osteotomy toward the anterior cortex.

displaced anteromedially along the osteotomy plane (Fig. 4-17). If advancement of the tuberosity is desired, a segment of the distal pedicle may be removed and the remaining fragment advanced slightly to compensate for patella alta. This may also be desirable if significant laxity of the patellar tendon is noted following anteromedialization or if there is patella alta. Once the best position for the tibial tuberosity is determined, a drill hole is made through the pedicle and into the posterior cortex of the tibia distal to the tuberosity, and a cortical lag screw is passed into the posterior cortex of the tibia, applying only slight compression (Fig. 4-18). The anterior tibial cortex must be overdrilled slightly to create a slight lag effect, and a second screw is added for additional stability, also using lag technique (Fig. 4-19). Anteriorization of the tibial tuberosity by about 15 mm is most desirable when there is a primary patellofemoral arthritis problem. In some patients, if subluxation persists, careful advancement of the medial patellofemoral ligament and vastus medialis obliquus may be desirable too selectively, but not so much that the patella is pulled posteriorly or a medial articular lesion is loaded.

When careful surgical technique is used, technical problems are uncommon. The surgeon must be careful to taper the distal osteotomy anteriorly so as not to remove too much of the tibial diaphyseal bone at the distal extent of the osteotomy. The osteotomy should be very flat, thereby maintaining excellent bone-to-bone contact on transfer of the bone pedicle. All drill holes must be made very carefully, taking care to avoid the deep peroneal nerve and anterior tibial artery just behind the proximal posterolateral tibia. Once the bone pedicle has been shifted in an anteromedial direction, it must be held securely in the corrected position both while making the initial drill hole and subsequently. Shifting of the transferred pedicle may make engagement of the posterior cortex difficult and necessitate extra drill holes, thereby weakening the posterior tibia. Once the first screw is secured to the posterior cortex, the pedicle is quite secure and the second screw is easy to place.

The surgeon may choose to use an "offset bone graft" (Fig. 4-20) if straight anterior displacement of the tibial tubercle is needed. By placing a 4- to 5-mm–thick section of corticocancellous auto- or

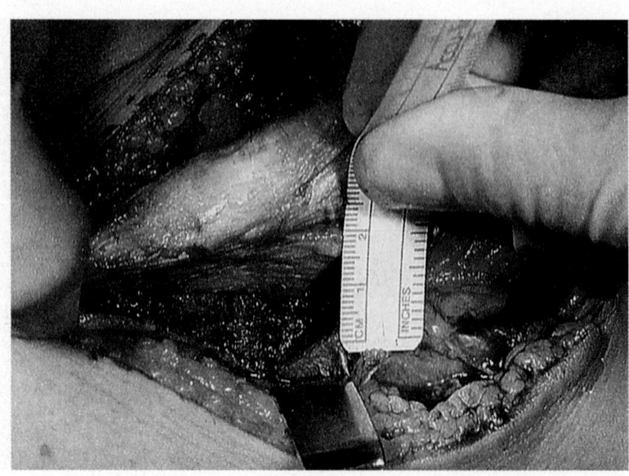

FIGURE 4-17

The bone pedicle will be displaced in an anteromedial direction, usually giving 12 to 17 mm of anteriorization as well as some medialization, depending on the obliquity of the osteotomy.

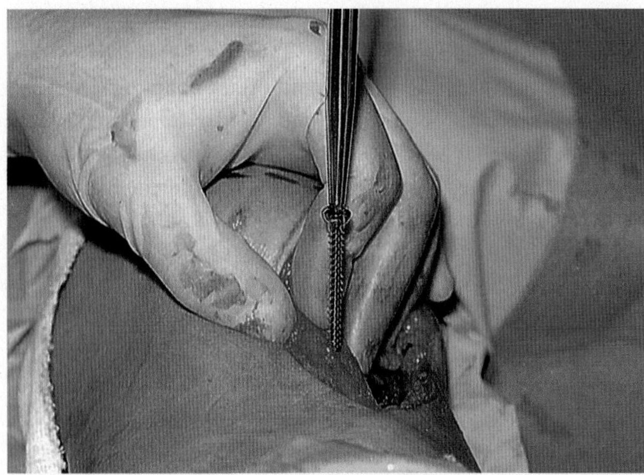

FIGURE 4-18

Cortical lag screws are used to lock the pedicle in the corrected position, placing the screws into the posterior tibial cortex for secure fixation. Keep the proximal screw at least 1 to 2 cm distal to the patella tendon insertion.

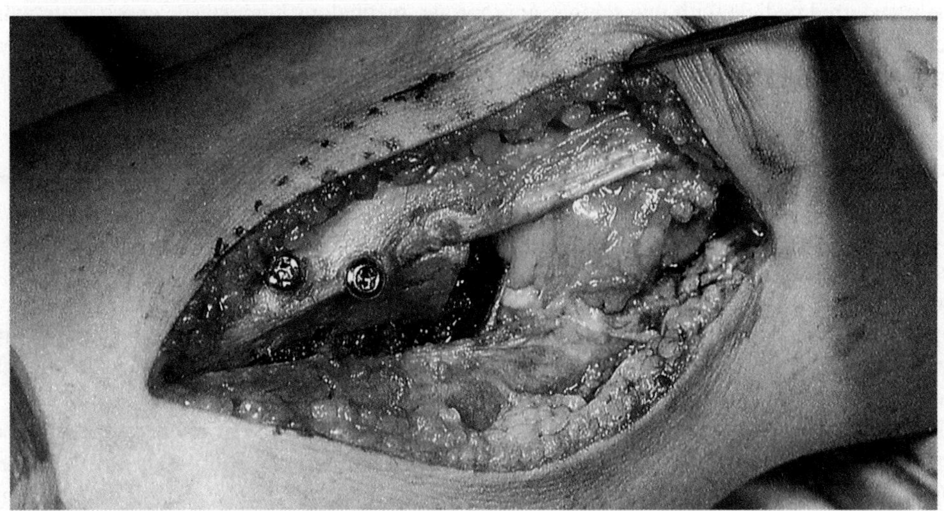

FIGURE 4-19

In most cases, two cortical lag screws are used to give firm fixation of the transferred bone pedicle.

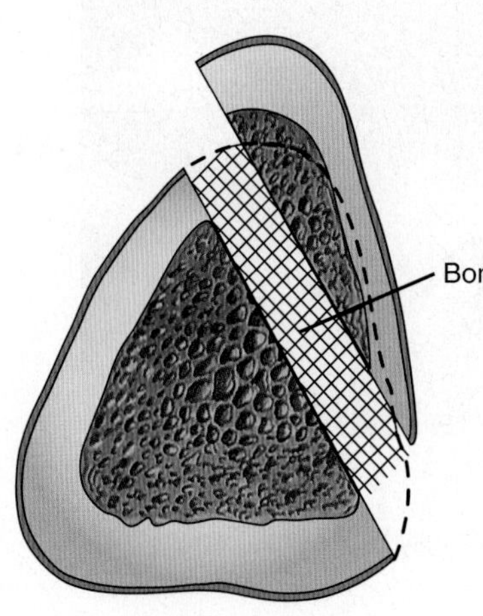

FIGURE 4-20

A local bone graft taken from the tibial metaphysis may be placed in the osteotomy plane, thereby displacing the osteotomy in an anterolateral direction, producing net anterior displacement of the tibial tubercle. Direct anteriorization with less bone graft can be achieved using this technique. A sagittal cut in the tibia as described in the text will also permit straight anteriorization.

allograft bone in the oblique osteotomy plane, any medial displacement of the tibial tubercle will be "offset" and slight additional anteriorization of the tubercle achieved. If the patella appears to be located too medially following anteromedial tibial tubercle transfer, an offset bone graft may be added. Also, because this gives additional anteriorization, the offset bone graft may be used selectively if there is need to further unload the distal, medial portion of the patella. Care must be used when an offset bone graft is added in the osteotomy site. Because this adds to anteriorization, the surgeon must be careful not to anteriorize excessively. In our experience, 2 cm of anteriorization is maximal to avoid undue "tenting" of the skin and risk of skin slough. In a consecutive series of over 600 anteromedial tibial tubercle transfers, I have not had a skin slough.

Another option for achieving straight anteriorization is to make a sagittal plane cut into the tibia, followed by a back cut from the lateral side, both tapered to an anterior point distally, thereby permitting a straight anterior transfer of the tibial tubercle along the osteotomy plane. This transferred bone pedicle can then be fixated with medial-lateral cortical screws.

The skin should close without tension, provided that no bone graft is added. We use a full subcutaneous closure with 2-0 absorbable suture, followed by skin clips or subcuticular closure and the application of full-length 0.5-in Steri-Strips, followed by infiltration with 0.5% Marcaine. A suction drain may be used but is not usually necessary. If one anteriorizes more than 2 cm, one may wish to consult preoperatively with a plastic surgeon.

Using careful surgical technique; a precise oblique osteotomy tapered anteriorly; secure fixation of the transferred pedicle with two screws; appropriate, meticulous hemostasis; appropriate patient selection; early range of motion; and good postoperative rehabilitation, anteromedial tibial tubercle transfer will give uniformly good results.

POSTOPERATIVE MANAGEMENT

Assuming secure two-screw fixation of the transferred bone pedicle (as described), patients are started on immediate, once-daily active and passive range-of-motion exercises of the knee but are maintained in a knee immobilizer for 4 weeks on crutches. Continuous passive motion has not been necessary except in unusual circumstances, such as concomitant release of arthrofibrosis. Cryotherapy is helpful in the immediate postoperative period. A Cryo/Cuff is applied immediately after surgery (Fig. 4-21) and maintained for 3 to 4 days. This has helped diminish pain and facilitate early mobilization by minimizing swelling and pain.

Elevation is encouraged for the first 72 hours, and patients are allowed to ambulate with toe-touch weight bearing, using crutches. The drain, if used, is removed at 18 to 24 hours after surgery if bleeding has subsided. Most patients are given antibiotic coverage preoperatively, and this may be continued for 5 days selectively. We recommend postoperative aspirin daily for 6 to 8 weeks. Most patients can be discharged the day of surgery as long as they are mobile, swelling and pain are controlled, and

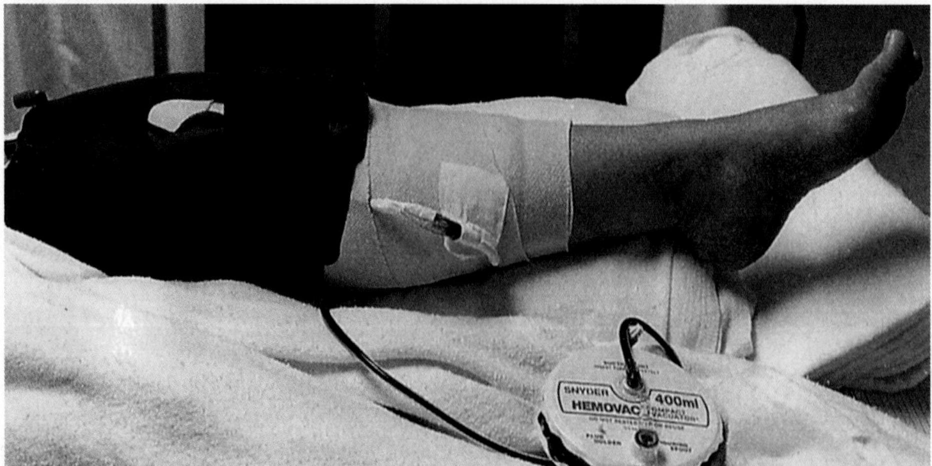

FIGURE 4-21

Cryotherapy will help reduce swelling and pain postoperatively. A Hemovac may be left in the wound for 2 to 24 hours, as needed.

there is no evidence of fever, calf tenderness, or any complication. Most patients need only a light dressing and knee immobilizer (4 weeks) over the wound as long as they are competent and appropriately cautious on crutches. The immobilizer should be taken off once each day to permit knee flexion. After 4 weeks, the patient may switch to a patellofemoral brace. Eighty-nine to ninety percent of patients have an objectively good or excellent result (11). Those patients with more advanced articular breakdown, however, can expect a 75% chance of a good result. Excellent results appear to be uncommon in patients with extensive articular breakdown. With 5 years minimum follow-up, results are maintained in most patients. Follow-up for 8 to 10 years has shown sustained improvement.

Some patients complain of discomfort along the anterior aspect of the tibia. Generally, this resolves by 6 to 12 months from the time of surgery. Some patients have some tenderness from the screws, and removal of the screws at 6 to 12 months after surgery is common. Most patients benefit from physical therapy, but some can recover on a home program, progressing to exercise bicycling, swimming, and progressive physical activity as tolerated after healing of the transferred bone pedicle. Active and passive motion are important in the first few weeks after surgery, and full range of motion of the knee should be achieved by 4 to 8 weeks from the time of surgery. Physical therapy may be very helpful to those patients with less motivation or who are progressing slowly. Full active work on quadriceps strengthening will generally start at 8 to 12 weeks from the time of surgery, but light quadriceps exercise, leg lifts, and range-of-motion exercises may be started immediately after surgery.

AVOIDING COMPLICATIONS, PEARLS, AND PITFALLS

Serious complications after properly performed anteromedial tibial tubercle transfer have been very uncommon. Proper indications are most important. The surgeon should of course watch carefully for evidence of infection or thrombophlebitis. Although aspirin prophylaxis is routine, the threshold for initiating Coumadin or a volume expander (e.g., Lovenox) should be low if there is any concern about elevated thrombophlebitis risk. Since the anterior compartment is not closed, anterior compartment syndrome has never occurred in the experience of the author, but a low threshold for performing fasciotomy must be maintained if a compartment syndrome is suspected.

Technical complications include fracture through a screw hole, nonunion, tibial fracture, neurovascular injury, deep venous thrombosis, overcorrection, skin slough, undercorrection, and incisional neuroma. Another potential complication is failure to achieve pain relief because of extensive articular degeneration. In fact, such complications are very rare when the surgery is done properly.

Fracture of the tibia is avoidable by using proper technique and rehabilitation, but will require open reduction and internal fixation if it does occur.

In the event of undercorrection, the tubercle transfer procedure can be repeated at 6 to 12 months after the initial operation, with additional anteriorization and/or medialization. After removing the screws, the operative technique is the same as that used initially. It is best to avoid cancellous lag screws, which can be difficult or near impossible to remove.

In the event of overcorrection, careful lateral transfer of the healed tibial tubercle may be necessary. This should not be undertaken until 6 to 12 months from the time of the initial surgery, and it is best to watch the patellar tracking carefully, with femoral nerve stimulation used at the time of surgery to balance the patella in the trochlea.

Medial subluxation, as a dynamic complication of patella realignment surgery, is possible, if the tubercle is moved too far medially. Such patients may not have an obvious medial alignment of the patella. Instead, they express a devastating and very painful feeling of the patella jumping out of place (from too far medial back into the trochlea) upon early knee flexion in gait. The astute examiner will detect this by holding the patella medially with the knee extended and then abruptly flexing the knee while releasing the patella simultaneously. This reproduces the event that the afflicted patient experiences. This complication can be controlled by using a patella-stabilizing brace holding the patella from medial to lateral (buttress pad medial). If necessary, a repair of released lateral tissues, with or without a tenodesis on the lateral side, can control this problem, but moving the tubercle back to proper alignment may be rarely necessary.

Nonunion of the transferred pedicle may be treated by removal of the fixation screws, debridement of fibrous tissue in the osteotomy site, exposure of bleeding bone, flattening of the osteotomy plane to allow improved apposition of the pedicle to underlying bone, cancellous bone grafting, and refixation with two cortical lag screws. This complication is almost nonexistent when the osteotomy is flat and the fixation secure.

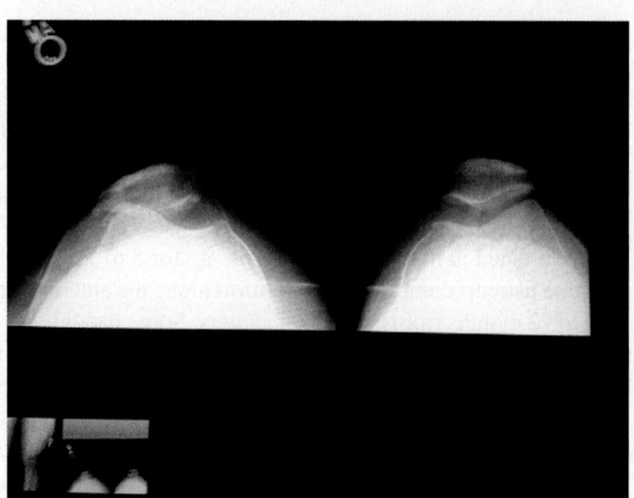

FIGURE 4-22
Long-term benefit of anteromedial tibial tubercle transfer compared to an unoperated knee.

Although stiffness is uncommon with the use of immediate postoperative range-of-motion exercises and ambulation, it may be treated if necessary by postoperative manipulation at 8 to 12 weeks after surgery, followed by physical therapy.

An important key to success with anteromedial tibial tubercle transfer osteotomy is to taper a precise osteotomy cut, at its distal extent, toward the **anterior** tibial cortex (avoid notching the anterior tibia). Also, the surgeon should not extend the proximal posterior corner of the osteotomy into the posterior tibia. In other words, do not let the osteotomy extend into or past the posterior, lateral corner of the tibia. Excellent visualization and a precise, flat, single plane osteotomy are of paramount importance in achieving the optimal osteotomy so as to avoid complication. Furthermore, excellent bone-bone contact and secure fully threaded, cortical screw fixation (do not use cancellous lag screws), well seated into good bone, using excellent technique (lag effect, countersinking screw heads, precise drill holes with secure grasp of posterior cortex) will assure stable fixation and freedom from complication. Proper technique permits early motion, outpatient surgery, earlier full weight bearing, primary bone-bone healing quickly, an excellent result, and a happy patient. Complications are rare when AMZ is done properly. This picture depicts the long-term (>25 years) mechanical benefit of AMZ (left knee) versus a right knee on which the patient had not had surgery (Fig. 4-22).

REFERENCES

1. Fulkerson J. Awareness of the retinaculum in evaluating patellofemoral pain. *Am J Sports Med.* 1982;10:147.
2. Fulkerson J, Becker G, Meany J, et al. Anteromedial tibial tubercle transfer without bone graft. *Am J Sports Med.* 1990;18:490–497.
3. Fulkerson J, Gossling H. Anatomy of the knee joint lateral retinaculum. *Clin Orthop.* 1980;153:183–188.
4. Trillat A, Dejour H, Coutette A. Diagnostique et traitement des subluxations recidivantes de la routle. *Rev Chir Orthop.* 1964;50:813–824.
5. Carney J, Mologne T, Muldoon M, et al. Long-term evaluation of the Roux-Elmslie-Trillat procedure for patellar instability. *Am J Sports Med.* 2005;33(8):1220–1223.
6. Powers CM, Ward SR, Chen YJ, et al. The effect of bracing on patellofemoral joint stress during free and fast walking. *Am J Sports Med.* 2004;32(1):224–231.
7. Merchant A, Mercer R, Jacobsen R, et al. Roentgenographic analysis of patellofemoral congruence. *J Bone Joint Surg.* 1974;56A:1391–1396.
8. Goutallier D, Bernageau J, Lecudonnec B. The measurement of the tibial tuberosity patella groove distance: technique and results. *Rev Chir Orthop Reparatrice Appar Mot.* 1978;64:423–428.
9. Grawe B, Stein BS. Tibial tubercle osteotomy: indication and techniques. *J Knee Surg.* 2015;28(4):279–284.
10. Stephen JM, Dodds AL, Lumpaopong P, et al. The ability of medial patellofemoral ligament reconstruction to correct patellar kinematics and contact mechanics in the presence of a lateralized tibial tubercle. *Am J Sports Med.* 2015;43(9):2198–2207.
11. Fulkerson J. *Disorders of the patellofemoral joint.* Philadelphia: Lippincott Williams & Wilkins; 2004.

RECOMMENDED READINGS

Fulkerson J. Anteromedial tibial tubercle transfer. In: Espreguiera-Mendes G, Nakamura N, eds. *The patellofemoral joint.* Springer; 2014; Chapter 20.

Fulkerson J. *Patella Instability and Arthrosis.* Blu Ray DVD produced by and available from the Arthroscopy Association of North America and the American Academy of Orthopaedic Surgeons, 2013.

Post W, Fulkerson J. *Distal realignment of the patellofemoral joint.* In: Scott N, Scuderi G, eds. *Surgery of the knee.* Churchill Livingstone; 2011; Chapter 62.

Saleh K, Arendt E, Eldridge J, et al. Operative treatment of patellofemoral arthritis. *J Bone Joint Surg* 2005;87A:659–671.

5 Sulcus-Deepening Trochleoplasty

Vinícius Canello Kuhn, Paulo Renato Fernandes Saggin, and David Dejour

INDICATIONS/CONTRAINDICATIONS

Trochlear dysplasia is one of the major anatomical factors that lead to patellar instability. It is present in up to 96% of patients who had at least one episode of patellar dislocation (1). Normal trochleae are concave, while dysplastic trochleae are shallower than normal ones, flat, or convex. In trochlear dysplasia, the osseous constraint to patellar tracking is lost and instability may overcome.

Trochleoplasty is the procedure designed to correct trochlear dysplasia. Deepening trochleoplasty is indicated in patients with high-grade trochlear dysplasia with bump (grades B and D) who suffer recurrent patellar dislocations, often demonstrating abnormal patellar tracking (2–4) in active and/or passive motion. It can also be performed in patients after a first failed surgery for patellar instability, when high-grade trochlear dysplasia was present but not addressed (5). The main goals of trochleoplasty are to decrease the abnormal prominence of the trochlea and to create a new groove with normal depth and orientation. The procedure treats the essential cause of dislocation as it corrects the abnormal patterns underlying the different grades of trochlear dysplasia.

The procedure is contraindicated in patients with established patellofemoral osteoarthritis or open growth plates. It is not indicated to treat patellofemoral pain or subjective instability.

PREOPERATIVE PLANNING

Routine investigation of patellofemoral instability patients prior to surgery includes standard knee radiographs in three incidences (weight-bearing anteroposterior, lateral view, and axial view), computed tomography (CT) with the Lyon Protocol (1) (Table 5-1), and/or magnetic resonance imaging (MRI) of the knee using a patellofemoral protocol.

Trochlear dysplasia is one of the four main anatomical factors that lead to patellar instability: trochlear dysplasia, excessive tibial tubercle-trochlear groove (TT-TG) distance, patellar tilt, and patella alta. They all must be evaluated in every case and corrected one by one when present. No single procedure will be successful if other important factors are neglected.

TABLE 5-1 The Lyon Protocol for Patellofemoral Instability Evaluation

Measure	How to Measure (CT)	Patients with Atleast One Episode of Patellar Dislocation (Mean ± SD)	Controls (Mean ± SD)	OBS
Femoral anteversion	Angle between center of femoral head/neck and posterior condyles	15.6 ± 9.0 degrees	10.8 ± 8.7 degrees	
TT-TG	Distance between trochlear groove and tibial tuberosity in 2 overlapped cuts	19.8 ± 1.6 mm	12.7 ± 3.4 mm	Pathologic threshold = 20 mm
External patellar tilt	Angle formed by the transverse axis of the patella and posterior femoral condyles	28.8 ± 10.5 degrees Average increase of 6 degrees with quadriceps contraction	10 ± 5.8 degrees Average increase of 1.5 degrees with quad contraction	Pathologic threshold without quadriceps contraction = 20 degrees
External tibial torsion	Angle formed by the tangent to the posterior aspect of the plateau and the bimalleolar axis	33 degrees	35 degrees	Too much variation, no particular significance found

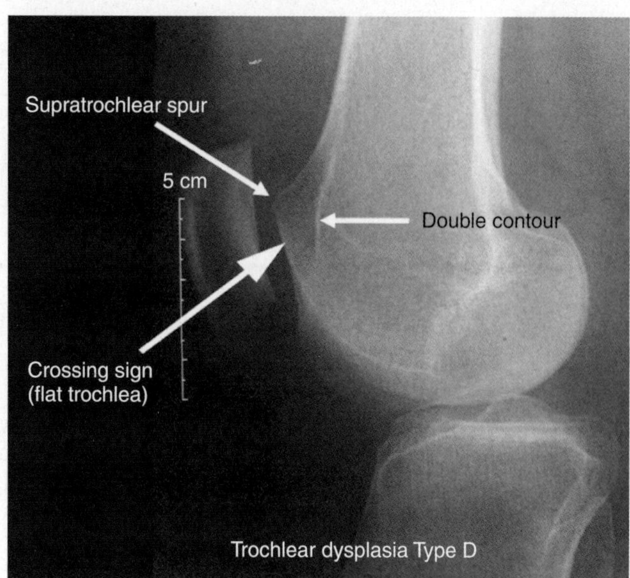

FIGURE 5-1

Adequate analysis of trochlear dysplasia requires a true profile, with perfect superimposition of the posterior femoral condyles. The three signs of trochlear dysplasia: (a) the crossing sign, (b) the supratrochlear spur, and (c) the double-contour ending below the crossing sign.

Preoperative planning starts with the radiographic studies evaluation. The anteroposterior view is less informative but already allows assessment of bone quality, knee alignment, femorotibial-associated pathologies, major patellar displacement, and loose bodies or bone fragments. On true lateral views (perfect superimposition of both posterior femoral condyles), trochlear dysplasia is diagnosed and classified (2,6) (Fig. 5-1), and patellar height is measured (Fig. 5-2). Dejour (Dejour, D.) classified the dysplasia in four types, depending on the presence of the crossing sign, supratrochlear spur, and the double contour (Figs. 5-3 and 5-4). The authors routinely utilize the Caton-Deschamps index to measure patellar height (7).

Axial radiographic views allow the evaluation of patellar inclination, articular congruence, cartilage thickness, and the possible presence of bone fragments from previous fractures and avulsions. In adequately performed axial views, the relation between the femoral trochlea and the patella can

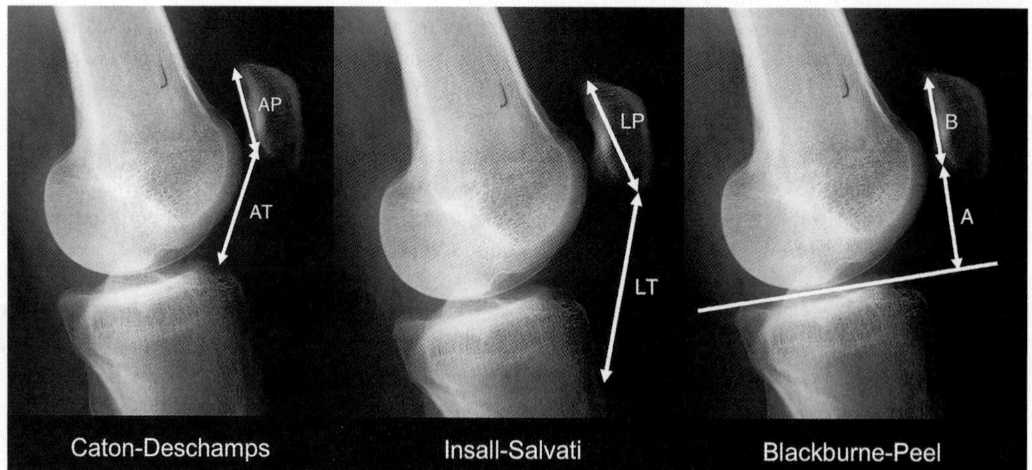

FIGURE 5-2

The Caton-Deschamps index (AT/AP) is the ratio between the distance from the lower edge of the patellar articular surface to the anterosuperior angle of the tibia outline (AT) and the length of the articular surface of the patella (AP); values equal or inferior to 0.6 determine patella infera and ratios superior to 1.2 indicate patella alta. The Insall-Salvati index (LT/LP) is the ratio between the length of the patellar tendon (LT) and the longest sagittal diameter of the patella (LP); ratio smaller than 0.8 indicates patella infera and greater than 1.2 patella alta. The Blackburne-Peel index (A/B) is the ratio between the length of the perpendicular line drawn from the tangent to the tibial plateau until the inferior pole of the articular surface of the patella (A) and the length of the articular surface of the patella (B); in patella infera, the ratio is smaller than 0.5, and in patella alta, it is greater than 1.

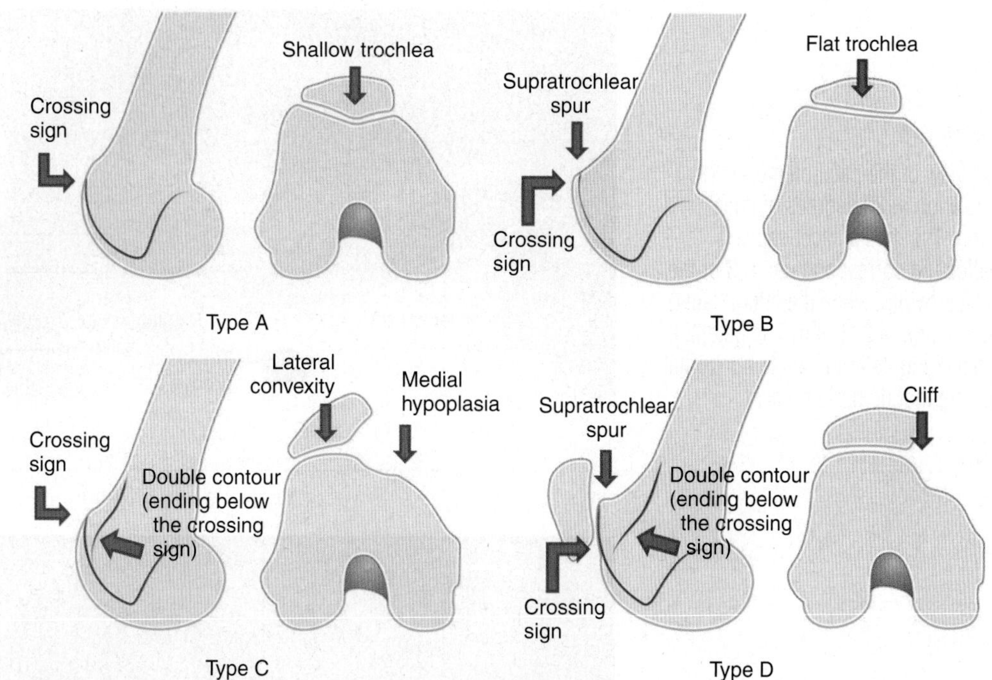

FIGURE 5-3

Trochlear dysplasia classification according to D. Dejour. **Type A:** presence of crossing sign in lateral true view. The trochlea is shallower than normal but still symmetric and concave. **Type B:** crossing sign and trochlear spur. The trochlea is flat or convex in axial images. **Type C:** presence of the crossing sign and the double-contour sign, representing the densification of the subchondral bone of the medial hypoplastic facet. In axial CT scan views, the lateral facet is convex. **Type D:** combines all the mentioned signs—crossing sign, supratrochlear spur, and double-contour sign going below the crossing sign. In axial CT scan views, there is a cliff pattern.

be effectively assessed: at 30 degrees of flexion, the trochlear lateral facet should compose approximately two-thirds of total trochlear width, and the patellar lateral facet should similarly represent two-thirds of the total patellar width (Fig. 5-5). Axial views obtained with 45 degrees of knee flexion (Merchant view) allow the measurement of the sulcus angle (Fig. 5-6). The mean normal value defined by Merchant was 138 degrees (standard deviation [SD] ± 6); angles superior to 150 degrees are considered abnormal. Dysplastic trochleae will show higher angles, some of which cannot even be measured because there is no sulcus.

On CT images with the Lyon Protocol, the TT-TG distance and patellar tilt are measured. TT-TG normal values should be inferior to 20 mm (Fig. 5-7), and the patellar tilt must not exceed

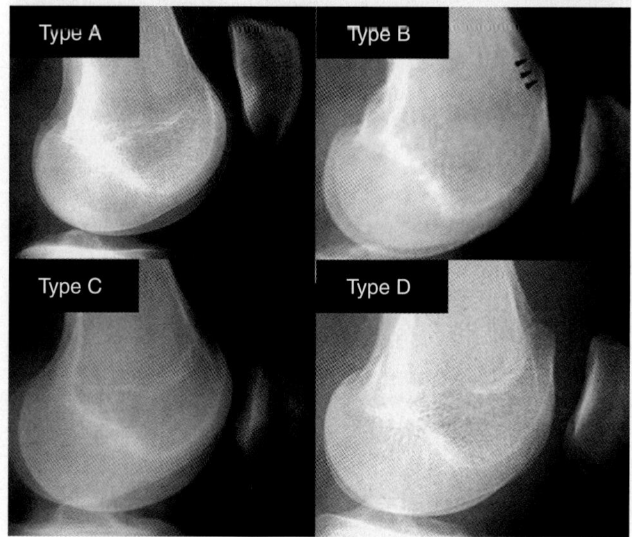

FIGURE 5-4

Trochlear dysplasia assessed in lateral views. The crossing sign, the supratrochlear spur, and the double-contour sign should all be assessed to classify it.

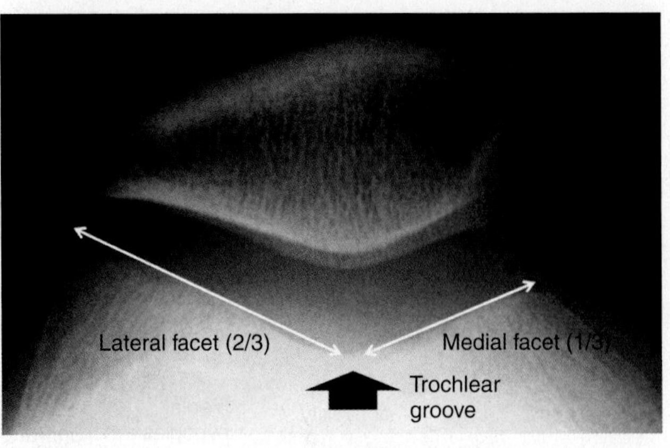

FIGURE 5-5

Axial view of the patellofemoral articulation at 30 degrees of knee flexion. The medial facet appears smaller and corresponds to 1/3 of the trochlear width, while the lateral facet corresponds to 2/3 of it. The patella is centered and its long axis is horizontal, meaning that no tilt is present.

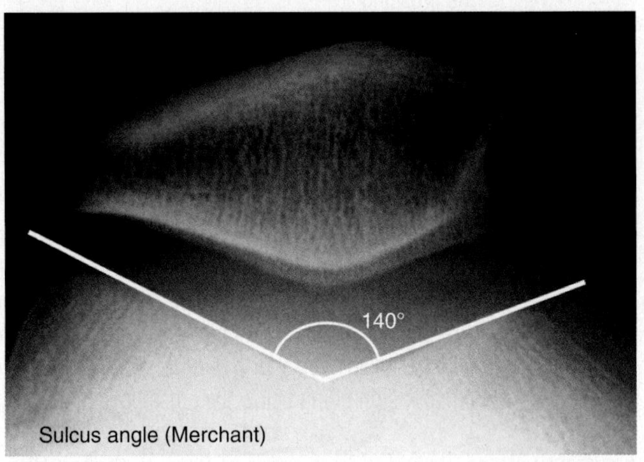

FIGURE 5-6

The sulcus angle defined by Brattström and popularized by Merchant is the angle formed by the two lines drawn from the deepest point of the trochlear groove to the highest point on the medial and lateral femoral condyles.

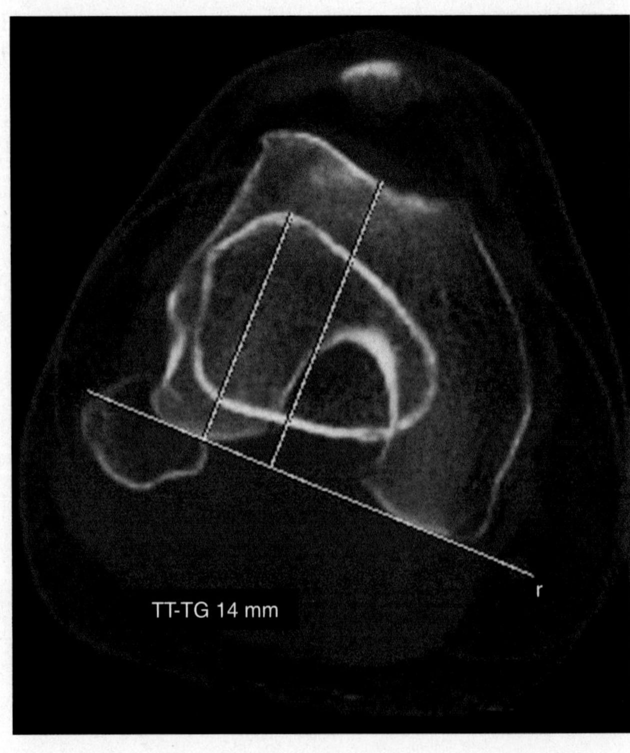

FIGURE 5-7

Tibial tubercle-trochlear groove distance. Two CT scan cuts are superimposed: one through superior part of the trochlea and other through the proximal patellar tendon tibial insertion. The deepest point of the trochlear groove and the tibial tubercle are projected on the posterior condylar line. The distance between them is the TT-TG value in millimeters.

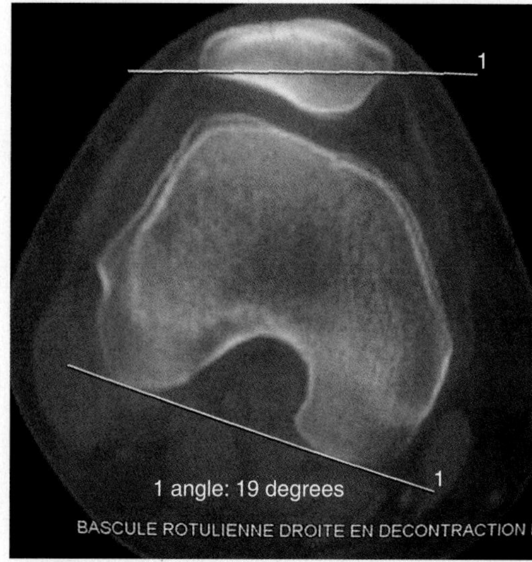

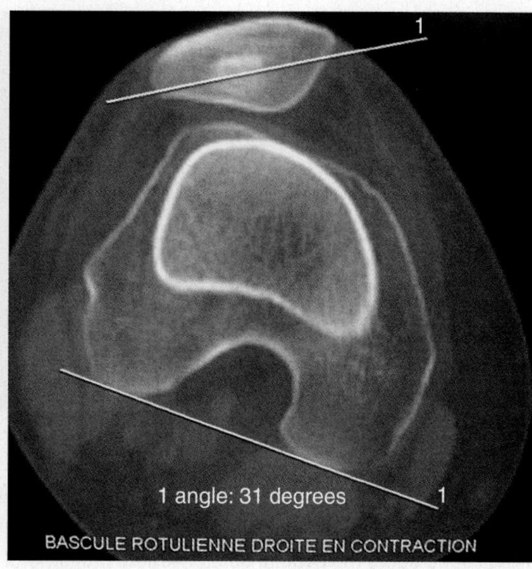

FIGURE 5-8
The patellar tilt measurement in CT scans (in extension) is performed drawing two lines: one tangent to the posterior femoral condyles and another through the patellar transverse axis. The angle between both lines is the patellar tilt angle. These CT scan images show the patellar tilt measurement with (**right figure**) and without (**left figure**) quadriceps contraction. The value increases from 19 degrees (within the normal range) to 31 degrees (abnormal) after the patient effectively contracts his or her quadriceps.

20 degrees (Fig. 5-8). In this specific protocol, femoral anteversion and external tibial torsion are also assessed. Finally, CT scan improves the visualization on the axial plane, and the sulcus angle can also be measured on this exam.

MRI provides superior anatomic and pathologic definition of soft tissues and articular cartilage (Fig. 5-9). It allows bony and cartilaginous shape assessment; because osseous and cartilaginous shapes do not match exactly, the true articulating surfaces can be revealed. The measures made on CT scan and x-ray can be applied to MRI. However, caution must be taken when measuring the TT-TG distance, which usually shows inferior values when compared to CT measures. Moreover, a threshold value for MRI TT-TG measurements has not yet been established. In sagittal MRI, the sagittal patellofemoral engagement (SPE) index (8) is measured, demonstrating the relationship between the patella and the trochlea, helping to establish the necessity of a distalization osteotomy of the tibial tubercle (Fig. 5-10).

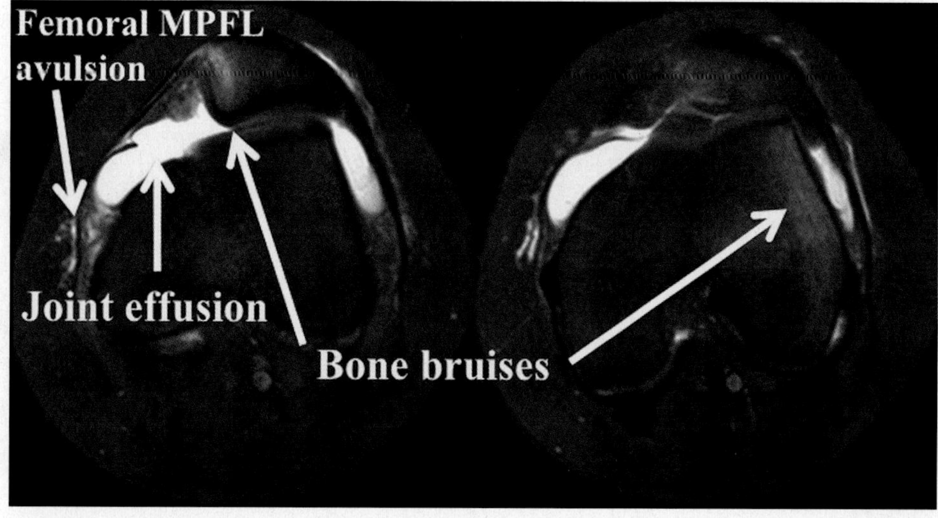

FIGURE 5-9
Several findings indicating acute dislocation of the patella.

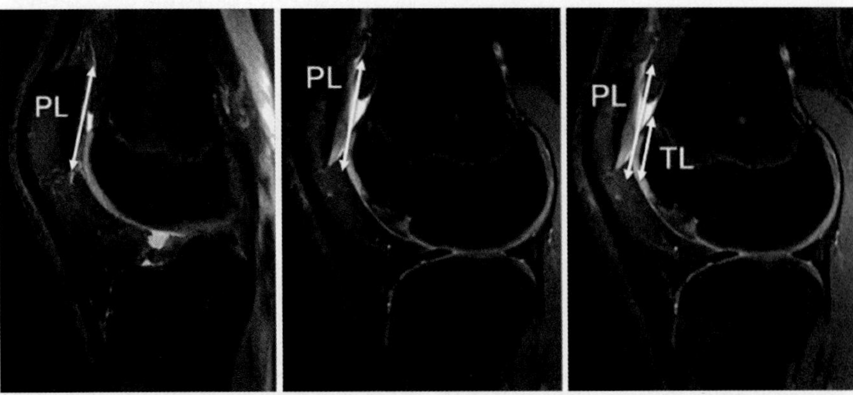

FIGURE 5-10

The SPE: the **left image** represents the MRI slice where the patella shows the longest articular cartilage. On this image, a patellar length (PL) line is drawn, measuring the entire length of the patellar articular cartilage. The second cut is the sagittal section where the femoral trochlear cartilage extends more proximally. On this slice, the PL line that has been previously copied is inserted (**middle image**). In the **right image**, a second line is drawn parallel to the PL, starting from the most proximal articular trochlear cartilage and finishing at the distal end of the PL, providing the trochlear length (TL) line. SPE is the ratio TL/PL. There is 95% probability that patients with patellar dislocation and SPE less than 0.45 have patella alta and insufficient functional sagittal PF engagement. Another 95% probability that a patient with patellar dislocation and SPE greater than 0.45 does not have patella alta and has adequate functional sagittal PF engagement.

The objective at the end of the surgery is to achieve a stable patella with a normal or type A trochlea. Regarding the other anatomical factors, the goal of patellar index value is 1, patellar tilt should be inferior to 20 degrees, and TT-TG distance should be between 10 and 15 mm. Trochleoplasty can lateralize the sulcus by 5 to 10 mm, acting as a proximal realignment, correcting the TT-TG distance, making a medial transfer of the tibial tubercle sometimes unnecessary.

SURGICAL PROCEDURE

The procedure can be performed under regional anesthesia and sedation. The patient is positioned supine. The entire extremity is prepared and draped. The incision is performed with the extremity flexed to 90 degrees; a straight midline skin incision is carried out from the superior patellar margin to the tibiofemoral articulation. The extremity is then positioned in extension and a medial full-thickness skin flap is developed. The arthrotomy is performed through a midvastus-adapted approach: medial retinaculum sharp dissection starting over the 1- to 2-cm medial border of the patella and blunt dissection of *vastus medialis obliquus* (VMO) fibers starting distally at the superomedial pole of the patella, extending approximately 4 cm into the muscle belly (Fig. 5-11).

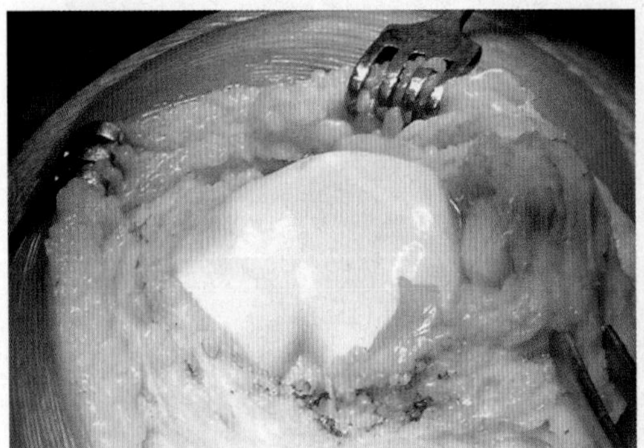

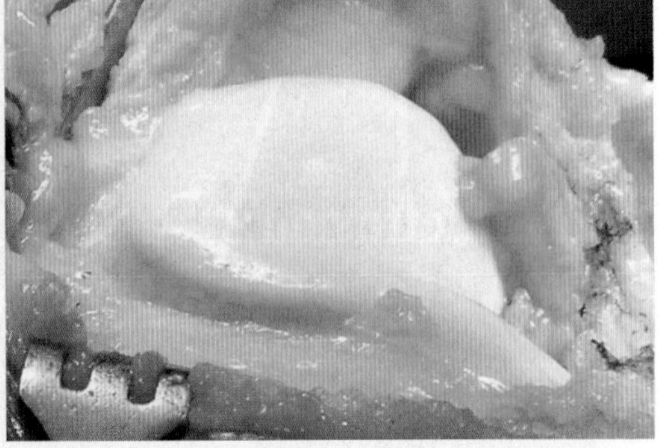

FIGURE 5-11

Trochlear dysplasia. Anterior (**left**) and lateral (**right**) view during surgical exposure showing the absence of the sulcus and the prominence of the trochlea in relation to the anterior femoral cortex.

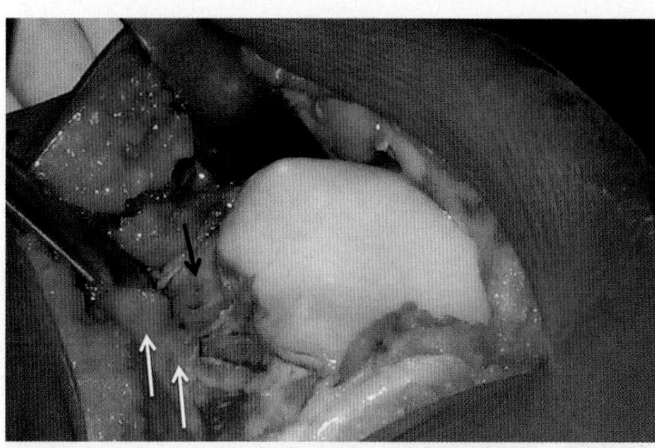

FIGURE 5-12

Surgical exposure. The periosteum is incised along the osteochondral edge and reflected away from the trochlear margin (*white arrows*). The anterior femoral cortex should be visible to guide the bone resection (*black arrow*).

The patella is briefly everted for inspection of chondral injuries and proper treatment (flap resection, microfracture, autologous chondrocyte implantation) if needed and then retracted laterally. The trochlea is exposed, and the peritrochlear synovium and periosteum are incised along their osteochondral junction and reflected from the field using a periosteal elevator. The anterior femoral cortex should be visible to determine the amount of deepening that should be undertaken (Fig. 5-12) (supratrochlear spur). Changing the knee's degree of flexion allows improved view of the complete operative field and avoids extending the incision.

Once the trochlea is fully exposed, the new one is planned and drawn with a sterile pen. The native trochlear groove is marked. Two additional divergent lines starting at the notch and going proximally through the condylotrochlear grooves (*sulcus terminalis*), representing the lateral and medial facet limits, are also traced. They should not enter the tibiofemoral articulation. Finally, the new trochlear groove is marked in a more lateral position according to the preoperative TT-TG value. The superior limit is the osteochondral edge and the inferior is the intercondylar notch (Fig. 5-13).

The next step is accessing the undersurface of the femoral trochlea. For this purpose, a thin strip of cortical bone is removed around the trochlea. The width of the strip is equal to the prominence of the trochlea from the anterior femoral cortex—that is, the bump formed. A sharp osteotome is used and gently tapped. A rongeur is used next to remove the bone (Fig. 5-14).

Subsequently, cancellous bone must be removed from the undersurface of the trochlea. An initial guide that is fixed onto the cartilage, anteriorly to the notch, is utilized to make multiple drill tunnels below the cartilage. This guide prevents the drill to trespass the cartilage since it blocks the advancement of the drill beyond 5 mm before reaching the tip of the guide (Fig. 5-15). After this, another drill with a depth guide set at 5 mm is used to ensure uniform thickness of the osteochondral flap, maintaining an adequate and uniform amount of bone attached to the cartilage (Fig. 5-16).

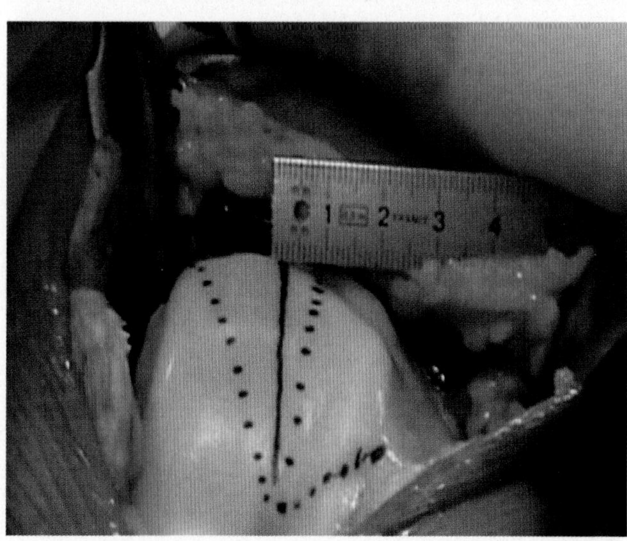

FIGURE 5-13

After surgical exposure, the new trochlea is drawn. From the intercondylar notch, the native trochlear groove and two divergent lines, representing the lateral and medial facet limits, are marked (*dashed lines*). The new trochlear groove is marked in a more lateral position according to the preoperative TT-TG value (*continuous line*).

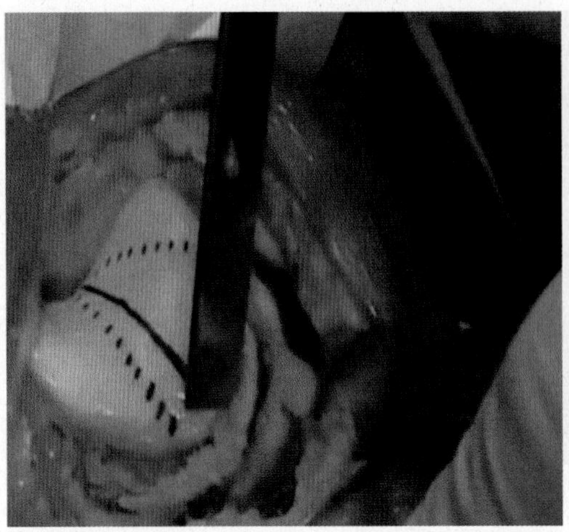
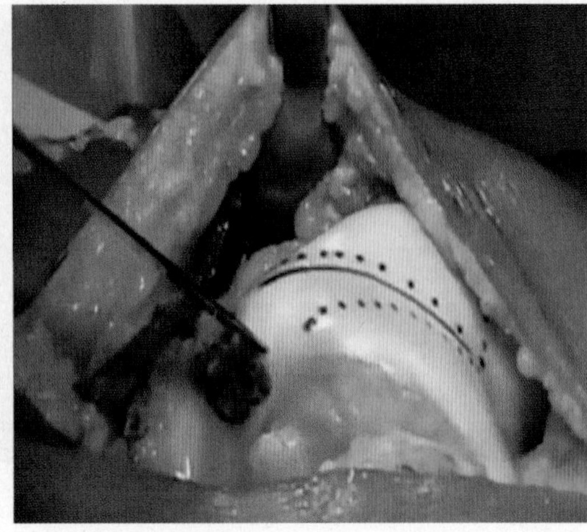

FIGURE 5-14
A sharp osteotome is used to remove a thin strip of cortical bone around the trochlea to access its undersurface.

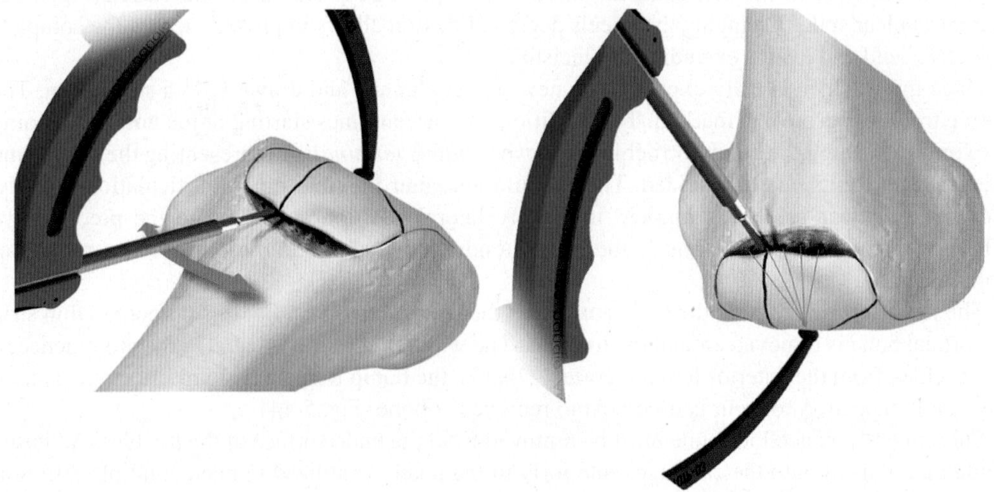

FIGURE 5-15
Drill with guide to initiate removing the cancellous bone under the cartilage of the trochlea. It is fixed anteriorly to the notch and prevents injuring the cartilage.

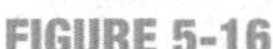

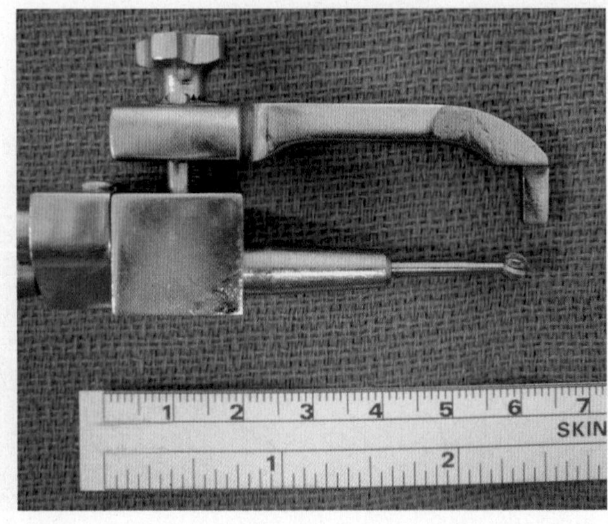

FIGURE 5-16
Drill with depth guide used to remove the cancellous bone from the trochlear under surface.

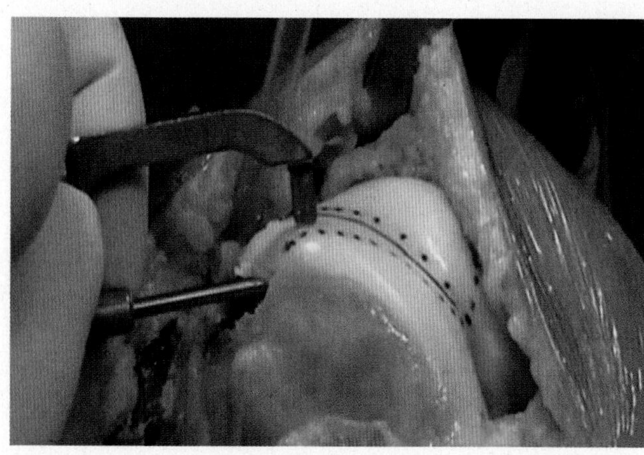

FIGURE 5-17
The guide avoids injuring the cartilage or getting to close to it. More bone is removed from the central portion.

The guide also avoids injuring the cartilage or getting too close to it, which could result in thermal injury. The shell produced must be sufficiently compliant to allow molding without being fractured. More cancellous bone is removed from the central portion of the trochlea, where the new groove will rest (Fig. 5-17).

Light pressure should be able to mold the flap to the underlying cancellous bone bed in the distal femur (Fig. 5-18). The groove, and sometimes the lateral facet external margin, should be cut to allow further molding, which is achieved gently tapping over a scalpel (Fig. 5-19). If the correction obtained is satisfactory, the new trochlea is fixated: one absorbable anchor is applied near the notch (vertex) (Fig. 5-20); one suture (doubled) spans each facet from the anchor in the notch until another anchor applied in the supratrochlear fossa, proximal to the end of the cartilage. The system employed precludes knots; the sutures are tensioned and fixated as the proximal anchors are inserted. Pressure is applied posteriorly while the sutures are being tensioned, ensuring that the prominence is removed and that the facets are flush with the anterior femoral cortex (Fig. 5-21). Patellar tracking is tested. Periosteum and synovial tissue are sutured to the osteochondral edge.

The authors always associate a soft tissue procedure to trochleoplasty. The medial patellofemoral ligament (MPFL) reconstruction is the procedure of choice using the surgeon's technique of choice (Fig. 5-22). In most cases, due to intense retraction of the lateral retinaculum, lateral release or lateral lengthening is required to allow the patella to relocate above the trochlea without tilt. If this procedure is needed, it must be done prior to the MPFL reconstruction.

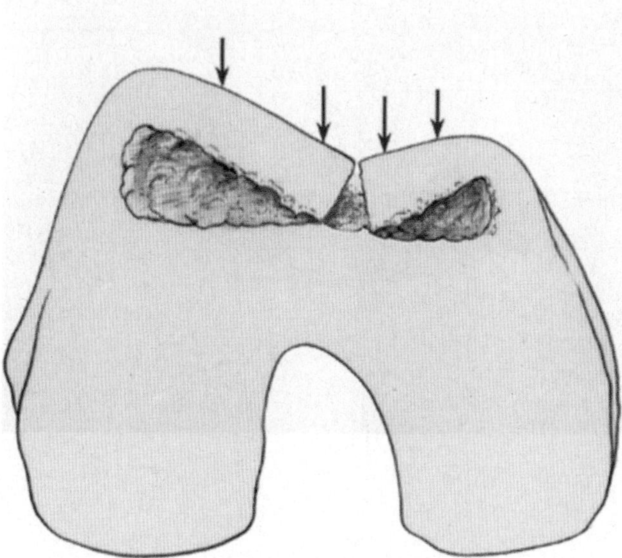

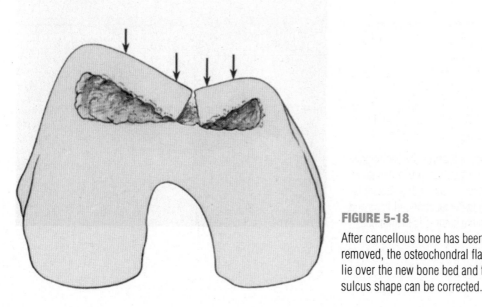

FIGURE 5-18
After cancellous bone has been removed, the osteochondral flaps can lie over the new bone bed and the sulcus shape can be corrected.

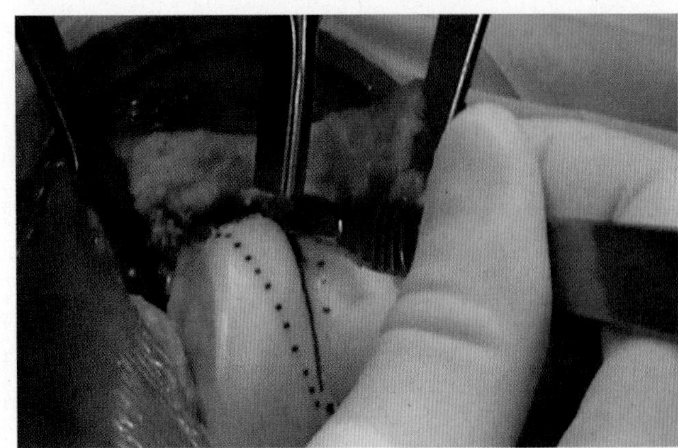

FIGURE 5-19

In order to allow further modeling to the underlying bone bed, the osteochondral flaps may be cut in the sulcus and facets lines.

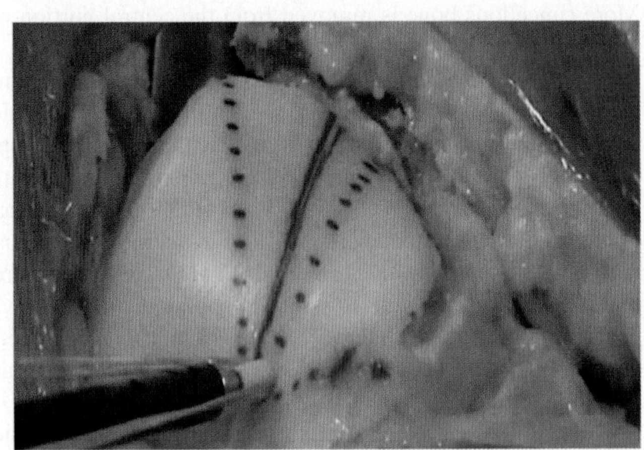

FIGURE 5-20

The first absorbable anchor is applied near the notch.

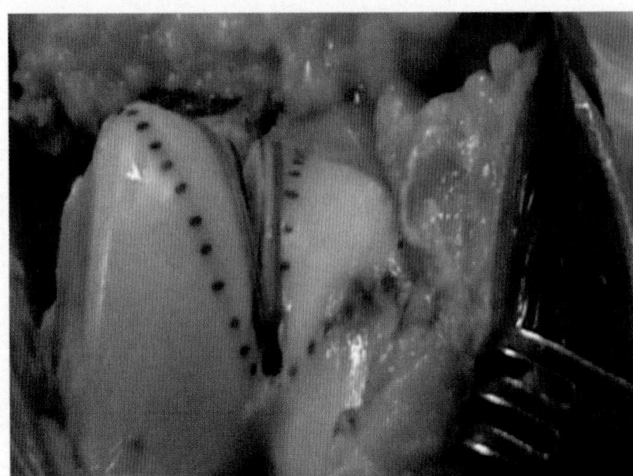

FIGURE 5-21

Final aspect of fixation. Two additional anchors were applied, one proximal to each facet, while posterior pressure is applied on the osteochondral flaps and tension on the sutures is maintained.

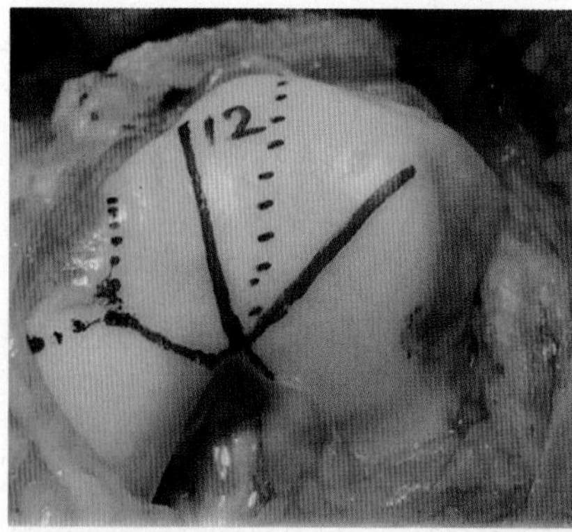

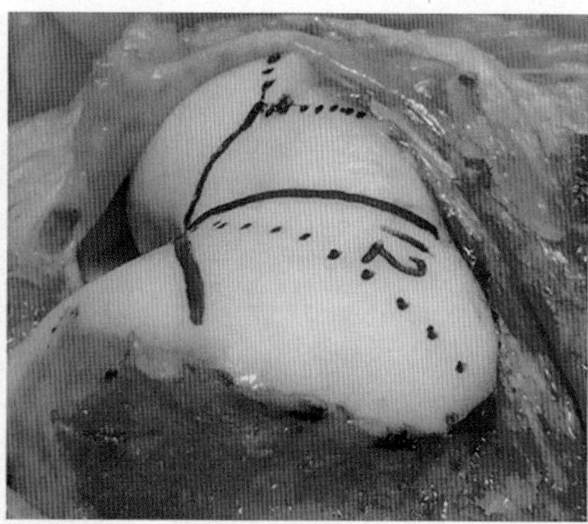

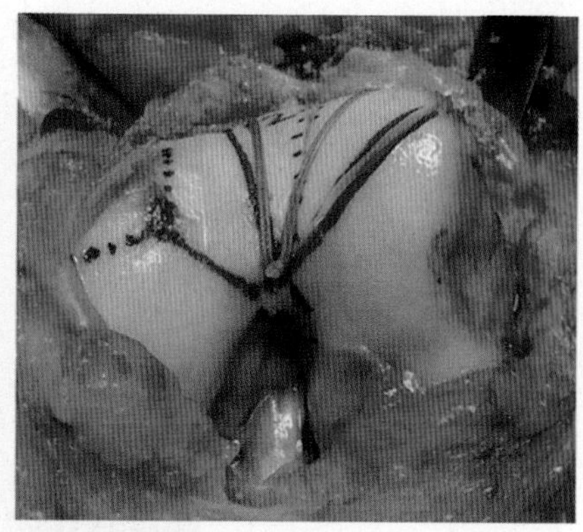

FIGURE 5-22

Illustrative case. High-grade trochlear dysplasia after exposure and planning; the new trochlea is planned 12 mm lateral to the native one (**left figure**). A thin strip of cortical bone around the trochlea is removed to access its undersurface (**middle figure**). After fixation with absorbable sutures, the new trochlea is flushed with the anterior femoral cortex, and the prominence presented before it is corrected (**right figure**).

POSTOPERATIVE MANAGEMENT

The main principles guiding rehabilitation have to respect the associated procedures, and rehabilitation must also apply to them. Trochleoplasty does not need weight protection or range-of-motion limitation. Movement may in fact improve cartilage healing and further molding of the trochlea; continuous passive movement (CPM) is usually employed during the first days. Partial weight bearing is allowed with an extension brace and aided by crutches in the first 15 days, when they can be discontinued if possible. The brace must be removed during the exercises.

During the first 6 weeks, patients are encouraged to perform exercises for range of motion as tolerated and isometric quadriceps and hamstring strengthening. Range of motion is gradually recovered, avoiding forced or painful postures. Quadriceps strengthening with weights on the feet or tibial tubercle is discouraged.

After 45 days, the rehabilitation protocol also includes closed chain and weight-bearing proprioception exercises. Cycling is usually possible, with weak resistance initially. Active ascension of the patella can be performed seated, with the leg extended, by static and isometric quadriceps contractions. Quadriceps strengthening with weights on the feet or tibial tubercle is still discouraged. The anterior and posterior muscular chains are stretched. Weight-bearing proprioception exercises are started when full extension is complete, first in bipodal stance and later in monopodal stance when there is no pain.

After 12 weeks, running can be initiated on a straight line. Closed kinetic chain muscular reinforcement between 0 and 60 degrees with minor loads but long series is allowed. Stretching of the anterior and posterior muscular chains is continued. The patient is encouraged to proceed with the rehabilitation on his or her own. After 6 months, sports on a recreational or competitive level can be resumed.

Six weeks postoperatively, radiographs, including AP, lateral view, and axial view in 30 degrees of flexion, are taken (Fig. 5-23). After 6 months, a CT scan is obtained to document the obtained correction (Fig. 5-24).

PEARLS AND PITFALLS

- Be alert for the indication—pain is not an indication.
- Positioning must allow full range of motion during procedure.
- Adequate exposure to access to the undersurface of the trochlea is essential.
- Intraoperative new trochlea planning—take your time.
- Adequate bone removal and achievement of a malleable osteochondral flap.
- Avoid cartilage damage during the osteochondral flap confection—keep a safe distance from the cartilage.
- Obtain a well-molded bone bed; otherwise, the new trochlea will not be adequately refashioned.

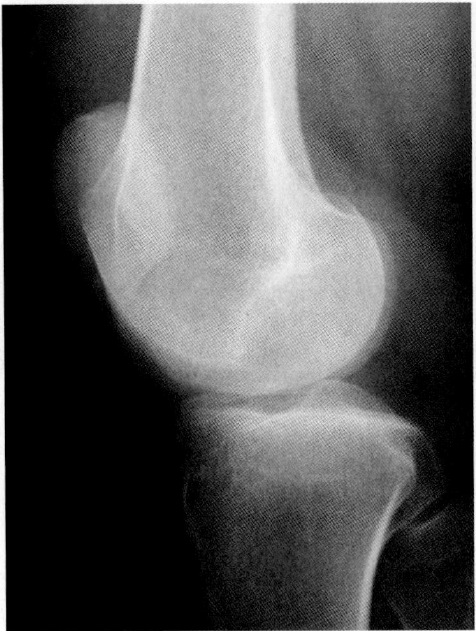

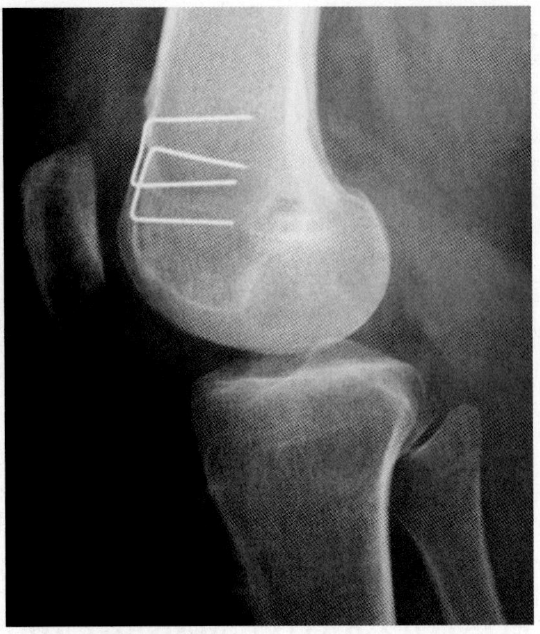

FIGURE 5-23

Pre- and postoperative lateral x-rays showing the resection of the supratrochlear spur and trochlear prominence correction. Additionally, patellar tilt is clearly improved. Fixation was achieved with staples.

- Correction of associated abnormalities is mandatory.
- Early rehabilitation; avoid prolonged immobilization (sometimes required for the associated procedures).

COMPLICATIONS TO AVOID

Patients submitted to trochleoplasty are at risk of the same complications inherent to any surgical procedure (e.g., infection, deep venous thrombosis), and routine measures employed to prevent them are similar to those employed in other orthopedic procedures.

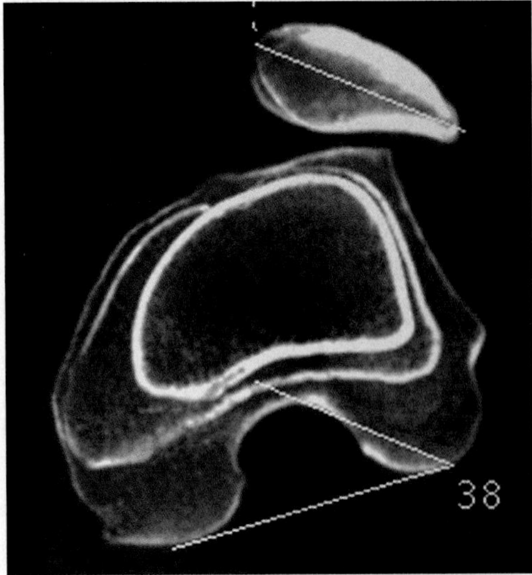

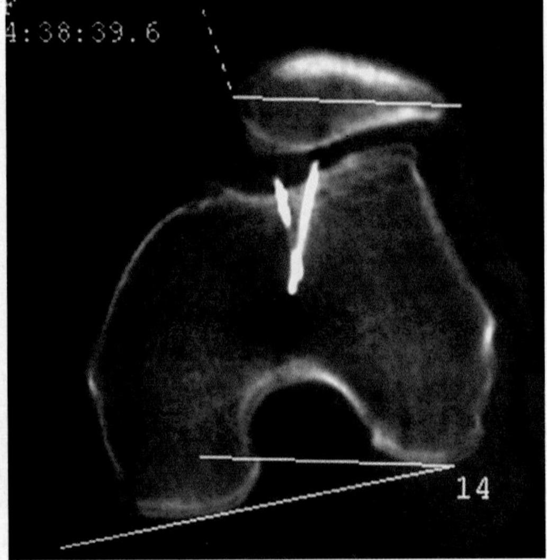

FIGURE 5-24

CT scan axial views before and after trochleoplasty. The trochlear sulcus is restored and patellar tilt is corrected. Patellar subluxation is also improved. Fixation was achieved with staples.

Specific complications of trochleoplasty are:

Recurrence of instability: It is very rare after such procedures and is more likely to result from missed associated abnormalities (5,9).

Trochlear necrosis/cartilage damage: There is a potential risk of cartilage damage while drilling the undersurface of the trochlear cartilage, when cutting the osteochondral flaps, and during the positioning of the new trochlea. The specific guides help to not trespass the cartilage and to maintain at least 5 mm of bone under the cartilage. During surgery, the assistant can slowly pour water with a syringe on the bone, to avoid thermal injury. The cuts on the cartilage have to be performed gently to avoid fracture. After drilling and cutting, the flaps must be easily manipulated with the surgeon's fingers to their new positions. Excessive force required to position the osteochondral flaps or failure to pressure down the flap generally indicate insufficient bone removal from the undersurface of the trochlea, which can lead to cartilage damage and osteochondral fracture.

Hypo- or hypercorrection: The new trochlear groove must be on the same level of the anterior femoral shaft, and the spur has to be totally removed. Ideally, the correction must achieve congruence between the patella and trochlea.

Pain: The results are not consistent regarding pain. A minority of patients may have intensity or frequency of pain increased after the procedure.

Loss of range of motion: Early beginning of physical therapy and orientations regarding range-of-motion restoration are of major importance in the postoperative period. Adequate analgesia must facilitate mobilization and cannot be overlooked.

There are some potential complications that are not yet well determined. Incongruence between the trochlea and the patella is a concern that needs longer follow-ups before any assumptions can be made about its consequences. Another issue of controversy is the development of osteoarthritis in the patients submitted to trochleoplasty. Osteoarthritis development and progression are multifactorial. Patients with patellofemoral instability are prone to develop osteoarthritis, and those patients operated for patellofemoral instability seem even more prone to degeneration than those treated conservatively.

In a systematic review performed by Song et al. (10), of the 329 patients who had undergone trochleoplasty procedures, 13.4% (44) had complications. Of these, 6.8% (3) were related to a redislocated patella, 27.3% (12) were related to a deficit of range of motion, and 65.9% (29) to increased patellofemoral pain level. Among 142 patients who were evaluated for patellofemoral osteoarthritis according to Iwano, 7.9% (13) were reported to present at least Iwano grade 2 at a mean follow-up of 69.9 months.

REFERENCES

1. Dejour H, Walch G, Nove-Josserand L, et al. Factors of patellar instability: an anatomic radiographic study. *Knee Surg Sports Traumatol Arthrosc.* 1994;2:19–26.
2. Dejour D, Le Coultre B. Osteotomies in patello-femoral instabilities. *Sports Med Arthrosc.* 2007;15:39–46.
3. Dejour H, Walch G, Neyret P, et al. Dysplasia of the femoral trochlea. *Rev Chir Orthop Reparatrice Appar Mot.* 1990;76:45–54.
4. Masse Y. Trochleoplasty. Restoration of the intercondylar groove in subluxations and dislocations of the patella. *Rev Chir Orthop Reparatrice Appar Mot.* 1978;64:3–17.
5. Dejour D, Byn P, Ntagiopoulos PG. The Lyon's sulcus-deepening trochleoplasty in previous unsuccessful patellofemoral surgery. *Int Orthop.* 2013;37:433–439.
6. Dejour D, Saggin P. The sulcus deepening trochleoplasty-the Lyon's procedure. *Int Orthop.* 2010;34:311–316.
7. Caton, J. Method of measuring the height of the patella. *Acta Orthop Belg.* 1989;55:385–386.
8. Dejour D, Ferrua P, Ntagiopoulos PG, et al.; French Arthroscopy Society (SFA). The introduction of a new MRI index to evaluate sagittal patellofemoral engagement. *Orthop Traumatol Surg Res.* 2013;99:S391–S398.
9. Ntagiopoulos PG, Byn P, Dejour D. Midterm results of comprehensive surgical reconstruction including sulcus-deepening trochleoplasty in recurrent patellar dislocations with high-grade trochlear dysplasia. *Am J Sports Med.* 2013;41:998–1004.
10. Song G-Y, Hong L, Zhang H, et al. Trochleoplasty versus nontrochleoplasty procedures in treating patellar instability caused by severe trochlear dysplasia. *Arthroscopy.* 2014;30:523–532.

6 Patellofemoral Replacement

Beth E. Shubin Stein, Lauren H. Redler, and Sabrina M. Strickland

INTRODUCTION

Isolated patellofemoral arthritis is seen in 9% of patients over 40 and 15% of those over 60 years old (1). In patients over 55, arthritis is more often isolated to the patellofemoral joint in women than in men (2). Since its introduction in 1955, patellofemoral arthroplasty (PFA) has evolved in sophistication and efficacy. Improved prosthetic design and patient selection have led to improved patient outcomes (3). Other surgical alternatives to PFA, including arthroscopic debridement with a cartilage restoration procedure (4) and patellectomy (5), have had limited success. Although total knee arthroplasty (TKA) may be an effective treatment option, PFA has many advantages over TKA for the treatment of isolated patellofemoral arthritis. It is less invasive, requires shorter tourniquet times, has a faster recovery, preserves native knee kinematics, is bone conserving, and has good clinical outcomes (6).

INDICATIONS/CONTRAINDICATIONS

The most important feature that influences success in PFA is appropriate patient selection. Patient factors including demographics, diagnosis, anatomy, and comorbidities influence a surgeons' decision to pursue nonsurgical versus surgical management, choose the appropriate operation, and plan the surgical approach. With any unicompartmental arthroplasty, there is always the risk for progressive degenerative joint disease (DJD) in the remainder of the knee. Survivorship of PFAs is tied to the etiology of the DJD—with posttraumatic, malalignment, and instability-related DJD faring better than primary osteoarthritis (OA) (3). It is important to recognize patella maltrackers early and perform PFA before significant erosion and patella acetabularization occurs (Fig. 6-1), and the patella becomes too thin on the lateral side with the remaining patella being too small to accommodate the prosthesis. PFAs are also very effective in the setting of trochlear dysplasia (6); it is important to remember that inlay designs are less appropriate than onlay designs in the setting of trochlear dysplasia because of the inability to change the version of the trochlear component.

Indications for PFA

- Primary OA
- Posttraumatic OA
- Instability-related OA
- Diffuse/bipolar disease not amenable to off-loading
- Patella maltracking and OA with early patella bone loss

Contraindications to PFA

- Inflammatory arthropathy
- Neuropathic arthropathy
- Tibiofemoral arthritis
- After history of infection in the affected joint (relative)
- Insufficient bone stock

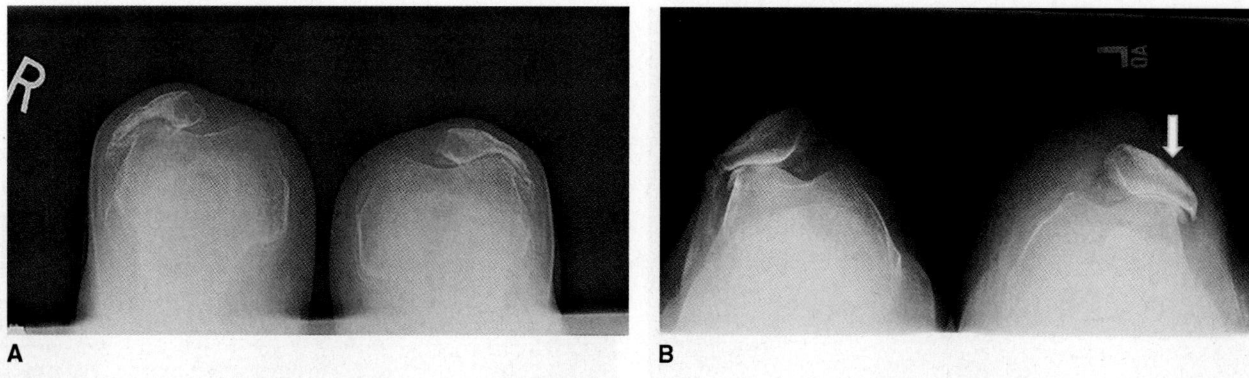

FIGURE 6-1
A merchant view showing (**A**) severe patellar bone loss and acetabularization of the patellae and (**B**) patellofemoral OA related to lateral maltracking.

Staged Procedure Required Prior to or Concomitant with PFA

- Significant patellofemoral instability
- TT-TG greater than 25 mm

Severe coronal deformity, if left uncorrected, can negatively affect patellar tracking and predispose to progression of tibiofemoral arthritis. Consider a staged or concomitant tibial tubercle transfer (TTT) in patients with severe maltracking or instability with a TT-TG greater than 25 mm. In patients with severe instability with a TT-TG less than 25 mm, a concomitant medial patellofemoral ligament (MPFL) reconstruction may be sufficient. Our preferred method of concomitant MPFL reconstruction is to use a partial thickness central third quadriceps tendon, 8 to 10 mm wide, 3 to 4 mm thick, and 90 to 100 mm in length, leaving the quadriceps tendon attached to the patella. The goal is to avoid any fixation in the patella. The quadriceps tendon works well as it has native attachments to the dorsal periosteum. We turn down the quadriceps tendon, bringing it out through a small incision in the soft tissue on the proximal medial side of the patella (anatomic position) and sew it in with a nonabsorbable suture to help it scar down. We then tunnel the graft between the capsule and medial retinaculum and fix it in a bone tunnel in the medial distal femur with a tenodesis screw in standard fashion.

PREOPERATIVE PLANNING

History and Physical Exam

A thorough history and meticulous physical exam are vital to appropriate patient selection. First, the hip joint and lumbar spine should be excluded as sources of the patient's pain with a history and a brief exam assessing range of motion. Other potential sources of anterior knee pain such as pes anserine bursitis, patellar tendonitis, and prepatellar bursitis should also be excluded.

Patellofemoral DJD typically presents as anterior knee pain that is worse with prolonged sitting, ascending or descending stairs, squatting/lunging, and walking on an incline. Pain with walking, particularly on a flat surface, is a red flag that the patient's DJD may not be isolated to the patellofemoral joint and should prompt further imaging to examine the tibiofemoral joint. On physical exam, patients will typically have patellofemoral crepitus with open chain knee flexion and extension, patellar facet and inferior pole tenderness, and reproducible pain with patellar compression. A careful examination for instability should be performed including patellar mobility both medially and laterally and an apprehension test. They should have no medial or lateral joint line tenderness, a negative McMurray's and Thessaly, as well as a stable ligament exam. It is important to note whether the patient's patella can be everted to neutral to decide if a concomitant lateral release should be done. Patellar tracking should also be assessed to determine the need for medialization of the patellar component.

Imaging

Weight-bearing radiographs are generally adequate for preoperative planning (Fig. 6-2A,B). The most important views are the lateral (Fig. 6-2C) and sunrise or merchant (Fig. 6-2D), which will demonstrate the presence of patellofemoral arthritis, patella alta/baja, patella tilt, or subluxation. However, if the patient has any history or positive physical exam findings of tibiofemoral symptoms or any

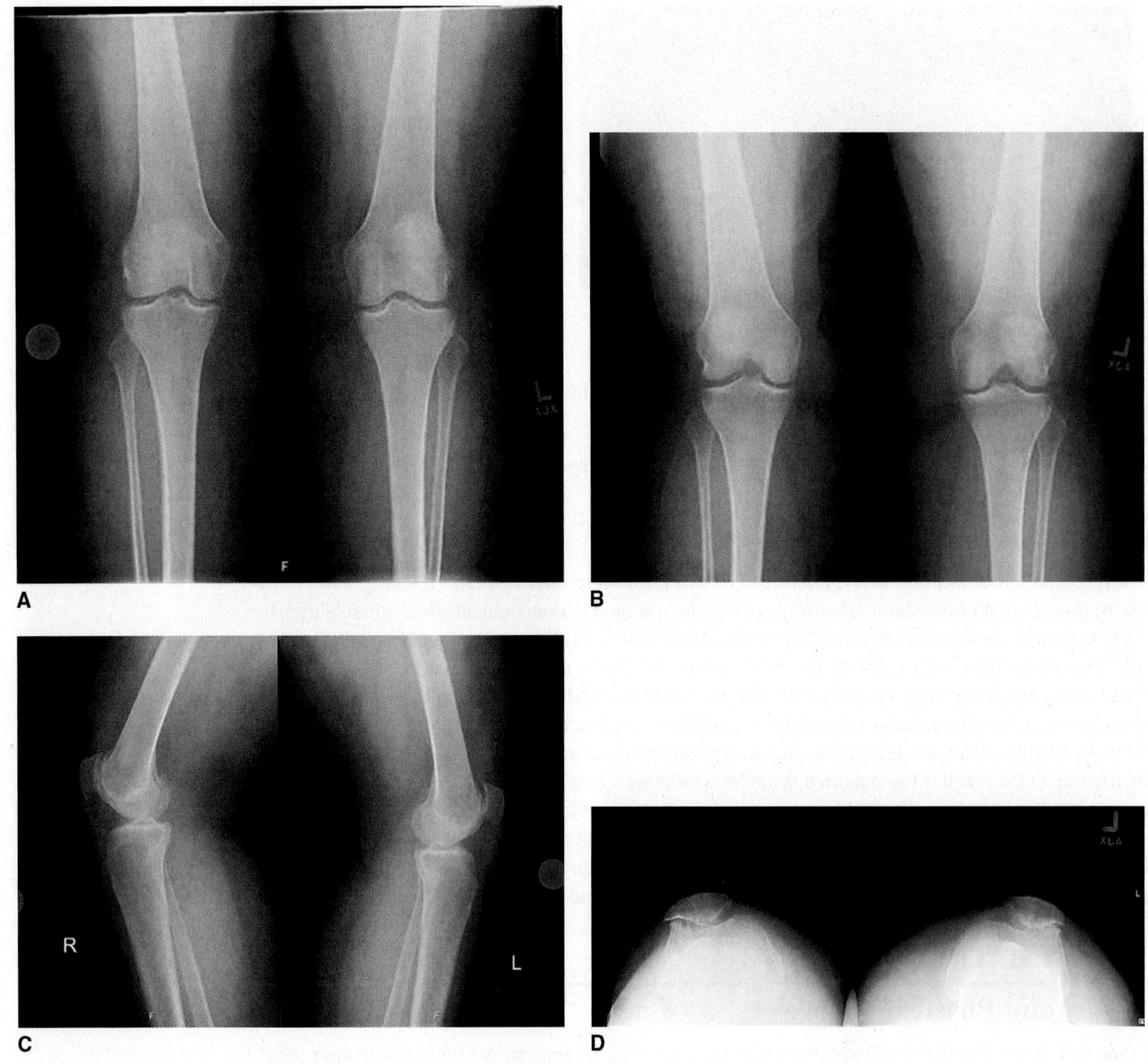

FIGURE 6-2

A: Preoperative standing AP, (**B**) midflexion posteroanterior (PA), (**C**) lateral, and (**D**) merchant view x-rays of bilateral knees show isolated patellofemoral arthritis.

radiographic evidence for concern, have a low threshold to perform a magnetic resonance imaging (MRI) of their knee to better evaluate the tibiofemoral joint. One benefit of preoperatively assessing the chondral surfaces of the femur and tibia with an MRI is avoiding this unnecessary step intraoperatively and therefore affording the ability to perform the PFA through a smaller, more cosmetic incision.

SURGICAL TECHNIQUE

Compared to first-generation PFAs, newer designs have features that optimize patellar tracking, which has solved some of the earlier problems. Most notably, there is a longer proximal trochlear component, which prevents the patella from traveling from the native femur and jumping onto the trochlear component. Currently, there are two styles of PFA: inlay and onlay. We prefer to use an onlay-style PFA as it allows the surgeon to change the rotation of the femoral component to some degree, which can be very helpful in cases of PF OA due to instability. As opposed to the onlay prosthesis, which is implanted flush to the anterior femoral cortex, the inlay-style component is inset into the anterior trochlear surface. Though the inlay design resects less bone, it does not allow for any change in rotation of the trochlear component. This prevents it from being able to accommodate all trochlear morphologies

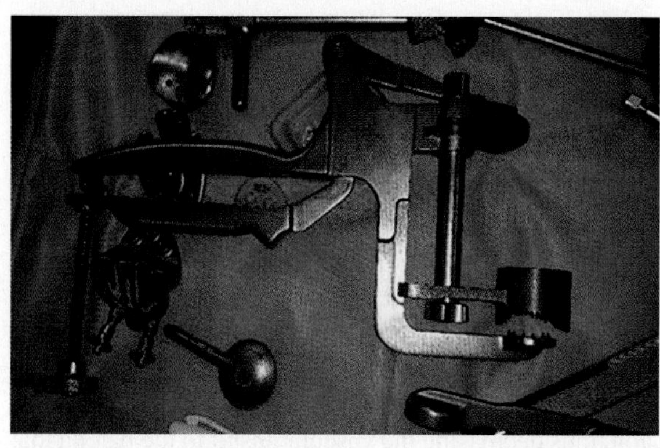

FIGURE 6-3
Various instruments used for PFA.

and has a higher tendency for patellar maltracking (7). In cases of severe trochlear dysplasia, both onlay and inlay components allow for creation of a trochlear groove when the native femur lacks a groove.

A short-acting spinal block with light sedation is our preferred anesthetic approach as this yields successful pain management, which can help with immediate weight bearing postoperatively. After induction of anesthesia, the patient is positioned in the supine position, with a small bump placed securely at the end of the table to allow the foot to be placed stably with the knee at 45 degrees of flexion, and a lateral post is used to prevent rotation and abduction. If the knee is flexed past 45 degrees, the proximal portion of the trochlea cannot be seen through a minimally invasive incision. A well-padded nonsterile tourniquet is placed about the proximal thigh.

Prior to starting the procedure, ensure that all necessary instruments are available and ready (Fig. 6-3). The lower extremity is prepped and draped in the usual sterile fashion, and the planned midline incision is marked out before covering the operative site with impermeable adherent wrap. We favor giving tranexamic acid 1 g intravenously 5 minutes prior to elevating the tourniquet to help reduce blood loss. This same dose is also sufficient for bilateral PFAs. Alternatively, 3 g of tranexamic acid can be diluted in 350 mL of saline and placed directly into the joint at the end of the procedure for 5 minutes after the wound has been thoroughly irrigated. If this method is elected, the tourniquet is not released until the tranexamic acid has sat for the full 5 minutes. Following the tranexamic acid, no further deep irrigation is performed.

After exsanguinating the limb either with gravity or an Esmarch elastic, the tourniquet is elevated to 250 mm Hg. A standard midline incision (Fig. 6-4) is used spanning one to two finger-breadths above and below the patella, depending on the patient's body habitus. To be able to perform a PFA through a minimally invasive incision, you must release the soft tissue deep to the incision such that you are able to move

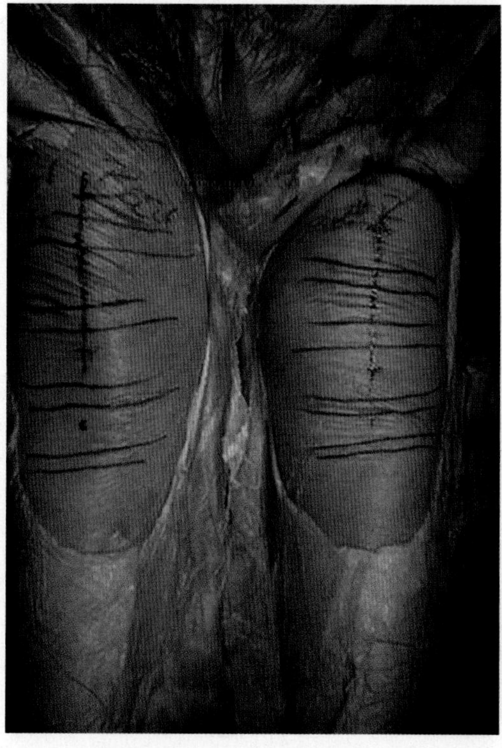

FIGURE 6-4
Draping and skin markings for bilateral PFAs.

the incision over the areas where you need to work. Initially, we used a midvastus approach, but found that it obscured our visualization and often required lengthening the incision in order to adequately see the lateral margin of the trochlea. Visualizing this area is critical to ensure the trochlear component is flush and not overhanging the underlying bone. We now perform a standard medial parapatellar arthrotomy, which affords better exposure, and we have not seen a change in quadriceps recovery during rehabilitation postoperatively. During the arthrotomy, it is important to protect the menisci and intermeniscal ligament. Partial resection or release of the infrapatellar fat pad at this point can facilitate exposure and aid with patellar eversion. If a partial resection of the fat pad is required to allow visualization, take care to protect the patellar tendon. Preoperatively, if the patella was not able to be everted to neutral, or in cases of severe lateral maltracking, we have used a lateral parapatellar arthrotomy instead of a medial one. We have done a lateral lengthening (step cutting the retinaculum separately from the capsule) in order to close the lateral side at the end of the case without tension, thus decreasing the vascular insult to the patella that would be required from a medial arthrotomy and lateral release (Fig. 6-5).

Patellar Preparation

- Kocher clamps placed on the quadriceps and patellar tendons and a sweetheart clamped to the intra-articular surface of the lateral retinaculum aid in patellar eversion (Fig. 6-6).

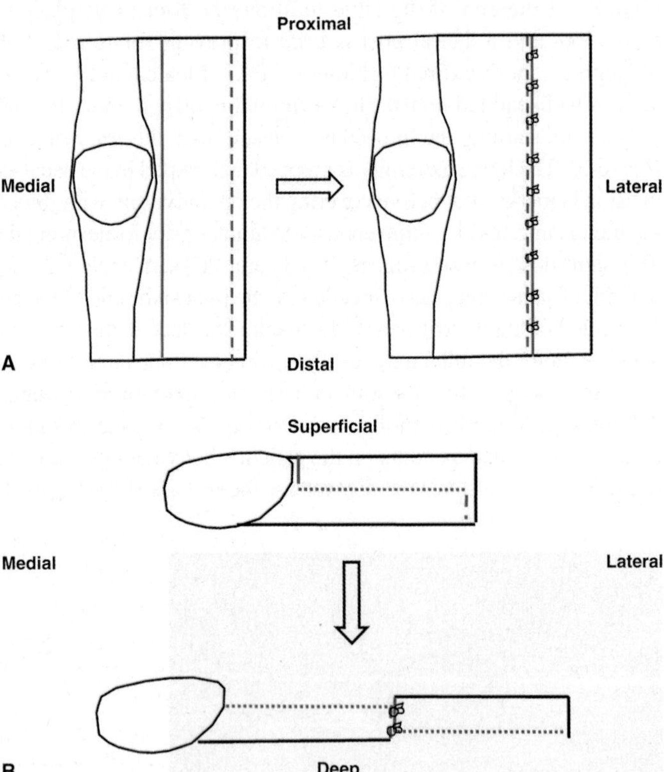

FIGURE 6-5

Lateral retinacular step-cut lengthening. (**A**) A coronal view and (**B**) an axial view. The superficial oblique fibers of lateral retinaculum are incised (*solid line*) and elevated from the deeper transverse fibers (*dotted line*). The superficial fibers are reflected and the deeper transverse fibers are then cut (*dashed line*) approximately 1.5 cm posterior to the patella. These two layers are then reapproximated, allowing for approximately 1.5 cm of lengthening of the lateral side and closure without any tension.

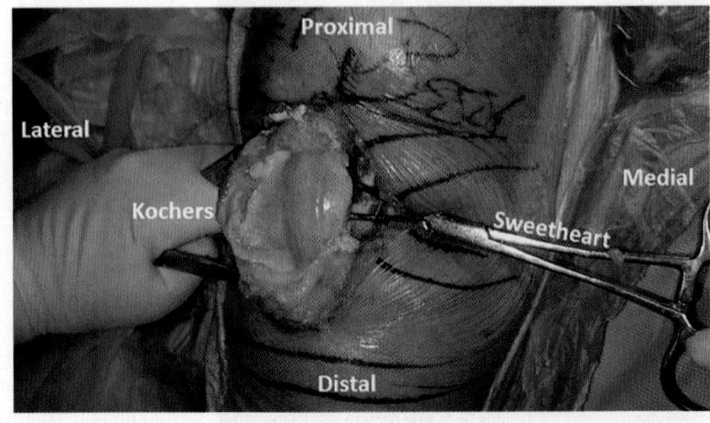

FIGURE 6-6

Patella eversion is aided with Kocher clamps placed on the patella and quadriceps tendons and a sweetheart clamp on the articular side of the lateral retinaculum.

- Measure patellar thickness with a caliper. Typically, the remaining patellar bone should be 12 to 15 mm thick depending on its original dimension. The goal is to restore normal patellar thickness as opposed to native thickness, as these patients often have significant bone loss prior to surgery from maltracking.
- Patella-reaming guide is clamped on, placed medially to aid in tracking of the patellar component (Fig. 6-7A).
- The reamer has automatic stops at 16, 14, and 12 mm (Fig. 6-7B). We prefer to use a reaming guide over freehand patellar resection, especially in patients with eccentric patellar wear and sclerotic bone as it allows more even bone resection.
- Remove the prominent bone surrounding the reamed patella (Fig. 6-8). This is especially important on the lateral side where the lateral patellar facet and prominent osteophytes will not be covered by the patellar component and can cause impingement if left behind.
- Place the patellar sizing/drill guide on the medial aspect of the patella (Fig. 6-9), ensuring that it does not overhang beyond the margins of the bone, and drill the three lug holes.
- Trial patella component is placed. The goal should be to restore "normal" patellar thickness, 1 to 2 mm thicker than the patient's starting patella thickness if there was bone loss present.
- A sagittal saw is used to bevel the lateral edge and remove osteophytes to prevent bony impingement.

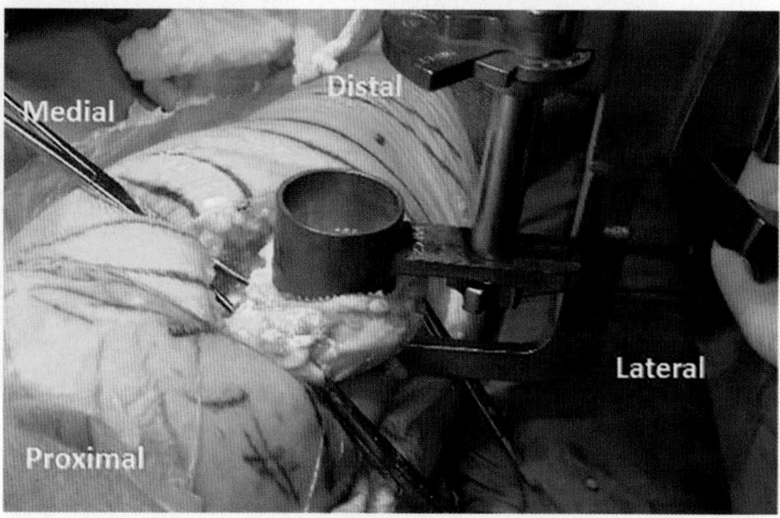

A

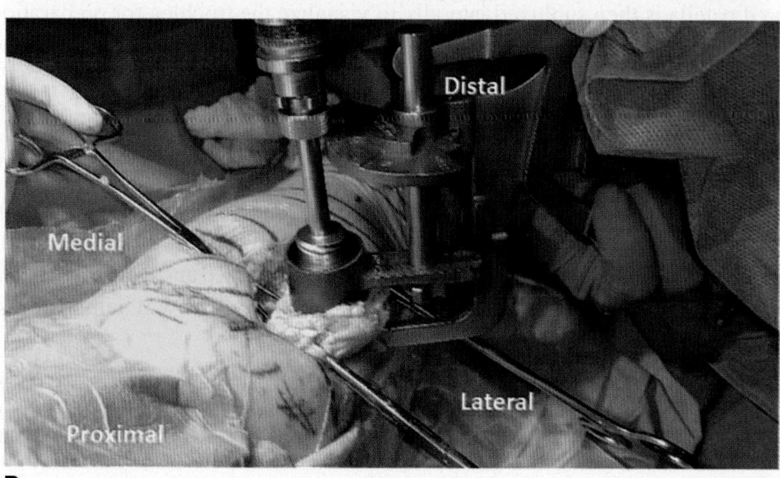

B

FIGURE 6-7

A: The patella reaming guide is clamped onto the patella, and the patella is (**B**) reamed until the stop collar on the reamer.

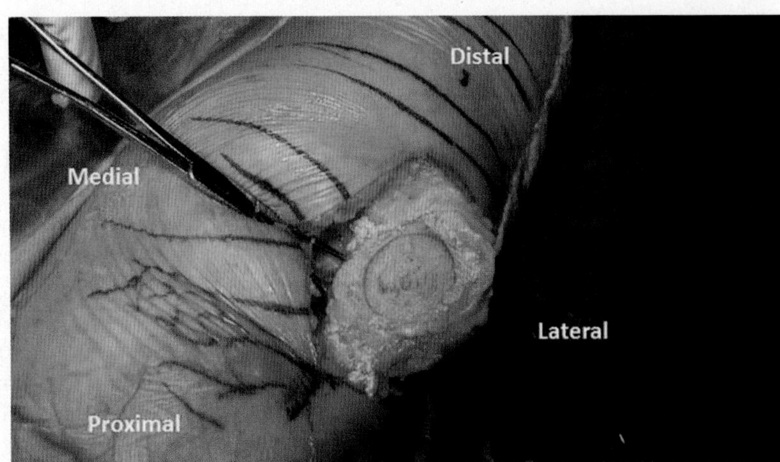

FIGURE 6-8

The patella appearance after reaming. The prominent bone surrounding the reamed area is removed with a rongeur.

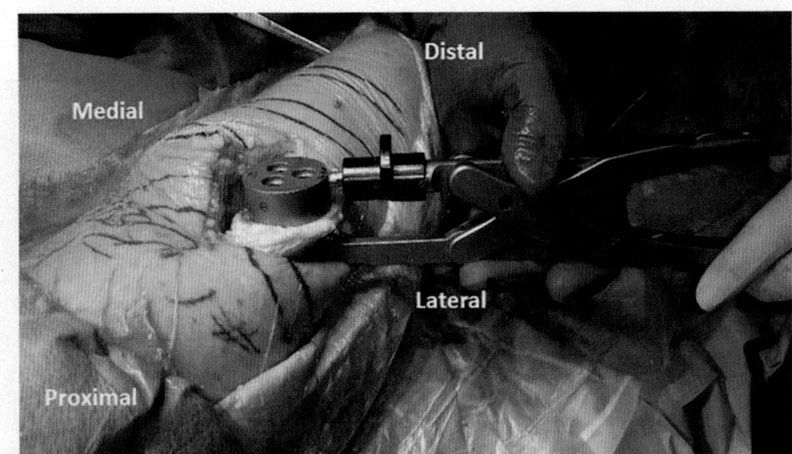

FIGURE 6-9

The patella sizing/drill guide is applied to the medial edge of the patella, and three lug holes are drilled.

- The prepared patella is then subluxed laterally to visualize the trochlea for preparation.
- *Tip*: Placing two retractors, one above and one below the patella, will help reduce the chance of bony damage to the prepared patella.

Mark Femoral Landmarks

- A Paulson retractor placed medially and laterally and an army-navy retractor proximally gives excellent exposure of the trochlea for preparation (Fig. 6-10).
- Use electrocautery to demarcate the proximal extent of the trochlea and excise an area of synovium so that you are able to palpate the anterior cortex of the femur. This will help to adjust the height of the guide to avoid notching the femur.
- Mark the anteroposterior (AP) axis, Whiteside line, from the lowest part of the trochlea to the highest part of the intercondylar notch. Mark two lines parallel to Whiteside's, one medially and one laterally, as Whiteside line will be obscured by the intramedullary cutting guide (Fig. 6-11).

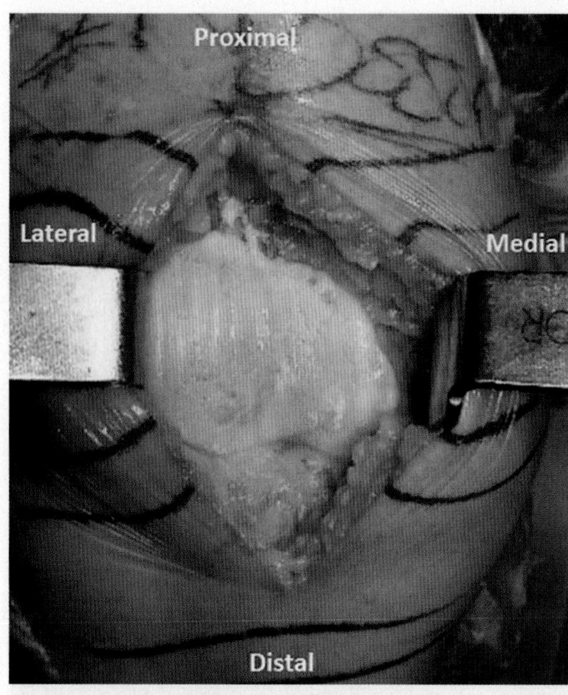

FIGURE 6-10

Advanced trochlear degeneration is noted, particularly laterally.

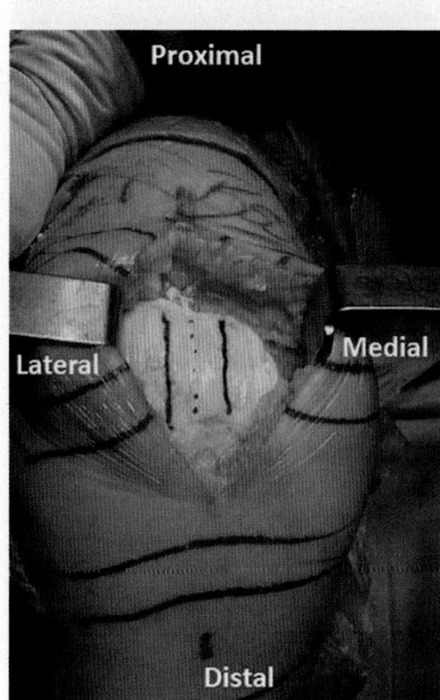

FIGURE 6-11

The AP axis of the femur (Whiteside line = *dashed line*) has been drawn from the lowest point of the trochlear sulcus to the roof of the intercondylar notch. This line will be obscured by the cutting guide so two parallel lines (*solid lines*) are drawn for later reference.

Femoral Anterior Cut

- Ream the femoral canal with the 6-mm intramedullary drill (Fig. 6-12). This should be 1 to 2 mm above the notch so that the trochlear component does not impinge on the notch.
- Insert the intramedullary anterior cutting guide with the attached telescoping boom (Fig. 6-13). This can be done by hand or with the insertion handle attached. The guide should be inserted until the proximal aspect of the guide just contacts the distal femoral sulcus.

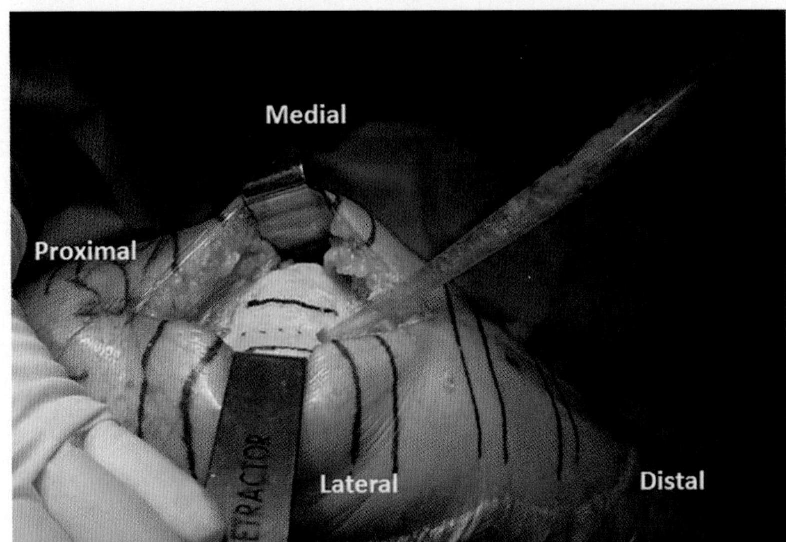

FIGURE 6-12

An entry hole for the intramedullary anterior trochlear cutting guide is drilled in the center of the trochlear groove, 1 to 2 cm above the roof of the intercondylar notch.

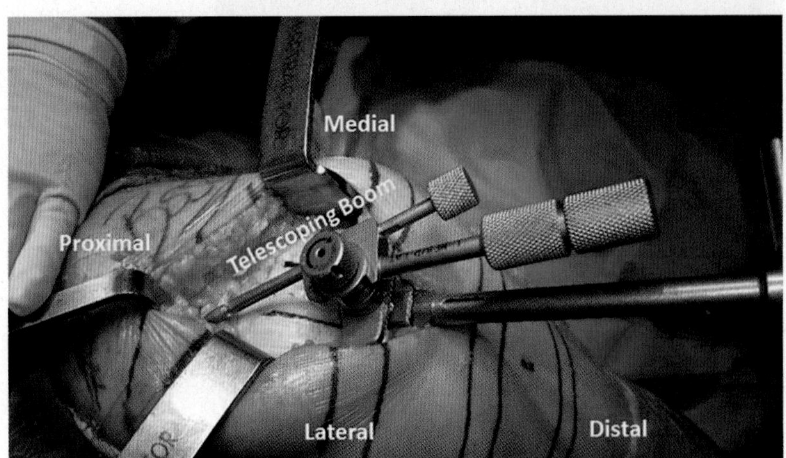

FIGURE 6-13

The intramedullary anterior cutting guide with the attached telescoping boom.

- Externally rotate the guide until the lines on the guide are parallel to the two lines parallel to Whiteside line (Fig. 6-14A,B). If there is significant trochlear dysplasia, using the transepicondylar axis will be more reliable, particularly if the sulcus of the trochlear groove is indeterminable. A slightly more extensile incision may be necessary to identify the medial and lateral epicondyles. Rotate the guide until the vertical lines on the guide are perpendicular to the marked transepicondylar axis. This is the point where adjustments can be made to increase external rotation of the trochlear component to aid in tracking, which can be very helpful especially in patients with a history of significant instability or severe trochlea dysplasia.
- *Tip*: Extending the knee slightly at this point will aid visualization of the anterior femur.
- With the rotation set, move the telescoping boom tip onto the anterior lateral femoral cortex. This is the planned resection level. Adjust the AP height of the cutting guide by turning the adjustment knob until the boom tip just contacts the cortex. By lining the boom tip up with the anterior cortex, it will help avoid notching. The goal is to create a cut flush with the anterior cortex.
- *Tip*: The height of the anterior cut can be checked at this stage with the angel-wing resection guide.
- Secure the cutting guide in place and remove the telescoping boom.
- Make the anterior femoral cut with an oscillating saw and then remove the anterior cutting guide.
- *Tip*: After resection, the anterior femur should look like a baby grand piano (8) (Fig. 6-15).

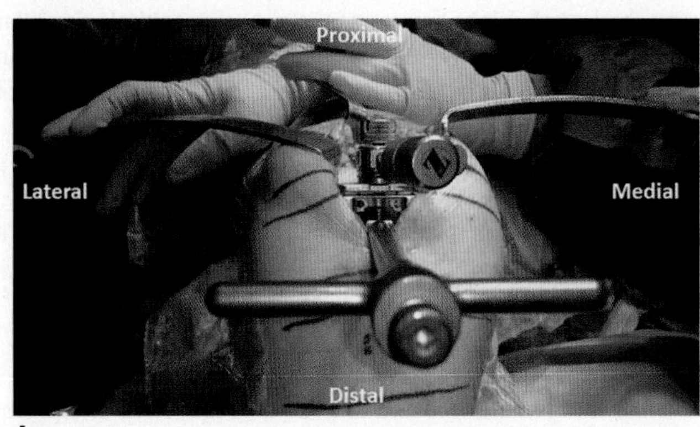

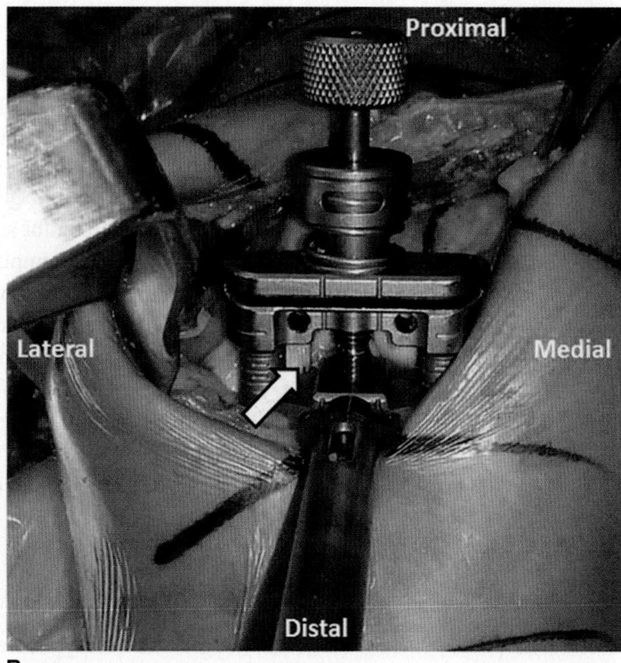

A B

FIGURE 6-14

A: The anterior cutting guide is externally rotated until (**B**) the lines on the guide are parallel to the two lines visible (*arrow*), which were drawn parallel to Whiteside line. This will ensure that the cutting slot is perpendicular to the AP axis of the femur and thus appropriate external rotation of the trochlear component.

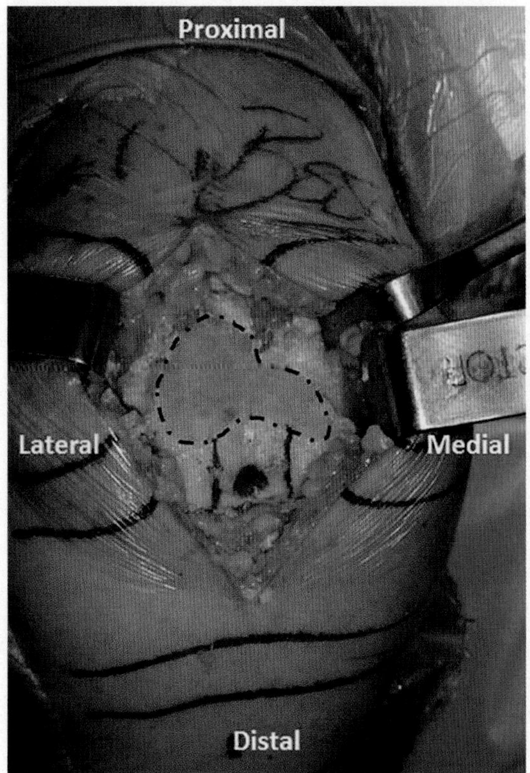

FIGURE 6-15

The prepared anterior cortex of the femur after the sagittal saw is used to resect the anterior trochlear surface. Note the appearance of a baby grand piano (*dashed lines*).

Trochlear Sizing

- Choose the appropriate size and side milling guide. Ensure that the feet are in the middle "set" position. Depress and hold the spring-loaded button to change the position of the feet. If the feet are in the "up" or "down" position, you will over- or under-resect, respectively.
- *Tip*: When the feet are in the appropriate position, the gold bar in the middle will not be visible.
- Place the sizing/milling guide and secure in place. Ensure that the anterior flange is sitting flush to the anterior cortex of the femur and both feet are in contact with the femoral condyles (Fig. 6-16A).
- Medial lateral widths of the implants are in 4- to 5-mm increments. Ideally, the implant maximally covers the trochlea without overhang on the lateral side to minimize the risk of capsular/retinacular irritation. Ensure acceptable proximal coverage as well as intercondylar notch clearance. You can estimate the notch clearance by inserting the angel-wing resection guide into the tail verification slot of the milling guide.
- Secure the milling guide by placing the pins into the anterior flange of the guide in the following order: central, lateral, medial.
- Patients with extremely soft bone may require additional stabilization of the milling guide with a tamp held on the guide.

Trochlear Preparation

- Ensure that the burr is fully seated in the milling handpiece and that the burr is locked into place. When the burr is fully secure, the red dots will be aligned.
- Hold the milling handpiece on the lower half, close to the tip, similar to holding a pencil (Fig. 6-16B).
- Place the burr guard into the track before initiating power.
- Positioning of the burr is crucial to this step. It must be perpendicular to the guide or it will get caught.
- *Tip*: Always run the burr at full throttle. If it catches or stalls at any point, keep it at full throttle but move through the track more slowly and check to ensure it is perpendicular to the guide.
- The tracks should be burred in the following order: central, lateral, medial.
- Before milling the lateral track, depress and hold the spring-loaded button on the lateral foot to raise it to the "mill" position. The gold band will now be visible above the guide. This allows the milling burr to pass under the raised foot.

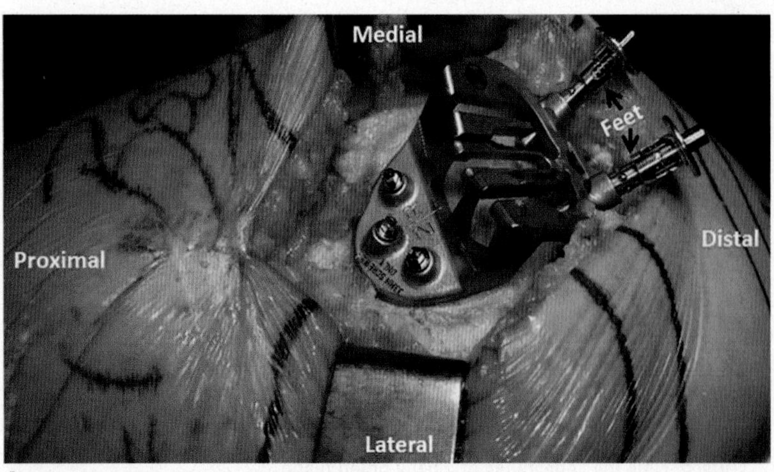

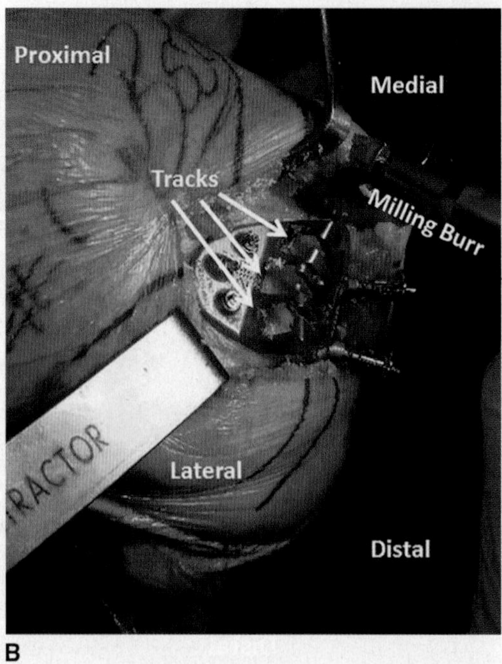

FIGURE 6-16

A: The sizing/milling guide is pinned in place. A view from above that the anterior flange and both feet are in contact with the femur. **B:** The milling burr should be held like a pencil and is placed into the track before initiating power, and the tracks are milled: central, lateral, then medial.

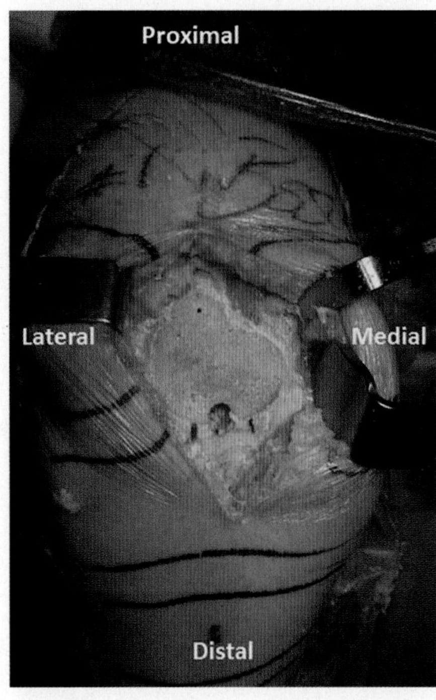

FIGURE 6-17
Trochlear bone preparation has been completed.

- After milling the complete lateral track, push the lateral foot into its down "stabilized" position. The gold band will now be visible below the guide. This will ensure stability of the guide when milling the medial track.
- Repeat these steps for the medial track.
- After all tracks of the distal bone preparation are milled, remove the screws and milling guide and irrigate to remove all bone and cartilage debris (Fig. 6-17).
- A small area of bone will remain distally but will be removed during tail preparation. Do not remove freehand.

Peg and Tail Holes

- Select the appropriate size and side peg/tail guide. This guide matches the outside geometry and thickness of the trochlear implant. This will be the same size as the milling guide.
- Make sure the guide is fully seated against the distal surface of the prepared trochlea, flush to femoral condyles, and secure with three screws.
- Drill the anterior, medial, and lateral peg holes (Fig. 6-18A). Drill the full depth until the shoulder of the drill stops against the boss for each drill hole.
- Drill the tail slot. Once the upper shoulder on the drill reaches the boss on the guide, continue drilling while sliding it side to side. The drill's shoulder must remain flush with the boss during this side to side drilling.
- *Tip*: Using the handle/loop of a Kocher can aid the side-cutting action of the drill especially in patients with hard bone (Fig. 6-18B).

Trial and Final Prosthesis

- Insert the trial trochlear prosthesis onto the femur (Fig. 6-19), taking care to properly align the pegs and tail with the holes. The pegs should engage into the holes at the same time.
- Use the impactor until the trial is fully seated. The impaction force should be delivered in the direction of the pegs' axis.
- The component edges must be flush with the adjacent articular cartilage, most importantly on the lateral side.
- Be careful to avoid damaging cartilage at the transition area during impaction.
- Place the appropriately sized patellar trial component.
- Evaluate patellar tracking throughout a range of motion. The patella should transition smoothly throughout, particularly at the transition from the trochlear component to the femoral condyles in

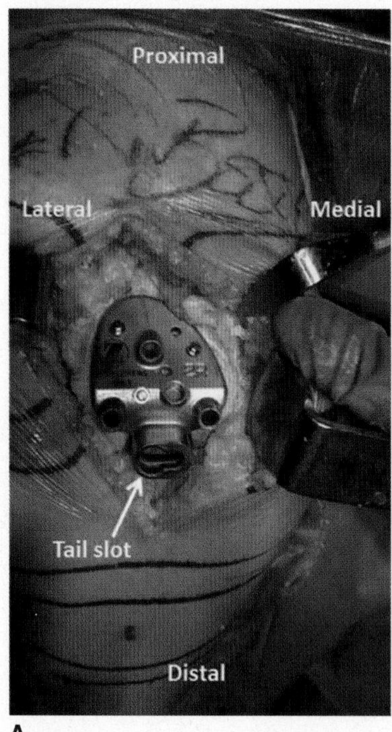

A

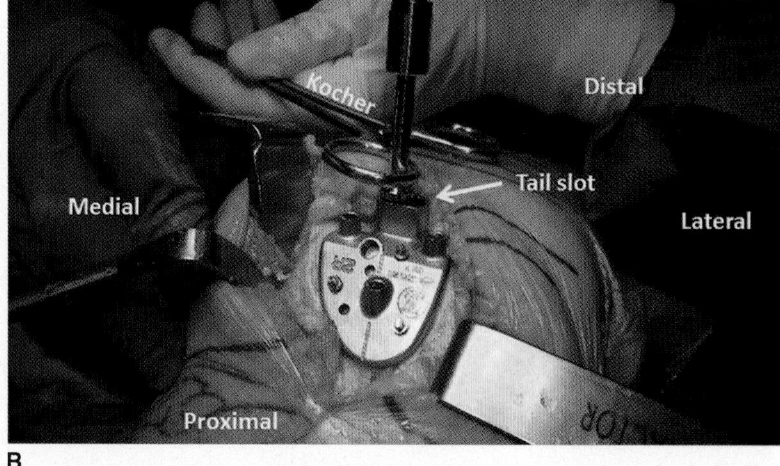

B

FIGURE 6-18

A: The correct size and side trochlear drill guide is pinned in place on the prepared trochlear surface, and the trochlear lug holes are drilled. **B:** When drilling the tail slot, using the back end of a Kocher can aid the side-cutting action of the drill.

flexion and onto the anterior femoral cortex in extension. Assess for tilt, subluxation, and catching. This is the time to check the tracking and adjust soft tissue balance.

- Remove the trial prostheses. Do not rock the trochlear trial back and forth during removal as this could compromise the bone preparation, peg hole preparation, surrounding cartilage, and the implant's fit. Copiously wash all bony surfaces with pulse lavage.

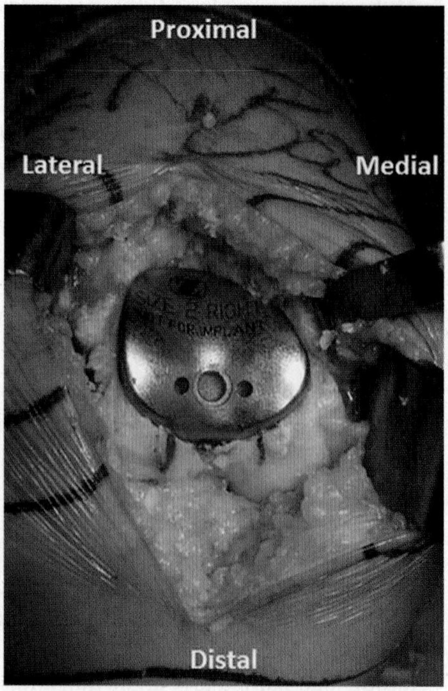

FIGURE 6-19

The trial trochlear component is in place. It is imperative at this stage to ensure that the edges are flush with the surrounding articular cartilage or recessed 1 mm and that there is no overhang, especially laterally on the anterior surface, which could lead to synovial irritation.

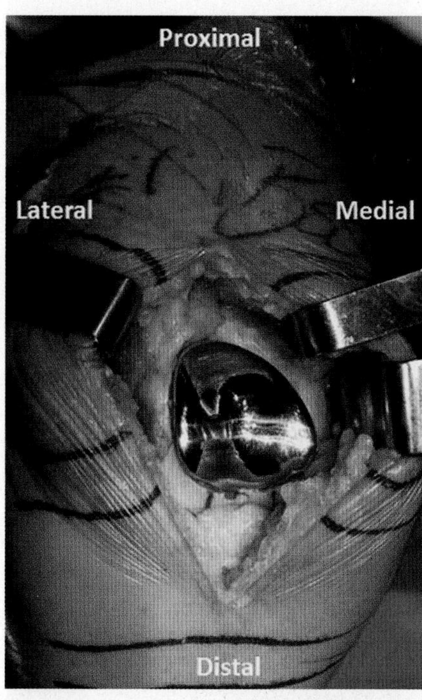

FIGURE 6-20

Intraoperative photograph of the trochlear component after cementation shows appropriate positioning.

- Apply bone cement to the undersurface of the trochlear component in the cement pockets and to the anterior surface of the femur. Mark the location of the peg holes on the femur by pushing cement down into the holes to aid in positioning the implant during peg insertion.
- Implant the trochlear component in place (Fig. 6-20), taking care to properly align the pegs and tail. Impact until it is fully seated, again ensuring that the force is in the same direction as the pegs' axis. Carefully remove excess cement and apply pressure to the component until the cement is cured.
- The patellar component is cemented in place and held in place with the compression clamp at maximum pressure (Fig. 6-21).
- Ensure the surgical site is clear of all bone and cement debris as foreign particles at the articular surface may cause inflammation and mechanical symptoms.
- Release the tourniquet (unless tranexamic acid is placed in the wound at this stage) and use electrocautery to achieve hemostasis.
- Copiously irrigate the wound (prior to placing tranexamic acid if used at this stage).

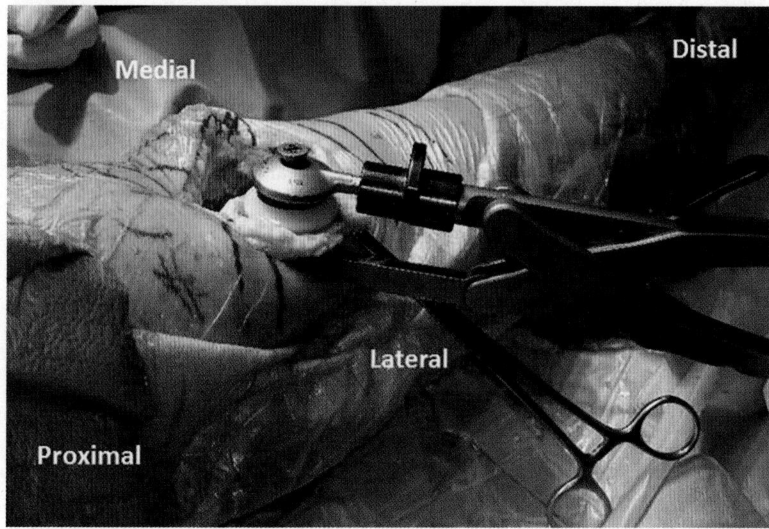

FIGURE 6-21

The patella component is clamped in place until the cement has cured.

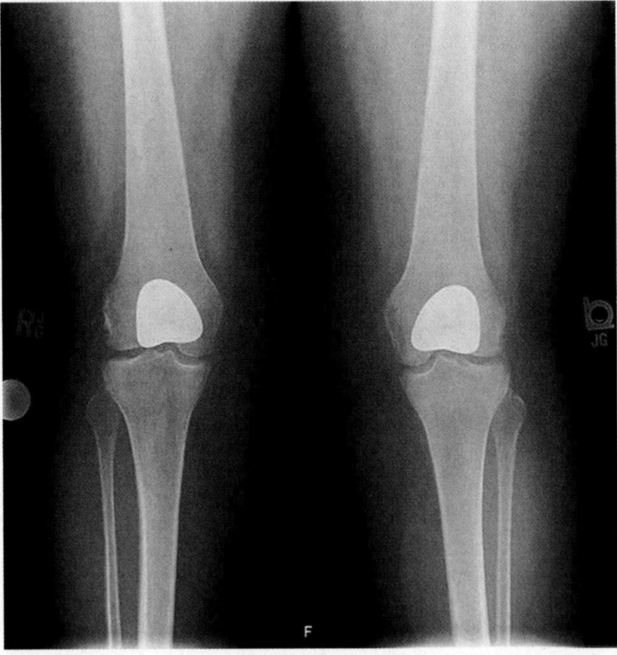
A

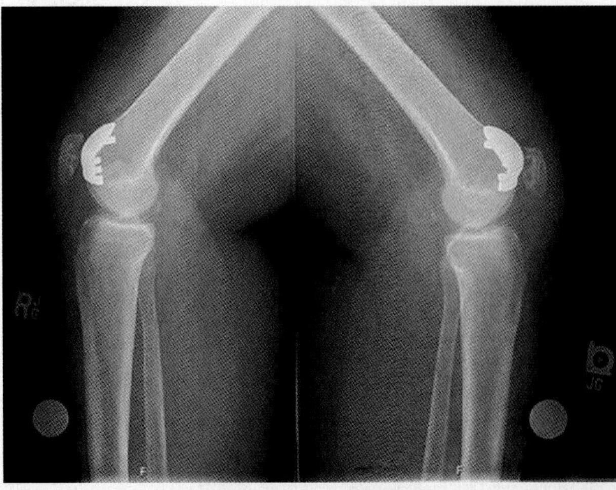
B

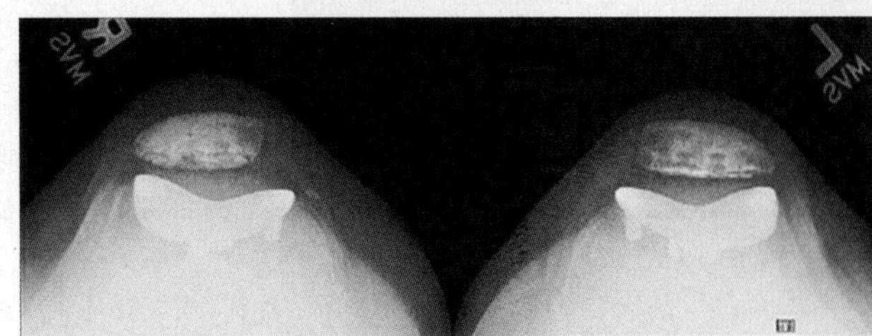
C

FIGURE 6-22

A: AP, (**B**) lateral, and (**C**) merchant postoperative standing x-rays showing a successful PFA.

- Close the arthrotomy in 30 to 40 degrees of flexion and the remainder of the wound in layers
- Postoperative radiographs confirm implant position and alignment (Fig. 6-22).

PEARLS AND PITFALLS

- An onlay design is very helpful in the setting of trochlear dysplasia or a history of patellar instability
- Slight lateral patellar tilt can usually be addressed effectively with a lateral retinacular release, medialization of the patellar component, and resection of the far lateral aspect of the lateral patellar facet.
- If a lateral release is needed, it is prudent to look for the vessels laterally and preserve them to prevent patellar avascular necrosis (AVN).
- The epicondylar axis is more important in patients with trochlear dysplasia because Whiteside line will not be as accurate.
- The goal is to restore normal patellar thickness. Patients requiring PFA secondary to maltracking and OA can have significant patellar bone loss so the end thickness of the patella + component will be greater than what they start with.
- Overstuffing is not usually an issue in PFAs. Reestablishing normal patellar height can help to restore the vector force on the quadriceps and improve the ability of the quadriceps to function
- Beveling the lateral facet of the patella beyond the edge of the patellar component is especially important in patients who were lateral overloaders preoperatively and are therefore at greatest risk for bony impingement on the lateral side.
- Ensure the anterior cutting guide is appropriately externally rotated before the anterior rough cut is made.
- The order the pins should be placed in the milling guide is the same as the order in which the tracks should be milled: central, lateral, medial. This order is also alphabetical.

POSTOPERATIVE MANAGEMENT

Immediate weight bearing and range of motion are encouraged. A continuous passive motion (CPM) machine may be used to aid in early range of motion at the surgeon's discretion though we have found this unnecessary as these patients are quick to regain their motion and that stiffness after PFA is not a significant problem. Prophylactic antibiotics are given for 24 hours and for patients without risk factors for DVT; aspirin is given for thromboembolic prophylaxis for 2 weeks. Isometric exercises isolating the quadriceps are started immediately. Assistive devices can be discontinued once quadriceps strength has recovered. In our experience, PFA patients achieve full range of motion earlier than TKA patients, but they take an equal amount of time before they are able to reciprocate stairs. Appropriate antibiotic prophylaxis for dental procedures is advised. Patients are allowed unrestricted activities with the recommendation to avoid excessive loading in deep flexion and high-impact activities.

COMPLICATIONS

Contemporary PFA designs have substantially reduced the tendency for patellar maltracking. A small percentage of patients will have mild anterior knee pain. Pain, snapping, and patellar subluxation can generally be avoided with careful attention to patient selection and surgical technique along with proper implant selection. There are no reported data on patellar AVN; however, this is a theoretical risk when combining a medial parapatellar arthrotomy and a lateral retinacular release, as may be necessary in patients with persistent lateral patellar subluxation during PFA. Late failures from component subsidence, polyethylene wear, or loosening occur in less than 1% of published cases combined (3). As with any arthroplasty procedure, infection and thromboembolism are potential complications that should be addressed with appropriate prophylaxis.

RESULTS

PFA can produce consistently good-quality functional results in the appropriately selected patient. Numerous patient factors influence functional prognosis including patient age, comorbidities, athletic status, mental health, pain, functional limitations, excessive caution and "artificial joint"–related worries, and rehabilitation protocol (9).

Beyond 10 to 15 years, tibiofemoral arthritis may be the primary failure mechanism after PFA (3). Still, a recent meta-analysis comparing modern second-generation PFA to standard TKA for patellofemoral arthritis showed that there was no significant difference in reoperation, revision, pain, or mechanical complications, even in older patient groups (10).

REFERENCES

1. Davies AP, Vince AS, Shepstone L, et al. The radiologic prevalence of patellofemoral osteoarthritis. *Clin Orthop Relat Res.* 2002(402):206–212. PMID:12218486.
2. McAlindon TE, Snow S, Cooper C, et al. Radiographic patterns of osteoarthritis of the knee joint in the community: the importance of the patellofemoral joint. *Ann Rheum Dis.* 1992;51(7):844–849. PMID:1632657.
3. Lonner JH, Bloomfield MR. The clinical outcome of patellofemoral arthroplasty. *Orthop Clin North Am.* 2013;44(3):271–280, vii. PMID:23827831.
4. Federico DJ, Reider B. Results of isolated patellar debridement for patellofemoral pain in patients with normal patellar alignment. *Am J Sports Med.* 1997;25(5):663–669. PMID:9302473.
5. Dinham JM, French PR. Results of patellectomy for osteoarthritis. *Postgrad Med J.* 1972;48(564):590–593. PMID:5079175.
6. Lonner JH. Patellofemoral arthroplasty. *J Am Acad Orthop Surg.* 2007;15(8):495–506. PMID:17664369.
7. Lonner JH. Patellofemoral arthroplasty: the impact of design on outcomes. *Orthop Clin North Am.* 2008;39(3):347–354, vi. PMID:18602563.
8. Moyad TF, Hughes RE, Urquhart A. "Grand piano sign," a marker for proper femoral component rotation during total knee arthroplasty. *Am J Orthop (Belle Mead NJ).* 2011;40(7):348–352. PMID:22013571.
9. Papalia R, Del Buono A, Zampogna B, et al. Sport activity following joint arthroplasty: a systematic review. *Br Med Bull.* 2012;101:81–103. PMID:21565802.
10. Dy CJ, Franco N, Ma Y, et al. Complications after patello-femoral versus total knee replacement in the treatment of isolated patello-femoral osteoarthritis. A meta-analysis. *Knee Surg Sports Traumatol Arthrosc.* 2012;20(11):2174–2190. PMID:21987361.

PART II
MENISCUS SURGERY

7 Meniscectomy

Matthew J. Matava and Simon Görtz

INDICATIONS

Meniscal tears are among the most common clinical conditions experienced by active patients. The incidence of isolated meniscal tears resulting in meniscectomy is 61 per 100,00 patients with a male-to-female ratio of 3:1 (1). The majority of all tears involve the medial meniscus. Meniscal tears are classified by their gross appearance (Fig. 7-1), anatomic location within the meniscus (e.g., posterior horn, midbody, or anterior horn), and blood supply. Only the peripheral 10% to 20% of the meniscus is vascularized (Fig. 7-2). Tears located in the meniscal periphery are described as "red-red" tears where there are (at least, theoretically) blood vessels present on both sides of the tear. "Red-white" tears are located at the junction of the vascularized and nonvascularized regions. "White-white" tears are located within the inner one-third of the meniscus where there is an absence of blood vessels. Intraoperatively, it is often difficult to know the vascular status of a meniscal tear when assessing its reparability. Only 20% of all meniscal tears are considered reparable; therefore, the majority of meniscal tears encountered will require excision. These are located in the avascular region and/or have significant traumatic damage that make repair either biologically not feasible or technically impossible. Patient age often predicts the chance of reparability in that older patients (over 40 years of age) typically have nonreparable tears requiring excision. Some patients may have a reparable tear, yet refuse a repair due to the lengthy and restrictive rehabilitation associated with a meniscal repair.

Typical symptoms of meniscal injury include joint line pain in the involved compartment (medial or lateral), a variable effusion that develops within 24 hours, mechanical symptoms (locking, catching, and/or giving-way), and increasing pain with deep knee flexion. The patient's physical examination should correlate with the location of the tear with point tenderness over the involved joint line, pain with hyperflexion of the knee, and a painful palpable "click" with flexion and rotation (McMurray test). The Thessaly maneuver often leads to joint line–specific discomfort and a sense of catching with internal and external rotation of the knee while weight bearing with the knee at both 5 and 20 degrees of flexion (2).

Meniscal surgery is indicated in those patients who fail nonoperative treatment of relative rest, nonsteroidal anti-inflammatory medications, corticosteroid injection, and physical therapy. In addition, surgery is indicated in those patients with mechanical symptoms or whose activity level is significantly impaired by the tear.

CONTRAINDICATIONS

Contraindications to meniscectomy include those patients with minimal symptoms, those with pain that does not correlate with the tear location, or patients with significant degenerative changes in the involved compartment without mechanical symptoms. Patients with associated comorbidities whose medical condition precludes surgery are also not candidates for this procedure.

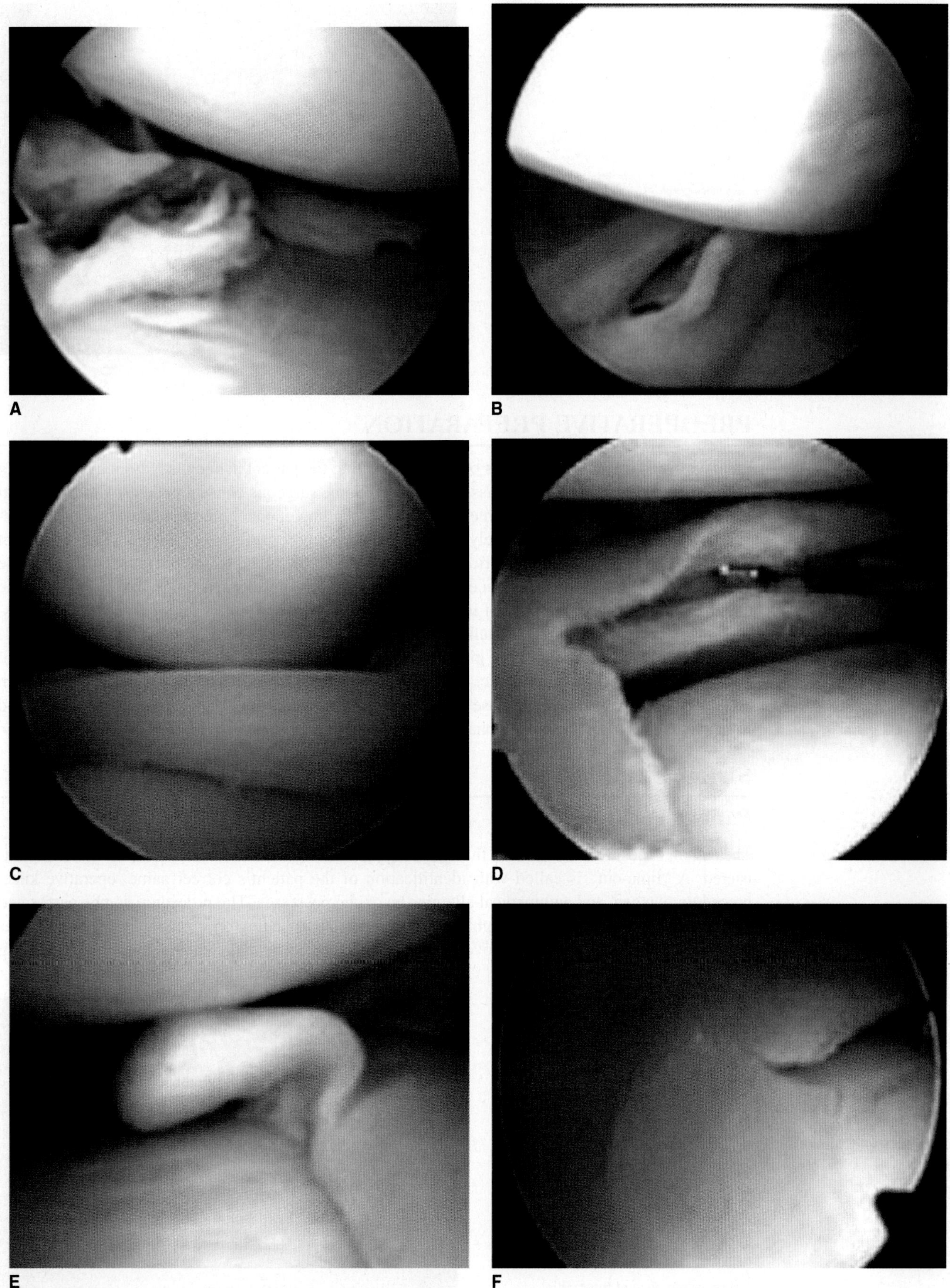

FIGURE 7-1

Types of meniscal tears based on tear configuration. **A:** Complex tear. **B:** Longitudinal tear. **C:** Bucket handle tear. **D:** Horizontal cleavage tear. **E:** Parrot beak tear. **F:** Radial tear.

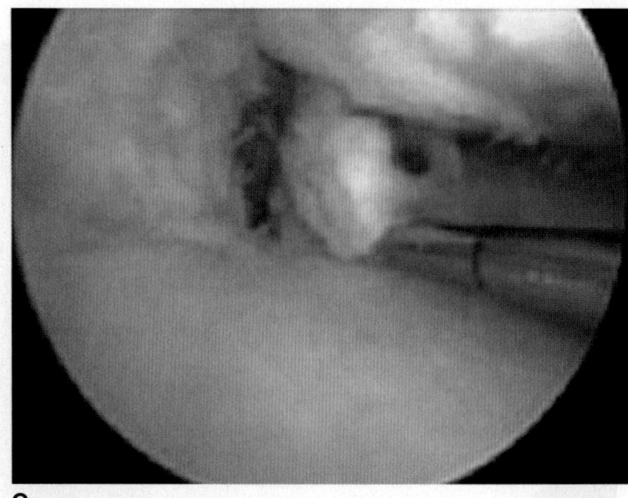

G

FIGURE 7-1 (*Continued*)
G: Root tear.

PREOPERATIVE PREPARATION

Preoperatively, informed consent is obtained indicating the patient acknowledges an understanding of the proposed procedure and its associated risks. Some surgeons consent patients with a meniscal tear for either a meniscal repair or meniscectomy depending upon the intraoperative findings as preoperative imaging is only moderately accurate at predicting reparability of the tear (3). The correct knee, as confirmed by the patient prior to sedation, should be signed by the operating surgeon in the preoperative holding area. The choice of general or regional anesthesia is left to the discretion of the anesthesiologist. The routine use of intravenous prophylactic antibiotics for an arthroscopic meniscectomy is debatable due to the small incisions needed and the absence of implantable hardware. If antibiotics are used, they should be given within 1 hour of the designated surgery time. One gram of a first-generation cephalosporin (i.e., cefazolin) is routinely given to patients who weigh less than 80 kg; 2 g is recommended for those over 80 kg. Clindamycin (600 to 900 mg) may be substituted if the patient has a penicillin or cephalosporin allergy (4).

SURGICAL SETUP

Patient Positioning

The patient is positioned supine on the operating table, and general anesthesia (if utilized) is administered. A "time-out" is called with identification of the patient's correct name, operative knee, procedure planned, and any medical allergies he or she possesses. The procedure can be performed with the foot of the bed either straight or bent 90 degrees depending on surgeon preference. I prefer to have the lower extremity flexed over the edge of the operating table with the thigh placed in a leg

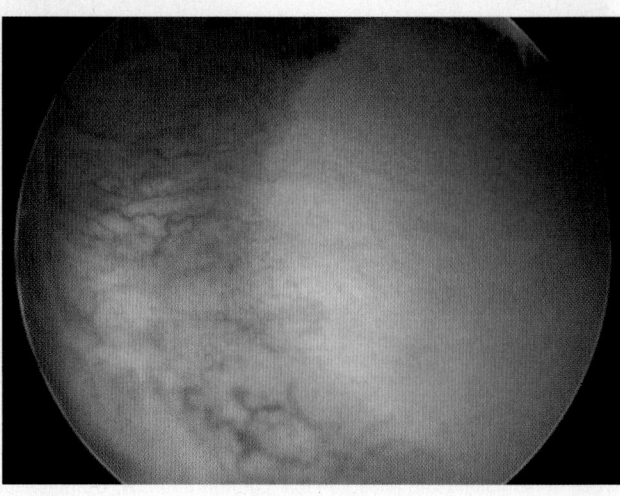

FIGURE 7-2
Arthroscopic view of the medial meniscus of the left knee showing its peripheral blood supply.

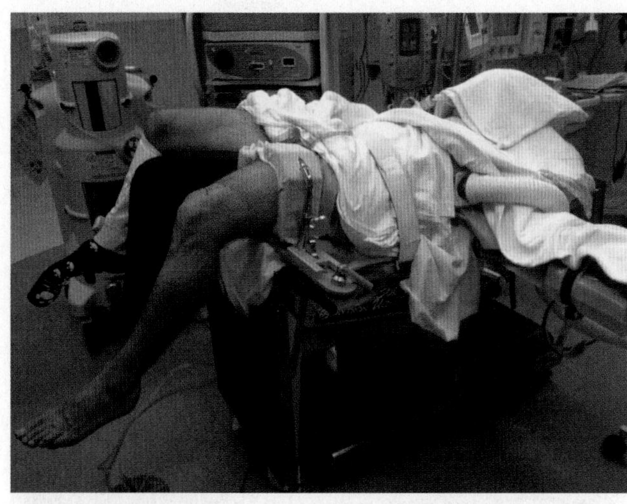

FIGURE 7-3

The patient is positioned with the operative knee (*left side*) suspended in a leg holder at the break of the operating table.

holder located at the edge of the table break (Fig. 7-3). A tourniquet is applied around the midthigh and may be inflated at the surgeon's discretion. The contralateral lower extremity is supported by a well-leg holder and/or blankets to flex the hip so as to reduce the tension on the femoral nerve and strain on the anterior hip capsule (Fig. 7-4). A TED hose and sequential compression device are placed on the well leg to reduce the risk of deep venous thrombosis. Placing the table in the Trendelenburg position elevates the operative knee to be optimally positioned at the level of the surgeon's umbilicus to facilitate arthroscopic manipulation.

Operating Room Setup

Once the patient is properly positioned with the skin prepped and the lower extremity draped, the video screen is positioned at the head of the table at the level of the patient's contralateral shoulder (Fig. 7-5). Most video screens can be freely moved to enhance viewing at the discretion of the surgeon. Some surgery centers independently suspend the viewing screen from the ceiling. Most arthroscopic towers possess control units for the fluid pump, shaver, and electrocautery either

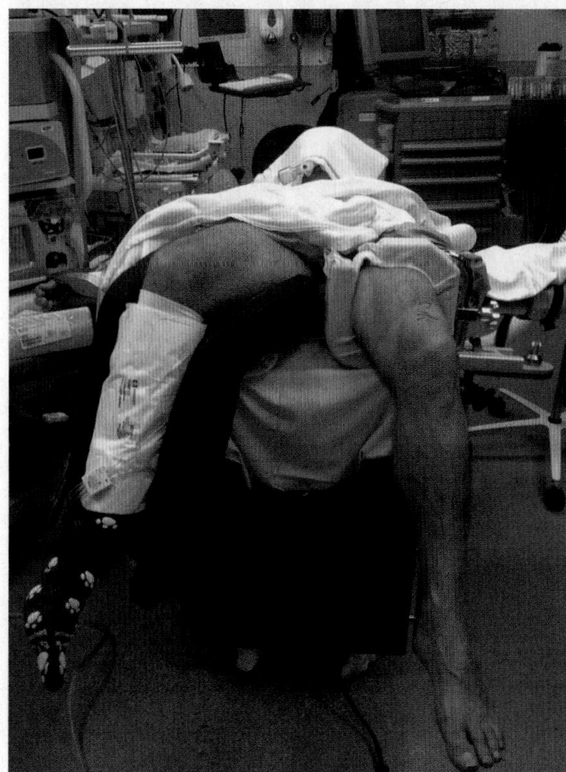

FIGURE 7-4

The contralateral lower extremity (*right side*) is supported by a well-leg holder to flex the hip in order to reduce tension on the femoral nerve and strain on the anterior hip capsule. Note the presence of a sequential compression device placed on the well leg to reduce the risk of deep venous thrombosis.

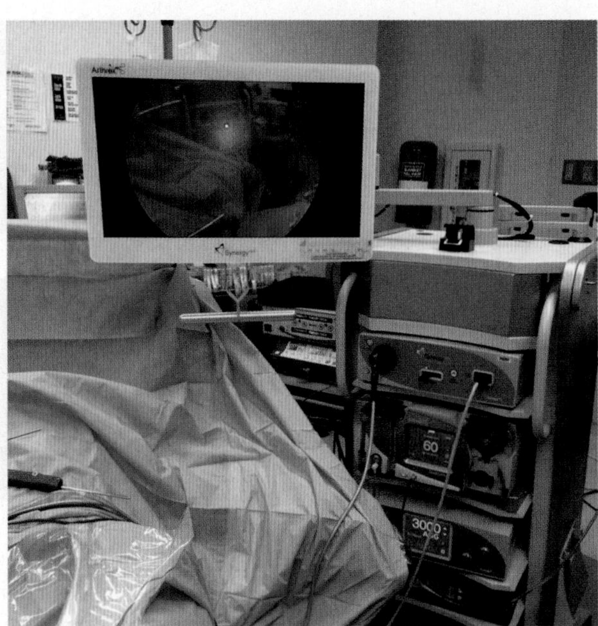

FIGURE 7-5

The video screen is positioned at the head of the table at the level of the patient's contralateral shoulder. The adjacent tower contains control units for the fluid pump, shaver, and electrocautery.

separately or as a single unit. Modern arthroscopic pumps coordinate fluid flow and pressure to optimize hemostasis to enhance arthroscopic viewing. I prefer to have the room lights out and the overhead operating room lights on as I feel that the arthroscopic video is best viewed with the room dark in order to provide greater contrast to the video screen.

It is imperative that the surgeon become familiar with the different types of arthroscopes commonly used (i.e., 30 degrees, 70 degrees) and have more than one of each type available in the event that damage occurs (typically to the optical lens) to one of them. Related to this is the need for various arthroscopic basket punches (straight, up-biting, left- and right-curved, 90-degree side-biting, and back-biting) (Fig. 7-6), graspers, and 4.5-mm rotary shavers (straight, curved, and tapered

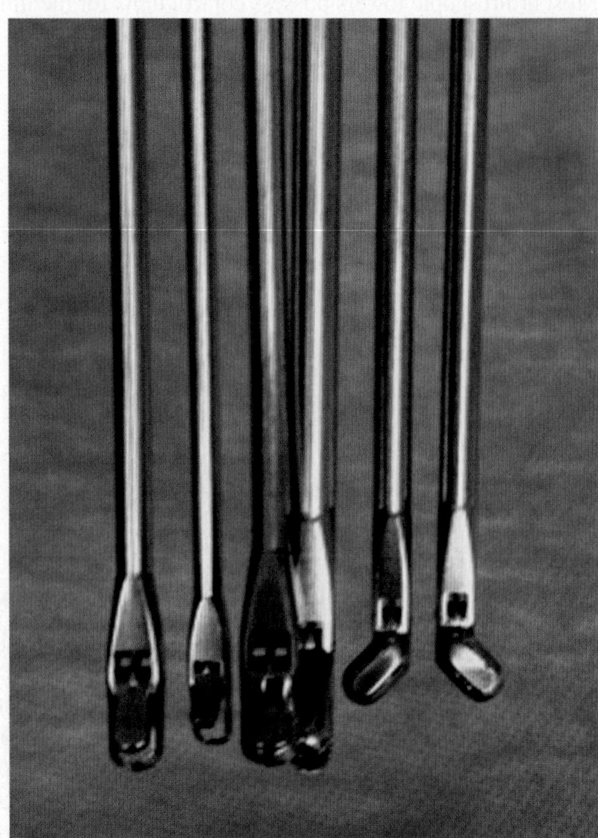

FIGURE 7-6

Various arthroscopic basket punches and graspers for meniscal excision.

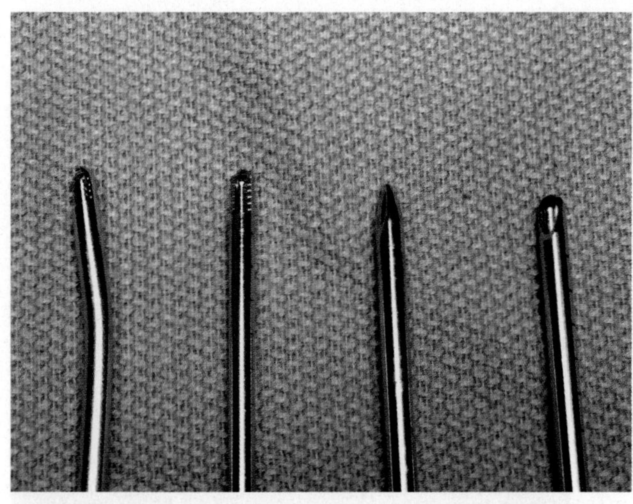

FIGURE 7-7
Variety of shavers (straight, curved, and tapered) for meniscal contouring. (Courtesy Arthrex Inc., Naples, FL.)

varieties) (Fig. 7-7). Narrow (3.5 mm) shavers are extremely helpful in the navigation of tight compartments of the knee—especially the medial compartment in older male patients and in younger patients with smaller knees.

My preference for arthroscopic fluid is to use lactated Ringer's solution due to its more favorable physiologic profile compared to normal saline. An arthroscopic pump is used to maintain joint distention. Improved visualization in the presence of intra-articular bleeding may be obtained by either an increase in fluid pressure, use of epinephrine in the fluid (1 mg epinephrine/3-L bag [0.33 mg/L]), or through the inflation of the tourniquet.

DIAGNOSTIC ARTHROSCOPY

As with any operative procedure, it is important that the surgeon develop a routine sequence in which to perform the procedure so as not to miss any relevant pathology. All portals are created with a no. 11 scalpel through just the skin and subcutaneous tissue. A blunt trochar is used for synovial penetration. A superomedial outflow portal is created at the junction of the superior pole of the patella and patellofemoral joint. The knee is passively flexed to 90 degrees, and the anterolateral and anteromedial portals are similarly created. These portal incisions are made with the blade facing superiorly and directed at a 45-degree angle from midline through the fat pad toward the intercondylar notch. In general, the anteromedial portal is positioned approximately 5 to 10 mm more proximal than the anterolateral portal (Fig. 7-8). Therefore, all three standard knee portals are made at the beginning of the procedure so that instrumentation (i.e., probe, shaver, and basket forceps) can be inserted into the joint as needed. Some surgeons prefer to make the anteromedial portal under direct visualization from inside the joint. It is my preference to treat each associated pathologic process (i.e., patellar chondroplasty, loose body removal) as it is viewed in order to most efficiently complete the operative procedure without making redundant passes around the knee.

The diagnostic arthroscopy is performed, initially, with the 30-degree arthroscope placed in the anterolateral portal with the fluid inflow through the arthroscopic cannula in order to "blow away" any joint material (i.e., cartilaginous debris, synovium) that may impair the surgeon's view. The medial and lateral gutters are evaluated to make sure there is no displaced meniscal fragment not visualized in the involved compartment (Fig. 7-9).

The knee is placed into approximately 20 degrees of flexion and 10 degrees of external rotation, as a valgus force is applied to the leg with the patient's foot locked onto the surgeon's hip or anterior pelvis in order to allow visualization of the medial compartment (Fig. 7-10). The medial meniscus should be probed from both the superior and inferior surfaces to assess its stability, determine the presence of any tears, and to make sure there are no loose bodies entrapped between it and the tibial plateau (Fig. 7-11). Moving the knee into near-full extension can enhance visualization of the posterior horn and root in a tight knee. External pressure on the posteromedial aspect of the knee can help deliver the posterior horn into view.

In order to view the lateral compartment, the knee is placed at approximately 20 degrees of flexion with internal rotation and varus load applied. Once in the lateral compartment, the surgeon should

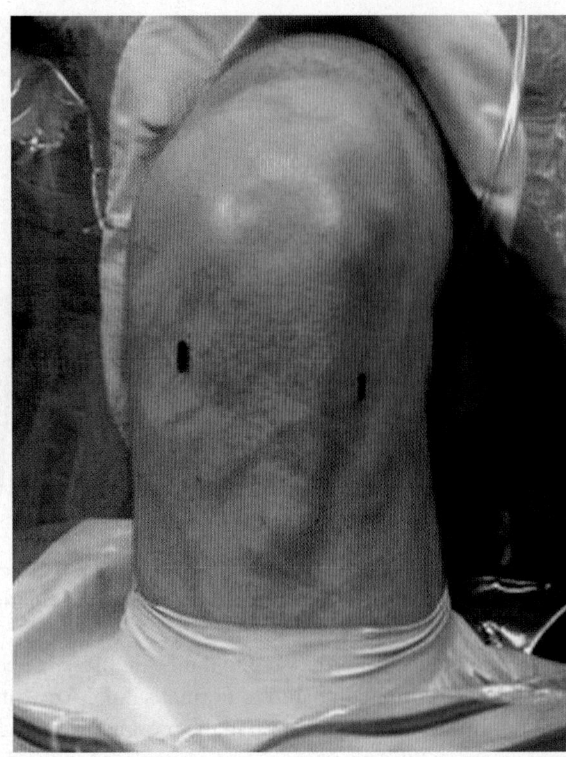

FIGURE 7-8

View of the left knee with anteromedial and anterolateral portals marked. Note that the anteromedial portal is typically 5 to 10 mm proximal to the anterolateral portal.

carry out a systematic evaluation starting with the posterior horn of the lateral meniscus. The popliteal hiatus should then be probed superiorly and inferiorly and inspected for any displaced meniscal fragments or occult loose bodies (Fig. 7-12). The midbody of the lateral meniscus should be evaluated for any tears by moving the camera laterally and aiming the arthroscope inferiorly (Fig. 7-13). This maneuver is facilitated by a rotating motion so as not to damage the articular surface of the lateral femoral condyle. Switching the arthroscope to the anteromedial portal and placing the instruments in the anterolateral portal can facilitate excision of a far posterior root tear that is often difficult to reach from an anteromedial working portal because of the prominence of the tibial spines.

The posteromedial and posterolateral compartments should both be visualized from the contralateral anterior portals by traversing through the intercondylar notch with the knee at 90 degrees of flexion (Gillquist maneuver). The arthroscopic cannula with blunt trochar is introduced through the anterolateral portal, posteriorly and inferiorly along the medial wall of the intercondylar notch, under the posterior cruciate ligament, and into the posteromedial compartment (Fig. 7-14).

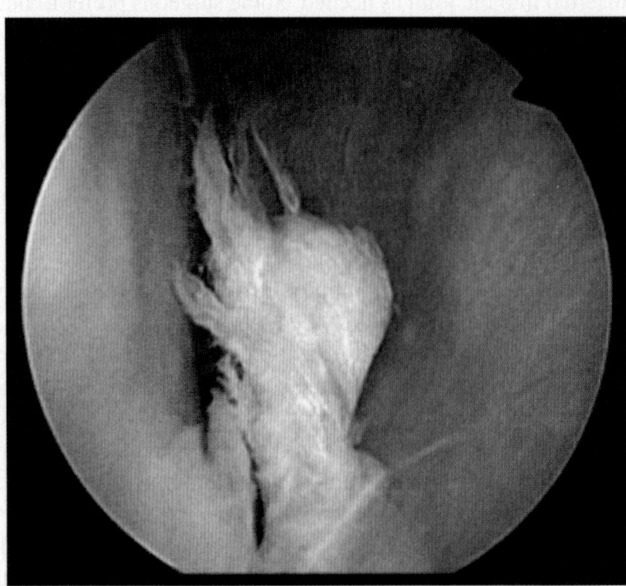

FIGURE 7-9

Displaced meniscal fragment located in the lateral gutter.

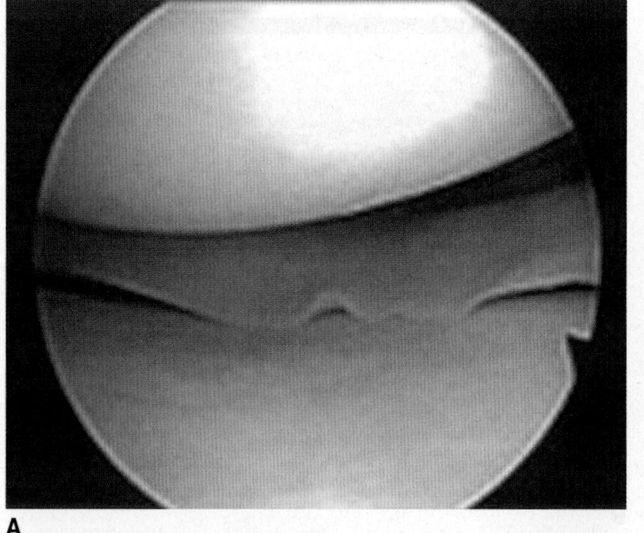

A

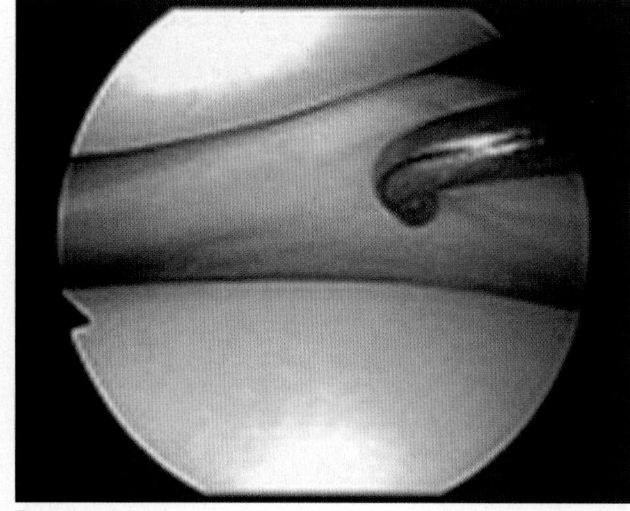

B

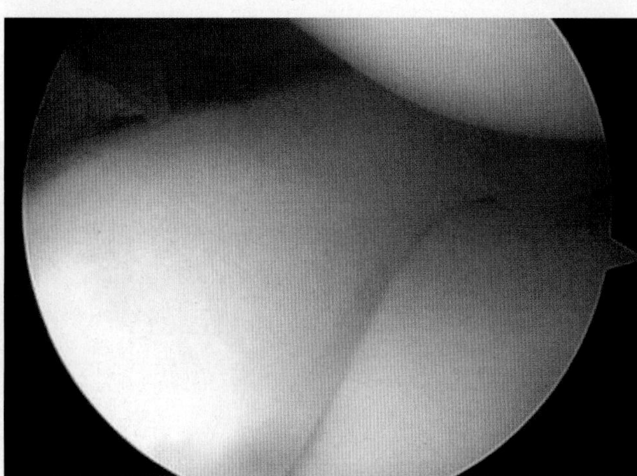

C

FIGURE 7-10

Visualization of the medial meniscus with the 30-degree arthroscope. **A:** Posterior horn probed on the superior surface. **B:** Undersurface of posterior horn inspected. **C:** Midbody of the medial meniscus.

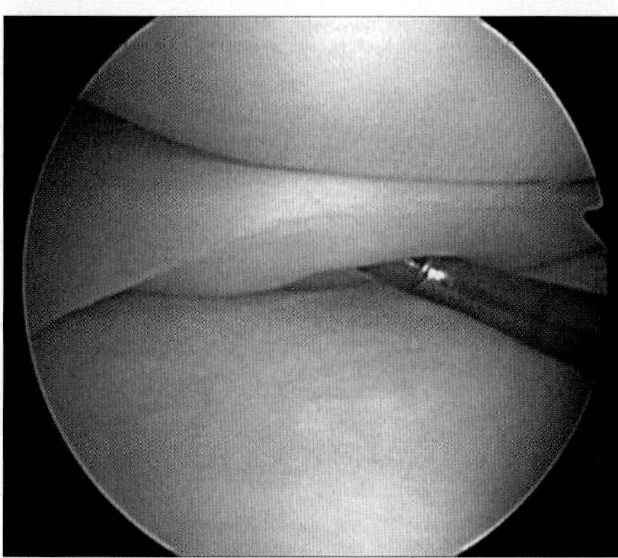

FIGURE 7-11

Posterior horn of medial meniscus probed with increased excursion consistent with an occult tear.

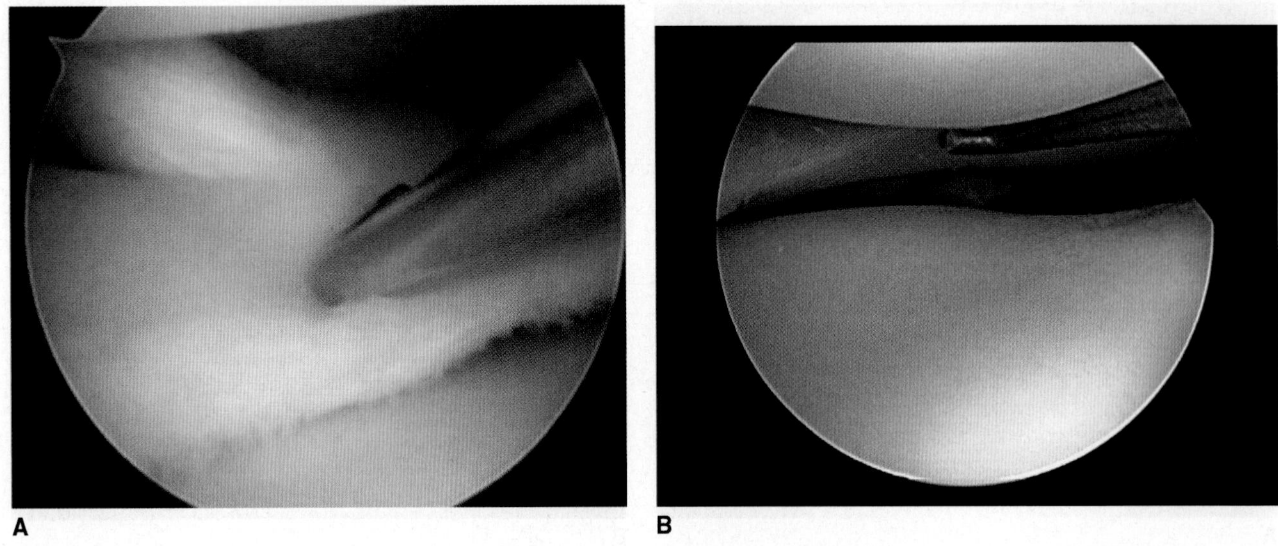

FIGURE 7-12

The popliteal hiatus is viewed from the superior (**A**) and inferior surface (**B**) of the lateral meniscus and probed for any tears or loose bodies.

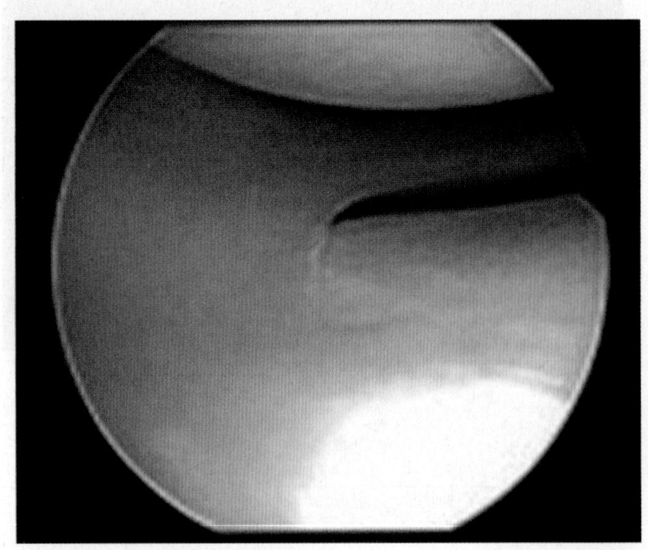

FIGURE 7-13

Midbody of the lateral meniscus.

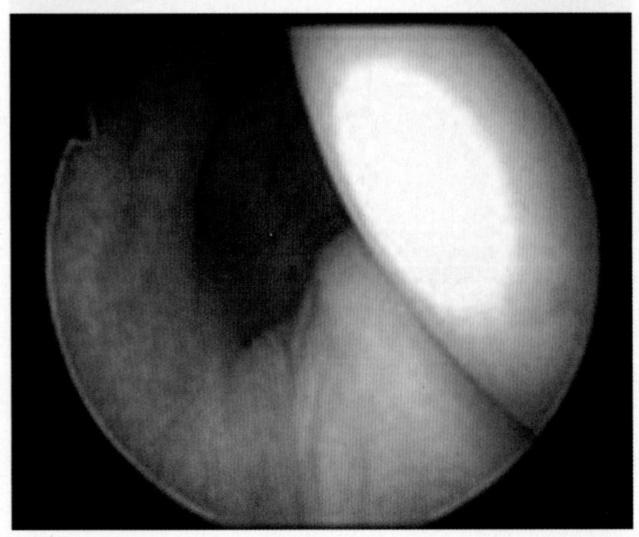

FIGURE 7-14

Posteromedial compartment viewed through the intercondylar notch with a 70-degree arthroscope placed in the anterolateral portal.

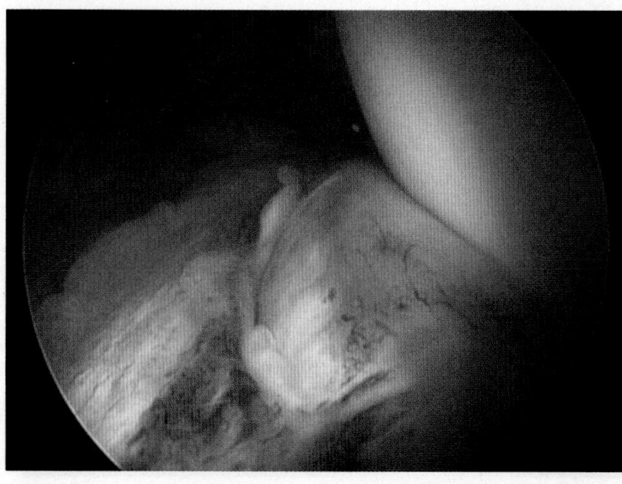

FIGURE 7-15
Meniscal tear identified in the posteromedial compartment with a 70-degree arthroscope.

The 70-degree arthroscope will provide an excellent view of any displaced meniscal flaps and reveal how much of the meniscus remains following debridement. If a meniscal tear is identified (Fig. 7-15), the surgeon must be prepared to make an accessory posteromedial portal for instrumentation. This portal is created by first transilluminating the skin over the posteromedial corner of the knee with the light from the arthroscope. An 18-gauge spinal needle is then inserted into the compartment 2 cm above the medial joint line just posterior to the medial femoral condyle (Fig. 7-16). A longitudinal stab incision is made with a no. 11 scalpel with care taken to avoid both the saphenous nerve and vein. A trochar is then advanced through this incision while puncturing the posteromedial capsule under direct visualization. Operating instruments can then be inserted as necessary (Fig. 7-17).

The posterolateral compartment can be entered in the same fashion as the posteromedial compartment but is typically easier to reach. The surgeon starts with the knee in 90 degrees of flexion with the blunt trochar and cannula placed in the anteromedial portal and directed posterolaterally along the medial wall of the lateral femoral condyle above the anterior cruciate ligament until a giving-way sensation is perceived indicating successful navigation through the intercondylar notch (Fig. 7-18). From this view, the posterolateral compartment is similarly evaluated for loose bodies or displaced meniscal fragments. If necessary, a posterolateral portal is created in a similar fashion to the posteromedial portal.

Tear Examination—Medial Meniscus

Most tears of the medial meniscus are identified once the 30-degree arthroscope is placed in the medial compartment and are located in the posterior horn. The meniscus should be sequentially probed starting at the posterior root moving anteriorly. The anterior horn of the medial meniscus is uncommonly injured due to its relatively diminutive size compared to the posterior horn and its attachment that is located on a non–weight-bearing region of the tibial plateau. Once a tear is

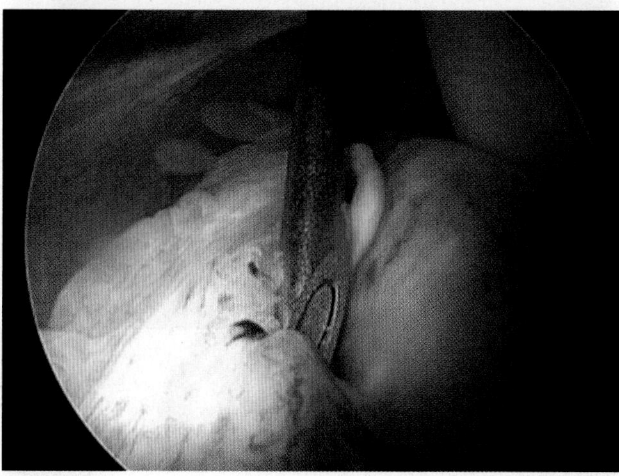

FIGURE 7-16
An 18-gauge spinal needle is then inserted into the posteromedial compartment 2 cm above the medial joint line just posterior to the medial femoral condyle.

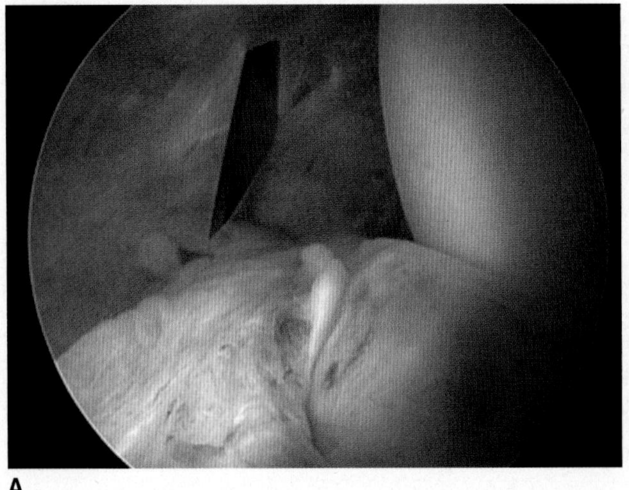

A

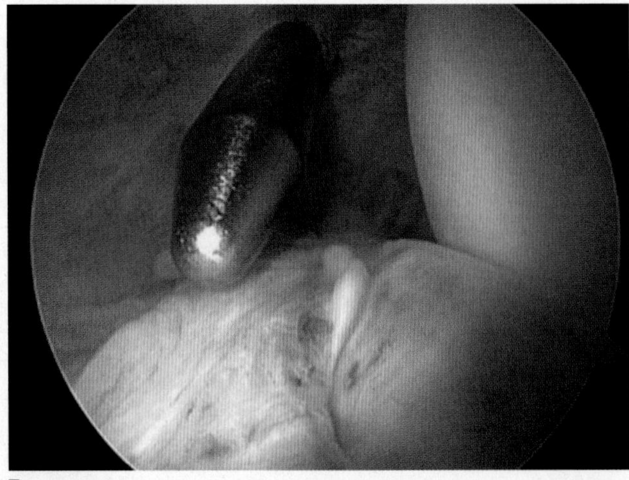

B

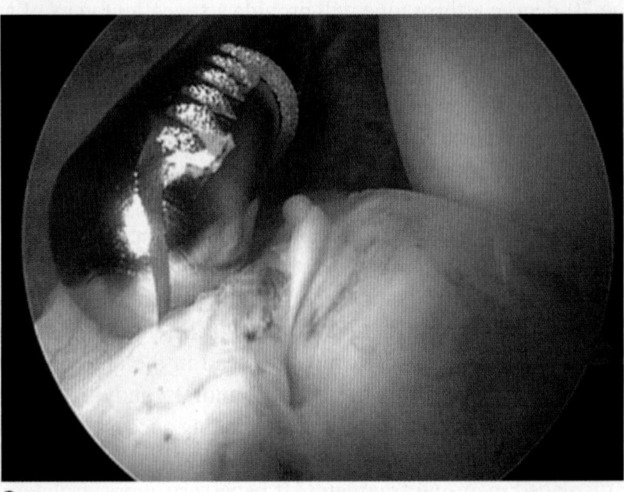

C

FIGURE 7-17

Creation of a posteromedial portal. **A:** A longitudinal stab incision is made in the posteromedial capsule with a no. 11 scalpel to place instruments in the posteromedial compartment. **B:** A trochar is then advanced through this incision while puncturing the posteromedial capsule. **C:** Arthroscopic shaver inserted into the posteromedial compartment to debride the meniscal tear shown in Figure 7-13.

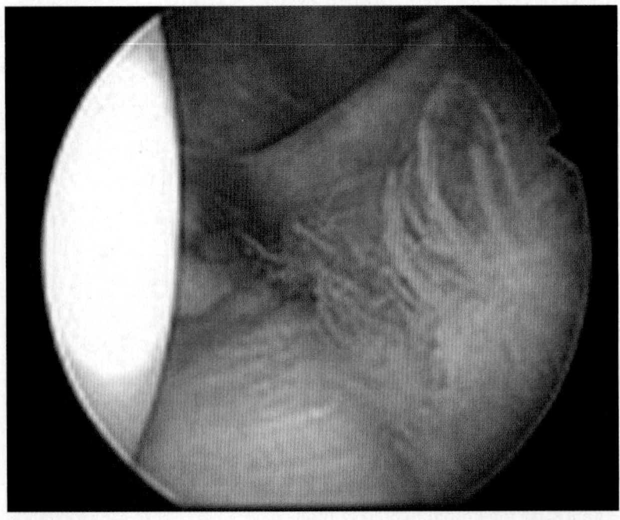

A

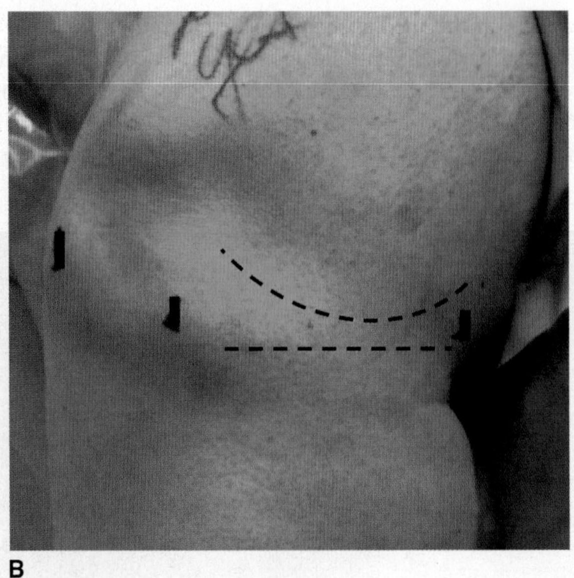

B

FIGURE 7-18

A: Posterolateral compartment viewed through the intercondylar notch with a 70-degree arthroscope placed in the anteromedial portal. **B:** Portal placement to access the posterolateral compartment.

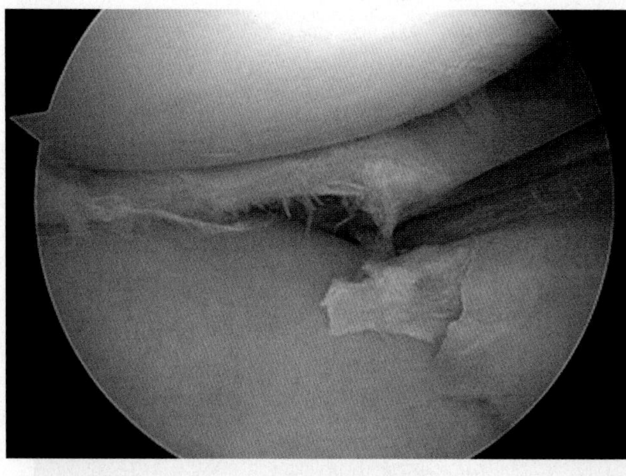

FIGURE 7-19

A displaced meniscal fragment is flipped back into the medial compartment after being entrapped under the meniscus behind the tibial plateau.

identified, it is probed on both the superior and inferior surfaces using a 4-mm probe to determine the degree of instability. Occasionally, there will be more than one tear present with the more peripheral tear obscured by the inner tear. Even though the inner tear is likely not reparable, the more peripheral tear may be reparable. It is important to account for all meniscal tissue in those tears that have not been previously debrided. If a segment of meniscal tissue is not visualized, it is important to ascertain if a displaced meniscal fragment is flipped backward into the posteromedial compartment or entrapped under the meniscus behind the tibial plateau (Fig. 7-19). Sweeping the probe across the superior and inferior meniscal surface will reveal the presence of a displaced fragment. The remainder of the midbody should be similarly probed.

Tear Examination—Lateral Meniscus

In a similar fashion, the lateral meniscus is thoroughly probed on both surfaces beginning at the posterior root and moving anteriorly. The anterior horn of the lateral meniscus is more substantial and located on the weight-bearing surface of the lateral tibial plateau due to its C-shaped configuration. Most lateral meniscus tears occur at the posterior horn and midbody, although complex degenerative tears are commonly seen in the anterior horn of older patients. Avulsion of the posterior root of the lateral meniscus is not as common as in the medial meniscus, but can still occur. Longitudinal and oblique tears of the posterior horn may involve the popliteal hiatus, which can increase the degree of instability (Fig. 7-20). Horizontal cleavage tears of the posterior horn are frequently located anterior

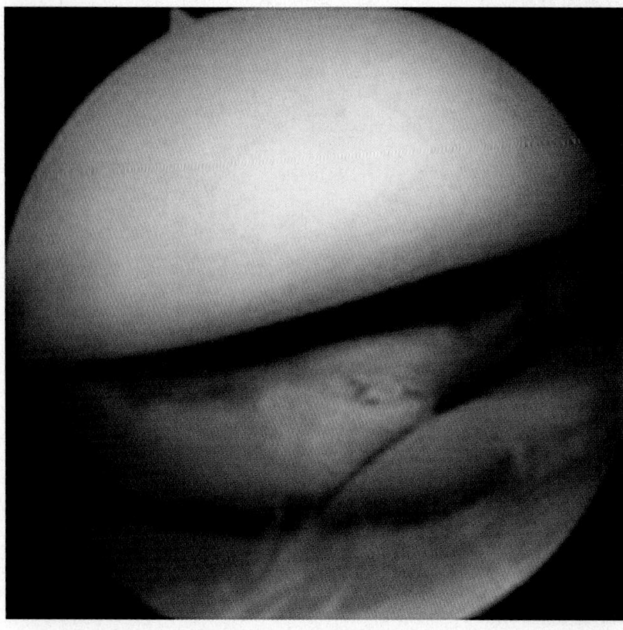

FIGURE 7-20

Oblique tear of the posterior horn of the lateral meniscus.

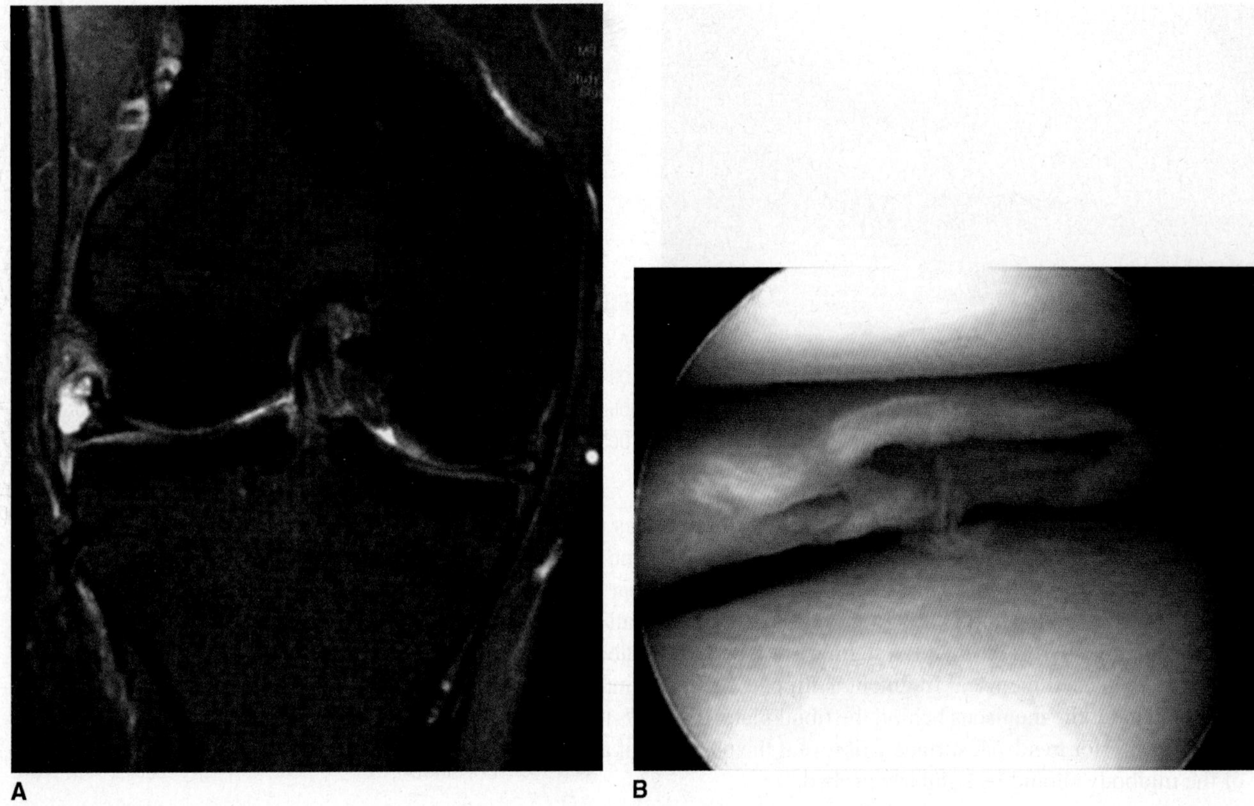

A B

FIGURE 7-21

A: Coronal T2 MRI of the right knee with a lateral meniscal cyst and associated horizontal tear of the lateral meniscus. **B:** Horizontal tear of lateral meniscus associated with a meniscal cyst. Note the cyst fluid expressed from the tear.

to the popliteus tendon and extend posteriorly into the hiatus. Horizontal cleavage and radial tears of the midbody are most likely to be associated with meniscal cysts caused by the peripheral extravasation of synovial fluid (Fig. 7-21) (see below).

Palpation of the posterior root of the lateral meniscus in its entirety may be technically difficult due to the presence of the tibial spine. In these cases, the 30-degree arthroscope can be moved to the anteromedial portal viewing laterally with instruments inserted through the anterolateral portal (Fig. 7-22). Alternatively, the 70-degree arthroscope can be placed in either the anterolateral or anteromedial portal to facilitate visualization of the anterior horn.

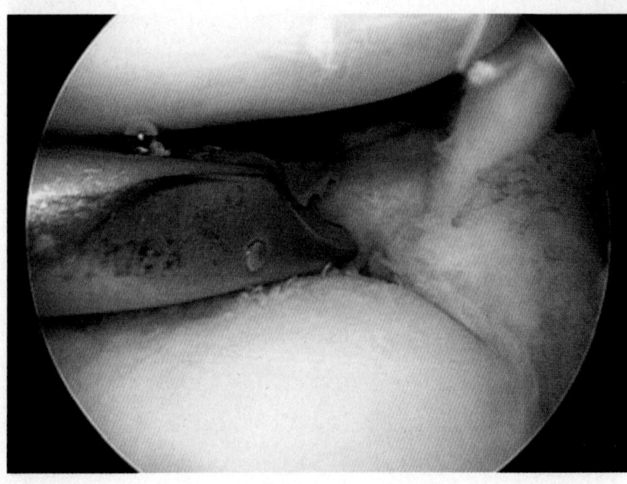

FIGURE 7-22

Root tear of the right lateral meniscus viewed with the 30-degree arthroscope from the anteromedial portal with instruments inserted through the anterolateral portal.

MENISCECTOMY TECHNIQUE FOR SELECTED MENISCAL TEARS

General Principles

The goal of a meniscectomy, irrespective of the involved side or type of tear, is to excise only the unstable meniscal segment. All mobile fragments that can be pulled past the inner meniscal margin into the center of the compartment should be removed. As much of the remaining peripheral rim of meniscal tissue as possible should be left. Segmental resection of a portion of the meniscus is essentially equivalent to a complete meniscectomy. Related to this is the goal to retain as much of the posterior meniscal root attachment as is feasible in order to maintain some degree of load transmission of the remaining meniscal segment. Both manual and motorized instruments exist to resect and contour essentially any tear configuration that may be encountered in either meniscus. It is imperative that the surgeon avoid iatrogenic damage to the articular cartilage of the femoral condyle while trying to resect the torn meniscus. Occasionally, an improved view of the torn meniscus and ease of resection are best accomplished by switching portals from which to view and insert instruments. Despite the fact that an arthroscopic partial meniscectomy is often considered a technically simple procedure, some tears present in relatively tight knees can pose a technical challenge that require adept arthroscopic skills in order to complete the procedure in a safe and efficient manner. Technical aspects of certain meniscal tear types are discussed below to aid both the novice and experienced arthroscopic surgeon.

Complex Meniscal Tears

Complex meniscal tears are accordingly named because of the complex configuration of the tear that occurs in multiple planes. These tears are initially debrided with an arthroscopic shaver since a basket forceps cannot easily debride the shredded tissue (Fig. 7-23). Once the obvious torn tissue is removed, a probe can be used to palpate the remaining meniscal tissue to confirm adequate debridement. Complex tears of the anterior horn of the lateral meniscus can be debrided with a curved shaver

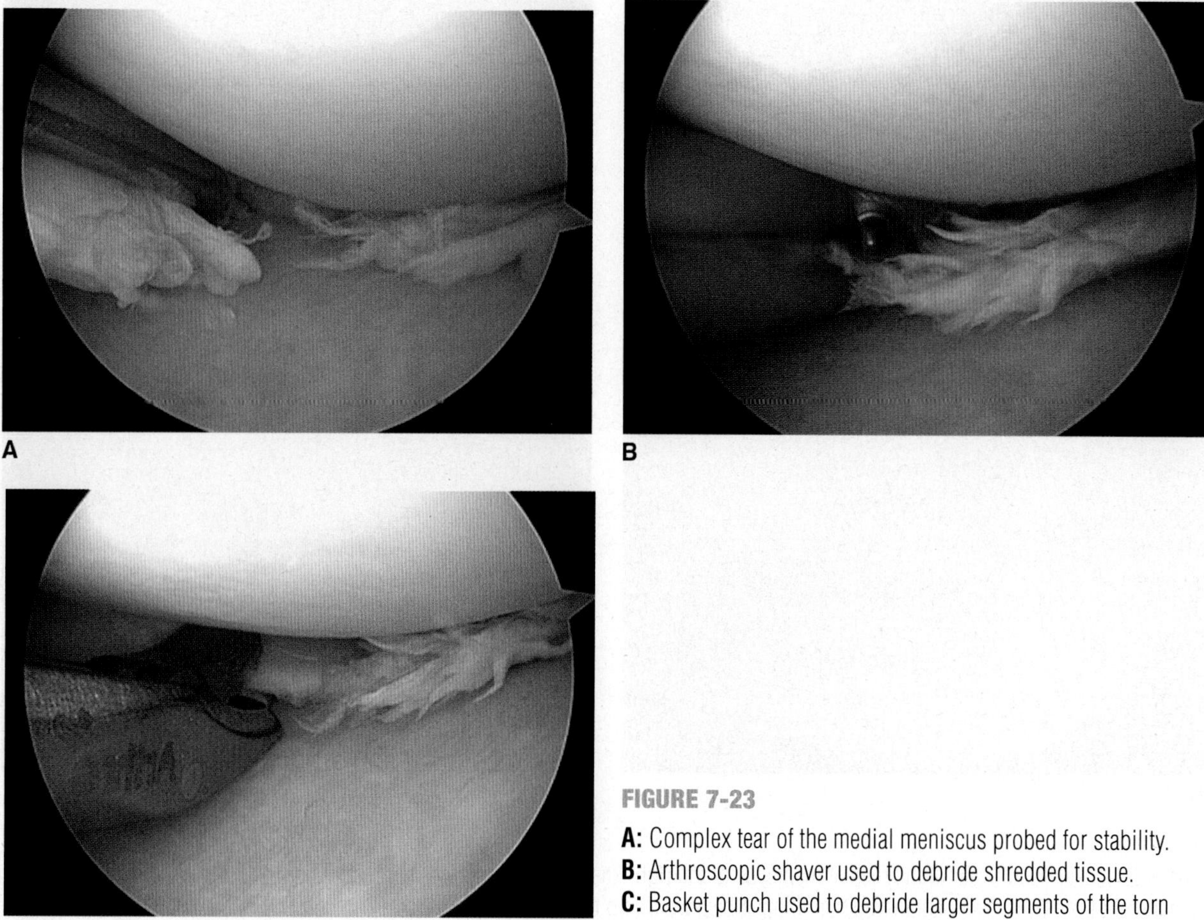

FIGURE 7-23

A: Complex tear of the medial meniscus probed for stability.
B: Arthroscopic shaver used to debride shredded tissue.
C: Basket punch used to debride larger segments of the torn meniscus after the shaver removes more shredded tissue.

through the anteromedial portal. Alternatively, a back-biting meniscal punch can be used for complex anterior horn tears of the lateral meniscus while viewing through the anteromedial portal.

Bucket Handle Tears

Bucket handle meniscal tears may be irreparable because of poor tissue quality, deformation, or avascularity. It is helpful to reduce the tear to assess its length and location. If a meniscectomy is indicated, the posterior horn attachment should be released first. Otherwise, the bucket handle fragment can displace into the posterior compartment if the anterior attachment is released first (Fig. 7-24). It is occasionally helpful to enlarge the ipsilateral portal with a hemostat to facilitate removal of the torn piece. The entire fragment should be visualized as it is removed through the anterior portal to ensure the piece is not left within the fat pad adjacent to the portal. A meniscal shaver is useful to smooth the remaining meniscus.

Posterior Root Tears

Tears of the posterior meniscal root usually involve the medial meniscus and are most common in overweight, middle-aged females with associated arthritis of the medial femoral condyle (Fig. 7-25).

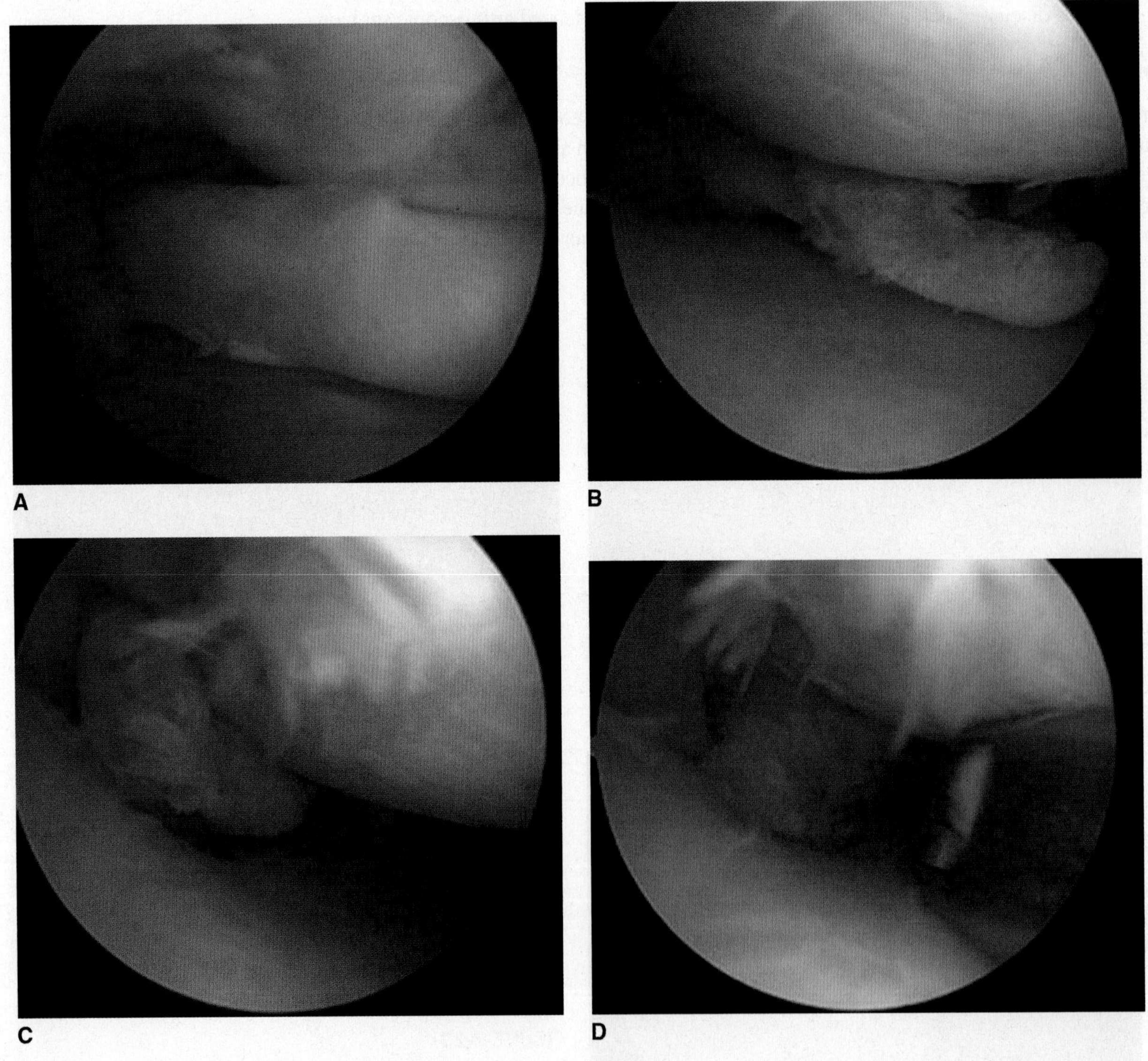

FIGURE 7-24

A: Irreparable bucket handle tear of the medial meniscus of the right knee. **B:** The torn fragment was incorrectly released from its anterior horn attachment first. **C:** Bucket handle fragment flipped backward into the posteromedial compartment. **D:** Final resection of the entire fragment after the posteriorly displaced piece was pulled anteriorly.

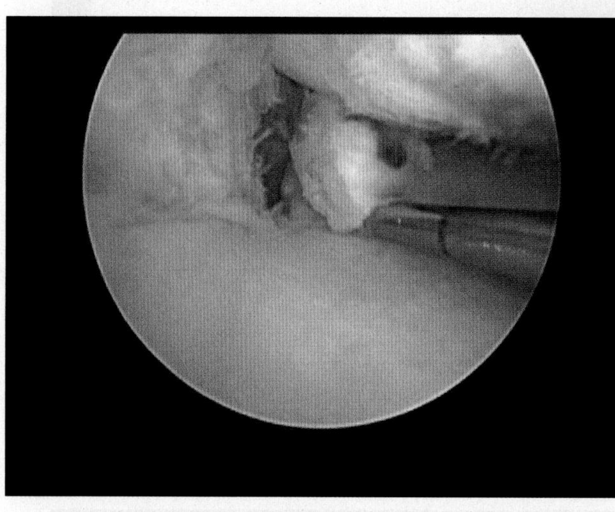

FIGURE 7-25
Irreparable root tear of the medial meniscus in a middle-aged female with associated osteoarthritis.

Root tears are also very common in Asian populations that frequently squat with activities of daily living. Reparable tears are occasionally found in young patients who have a coexistent tear of the anterior cruciate ligament. Irreparable root tears typically result in a nonfunctional meniscus due to extravasation of the meniscus body and corresponding loss of hoop stress (Fig. 7-26). Surgical excision of a root tear should attempt to contour any abrupt edges. Given the fact that these patients usually have associated arthritis of the femoral condyle and are above their ideal body weight, the outcome following excision of a root tear is not uniformly favorable as the remaining meniscal body is still in an extravasated position (Fig. 7-27).

Horizontal Cleavage Tears

Horizontal cleavage tears are commonly encountered in both menisci and typically require excision rather than repair. Similar to other nonreparable tears, only the unstable portion should be excised. One or both leafs may require excision as it can be difficult to determine the most functional and least symptomatic leaf (Fig. 7-28). If one leaf possesses the majority of the meniscal tissue, then it is usually preserved in favor of the lesser leaf. The surgeon should be mindful of the quality of tissue left behind. Debridement of the tear is often facilitated by the use of left- or right-angled basket punches. Degenerative tissue is often found within the center of the tear following debridement.

Discoid Meniscus Tears

Discoid menisci occur in 3% to 5% of the US population and in approximately 15% of the Japanese population (5), though the true incidence of asymptomatic discoid menisci is unknown. The vast

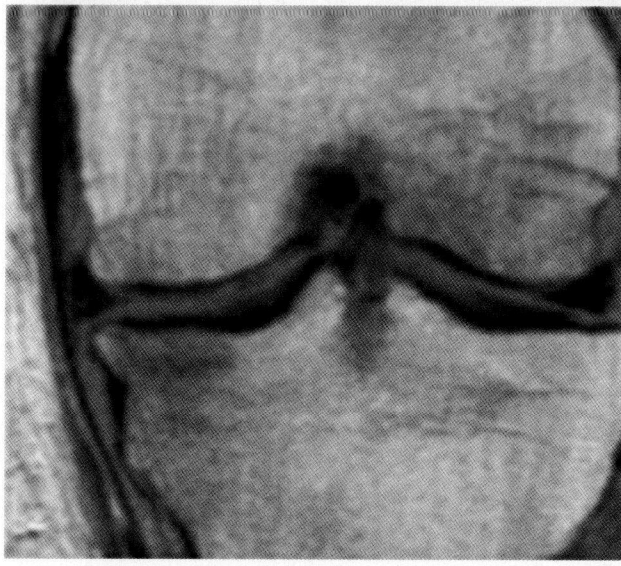

FIGURE 7-26
T1 MRI in coronal plane showing the extravasated medial meniscus associated with a degenerative tear of the posterior root of the medial meniscus.

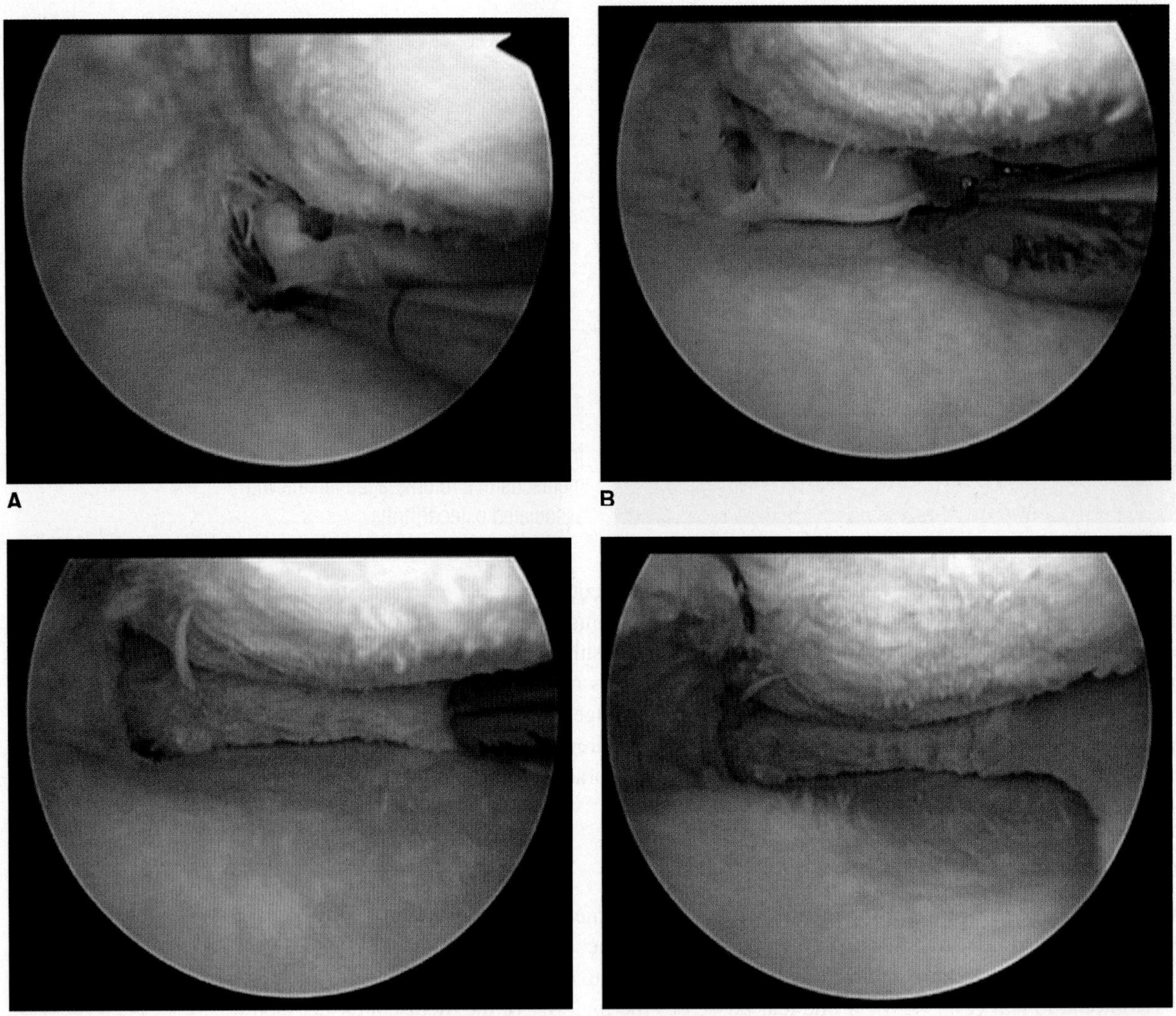

A B

C D

FIGURE 7-27

A: Irreparable tear of the posterior root of the medial meniscus. **B:** Basket punch used to debride the unstable root segment. **C:** Arthroscopic 4.5 shaver used to contour the remaining posterior horn. **D:** Posterior horn of the meniscus following debridement of the root tear. Note the degree of chondrosis of the medial femoral condyle.

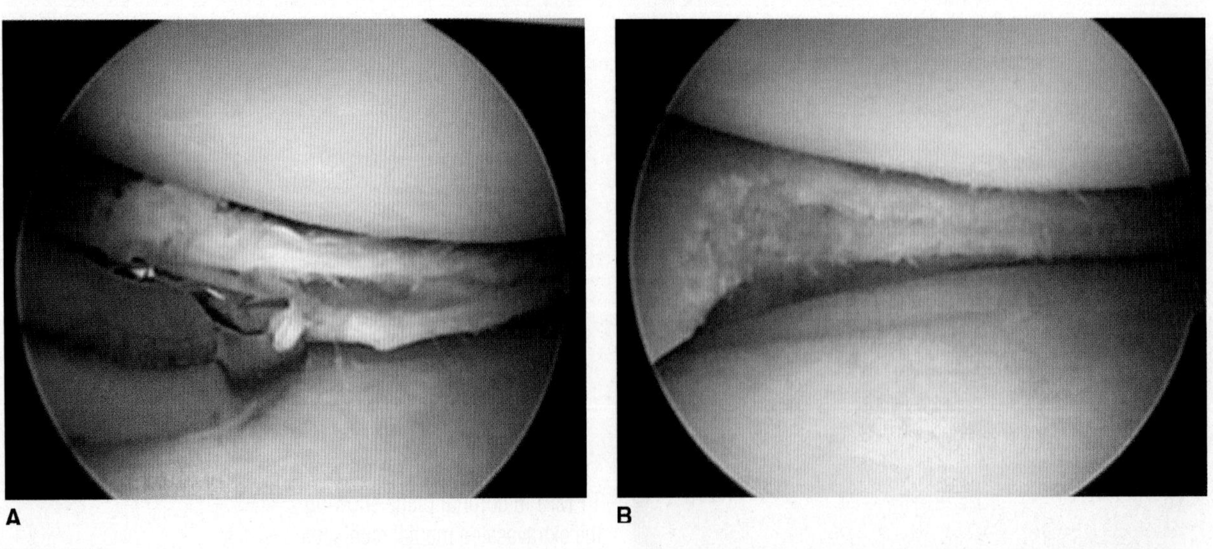

FIGURE 7-28

A: Horizontal tear of the medial meniscus. **B:** Remaining meniscus following the debridement of both the superior and inferior meniscal leafs.

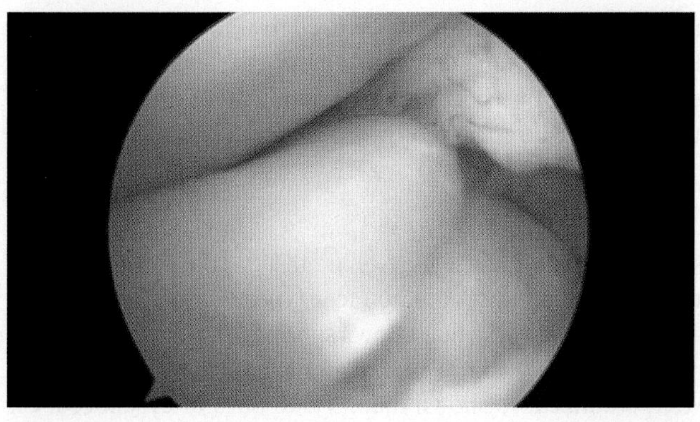

FIGURE 7-29

Complete discoid lateral meniscus of the right knee.

majority of discoid menisci involve the lateral meniscus (Fig. 7-29). The Watanabe classification subdivides discoid menisci into either stable (type I—complete or type II—incomplete) based on whether the discoid meniscus completely covers the tibial plateau or as unstable (type III—Wrisberg variant) where the posterior horn is attached solely by the meniscofemoral (Wrisberg) ligament (6). An asymptomatic discoid meniscus found incidentally during knee arthroscopy should not be surgically excised as this may lead to a symptomatic tear postoperatively.

Treatment of a symptomatic torn discoid meniscus involves an arthroscopic saucerization to debride the torn central segment and sculpt the remaining meniscus to recreate the normal C-shaped configuration. When possible, a 3.5-mm arthroscope is used, but smaller knees in children may require a 2.7-mm arthroscope. Low-profile straight and curved arthroscopic basket punches and small straight and curved shavers are used for meniscal contouring in order to leave a 6- to 8-mm peripheral rim of meniscal tissue. It can be difficult to precisely duplicate the normal wedge-shaped configuration of the lateral meniscus. Placement of the 30-degree arthroscope in the anteromedial portal or use of the 70-degree arthroscope through the anterolateral portal can facilitate visualization of the entire lateral meniscus. It is often easiest to begin the saucerization by placing the knee in the figure-of-four position. A low-profile straight basket punch is used to debride the central portion of the discoid meniscus, followed by the posterior portion. For the midbody, a side-basket punch can be useful for trimming (Fig. 7-30). A back-biter or electrocautery device can be used to contour the

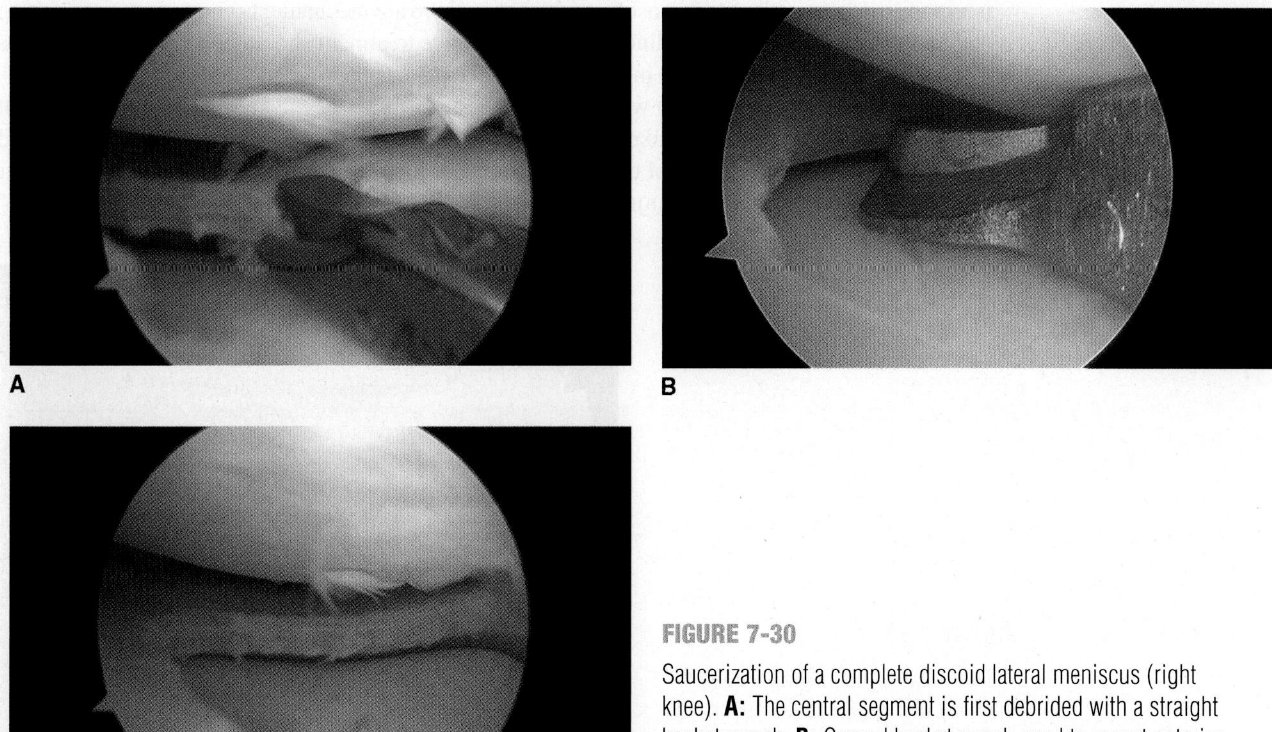

FIGURE 7-30

Saucerization of a complete discoid lateral meniscus (right knee). **A:** The central segment is first debrided with a straight basket punch. **B:** Curved basket punch used to resect anterior segment of the discoid lateral meniscus. **C:** Final appearance of the lateral meniscus following arthroscopic saucerization.

inner rim of the remaining anterior horn. An oscillating shaver can be used to smooth the remaining inner rim. Caution must be taken not to completely excise the entire meniscus, though if the tear extends to the periphery, this may be necessary. For Wrisberg variants, stabilization of the posterior horn can be performed similar to a standard meniscal repair.

Meniscal Cysts

Meniscal tears have been reported in association with meniscal cysts in 50% to 100% of cases with complex horizontal cleavage or radial tears being the most common tear types (7,8). The meniscus tear results in a rent in the capsule creating a one-way valve that allows synovial fluid to collect in an extra-articular location. Most clinically relevant cysts occur in association with the lateral meniscus, though magnetic resonance imaging (MRI) studies have shown that 59% to 66% of cysts occur on the medial side (7,8).

Treatment of a meniscal cyst necessitates standard excision or repair of the associated meniscal tear (when present). The cyst can be "decompressed" with a shaver through the torn segment of the meniscus to allow evacuation of the cyst fluid into the knee. However, arthroscopic debridement alone may result in a 50% risk of cyst recurrence (9). My preference is to perform an open debridement of the cyst in conjunction with the arthroscopic meniscectomy as recurrence of the cyst is reduced to 20% with the associated open cystectomy (9).

WOUND CLOSURE

The portals may be closed with interrupted absorbable or nonabsorbable suture or staples at the surgeon's discretion. Local anesthetic (5 to 10 mL of 0.5% bupivacaine) is injected into the portal sites, and a sterile dressing is applied with a compressive wrap. Intra-articular injection of anesthetic is not typically needed and is not recommended because of a concern for chondrotoxicity (10). A cold compression unit can be very helpful to reduce the amount of postoperative swelling.

PEARLS AND PITFALLS

- It is difficult to completely discern the cause of pain in patients with meniscal pathology and coexistent osteoarthritis in the same compartment (Fig. 7-31). The results following a partial meniscectomy in these patients are most favorable when there are mechanical symptoms (i.e., catching and locking) in addition to joint line pain. Nonoperative treatment should be emphasized in those patients with osteoarthritis and a meniscal who have pain as their only symptom.
- Patients (especially older males) with associated osteoarthritis of the knee often have very tight medial compartments that can make visualization difficult. Overly aggressive valgus force needed for exposure can lead to rupture of the medial collateral ligament, or worse, a fracture of the femur or tibia. Iatrogenic ligamentous injury or fracture is less common with varus stress.

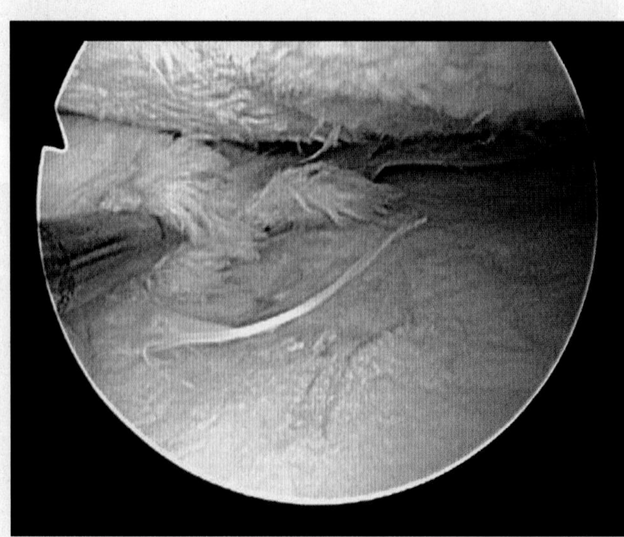

FIGURE 7-31

Complex tear of the posterior horn and midbody of the right medial meniscus in conjunction with osteoarthritis of the medial compartment.

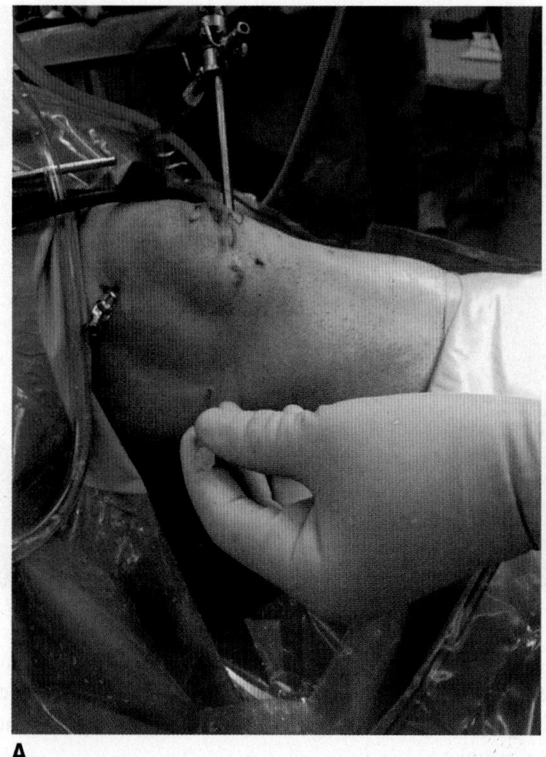

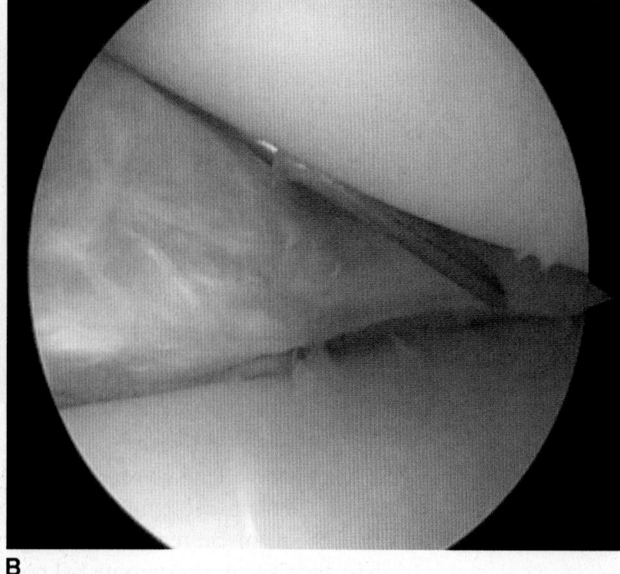

A B

FIGURE 7-32

Percutaneous "pie-crusting" of the superficial medial collateral ligament in order to improve posterior horn visualization. **A:** An 18-gauge needle is inserted multiple times through a single skin puncture just above the joint line in the posteromedial aspect of the knee. **B:** An 18-gauge needle used to "pie-crust" the medial collateral ligament as viewed inside the knee.

- In patients with tight medial compartments, a simple percutaneous "pie-crusting" can be performed with an 18-gauge needle inserted just above the joint line in the posteromedial aspect of the knee (Fig. 7-32). The medial collateral ligament can be perforated at multiple sites at its insertion on the medial femoral condyle through a single percutaneous stick. The medial compartment can then be sequentially "opened" with a gentle valgus force applied to the knee to the degree necessary to fully visualize the posterior meniscal structures.
- The intact medial meniscus has a typical fold (flounce) at the junction of the posterior horn and midbody that is usually indicative of an intact meniscus (Fig. 7-33). Absence of flounce is highly associated with a medial meniscal tear.

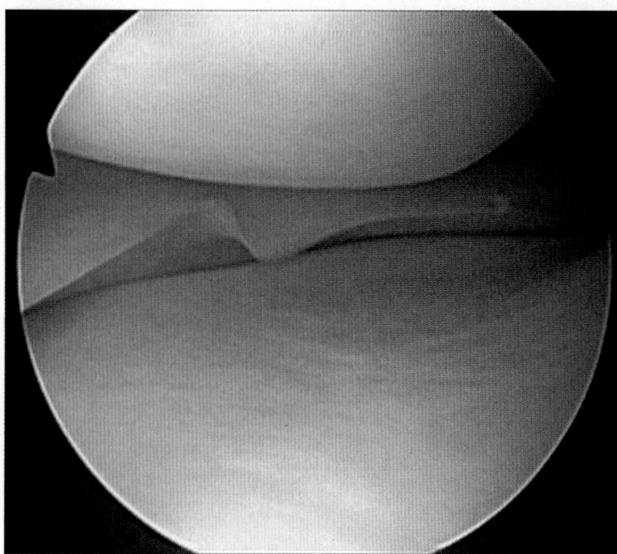

FIGURE 7-33

Meniscal flounce suggestive of an intact medial meniscus.

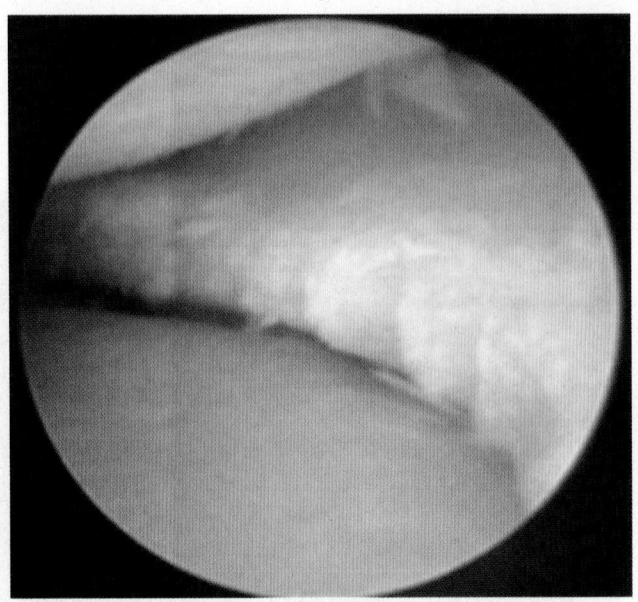

FIGURE 7-34

The inner edge of the medial meniscus following a partial meniscectomy. Note the absence of a completely smooth inner edge. This edge will smooth out over time.

- Bucket handle tears are best removed by first releasing the posterior horn insertion so that the displaced meniscal remnant floats anteriorly for ease of removal. If the anterior horn is released first, the meniscal remnant will likely become displaced in the posteromedial compartment that will necessitate a posteromedial portal to remove.
- An accessory transpatellar tendon portal can be used to access various parts of the meniscus if it cannot be achieved through the standard portals.
- It is important not to blindly "bite" the posterior meniscal root so as not to inadvertently damage the adjacent extra-articular neurovascular structures, especially the popliteal artery.
- A perfectly smooth inner rim is not necessary when performing a meniscectomy as this edge will smooth out over time (Fig. 7-34).
- An up-biting basket punch can be used to debride the posterior horn of either meniscus in a tight knee. The curved punch follows the contour of the femoral condyle (Fig. 7-35). A straight punch in this situation would be directed into the posterior tibial plateau.
- The surgeon should become adept at accessing the posteromedial and posterolateral compartments with the 70-degree arthroscope through the intercondylar notch (Gillquist maneuver). If a meniscal fragment is displaced into the posterior compartment (medial or lateral), it can be removed via a posteromedial or posterolateral portal.
- Corticosteroids should not be injected intraoperatively at the conclusion of the procedure as this practice has been associated with the development of deep infections following knee arthroscopy (11).

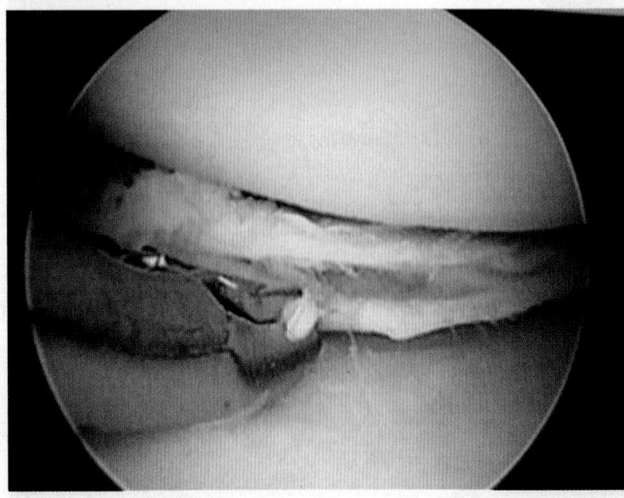

FIGURE 7-35

An up-biting basket punch is used to debride the posterior horn of the medial meniscus in a tight knee.

POSTOPERATIVE MANAGEMENT

Patients are given oral pain medications for a limited time following surgery, though they typically do not require strong narcotics for prolonged periods of time. Either formal physical therapy or a home exercise program is initiated soon after the procedure. Patients are allowed to weightbear as tolerated as most patients do not require the use of crutches. The postoperative dressing is left in place for 3 days, and the patient is allowed to shower and get the portals wet. Submersion of the knee underwater is not allowed for 2 weeks following surgery. Ice or a commercially available cooling unit is used intermittently throughout the day (especially following physical therapy exercises) for 15 to 20 minutes. Longer periods of icing may cause thermal injury to the skin and/or an increase in knee swelling. Range of motion is encouraged to the patient's tolerance. Quadriceps and hamstring strengthening exercises and patellar mobilization are initiated with electrical stimulation or other modalities used as necessitated by the patient's clinical condition. Progression to a stationary cycle for range of motion and aerobic conditioning is usually possible within the first 2 to 3 weeks. Sports-specific drills or work-related conditioning are instituted depending on the patient's goals. Most patients are able to return to full sports participation within 6 weeks following surgery.

COMPLICATIONS

Complications following arthroscopic meniscectomy are relatively rare. Deep infection occurs in approximately 1 in 500 patients irrespective of the use of prophylactic antibiotics and is treated with arthroscopic irrigation and debridement followed by 6 weeks of intravenous antibiotics. Superficial cellulitis or localized portal infections require less extensive treatment with oral antibiotics alone. Deep venous thrombosis has been recognized following this procedure and is manifested by calf or thigh pain, leg swelling, erythema, and pain with passive ankle dorsiflexion (Homan's sign). This condition is diagnosed by Doppler ultrasound or venography and is treated with 3 to 6 months of anticoagulation. Persistent or worsening knee pain can be seen in those patients who have coexistent osteoarthritis. The possibility of persistent pain should be addressed with the patient preoperatively. An intra-articular corticosteroid injection can be administered to these patients for symptomatic relief. Persistent or worsening pain should prompt the surgeon to consider postarthroscopic osteonecrosis as part of the differential diagnosis. This is typically seen in older patients who undergo a medial meniscectomy and is theorized to be secondary to altered weight-bearing mechanics on the femoral condyle following an excision of meniscal tissue (12).

RESULTS

While long considered a benign intervention, several basic science studies have since demonstrated the detrimental effects of total meniscectomy (13,14). Partial meniscectomy is now the widely accepted standard of care as knee function appears to be inversely related to the amount of meniscal tissue resected. Several studies have documented favorable clinical and radiological outcomes over total meniscectomy (15–17). It has been postulated that many arthroscopic partial meniscectomies may functionally represent a total meniscectomy, as the disruption of circumferential collagen fibers—as encountered in radial tears—prevents hoop stress formation, making the remaining meniscus functionless (18).

Several studies (16,19–21) have reported worse outcomes after lateral compared to medial meniscectomy. This likely reflects the meniscal-dependent nature of the lateral compartment due to its bicondylar convexity, with subsequent point loading leading to increased peak contact pressures. In a 30-year longitudinal study, McNicholas et al. (21) reported 80% good or excellent results following medial meniscectomy compared to 47% good or excellent results after lateral meniscectomy. Similarly, Nawabi et al. (22) found a significantly longer time to return to preinjury level of competition, a greater number of adverse events, and an increased reoperation rate in lateral versus medial meniscectomies in 90 elite soccer players. Scheller et al. noted that 78% of 75 patients who underwent a partial lateral meniscectomy developed Fairbank's signs of osteoarthritis between 5 and 15 years postoperatively (23). Preexisting degenerative changes (24), ligamentous instability (25), and axial malalignment (26) have all been found to negatively impact the outcome following a meniscectomy and should be discussed with the patient preoperatively.

REFERENCES

1. Baker B, Peckham A, Pupparo F, et al. Review of meniscal injury and associated sports. *Am J Sports Med.* 1985;13:1–4.
2. Karachalios T, Hantes M, Zibis A, et al. Diagnostic accuracy of a new clinical test (the Thessaly test) for early detection of meniscal tears. *J Bone Joint Surg Am.* 2005;87-A:955–962.
3. Matava M, Eck K, Totty W, et al. Magnetic resonance imaging as a tool to predict meniscal reparability. *Am J Sports Med.* 1999;27:436–443.
4. Kurzweil P. Antibiotic prophylaxis for arthroscopic surgery. *Arthroscopy.* 2006;22:452–454.
5. Jordan M. Lateral meniscal variants: evaluation and treatment. *J Am Acad Orthop Surg.* 1996;4:191–200.
6. Watanabe M, Takeda S, Ikeuchi H. *Atlas of arthroscopy*. 3rd ed. Tokyo, Japan: Igaku-Shoin; 1979:75–130.
7. Campbell S, Sanders T, Morrison W. MR imaging of meniscal cysts: incidence, location, and clinical significance. *Am J Roentgenol.* 2001;177:409–413.
8. De Smet A, Graf B, del Rio A. Association of parameniscal cysts with underlying meniscal tears as identified on MRI and arthroscopy. *Am J Roentgenol.* 2011;196:W180–W186.
9. Reagan W, McConkey J, Loomer R, et al. Cysts of the lateral meniscus: arthroscopy versus arthroscopy plus open cystectomy. *Arthroscopy.* 1989;5:274–281.
10. Dragoo J, Braun H, Kim H, et al. The in vitro chondrotoxicity of single-dose local anesthetics. *Am J Sports Med.* 2012;40:794–799.
11. Marmor S, Farman T, Lortat-Jacob A. Joint infection after knee arthroscopy: medicolegal aspects. *Orthop Traumatol Surg Res.* 2009;95:278–283.
12. Mont M, Marker D, Zywiel M, et al. Osteonecrosis of the knee and related conditions. *J Am Acad Orthop Surg.* 2011;19:482–494.
13. Baratz M, Fu F, Mengato R. Meniscal tears: the effect of meniscectomy and of repair on intraarticular contact areas and stress in the human knee. *Am J Sports Med.* 1986;14:270–274.
14. Ihn J, Kim S, Park I. In vitro study of contact area and pressure distribution in the human knee after partial and total meniscectomy. *Int Orthop.* 1993;17:214–218.
15. Northmore-Ball M, Dandy D, Jackson R. Arthroscopic, open partial, and total meniscectomy: a comparative study. *J Bone Joint Surg Br.* 1983;65-B:400–404.
16. Hede A, Larsen E, Sandberg H. The long term outcome of open total and partial meniscectomy related to the quantity and site of the meniscus removed. *Int Orthop.* 1992;16:122–125.
17. Andersson-Molina H, Karlsson H, Rockborn P. Arthroscopic partial and total meniscectomy: a long-term follow-up study with matched controls. *Arthroscopy.* 2002;18:183–189.
18. Hoser C, Fink C, Brown C, et al. Long-term results of arthroscopic partial lateral meniscectomy in knees without associated damage. *J Bone Joint Surg Br.* 2001;83:B513–B516.
19. Johnson R, Kettelkamp D, Clark W, et al. Factors effecting late results after meniscectomy. *J Bone Joint Surg Am.* 1974;56-A:719–729.
20. Jorgensen U, Sonne H, Lauridsen F, et al. Long-term follow-up of meniscectomy in athletes: a prospective longitudinal study. *J Bone Joint Surg Br.* 1987;69-B:80–83.
21. McNicholas M, Rowley D, McGurty D, et al. Total meniscectomy in adolescence: a thirty-year follow-up. *J Bone Joint Surg Br.* 2000;82-B:217–221.
22. Nawabi D, Cro S, Hamid I, et al. Return to play after lateral meniscectomy in Elite professional Soccer players. *Am J Sports Med.* 2014;42:2193–2198.
23. Scheller G, Sobau C, Bulow JU. Arthroscopic partial lateral meniscectomy in an otherwise normal knee: clinical, functional, and radiographic results of a long-term follow-up study. *Arthroscopy*. 2001;17:946–952.
24. Schimmer R, Brulhart K, Duff C, et al. Arthroscopic partial meniscectomy: a 12-year follow-up and two-step evaluation of the long-term course. *Arthroscopy.* 1998;14:136–142.
25. Sherman M, Warren R, Marshall J, et al. A clinical and radiographical analysis of 127 anterior cruciate insufficient knees. *Clin Orthop.* 1988;227:229–237.
26. Jaureguito J, Elliot J, Lietner T, et al. The effects of arthroscopic partial lateral meniscectomy in an otherwise normal knee: a retrospective review of functional, clinical, and radiographic results. *Arthroscopy.* 1995;11:29–36.

8 Meniscal Root Repair

Jay V. Kalawadia, Edward S. Chang, and Christopher D. Harner

INTRODUCTION

The menisci are semilunar fibrocartilage structures that serve a role in tibiofemoral joint congruity, stability, shock absorption, and proprioception (1–4). During gait, the menisci convert compressive forces into hoop stresses, which are transferred to the tibial plateau via the peripheral meniscal attachments and the meniscal roots (1,4). The meniscal roots link the fibrocartilage tissue to the subchondral bone via fibrous tissue composed of collagen, proteoglycans, and glycoproteins, which transmit tensile, compressive, and shear forces (5).

The four meniscal roots possess differing mechanical properties and see different forces during normal gait. The anterior roots have a more linear elastic modulus than the posterior roots, which leads to greater anterior root mobility (6–9). In addition, Kopf et al. (4) demonstrated that native anteromedial meniscal root is weaker and requires significantly less force to fail than the anterolateral, posterolateral, and posteromedial roots. The force each meniscal root sees during gait also varies. Internal pressure measurement studies demonstrate higher forces experienced by the posterior roots, especially the posterior medial root (10).

Meniscal root injury significantly affects knee kinematics, resulting in accelerated degenerative wear of the articular cartilage (1,3,4,11–13). Using high-speed, biplanar radiography, Marsh et al. (14) demonstrated that a posterior horn medial meniscal root tear results in increased lateral tibial translation with all dynamic activities compared to the uninjured limb. The medial compartment also demonstrated increased joint mobility than the ipsilateral lateral compartment. Guermazi et al. (15) studied the progression of osteoarthritis in 596 patients as measured by the Whole-Organ Magnetic Resonance Imaging Score system in those with a medial meniscal root tear, those with medial meniscal tear without root involvement, and those without any meniscal pathology. They found the presence of an untreated medial meniscal root tear led to increased tibiofemoral cartilage damage at the 30-month follow-up. Schillhammer et al. (16) evaluated the effects of a lateral meniscal tear in a cadaveric biomechanical study. They found a lateral posterior meniscal root tear increased tibiofemoral contact from 2.8 to 4.2 MPa and decreased contact area from 451 to 304 mm^2. After the lateral meniscal root was repaired, the peak contact pressure and maximum contact area returned close to baseline.

The goal for meniscal root repair is to restore its native biomechanical and kinematic functions. Precise knowledge of the meniscal root insertions is critical to restoring the function of the native meniscus including proper knee kinematics and shock absorption. Nonanatomic repair has been shown to increase the tension in the repair and consequently lead to local stress-induced deformation of the articular cartilage (17). Following successful repair, the repaired meniscal function improves to that of the uninjured meniscus (18).

Kim et al. (19) demonstrated that at 2-year postsurgical follow-up, patients with meniscal root repair demonstrated improved function, decreased meniscal extrusion, and better Kellgren-Lawrence grades compared to those who retore. The surgical technique, suture anchor, or pullout suture did not demonstrate any difference. Lee et al. (20) demonstrated similar clinical outcomes with a Modified Mason-Allen stitch and simple stitches at 2 years. Several other studies have demonstrated improved outcome following meniscal root repair as well (19,21–27).

HISTORY AND PHYSICAL EXAMINATION

Medial meniscal root tears can present acutely or chronically. Acute tears result from a sudden hyperflexion or squatting mechanism and are often associated with other ligamentous involvement

TABLE 8-1 Demographics

Medial Meniscal Root Tears	Lateral Meniscal Root Tears

• Middle-aged patients
  • Often high BMI
  • Often female
• Associated with minor trauma
• Posterior medial knee pain
• Usually some degree of chondrosis (grade II–IV)
• Usually not associated with other injuries, but when present:
  • PCL
  • Multiple ligament injured knee
	• Almost always seen in association with ACL injuries
	• About 50% are soft tissue avulsions of bone
	• About 50% are peri-insertional radial tears (within 1 cm of insertion)
	• Not all are repairable

(3% incidence) (1,3,11,28,29). Because the posterior horns receive more force transmission in the hyperflexed knee, the posterior horn is injured more often (26,30,31). Furthermore, the medial meniscal posterior horn has the least mobility, which contributes its greater incidence of root tears (about 10% to 21% of arthroscopic meniscal repairs or meniscectomy have root involvement) (26,32–34). Risk factors for medial meniscal posterior root tears include older age, female gender, and higher body mass index. (1,33,34) Patients will often complain of posteromedial knee (not joint line) pain, pain with weight bearing, and locking of the knee (Table 8-1).

The lateral meniscus is more mobile and almost always found to be injured in conjunction with other ligamentous injuries. Studies have observed an 8% to 9.8% incidence of lateral meniscal posterior root tears in association with anterior cruciate ligament (ACL) injury (35,36). The only risk factor shown for a lateral meniscal injury is a contact injury (37). Patients will have similar complaints and physical exam to those seen with an ACL injury.

IMAGING

Bilateral posteroanterior 45 degrees of flexion weight-bearing views, bilateral standing anteroposterior weight-bearing views, lateral, and Merchant views should be obtained in all patients. Standing long-leg cassette films should be obtained to determine the mechanical axis. When there is meniscal root injury, there may exist tibiofemoral subluxation and possible joint space narrowing.

Magnetic resonance imaging is helpful to confirm the diagnosis of a meniscal root injury. Injury to the meniscal root (avulsion, adjacent radial tear, or degenerative tear) leads to meniscal extrusion, visible as meniscal overhang on the tibial plateau seen on MRI (38). A high clinical suspicion must exist as MRI has been shown to be only 72.9% to 93.3% sensitive for posterior medial meniscal root (26,33,36,39,40). The MRI should also be used to determine the degree of chondrosis and associated ligamentous injury (Table 8-2).

CLASSIFICATION (TABLE 8-3)

INDICATIONS/CONTRAINDICATIONS

Medial Meniscal Root Repair Indications

- Pain with activities of daily living that interferes with quality of life
- Failure of nonoperative treatment (anti-inflammatories, physical therapy, activity modification, intra-articular injections, bracing)

TABLE 8-2 Standard Imaging for Meniscal Root Tear

- Bilateral posteroanterior 45 degrees of flexion weight-bearing view
- Bilateral standing anteroposterior weight-bearing view
- Lateral view
- Bilateral Merchant view
- ± Long-leg standing cassette (for alignment)
- MRI (noncontrast) of affected knee

TABLE 8-3 Classifying the Meniscal Root Tear

- Timing of injury
  - Acute (seen in younger patients with trauma)
  - Chronic (seen in middle-aged individuals, typically female and overweight)
- Tear pattern
  - Bony avulsion (rare)
  - Soft tissue avulsion (most common)
  - Peri-insertional radial tear (most problematic to repair)
- Meniscal quality
  - Healthy, high-quality tissue (use two-loop sutures)
  - Macerated, poor-quality tissue (use one-loop suture if repairable at all)
- Meniscal location
  - Retracted
  - Nonretracted
- Articular cartilage status in affected compartment
  - Minimal chondrosis (continue with procedure)
  - Significant chondrosis (abort root repair attempt)

- Acute injury with sudden onset of pain and symptoms
- Normal mechanical axis alignment
- Repairable meniscal properties (no maceration or minimal extrusion)

Medial Meniscal Root Repair Contraindications

- Greater than or equal to Kellgren-Lawrence grade III
- Macerated, poor quality, or irreducible meniscal root tissue

Lateral Meniscal Root Repair Indications

- Typically seen in setting of concomitant ACL tear. Should be recognized and addressed at time of ACL reconstruction

Lateral Meniscal Root Repair Contraindications

- Partial tear in setting of intact meniscofemoral ligaments

SURGERY (TABLE 8-4)

Setup and Positioning

Following induction of general anesthesia (with or without a regional block), the patient is positioned supine on the operating table. A bump is placed under the hip of the operative knee to reduce external rotation of the operative limb. A lateral post is placed at the level of the greater trochanter. The senior author does not employ the use of a tourniquet.

An examination under anesthesia is then performed on both the operative and contralateral leg. Range of motion and ligamentous stability are documented on both extremities. The relevant

TABLE 8-4 Standard Required Equipment

- 30- and 70-degree arthroscopic lenses
- 4.5-mm full radius resector (straight and curved)
- Leg positioning device (i.e., SPIDER, Smith & Nephew, Andover, MA)
- ACL drill guide with guide pin (3/32-in Kirschner wire)
- Meniscal rasp
- 70-degree hooked suture–passing device (i.e., ACCU-PASS suture shuttle, Smith & Nephew, Andover, MA)
- Arthroscopic knot pusher
- Hewson suture passer
- 8-mm clear cannula
- No. 2 nonabsorbable braided suture
- 4.5 AO cancellous screw with washer

anatomy and planned incisions are marked out. The arthroscopic portals employed are the anterolateral, anteromedial, and posteromedial portals along with a superolateral outflow portal. Just distal to Gerdy tubercle, a 3-cm oblique incision following Langer skin lines is placed on the flare of the anterolateral aspect of the proximal tibia (Fig. 8-1A–C).

The incisions are then scrubbed with Betadine and then preinjected with a local anesthetic (bupivacaine with epinephrine [1:100,000]). The operative extremity is then prepped and draped (Fig. 8-2A,B). We utilize a SPIDER Limb Positioner (Smith & Nephew, Andover, MA) and begin the procedure with the knee flexed at 90 degrees.

Diagnostic Arthroscopy

The arthroscope is placed in the anterolateral portal, and a careful diagnostic arthroscopy is performed, making note of the status of the chondral surfaces, as well as any additional pathology. The medial meniscus is then carefully examined and probed. It is especially important to probe the posterior root because often times the meniscus can appear normal (Figs. 8-3 and 8-4).

To better visualize the meniscal root, we switch to a 70-degree arthroscope and drive the camera into the posteromedial compartment utilizing the Gillquist maneuver (Fig. 8-5). We routinely perform a limited reverse notchplasty of the posterior-inferior medial femoral condyle with a 4.5-mm full radius resector to provide easier access to the posteromedial compartment as well as the necessary space to pass instruments. The arthroscope is then driven through the intercondylar notch,

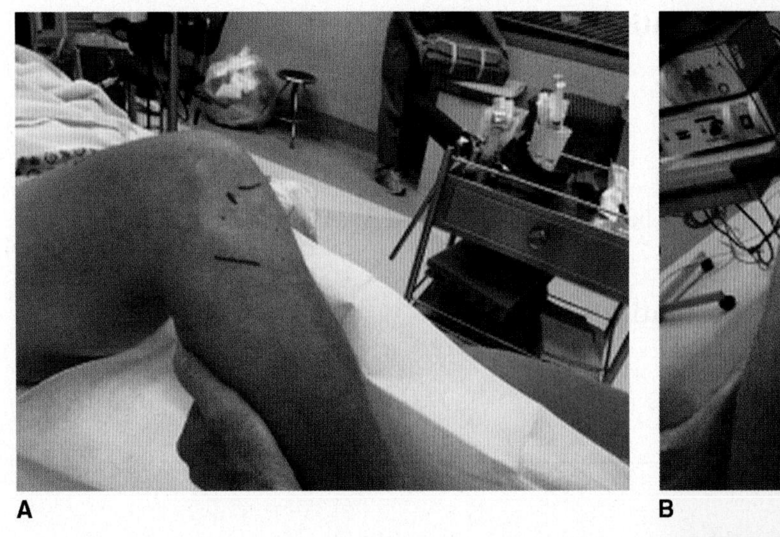

A

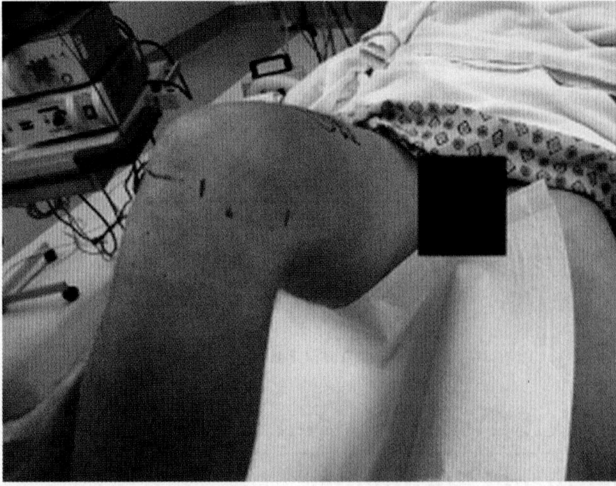

B

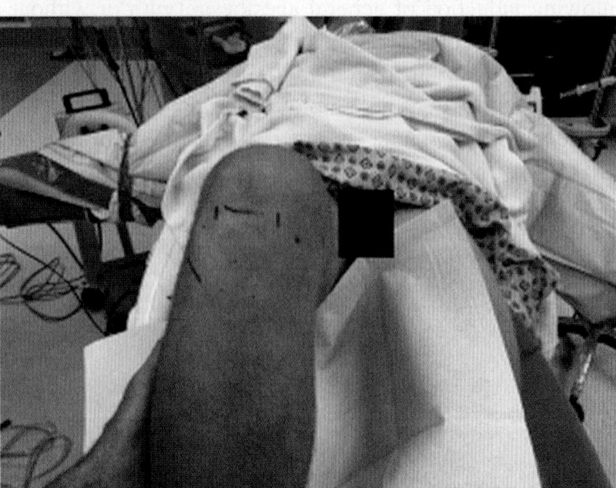

C

FIGURE 8-1

Anatomic landmarks (**A**), proposed skin incisions (**B**), and portal sites (**C**).

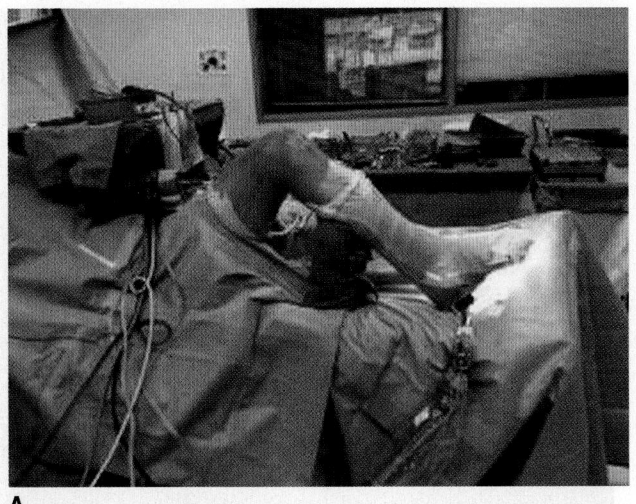

A

B

FIGURE 8-2

A, B: Operating room setup and positioning.

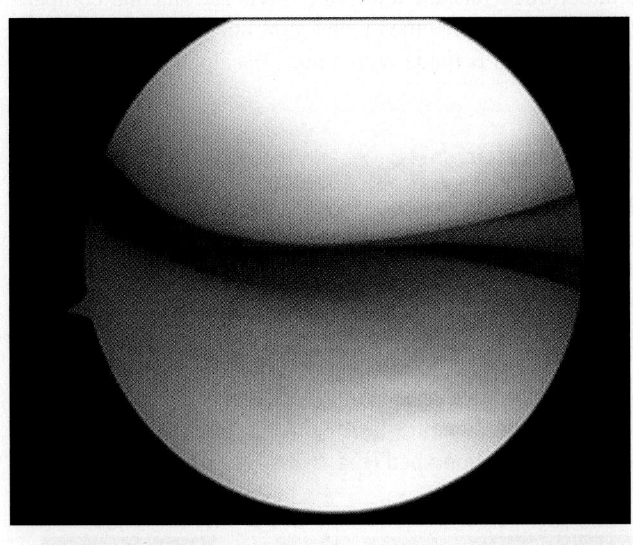

FIGURE 8-3

Diagnostic arthroscopy of the medial compartment revealing an otherwise normal compartment.

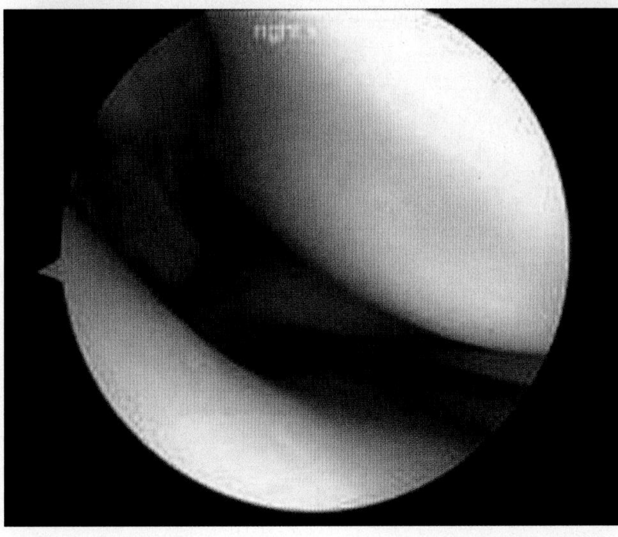

FIGURE 8-4

An arthroscopic probe placed through the anteromedial portal showing hemorrhage at the meniscal root.

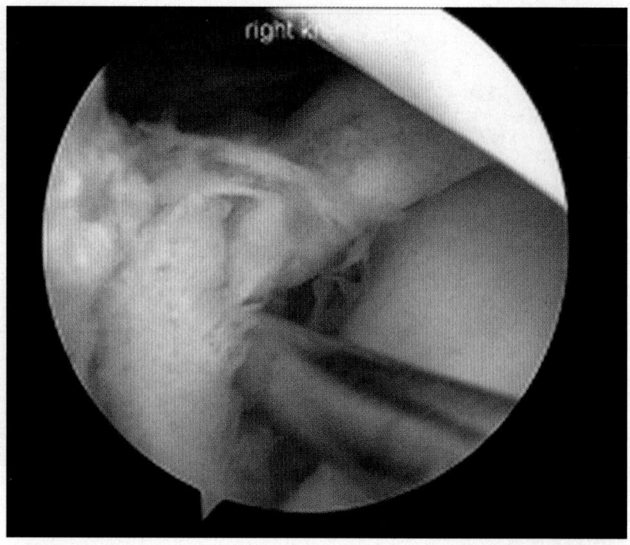

FIGURE 8-5

Gillquist view of the posteromedial compartment. The 70-degree arthroscope is passed between the PM bundle of the PCL and the medial femoral condyle, allowing direct visualization of the meniscal root insertion site.

staying lateral to the medial femoral condyle and under the posteromedial bundle of the posterior cruciate ligament.

An 18-gauge spinal needle is placed under direct visualization into the posteromedial compartment (Fig. 8-6A). This is typically placed 10 mm proximal the medial joint line and 5 mm posterior the medial femoral condyle. A vertical stab incision is made with a no. 11 scalpel, cutting into the capsule under direct visualization (Fig. 8-6B).

Preparation of Meniscus and Insertion Site

The surgeon should be well aware of the meniscal root insertions as shown in Figure 8-7. Johnson et al. (41) defined the size and geometry of the root insertions, and LaPrade et al. (42) further defined these roots in relation to other intra-articular structures. They demonstrated the anteromedial root is about 27.5 mm anterior to the medial tibial spine. The anterolateral root is about 14.4 mm anteromedial to the lateral tibial spine and 5.0 mm anterolateral to the center of the ACL. If desired, fluoroscopy can be used to help identify the insertion sites as described by James et al. (43).

Once the insertion site is identified, a curved 4.5-mm shaver is introduced through the posteromedial portal, and the site is prepared down to bleeding bone for healing. An arthroscopic rasp is also used to help facilitate the preparation of the bleeding bony bed (Fig. 8-8A,B).

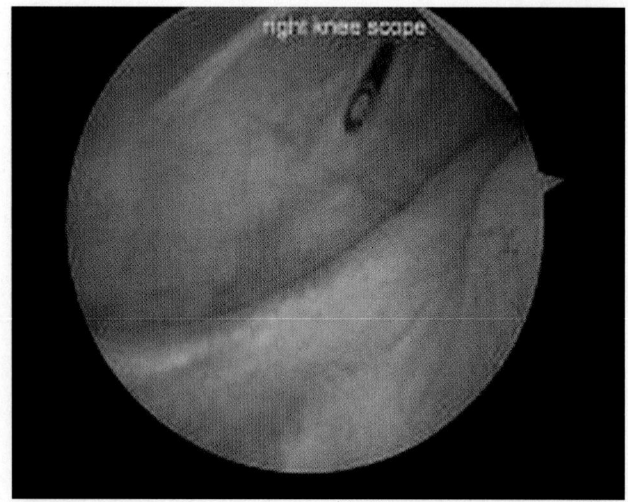

A

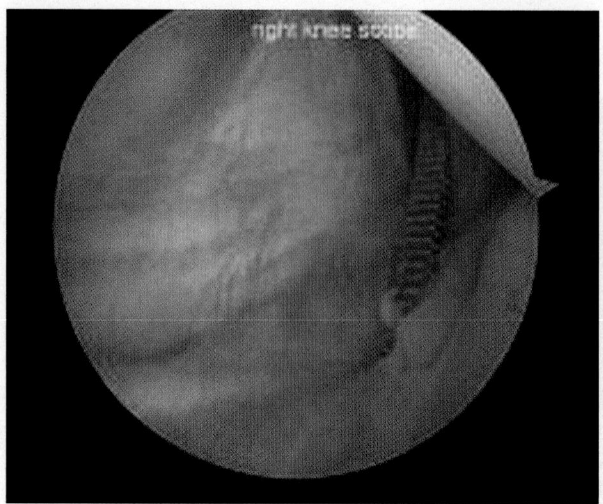

B

FIGURE 8-6

A, B: The posteromedial portal is placed under direct visualization.

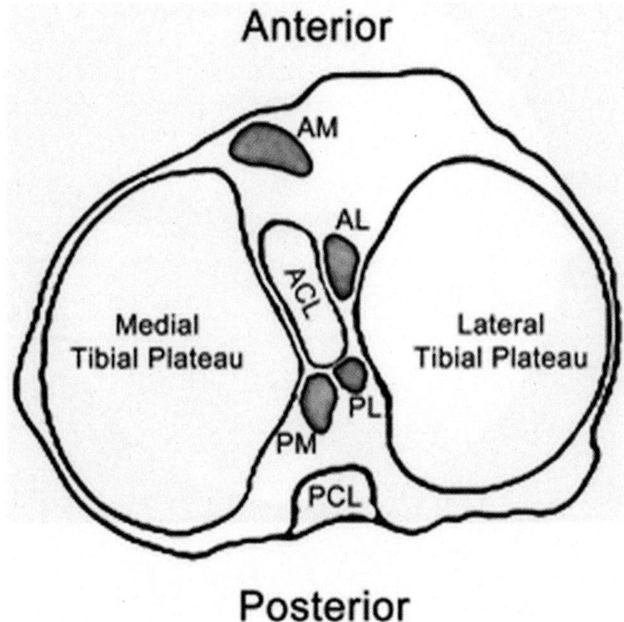

FIGURE 8-7

Diagram depicting the root insertion sites of the medial and lateral menisci.

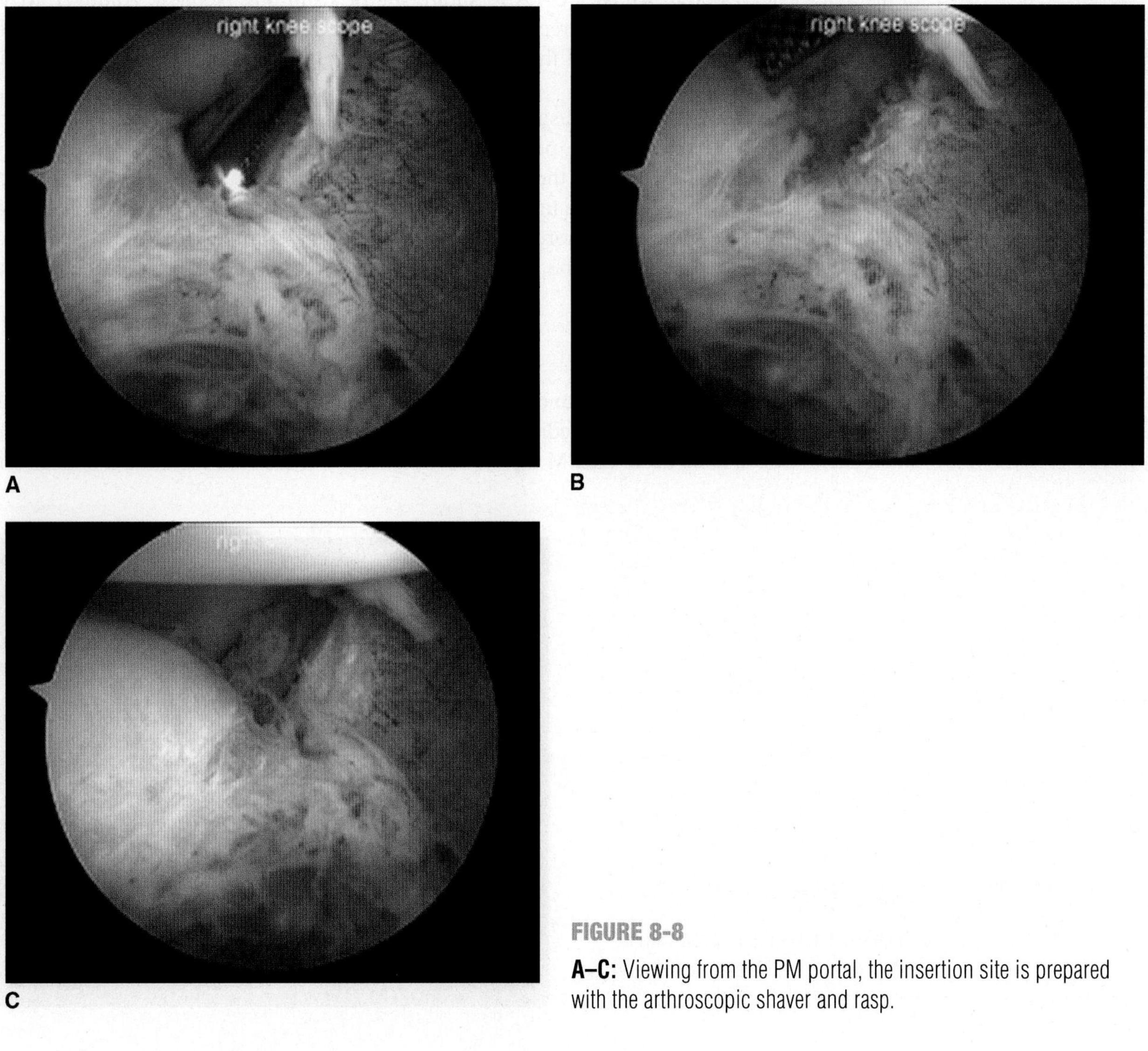

A

B

C

FIGURE 8-8

A–C: Viewing from the PM portal, the insertion site is prepared with the arthroscopic shaver and rasp.

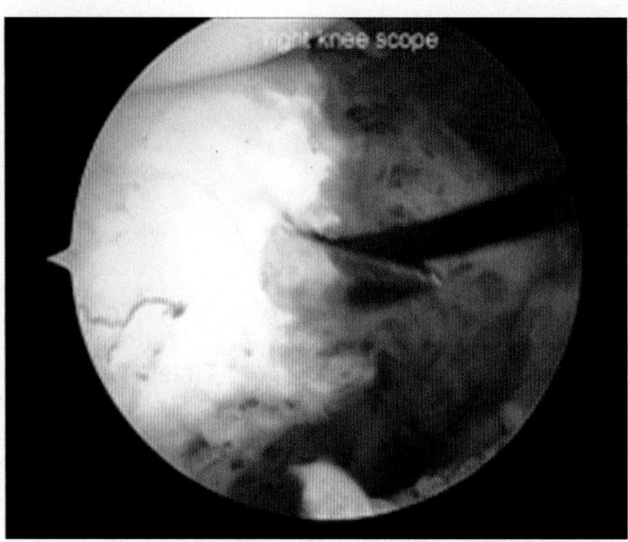

FIGURE 8-9

The free ends of the Ultrabraid suture are then placed through the loop and passed through the meniscus.

Suture Passage

The arthroscope is placed in the posteromedial portal (Fig. 8-8C). In our experience, suture passage is most easily accomplished through the anterolateral portal. An 8-mm cannula is first placed in the anterolateral portal. An ACCU-PASS suture shuttle (Smith & Nephew, Andover, MA) is placed through the cannula and pierces the meniscal tissue that is closest to the root insertion. The monofilament is advanced, and the looped end is retrieved and pulled through the cannula (Figs. 8-9 and 8-10).

The two ends of a 2-0 Ultrabraid suture (Smith & Nephew, Andover, MA) are subsequently placed in the looped monofilament, pulled through the meniscal root and back out through the cannula (Fig. 8-11). The ends are then placed through the loop of the 2-0 Ultrabraid suture and pulled tight to create a luggage tag construct. These steps are then repeated with a second 2-0 Ultrabraid suture to pass the more medial of the two-loop stitches (Fig. 8-12). Two transtibial sutures have been shown to be better than one with regard to stiffness, elongation, and failure load (44).

Tunnel Preparation

The tibial tunnel can be drilled prior to or after passage of the sutures. The meniscal root insertion is best visualized through the posteromedial portal. An ACUFEX ACL tip guide is passed through the anterolateral portal, underneath the PM bundle of the PCL and toward the insertion site (Fig. 8-13).

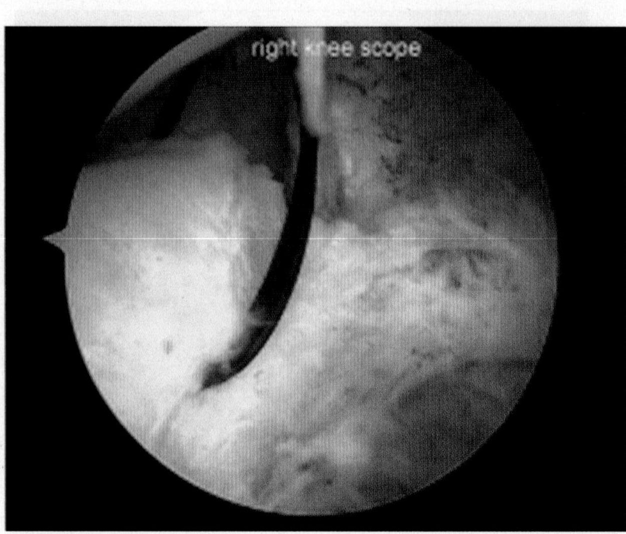

FIGURE 8-10

The meniscal root is pierced with a suture passer, and the monofilament loop is pulled through the AL portal.

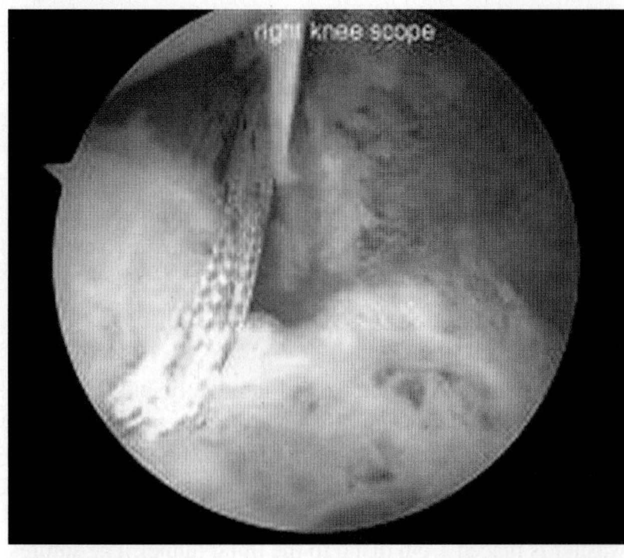

FIGURE 8-11

The free ends of the Ultrabraid suture are then passed through the loop and the meniscal root.

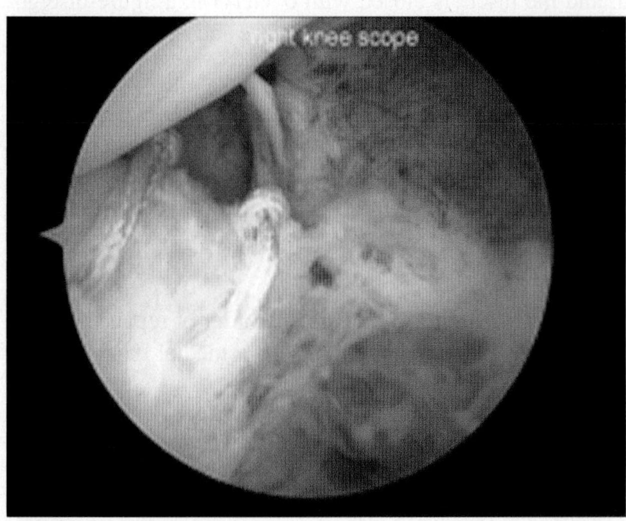

FIGURE 8-12

The loop is then cinched down via the "luggage tag" technique, and these steps are repeated again for a second suture.

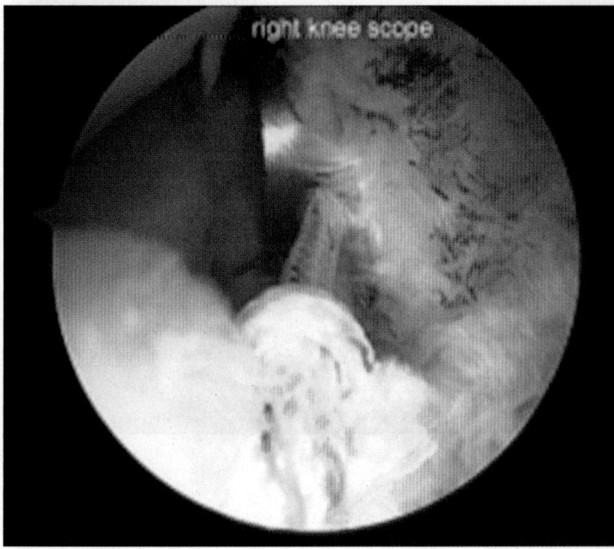

FIGURE 8-13

An ACL tip guide is placed through the AL portal at the anatomic insertion site. The guide is seated externally just distal to the lateral flare of the tibia.

The drill sleeve is then placed through the tip guide, and its position on the skin in relation to the proposed incision mark is confirmed.

A 3-cm incision over the previous mark is then made, and sharp dissection is carried down to the periosteum. The periosteum is sharply incised and elevated off the tibia to accommodate the ACUFEX drill sleeve and placement of a 6.5-mm AO cancellous screw and washer, which will serve as final fixation.

The drill sleeve is then placed onto the exposed lateral tibia and under direct arthroscopic visualization; a 3/32-in. guide pin is drilled to (but not through) the far cortex. The tunnel is completed with controlled, gentle tapping of the guide pin with a mallet.

Fixation

A Hewsen suture passer (Smith & Nephew, Andover, MA) is introduced into the tibial tunnel. The arthroscope is then placed in the anteromedial portal and through the anterolateral portal; a suture retriever is used to pull the Hewsen loop into the anterior aspect of the intercondylar notch. The suture strands are placed through the Hewsen loop, and then the loop is pulled through the tunnel (Fig. 8-14A,B).

A 6.5-mm AO cancellous screw and washer is placed 1 cm distal to the tibial tunnel. The sutures are then tied down over the screw/suture post with the knee in 30 degrees of flexion. The arthroscope is placed back into posteromedial portal to confirm reduction of the meniscal root (Fig. 8-15A,B). The wound is then thoroughly irrigated, and the fascia is closed with 0 Vicryl in a figure-of-eight fashion, followed by 2-0 Vicryl and 3-0 Monocryl for the subcutaneous tissue and skin, respectively.

Medial Meniscal Root Tear Specifics

- Visualization for medial meniscal root repair is improved through the creation of a posteromedial portal large enough to accommodate the arthroscope and for instruments to be passed.
- The reverse notchplasty as described above is especially helpful for passage of the instruments.

Lateral Meniscal Root Tear Specifics

As lateral meniscal root tears are seen almost entirely with ACL tears, the order of repair is important. The remainder of the procedure is otherwise performed similarly to a medial meniscal root repair with the following exceptions.

- Following the diagnostic arthroscopy, the ACL graft should be harvested, and the torn ligament is subsequently debrided using a full radius resector. Once completed, the lateral meniscal root tear is addressed next (Fig. 8-16A,B).

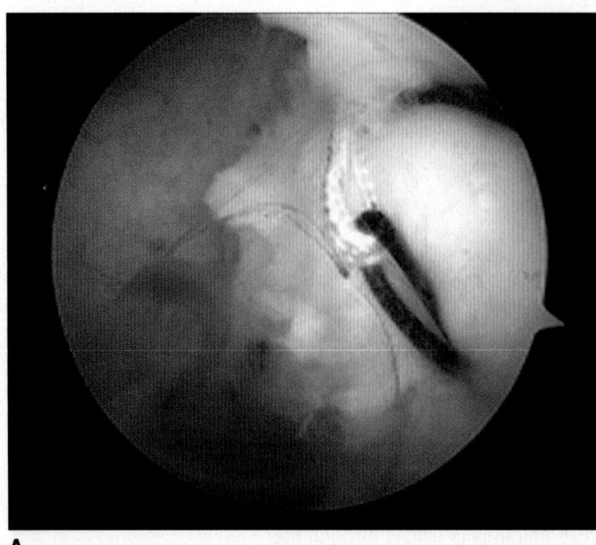

A

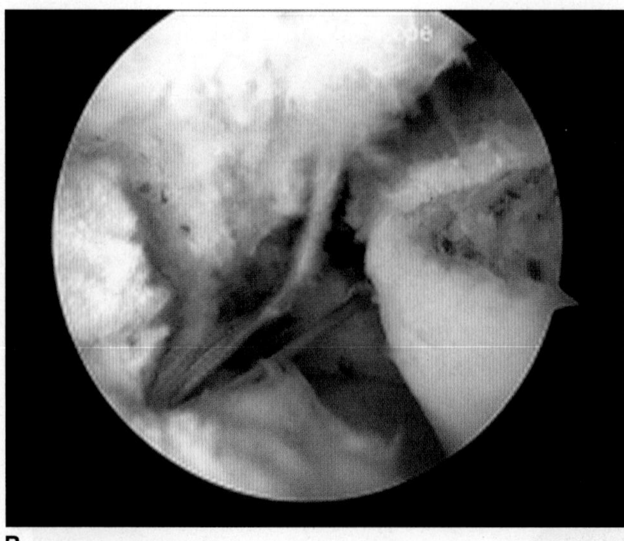

B

FIGURE 8-14

A, B: Following drilling of the tunnel with a 3/32-in. guide pin, a Hewsen suture passer is used to shuttle the suture through the tibial tunnel.

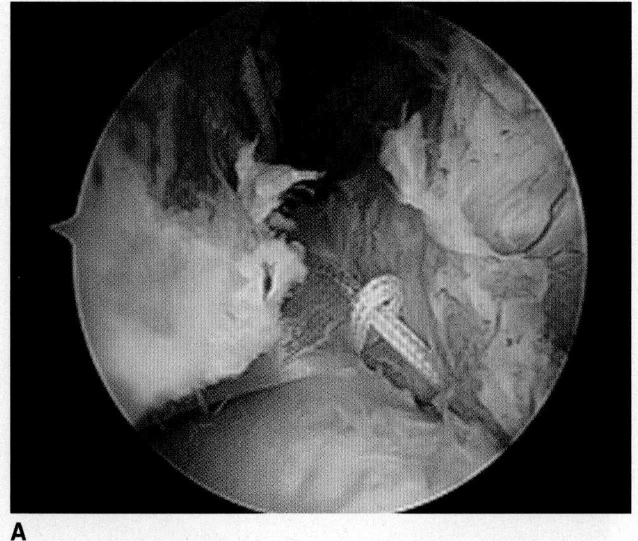
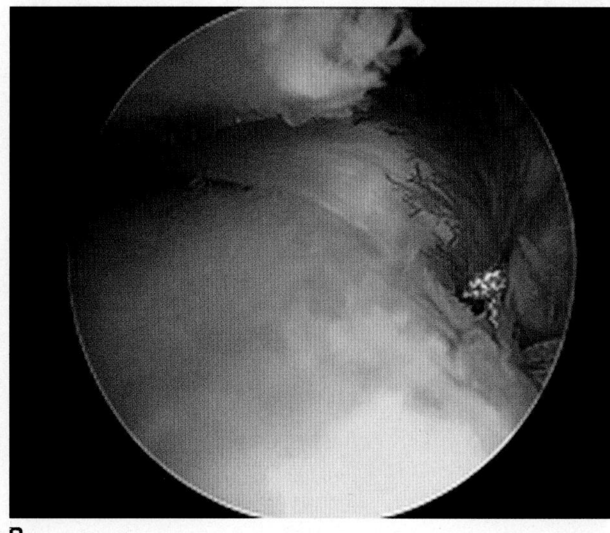

A B

FIGURE 8-15

A, B: PM view of the meniscal root unreduced and reduced.

- A figure-of-four position helps open the lateral compartment. Placing the arthroscope in the anterolateral portal will aid in visualization.
- The ACL tip targeting guide is introduced through the anteromedial portal. With the ACL debrided away, there should be adequate space to place the ACL targeting guide in the appropriate anatomic location (Fig. 8-17).
- The same tibial incision used for ACL graft harvest (anteromedial tibia) can be undermined and expanded to allow for the lateral meniscal root tunnels, which will be more posterior to the ACL tunnel. This should prevent tunnel intersection, although one can ensure this by pulling on the meniscal root sutures and viewing intra-articular with the arthroscope to make sure the sutures have not been cut.
- An 8-mm clear cannula can be placed through the anteromedial portal. Through this portal, the suture shuttling device is passed so that a soft tissue bridge does not develop between the sutures (Fig. 8-18).
- The lateral meniscal root repair is tensioned and secured with the knee in 30 degrees of flexion. This is done after the ACL graft has been passed, but prior to fixation of the ACL on the tibia. The sutures can be secured over a 4.5-mm cancellous screw used for ACL fixation or over a separate button (Fig. 8-19).
- If the tear is a peri-insertional radial tear (A), a standard meniscal repair technique can be employed (B) (Fig. 8-20).

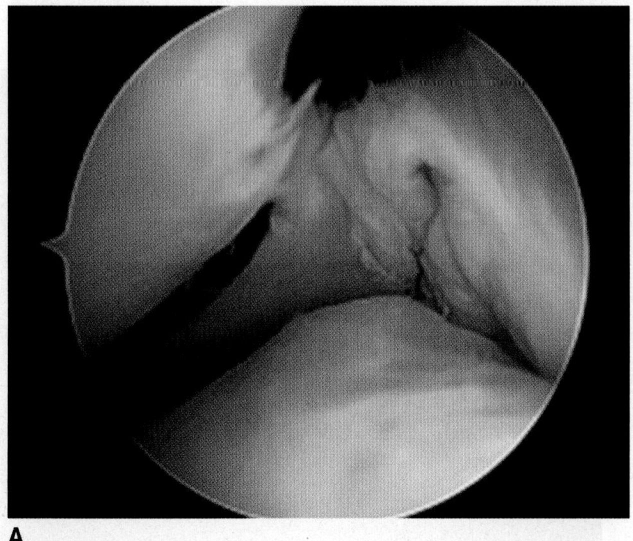
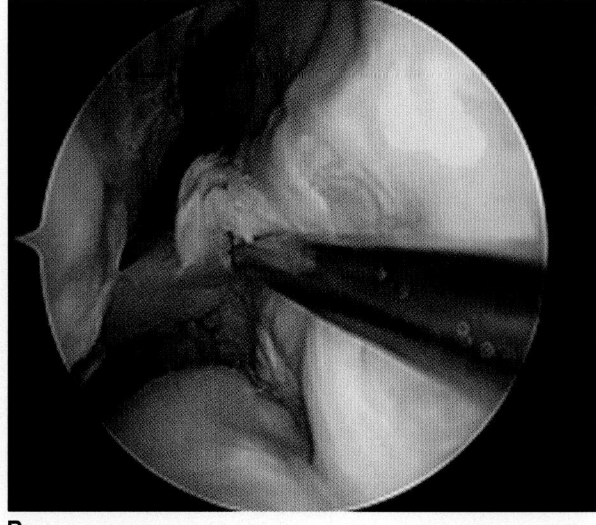

A B

FIGURE 8-16

A, B: With the ACL debrided, the lateral meniscal root can easily be probed and examined.

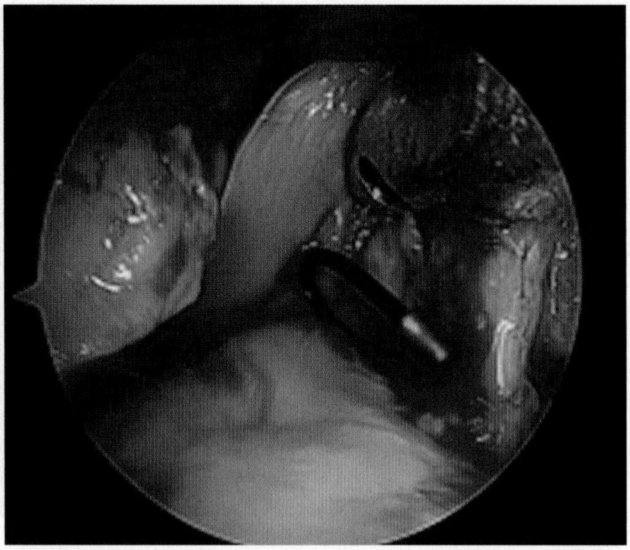

FIGURE 8-17

A Hewson suture passer is pushed through the posterior root tunnel. The tunnels are created prior to suture passage.

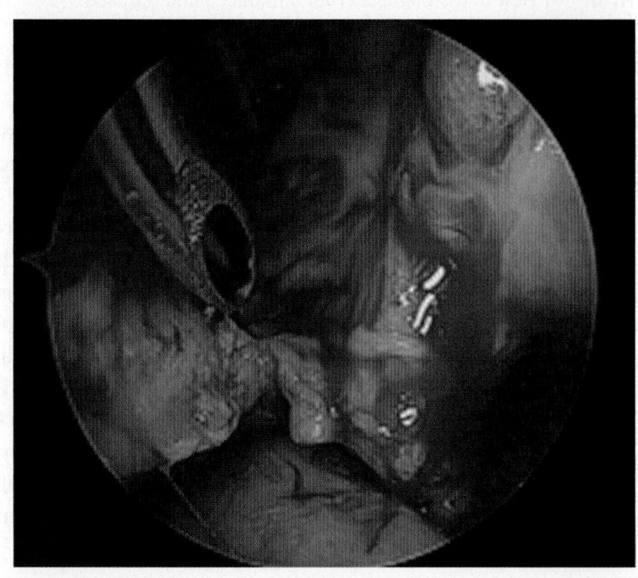

FIGURE 8-18

The suture-passing device is entered through the anteromedial portal.

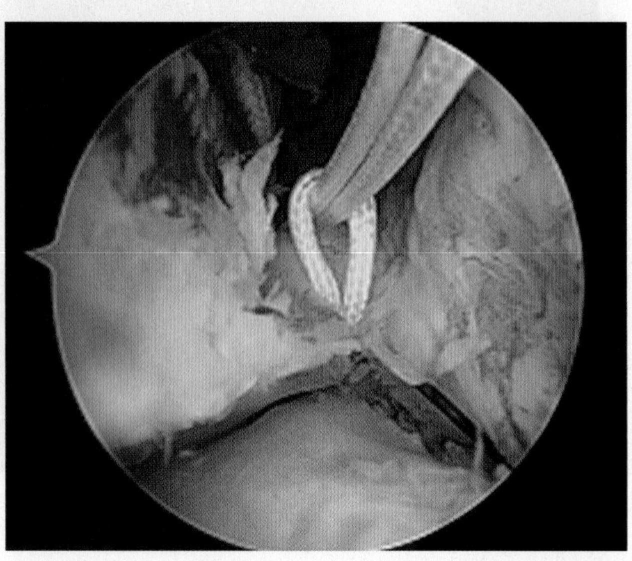

FIGURE 8-19

A luggage tag knot is created through the posterior root.

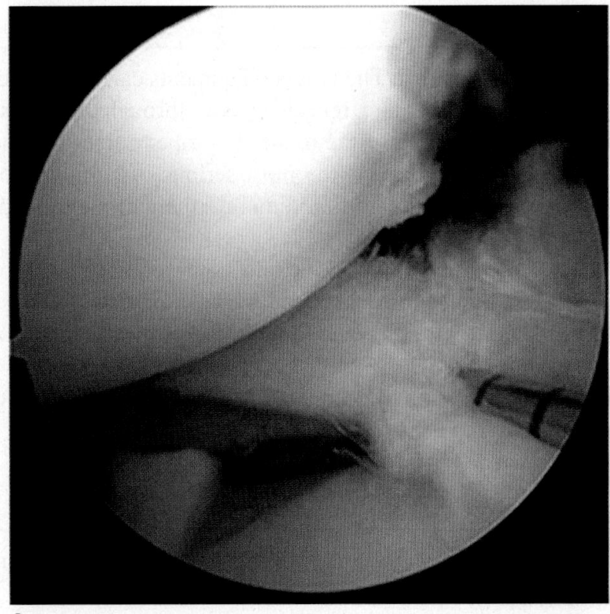

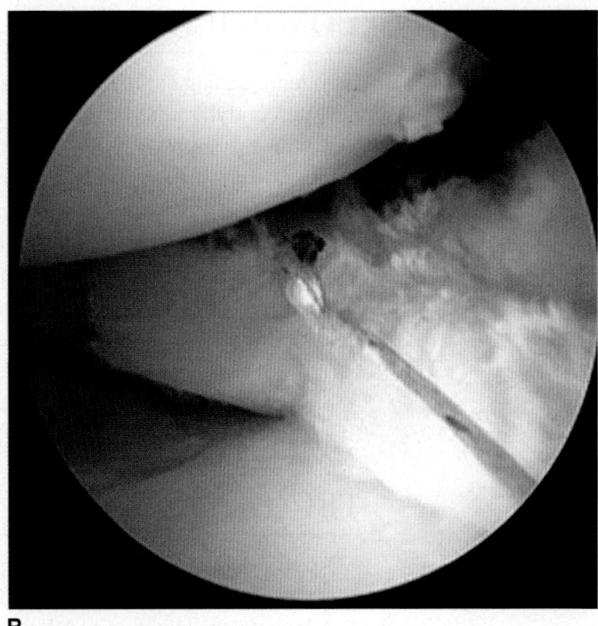

FIGURE 8-20
Peri-insertional radial split lateral meniscal tear (**A**). In this scenario, a standard meniscal repair technique can be employed (**B**).

Rehabilitation

Kopf et al. (4) demonstrated regardless of fixation type used; without proper healing, none of the constructs recreated the strength of the native roots (about 100 N vs. 600 N). Moreover, the strength of the repair is less than the native strength during initial healing as the AM, PM, PL roots have supplemental fibers, which are not surgically repaired. These supplemental fibers have been shown to contribute substantially to the ultimate failure strength (45). For all these reasons, rehabilitation must be performed cautiously to allow for proper healing prior to stressing the repair.

After repair, the medial meniscal posterior root experiences higher forces with internal rotation and flexion (46). These positions should be avoided during rehabilitation. Cyclical loading should also be avoided during rehabilitation (47). After proper healing is completed, studies have demonstrated improvement in tibiofemoral contact forces (18).

Our postoperative rehabilitation protocol is summarized in Table 8-5.

TABLE 8-5 Postoperative Rehabilitation Protocol

- Immediately after surgery
  - Non–weight-bearing using crutches
  - Hinged knee brace locked in 20 degrees of knee flexion
- Weeks 1–6 postsurgery
  - Range-of-motion exercises from 0 to 90 degrees of knee flexion
  - ± Continuous passive motion machine
  - Isometric quadriceps exercises (straight leg raises and quadriceps sets)
  - Calf pumps
  - Heel slides to 90 degrees
- Weeks 6–8 postsurgery
  - Begin progression to full weight bearing and wean off crutches under supervision of a physical therapist
  - Develop normal gait pattern
- Weeks 8–16 postsurgery
  - Begin functional exercises
  - Continue to work on restoring quadriceps strength
- 4 months postsurgery
  - Allow return to sports (for isolated meniscal root repair) depending on restoration of quadriceps strength, range of motion, and ability to perform sport-specific tasks
  - Avoid deep knee flexion to avoid retearing the meniscal root

COMPLICATIONS

Iatrogenic damage at the time of surgery must be avoided. The cruciate ligaments can be injured in the intercondylar notch with instrument passage. Furthermore, repeated passes through the meniscal root with the suture-passing device can cause weakening of the tissue. Improper guide pin placement can injure the popliteal neurovascular structures and is the most serious of complications. Nonanatomic repair of the meniscal root can lead to altered tibiofemoral kinematics and lead to accelerated progression of osteoarthritis.

When a proper repair is performed, other complications can include suture creep and/or abrasion within the tunnels causing root fixation failure. Furthermore, in the case of lateral meniscal root repair, the meniscal root tunnels can intersect with the ACL tibial tunnel if the surgeon is not careful.

Similar to any knee arthroscopic procedure, other complications include infection, deep venous thrombosis, postoperative knee stiffness, and wound dehiscence.

TECHNICAL PEARLS

- Appropriate patient indications, amenable root tear characteristics, and healthy articular cartilage status are a must for all patients undergoing surgery.
- Adequate visualization and detailed understanding of root insertion anatomy are the keys to success.
- For medial meniscal root repair, an accessory posteromedial portal should be utilized for improved visualization and instrumentation.
- A reverse notchplasty (interval between PCL and the medial femoral condyle) will allow for ease in instrumentation (suture passage, tunnel creation, etc.) in medial meniscal root repair.
- Defining the posterior edge of the meniscus by clearing away synovium and soft tissue will aid in suture passage.
- Two-loop sutures are preferable to one (able to perform in 80% of cases). In degenerative tissue, only one looped suture may be possible without damaging the tissue.
- If using two sutures, pass the suture closer to the root first. By pulling on the loop suture, it will translate the root anteriorly and increase tension across the tissue thereby facilitating ease in passage of the second loop suture.
- In lateral meniscal root repair with concurrent ACL injury, perform the root repair (with exception of tying it down) prior to passing the ACL graft.
- In lateral meniscal root repair with concurrent ACL injury, make sure the tunnels of the meniscal root repair and the ACL do not intersect.
- Patients should be made aware that deep flexion will be restricted permanently to avoid retearing the repair.

REFERENCES

1. Bhatia S, LaPrade CM, Ellman MB, et al. Meniscal root tears: significance, diagnosis, and treatment. *Am J Sports Med.* 2014;42(12):3016–3030.
2. Fithian DC, Kelly MA, Mow VC. Material properties and structure-function relationships in the menisci. *Clin Orthop Relat Res.* 1990(252):19–31.
3. Koenig JH, Ranawat AS, Umans HR, et al. Meniscal root tears: diagnosis and treatment. *Arthroscopy.* 2009;25(9):1025–1032.
4. Kopf S, Colvin AC, Muriuki M, et al. Meniscal root suturing techniques: implications for root fixation. *Am J Sports Med.* 2011;39(10):2141–2146.
5. Shaw HM, Benjamin M. Structure-function relationships of entheses in relation to mechanical load and exercise. *Scand J Med Sci Sports.* 2007;17(4):303–315.
6. Abraham AC, Moyer JT, Villegas DF, et al. Hyperelastic properties of human meniscal attachments. *J Biomech.* 2011;44(3):413–418.
7. Hauch KN, Villegas DF, Haut Donahue TL. Geometry, time-dependent and failure properties of human meniscal attachments. *J Biomech.* 2010;43(3):463–468.
8. Yao J, Lancianese SL, Hovinga KR, et al. Magnetic resonance image analysis of meniscal translation and tibio-meniscofemoral contact in deep knee flexion. *J Orthop Res.* 2008;26(5):673–684.
9. Vedi V, Williams A, Tennant SJ, et al. Meniscal movement. An in-vivo study using dynamic MRI. *J Bone Joint Surg Br.* 1999;81(1):37–41.
10. Abraham AC, Villegas DF, Kaufman KR, et al. Internal pressure of human meniscal root attachments during loading. *J Orthop Res.* 2013;31(10):1507–1513.
11. Papalia R, Vasta S, Franceschi F, et al. Meniscal root tears: from basic science to ultimate surgery. *Br Med Bull.* 2013;106:91–115.

12. Sung JH, Ha JK, Lee DW, et al. Meniscal extrusion and spontaneous osteonecrosis with root tear of medial meniscus: comparison with horizontal tear. *Arthroscopy.* 2013;29(4):726–732.
13. Allaire R, Muriuki M, Gilbertson L, et al. Biomechanical consequences of a tear of the posterior root of the medial meniscus. Similar to total meniscectomy. *J Bone Joint Surg Am.* 2008;90(9):1922–1931.
14. Marsh CA, Martin DE, Harner CD, et al. Effect of posterior horn medial meniscus root tear on in vivo kinematics. *Orthop J Sports Med* 2014 2014;2(7). doi: 10.1177/2325967114541220.
15. Guermazi A, Hayashi D, Jarraya M, et al. Medial posterior meniscal root tears are associated with development or worsening of medial tibiofemoral cartilage damage: the multicenter osteoarthritis study. *Radiology.* 2013;268(3):814–821.
16. Schillhammer CK, Werner FW, Scuderi MG, et al. Repair of lateral meniscus posterior horn detachment lesions: a biomechanical evaluation. *Am J Sports Med.* 2012;40(11):2604–2609.
17. Starke C, Kopf S, Grobel KH, et al. The effect of a nonanatomic repair of the meniscal horn attachment on meniscal tension: a biomechanical study. *Arthroscopy.* 2010;26(3):358–365.
18. Kim JG, Lee YS, Bae TS, et al. Tibiofemoral contact mechanics following posterior root of medial meniscus tear, repair, meniscectomy, and allograft transplantation. *Knee Surg Sports Traumatol Arthrosc.* 2013;21(9):2121–2125.
19. Kim JH, Chung JH, Lee DH, et al. Arthroscopic suture anchor repair versus pullout suture repair in posterior root tear of the medial meniscus: a prospective comparison study. *Arthroscopy.* 2011;27(12):1644–1653.
20. Lee DW, Kim MK, Jang HS, et al. Clinical and radiologic evaluation of arthroscopic medial meniscus root tear refixation: comparison of the modified Mason-Allen stitch and simple stitches. *Arthroscopy.* 2014;30(11):1439–1446.
21. Jung YH, Choi NH, Oh JS, et al. All-inside repair for a root tear of the medial meniscus using a suture anchor. *Am J Sports Med.* 2012;40(6):1406–1411.
22. Kim SB, Ha JK, Lee SW, et al. Medial meniscus root tear refixation: comparison of clinical, radiologic, and arthroscopic findings with medial meniscectomy. *Arthroscopy.* 2011;27(3):346–354.
23. Lee DH, Lee BS, Kim JM, et al. Predictors of degenerative medial meniscus extrusion: radial component and knee osteoarthritis. *Knee Surg Sports Traumatol Arthrosc.* 2011;19(2):222–229.
24. Lee JH, Lim YJ, Kim KB, et al. Arthroscopic pullout suture repair of posterior root tear of the medial meniscus: radiographic and clinical results with a 2-year follow-up. *Arthroscopy.* 2009;25(9):951–958.
25. Nicholas SJ, Golant A, Schachter AK, et al. A new surgical technique for arthroscopic repair of the meniscus root tear. *Knee Surg Sports Traumatol Arthrosc.* 2009;17(12):1433–1436.
26. Ozkoc G, Circi E, Gonc U, et al. Radial tears in the root of the posterior horn of the medial meniscus. *Knee Surg Sports Traumatol Arthrosc.* 2008;16(9):849–854.
27. Shelbourne KD, Roberson TA, Gray T. Long-term evaluation of posterior lateral meniscus root tears left in situ at the time of anterior cruciate ligament reconstruction. *Am J Sports Med.* 2011;39(7):1439–1443.
28. Pagnani MJ, Cooper DE, Warren RF. Extrusion of the medial meniscus. *Arthroscopy.* 1991;7(3):297–300.
29. Kim YJ, Kim JG, Chang SH, et al. Posterior root tear of the medial meniscus in multiple knee ligament injuries. *Knee.* 2010;17(5):324–328.
30. Fox AJ, Bedi A, Rodeo SA. The basic science of human knee menisci: structure, composition, and function. *Sports Health.* 2012;4(4):340–351.
31. Walker PS, Erkman MJ. The role of the menisci in force transmission across the knee. *Clin Orthop Relat Res.* 1975(109):184–192.
32. Thompson WO, Thaete FL, Fu FH, et al. Tibial meniscal dynamics using three-dimensional reconstruction of magnetic resonance images. *Am J Sports Med.* 1991;19(3):210–215; discussion 215–216.
33. Bin SI, Kim JM, Shin SJ. Radial tears of the posterior horn of the medial meniscus. *Arthroscopy.* 2004;20(4):373–378.
34. Hwang BY, Kim SJ, Lee SW, et al. Risk factors for medial meniscus posterior root tear. *Am J Sports Med.* 2012;40(7):1606–1610.
35. Brody JM, Lin HM, Hulstyn MJ, et al. Lateral meniscus root tear and meniscus extrusion with anterior cruciate ligament tear. *Radiology.* 2006;239(3):805–810.
36. De Smet AA, Blankenbaker DG, Kijowski R, et al. MR diagnosis of posterior root tears of the lateral meniscus using arthroscopy as the reference standard. *AJR Am J Roentgenol.* 2009;192(2):480–486.
37. Feucht MJ, Bigdon S, Mehl J, et al. Risk factors for posterior lateral meniscus root tears in anterior cruciate ligament injuries. *Knee Surg Sports Traumatol Arthrosc.* 2015;23(1):140–145.
38. Lerer DB, Umans HR, Hu MX, et al. The role of meniscal root pathology and radial meniscal tear in medial meniscal extrusion. *Skeletal Radiol.* 2004;33(10):569–574.
39. Choi SH, Bae S, Ji SK, et al. The MRI findings of meniscal root tear of the medial meniscus: emphasis on coronal, sagittal and axial images. *Knee Surg Sports Traumatol Arthrosc.* 2012;20(10):2098–2103.
40. Harper KW, Helms CA, Lambert HS III, et al. Radial meniscal tears: significance, incidence, and MR appearance. *AJR Am J Roentgenol.* 2005;185(6):1429–1434.
41. Johnson DL, Swenson TM, Livesay GA, et al. Insertion-site anatomy of the human menisci: gross, arthroscopic, and topographical anatomy as a basis for meniscal transplantation. *Arthroscopy*. 1995;11(4):386–394.
42. LaPrade CM, Ellman MB, Rasmussen MT, et al. Anatomy of the anterior root attachments of the medial and lateral menisci: a quantitative analysis. *Am J Sports Med.* 2014;42(10):2386–2392.
43. James EW, LaPrade CM, Ellman MB, et al. Radiographic identification of the anterior and posterior root attachments of the medial and lateral menisci. *Am J Sports Med.* 2014;42(11):2707–2714.
44. Rosslenbroich SB, Borgmann J, Herbort M, et al. Root tear of the meniscus: biomechanical evaluation of an arthroscopic refixation technique. *Arch Orthop Trauma Surg.* 2013;133(1):111–115.
45. Ellman MB, LaPrade CM, Smith SD, et al. Structural properties of the meniscal roots. *Am J Sports Med.* 2014;42(8):1881–1887.
46. Starke C, Kopf S, Lippisch R, et al. Tensile forces on repaired medial meniscal root tears. *Arthroscopy.* 2013;29(2):205–212.
47. Cerminara AJ, LaPrade CM, Smith SD, et al. Biomechanical evaluation of a transtibial pull-out meniscal root repair: challenging the bungee effect. *Am J Sports Med.* 2014;42(12):2988–2995.

9 Meniscal Repair Using an All-Inside Technique

Andrew A. Millis and Richard D. Parker

The meniscus plays an important chondroprotective role in the long-term health of the knee. The long-term clinical results of meniscectomy suggest that meniscal removal increases the chances of developing osteoarthritis secondary to increased contact forces seen by the knee articular cartilage. Therefore, a trend toward meniscal repair and preservation has occurred over the past few decades in an attempt to preserve the native anatomy and biomechanics of the knee joint. Technological advances have allowed meniscal repair to be performed through an all arthroscopic technique discussed in this chapter—an all-inside meniscal repair. These devices allow for easier repair without an extensive open approach.

Meniscal repair techniques and devices have evolved over time. The first meniscal repairs were performed through an open approach to repair peripheral meniscal tears at the meniscal-capsular junction (1). With the advancement of arthroscopically assisted repairs, the inside-out technique was described by Henning in 1983 (2) and used to repair intrasubstance tears of the meniscus. The inside-out technique remains the gold standard by which all other meniscal repair techniques are compared. However, addressing posterior horn meniscal tears remained difficult using the inside-out technique. To address this issue, Morgan developed the "all-inside" meniscal repair technique using arthroscopic instruments to place vertically oriented sutures into longitudinal tears of the posterior horn. The technique uses arthroscopic knot tying and can be technically demanding, utilizing accessory posterior portals and curved suture passers. Morgan also described more anterior meniscal tears as a relative contraindication to his all-inside technique.

In response to the technical difficulties and limitations of the all-suture technique (first-generation all-inside repairs), various all-inside repair devices have been developed over the past 25 years and allowed expansion of indications for all-inside meniscal repair techniques. Second-generation all-inside meniscal repair devices eliminated the need for accessory posterior portals. These devices were composed of a nonabsorbable suture attached to a polyethylene bar that was inserted via a cannula and used a needle to pierce the meniscus and capsule (Smith & Nephew FasT-Fix, Andover, MA). After the polyethylene was placed through the meniscus and capsule, it was used as a backstop to arthroscopically tie the suture and secure the meniscal repair. These devices represented a large advancement as now all-inside meniscal repair could safely be performed through standard anterior arthroscopic portals. Additionally, these devices showed minimal risk to surrounding neurovascular structures by allowing the surgeon to adjust depth of penetration. However, a large disadvantage of these devices was difficulty tensioning the repair and inability to adjust the tension after knot placement.

Third-generation all-inside repair devices represented a shift away from the suture fixation of meniscus tears. These new devices included bioabsorbable screws, darts, staples, and arrows made of poly-L-lactic-acid (PLLA), a rigid polymer, that were placed across the tear and through the capsule. The Meniscal Arrow (Linvatec, Largo, Florida) was the most common third-generation device used. Initial short-term results with these devices were good, showing over a 90% clinical success rate at 2-year follow-up. However, several studies reported poor midterm follow-up clinical results with 28% to 42% failures at between 4- and 6-year follow-up. Additionally, the PLLA polymer proved not to be benign to the knee joint. Numerous case reports of inflammatory processes have been described, including cysts and inflammatory synovitis. The devices can also fail and migrate into the joint producing chondral damage.

Fourth-generation all-inside meniscal repair devices were developed to address the limitations of the second- and third-generation devices. This current set of all-inside repair devices is most similar to the

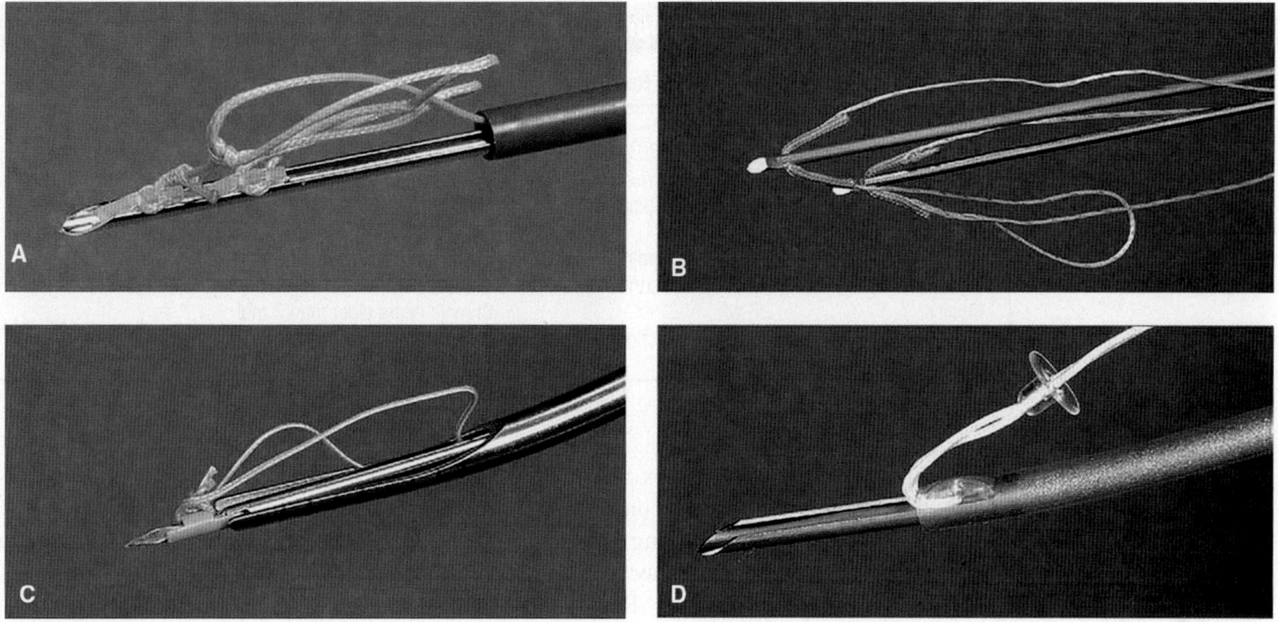

FIGURE 9-1
Fourth-generation, all-inside suture repair systems (**A**) Smith & Nephew FasT-Fix, (**B**) Biomet MaxFire, (**C**) Arthrex Meniscal Cinch, (**D**) DePuy Mitek RapidLoc. (From Starke C, Kopf S, Petersen W, et al. Meniscal repair. *Arthroscopy.* 2009;25(9):1033–1044, with permission.)

second-generation, suture-and-anchor devices and includes the FasT-Fix (Smith & Nephew, Andover, MA), RapidLoc (DePuy Mitek, Westwood, MA), Meniscal Cinch (Arthrex, Naples, FL), and the MaxFire (Biomet, Warsaw, IN) (Fig. 9-1A–D). However, unlike the second-generation devices, these new devices do not require arthroscopic suture knot tying and allow compression and re-tensioning of the repair as well as placement of vertical and horizontal mattress-type sutures. Our preferred fourth-generation device is the FasT-Fix 360, which is composed of two 5-mm anchors that are connected by a suture with a pretied sliding, locking knot. This eliminates the need to tie an arthroscopic knot.

These fourth-generation devices have shown good biomechanical results. Several studies have shown that these devices have load-to-failure strength comparable to inside-out mattress constructs and significantly improved load-to-failure strength compared to second-generation devices. However, other biomechanical studies still show 3.2 to 4.6 mm displacement with cyclic loading for these all-inside meniscus repair devices. As such, we recommend a small amount of overtightening at the time of insertion as some slippage is expected with loading.

Clinical studies have also shown successful outcomes of fourth-generation all-inside meniscal repair devices. Follow-up data are limited, but meniscal repairs with these devices appear more durable than the third-generation repair devices. A recent study by Bogunovic (3) showed a 16% failure rate for meniscal repair at a minimum of 5-year follow-up. These patients also reported favorable patient-based outcome measures including Knee injury and Osteoarthritis Outcome Score (KOOS), International Knee Documentation Committee (IKDC) score, and Marx activity scores. There was also no significant difference in the failure rate of meniscal repair between isolated repairs (12% failure) and meniscal repairs performed with concurrent anterior cruciate ligament (ACL) reconstruction (18% failure). As such, these fourth-generation devices are our implant of choice for the majority of meniscal repairs.

INDICATIONS/CONTRAINDICATIONS

Meniscal tears vary, and many factors dictate whether repair or meniscectomy is our preferred treatment. Table 9-1 shows factors that guide our decision making on whether to repair a meniscal tear. Our preferred meniscal tear to repair is a 1- to 4-cm longitudinal tear in the red-red zone of a younger patient with normal articular cartilage in the setting of an ACL reconstruction. Again,

TABLE 9-1 Indications for Meniscal Repair Versus Meniscectomy

	Meniscal Repair	Meniscectomy
Size	1–4 cm length	Larger than 4 cm, bucket-handle type tears
Patient age	Younger than 30 years old	Older than 50 years old
Articular cartilage	No arthritis	Grade III or IV articular surface changes
Alignment	Normal mechanical axis	Malalignment—consider correction of mechanical axis if repair attempted
Tear pattern	Vertical, longitudinal	Radial, complex/degenerative
Location	Peripheral—red/red zone	White zone
Acuity	<6 wk	Chronic (tears older than 3 mo)
Other injuries	ACL reconstruction	Articular cartilage damaged

these factors are more guidelines than dogma, and the individual patient, his/her activities, and tear personality/biology all contribute to our decision. It should be noted that small tears (<1 cm) that are stable to probing can generally be left alone and allowed to heal without operative fixation. These tears may be rasped or trephinated to encourage healing or left alone depending on surgeon preference. Regardless of repair technique, the indications for repair do not change.

Once the decision has been made to perform a meniscal repair, the tear location and type dictate our decision of repair technique to utilize. All-inside is our preferred technique for most tears. These tears tend to be 1 to 4 cm in size and in the posterior horn or body of the meniscus. Isolated anterior tears are more easily addressed with an outside-in technique. The gold standard inside-out repair is utilized most frequently for a larger, isolated tear or for fixation of meniscal allograft. In these cases, a mixed technique of using all-inside devices for the posterior horn and then inside-out sutures for the posterior body coming anteriorly has worked well for us.

For meniscal root avulsion tears, we prefer to repair the root back onto its insertion on the proximal tibia utilizing a transosseous suture technique. A FlipCutter (Arthrex, Naples, FL) is used to drill from the anterior proximal tibia onto the meniscal root insertion site of the posterior tibial joint line. A FlipCutter ACL guide is positioned and visualized during drilling using arthroscopic guidance. Once the FlipCutter has been passed through the tibia and the tip into the posterior knee joint, the FlipCutter is flipped and pulled down into the bone at the native site of meniscal root insertion to create a small approximately 5-mm deep trough to pull the root down into. We prefer to use the smallest available FlipCutter size (6.0 mm). The device is then "flipped" back into a straight drilling pin and removed. Suture is then passed through the meniscal root. We prefer to use an intra-articular Scorpion (Arthrex) suture passer through a cannula to do this. Then, the meniscal root suture is retrieved through the bone tunnel and tied over a button or tensioned and fixed with a PushLock anchor (Arthrex) into the anterior tibia. A summary of our technique preferences for meniscal tears is presented in Table 9-2.

TABLE 9-2 Preferred Meniscal Repair Technique Based on the Setting of the Repair

Repair Situation	Repair Technique Preferred
Concomitant ACL reconstruction	All-inside
Posterior horn	All-inside
Meniscal body	All-inside
Anterior horn	Outside-in
Meniscal root avulsion	Transosseous suture technique utilizing suture through the proximal tibia to reduce the root back onto its insertion
Larger circumferential/bucket-handle tears	Mixed technique using all-inside for the posterior horn and inside-out sutures for the remaining repair
Meniscal allograft	Mixed technique using all-inside for the posterior horn and inside-out sutures for the remaining repair

PREOPERATIVE PREPARATION

The most important part of the preoperative process is appropriately counseling the patient regarding the postoperative rehabilitation for both a meniscal repair and a meniscal debridement. We also then explain to the patient the likelihood of performing one versus the other as it drastically alters expectations for timing of return to work or athletic activities. We routinely obtain magnetic resonance imaging (MRI) scans for all planned meniscal surgeries in order to better counsel our patients preoperatively. The MRI scan allows us to characterize tear pattern, location, and concomitant injuries that may lean us toward meniscal repair rather than meniscectomy. Additionally, having an idea that the surgeon may perform a meniscal repair helps the operating facility and staff be prepared with appropriate setup, implants, and case length. Finally, if an open approach is planned near major neurovascular structures for the meniscal repair, having a vascular surgeon available is appropriate.

SURGICAL TECHNIQUE

Patient Positioning

We prefer to have the patient supine on the operating room table and raise the table and drop the foot of the bed. The operative leg is placed in an arthroscopic leg holder at the level of the distal femur, approximately 8 cm (one hand breadth) above the superior pole of the patella with the knee in full extension. This leg holder allows varus and valgus stress to be placed on the knee during the case for ease of visualization. A tourniquet can be applied to the thigh but is not routinely inflated for an isolated meniscus repair arthroscopic surgery.

Meniscal Preparation

Once a full diagnostic arthroscopy has been performed and a decision has been made to perform a repair of a meniscal tear, the meniscal tissue must be probed and investigated thoroughly to determine the best strategy for repair. Before beginning an all-inside repair, the meniscal tissue should be prepared to encourage healing. We prefer to use an arthroscopic rasp to roughen both edges of the meniscal tear (Fig. 9-2A,B). Additionally, if the capsular side of the tear does not have hemorrhagic or bleeding tissue, then an arthroscopic shaver or rasp can be used to debride underneath the tear to encourage a bleeding response (Fig. 9-2C). We do not routinely use trephination; however, this remains an appropriate option for creating vascular channels to more peripheral tears.

We do not typically utilize any fibrin clot or other biologic augmentation of the repair surface. Some case series report improved healing rates with adjunct fibrin clot use in the setting of isolated meniscal repairs (4). However, no randomized comparison of fibrin clot use to other meniscal repair preparation methods exists. Because clot use can be technically demanding and often leads to extra suture bulk at the repair site due to fixation of the clot to the undersurface of the repair, we do not recommend its use until more literature is available to confirm its improved healing potential. We have similar thoughts concerning platelet-rich plasma (PRP) and other current biologic augments and, thus, do not routinely use these adjuncts with our repairs.

Implant Insertion and Repair

Once the meniscal tear has been prepared, attention is then turned toward stable fixation of the tear. Our preferred device for an all-inside meniscal repair is the FasT-Fix 360 (Smith & Nephew). The device comes in three types: a straight needle, a 22-degree curved needle, and a reverse-curved 22-degree needle. Generally, we prefer the curved or reverse-curved device as it allows for easier implant deployment into the posterior meniscus. The curve allows for the surgeon to get underneath the femoral condyle easily without damaging the articular cartilage. Additionally, the curved and reverse-curved devices allow the surgeon to direct the needle away from neurovascular structures that may be immediately behind the repair location. The reverse-curved needle is also technically easier to use for fixation of a meniscal tear as the tear moves more anteriorly in the knee.

When inserting the FasT-Fix 360 device into the knee, a slotted cannula is used to facilitate easier passage of the device through the soft tissues and fat pad. After insertion into the knee, the cannula can be removed (Fig. 9-3). The needle-tipped inserter is then used to pierce the meniscus and/or capsule. The device has a depth of penetration limiter, which can be adjusted based on tear location in the knee. The limiter can be set from 10 to 18 mm. We generally set the limiter to 12 or

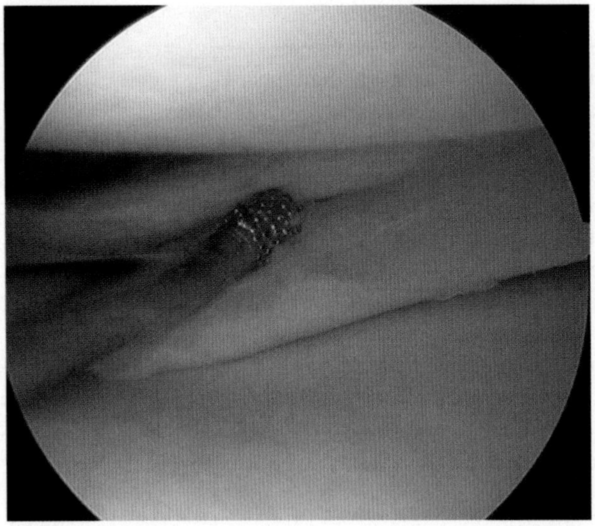

A

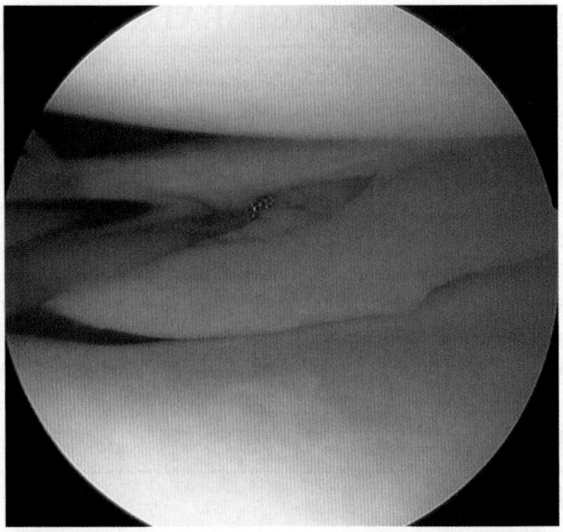

B

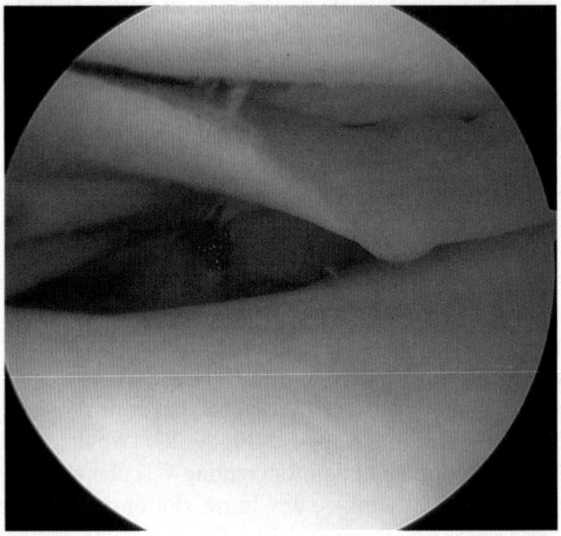

C

FIGURE 9-2

A, B: An arthroscopic rasp being used to prepare the edges of the meniscal tear prior to repair. **C:** The rasp being used to encourage bleeding from the capsule adjacent to the tear.

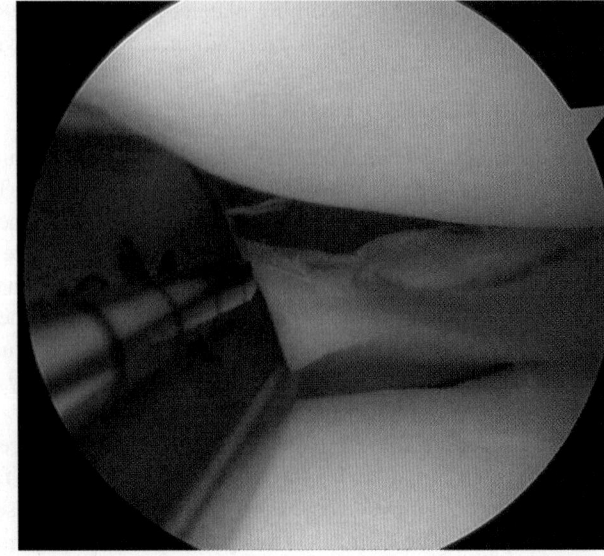

FIGURE 9-3

An insertion sled is used to facilitate passage of the FasT-Fix 360 needle system (Smith & Nephew) into the knee joint through an anterior portal. The sled may be removed after device insertion.

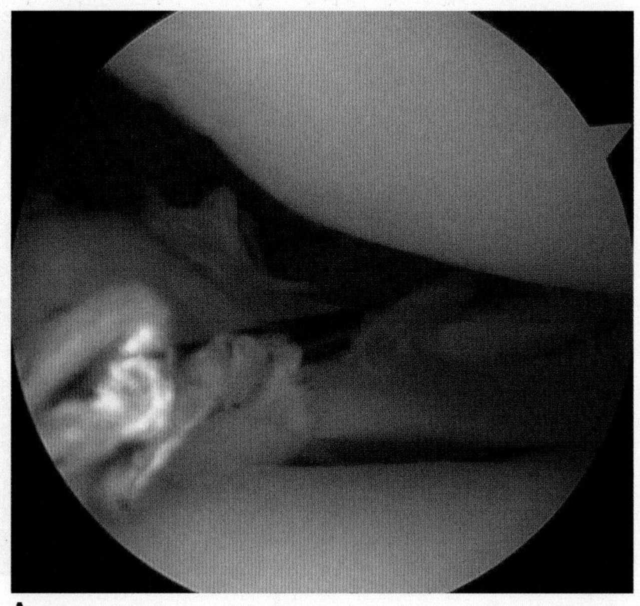
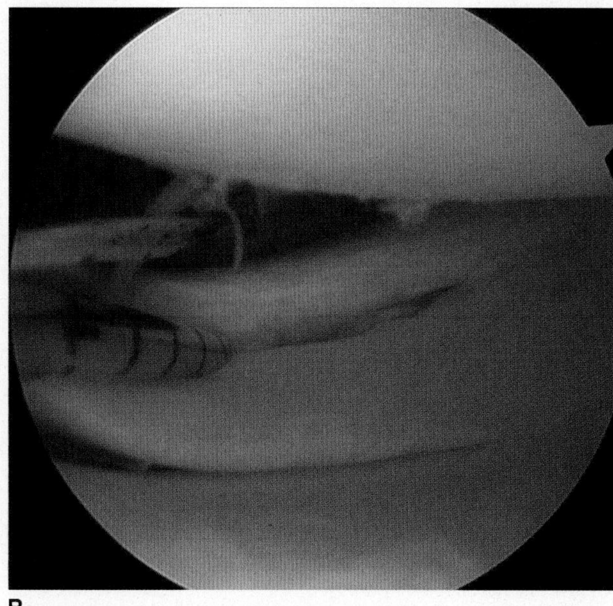

A B

FIGURE 9-4

A: Immediately prior to advancement of the first anchor through the meniscal and capsule tissue. **B:** After deployment of the first anchor onto the posterior aspect of the capsule.

13 mm, which is of sufficient depth to grab the tear tissue and capsule but also safe in relation to surrounding neurovascular structures. The first 5-mm anchor is then placed by passing the delivery needle through the meniscus and/or capsule and advancing the deployment slider. A backstop has been created by the first anchor. The deployment slider is then pulled back. The suture remains in the needle, which is now ready for its second pass (Fig. 9-4A,B).

The next pass with the needle determines the repair type. Both horizontal and vertical mattress stitches can be achieved with the FasT-Fix 360 device. Vertical mattress stitches are generally regarded as the strongest fixation and remain the gold standard for meniscal repair. However, horizontal mattress sutures are strong as well and may fit certain tear patterns better. We tend to utilize a mix of horizontal and vertical mattress sutures in our repairs depending on tear pattern.

After a type of stitch is selected, the needle is reinserted through the "free" edge of the tear, and the deployment slider is advanced forward a second time to deploy the second anchor (Fig. 9-5). It is very important to keep in mind the design of the device when placing these stitches. For the FasT-Fix system, the tensioning will draw the tissue *toward the second anchor*. After the second anchor is placed, the needle inserter is removed and the pretied sliding knot is now ready for tensioning.

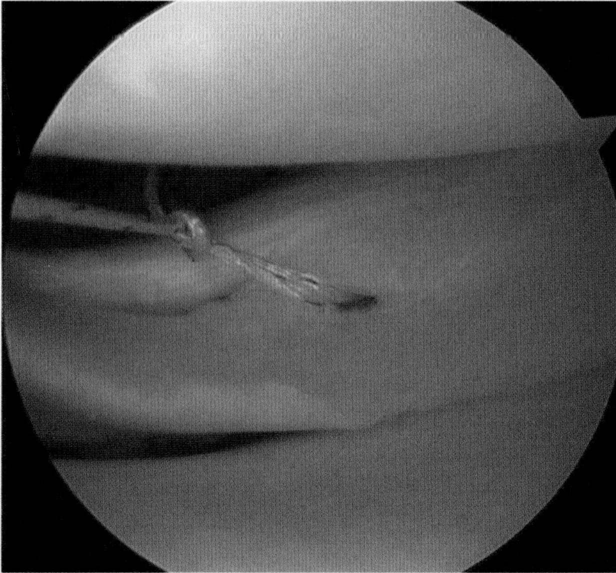

FIGURE 9-5

The second anchor has now been deployed, and the sliding knot is ready for tensioning the repair.

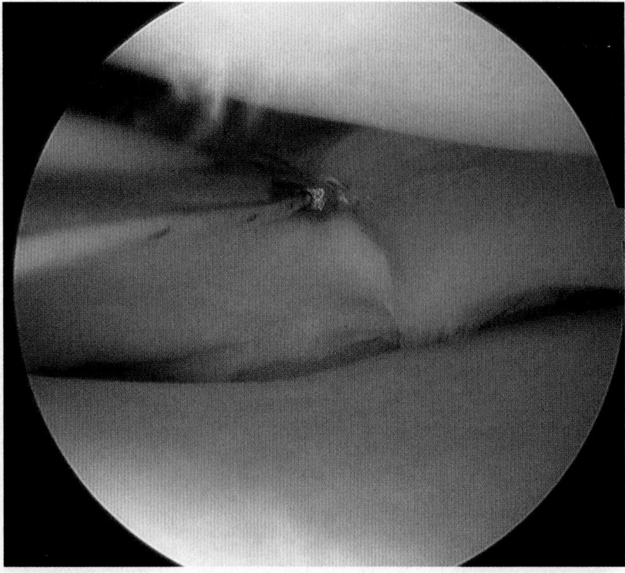

FIGURE 9-6

Tensioning the repair with the knot pusher/suture cutter. A "pucker" of the meniscus signifies appropriate tension prior to cutting the suture.

We *do not* recommend pulling too hard on the suture to advance the knot as this can pull the anchor back through the repair and capsule. This error makes this device ineffective and requires removal of the implant and starting over with a new all-inside device. Rather, utilize the knot pusher/suture cutter to advance the knot and tension the repair (Fig. 9-6). All of the available fourth-generation all-inside devices have been shown to slip at least several millimeters with repetitive loading in biomechanical studies (3.2 mm for the FasT-Fix and 4.6 mm for the RapidLoc used in vertical mattress fashion). Therefore, it is our preference to slightly over tension the repair with the assumption it will loosen with loading over time; we like to see the knot dimple or pucker the meniscal surface. Once tensioned, the trigger of the knot pusher/suture cutter device is advanced to cut the suture. Care is taken to make sure the device is directly against the knot to avoid leaving an excessively long suture tail in the joint.

This process is repeated until the tear is effectively stabilized. Periodic probing of the tear for gapping after each stitch placed is recommended to assess for tear fixation stability. The exact number of stitches needed depends mostly on tear length and tear pattern. However, using horizontal mattress stitches may also decrease the number of devices used. In general, we allow about 5 mm of space between stitches (Fig. 9-7A,B). Therefore, a 1-cm tear may only require one device placed in

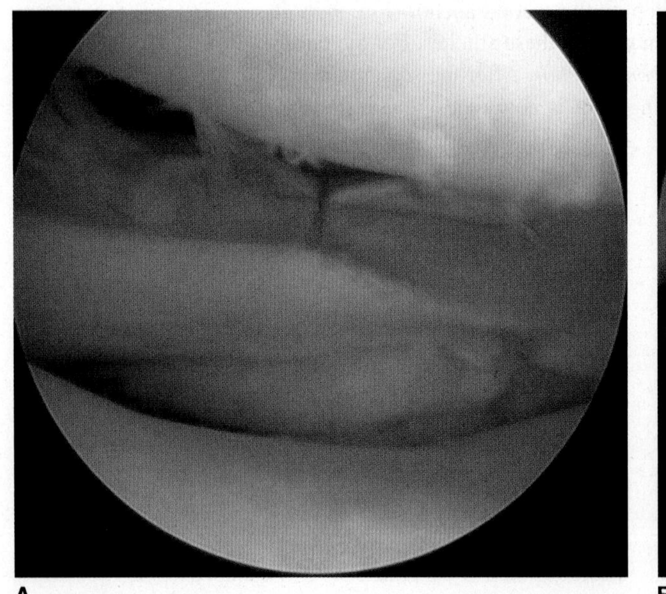

A

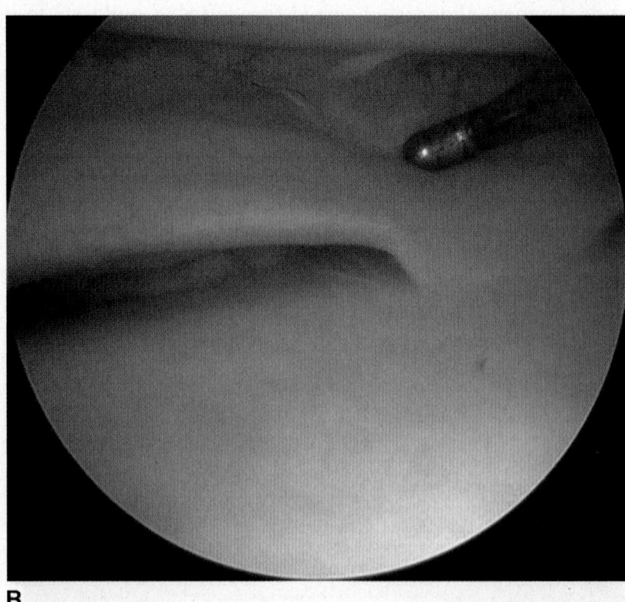

B

FIGURE 9-7

A: A completed all-inside repair. Note the stitches placed about 5 mm apart with no gapping in the repair. **B:** The repair is probed looking for any gapping of the repair.

the center of the tear using a vertical mattress stitch and so forth. After the repair has been stabilized, the knee is taken through a cycle of knee flexion and extension with the arthroscopic observing the repair for any gapping or displacement into the joint.

PEARLS AND PITFALLS

- All-inside devices are tools, and knowing how to use the tool you choose is critical. For example, knowing the direction of pull of the knot can affect the ability to appropriately reduce a displaced tear. Therefore, we recommend getting comfortable with one device and using it rather than utilizing several different all-inside devices.
- Biology is important for healing. Do not neglect preparation of the meniscal tear edges as this can be as critical to healing as tear fixation.
- Utilize *vertical mattress* stitches when able to.
- Place sutures approximately 5 mm apart until the tear is stable to probing.
- Use the inserter cannula for needle passage into the knee to avoid getting soft tissue and fat pad caught in the device.
- Slightly *over-tighten* the repair creating a "dimple" or "pucker."
- Do not be afraid to switch viewing and working portals. To continue placing all-inside stitches in a more anterior tear, it is often required to insert the device from the opposite portal to get the correct angle. Accessory portals can also be helpful.
- Know the limitations of all-inside repair and utilize other repair techniques when appropriate (Table 9-2).

POSTOPERATIVE MANAGEMENT

Biomechanical studies have shown all-inside meniscal repairs performed with fourth-generation suture–based devices to have similar biomechanical properties to the gold standard inside-out repair. Therefore, we do not adjust our rehabilitation protocol for all-inside repairs compared with inside-out or other repair techniques.

We use a brace for the first 4 weeks after surgery. The brace is locked in extension for ambulation for the first 4 weeks. The brace is unlocked from 0 to 90 degrees for range-of-motion exercises when not ambulating. The brace may be discontinued at 4 weeks if adequate quadriceps control is achieved in therapy. The patient is partial weight bearing for the first 4 weeks after surgery. For the first 2 weeks, the patient is 0% to 50% weight bearing. For weeks 2 to 4, the patient gradually advances to 75% weight bearing. It is important for the therapist to instruct them with percentage weight bearing utilizing a scale to avoid overzealous stress to the repair. At 1 month, the patient is made weight bearing as tolerated and active range of motion as tolerated. Tear pattern can delay progression. Generally, larger tears, more complex tears, and more central tears with less healing potential would favor a slower rehabilitation protocol, delaying full weight bearing and deep flexion for 6 to 8 weeks after repair. As the patient progresses with quadriceps strengthening, stretching, range of motion, and functional activities, return to sport can be considered. Generally, this will occur at 4 to 6 months after repair. Also, deep squatting especially with heavy weight is avoided for at least 4 months after repair.

COMPLICATIONS

There are numerous case reports in the literature regarding complications with all-inside meniscal repair devices. The most devastating complication with any meniscal repair is injury to neurovascular structures. This is extremely rare in the setting of an all-inside meniscal repair. However, proper technique utilizing the depth limiter of fourth-generation devices (set at <15 mm) and knowledge of anatomy around the knee joint can prevent these complications. Most reported complications with all-inside repairs involved articular cartilage damage secondary to third-generation meniscal repair devices like to be meniscal arrow. The head of the arrow device can score the articular cartilage during the motion. (The newest generation of the arrow has a less prominent head to minimize this complication.) There are also reports of the area devices becoming loose bodies and floating in the knee, damaging articular cartilage as well.

RESULTS

Our experience with newer generation all-inside repair devices has yielded satisfactory results. Our published data from the Multicenter Orthopaedic Outcomes Network (MOON) study group showed that meniscal repair in the setting of ACL reconstruction yielded an 86% survival at an average of 6 years after repair and ACL reconstruction. This is a heterogeneous group of surgeons with most utilizing third- or fourth-generation all-inside or inside-out meniscus repair techniques (5). A total of 235 (82.2% follow-up) meniscal repairs with ACL reconstruction were available for follow-up at 6 years post-op. Of these repairs, 154 were medial meniscus repairs, 72 lateral repairs, and 9 combined medial and lateral repairs. The predominant repair technique was all-inside repair: 90.3% (65/72) of lateral meniscus repairs were all-inside and 87.7% (135/154) of medial meniscal repairs used all-inside technique. 10/65 (15.4%) of all-inside lateral meniscus repairs had failed at 6 years. 19/135 medial all-inside repairs had failed at 6 years post-op. Of these failures, 9 of the 29 all-inside repair failures occurred in the setting of a revision ACL reconstruction, and the meniscal failures were addressed at the same revision surgery. Overall, all-inside technique was utilized in 88.5% of patients and had a 14.9% failure rate at 6 years.

Additionally, our data suggest that these all-inside techniques do well clinically in the setting of ACL reconstruction. The same group of patients from our MOON group showed sustained, improved IKDC scores 6 years after meniscal repair and ACL reconstruction. The median IKDC score at 6 years was 87.4 (74.7 to 95.4). There was no significant difference noted between IKDC scores at 2 and 6 years. This trend in sustained clinical outcomes held true for KOOS and Western Ontario and McMaster Universities Osteoarthritis Index score as well (5). These good midterm results with newer all-inside devices represent an improvement over prior deterioration of midterm results with third-generation devices like the meniscal arrow.

ACKNOWLEDGMENTS

We would like to acknowledge the Cleveland Clinic Foundation for its support of our education and research endeavors.

REFERENCES

1. DeHaven KE, Hales W. Peripheral meniscus repair: an alternative to meniscectomy. *Orthop Trans.* 1981;5:399–400.
2. Henning CE. Arthroscopic repair of meniscus tears. *Orthopedics.* 1983;6:1130–1132.
3. Bogunovic L, Kruse LM, Haas AK, et al. Outcome of all-inside second-generation meniscal repair: minimum five-year follow-up. *J Bone Joint Surg Am.* 2014;96:1303–1307.
4. Henning CE, Lynch MA, Yearout KM, et al. Arthroscopic meniscal repair using an exogenous fibrin clot. *Clin Orthop Relat Res.* 1990;252:64–72.
5. Westermann RW, Wright RW, Spindler KP, et al. Meniscal repair with concurrent anterior cruciate ligament reconstruction: operative success and patient outcomes at 6-year follow-up. *Am J Sports Med.* 2014;42(9):2184–2192.

RECOMMENDED READINGS

Barber FA, Herbert MA, Richards DP. Load to failure testing of new meniscal repair devices. *Arthroscopy.* 2004;20:45–50.

Kocabey Y, Chang HC, Brand JC, et al. A biomechanical comparison of the FasT-Fix meniscal repair suture system and the RapidLoc device in cadaver meniscus. *Arthroscopy.* 2006;22:406–413.

Kotsovolos ES, Hantes ME, Mastrokalos DS, et al. Results of all-inside meniscal repair with the FasT-Fix Meniscal Repair System. *Arthroscopy.* 2006;22(1):3–9.

Kurzweil PR, Tifford CD, Ignacio EM. Unsatisfactory clinical results of meniscal repair using the meniscus arrow. *Arthroscopy.* 2005;21(8):905.e1–905.e7.

Morgan CD. The "all-inside" meniscus repair. *Arthroscopy* 1991;7:120–125.

Rosso C, Kovtun K, Dow W, et al. Comparison of all-inside meniscal repair devices with matched inside-out suture repair. *Am J Sports Med.* 2011;39(12):2634–2639.

Turman KA, Diduch DR, Miller MD. All-inside meniscal repair. *Sports Health.* 2009;1(5):438–444.

10 Meniscal Repair: Inside-Out/Outside-In

Cristin J. Mathew, Randy M. Cohn, and Nicholas A. Sgaglione

INDICATIONS

Specific types of tears and clinical presentations determine decision making regarding meniscal repair and preservation.

- Location
  - To be repairable, a meniscal tear should usually be in a vascularized region of the meniscus (red-red zone or red-white zone).
  - Attempted meniscal repairs in the central white-white zone are controversial, with potentially increased failure rates.
  - Tears within 2 mm of the meniscal rim have the highest healing potential; tears greater than 4 mm from the meniscal rim have higher failure rates with attempted repair.
- Size
  - The length of a meniscal tear affects its stability, with tears less than 1 cm in length often being stable without repair and tears greater than 4 mm in length having higher failure rates with attempted repair.
- Tear pattern
  - Vertical tear patterns (i.e., bucket-handle pattern) are most amenable to repair.
  - Radial tear patterns that extend the entire width of the meniscus may be indicated for repair of the peripheral portion of the meniscus to the capsule and excision of the central avascular portion of the meniscus.
- Timing
  - There is no consensus on the definition of an acute versus chronic meniscal tear, and time periods ranging from 3 months to greater than 1 year have been cited in the literature.
  - In several studies, tears repaired within 6 weeks of injury have higher healing rates; however, this is controversial.
  - Several studies have shown no difference in healing rates or incidence of reoperation based on the time from the index injury to meniscal repair.
  - Higher failure rates have been reported with attempted meniscal repair greater than 1 year from injury.
- Patient age
  - Some studies have demonstrated higher rates of success with meniscal repair in patients under age 40; however, this is not consistent in the literature.
- Concomitant injuries
  - Meniscal repair is indicated with concomitant anterior cruciate ligament (ACL) reconstruction, if there is a repairable pattern of meniscal tear (Table 10-1).

CONTRAINDICATIONS

- Location
  - Meniscal repair is relatively contraindicated in tears isolated to the white-white zone of the meniscus, as there is no blood supply for healing of the tear.

TABLE 10-1 Indications for Meniscus Repair

- Tear between 1 and 4 cm in length
- Red-red zone tears
- Vertical and red-white tears
- Acute tears within 6 wk
- Concomitant ACL reconstruction

  - Tears extending from the peripheral portion of the meniscus into the central white-white zone may be amenable to repair, with potentially higher failure rates than tears isolated to the peripheral vascularized portions of the meniscus.
- Size
  - Failure rate of attempted meniscal repair may be higher in larger-sized tears, especially those greater than 4 cm in length. However, tear size is not an absolute contraindication to attempted repair.
- Tear pattern
  - Meniscal repair is relatively contraindicated in radial tear patterns isolated to the central avascular portion of the meniscus. Repair may be attempted in radial tears extending from the avascular region into the vascularized portion of the meniscus.
  - Horizontal cleavage patterns are usually not amenable to attempted repair.
  - Degenerative meniscal tears should not be repaired.
- Timing
  - There is no absolute contraindication for time from injury to attempted repair, as long as there is a repairable tear pattern.
- Patient age
  - There is no absolute contraindication to patient age and attempted repair, although failure rate may be higher in patients over 40 years of age.
- Concomitant injuries
  - Attempted repair may be contraindicated in cases with malalignment, instability, or severe degenerative joint disease (Table 10-2).

PREOPERATIVE PREPARATION

A focused history and physical examination are essential. It is important to ascertain injury mechanism, as well as complaints associated with intra-articular pathology such as swelling, mechanical symptoms, or giving way. Plain radiographs are obtained to evaluate alignment, bony pathology, and associated concomitant pathology such as osteochondritis dissecans or Segond sign, consistent with concomitant ACL injury. Recommended images include 45-degree posteroanterior flexion weight-bearing view, true lateral view, notch view, and patella skyline view (Fig. 10-1).

MRI is used to evaluate meniscal pathology and concomitant injuries. Potentially repairable meniscal tear patterns may be identified with MRI (Fig. 10-2A,B).

Risks and benefits of meniscal repair versus partial meniscectomy must be discussed with the patient preoperatively so the patient can better understand the short- and long-term natural history and consequences of meniscal surgery. The patient should be counseled preoperatively about the different rehabilitation protocols with meniscal repair versus partial meniscectomy.

A thorough examination under anesthesia is essential to detect associated patholaxity before beginning the procedure.

TABLE 10-2 Contraindications to Meniscus Repair

- Tears >4 mm from the rim (white-white zone)
- Tears <1 cm or >4 cm
- Horizontal degenerative tears
- Maligned, unstable, or degenerated joints

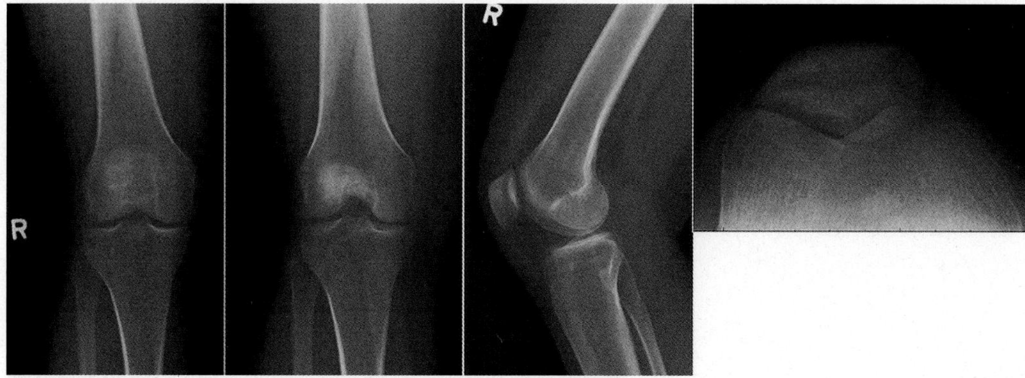

FIGURE 10-1

Radiographs of a 20-year-old female patient with a bucket-handle tear of the medial meniscus. Recommended radiographs include 45-degree posteroanterior flexion weight-bearing view, notch view, true lateral view, and patella skyline view.

TECHNIQUE

- Patient is placed in the supine position.
- A knee holder or lateral post is used to be able to provide valgus stress to the knee.
  - With use of a knee holder, the end of the table is dropped to allow the knee to flex. A knee holder also allows for application of varus stress when addressing the lateral meniscus.
  - With use of a lateral post, the knee is flexed by placing the leg off the side of the table.

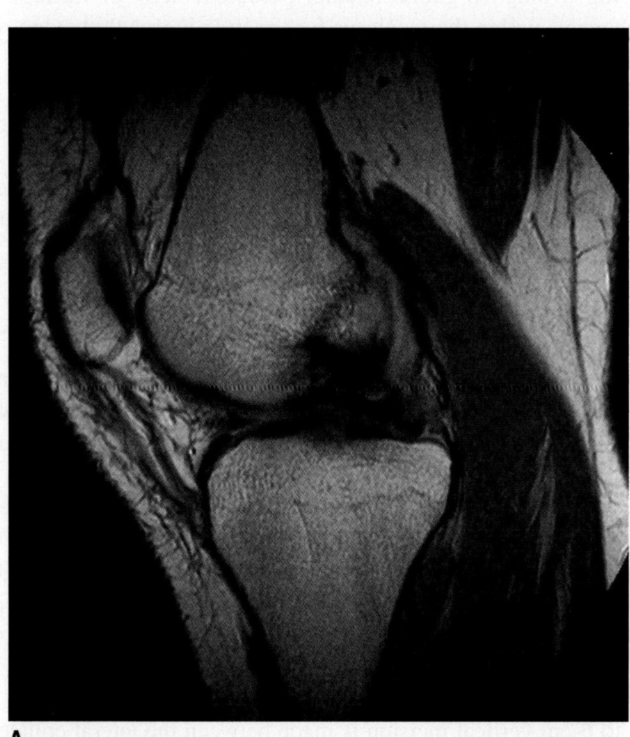

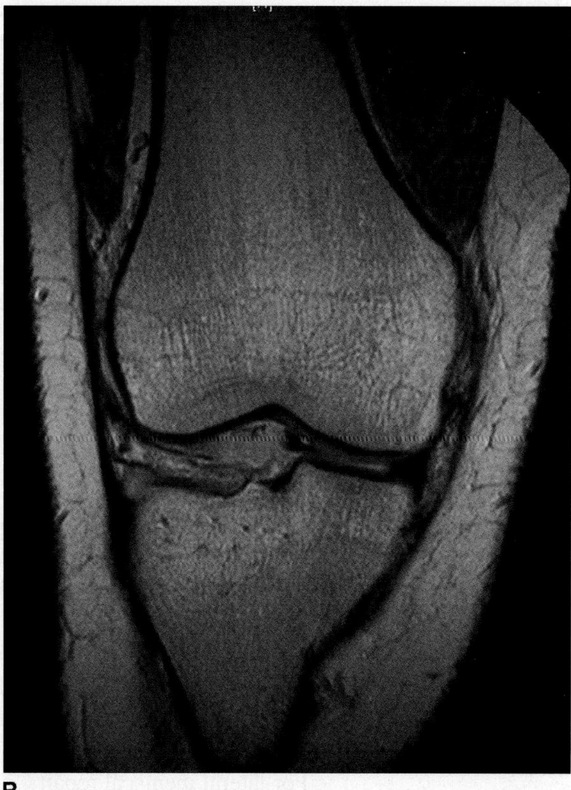

FIGURE 10-2

A: T1-weighted sagittal MRI cut depicting the "double PCL" sign, indicating a bucket-handle tear of the medial meniscus that is flipped centrally into the intercondylar notch. **B:** A T1-weighted coronal MRI cut again depicting a bucket-handle tear pattern. The medial meniscus appears truncated with the bucket-handle fragment flipped into the notch.

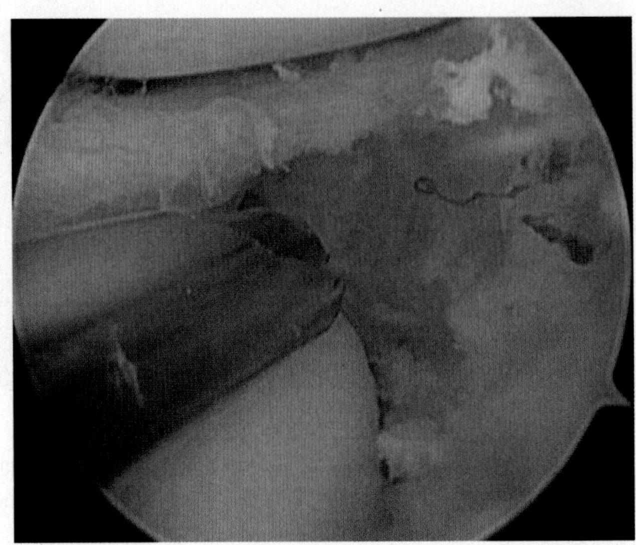

FIGURE 10-3

An arthroscopic photograph depicting the bleeding knee capsule after abrasion with an arthroscopic shaver. (Image courtesy of Dr. Andrew Goodwillie.)

- Prior to prepping and draping, the knee is taken through a range of motion to ensure that appropriate positioning has been achieved.
- A thigh tourniquet may be used to control intraoperative bleeding.
- The contralateral leg and all bony prominences are well padded.
- Standard anterolateral and anteromedial portals are used in the majority of meniscal repairs.
- Superomedial, superolateral, posteromedial, posterolateral, midpatellar, central, and far medial or lateral accessory portals may be used, as necessary.
- Rasping and trephination of meniscus tears may help stimulate vascular ingrowth and healing.
  - Rasping can be done with a meniscal rasp or arthroscopic shaver that lightly abrades the edges of tear site and meniscocapsular junction (Fig. 10-3).
  - Trephination is performed using a long 18-gauge needle, percutaneously or through an arthroscopic portal, to create channels within the meniscus for vascular ingrowth that are perpendicular to the meniscal circumferential fiber band.
- It is important to avoid overperforation of the femoral and tibial meniscal surfaces.
- In cases with a tight medial compartment in response to valgus stress opening, pie crusting of the medial collateral ligament (MCL) can be performed to avoid articular cartilage injury. An arthroscopic awl or 18-gauge spinal need can be used to create multiple punctures in the deep MCL with an applied valgus force. Begin posteriorly and proceed in an anterior direction until adequate visualization is achieved.

Inside-Out

This technique is best used for certain posterior horn, middle third, peripheral capsule and bucket-handle tear patterns (Fig. 10-4). The technique involves use of long flexible needles with nonabsorbable suture passed through contoured suture cannulas that pierce the meniscus and exit and captured through accessory posteromedial and posterolateral incisions (Fig. 10-5A,B).

Prior to suture passage, a posteromedial or posterolateral skin incision is made (based on side of meniscal repair) to capture needles and protect neurovascular structures.

For medial meniscal repairs, a 4- to 6-cm vertical incision is made just posterior to the MCL extending approximately one-third above and two-thirds below the joint line. Dissection proceeds anterior to the sartorius and semimembranosus muscles and deep to the medial head of the gastrocnemius. The knee is held in 20 to 30 degrees of flexion for suture passage to avoid tethering of the posteromedial capsule.

For lateral meniscal repairs, a 4- to 6-cm vertical incision is made between the lateral collateral ligament and biceps femoris tendon, with one-third above and two-thirds below the joint line.

This posterolateral incision is made with the knee in 90 degrees of flexion to increase the distance from the incision to the peroneal nerve, popliteus tendon, and inferior lateral geniculate artery.

Dissection is carried out between the iliotibial band and biceps tendon and then proceeds anterior and deep to the lateral head of the gastrocnemius. Once the capsule is exposed, a popliteal

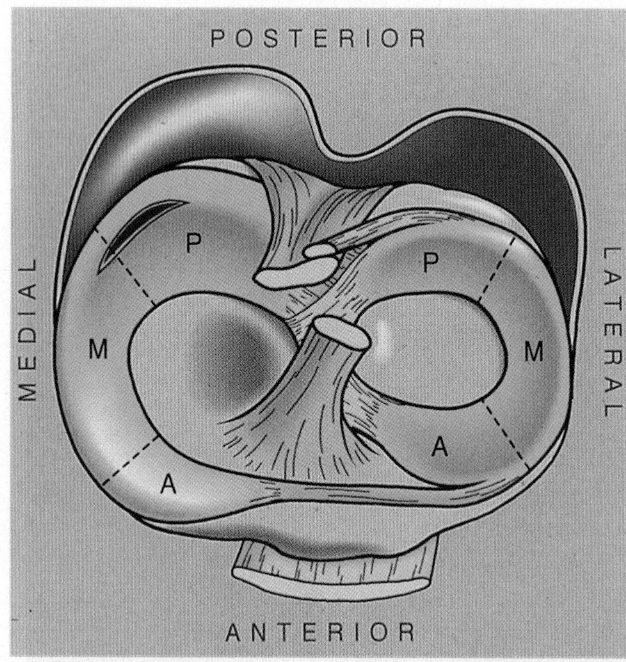

FIGURE 10-4

Illustration of a vertical meniscal tear in the posterior horn and body of the medial meniscus. This pattern is ideally suited for meniscal repair with an inside-out technique. (Image courtesy of ConMed.)

retractor or proprietary spoon is inserted posteriorly and used to retract the posterior midline structures including the neurovascular bundle (Fig. 10-6).

Several proprietary needle delivery devices exist to facilitate inside-out meniscal repair (i.e., Zone Specific II Meniscal Repair System, Conmed Linvatec, Edison, NJ; Meniscal Repair Joystick System, Arthrex, Naples, FL). Meniscal repair cannulas are passed through the arthroscopic portals to the region of the tear. Cannulas can be single or double lumen.

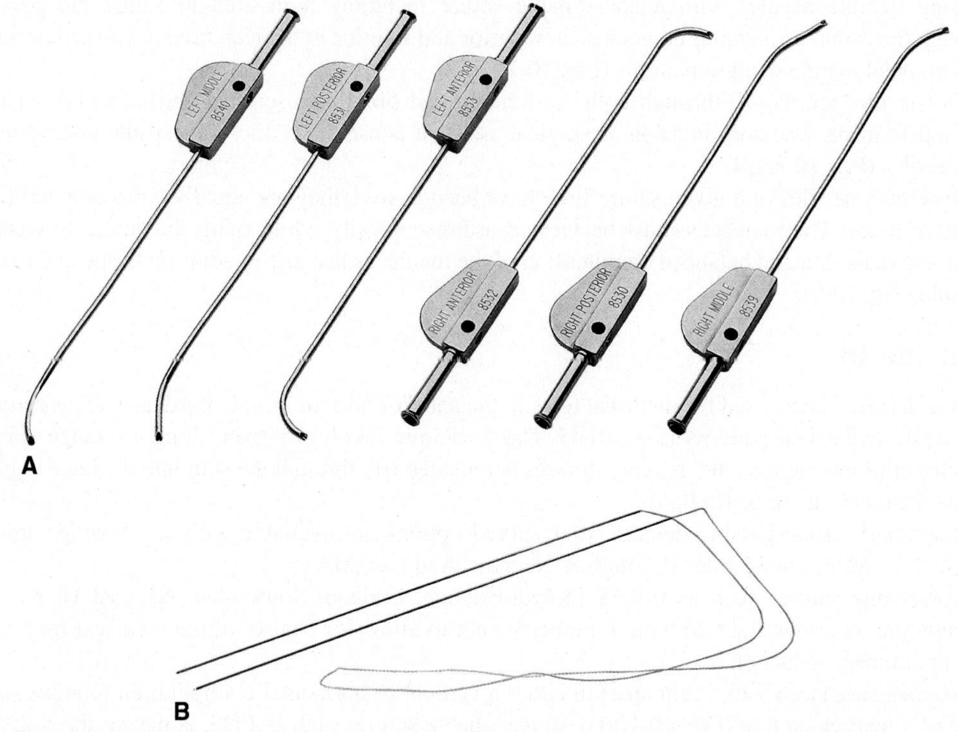

FIGURE 10-5

A: Precontoured cannulas for inside-out meniscal repair. The cannulas are specifically designed to target the anterior, middle, and posterior third of each meniscus. **B:** Long flexible double-armed needles with nonabsorbable suture ideally suited for meniscal repair. (Images courtesy of ConMed.).

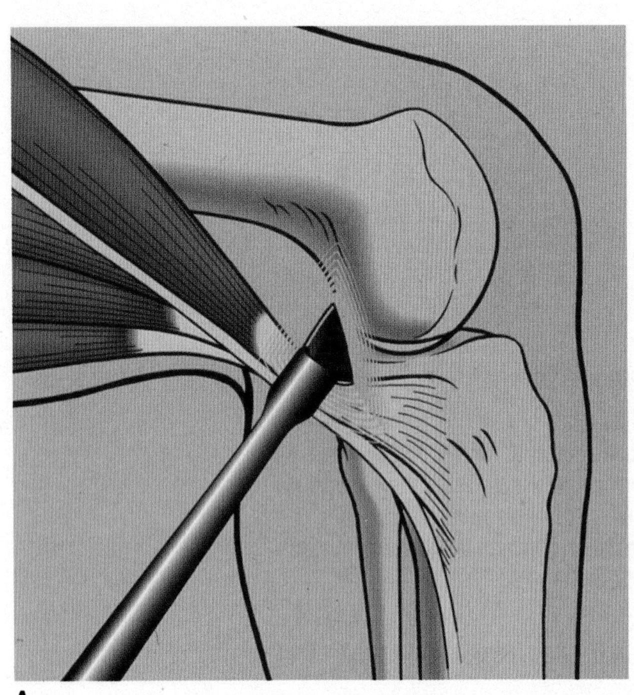

A

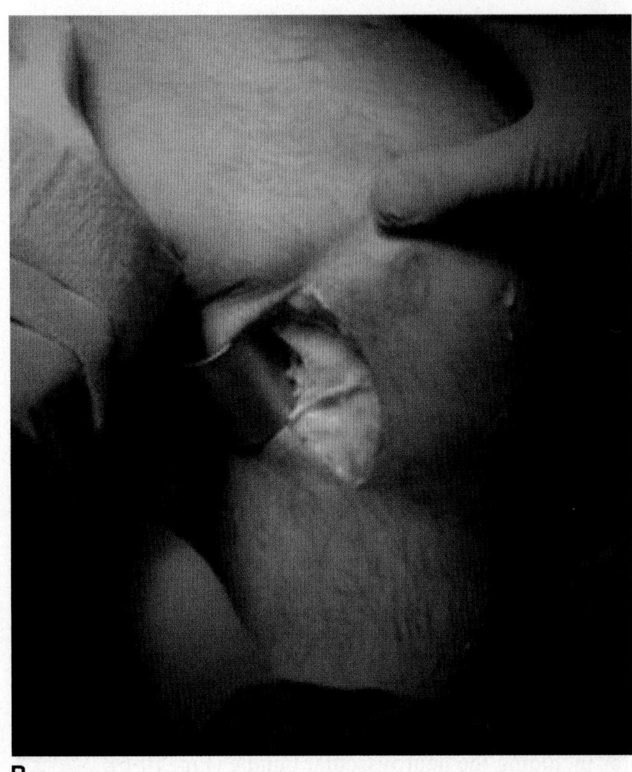

B

FIGURE 10-6

A: Illustration of a lateral meniscal repair. The popliteal retractor has been placed to protect the neurovascular bundle. (Image courtesy of ConMed.) **B:** Placement of a popliteal retractor with exposure to the capsule.

Long flexible needles with nonabsorbable suture including high-strength suture are passed through the cannulas piercing the meniscus superior and inferior to the tear, creating a vertical and/or horizontal mattress suture patterns (Fig. 10-7A–E).

The needles are passed through both the femoral and tibial meniscal tear surfaces and out the previously made accessory incision. A surgical assistant is used to retract the capsule and retrieve the needles (Fig. 10-8A,B).

Once both needles of a given suture limb have been passed, they are equally tensioned and tied to the capsule. The meniscus must be viewed arthroscopically while tying the suture to ensure anatomic reduction and balanced compression of the meniscus tear site to adjacent tissue and to the capsule (Fig. 10-9).

Outside-In

This technique is best used for meniscal tears in the anterior horn or middle third, as well as certain repairable radial tear patterns (Fig. 10-4). The technique involves passing long 18-gauge spinal needles or proprietary needle delivery devices percutaneously through the skin into the knee to perforate the meniscus (Fig. 10-10A).

Proprietary suture-passing devices offer curved options not available with an 18-gauge spinal needle (i.e., Meniscus Mender II, Smith & Nephew, Andover, MA).

Absorbable sutures such as 0-PDS (polydioxanone, Ethicon, Somerville, NJ) can be passed through the meniscus and tied with a mulberry knot to allow for control of the meniscal fragment and preliminary reduction.

Needles are placed 3 to 5 mm apart in either a vertical or horizontal configuration to allow passage of a mattress suture (Fig. 10-10B). An absorbable suture, such as PDS, is passed through the needle into the joint and used to shuttle a high-strength nonabsorbable suture used for the meniscal repair. A small wire retriever (3-0 wire suture) is passed through a second needle and used to retrieve the other end of the nonabsorbable suture (Fig. 10-10C). After suture passage, the spinal needles are removed, and the suture is tensioned (Fig. 10-10D).

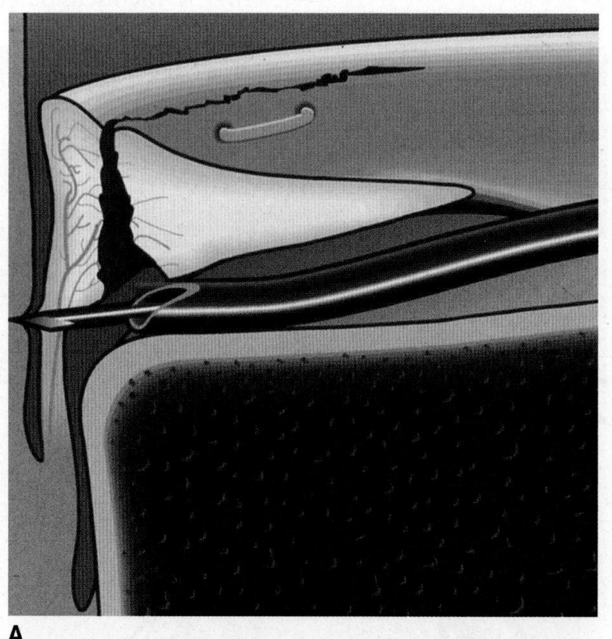

A

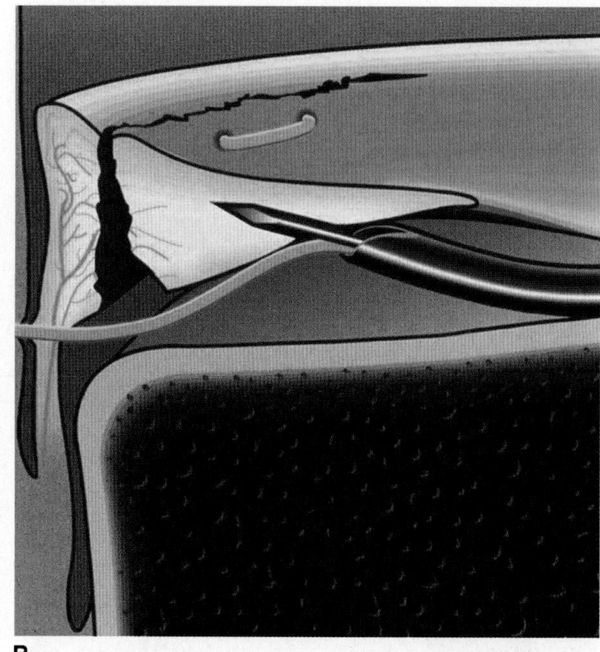

B

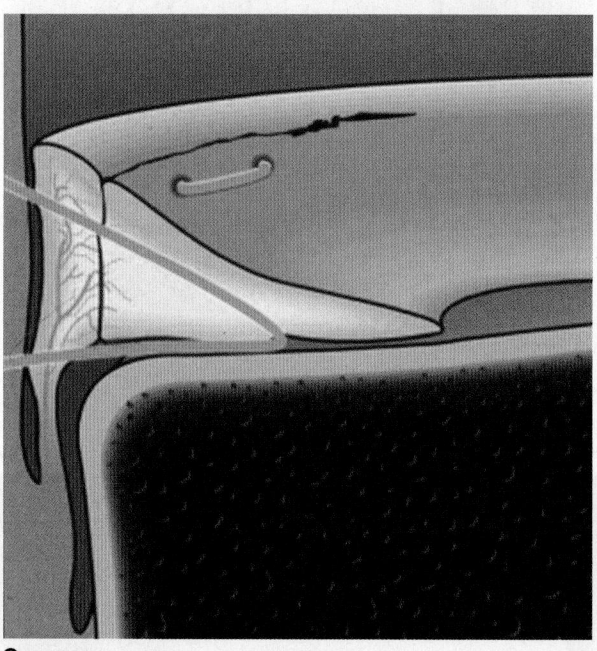

C

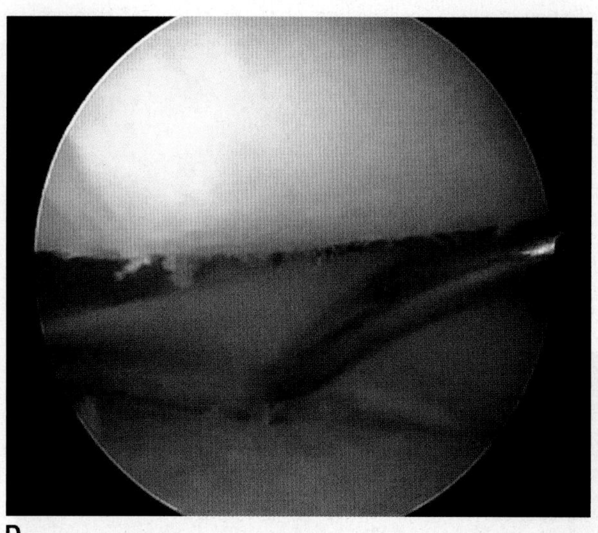

D

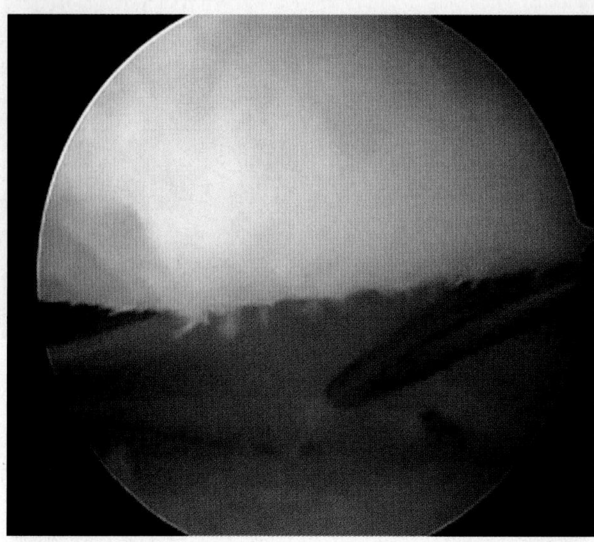

E

FIGURE 10-7

A: Illustration of a precontoured cannula with a double-armed needle piercing the knee capsule. A previously placed horizontal mattress suture is depicted, as well. **B:** The suture has been passed through the capsule. The needle is shown piercing the meniscus. **C:** A vertical mattress suture is depicted after passage of both long flexible needles. (Images courtesy of ConMed.) **D:** Demonstrates an arthroscopic placement o the cannula with needle direction inferior to the meniscus into the capsule. **E:** Demonstrates an arthroscopic placement of the cannula with needle direction into the inferior rim of the meniscus.

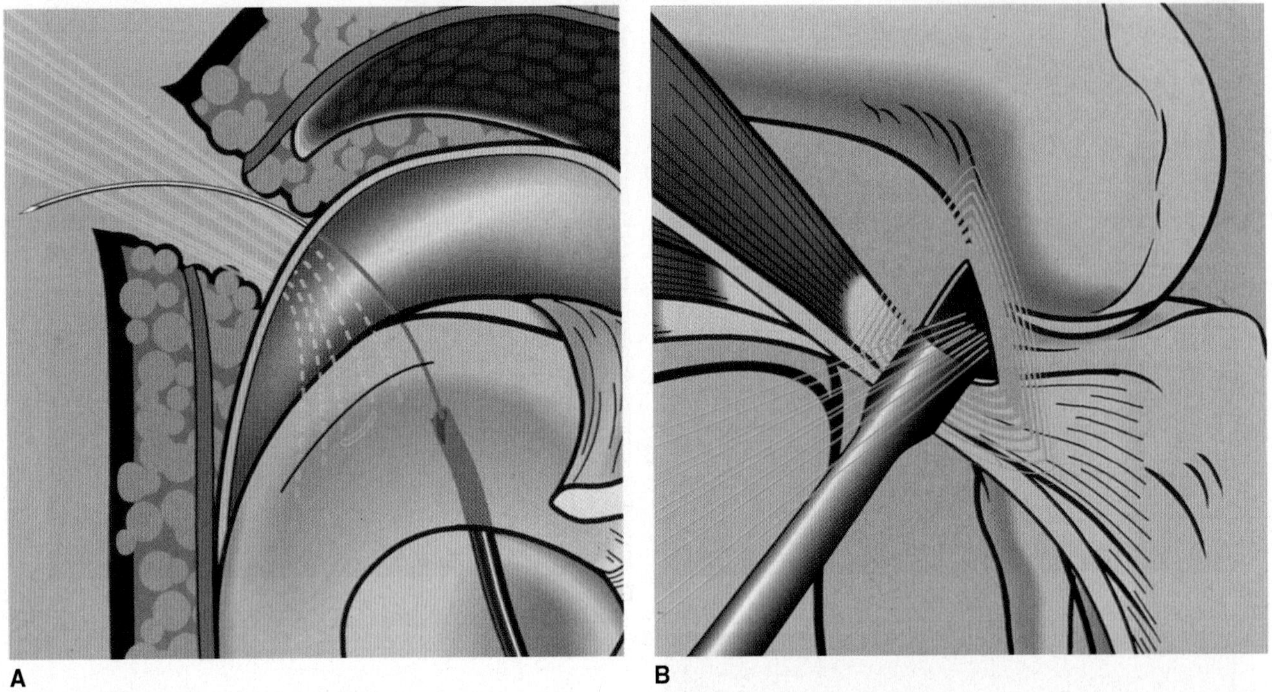

FIGURE 10-8

A: Illustration of suture passage through the precontoured meniscal repair cannula. Several sutures have already been placed. **B:** Illustration of the sutures exiting the knee through the lateral incision. A retractor is in place protecting the posterior structures. (Images courtesy of ConMed.)

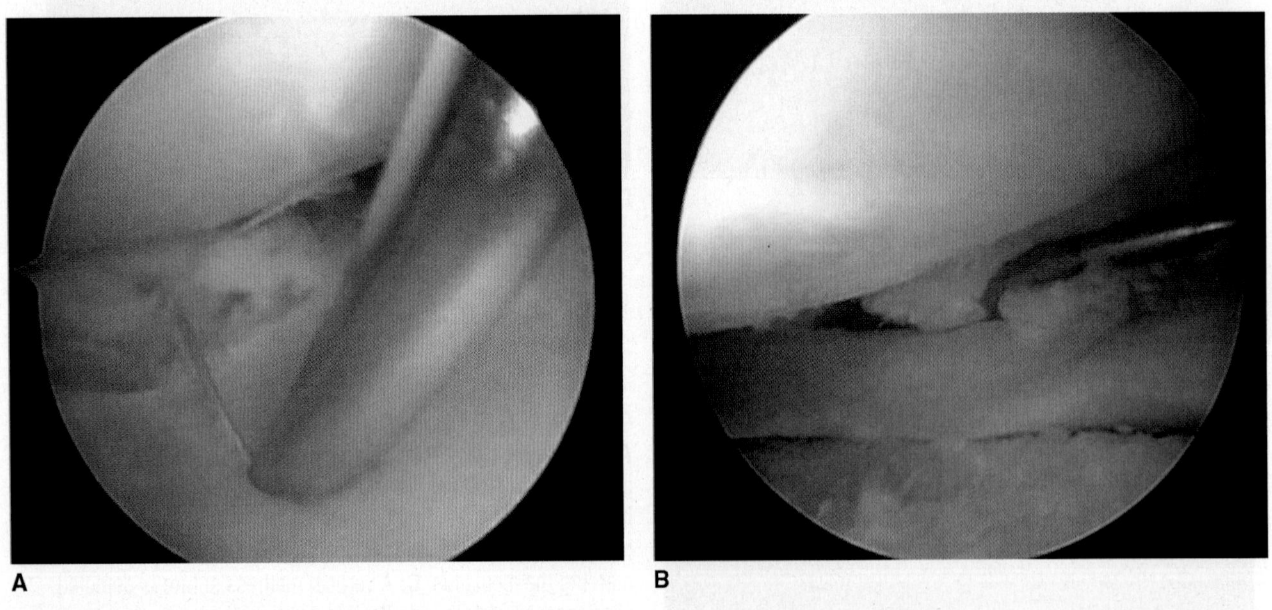

FIGURE 10-9

A: Arthroscopic photograph of the second arm of suture being placed at the superior margin of the meniscus in vertical mattress configuration. **B:** Arthroscopic photograph of an intraoperative exam after inside-out repair of the medial meniscus. Sutures were placed in a vertical mattress configuration.

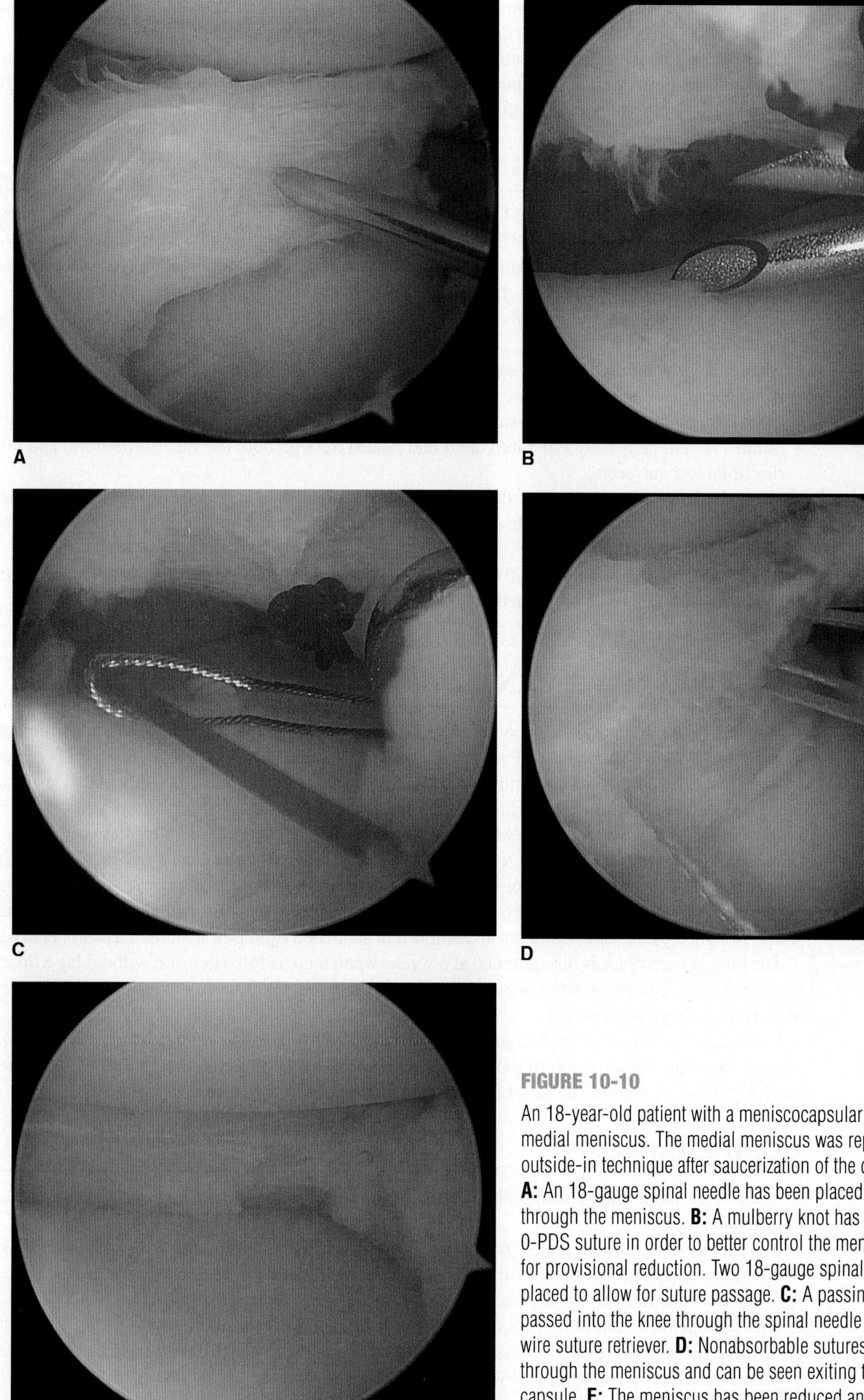

FIGURE 10-10

An 18-year-old patient with a meniscocapsular tear of a discoid medial meniscus. The medial meniscus was repaired with an outside-in technique after saucerization of the discoid meniscus. **A:** An 18-gauge spinal needle has been placed from outside-in through the meniscus. **B:** A mulberry knot has been tied with 0-PDS suture in order to better control the meniscus and allow for provisional reduction. Two 18-gauge spinal needles have been placed to allow for suture passage. **C:** A passing suture has been passed into the knee through the spinal needle and through the wire suture retriever. **D:** Nonabsorbable sutures have been passed through the meniscus and can be seen exiting through the knee capsule. **E:** The meniscus has been reduced and sutures tied through the incision on the medial aspect of the knee. (Images courtesy of Dr. Andrew Goodwillie.)

A 3- to 5-mm skin incision is made adjacent to and/or between the suture strands, and blunt dissection with a hemostat is performed down to the capsule. Both limbs of the suture are retrieved through the skin incision, and the sutures are tied down to the capsule. Care must be taken to ensure no contiguous neurovascular structures are incarcerated by the sutures. The meniscus is visualized arthroscopically to ensure an anatomic reduction of the meniscus (Fig. 10-10E).

PEARLS AND PITFALLS

- Meniscus repair is best indicated for unstable peripheral tears in the red-red or red-white zones.
- Concurrent pathology, such as ACL tear, should be addressed along with meniscal repair.
- The tear should be approached from whichever portal allows perpendicular delivery of the suture while also projecting away from the neurovascular bundle.
- Preparation of the tear site with abrasion or trephination is essential to facilitate vascular ingrowth and healing.
- Anatomic reduction of the meniscus is necessary to facilitate repair and healing.
- An anchoring stitch may facilitate provisional tear reduction.
- Accessory portals are often necessary to improve access and facilitate optimal suture configuration.
- Sutures should be placed 3 to 5 mm apart and placed through both the superior femoral and inferior tibial tear surfaces.
- Vertical mattress sutures provide the most stable and biomechanically superior fixation construct.
- Sutures are placed with the knee in 20 degrees of flexion for medial meniscal repairs and 90 degrees of flexion for lateral tears.
- Rehabilitation programs are individualized for each patient based on tear pattern and repair construct with emphasis on immediate range of motion and potential modified weight bearing in extension.

POSTOPERATIVE MANAGEMENT

Postoperative rehabilitation must be individualized based on the tear pattern, repair construct, and concomitant surgical procedures. Patients are placed in a knee immobilizer or hinged knee brace locked in full extension during ambulation for the first 4 weeks. Patients with isolated meniscal repair are made partial weight bearing for the first month.

Passive and active-assisted range of motion is initiated on the first postoperative day, with range of motion limited from full extension to 90 degrees of flexion for the first 3 to 4 weeks. Hyperflexion greater than 90 degrees is limited for up to 4 to 6 weeks with repair of larger bucket-handle patterns. Tibial rotation is avoided for the first 6 weeks after meniscal repair. Quadriceps and hamstring sets, heel slides, straight leg raises and isometric abduction, and adduction exercises are initiated postoperatively.

The hinged knee brace is discontinued at 6 weeks when there is full extension without lag. Closed-chain exercises, hamstring strengthening, lunges, and leg presses from full extension to 90 degrees of flexion are begun at 6 weeks.

Full weight bearing with normal gait pattern is expected by 12 to 16 weeks, and light jogging may begin at this time. Gradual return to sports activity is permitted by 4 to 6 months, when the patient has full extension, painless terminal flexion, no point tenderness, or effusion.

COMPLICATIONS

- The complication rate of meniscal repair is higher than meniscus resection, including incidence of reoperation.
- The incidence of infection after meniscus repair is 0.23% to 0.42% and associated with longer operating time, history of prior surgeries, and multiple concurrent procedures.
- Prophylactic antibiotics are routinely given prior to surgery; however, a reduction in infection rate with perioperative antibiotics has not been validated in high-level studies.
- The incidence of deep venous thrombosis after meniscal repair ranges from 1.2% to 4.9%. There is no consensus on optimal prophylactic measures; however, the use of enteric-coated aspirin for 4 weeks following surgery is more clearly indicated in patients who are stratified for thromboembolic risks.

- Vascular injuries are a potentially devastating complication of meniscus repair with incidence ranging from 0.54% to 1.0%.
  - The popliteal artery is in close proximity to the posterior knee adjacent to the posterior horn of the lateral meniscus and is at risk with repair of the posterior horns of the medial and lateral menisci.
  - Injuries to the popliteal artery including hematoma, aneurysm, pseudoaneurysm, and arteriovenous fistula have been described.
- Neurologic complications after meniscus repair range from 0.06% to 2.0%.
  - The saphenous nerve and its associated branches are at risk with medial meniscus repair, and injuries ranging from transient paresthesia to complete neuropathy have been reported.
- Chondral injury is a potential complication of meniscus repair, although incidence may be lower with outside-in or inside-out technique versus use of all-inside repair devices.
- A low threshold should be considered for MCL pie crusting to "open" up a tight medial compartment and avoid articular cartilage scuffing.

RESULTS

- The long-term success of meniscal repair range from 75% to 85% in most series.
- A systematic review of 145 patients with greater than 10-year follow-up found a 24% reoperation rate with isolated meniscus repair versus 14% reoperation rate with meniscal repair and ACL reconstruction.
- A recent systematic review of 566 patients with 5-year follow-up found a failure rate ranging from 22.3% to 24.3%. The failure rate was similar between medial and lateral meniscal repair and regardless of reconstruction of the ACL.
- A prospective study of outside-in meniscal repairs found a failure rate of 12% (5 of 41 subjects) with an average Lysholm score of 87.3 in the 36 successful meniscal repairs at 11.7-year follow-up.
- Several studies have shown no difference in healing rates between outside-in and all-inside repair techniques.
- Similar outcomes have been reported with outside-in compared to other meniscal repair techniques. One study had an 88% success rate at 27-month follow-up in 41 patients with improvement in Lysholm scores from 34 to 88 and International Knee Documentation Committee scores from 25 to 88.
- A systematic review of meniscal repairs in the red-white zone found a clinical healing rate of 81% with inside-out repairs, and failure was not influenced by patient age, chronicity of injury, involved tibiofemoral compartment, gender, and concurrent ACL reconstruction.
- Successful meniscal repair has been reported in tears extending into the central avascular portion of the meniscus. One study of active patients under the age of 20 showed a clinical healing rate of 75% with an inside-out vertical divergent suture technique. The same authors found a clinical healing rate of 87% in patients 40 years of age and older with the same tear pattern extending into the avascular zone.

RECOMMENDED READINGS

Abdelkafy A, Aigner N, Zada M, et al. Two to nineteen years follow-up of arthroscopic meniscal repair using the outside-in technique: a retrospective study. *Arch Orthop Trauma Surg.* 2007;127:245–252.

Barber-Westin SD, Noyes FR. Clinical healing rates of meniscus repairs of tears in the central-third (red-white) zone. *Arthroscopy.* 2014;30:134–146.

Choi NH, Kim TH, Victoroff BN. Comparison of arthroscopic medial meniscal suture repair techniques: inside-out versus all-inside repair. *Am J Sports Med.* 2009;37:2144–2150.

Goodwillie A, Myers K, Sgaglione N. Current strategies and approaches to meniscal repair. *J Knee Surg.* 2014;27(6):423–434.

Grant JA, Wilde J, Miller BS, et al. Comparison of inside-out and all-inside techniques for the repair of isolated meniscal tears: a systematic review. *Am J Sports Med.* 2012;40:459–468.

Kessler MW, Sgaglione NA. All-arthroscopic meniscus repair of avascular and biologically at-risk meniscal tears. *Instr Course Lect.* 2011;60:439–452.

Laible C, Stein DA, Kiridly DN. Meniscal repair. *J Am Acad Orthop Surg.* 2013;21:204–213.

Nepple JJ, Dunn WR, Wright RW. Meniscal repair outcomes at greater than five years: a systematic literature review and meta-analysis. *J Bone Joint Surg Am.* 2012;94:2222–2227.

Noyes FR, Barber-Westin SD. Arthroscopic repair of meniscus tears extending into the avascular zone with or without anterior cruciate ligament reconstruction in patients 40 years of age and older. *Arthroscopy.* 2000;16:822–829.

Noyes FR, Barber-Westin SD. Arthroscopic repair of meniscal tears extending into the avascular zone in patients younger than twenty years of age. *Am J Sports Med.* 2002;30:589–600.

Noyes FR, Barber-Westin SD. Repair of complex and avascular meniscal tears and meniscal transplantation. *J Bone Joint Surg Am.* 2010;92:1012–1029.

Paxton ES, Stock MV, Brophy RH. Meniscal repair versus partial meniscectomy: a systematic review comparing reoperation rates and clinical outcomes. *Arthroscopy.* 2011;27:1275–1288.

Sobhy MH, AbouElsoud MM, Kamel EM, et al. Neurovascular safety and clinical outcome of outside-in repair of tears of the posterior horn of the medial meniscus. *Arthroscopy.* 2010;26:1648–1654.

11 Meniscal Allograft Reconstruction: Indications, Surgical Technique, and Clinical Outcomes

Kirk A. Campbell, Annemarie K. Tilton, and Brian J. Cole

INTRODUCTION

Partial or complete meniscectomy leads to biomechanical and biological consequences that can negatively impact knee function (1–6). In a healthy knee, the menisci contribute to mechanical protection of the joint through shock absorption and load transmission and also contribute to tibiofemoral stability though joint lubrication and joint congruency (7–9). In flexion and extension, approximately 90% and 50%, respectively, of the load through the knee is transmitted through the menisci (10,11). Because the menisci increase the articular contact area and dissipate the force across the joint, loss of all or part of the menisci increases the load and contact forces on the articular cartilage and contributes to degenerative changes in the joint.

Due to altered contact pressures and the resulting degenerative changes, patients often experience pain, recurrent effusions, and functional limitations following meniscectomy (12,13). However, in cases where meniscal preservation was not possible, meniscal allograft transplantation (MAT) can restore near-normal knee function and anatomy, thus relieving pain and improving function for patients with symptomatic meniscal deficiency (12,13).

Meniscal transplant techniques continue to develop, and several techniques are in use today with fixation achieved through bony fixation, sutures, or a combination of both. Allografts can be anchored with a bone bridge that rigidly fixes the distance between the anterior and posterior horns or by using separate bone plugs on the anterior and posterior horns. For lateral meniscus transplants, the bone bridge is typically used because the short distance between the anterior and posterior horns risks tunnel communication when bone plugs are used. On the medial side, either technique can be used. The senior author prefers the bridge-in-slot technique for both lateral and medial meniscal transplantation because of the ease of performing the procedure, its reproducibility, stable bony fixation, compatibility with concomitant procedures, and, more importantly, the fact that it maintains the native anterior and posterior horn attachments and relationship to each other.

The ideal MAT patient is a nonobese patient following a meniscectomy with pain in the involved compartment with minimal articular cartilage degeneration, normal or corrected malalignment, normal or corrected ligament status, and the willingness to consider limiting postrestoration activities that could compromise the transplant tissue. Studies have shown that such patients experience symptomatic relief and may potentially have attenuation of degenerative changes following MAT, which are likely secondary to lowered contact pressures in the involved compartment (14–16).

Clinical outcome studies have shown good to excellent results in the short-term to midterm; however, long-term results suggest that outcomes diminish over time (17–24).

PATIENT EVALUATION

History and Physical

The patient history is important and should include the mechanism of injury, related injuries, and prior treatment, including ligamentous reconstruction or cartilage procedures. Patients typically report an acute traumatic knee injury followed by multiple surgeries, including meniscus repair, meniscectomy, or both. Many patients undergo one or more meniscectomies with initial improvement, but subsequently experience continued symptoms, such as joint line pain and swelling with activity. Giving way is occasionally reported.

On physical exam, range of motion (ROM) is usually preserved, and effusion may be present. Patients may exhibit joint line tenderness with palpation of the affected compartment. The physical exam must include evaluation of gait, alignment, and ligamentous stability to assess for concomitant pathology that could affect surgical planning. The patient's knee must be stable with normal alignment and intact cartilage prior to meniscus allograft transplant. Concomitant or staged procedures can be performed to correct these pathologies along with meniscal transplant.

Imaging

Radiographs (required):

- Weight-bearing anteroposterior (AP) in full extension
- Weight-bearing posteroanterior 45° flexion to identify joint space narrowing that might be missed on extension
- Non–weight-bearing 45° flexion lateral
- Axial view of the patellofemoral joint
- Long mechanical axis films to assess for malalignment

MRI:

- Assess ligamentous deficiency
- Articular cartilage damage
- Extent of meniscectomy
- Presence of subchondral edema in affected compartment

Indications

- Less than 50 years old.
- Previous functional meniscectomy.
- Persistent pain in the meniscus-deficient compartment.
- Coronal malalignment (low threshold for correcting malalignment, correct to neutral or slightly beyond), ligamentous instability, or focal chondral defects (ICRS grade III or above) can be addressed concomitantly.

Contraindications

- Diffuse arthritic changes
- Radiographic joint space narrowing
- Radiographic femoral or tibial flattening
- Significant osteophyte formation
- Tibiofemoral subluxation
- Synovial disease
- Skeletal immaturity
- Inflammatory arthritis
- Prior joint infection
- Obesity (BMI > 32 to 34)

PREOPERATIVE PREPARATION

Meniscal Allograft Sizing

The transplanted meniscus allograft is both size and compartment specific. The preoperative sizing of the allograft is one of the most critical aspects of the procedure and the importance of this has been highlighted by the fact that oversized meniscal allografts lead to greater forces across the articular cartilage and may result in extrusion of the graft with abnormal transmission of compressive loads across the joint. Similarly, undersized allografts may result in poor congruity with the femoral condyle and result in excessive load transmission (25–27).

The most commonly used method for sizing the allograft is the plain film radiographic method proposed by Pollard et al. (28) in which preoperative measurements are obtained from AP and lateral radiographs that have been taken with a magnification marker placed on the skin at the level of the joint line. After the magnification has been accounted for, the AP radiograph is used to determine the meniscal width that will be needed by measuring from the edge of the ipsilateral tibial spine to the edge of the tibial plateau (Fig. 11-1B). The length of the meniscal allograft that will be needed is determined by using the lateral radiograph (Fig. 11-1A). Meniscal length is calculated by multiplying the depth of the tibial plateau that is measured from the lateral radiograph by 0.8 for the medial meniscus or 0.7 for the lateral meniscus (Fig. 11-1). An MRI-based measurement has also been developed by Haut et al. (29), and its accuracy was later confirmed by Prodromos et al. (30). Additionally, the senior author and colleagues (31) have also shown in a validated regression model that the use of gender, height, and weight accurately predicts the meniscal allograft size that would be needed and that this method is more accurate than both the radiographic and MRI sizing techniques.

Meniscal Graft Procurement and Processing

The use of a rigorous donor selection process, which includes screening donors with comprehensive medical record and social history review, has led to the continued procurement of disease-free allograft tissue. Furthermore, the risk of disease transmission is further decreased by testing for hepatitis B and C, human immunodeficiency virus, human T-cell lymphotropic virus, and syphilis. The grafts may also be cultured for aerobic and anaerobic bacteria, and lymph nodes may be

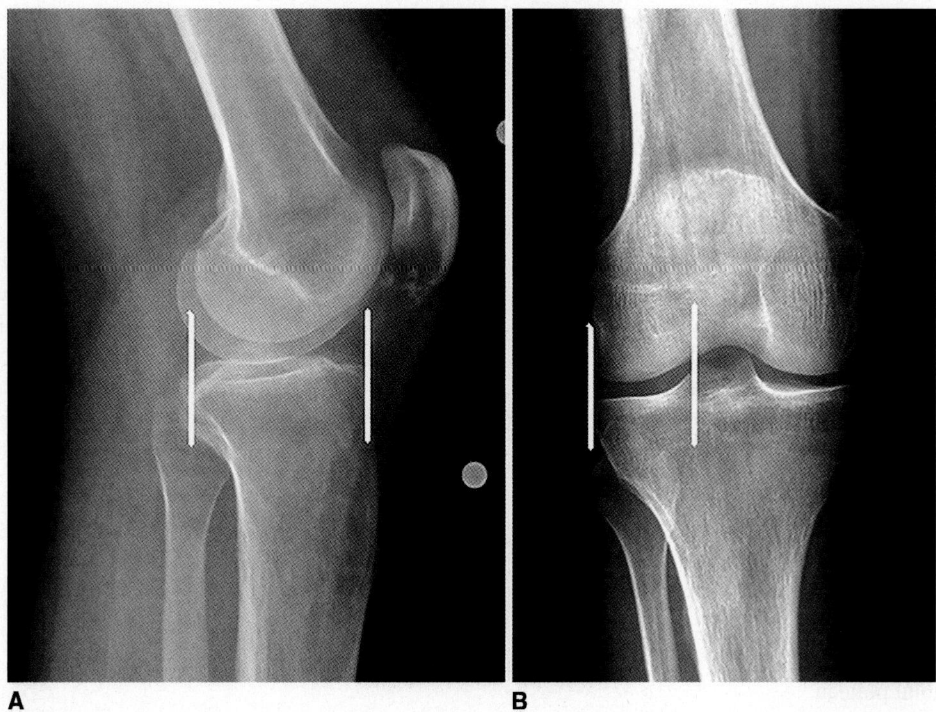

FIGURE 11-1
Graft sizing on the AP and lateral radiographs.

sampled to further decrease the risk of disease transmission. Several tissue banks have also utilized other sterilization techniques, such as ultrasonic-pulsatile washing or ethanol, to denature proteins to further lower the risk of disease transmission (32).

The meniscal allografts are harvested aseptically and frozen using sterile surgical technique, which is ideally done within 24 hours after the donor is deceased. Unlike fresh osteochondral allografts (OAs), meniscal allografts do not rely on cell viability for their morphological or biomechanical characteristics, and as a result, either fresh-frozen (to −80°C) or cryopreserved grafts can be implanted. The other graft preservation methods include fresh and freeze-dried allografts; however, the fresh-frozen grafts are the most commonly used and this is the preferred graft choice.

It has been shown that grafts from donors under 45 years old have similar tissue properties regardless of exact age; therefore, any graft from a patient under 45 years old will work well (33).

SURGICAL TECHNIQUE

A variety of techniques for meniscus transplantation are commonly used. These techniques generally rely on either suture or bony fixation of the meniscal allograft, and sometimes a combination of the two techniques is used to fix the graft to the tibial plateau. In terms of the bony fixation options, the anterior and posterior horns can be secured with separate bone plugs or with a bone bridge (bridge-in-slot, dovetail, keyhole, and trough techniques). Due to the anatomy of the anterior and posterior horns of the medial meniscus, either the separate bone plug or one of the bone bridge techniques may be used. However, because of the close proximity of the anterior and posterior horns of the lateral meniscus, lateral meniscus transplants are done with one of the bone bridge techniques to maintain this relationship.

Our preference is to perform the bridge-in-slot technique (34) for both the medial and lateral meniscus transplants due to the secure bony fixation, simplicity of performing concomitant procedures, such as an osteotomy or anterior cruciate ligament (ACL) reconstruction, and the ability to maintain native anterior and posterior horn attachments.

Equipment

The surgeon should have available and be comfortable with the instrumentation necessary to perform their preferred meniscal transplantation technique. Additionally, a workstation, which may be provided by the company that supplied the meniscal allograft, may be utilized to prepare the transplanted meniscus to the correct size. Zone-specific cannulas and double-armed needles are required for the meniscocapsular repair.

Anesthesia and Positioning

The type of anesthesia is selected for the procedure is based on a consensus between the surgeon, anesthesiologist, and patient which incorporates patient-risk factors such as age and medical comorbidities. The meniscal transplantation can be performed under regional, spinal, general anesthesia, or a combination of these techniques. The patient is positioned supine on a standard operating room table with the leg of the bed down. A thigh tourniquet is utilized to aid in visualization, and the leg is placed in a thigh holder that allows for knee hyperflexion (Fig. 11-2). The contralateral leg is placed in a well-leg holder in flexion, abduction, and external rotation. It is important to ensure that the posteromedial and posterolateral corners of the knee are easily accessible for the inside-out meniscal repair that will be required to secure the graft.

Surgical Landmarks, Incisions, and Portals

Landmarks

- Patella
- Patella tendon
- Tibial plateau
- Fibular head

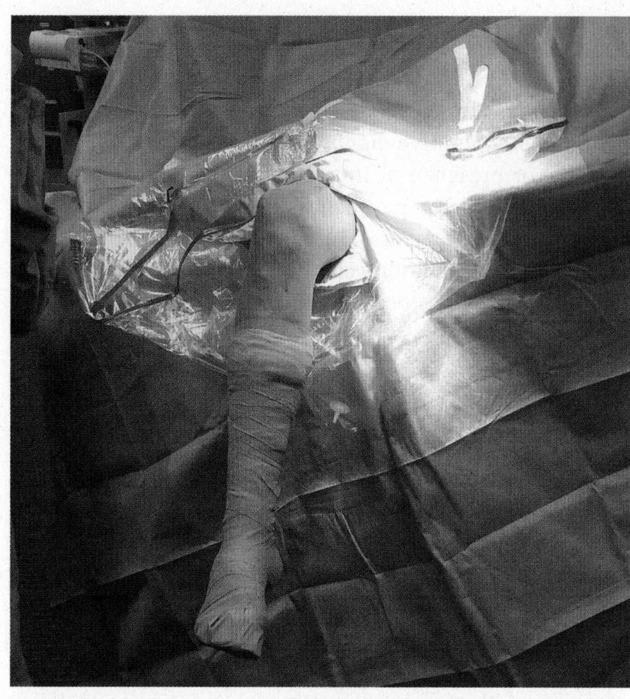

FIGURE 11-2

Patient positioning.

Portals

See Figure 11-3 for portals and approaches.

- Inferomedial portal
- Inferolateral portal
- Outflow portal as needed

Approaches

- For a medial meniscus transplant, the *Posteromedial approach* is utilized to secure the allograft to the capsule with inside-out sutures.
    - *Structures at risk:* Saphenous nerve and medial collateral ligament
- For a lateral meniscus transplant, the *Posterolateral approach* is utilized to secure the allograft.
    - *Structures at risk:* Peroneal nerve, lateral collateral ligament, and popliteus tendon
- Mini-arthrotomy through the ipsilateral side of the patellar tendon.
    - *Structure at risk:* Patella tendon

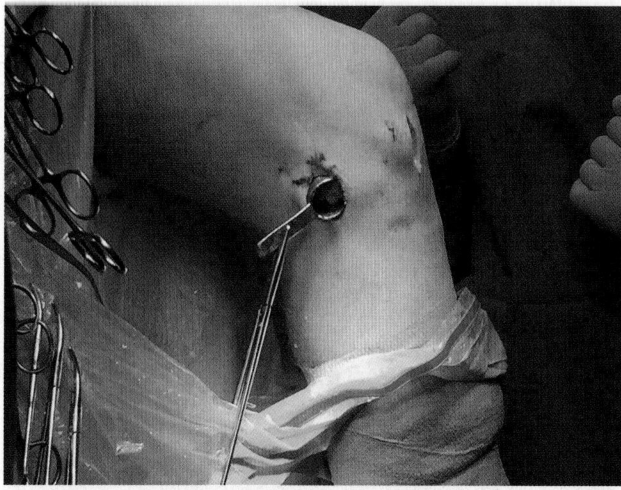

FIGURE 11-3

Portals, mini-arthrotomy, and accessory incisions.

Examination Under Anesthesia and Diagnostic Arthroscopy

Standard preoperative antibiotics are administered prior to making incisions, and an examination of the knee under anesthesia is performed to assess for ROM and ligamentous stability. A diagnostic arthroscopy is performed to confirm the preoperative diagnosis and evaluate any changes in articular cartilage, ligamentous deficiency, or presence of loose bodies. Diagnostic arthroscopy should confirm that any arthrosis in the affected compartment is limited to only grade I or II cartilage damage, which is acceptable at the time of meniscal transplantation. However, if a focal area of grade IV chondral damage is identified, then this can be treated with concomitant cartilage restoration procedure depending upon the size, location, and degree of bony involvement on MRI. Similarly, ligamentous deficiency, especially involving the ACL, should also be addressed.

Graft Preparation

The preparation of the meniscal allograft can commence either during anesthesia induction or following the preparation of the tibial slot. Our preferred transplantation technique utilizes a bone bridge to secure the graft to the tibial plateau, and this is intentionally undersized by 1 mm to facilitate passage of the graft and reduce the risk of bone bridge fracture during graft insertion. The meniscal allograft tissue arrives as a hemiplateau with the attached meniscus and should be thawed in normal saline before preparation (Fig. 11-4). The insertions of the anterior and posterior meniscal horns on the graft are identified on the bone block, and any extraneous soft tissue is removed. The bone bridge is cut to a height of 1 cm and a width of 7 mm with removal of any bone posterior to the posterior horn attachment. The distance from the posterior tibia to the posterior meniscal insertion can be estimated intraoperatively with the use of a graduated guide, and this is used to determine the amount of bone that can remain on the posterior aspect of the allograft. However, excising all bone posterior to the posterior horn attachment will allow for easy anterior to posterior graft positioning at the time of insertion. It is important to preserve any extra bone anterior to the anterior horn attachment site, so that the integrity of the graft can be maintained during insertion. Although the remaining anterior and posterior meniscal attachment sites generally measure approximately 5–6 mm, occasionally, the anterior horn attachment can measure up to 9 mm. In this scenario, the anterior aspect of the bone bridge should be adjusted to match the larger size of the anterior meniscal attachment and then the rest of the bone bridge should be tapered back down to the desired 7-mm size throughout the rest of the bone block. The proper adjustments should also be made in the recipient slot on the tibia, and this should be similarly widened anteriorly to accommodate the larger anterior bone plug. Alternatively, elevation of the soft tissue attachment in a limited fashion, while maintaining the bulk of the anterior horn footprint, can allow a 7-mm wide block anteriorly without any additional modifications. After the correct size graft is fashioned, a No. 0 polydioxanone suture (Ethicon, Blue Ash, OH) is placed at the junction of the posterior and middle third of the meniscus in a vertical mattress fashion and is used as a traction suture to reduce the meniscus (Fig. 11-5).

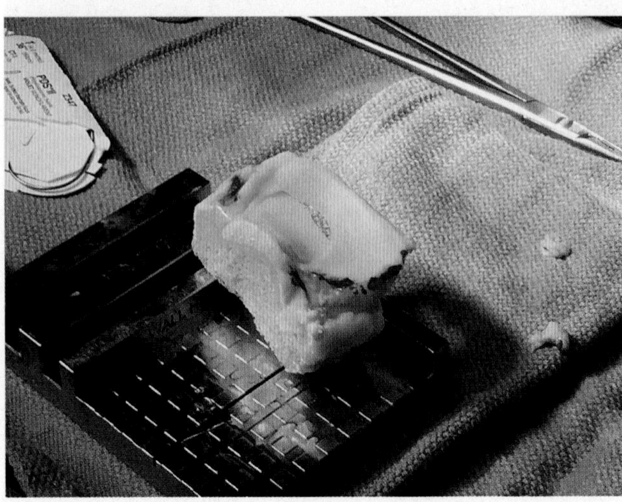

FIGURE 11-4
Meniscal allograft on the hemiplateau.

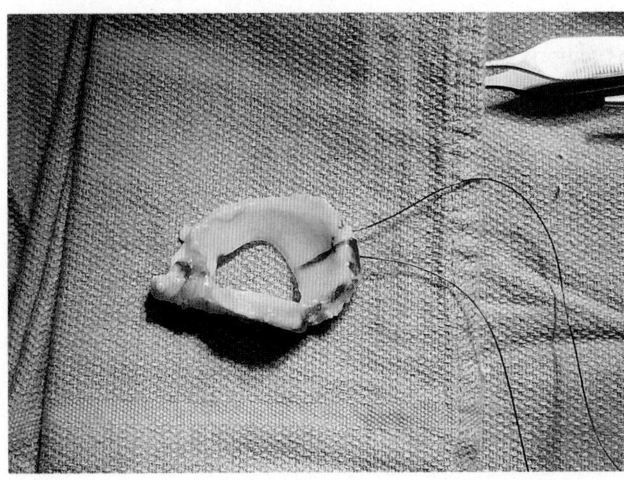

FIGURE 11-5

Prepared allograft with the traction suture in place.

Arthroscopic Preparation

A standard diagnostic arthroscopy is performed through the inferolateral and inferomedial portals as described above. The use of the bridge-in-slot technique for meniscal transplantation facilitates the use of the same steps for preparing the involved compartment. The most anterior part of the meniscus can be excised with the use of No. 11 scalpel through the respective anterior portal followed by the use of an aggressive arthroscopic shaver. The remnant of the native meniscus is debrided to a 1- to 2-mm peripheral rim until punctate bleeding occurs, but care should be taken to not penetrate the joint capsule (Fig. 11-6). The anterior and posterior horn insertions of the native meniscus can be maintained or should at least be noted, because they serve as useful markers for slot preparation. A limited notchplasty of the most inferior and posterior aspects of the ipsilateral femoral condyle is performed to improve visualization of the posterior horn and facilitate graft passage. While this is more useful in the medial compartment, it is typically not necessary for the bone trough technique. Additionally, for a medial meniscus transplant, a few of the most medial ACL fibers at the tibial insertion should be released to allow visualization of the medial tibial spine. In the ideal situation, the spine on the meniscal transplant will align with the location of the patient's native tibial spine.

Exposure

An 18-gauge spinal needle is used to localize the location of the transpatellar tendon mini-arthrotomy, which is performed in line with the anterior and posterior horn insertion sites of the involved meniscus. This facilitates correct orientation for the tibial slot preparation and subsequent graft introduction.

An ipsilateral (posteromedial or posterolateral) approach is required for the meniscal repair (Fig. 11-3). This accessory incision should extend approximately one-third above the joint line and two-thirds below the joint line and allow for adequate exposure to protect the posterior neurovascular structures during passage of the inside-out sutures for the meniscal repair. For a lateral meniscus

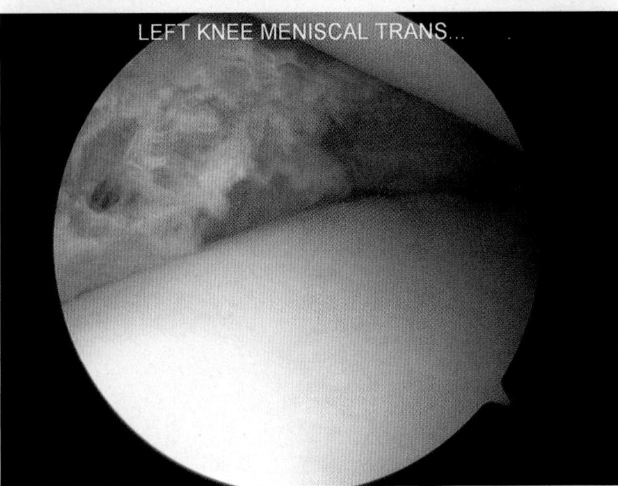

FIGURE 11-6

Meniscus debrided back to the stable 1- to 2-mm peripheral rim with punctate bleeding.

transplant, a posterolateral incision is made at the interval between the posterior edge of the iliotibial band and the anterior edge of the biceps femoris tendon. The gastrocnemius muscle-tendon junction is then elevated off the posterior capsule at the level of the joint line, and a meniscal retractor is placed anterior to the muscle in order to protect the neurovascular structures and soft tissue. Careful retraction allows suture tying beneath these structures to minimize the chances of causing a soft tissue tether to the knee during ROM.

For the medial meniscus transplant, a posteromedial incision is made just anterior to the semitendinosus and semimembranosus tendons. The infrapatellar branch of the saphenous nerve, when present, should be identified and protected. The sartorial fascia is then incised, and the hamstring tendons are retracted posteriorly. The interval is opened between the posteromedial aspect of the capsule just anterior to the gastrocnemius and semitendinosus tendons, and the gastrocnemius muscle-tendon junction is then elevated off the posterior capsule at the level of the joint line. A meniscal retractor is placed anterior to the muscle. Similarly, proper retraction here facilitates the passage, retrieval, and tying of the meniscal sutures while minimizing the potential for soft tissue tethering.

Tibial Slot Preparation

The orientation of the tibial slot follows the normal anatomy of the meniscus anterior and posterior horn attachment sites. An electrocautery device is used to create a line connecting the anterior and posterior horn attachment sites, which is then used as a guide for a 4.5-mm burr to create a superficial reference slot in the tibial plateau along this line. This slot follows the native slope of the tibial plateau and should measure the same width and height as the burr (Fig. 11-7). A hooked depth gauge is then placed in the reference slot to measure the AP length of the tibial plateau and as a reference for placement of a guide pin, which is placed just distal and parallel to the reference slot (Fig. 11-8). The guide pin is advanced up to, but not through, the posterior tibial cortex and is then over-reamed with an 8-mm cannulated reamer, without violating the posterior cortex. A box cutter is then used to create a tibial slot measuring 8-mm wide by 10-mm deep (Fig. 11-9), and this is then smoothed and refined with a three-sided rasp to ensure smooth passage of the meniscal allograft bone bridge in the tibial slot (Fig. 11-10).

Meniscus Allograft Insertion and Fixation

To facilitate insertion of the meniscal allograft, the arthroscope is placed into the ipsilateral portal for viewing and then a single-barrel, zone-specific meniscal repair cannula is placed into the contralateral portal.

The cannula is directed toward the capsular attachment site of the junction of the posterior and middle thirds of the meniscus, and a long, flexible nitinol suture passing wire is passed to the exit through the accessory posterolateral or posteromedial incision. The proximal end of the nitinol pin is pulled out through the anterior mini-arthrotomy, and the previously placed No. 0 PDS traction sutures from the allograft are passed through the loop of the nitinol wire. The wire and traction sutures are pulled through the posterior accessory incision and used to pull the meniscal allograft into

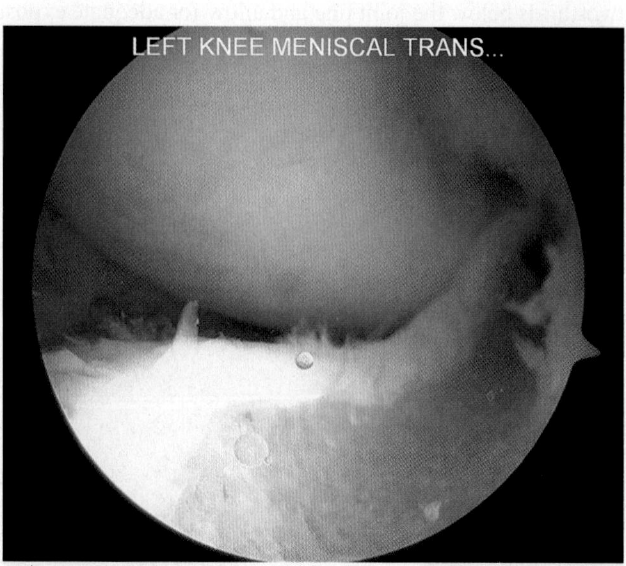

FIGURE 11-7

Reference slot created with the 4.5-mm burr.

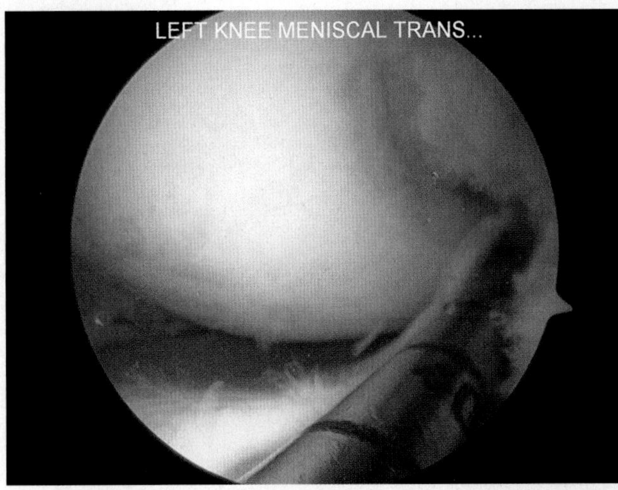

FIGURE 11-8

Hooked measuring guide in the reference slot.

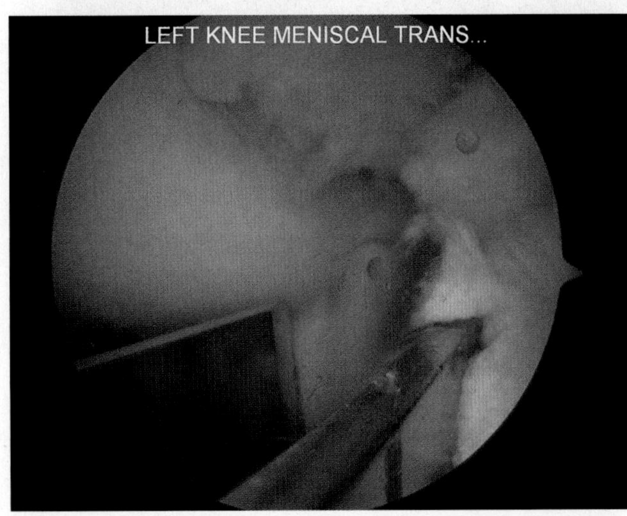

FIGURE 11-9

Box cutter deepening the reference slot in the tibia.

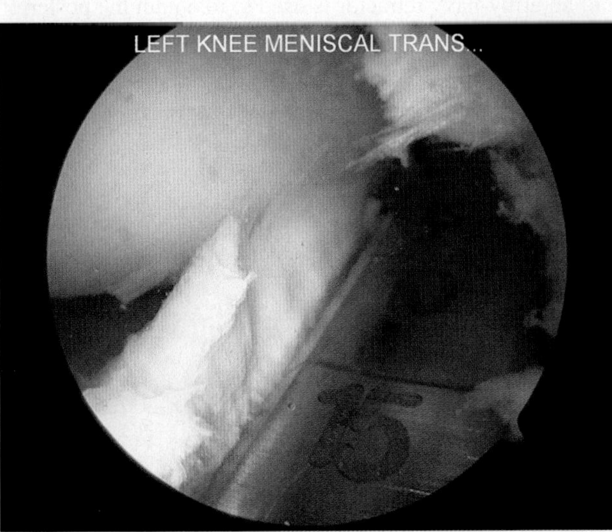

FIGURE 11-10

A rasp being used to smooth and refine the slot.

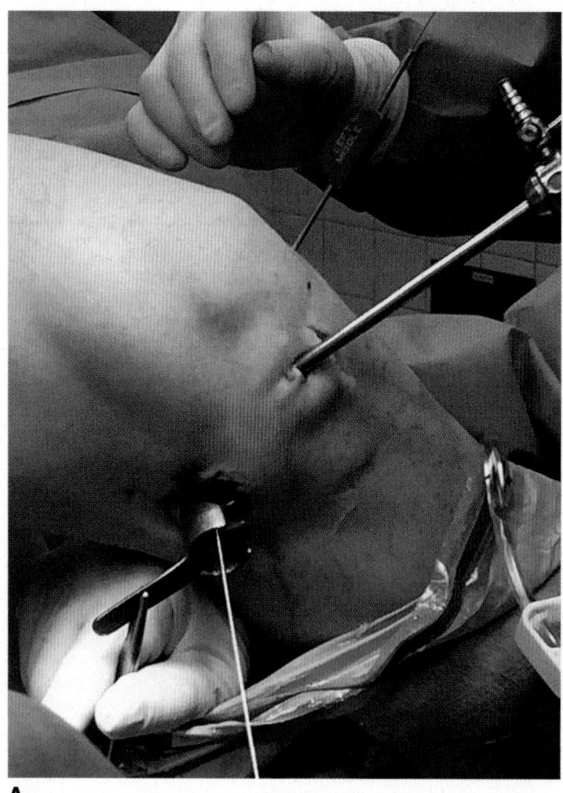

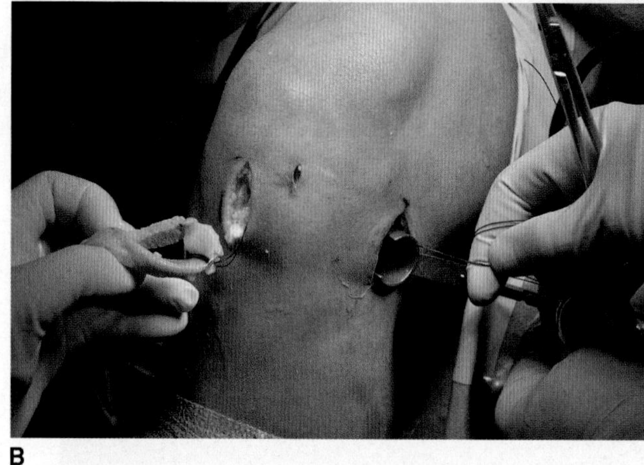

A B

FIGURE 11-11

A: The traction suture has been passed through the accessory incision with the nitinol pin and (**B**) the meniscus is being introduced through the mini-arthrotomy with traction suture being pulled.

the joint through the anterior mini-arthrotomy (Fig. 11-11A,B). The bone bridge is advanced into the tibial slot, and the meniscus is manually reduced under the ipsilateral femoral condyle with the use of a finger placed through the mini-arthrotomy. Additionally, varus or valgus stress may be required to open the ipsilateral compartment and facilitate the introduction of the graft. Knee hyperflexion is generally needed during the introduction, and hyperextension typically helps with the reduction, which is usually done under arthroscopic visualization. Once the meniscus has been reduced, the knee is cycled to seat the graft and ensure proper placement. With the knee in flexion, the bone bridge is secured in the tibial slot with a 7 × 23-mm bioabsorbable cortical interference screw under direct visualization against the far side of the bone bridge within the slot. More specifically, a guidewire is first inserted between the bone bridge and the notch, and a tap is inserted over the guidewire to create a path for the screw. A freer and the side of an army-navy retractor is used to maintain the posterior aspect of the bone plug in the trough during interference screw placement (Fig. 11-12).

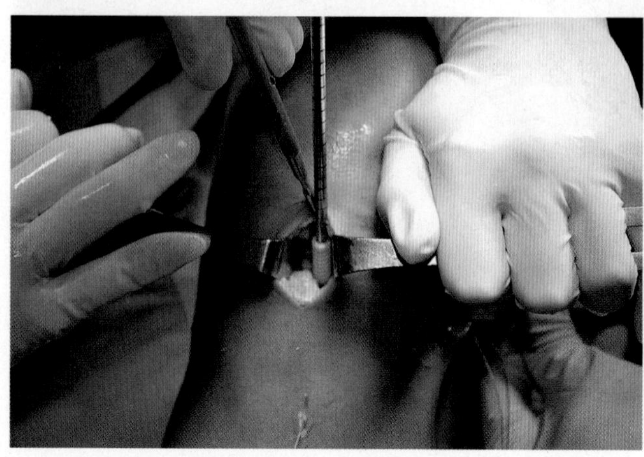

FIGURE 11-12

Bony fixation of the meniscus in the tibial slot. The freer and army-navy retractor help to maintain the allograft in the slot and as the bioabsorbable interference screw is introduced.

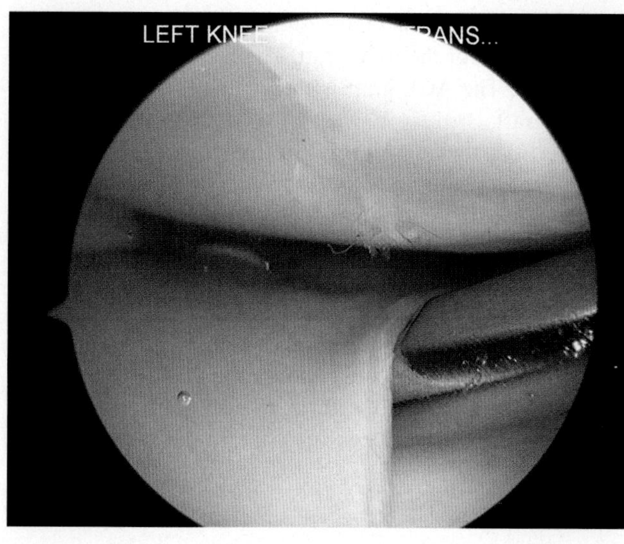

FIGURE 11-13

The reduced meniscus being repaired to the capsule with inside-out vertical mattress sutures.

The meniscus allograft is then repaired to the capsule using inside-out vertical mattress sutures in the standard fashion (Fig. 11-13). The sutures should be placed peripherally in the meniscus because sutures placed in the middle or inner third of the meniscus can weaken the implant. The meniscal stitches are generally started at the site of the traction sutures and are placed sequentially superiorly and inferiorly to ensure correct tension. In general, 8 to 10 sutures are required and are placed equally on the superior and inferior surfaces of the meniscus to create balance and decrease the amount of graft eversion. Although not always necessary, an all-inside meniscal fixation device may be placed posteriorly and outside-in techniques may be used anteriorly.

Closure

The mini-arthrotomy, portal, and accessory incisions are then closed in the standard fashion, and the knee is immobilized in a hinged knee brace that is locked in extension.

CONCOMITANT PROCEDURES

Cartilage Repair

In the presence of a focal cartilage defect that is indicated for a cartilage restoration procedure, such as autologous chondrocyte implantation (ACI) or an OA, all steps of the MAT should be performed prior to the cartilage procedure. It is important to take great care when making the arthrotomy for the placement of osteochondral grafts in order to avoid damage to the anterior horn of the transplanted meniscus. It is recommended that the meniscal sutures are not placed in the anterior horn until after the OA graft has been placed. The anterior sutures can then be placed through the anterior arthrotomy at the end of the procedure. Additionally, in order to avoid damage to the meniscus graft, it is recommended that the knee is flexed and retractors are used to facilitate visualization while performing the cartilage procedure.

Anterior Cruciate Ligament Reconstruction

A ligamentously stable joint and normal axial alignment are required for the optimal functioning of a meniscal transplant because ACL deficiency and untreated limb malalignment have been shown to lead to a high failure rate after meniscus allograft transplantation. In cases where a concomitant ACL reconstruction is indicated, a modified bridge-in-slot technique can be used with some modification to your preferred ACL reconstruction technique. One major change in the technique is the use of two smaller bone blocks instead of the one long bridge, which allows the ACL graft to be passed between the bone blocks. The use of a soft tissue graft (hamstring autograft or allograft, tibialis anterior allograft, or Achilles tendon allograft) for the ACL reconstruction is necessary because this will facilitate the use of the smallest tibial tunnel possible, while also avoiding possibility of unseating the meniscal allograft blocks during graft passage.

The sequence of events should start with drilling of the tibial tunnel for the ACL graft as obliquely as possible followed by drilling of the femoral tunnel for the ACL graft. The meniscal slot can then be prepared in the usual fashion described above. The ACL graft is then passed and fixed on the femoral side before preparing the meniscal allograft.

To prepare the meniscal transplant for insertion, the central third of the meniscal bone block is removed to create separate anterior and posterior bone blocks. The ACL tibial aiming guide is then used to drill two transtibial tunnels that exit inside the prepared meniscal slot and to create two transosseous tunnels that can be used to retrieve sutures passed within the anterior and posterior soft tissue attachments and subsequently passed through the bone block. A suture passing device is used to pass these sutures through their respective tibial tunnels and the graft is inserted and reduced, ensuring that both bony and soft tissue components are in appropriate position. The sutures are then tied over a bony bridge on the tibia and the tibial side of the ACL graft is fixed. The meniscus is then repaired to the capsule with inside-out vertical mattress sutures placed in the standard fashion and tied through the accessory posteromedial or posterolateral incision.

Osteotomy

Concomitant correction of the malalignment is recommenced if the weight-bearing line is less than 45% (varus) or greater than 55% (valgus), which represents a 2 to 3° change from normal alignment. In cases of a medial meniscus deficiency and varus alignment, all steps of the meniscus transplantation should be completed first and a concurrent high tibial osteotomy (HTO) should be performed to correct coronal malalignment. The opening wedge osteotomy should be performed such that the osteotomy line passes at least 1.5 cm below the bottom of the tibial slot. Great care is taken to avoid the risk for fracture propagation into the tibial slot during when opening and distracting the osteotomy surfaces. In cases of lateral meniscus deficiency and valgus alignment, a distal femoral osteotomy (DFO) is indicated, and as above, all steps for meniscal transplantation should be completed before performing the osteotomy.

PEARLS AND PITFALLS

- Meniscal transplants are indicated for symptomatic compartment overload in patients younger than 50 years old.
- ACL deficiency and malalignment should be addressed with concomitant ACL reconstruction and/or an osteotomy.
- Have a careful discussion with the patient informing him or her that the meniscal transplant may be postponed if the meniscal allograft that was obtained is not acceptable (the size and side should be confirmed prior to anesthesia induction) and/or if the examination under anesthesia and diagnostic arthroscopy identifies unexpected joint pathology (such as a large bipolar cartilage defect or joint instability) that may need to be addressed.
- A transpatellar mini-arthrotomy and an accessory posteromedial or posterolateral incisions are necessary for tibial slot alignment, preparation, and graft insertion as well as for graft fixation.
- Meniscal allograft arrives as a hemiplateau with attached meniscus; insertions of the anterior and posterior meniscal horns are identified on the bone block and any extraneous soft tissue is removed.
- The allograft's bone bridge is cut to a height of 1 cm and a width of 7 mm with removal of any bone posterior to the posterior horn attachment.
- No. 0 PDS suture is used as a traction suture and is placed at the junction of the posterior and middle third of the meniscus in a vertical mattress fashion.
- A 1- to 2-mm peripheral rim of native meniscus tissue should be maintained in order to facilitate the repair of the meniscal allograft to the meniscocapsular junction. Care should be used to avoid violating the capsular layer while preparing the peripheral rim.
- The anterior and posterior horn insertions of the native meniscus should be maintained because they serve as useful markers for slot preparation.
- A limited notchplasty of the most inferior and posterior aspects of the ipsilateral femoral condyle aids in visualization of the posterior horn and facilitates graft passage.

- Orientation of the tibial slot follows normal anatomy of the meniscus anterior and posterior horn attachment sites. An electrocautery device and a 4.5-mm burr are to create a superficial reference slot in the tibial plateau.
- Use of appropriate varus or valgus stress combined with knee hyperflexion followed by extension facilitates the insertion of the meniscal allograft.
- The freer and army-navy retractor should be used to help maintain the allograft in the slot as the bioabsorbable interference screw is introduced.
- In general, 8 to 10 inside-outside vertical mattress meniscal sutures are required to secure the graft, and these are placed equally on the superior and inferior surfaces of the meniscus to create balance and decrease the amount of graft eversion. Occasionally, an all-inside suture device may be needed to repair the posterior aspect of the allograft, and an outside-in technique may be needed anteriorly.
- Care should be taken not to damage the articular cartilage while performing the transplantation.
- It is important to make sure that the graft is appropriately sized because undersized grafts may complicate capsular repair and are likely to behave biomechanically inferior to appropriately sized grafts.
- A soft tissue ACL graft is required for concomitant ACL reconstruction. The tibial tunnel for the ACL should be created prior to the tibial slot preparation. The femoral side of the ACL graft should be passed and fixed prior to inserting the meniscal allograft.
- All aspects of the meniscal transplant should be performed prior to performing an HTO or DFO. HTO should be performed at least 1.5 cm below the bottom of the tibial slot to decrease the risk of the osteotomy propagating into the tibial slot.
- For an OA or an ACI procedure that requires an arthrotomy, consideration should be given for not passing the anterior-most meniscal sutures until after the cartilage restoration procedure has been concluded.
- Patients should be counseled that the rate of reoperation after MAT ranges from 32% to 50% (23,35); however, a majority of cases only require a simple arthroscopic debridement.

POSTOPERATIVE MANAGEMENT

Patients are Typically Seen for Follow-Up at 7 to 10 days after Surgery for Suture Removal and Postoperative Radiographs. The Typical Rehab Protocol for an Isolated Meniscal Transplant is as Follows:	
0–2 wk	Partial weight bearing; hinged brace, locked in extension ROM 0–90 degrees, only without weight bearing
3–8 wk	Full weight bearing as tolerated >90 degrees of flexion full weight bearing
9 wk	Full weight bearing without brace
16 wk	In line running
6–9 mo	Full return to activity if full pain-free motion with minimum 80%–85% strength compared to contralateral leg; return to pivoting/cutting sports is discouraged

COMPLICATIONS

The complications that occur with MAT are similar to those encountered with a standard meniscal repair, and recent systematic reviews found that the overall rate of complication ranged from 10.6% to 13.9% (36,37). These complications include incomplete healing of the sutured meniscal allograft to the capsule, infection, arthrofibrosis, and saphenous or peroneal nerve injury. It should be noted that the meniscus allograft is at a higher risk of injury than the native meniscus, and these injuries are treated with standard arthroscopic meniscal repair or partial meniscectomy as indicated.

RESULTS

MAT has been in clinical use to address the adverse effects of postmeniscectomy syndrome since 1984 (38), and over the last several decades, the available literature has shown that it is a safe and reliable procedure resulting in roughly 85% good to excellent results (35–37,39–41). Unfortunately, there is a lack of high-quality level I or II studies available on the outcomes of MAT, and the majority of the current literature is from small retrospective studies or case series, which makes it difficult to draw definitive conclusions about the outcomes of MAT. Despite these limitations, there have been several recent systematic reviews that have provided an excellent consolidation of the best available evidence on the outcomes of MAT and have confirmed the findings of good to excellent short-short and midterm outcomes after MAT (35,37,39,42,43). See Table 11-1 for a concise summary of the clinical outcomes of MAT.

In one of two of the most recent systematic reviews on MAT published in 2015 by Smith et al. (37), it was shown in an a analysis of 35 studies, with a mean follow-up of 5.1 years and involving 1,332 (1,374 knees) patients, that MAT led to significant improvements in the Lysholm, International Knee Documentation Committee (IKDC), and Tegner outcome scores from preoperative values compared to postoperative values. Additionally, it was shown that mean failure rate across all studies was 10.6% at 4.8 years and that the complication rate was 13.9% at 4.7 years. It was highlighted that there was a high risk of bias across the many different studies due to heterogeneity in study design, outcome measures, and reported data. Nevertheless, this study showed that MAT is an effective intervention for patients with a symptomatic meniscal-deficient knee (37). In an interesting systematic review evaluating the potential chondroprotective role of MAT, Smith et al. (43) evaluated 38 studies that included a total of 1,056 allografts and showed that the weighted mean joint space loss was 0.032 mm at 4.5 years in the 11 studies that reported these values. They similarly found that in the 2 studies that used the contralateral knee as a control, there were no significant differences in joint space changes between the MAT and control. A high rate of meniscal extrusion was shown; however, this did not affect clinical outcomes. Furthermore, it showed that the rate of meniscal healing was high; however, the size, shape, and signal intensity of the allografts were commonly altered from that of the native meniscus on imaging. Despite the low level of evidence of the included studies, they were able to show that there is some evidence that MAT may reduce the progression of osteoarthritis and thus serve a chondroprotective role in the postmeniscectomized patient. However, the meniscus allograft is unlikely to be as effective as the native meniscus. Rosso et al. (36) in a systematic review of 55 studies also showed that MAT provided good clinical results at short-term and midterm follow-up. They showed that it resulted in improvements in knee function and had an acceptable complication and failure rate.

In the past, the different types of graft processing (fresh, fresh-frozen, cryopreserved, or lyophilized) and different graft fixation techniques (suture fixation vs. bony fixation) have made the interpretation of outcome studies more difficult. However, as shown in the recent systematic review by Smith et al. (37), there has been a trend toward using more fresh-frozen allografts, and all studies included in their review that were published after 2010, only used fresh-frozen allografts. Therefore, the removal of the heterogeneity introduced by the different graft preservation techniques will afford a better assessment of outcomes in the future. Additionally, consideration should be given toward using bony fixation rather than suture-only fixation given the finding by Abat et al. (44) that suture-only fixation resulted in a higher rate of meniscus extrusion, although it should be highlighted that the clinical significance of this finding has still not been determined. In terms of limiting the heterogeneity introduced by the use of suture versus bony fixation in different studies, Hergan et al. (39) reviewed 14 studies that documented bony fixation of the allograft meniscal horns that each had a minimum follow-up of 2 years. They were able to show that MAT results in pain relief, improved function, and good patient outcomes. It was shown that there are no differences between medial and lateral MAT procedures, and no differences between patients undergoing isolated MAT and those undergoing MAT with concomitant procedures

Harris et al. (35) published a systematic review of the clinical outcomes of patients undergoing MAT concomitantly with articular cartilage procedures, osteotomy, and/or ACL reconstruction. Results showed improved clinical outcomes at a mean of 36 months after surgery. However, there was a 50% reoperation rate on the 110 patients in the study, and the failure rate was 12%. Similarly, in the largest MAT outcome study to date, McCormick et al. (23) showed that at an average follow-up of 59 months, the 172 patients in their study who had undergone either isolated MAT (40% of cohort) or MAT with concomitant procedures (such as articular cartilage repair, corrective osteotomies, and/or ACL reconstruction) had an overall survival rate of 95% at an average 5-year follow-up. However, there was a 32% reoperation rate, but the majority of patients only required a debridement. The failure rate (revision MAT or arthroplasty) was found to be 5%. Again, this study shows that patients undergoing MAT could expect good/excellent short-term to midterm clinical outcomes.

TABLE 11-1 Clinical Outcomes of MAT (13,17–19,22,23,44–76)

Author	Study Type/ Level of Evidence	Pts No. (Grafts No.)	Mean Age (y)	Mean Follow-up (mo)	No. of Medial MAT	No. of Lateral MAT	Concomitant Procedures	Subjective Outcome Scores	Summary of Outcomes	Failures/ Complications, Time to Failure
Abat (2012)	2	88 (88)	37.7	60	40	48	Not listed	Lysholm improvement	MAT fixed with suture-only technique had significantly higher degree of extruded meniscal body than with bony fixation; higher graft tear rate in suture-only group but not statistically significant	47 (53.4%) with graft extrusion; 7 graft tears in suture-only fixation group; 4 graft tears in bone plug group
Alentorn-Geli (2010)	4	35 (37)	27.2	38.6	24	13	Not listed	Decreased Lysholm score in 3/35 patients compared to preoperative scores, no change in Lysholm in 2/35 patients; 3 patients worsened on IKDC, 1 showed no change; all patients improved on VAS except for 2 with no change	MAT without bone plugs improved knee function and symptoms after partial or total meniscectomy	2 failures (3%)
Bhosale (2007)	4	8 (8)	42	38	2	6	8 ACI (6 bipolar)	Lysholm 49–64	63% satisfied; combination of ACI with MAT is effective	Aseptic synovitis in 2/8; 3/8 failures (35%) in the first 2 y
Chalmers (2013)	4	13 (13)	19.8	39.6	3	10	2 ACLR, 3 OA graft, 1 DFO, 1 MFX	KOOS 76, IKDC 77, Lysholm 80	High-level athletes with symptomatic "postmenisectomy" syndrome can return to desired level of play	2 (23%) needing further surgery including 1 rMAT, 1 MXR, 1 MX
Chang (2008)	4	12 (12)	26.7	17	5	7	3 ACLR, 1 MCLR	Significant improvement in pain, Tegner, Lysholm, and IKDC scores	Symptomatic relief and improvement in knee function following MAT	None
Cole (2006)	4	40 (40)	31	34	25	15	6 OA/allograft, 2 MFX, 2 OCD fixation, 1 ACI, 1 chondral debridement, 6 ligament reconstruction, 1 osteotomy	Significant improvements in Lysholm, Tegner, Noyes, IKDC	78% mostly or completely satisfied, 88% of successes would repeat surgery	7/43 failures (3/7 in 1st year, 7% total patients)

(*Continued*)

TABLE 11-1 Clinical Outcomes of MAT (13,17–19,22,23,44–76) (*Continued*)

Author	Study Type/ Level of Evidence	Pts No. (Grafts No.)	Mean Age (y)	Mean Follow-up (mo)	No. of Medial MAT	No. of Lateral MAT	Concomitant Procedures	Subjective Outcome Scores	Summary of Outcomes	Failures/ Complications, Time to Failure
Farr (2007)	4	29 (29)	37	52	21	8	29 ACI (4 bipolar), 6 HTO, 1 TT medialization, 1 TTO with ACL, 7 ACLR, 1 AMZ	Lysholm 58–78, Cincinnati 4–6, no differences between medial vs. lateral, isolated vs. concomitant, unipolar vs. bipolar	40% good to excellent, including 4 early failures; overall MAT with ACI results in improved symptoms and knee function, but these improvements were less than literature-reported outcomes with isolated procedures	68% of nonfailures in the first 2 y required at least 1 additional procedure; 56% fair/poor by use of Lysholm; 4/33 in the first 2 y
Felix (2003)	4	36 (36)	28.5	62	20	16	18 ACLR, 2 osteotomies, 4 ACLR + osteotomy	Patients report function (0–10) improved from 5.2 preoperatively to 7.3 postoperatively	80% satisfaction; MAT is effective in at least partially replacing functions of the normal meniscus with significant improvement in pain, swelling, and knee function in the short term	6 failures (17%); 10 arthrofibrosis requiring manipulation (3 treated with repair, 1 treated with subsequent meniscectomy); 1 partial meniscectomy of anterior horn, 1 peroneal neuropraxia, 1 hep C possibly related to MAT or ACL graft
Fukushima (2004)	4	40 (40)	37.3	12	29	12	8 ACLR, 1 HTO	Pain and swelling decreased after surgery compared to before surgery	95% satisfaction, pain (5%) and swelling (10%)	1 TKA 12 mo after MAT, 1 HTO 12 mo after MAT; 1 retear 15 mo after MAT
Gonzalez-Lucena (2010)	4	33 (33)	39	78	14	19	8 ACLR, 8 MFX, 9 chondral shaving	Lysholm 65–89, with 69% of scores good or excellent; Tegner 3.1–5.5, VAS 6.4–1.5	No differences between lateral/ medial; no differences between concomitant vs. isolated	33% complication rate
Graf (2004)	4	8 (8)	33	115	8	0	All ACLR (staged or concomitant)	100% of patients were satisfied; no normal IKDC scores: 1 nearly normal, 4 abnormal, 3 severely abnormal	Medial MAT with ACLR can significantly improve knee function in ligamentously unstable, medial meniscus–deficient knees	1 ACLR with allograft requiring revision 6 mo post-op secondary to trauma; 1/9 failures in the first 2 y (due to low-grade infection vs. immune reaction)
Ha (2011)	4	22 (22)	36	25	22	0	2 osteotomy, 15 ACLR, 2 PCL, 4 PLC	Lysholm 68–90, IKDC 60–85	MAT with modified bone plug method is effective; meniscal extrusion not correlated with clinical outcomes	1 case of posterior root graft "failure" on postoperative MRI and second look arthroscopy

Hommen (2007)	4	22 (22)	32	141	14	8	Multiple	90% improvement in Lysholm and pain scores, with no difference between medial vs. lateral, or between bone plug vs. soft tissue fixation	30% good to excellent, 2 worse (both lateral)	40 subsequent procedures; 7/20 total failures (4/8 lateral, 3/12 medial; as determined by Lysholm and pain scores) at mean follow-up of 11.8 y; 55% failure rate if also considering MRI, second-look surgery, and surveys; 85% underwent subsequent procedures
Jang (2011)	3	36 (36)	33.3	14.4	15	21	13 ACLR, 3 PCLR, 4 MFX or ACI	Lysholm increased in all patients	Reducing MAT graft by 5% from the Pollard method decreases the percentage of meniscal extrusion following MAT without any adverse clinical or radiographic outcomes	None
Jang (2013)	4	13 (13)	33	21	0	13	5 MFX	Lysholm 85, IKDC 80, Tegner 6: all significantly improved	This "novel" technique is safe and effective for lateral MAT	None
Kim (2011)	4	29 (29)	30	54	0	29	None	Lysholm 70–90, HSS 15–27; 69% satisfactory, 17% fair, 14% poor	Acceptable subjective and objective findings at short-intermediate follow-up	14% (4 cases)
Kim (2012)	4	106 (110)	33	49	27	83	Unclear (22 ACLR, 4 OCD, 1 ACL/PLC, 1 PCL)	Lysholm 73–92, KSS pain score 33–48	MAT with bone fixation is effective; the authors recommend MRI or arthroscopy to evaluate outcomes in addition to clinical assessment	11% with poor outcomes (failures)
Koh (2012)	4	99 (99)	35	32	26	73	15 ACL, 9 OAT	Lysholm 86–89	No clinical differences between medial and lateral MAT; lateral meniscal transplants extrude further	None
LaPrade (2010)	4	40 (4)	25	30	19	21	6 ACLR, 4 revision ACLR, 4 ROH, 5 MFX, 3 OA allograft, 3 DFO	IKDC 55–72, Cincinnati 55–75	35/40 (88%) successful, 91% improved pain and function	5 with retears requiring partial meniscectomy; 1 infection

(*Continued*)

TABLE 11-1 Clinical Outcomes of MAT (13,17–19,22,23,44–76) (*Continued*)

Author	Study Type/ Level of Evidence	Pts No. (Grafts No.)	Mean Age (y)	Mean Follow-up (mo)	No. of Medial MAT	No. of Lateral MAT	Concomitant Procedures	Subjective Outcome Scores	Summary of Outcomes	Failures/ Complications, Time to Failure
Lee (2010)	4	43 (43)	34	61	7	36	n/a	Lysholm 72–92,	No correlation of graft extrusion with Lysholm score improvement	None
Lee (2011)	4	43 (43)	36	32	6	37	n/a	Lysholm 72–88, but not related to signal intensity on MRI	Transplanted menisci have higher MRI signal intensities than native menisci; signal intensity on MRI not related to clinical outcome	2% with fair outcomes on Lysholm; no failures or complications
Marcacci (2012)	4	32 (32)	36	40	16	16	4 ACLR, 3 HTO, 3 DFO	Significant improvements in VAS, SF-36, Tegner, Lysholm, IKDC	No differences between medial and lateral; no differences between isolated MAT and combined MAT	2 failed (6%), due to lack of benefit
Marcacci (2014)	4	12 (12)	25	36	6	6	2 ACLR, 3 MFX, 1 chondrocyte harvesting, 1 osteochondral scaffolding	Tegner 8–10, Lysholm 67–92, IKDC 62–85, WOMAC 77–92	11/12 professional soccer players returned to play, with 9 (75%) at the professional level at 3 y	1 infection (8%); 3 (25%) with second surgeries not related to MAT and considered successes
McCormick (2014)	4	200	34.3	59	128	72	74 cartilage procedure, 14 cartilage procedure + osteotomy, 23 ACLR, 8 osteotomy	n/a	MAT has a 32% reoperation rate with debridement being the most common subsequent procedure; 95% allograft survival at 5 y, 88% graft survival rate and increased risk of failure in those requiring additional surgery	8/172 failures (4.7%) and required revision MAT or total knee replacement; 64 (32%) had subsequent surgery at mean 21 mo, 44/64 subsequent surgeries were for hardware removal or debridement
Noyes (2005)	4	38 (40)	30	40	20	20	16 osteochondral autograft, 7 ACLR, 1 MCLR, 1 PCL, 1 ACL/PCL	89% pain free with ADLS	MAT improves short-term function and decreases knee pain	4 limited flexion requiring manipulation; 4 allografts failed 8 wk–18 mo requiring removal; 11 (28%) failed, lateral at mean 53 m, medial at mean 25 m; 12 (30%) altered characteristics based on MRI, second-look arthroscopy, and clinical examination

Rath (2001)	4	18 (22)	30	52	15	7	11 ACLR, 3 mx of opposite compartment meniscus, 1 AMZ	Mean IKDC 54, significant improvement in SF-36, including improved scores in patients who had retears allograft	14/22 (64%) successful	1 arthrofibrosis requiring repeat arthroscopy, 8 retears, 1 patellofemoral pain; 8/26 failures (36%) with symptomatic retear at mean 31 mo, resulting in 6 partial and 2 total meniscectomies (4 of these patients had concomitant ACLR, with ACL intact at time of second arthroscopy)
Roumazeille (2013)		22 (22)	37	53	2	20	5 ACLR	Significant improvements in KOOS, IKDC	MAT without bone plugs is effective, and the graft heals in "most" cases at 6 mo	No revisions, 2 second-look scopes
Rue (2008)	4	30 (31)	30	37	20	11	16 ACI, 15 OATS	48% normal/near-normal IKDC	76% mostly or completely satisfied, 90% would repeat surgery	2/29 failed (6.9%) at 2.4 and 3 y
Rueff (2006)	3	8 (8)	51	65	8	0	All with ACLR	IKDC improved from 61 to 90, Lysholm significantly improved	88% would repeat procedure	None reported
Ryu (2002)	4	25 (26)	35	33	10	16	12 ACLR	83% satisfied; significant improvements in IKDC, Lysholm	MAT improves early-term and midterm function and decreases knee pain; isolated MAT and MAT with ACLR with similar outcomes	No complications, 1 clinical failure
Saltzman (2012)	4	22 (22)	33	108	13	9	5 ACI, 3 ACL revision, 2 MFX, 4 osteochondral autograft/allograft, 3 ROH, 1 thermal shrinkage	86% near-normal or normal IKDC	Survivorship 88%; all patients completely or mostly satisfied	12% failures
Sekiya (2003)	4	28 (31)	35	32	7	24	19 ACLR, 9 revision ACLR, 2 lateral closing wedge HTO	93% somewhat or greatly improved; 86% near-normal or normal IKDC with SF-36 components higher than age/sex-matched populations	MAT with ACLR can be beneficial in properly selected patients with ACL and meniscal deficiency	1 pt felt worse

(Continued)

TABLE 11-1 Clinical Outcomes of MAT (13,17–19,22,23,44–76) (*Continued*)

Author	Study Type/ Level of Evidence	Pts No. (Grafts No.)	Mean Age (y)	Mean Follow-up (mo)	No. of Medial MAT	No. of Lateral MAT	Concomitant Procedures	Subjective Outcome Scores	Summary of Outcomes	Failures/ Complications, Time to Failure
Sekiya (2006)	4	25 (25)	30	39	0	25	None	SF-36 higher than age/sex-matched controls; 96% improved function and activity level; bony fixation with better ROM compared to suture fixation	Isolated lateral MAT is a beneficial procedure in properly selected patients; bony fixation may have benefit over suture fixation	Not defined, 1/25 unsatisfied
Stollsteimer (2000)	4	22 (23)	31	40	11	12	n/a	Overall reduction of pain; significant improvements in Tegner, IKDC, and Lysholm	78% with pain improvement, but allograft shrinkage on MRI remains a concern	1 infection, 1 hemarthrosis, 2 synovitis requiring synovectomy, 1 loosened bone plug, 6 meniscal tears requiring surgery (5 partial meniscectomies and 1 repair); failure not defined, 1 infection requiring graft removal
Stone (2010)	4	115 (119)	46.9	69.6	85	34	67 cartilage paste grafting, 69 MFX, 15 medial opening tibial osteotomy, 10 ACLR with bone-patellar tendon-bone allograft, 6 ACLR with middle-third patellar tendon autograft, 1 ACLR with Achilles tendon allograft	Significant improvements at all periods of follow-up in Tegner, IKDC, and WOMAC with the exception of the 7-y Tegner index score	Survival of transplant not affected by gender, severity of cartilage damage, axial alignment, degree of joint space narrowing, or medial vs. lateral transplant	8 (6.7%) requiring revision MAT (1 required 2 revisions) at mean 7 mo; 18 progressed to knee replacement at mean 5.1 y

van der Wal (2009)	4	63 (57)	39.4	165.6	23	40	8 ACLR	Overall Lysholm scores significantly improved at long-term follow-up. All subgroups had poor scores at mean follow-up of 13.8 y, except the male patients group, which had a fair score. Short-term Lysholm scores were 79 ± 19 at 3.1 ± 1.5 y. All subgroups demonstrated a significant difference between short- and long-term Lysholm scores	Open MAT is a good salvage treatment option for postponing TKA in the young patient with postmeniscectomy arthritis; patients <50 year old with normally aligned, stable knee joints with sufficient ACLs are the best candidates for MAT	18 (29%) failures (8 medial, 10 lateral), mean time to failure = 123 mo
Verdonk (2005)	4	100 (100)	35	86	39	61	3 ACLR, 15 HTO, 2 DFO, 4 OA transfer, 3 MFX	Significant improvements in modified HSS scores	74% medial, 70% lateral survived, increased survived when osteotomy performed	21 failed grafts (11 medial, 10 lateral)
Vundelinckx (2010)	4	34 (35)	33	105	13	22	1 alignment correction with Ilizarov correction system, 2 HTO, 2 MFX, 5 ACLR	Significant and clinically relevant increase on all scales: VAS, KOOS, all KOOS subscales, Lysholm, and SF-36	All but 1 would undergo the procedure again; the more severe the osteoarthritis, the less the improvement following MAT ($p < 0.001$) increase in osteoarthritis in 42% of the patients (14 of 33), as scored following the Kellgren-Lawrence classification	5 failures ~10 y post-MAT; 1 arthrofibrosis requiring mobilization, 1 reinsertion of anterior horn of the allograft 15 mo post-MAT and partial meniscectomy 24 mo post-MAT; 1 patient required graft removal
Wirth (2002)	3	23 (23)	29.6	168	23	0	23 ACLR	Lysholm score was 84 ± 12 points at 3 y postoperatively and 75 ± 23 points at 14 y	All showed degenerative changes by radiography; no differences between transplanted vs. meniscectomy control group	n/a

(*Continued*)

TABLE 11-1 Clinical Outcomes of MAT (13,17–19,22,23,44–76) (*Continued*)

Author	Study Type/ Level of Evidence	Pts No. (Grafts No.)	Mean Age (y)	Mean Follow-up (mo)	No. of Medial MAT	No. of Lateral MAT	Concomitant Procedures	Subjective Outcome Scores	Summary of Outcomes	Failures/ Complications, Time to Failure
Yoldas (2003)	3	31 (34)	28	33	19	15	20 ACLR (12 primary, 8 revision)		97% somewhat or greatly improved, 97% knee function near-normal or normal	
Yoon (2014)	3	91 (91)	34	40	35	56	Medial: 18 ACLR, 10 ACI, 4 MFX, 2 HTO; lateral: 11 ACLR, 2 PCL, 11 ACI, 12 MFX	VAS 5–3, IKDC 52–67, Lysholm 64–77, Tegner 2–4	No differences between medial and lateral; isolated MAT group with higher VAS and Lysholm than combined group	Unclear, but 27 second-look scopes for "painful knee with suspected meniscal tear"
Zhang (2011)	3	18 (18)	37	25	7	11	10 (ACLR, osteotomies)	Significant improvements in Lysholm, KOOS, VAS	No differences between medial and lateral; no differences between isolated and combined	11% ($n = 2$)

ACI, autologous chondrocyte implantation; ACL, anterior cruciate ligament; ACLR, anterior cruciate ligament repair; AMZ, anteromedialization; HTO, high tibial osteotomy; MCLR, medial collateral ligament repair; MFX, microfracture; N/A, data not available; OATS, osteochondral autograft transplant system; OCD, osteochondritis dissecans; PCLR, posterior cruciate ligament repair; TTO, tibial tubercle osteotomy.

Furthermore, although patients with the desire to return to high-impact activities are cautioned about the risk of graft tearing and failure, some recent studies (45,46) have shown that patients are able to return to competitive sports after MAT. In a study by Chalmers et al. (46) in which our preferred bridge-in-slot technique was used, they reported on 13 high-level athletes (high school through professional level) with a mean follow-up of 3.3 years. Seventy-seven percent of the athletes were able to return to play at a mean of 17 months after surgery. There were significant improvements in nearly all outcomes scales, including IKDC, Lysholm, knee injury and osteoarthritis outcome score, and patient satisfaction. Similarly, Marcacci et al. (45) showed that 11/12 professional soccer players were able to return to competition after MAT and that 75% of patients reported that they were playing at their preinjury level.

In the small cohort of patients who have a failed MAT and still meet all of the criteria to be indicated for MAT, consideration should be given for a revision MAT procedure. Yanke et al. (20) recently reported on the clinical and radiographic outcomes after revision MAT in 12 patients and found that at a mean follow-up of 3.83 ± 1.3 years, revision MAT resulted in high patient satisfaction and significant improvements on validated outcome scores. It should be highlighted that correctable causes of MAT failure should be addressed either prior to or simultaneously with the revision MAT to decrease the chances of another failed procedure.

CONCLUSIONS

MAT is a safe and effective procedure for a patient with a meniscus-deficient knee. The procedure has resulted in roughly 85% good to excellent outcomes in short-term to midterm follow-up studies, and patients have enjoyed significant pain reduction and increased activity. Further studies will be needed to determine the long-term clinical outcomes of MAT and its possible chondroprotective effect, as well as the potential future roles of synthetic scaffolds and tissue-engineered meniscal grafts.

ACKNOWLEDGMENTS

The authors would like to thank Maggie Smith for her assistance with this manuscript.

REFERENCES

1. Baratz ME, Fu FH, Mengato R. Meniscal tears: the effect of meniscectomy and of repair on intraarticular contact areas and stress in the human knee. A preliminary report. *Am J Sports Med.* 1986;14:270–275.
2. Chatain F, Robinson AH, Adeleine P, et al. The natural history of the knee following arthroscopic medial meniscectomy. *Knee Surg Sports Traumatol Arthrosc.* 2001;9:15–18.
3. Allen PR, Denham RA, Swan AV. Late degenerative changes after meniscectomy. Factors affecting the knee after operation. *J Bone Joint Surg Br.* 1984;66:666–671.
4. Yoon KH, Lee SH, Bae DK, et al. Does varus alignment increase after medial meniscectomy? *Knee Surg Sports Traumatol Arthrosc.* 2013;21:2131–2136.
5. Mow VC, Ratcliffe A, Poole AR. Cartilage and diarthrodial joints as paradigms for hierarchical materials and structures. *Biomaterials.* 1992;13:67–97.
6. McGinity JB, Geuss LF, Marvin RA. Partial or total meniscectomy: a comparative analysis. *J Bone Joint Surg Am.* 1977;59:763–766.
7. MacConaill MA. The movements of bones and joints; the synovial fluid and its assistants. *J Bone Joint Surg Br.* 1950;32-B:244–252.
8. Levy IM, Torzilli PA, Warren RF. The effect of medial meniscectomy on anterior-posterior motion of the knee. *J Bone Joint Surg Am.* 1982;64:883–888.
9. Markolf KL, Mensch JS, Amstutz HC. Stiffness and laxity of the knee–the contributions of the supporting structures. A quantitative in vitro study. *J Bone Joint Surg Am.* 1976;58:583–594.
10. Walker PS, Erkman MJ. The role of the menisci in force transmission across the knee. *Clin Orthop Relat Res.* 1975:184–192.
11. Ahmed AM, Burke DL. In-vitro measurement of static pressure distribution in synovial joints–part i: tibial surface of the knee. *J Biomech Eng.* 1983;105:216–225.
12. Alford JW, Lewis P, Kang RW, et al. Rapid progression of chondral disease in the lateral compartment of the knee following meniscectomy. *Arthroscopy.* 2005;21:1505–1509.
13. Sekiya JK, West RV, Groff YJ, et al. Clinical outcomes following isolated lateral meniscal allograft transplantation. *Arthroscopy.* 2006;22:771–780.
14. Arnoczky SP, Warren RF, McDevitt CA. Meniscal replacement using a cryopreserved allograft. An experimental study in the dog. *Clin Orthop Relat Res.* 1990;252:121–128.
15. Jackson DW, Whelan J, Simon TM. Cell survival after transplantation of fresh meniscal allografts. DNA probe analysis in a goat model. *Am J Sports Med.* 1993;21:540–550.
16. Szomor ZL, Martin TE, Bonar F, et al. The protective effects of meniscal transplantation on cartilage. An experimental study in sheep. *J Bone Joint Surg Am.* 2000;82:80–88.

17. Cole BJ, Dennis MG, Lee SJ, et al. Prospective evaluation of allograft meniscus transplantation: a minimum 2-year follow-up. *Am J Sports Med.* 2006;34:919–927.
18. LaPrade RF, Wills NJ, Spiridonov SI, et al. A prospective outcomes study of meniscal allograft transplantation. *Am J Sports Med.* 2010;38:1804–1812.
19. Vundelinckx B, Bellemans J, Vanlauwe J. Arthroscopically assisted meniscal allograft transplantation in the knee: a medium-term subjective, clinical, and radiographical outcome evaluation. *Am J Sports Med.* 2010;38:2240–2247.
20. Yanke AB, Chalmers PN, Frank RM, et al. Clinical outcome of revision meniscal allograft transplantation: minimum 2-year follow-up. *Arthroscopy.* 2014;30:1602–1608.
21. Matava MJ. Meniscal allograft transplantation: a systematic review. *Clin Orthop Relat Res.* 2007;455:142–157.
22. Rue JP, Yanke AB, Busam ML, et al. Prospective evaluation of concurrent meniscus transplantation and articular cartilage repair: minimum 2-year follow-up. *Am J Sports Med.* 2008;36:1770–1778.
23. McCormick F, Harris JD, Abrams GD, et al. Survival and reoperation rates after meniscal allograft transplantation: analysis of failures for 172 consecutive transplants at a minimum 2-year follow-up. *Am J Sports Med.* 2014;42:892–897.
24. Ha JK, Jang HW, Jung JE, et al. Clinical and radiologic outcomes after meniscus allograft transplantation at 1-year and 4-year follow-up. *Arthroscopy.* 2014;30:1424–1429.
25. Alhalki MM, Hull ML, Howell SM. Contact mechanics of the medial tibial plateau after implantation of a medial meniscal allograft. A human cadaveric study. *Am J Sports Med.* 2000;28:370–376.
26. Dienst M, Greis PE, Ellis BJ, et al. Effect of lateral meniscal allograft sizing on contact mechanics of the lateral tibial plateau: an experimental study in human cadaveric knee joints. *Am J Sports Med.* 2007;35:34–42.
27. Yoon JR, Kim TS, Wang JH, et al. Importance of independent measurement of width and length of lateral meniscus during preoperative sizing for meniscal allograft transplantation. *Am J Sports Med.* 2011;39:1541–1547.
28. Pollard ME, Kang Q, Berg EE. Radiographic sizing for meniscal transplantation. *Arthroscopy.* 1995;11:684–687.
29. Haut TL, Hull ML, Howell SM. Use of roentgenography and magnetic resonance imaging to predict meniscal geometry determined with a three-dimensional coordinate digitizing system. *J Orthop Res.* 2000;18:228–237.
30. Prodromos CC, Joyce BT, Keller BL, et al. Magnetic resonance imaging measurement of the contralateral normal meniscus is a more accurate method of determining meniscal allograft size than radiographic measurement of the recipient tibial plateau. *Arthroscopy.* 2007;23:1174–1179.e1171.
31. Van Thiel GS, Verma N, Yanke A, et al. Meniscal allograft size can be predicted by height, weight, and gender. *Arthroscopy.* 2009;25:722–727.
32. Vangsness CT Jr, Garcia IA, Mills CR, et al. Allograft transplantation in the knee: tissue regulation, procurement, processing, and sterilization. *Am J Sports Med.* 2003;31:474–481.
33. Bursac P, York A, Kuznia P, et al. Influence of donor age on the biomechanical and biochemical properties of human meniscal allografts. *Am J Sports Med.* 2009;37:884–889.
34. Farr J, Meneghini RM, Cole BJ. Allograft interference screw fixation in meniscus transplantation. *Arthroscopy.* 2004;20:322–327.
35. Harris JD, Cavo M, Brophy R, et al. Biological knee reconstruction: a systematic review of combined meniscal allograft transplantation and cartilage repair or restoration. *Arthroscopy.* 2011;27:409–418.
36. Rosso F, Bisicchia S, Bonasia DE, et al. Meniscal allograft transplantation: a systematic review. *Am J Sports Med.* 2015;43(4):998–1007.
37. Smith NA, MacKay N, Costa M, et al. Meniscal allograft transplantation in a symptomatic meniscal deficient knee: a systematic review. *Knee Surg Sports Traumatol Arthrosc.* 2015;23:270–279.
38. Milachowski KA, Weismeier K, Wirth CJ. Homologous meniscus transplantation. Experimental and clinical results. *Int Orthop.* 1989;13:1–11.
39. Hergan D, Thut D, Sherman O, et al. Meniscal allograft transplantation. *Arthroscopy.* 2011;27:101–112.
40. Lee AS, Kang RW, Kroin E, et al. Allograft meniscus transplantation. *Sports Med Arthrosc.* 2012;20:106–114.
41. Verdonk R, Volpi P, Verdonk P, et al. Indications and limits of meniscal allografts. *Injury.* 2013;44(suppl 1):S21–S27.
42. Elattar M, Dhollander A, Verdonk R, et al. Twenty-six years of meniscal allograft transplantation: is it still experimental? A meta-analysis of 44 trials. *Knee Surg Sports Traumatol Arthrosc.* 2011;19:147–157.
43. Smith NA, Parkinson B, Hutchinson CE, et al. Is meniscal allograft transplantation chondroprotective? A systematic review of radiological outcomes. *Knee Surg Sports Traumatol Arthrosc.* 2016;24(9):2923–2935.
44. Abat F, Gelber PE, Erquicia JI, et al. Suture-only fixation technique leads to a higher degree of extrusion than bony fixation in meniscal allograft transplantation. *Am J Sports Med.* 2012;40:1591–1596.
45. Marcacci M, Marcheggiani Muccioli GM, Grassi A, et al. Arthroscopic meniscus allograft transplantation in male professional soccer players: a 36-month follow-up study. *Am J Sports Med.* 2014;42:382–388.
46. Chalmers PN, Karas V, Sherman SL, et al. Return to high-level sport after meniscal allograft transplantation. *Arthroscopy.* 2013;29:539–544.
47. Alentorn-Geli E, Seijas Vázquez R, García Balletbó M, et al. Arthroscopic meniscal allograft transplantation without bone plugs. *Knee Surg Sports Traumatol Arthrosc.* 2010. doi: 20390252.
48. Bhosale AM, Myint P, Roberts S, et al. Combined autologous chondrocyte implantation and allogenic meniscus transplantation: a biological knee replacement. *Knee.* 2007;14:361–368.
49. Farr J, Rawal A, Marberry KM. Concomitant meniscal allograft transplantation and autologous chondrocyte implantation: minimum 2-year follow-up. *Am J Sports Med.* 2007;35:1459–1466.
50. Felix NA, Paulos LE. Current status of meniscal transplantation. *Knee.* 2003;10:13–17.
51. Fukushima K, Adachi N, Lee JY, et al. Meniscus allograft transplantation using posterior peripheral suture technique: a preliminary follow-up study. *J Orthop Sci.* 2004;9:235–241.
52. González-Lucena G, Gelber PE, Pelfort X, et al. Meniscal allograft transplantation without bone blocks: a 5- to 8-year follow-up of 33 patients. *Arthroscopy.* 2010;26:1633–1640.
53. Graf KW, Sekiya JK, Wojtys EM, et al. Long-term results after combined medial meniscal allograft transplantation and anterior cruciate ligament reconstruction: minimum 8.5-year follow-up study. *Arthroscopy.* 2004;20:129–140.
54. Ha JK, Sung JH, Shim JC, et al. Medial meniscus allograft transplantation using a modified bone plug technique: clinical, radiologic, and arthroscopic results. *Arthroscopy.* 2011;27:944–950.
55. Hommen JP, Applegate GR, Del Pizzo W. Meniscus allograft transplantation: ten-year results of cryopreserved allografts. *Arthroscopy.* 2007;23:388–393.
56. Jang SH, Kim JG, Ha JG, et al. Reducing the size of the meniscal allograft decreases the percentage of extrusion after meniscal allograft transplantation. *Arthroscopy.* 2011;27:914–922.

57. Kim JM, Lee BS, Kim KH, et al. Results of meniscus allograft transplantation using bone fixation: 110 cases with objective evaluation. *Am J Sports Med.* 2012;40:1027–1034.
58. Kim CW, Kim JM, Lee SH, et al. Results of isolated lateral meniscus allograft transplantation: focus on objective evaluations with magnetic resonance imaging. *Am J Sports Med.* 2011;39:1960–1967.
59. Koh YG, Moon HK, Kim YC, et al. Comparison of medial and lateral meniscal transplantation with regard to extrusion of the allograft, and its correlation with clinical outcome. *J Bone Joint Surg Br.* 2012;94:190–193.
60. Lee DH, Kim SB, Kim TH, et al. Midterm outcomes after meniscal allograft transplantation: comparison of cases with extrusion versus without extrusion. *Am J Sports Med.* 2010;38:247–254.
61. Lee DH, Lee BS, Chung JW, et al. Changes in magnetic resonance imaging signal intensity of transplanted meniscus allografts are not associated with clinical outcomes. *Arthroscopy.* 2011;27:1211–1218.
62. Marcacci M, Zaffagnini S, Marcheggiani Muccioli GM, et al. Meniscal allograft transplantation without bone plugs: a 3-year minimum follow-up study. *Am J Sports Med.* 2012;40:395–403.
63. Noyes FR, Barber-Westin SD, Rankin M. Meniscal transplantation in symptomatic patients less than fifty years old. *J Bone Joint Surg Am.* 2005;87(suppl 1):149–165.
64. Rath E, Richmond JC, Yassir W, et al. Meniscal allograft transplantation. Two- to eight-year results. *Am J Sports Med.* 2001;29:410–414.
65. Roumazeille T, Klouche S, Rousselin B, et al. Arthroscopic meniscal allograft transplantation with two tibia tunnels without bone plugs: evaluation of healing on mr arthrography and functional outcomes. *Knee Surg Sports Traumatol Arthrosc.* 2015;23:264–269.
66. Rueff D, Nyland J, Kocabey Y, et al. Self-reported patient outcomes at a minimum of 5 years after allograft anterior cruciate ligament reconstruction with or without medial meniscus transplantation: an age-, sex-, and activity level-matched comparison in patients aged approximately 50 years. *Arthroscopy.* 2006;22:1053–1062.
67. Ryu RK, Dunbar V WH, Morse GG. Meniscal allograft replacement: a 1-year to 6-year experience. *Arthroscopy.* 2002;18:989–994.
68. Saltzman BM, Bajaj S, Salata M, et al. Prospective long-term evaluation of meniscal allograft transplantation procedure: a minimum of 7-year follow-up. *J Knee Surg.* 2012;25:165–175.
69. Sekiya JK, Giffin JR, Irrgang JJ, et al. Clinical outcomes after combined meniscal allograft transplantation and anterior cruciate ligament reconstruction. *Am J Sports Med.* 2003;31:896–906.
70. Stollsteimer GT, Shelton WR, Dukes A, et al. Meniscal allograft transplantation: a 1- to 5-year follow-up of 22 patients. *Arthroscopy.* 2000;16:343–347.
71. Stone KR, Adelson WS, Pelsis JR, et al. Long-term survival of concurrent meniscus allograft transplantation and repair of the articular cartilage: a prospective two- to 12-year follow-up report. *J Bone Joint Surg Br.* 2010;92:941–948.
72. van der Wal RJ, Thomassen BJ, van Arkel ER. Long-term clinical outcome of open meniscal allograft transplantation. *Am J Sports Med.* 2009;37:2134–2139.
73. Wirth CJ, Peters G, Milachowski KA, et al. Long-term results of meniscal allograft transplantation. *Am J Sports Med.* 2002;30:174–181.
74. Yoldas EA, Sekiya JK, Irrgang JJ, et al. Arthroscopically assisted meniscal allograft transplantation with and without combined anterior cruciate ligament reconstruction. *Knee Surg Sports Traumatol Arthrosc.* 2003;11:173–182.
75. Yoon KH, Lee SH, Park SY, et al. Meniscus allograft transplantation: a comparison of medial and lateral procedures. *Am J Sports Med.* 2014;42:200–207.
76. Zhang H, Liu X, Wei Y, et al. Meniscal allograft transplantation in isolated and combined surgery. *Knee Surg Sports Traumatol Arthrosc.* 2012;20:281–289.

PART III LIGAMENT INJURIES/ INSTABILITY

12 Graft Harvest Techniques for Knee Ligament Reconstruction

K. J. Hippensteel, Marcus A. Rothermich, and Rick W. Wright

INDICATIONS AND CONTRAINDICATIONS

Donor options for knee ligament reconstruction include various allograft or autograft harvests. Surgeon comfort level with particular grafts and patient characteristics such as age, lifestyle, sporting activity level, and prior knee injuries or surgical procedures to the knee affect decision making. Allografts are attractive options for knee ligament reconstructions secondary to their lack of harvest morbidity, decreased postoperative pain, and easier initial rehabilitation. Potential allograft sources include the tibialis posterior, tibialis anterior, Achilles tendon, and bone patellar tendon bone. However, the MOON (Multicenter Orthopaedic Outcomes Network) prospective longitudinal cohort determined that allograft primary anterior cruciate ligament (ACL) reconstructions had a four times higher odds of graft rupture compared to autografts when holding age constant at 2-year follow-up (1). When further analyzed, tissue bank, allograft type, and irradiation status were not found to be significant variables affecting allograft retear rate (1). Furthermore, the MARS (Multicenter ACL Revision Study) prospective longitudinal cohort showed that in the setting of revision ACL reconstructions, autografts had significantly improved sports function and activity levels as determined by patient-reported outcome measures at 2-year follow-up when compared to allografts (2). In addition, autografts were found to be 2.78 times less likely to endure a subsequent graft rupture (2). Interestingly, bone-patella-tendon-bone (BPTB) and soft tissue grafts did not differ in revision graft rerupture rate for either autograft or allograft in this study, but this may be due to the limited 2-year follow-up (2).

Potential autograft options for knee ligament reconstruction include BPTB, quadrupled hamstring, and quadriceps tendon grafts. All three graft options have advantages and disadvantages in their harvest. A systematic review comparing BPTB and hamstring grafts for ACL reconstruction found no differences in subjective or objective outcomes, return to activity, or failure rates (3). In the early postoperative time frame, the fixation of the graft to the bone rather than the ultimate tensile strength of the graft is the most significant variable affecting the structural characteristics of the graft (4,5). This weak link in regard to graft fixation persists for up to 4 to 12 weeks postoperatively (5).

Advantages of BPTB grafts include its comparable initial strength and stiffness to hamstring and quadriceps autografts that are also four times greater than a native ACL, its long-term stability, and the presence of a bone plug on each end of the tendon (4–7). This ensures bone-to-bone healing that is thought to occur more quickly when compared to soft tissue-to-bone healing (5,7). It also helps provide an interference fit within the tunnel that when combined with an interference screw helps provide sturdy fixation allowing for early rehabilitation (5). The main disadvantage of BPTB grafts is donor site morbidity, which can include loss of quadriceps strength, damage to the infrapatellar branch of the saphenous nerve, patellofemoral crepitus, loss of knee flexion, anterior knee pain, patella tendonitis, and kneeling knee pain (5). Careful surgical technique can help minimize complications such as patellar fracture and patella tendon rupture (3,5,7–9). While 10% to 40% of patients report anterior knee pain after BPTB harvest, it has been shown that this may occur regardless of graft choice (3,5,10). Kneeling pain has been shown in multiple randomized controlled trials to occur more frequently in 36% to 67% of patients with BPTB grafts compared to 15% to 26% of patients with hamstring grafts at 2- to 3-year follow-up (3,5,11–13).

Advantages of quadrupled hamstring grafts include the greatest initial strength and stiffness of all three grafts, a large surface area of collagen closer in size to a normal ACL, adaptability for precise positioning, less donor site morbidity, no risk of patella fracture or patella tendon rupture, ability to use in skeletally immature patients to avoid physeal damage, and avoidance of the knee extensor mechanism (4,5,7,14–16). Bone tunnels can be placed in the desired location and then completely filled with the collagenous soft tissue, while BPTB grafts require over drilling of the bone tunnels to fit the bone blocks on the proximal and distal ends (14). The main disadvantages of hamstring grafts include the unpredictable hamstring size or risk of amputation of graft during harvest and the risk of damage to or harvesting of the medial collateral ligament (MCL) (5,7–9,15,17). Other complications of hamstring grafts involve risk of damage to the saphenous nerve during harvest, pain from prominent fixation hardware, recurrence of knee ligamentous laxity, longer time to healing for soft tissue healing to bone, bone tunnel widening, and residual hamstring weakness, which can lead to a 10% loss in hamstring strength after recovery (5,7–9,15,17). While newer aperture fixation methods of hamstring graft fixation have addressed the bungee effect causing micromotion and tunnel widening seen in suspensory fixation, they still rely on soft tissue-to-bone healing, which does not occur as quickly as bone-to-bone healing (5,7). Animal models have shown that soft tissue tendon grafts do not fully incorporate to bone until at least 12 weeks postoperatively, while BPTB grafts have been noted to be histologically incorporated at 8 weeks postoperatively (18,19). This correlates with a case report that performed histological analysis on the tibial graft-bone interface for revision hamstring ACL reconstructions at 12 and 15 weeks postoperatively and found well-developed graft integration at these times (20).

Advantages of quadriceps grafts are a large surface area that provides about 50% more collagen than a BPTB graft, bone to bone fixation on one side of the graft (if using a patella bone plug), similar tensile strength to the other grafts, less donor site morbidity than BPTB grafts, an incision that avoids the infrapatellar branch of the saphenous nerve, and its utility in revision settings where BPTB and hamstring grafts have already been harvested (5,7,21). Disadvantages include a risk of patella fracture, a risk of entering the suprapatellar pouch during harvest causing loss of knee distention during arthroscopic ligament reconstruction, decreased graft stiffness, and a decrease of up to 20% in quadriceps strength postoperatively (5,7,21).

A contraindication to any of the grafts would be in the setting of revision surgery where this particular graft has already been harvested. Contraindications for BPTB grafts include a degenerative patellofemoral joint or prior patella fracture (14,17). A relative contraindication to BPTB would be any patient who repeatedly kneels for their occupation or sport as BPTB grafts have an increased risk of kneeling pain compared to other autograft options (3,5,12–14,17). A relative contraindication to hamstring grafts is athletes that do significant running backward such as football defensive backs.

PREOPERATIVE PLANNING

A patient's history, physical exam, and radiographic findings can help guide the surgeon on the graft to choose. While obtaining a history, one should identify the patient's age, occupation, prior knee surgeries or arthrosis, and athletic pursuits. Physical exam of the knee should determine if there is any patella maltracking or instability, an injury to the extensor mechanism, or any other associated knee ligamentous injuries (9). Prior surgical procedures on the knee should be confirmed to either rule out an ipsilateral graft as a potential option or to allow consideration of the contralateral extremity for graft harvest. Radiographic imaging of the knee is used preoperatively to evaluate for patellofemoral osteoarthritis, open physes, or patella baja or alta. If patella alta is determined on radiographs, many techniques are available to deal with a graft that will be longer than expected to help prevent external graft protrusion (9). In the operating room, a suitable table for graft preparation and all required instrumentation for graft harvest and fixation should be available. In the rare incidence that a graft is dropped on the surgical floor, consent for either another ipsilateral or contralateral autograft or an allograft should be obtained. Furthermore, the hardware required for alternative graft fixation should be verified before harvest, and allograft options should be available (9). However, this may not be practical in day-to-day practice. Therefore, one should be familiar with graft sterilizing techniques to salvage a graft if other autograft or allograft options are not available.

OPERATIVE TECHNIQUES

Patellar Tendon

Introduction

In the ligamentous reconstruction of the knee, the patellar tendon is a commonly used autograft. As discussed, the patellar tendon and hamstring tendons are the most frequently used autografts for reconstruction, and controversy remains over the ideal autograft for each individual patient. For patients in whom the patellar tendon has been chosen for reconstruction, we have developed a standardized technique for the harvest of the middle third of the tendon, reliably producing an adequate graft from knee ligament reconstruction.

Patient Positioning

For patellar tendon, hamstring tendon, and quadriceps tendon harvesting, patient positioning is uniform. The patient is positioned supine in all three harvesting scenarios with the leg supported by a thigh holder anterior and posterior. A nonsterile tourniquet is placed around the thigh as proximally as possible. The posterior thigh holder is positioned as distally as possible at the break in the bed, and the anterior thigh holder is placed below the nonsterile tourniquet as proximally as possible on the thigh. The contralateral thigh is padded, and the operative extremity is prepped and draped in standard fashion. General endotracheal anesthesia is preferred, although utilization of an epidural is possible if necessitated by patient comorbidities.

Technique

When beginning a patellar tendon graft harvest, the knee is flexed to 90 degrees to tighten the patellar tendon. Make a vertical incision through the skin from the inferior patellar pole to the tibial tubercle with a 15-blade. Open the peritenon with a 15-blade and elevate the peritenon with Metzenbaum scissors, elevating distally and laterally. Find the lateral edge of patellar tendon, which is more sharply defined than the medial edge. Measure 1 cm medially from the lateral edge of tendon using a ruler. With an 11-blade, incise the patellar tendon with the blade facing up in line with the tendon fibers (Fig. 12-1). As soon as resistance is felt on the patella, bring 11-blade distally 1 cm and flip to have the blade facing down. Incise the patellar tendon down to the tibial tubercle, and begin incising periosteum with the 11-blade perpendicular to the bone. Extend the knee when incising distal to the tibial tubercle, and incise approximately 3 cm down on the tibial tubercle. Flex the knee, and measure 1 cm medial to the first incision with the metal ruler (Fig. 12-2). Follow the same steps to make a second vertical incision in line with the fibers of the patellar tendon. After the second incision has been completed by incising the periosteum of the most proximal 3 cm of the tibial tubercle, transversely score the periosteum distally for the distal saw cut. Place the foot on a stand with the knee extended.

Drill two holes in the tibial tubercle bone plug with a 0.062-in Kirschner wire from anterior to posterior at 1 cm and 2 cm along the length of the 3-cm bone plug (Fig. 12-3). Mark the holes from this drilling with an indelible marking pen. Use a goiter retractor to retract the skin and the split tendon edge to expose the interface of the patellar tendon and the tibial tubercle. Use an oscillating saw to cut through the cortex of the tibial tubercle in line with the fibers of the patellar tendon for the entire 3 cm length of the bone plug at a 45-degree angle from the vertical (Fig. 12-4). Start the saw

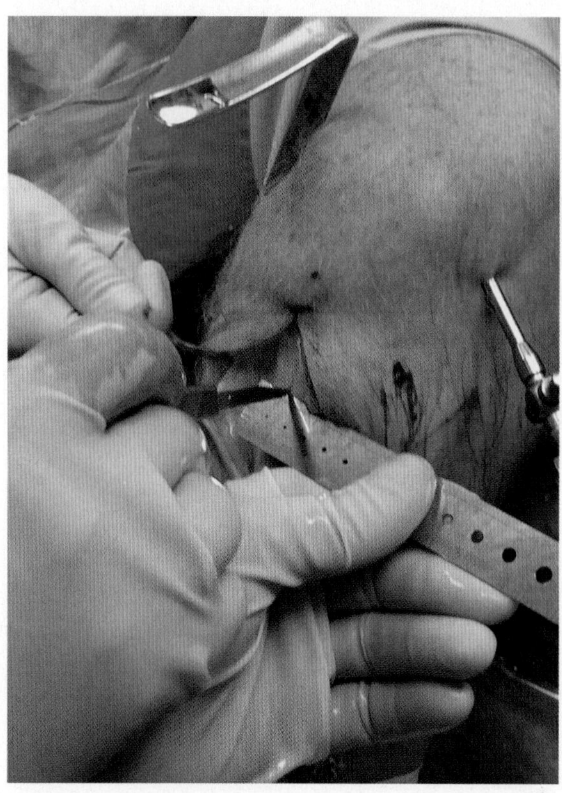

FIGURE 12-1

Incising patella tendon 1 cm medially from lateral edge of the tendon.

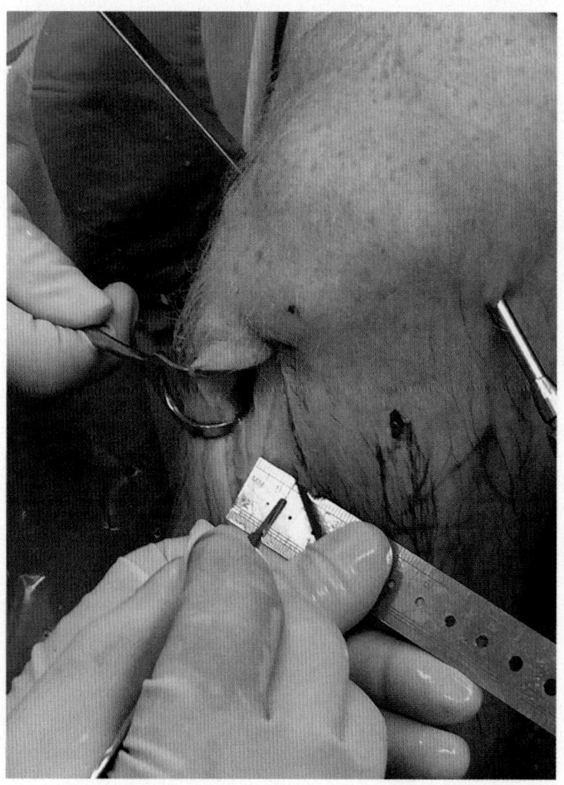

FIGURE 12-2

Measuring 1 cm medial to first patella tendon incision with ruler.

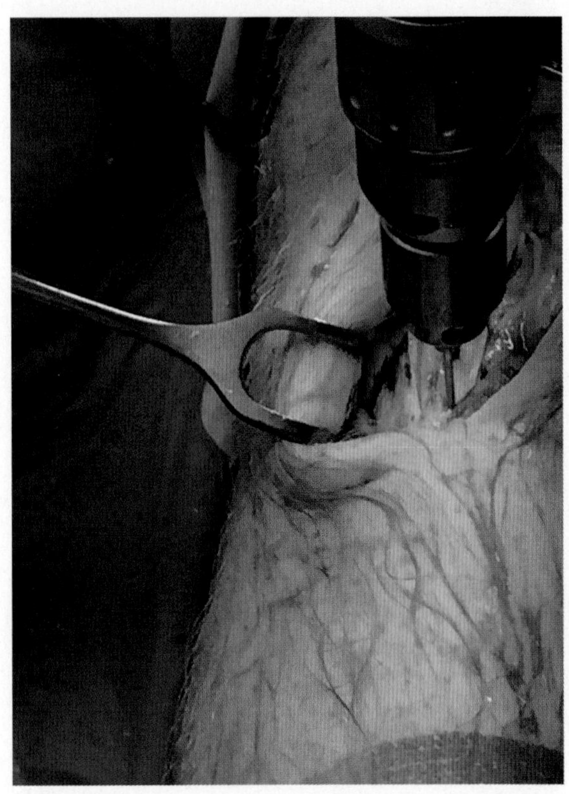

FIGURE 12-3

Drilling hole in the tibial tubercle bone plug with a 0.062-in Kirschner wire.

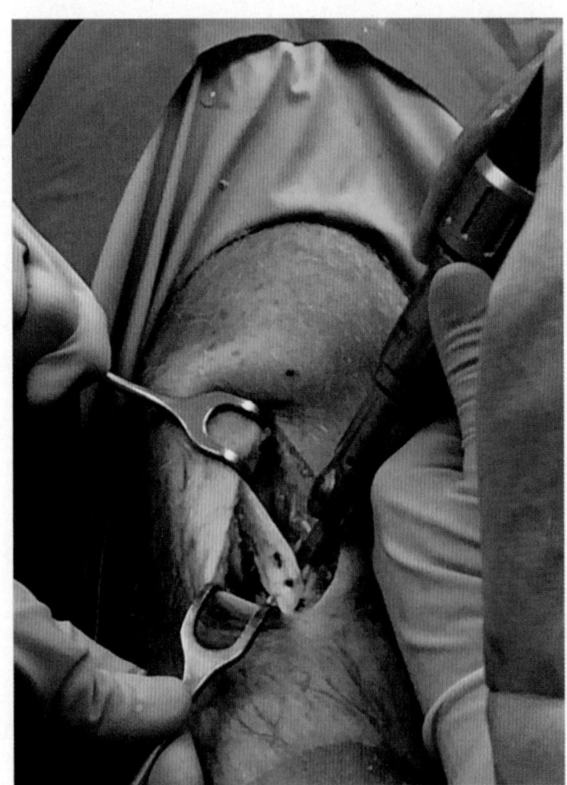

FIGURE 12-4

Oscillating saw cutting through the cortex of the tibial tubercle at a 45-degree angle from the vertical.

blade proximal to the tibial tubercle cortex to ensure that no tendon is left attached after the cut has been made. Cut only the cortex. After both longitudinal cuts have been made on the tibial tubercle, make the transverse cortical cut on the distal end of the tibial tubercle bone plug. Tap a ¼-in straight osteotome into distal saw cut and gently pry the bone plug out. If the plug does not come out easily, recut the bone.

Use a rongeur to shape the bone plug to slide easily through a 10-mm sizer. Pass a no. 2 Ethibond through the predrilled holes in the tibial tubercle bone plug. Cut the needle off of the suture and tie the two strands together in a single knot. Have an assistant pull distally on these sutures to place graft on tension and expose the patella.

Place a goiter proximally to help expose the patella. Use a 15-blade to score the distal 2/3 of the patella in line with the longitudinal split incisions in the patellar tendon. Predrill two holes for tagging sutures from anterior to posterior with a 0.062 Kirschner wire. Use an oscillating saw to cut through the cortex of the patella in line with the fibers of the patellar tendon along the scored markings at a 45-degree angle from the vertical. Carefully elevate the patellar bone plug with a ¼-in osteotome.

After the graft has been removed, use a rongeur to shape the autograft to fit the desired sizer. Place tagging sutures in the predrilled holes through the patellar bone plug. Measure the bone plugs and mark along the tendon with an indelible marking pen. The shorter plug is used in the femoral tunnel for an ACL reconstruction. The longer plug is used in the tibial tunnel for an ACL reconstruction, allowing for resection of additional bone at the distal end of the graft through the tibial tunnel if long.

Hamstring Tendons

Introduction

The gracilis and semitendinosus tendons are also commonly harvested for knee reconstruction procedures. In addition to the use of the hamstring tendons in ACL reconstructions, they are also often harvested for reconstruction of the posterior cruciate ligament (PCL), lateral collateral ligament (LCL), and MCL. Similarly to the harvesting of the patellar tendon autograft, the technique for hamstring tendon harvesting has been standardized to produce reliable autografts for various knee ligament reconstructions.

Technique

When beginning a harvest of the hamstring tendons for knee ligament reconstruction, flex the knee to loosen the hamstring tendons. Palpate the common tendon insertion of the sartorius, gracilis, and semitendinosus at the pes anserinus, 2 cm distal and 2 cm medial to the proximal portion of the tibial tubercle. Make a 4-cm longitudinal incision directly over the hamstring insertion with a 15-blade. Dissect through the subcutaneous tissue to the sartorial and deep crural fascia, either bluntly or with a Metzenbaum scissors. Place a goiter medially for retraction.

Palpate the superior border of the gracilis tendon as it travels diagonally and distally from the posteromedial knee toward the anterior tibia. Make an L-shaped incision through the sartorial fascia along the superior border of the gracilis and coming down along the distal insertion to expose the tendons from the undersurface of the sartorius. Pass a right-angle clamp around the gracilis to isolate it. Isolate the distal end of the gracilis tendon; tag it with several interlocking passes of a no. 2 Ethibond suture. Incise the distal end of the gracilis tendon. Release fibrous attachments to the semitendinosus and to the tibia with the Metzenbaum scissors under direct visualization (Fig. 12-5). Place the tendon stripper over the gracilis tendon and pass it proximally in line with the natural path of the tendon. Pass the tendon stripper to the hilt while aiming at the ischial tuberosity. When the tendon has been completely harvested, place it on a back table for preparation.

Isolate the semitendinosus tendon and incise the distal end of the tendon after tagging it with a no. 2 Ethibond suture. Place the tendon stripper over the semitendinosus tendon and pass it proximally in line with the natural path of the tendon (Fig. 12-6). Pass the tendon stripper to the hilt while aiming at the ischial tuberosity. When the tendon has been completely harvested, place it on a back table for preparation.

Clean the muscle fibers from the tendons with the edge of a scalpel or periosteal elevator (Fig. 12-7). Combine the two tendons to make a single-bundle autograft using the Krackow suture technique (Fig. 12-8).

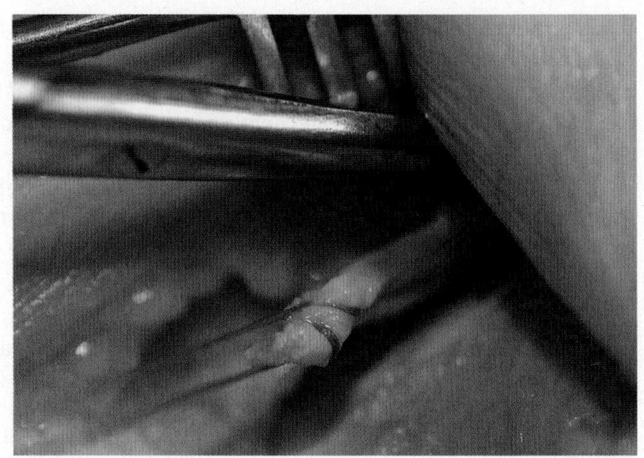

FIGURE 12-5

Releasing attachments to the tendon with Metzenbaum scissors under direct visualization.

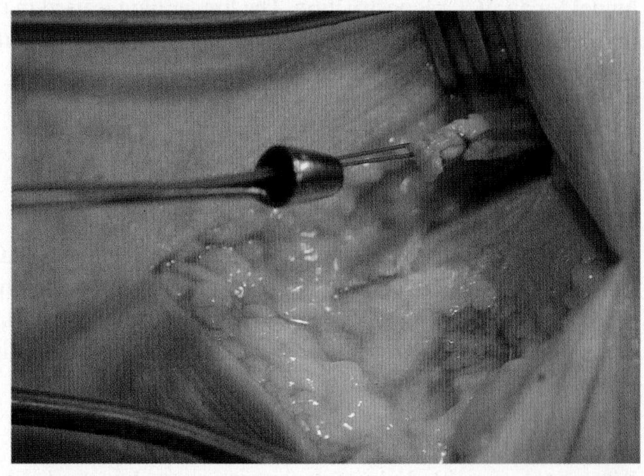

FIGURE 12-6

Placing the tendon stripper over the semitendinosus tendon and passing it proximally in line with the natural path of the tendon.

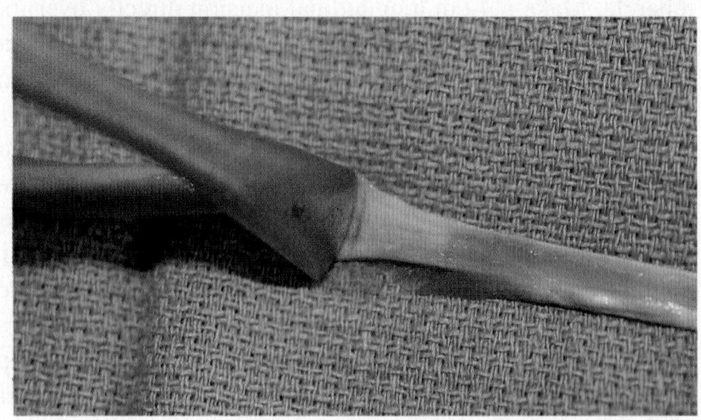

FIGURE 12-7

Cleaning the muscle fibers from the tendons with a periosteal elevator.

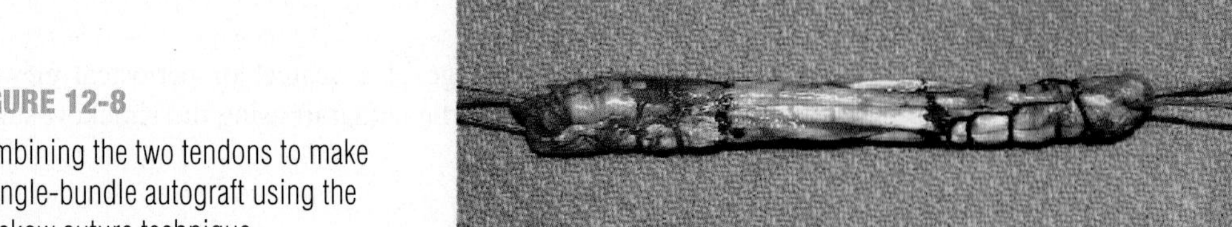

FIGURE 12-8

Combining the two tendons to make a single-bundle autograft using the Krackow suture technique.

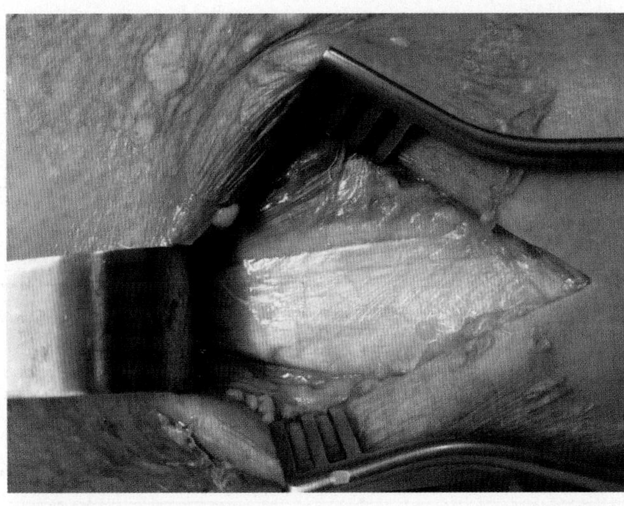

FIGURE 12-9

Placing a Weitlaner retractor to better expose the distal quadriceps tendon and an army-navy retractor proximally to expose the proximal end of the graft during harvesting.

Quadriceps Tendon

Introduction

A third and less often used option for autograft harvest in the ligamentous reconstruction of an injured knee is the quadriceps tendon. This autograft is typically used only when the patellar tendon and hamstring tendons are not available, but has been shown to be a valid graft for ACL reconstruction. In 2012, Lippe et al. (22) provided anatomic guidelines for harvesting the quadriceps tendon. This study demonstrated that the gross morphology of the quadriceps tendon is asymmetric and recommended a 1-cm wide graft centered 2 cm medial to the apex of the tendon (23).

Technique

When beginning a harvest of the quadriceps tendon, flex the knee to tighten the quadriceps tendon. Make a 4-cm longitudinal incision proximal to the superior pole of the patella at the midline with a 15-blade. Dissect bluntly through the subcutaneous tissue to expose the fascia overlying the quadriceps tendon. Place a Weitlaner retractor to better expose the distal quadriceps tendon. Place an army-navy retractor proximally to expose the proximal end of the graft during harvesting (Fig. 12-9).

Starting 2 cm proximal to the superior pole of the patella, identify the point 2 cm medial to the proximal apex of the tendon and incise transversely 5 mm medially and 5 mm laterally to this point. Then, incise proximally 8 cm for both the medial and lateral edges of the quadriceps tendon autograft at a depth of approximately 7 mm. Identify the distal end of the graft and tag with a no. 5 Ethibond suture. Incise the distal end of the graft.

Using the army-navy retractor, identify the proximal end of the graft. Incise the proximal end of the graft, and carry the autograft to the back table for preparation (Fig. 12-10). Prepare the graft by using the Krackow suture technique on both the proximal and distal ends of the graft (Fig. 12-11). While Lippe's (22) description of quadriceps tendon harvest shown above only harvests a soft tissue graft, it can also be harvested with a 10-mm wide, 20-mm long, and 7-mm deep patella bone plug as described by Fulkerson et al. (21).

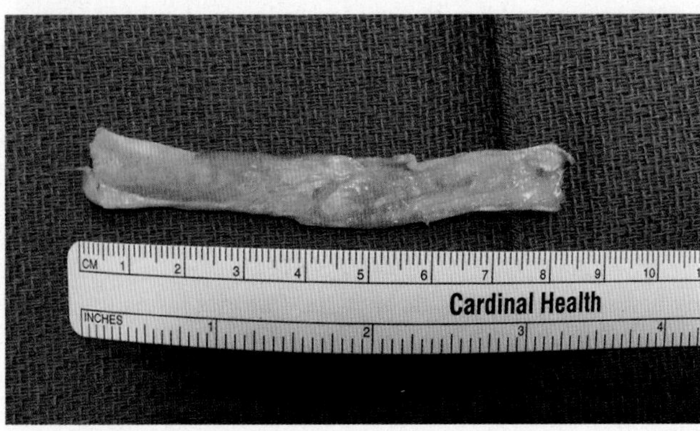

FIGURE 12-10

Quadriceps autograft harvested and on back table.

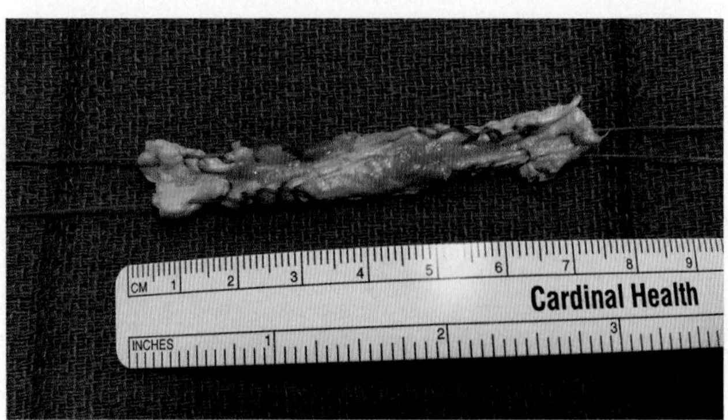

FIGURE 12-11

Prepared graft using the Krackow suture technique on both the proximal and distal ends of the graft.

PEARLS AND PITFALLS

Bone-Patella-Tendon-Bone Graft

- Minimize risk of patella fracture and damage to patella articular surface by using an oscillating saw guide with a depth stop of 8 mm at 45- to 60-degree angle for 2.5 cm proximally and distally for patella and tibia longitudinal cuts, respectively.
- Prevent stress risers in patella and tibia by not extending saw cuts past corners of bone plug. Also, do not forcefully lever patella bone plug out of donor site.
- Avoid fat-pad laceration by carefully dissecting patella tendon with 11-blade. This complication will lead to fluid extravasation during the arthroscopic part of the procedure and can lead to fat-pad fibrosis and patella baja, which can significantly decrease post-op knee flexion. If this happens intraoperatively, use suture to repair fat pad to create a water-tight seal to the extensor mechanism (9).
- There is no evidence to confirm that postoperative pain or fracture risk is decreased or that there is improved healing of the patella defect by filling patella bone defect at the end of the case before wound closure with bone chips saved from graft tunnel preparation. Thus, this is not done by the surgeon at our institution.
- Augment abnormally low-interference screw insertion torque by using the next larger diameter screw size, by using a second screw of same size, or by adding supplemental fixation with an Arthrex SwiveLock device.
- Avoid graft protrusion by keeping tibial angle between 55 and 60 degrees to the tibial plateau. If graft is still too long, options include drilling the femoral tunnel an additional 5 mm deeper, rotating the graft to shorten graft length, folding the tibial bone plug backward before interference screw fixation, or by creating a trough in tibial metaphysis and fixing the bone plug to tibia with staples (9). This is usually not an issue when performing a 2-incision technique, but can occur with the endoscopic method.

Hamstring Graft

- Avoid premature graft amputation by releasing all tendinous bands from the hamstring grafts to the gastrocnemius as well as any accessory semitendinosus bands to the tibia with blunt finger dissection (Fig. 12-12) and Metzenbaum scissors. Also, the tendon stripper should be aimed toward the ipsilateral ischial tuberosity to proceed along the native course of the tendons. Do NOT advance stripper if resistance is met. Instead, remove the stripper and palpate for additional fascial bands or accessory insertions that need to be released.
- Pes anserinus insertion is 19 mm (10 to 25 mm) distal and 22.5 mm (10 to 25 mm) medial to apex of tibial tubercle with width of 20 mm (15 to 34 mm) (15). Gracilis and semitendinosus tendons become separate structures 18 mm (10 to 25 mm) proximal to combined insertion site (15).
- Avoid MCL harvest deep to tendons by carefully dissecting through the sartorial fascia to expose the gracilis and semitendinosus tendons.
- Minimize the risk of saphenous nerve laceration by placing knee in 90-degree flexed or figure-of-four position. This relaxes tension on the nerve, which crosses superficial to the gracilis tendon at the posteromedial joint line.

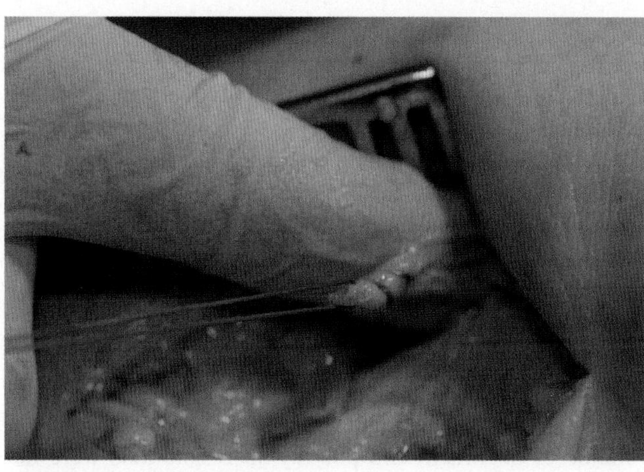

FIGURE 12-12

Releasing all tendinous bands from the hamstring graft to the gastrocnemius as well as any accessory semitendinosus bands to the tibia with blunt finger dissection.

Quadriceps Graft

- Avoid entrance into the suprapatellar pouch by using direct visualization and careful dissection during graft harvest. Also, a bone block of 6 to 8 mm thickness should be freed leaving 2 mm of vastus intermedius tendon attached to patella and underlying suprapatellar pouch.

POSTOPERATIVE MANAGEMENT

For most cases of knee ligament reconstruction, we use a standardized rehabilitation protocol that was developed in collaboration with the other institutions participating in the MOON Group. This protocol was primarily intended for patients recovering from ACL reconstruction, but the basic principles can be applied to other knee ligament reconstruction scenarios as well (24). The rehabilitation program structure is identical for all patients, regardless of the graft harvest used for the procedure. It is intended to service the spectrum of ACL patients and thus should be tailored to match each individual patient's particular abilities and needs.

An important element of postoperative rehabilitation following knee ligament reconstruction includes an adequate preoperative therapy program to optimize patient results postoperatively. Preoperative recommendations include a normal gait, active range of motion (AROM) of 0 to 120 degrees, minimal effusion of the knee, adequate strength to achieve 20 degrees of elevation from the examination table in a straight leg raise, and proper education regarding postoperative therapy and rehabilitation expectations.

The first phase of postoperative recovery from knee ligament reconstruction includes the immediate postoperative period, typically the first 2 weeks following surgery. During this period, full knee extension is critical. Also, minimizing pain and swelling are important goals. The patient should walk with a normal gait during this phase, and ACL patients should demonstrate good quadriceps control. No knee immobilizers or braces are used for cruciate reconstructions, but may be necessary for patients following collateral ligament reconstruction.

The rehabilitation phases after the immediate postoperative period are quite variable depending on the nature of the knee ligament reconstruction and individual patient progress, but the phase progression is widely uniform for most patients. Following the immediate postoperative period, the early rehabilitation phase includes full range of motion about the knee with improved muscle strength and a progression in neuromuscular retraining. This includes cardiopulmonary training to ensure that the overall patient fitness level is maintained in the early rehabilitation phase. Progression to the strengthening and control phase allows the patient to run and hop as long as range of motion is preserved and no pain or swelling accompanies these activities. After the patient successfully progresses through a period of strengthening and control of the knee, advanced training includes running patterns and jumping without difficulty. These are required phases of rehabilitation before the patient enters into the final phase, the return-to-sport phase. To achieve a full rehabilitation of the knee and to begin advanced training in preparation for a return to play, the patient should demonstrate 85% of the contralateral strength and control and should be able to participate in sport-specific training without pain or swelling. To complete the rehabilitation process for all knee ligament reconstructions, the patient must have no functional complaints and must demonstrate confidence when running, cutting, and jumping at full speed.

COMPLICATIONS

Complications that occur postoperatively no matter the graft choice comprise infection, arthrofibrosis, and graft failure (7). The dreaded intraoperative complication of any type of graft is the dropped graft onto the surgical floor. Ways to help avoid this complication include placing the arthroscopic fluid collection bag under the harvest site during removal of the graft, placing the graft in a basin before transfer to the back table, drilling the suture holes for a BPTB graft before the graft is harvested or securing the BPTB graft with a towel clip while drilling on a back table, and placing the basin holding the graft in a location not close to the table containing most of the more commonly used surgical instruments during the case (9). If a graft is dropped, the use of an alternative graft should be strongly considered. However, if this is not possible, a 30-minute soak in 4% chlorhexidine gluconate followed by a 30-minute soak in triple antibiotic solution has been shown in a rabbit BPTB graft study to provide 100% graft sterility after being contaminated with six common virulent organisms (25). Use of 10% povidone-iodine or bacitracin and polymyxin B solutions were not 100% effective in obtaining graft sterility in either rabbit or cadaver BPTB grafts (25,26).

Complications associated with BPTB harvests include acute and delayed patella fracture, damage to the infrapatellar branch of the saphenous nerve, patella tendon rupture, patella tendonitis, infrapatellar contracture syndrome, fat-pad laceration, postoperative quadriceps loss of strength, patellofemoral crepitation, anterior knee pain, and kneeling pain (3,5,7–9,14). Some of these can be avoided by meticulous surgical technique.

Acute and delayed patella fracture can be minimized by avoiding stress risers created when saw cuts extend beyond the corners of the patella plug, when saw cuts extend too deeply into the patella, by avoiding levering the patella bone plug out of the donor bone too firmly, or by avoiding forced hyperflexion of the knee postoperatively before the donor site is completely healed (9,14,17). Patella cuts should be limited to a depth of 8 mm and can be prevented by using a saw blade with a manual stop on the blade or by angling the saw blade to 45 to 60 degrees (9,17).

Complications associated with hamstring harvests include micromotion of the graft in the tunnels leading to tunnel widening, amputation of the graft during harvest or lack of adequate tissue, dissection through or harvest of the superficial MCL, injury to the saphenous nerve, concerns about recurrent knee laxity, and residual hamstring weakness of 10% (5,7–9,15,17).

It is crucial to release all attachments of the hamstring tendon to the medial head of the gastrocnemius so that the tendon stripper has a clear path to the hamstring muscle belly. If this is not done, then either amputation of the graft or a harvest of insufficient length may be obtained. A minimum length of 20 cm of both tendons is needed for a doubled four-stranded graft so that at least 2 cm of collagenous tissue is present in both the femoral and tibial tunnels (9,16). Blunt dissection with fingertips or Metzenbaum scissors can help release these tendinous bands, which can number up to 5 between the gracilis/semitendinosus and the gastrocnemius (15,17). Finally, placing the leg in a figure-of-4 position minimizes tension on the saphenous nerve and decreases the risk of cutting this while harvesting the hamstring graft (15).

Complications associated with quadriceps harvests include acute and delayed patella fracture, violating the suprapatellar pouch during harvest that can lead to loss of knee distention during arthroscopic ACL reconstruction, and a decrease of up to 20% in quadriceps strength postoperatively (5). A crucial step during harvest of the quadriceps tendon is to attain direct visualization and use careful dissection to avoid entering the suprapatellar pouch (21). Similar to a BPTB harvest, a patella cut depth of less than 8 mm should be used, but only a 6 mm depth of the quadriceps tendon should be harvested (21). This leaves 2 mm of vastus intermedius attached to the patella and the suprapatellar pouch deep to this and intact (21).

ACKNOWLEDGMENTS

We acknowledge Dr. Matthew Matava at Washington University School of Medicine in Saint Louis, MO, for providing pictures related to hamstring graft harvesting.

REFERENCES

1. Kaeding CC, Aros B, Pedroza A, et al. Allograft versus autograft anterior cruciate ligament reconstruction: predictors of failure from a MOON prospective longitudinal cohort. *Sports Health.* 2011;3(1):73–81.
2. Group M, Group M. Effect of graft choice on the outcome of revision anterior cruciate ligament reconstruction in the Multicenter ACL Revision Study (MARS) Cohort. *Am J Sports Med.* 2014;42(10):2301–2310.

3. Spindler KP, Kuhn JE, Freedman KB, et al. Anterior cruciate ligament reconstruction autograft choice: bone-tendon-bone versus hamstring: does it really matter? A systematic review. *Am J Sports Med.* 2004;32(8):1986–1995.
4. Fu FH, Bennett CH, Lattermann C, Ma CB. Current trends in anterior cruciate ligament reconstruction. Part 1: Biology and biomechanics of reconstruction. *Am J Sports Med.* 1999;27(6):821–830.
5. Johnson DL, Mair SD. *Clinical sports medicine*. Philadelphia: Mosby Elsevier; 2006.
6. Miller SL, Gladstone JN. Graft selection in anterior cruciate ligament reconstruction. *Orthop Clin North Am.* 2002;33(4):675–683.
7. Schepsis AA, Busconi BD. *Sports medicine*. Philadelphia: Lippincott Williams & Wilkins; 2006.
8. Freedman KB, D'Amato MJ, Nedeff DD, et al. Arthroscopic anterior cruciate ligament reconstruction: a metaanalysis comparing patellar tendon and hamstring tendon autografts. *Am J Sports Med.* 2003;31(1):2–11.
9. Matava MJ, Muller MS, Clinton CM, et al. Complications of anterior cruciate ligament reconstruction. *Instr Course Lect.* 2009;58:355–375.
10. Bynum EB, Barrack RL, Alexander AH. Open versus closed chain kinetic exercises after anterior cruciate ligament reconstruction. A prospective randomized study. *Am J Sports Med.* 1995;23(4):401–406.
11. Aglietti P, Giron F, Buzzi R, et al. Anterior cruciate ligament reconstruction: bone-patellar tendon-bone compared with double semitendinosus and gracilis tendon grafts. A prospective, randomized clinical trial. *J Bone Joint Surg Am.* 2004;86-A(10):2143–2155.
12. Aune AK, Holm I, Risberg MA, et al. Four-strand hamstring tendon autograft compared with patellar tendon-bone autograft for anterior cruciate ligament reconstruction. A randomized study with two-year follow-up. *Am J Sports Med.* 2001;29(6):722–728.
13. Feller JA, Webster KE. A randomized comparison of patellar tendon and hamstring tendon anterior cruciate ligament reconstruction. *Am J Sports Med.* 2003;31(4):564–573.
14. Jackson DW. *Reconstructive knee surgery*. 3rd ed. Philadelphia: Lippincott Williams & Wilkins; 2007.
15. Solman CG Jr, Pagnani MJ. Hamstring tendon harvesting. Reviewing anatomic relationships and avoiding pitfalls. *Orthop Clin North Am.* 2003;34(1):1–8.
16. Gobbi A. Single versus double hamstring tendon harvest for ACL reconstruction. *Sports Med Arthrosc.* 2010;18(1):15–19.
17. McGuire DA, Hendricks SD. Anterior cruciate ligament reconstruction graft harvesting: pitfalls and tips. *Sports Med Arthrosc.* 2007;15(4):184–190.
18. Clancy WG Jr, Narechania RG, Rosenberg TD, et al. Anterior and posterior cruciate ligament reconstruction in rhesus monkeys. *J Bone Joint Surg Am.* 1981;63(8):1270–1284.
19. Rodeo SA, Arnoczky SP, Torzilli PA, et al. Tendon-healing in a bone tunnel. A biomechanical and histological study in the dog. *J Bone Joint Surg Am.* 1993;75(12):1795–1803.
20. Pinczewski LA, Clingeleffer AJ, Otto DD, et al. Integration of hamstring tendon graft with bone in reconstruction of the anterior cruciate ligament. *Arthroscopy.* 1997;13(5):641–643.
21. Fulkerson JP, Langeland R. An alternative cruciate reconstruction graft: the central quadriceps tendon. *Arthroscopy.* 1995;11(2):252–254.
22. Lippe J, Armstrong A, Fulkerson JP. Anatomic guidelines for harvesting a quadriceps free tendon autograft for anterior cruciate ligament reconstruction. *Arthroscopy.* 2012;28(7):980–984.
23. Fulkerson JP. Central quadriceps free tendon for anterior cruciate ligament reconstruction. *Oper Techn Sport Med.* 1999;7(4):195–200.
24. Wright RW, Haas AK, Anderson J, et al. Anterior cruciate ligament reconstruction rehabilitation: MOON guidelines. *Sports Health.* 2014. doi:10.1177/1941738113517855.
25. Goebel ME, Drez D Jr, Heck SB, et al. Contaminated rabbit patellar tendon grafts. In vivo analysis of disinfecting methods. *Am J Sports Med.* 1994;22(3):387–391.
26. Cooper DE, Arnoczky SP, Warren RF. Contaminated patellar tendon grafts: incidence of positive cultures and efficacy of an antibiotic solution soak–an in vitro study. *Arthroscopy.* 1991;7(3):272–274.

13 ACL Reconstruction in the Skeletally Immature: Transphyseal, All-Epiphyseal, Over-the-Top

Allen F. Anderson and Christian N. Anderson

INDICATIONS/CONTRAINDICATIONS

Anterior cruciate ligament (ACL) tears in children and adolescents are relatively rare injuries. Even so, ACL reconstructions in this population have increased considerably over the last two decades (1). Historically, these injuries have been treated nonoperatively or with delayed surgical management until skeletal maturity to avoid risking iatrogenic growth disturbance. However, studies evaluating the efficacy of conservative treatment generally demonstrate poor outcomes, including high rates of recurrent instability, meniscal tearing, chondral damage, and sports-related disability (2,3). Noncompliance and significantly higher activity levels observed in children are likely contributing factors to the poor results observed with conservative treatment. Consequently, surgical reconstruction is the preferred treatment method in skeletally immature patients and has been shown to be effective at restoring normal knee function and stability (4).

There are very few contraindications to ACL reconstruction in active and healthy skeletally immature patients. Infection about the knee is an absolute contraindication to surgery. ACL insufficiency from a displaced ACL avulsion fracture should be treated with arthroscopic reduction and internal fixation of the bony avulsion. Patients unable to participate in postoperative rehabilitation due to polytrauma or noncompliance are not appropriate candidates for ACL reconstruction. It is important for the patient to have regained knee extension and have near-normal flexion before surgery to minimize the risk of postoperative arthrofibrosis.

PREOPERATIVE PLANNING

History, Physical Exam, and Radiographic Evaluation

The diagnosis of an ACL injury in pediatric patients begins with a thorough history and physical examination. The majority of ACL tears in this population occur with a noncontact mechanism of injury during sports participation. Patients commonly hear an audible pop at the time of injury and may present with an acute hemarthrosis. Physical examination should include a thorough musculoskeletal evaluation of the knee, as well as a complete neurovascular exam of the lower extremity.

Radiographic evaluation begins with anteroposterior (AP) and lateral radiographs of the knee to rule out ACL avulsion fracture or other osseous trauma. Magnetic resonance imaging (MRI) is the preferred imaging modality to confirm ACL injury and to evaluate associated pathology of the menisci, articular cartilage, or collateral ligaments.

Once the diagnosis of an intrasubstance ACL injury has been confirmed, the skeletal age of the patient, a direct indicator of the amount of knee growth remaining (5), is determined by comparing posteroanterior hand radiographs to a Greulich and Pyle atlas (see Fig. 13-17C). In determining the skeletal maturity, the relative risk and potential consequences of iatrogenic physeal injury can be estimated, and the appropriate surgical technique can be selected to minimize the chance of growth deformity.

Risk Stratification and Treatment Algorithm

Patients are risk stratified based on skeletal maturity at the time of presentation. Females with a bone age less than 12 years old and males less than 13 years old and are placed in a high-risk category because they have substantial knee growth remaining (5) and the effects of growth arrest would be severe. Females with a bone age from 12 to 13 years and males from 13 to 15 years have at least 1 to 2 cm of knee growth remaining (5) and are consequently placed in an intermediate-risk category. Females with bone age greater than 13 years and males greater than 15 years old are placed in a low-risk category because they have 1 cm or less of knee growth remaining (5), and iatrogenic physeal damage would likely result in no significant growth disturbance.

Surgical reconstruction options include transphyseal, physeal sparing, and hybrid techniques. Transphyseal and hybrid techniques require drilling through one or both of the growth plates, risking physeal damage and growth deformity in patients with substantial growth remaining. Consequently, we prefer to treat patients categorized as high risk with all-epiphyseal reconstruction using suspensory fixation on the tibial side and shielded screw fixation on the femoral side (OrthoPediatrics, Warsaw, IN; Figures X and Y). This procedure follows the generally accepted principles of ACL reconstruction in adults but relies on anatomic drill tunnels placed completely within the epiphyses, thereby theoretically minimizing the chance of growth disturbance by not transgressing either the tibial or femoral physis. Furthermore, fixation of the graft is completely within the epiphyses, allowing unimpeded growth of the knee on both the tibial and femoral sides. Alternatively, surgeons concerned with the technical difficulty of transepiphyseal drilling can perform physeal sparing "over-the-top" reconstruction, as described by Micheli et al. (6), for high-risk patients (see Fig. 13-11A,B). While clinical results of this procedure are favorable (6,7), the graft is not anatomic, lacks isometry, and relies on metaphyseal fixation, which can theoretically tether the physis.

Younger patients in the intermediate group (males with bone age 13 to 14 years and females 12 years old) may be treated either with transepiphyseal (4) or all-epiphyseal reconstruction. Similar to all-epiphyseal reconstruction, the transepiphyseal technique relies on epiphyseal drill tunnels that do not violate the physis; however, graft fixation on the tibial side occurs on the metaphysis. The theoretical tethering effect on the physis from metaphyseal graft fixation is likely minimized in this age group given the intermediate knee growth remaining, and clinical results of this technique in patients with substantial postoperative growth have not demonstrated growth deformity (4).

Older patients in the intermediate group (males with bone age 14 to 15 years old and females 13 years old) may be treated with transphyseal reconstruction using quadruple hamstring grafts and a modified vertical femoral tunnel. Patients classified as low risk undergo adult-type reconstruction with quadrupled hamstring autografts and anatomic femoral tunnel drilling through the anteromedial portal.

SURGICAL TECHNIQUE

All-Epiphyseal Reconstruction

Setup

The patient is positioned supine on the operating table. The operative leg is placed in an arthroscopic leg holder one handbreadth above the patella. The leg holder is then raised to elevate the operative knee above the contralateral extremity. Raising the leg holder facilitates visualization in the lateral plane while using fluoroscopy. The C-arm is placed on the side of the table opposite the injured knee, with the monitor at the head of the table on the same side as the operative extremity. Before the leg is prepared and draped, the tibial and femoral physes should be visualized in both AP and lateral planes. The C-arm is then rotated 30 degrees to visualize the extension of the tibial physis into the tibial tubercle on the lateral view of the tibia.

Graft Harvesting and Preparation

The hamstrings are harvested through a 3- to 4-cm oblique incision made at the level of the pes anserinus. The semitendinosus and gracilis tendons are isolated from the undersurface of the sartorius with a 90-degree hemostat and dissected free of any adhesions proximally. Then, a standard tendon stripper is used to detach the tendons at the musculotendinous junction. The tendons are then sharply removed from their distal insertion. Next, the tendons are doubled and a no. 2 FiberWire suture (Arthrex, Naples, FL) is placed in the ends using a locking whipstitch. The doubled tendons are then placed on the back table under 4.5 kg of tension using the Graft Master device (Acufex-Smith Nephew, Andover, MA).

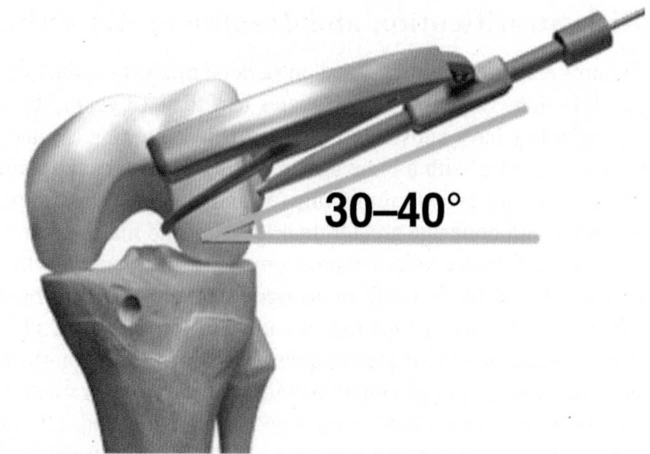

FIGURE 13-1

The femoral guide. The handle of the guide should be elevated approximately 30 to 40 degrees to avoid damaging the lateral collateral ligament and popliteus tendon during reaming. (Copyright 2013 OrthoPediatrics Corp., with permission.)

Diagnostic Arthroscopy and Notch Preparation

The arthroscope is introduced into the anterolateral portal, and a probe is inserted through the anteromedial portal. An intra-articular examination is then performed in a standard manner, and tears of the menisci can be repaired at this time. The ACL stump is then removed from the intercondylar notch so its anatomic footprint on the femur can be visualized.

Femoral and Tibial Tunnel Placement

The OrthoPediatrics all-epiphyseal ACL set is used for the case and has all the necessary instrumentation to perform each step. For femoral tunnel drilling, the arthroscope is placed in the anteromedial portal and the ACL drill guide in the anterolateral portal. The tip of the guide is placed in the center of the ACL footprint on the femur (Fig. 13-1). A minimal notchplasty may be required to visualize the footprint adequately. The handle of the guide is elevated 30 to 40 degrees anteriorly so the drill hole does not damage the lateral collateral ligament or popliteus tendon attachment. At this point, the C-arm is used in the AP plane to place the drill guide and guide wire distal to the femoral physis. Once adequate distance between the femoral physis and the guide wire is confirmed, the wire can be advanced across the femoral epiphysis (Fig. 13-2A,B). Using the arthroscope, the guide wire is then

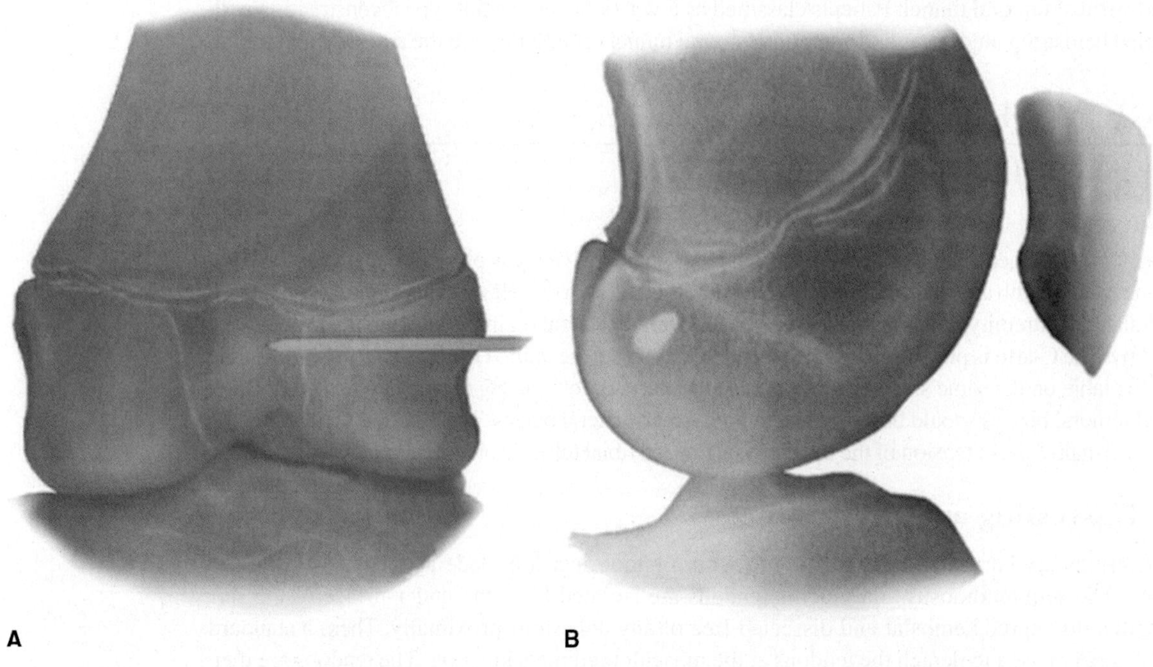

FIGURE 13-2

AP (**A**) and Lateral (**B**) fluoroscopic images demonstrating the position of the guide wire in the femoral epiphysis. (From Anderson AF, Anderson CN. Anterior cruciate ligament reconstruction in skeletally immature patients. In: Prodromos C, Brown C, Fu FH, et al., eds. *The anterior cruciate ligament: reconstruction and basic science.* Philadelphia: Saunders; 2008:464, with permission.)

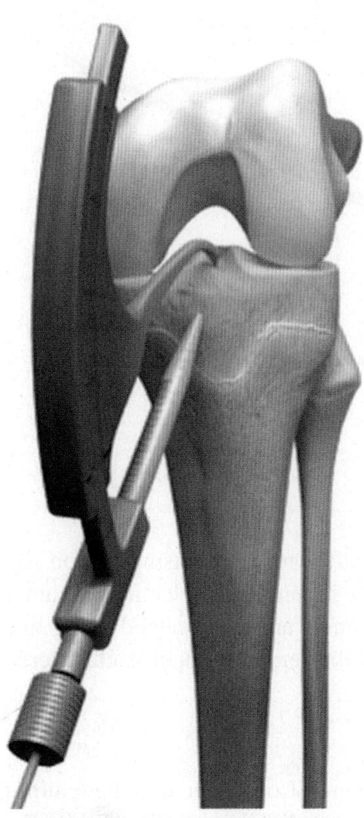

FIGURE 13-3

The tibial guide. The handle of the guide is positioned medial to the tibial tubercle to allow the guide wire to be advanced through the anteromedial epiphysis. (Copyright 2013 OrthoPediatrics Corp., with permission.)

visualized entering into the center of the anatomic footprint of the ACL on the femur. The appropriately sized reamer is then advanced over the guide wire to confirm the femoral tunnel will be distal to and not encroach upon the physis. The femoral guide wire is left in place, and the arthroscope is switched back to the anterolateral portal for tibial guidewire placement. To visualize the tibial physis extending into the tibial tubercle, the C-arm is rotated approximately 30 degrees from the lateral plane. The tip of the tibial drill guide is introduced into the anteromedial portal and positioned anterior to the free edge of the lateral meniscus in the footprint of the ACL (Fig. 13-3). The guide wire is positioned on the anteromedial tibial epiphysis between the physis and joint surface and advanced using real-time fluoroscopic imaging through the epiphysis into the tibial footprint (Fig. 13-4).

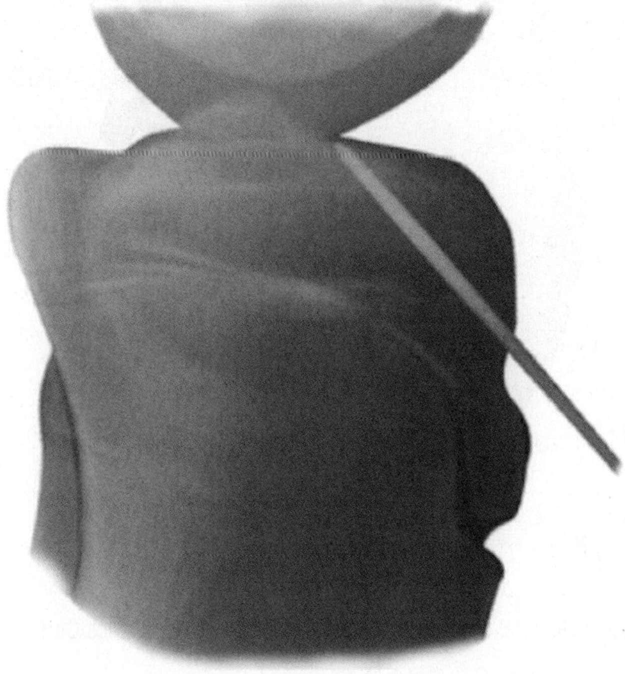

FIGURE 13-4

Lateral fluoroscopic image demonstrating the position of the tibial guide wire. (From Anderson AF, Anderson CN. Anterior cruciate ligament reconstruction in skeletally immature patients. In: Prodromos C, Brown C, Fu FH, et al., eds. *The anterior cruciate ligament: reconstruction and basic science.* Philadelphia: Saunders; 2008:464, with permission.)

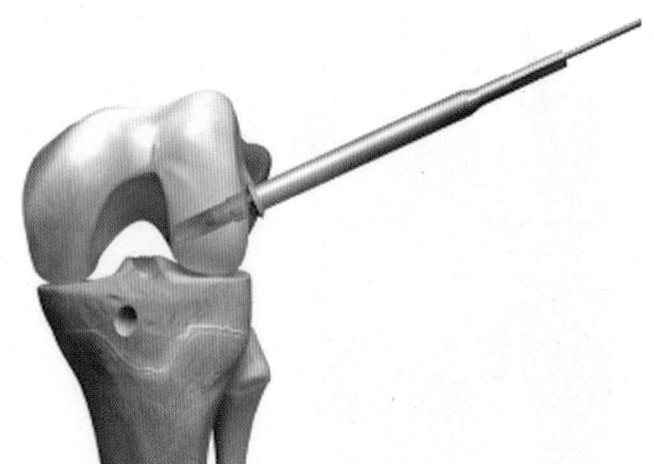

FIGURE 13-5

The counter bore reamer. (Copyright 2013 OrthoPediatrics Corp., with permission.)

Before proceeding, the diameter of the quadruple hamstring graft is measured using tendon sizers; these grafts typically range from 6 to 8 mm in diameter. We recommend selecting a reamer size that results in a tight fit for the graft in the tunnels. The tunnels are then reamed using live fluoroscopy. After reaming, the anterior intra-articular aspect of the femoral tunnel is chamfered using a rasp.

Graft Fixation

The first step in graft fixation on the femoral side is to insert the ShieldLoc sleeve into the femoral hole. The ShieldLoc sleeve is designed to protect the physis from radial pressure caused by the insertion of the interference screw. First, the counter bore reamer is inserted into the femoral hole until it bottoms out on the lateral femoral cortex (Fig. 13-5). During this step, the counter bore is inserted to a depth of 8 mm and increases the diameter of the femoral hole by 2 mm. The small amount of bone removal occurs rapidly. The iliotibial band should be retracted, and soft tissue immediately around the hole is removed to allow for clear placement of the ShieldLoc sleeve. The appropriately sized ShieldLoc sleeve is then screwed on to the insertion device (Fig. 13-6A) and gently tapped it into the femoral tunnel (Fig. 13-6B). The fluted fins on the outside of the ShieldLoc sleeve prevent the device from backing out of the femoral tunnel while removing the insertion device. After the ShieldLoc has been inserted, the Graft Passer from the Disposable Kit is placed through the femoral tunnel and retrieved through the tibial tunnel with an arthroscopic grasper. One of the free ends of both the semitendinosus and gracilis tendons is placed through

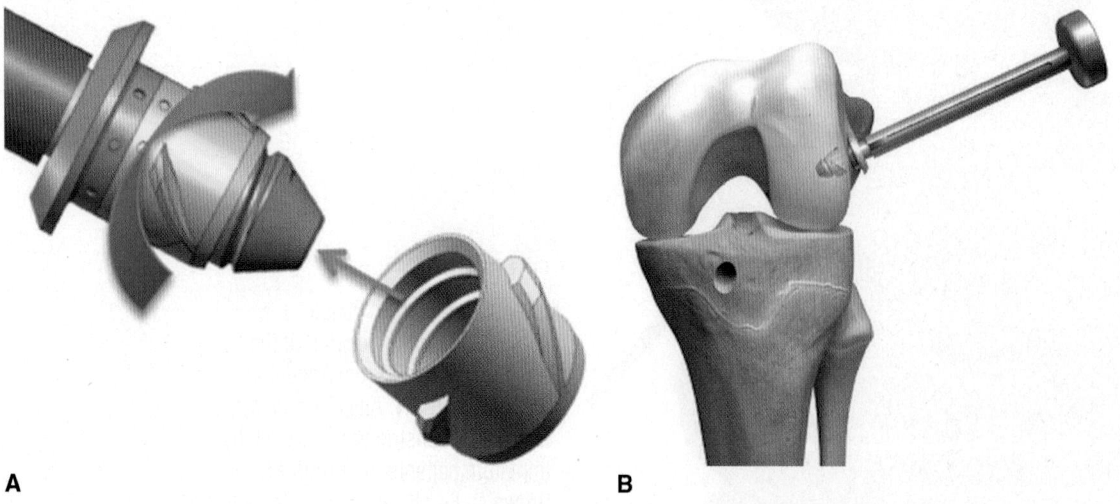

FIGURE 13-6

The ShieldLoc sleeve is screwed on the insertion device (**A**) and tapped into the femoral tunnel (**B**). (Copyright 2013 OrthoPediatrics Corp., with permission.)

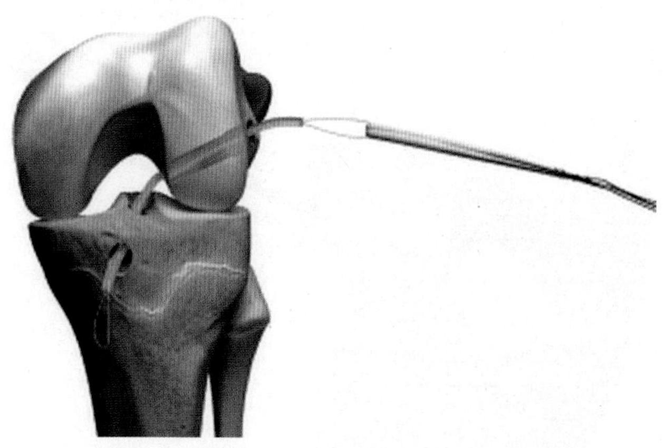

FIGURE 13-7

The Graft Passer loop is used to shuttle the graft through the femoral tunnel into the tibial tunnel. (Copyright 2013 OrthoPediatrics Corp., with permission.)

the Graft Passer loop on the femoral side (Fig. 13-7). The tibial end of the Graft Passer is pulled, bringing the graft through the femoral tunnel into the tibial tunnel. Approximately 1 to 2 cm of the graft is pulled outside of the anterior tibial cortex to allow installation of the ArmorLink implant. The ArmorLink provides suspensory fixation on the tibial side. A hemostat is used to pass the ArmorLink around the tendons (Fig. 13-8A). The free ends of the graft coming out of the femoral tunnel are pulled to seat the ArmorLink on the tibial cortex (Fig. 13-8B). The ArmorLink may be positioned in any orientation. Observe the ShieldLoc sleeve when pulling the free strands of the graft to make sure the ShieldLoc does not catch on the sutures in the free ends of the graft and become displaced. If the ShieldLoc sleeve moves when pulling the tendons through, it can be stabilized with a hemostat to prevent displacement. With the knee in approximately 20 to 30 degrees of flexion, tension is applied to the graft using a graft tensioner, and the corresponding screw is inserted into the ShieldLoc sleeve (Fig. 13-9). The graft is evaluated for intercondylar notch impingement, and the free ends of the semitendinosus and gracilis are trimmed after satisfactory stability is confirmed (Fig. 13-10A,B). The wounds are closed in a standard fashion.

Physeal Sparing "Over-the-Top" Reconstruction

The following technique described by Micheli et al. (6) is a modification of the MacIntosh and Darby intra-articular and extra-articular ACL reconstruction.

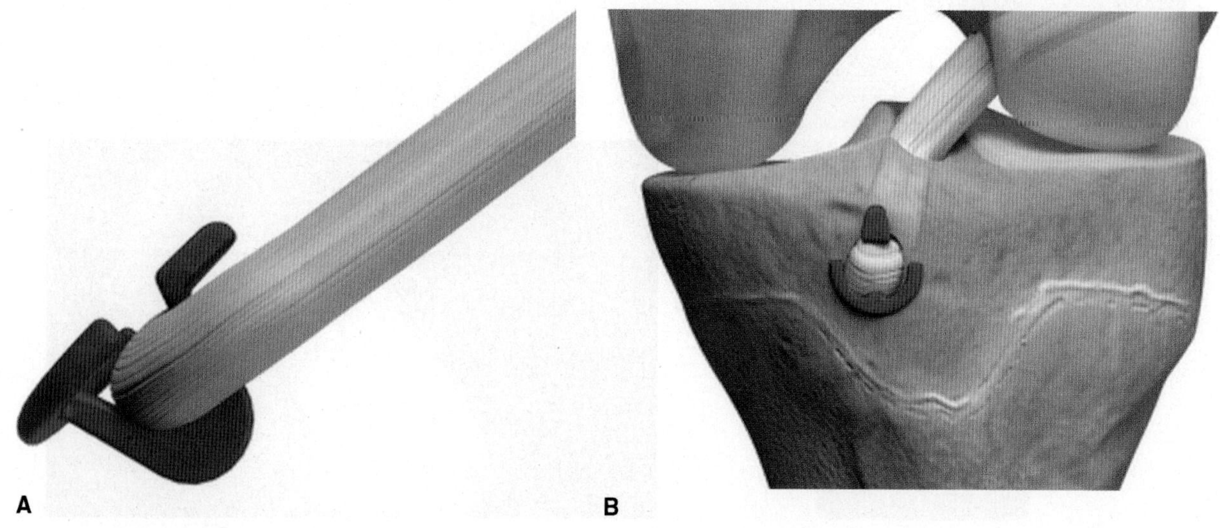

FIGURE 13-8

The ArmorLink device is passed around the loops formed from doubling over the hamstring tendons (**A**) and seated on the anteromedial tibia by pulling the free ends of the tendons proximally (**B**). (Copyright 2013 OrthoPediatrics Corp., with permission.)

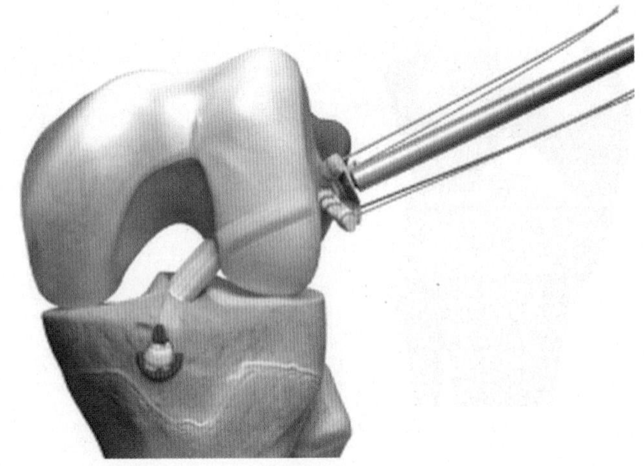

FIGURE 13-9

The interference screw is then inserted into the ShieldLoc with the knee in 20 to 30 degrees of flexion. (Copyright 2013 OrthoPediatrics Corp., with permission.)

Setup and Graft Harvesting/Preparation

The patient is placed supine, and a tourniquet is applied to the proximal thigh. After preparing and draping the leg, a 6- to 10-cm incision is made from the lateral joint line proximally along the superior border of the iliotibial band. A Cobb elevator is used to elevate adherent subcutaneous tissue off the iliotibial band proximally. The iliotibial band is then incised on both its superior and inferior margins from Gerdy tubercle for a distance of 15 to 20 cm proximal to the joint line, depending on the patient's size. The iliotibial band is detached proximally, dissected free from the lateral capsule, and tubularized with a whipstitch using a no. 2 FiberWire suture (Arthrex, Naples, FL).

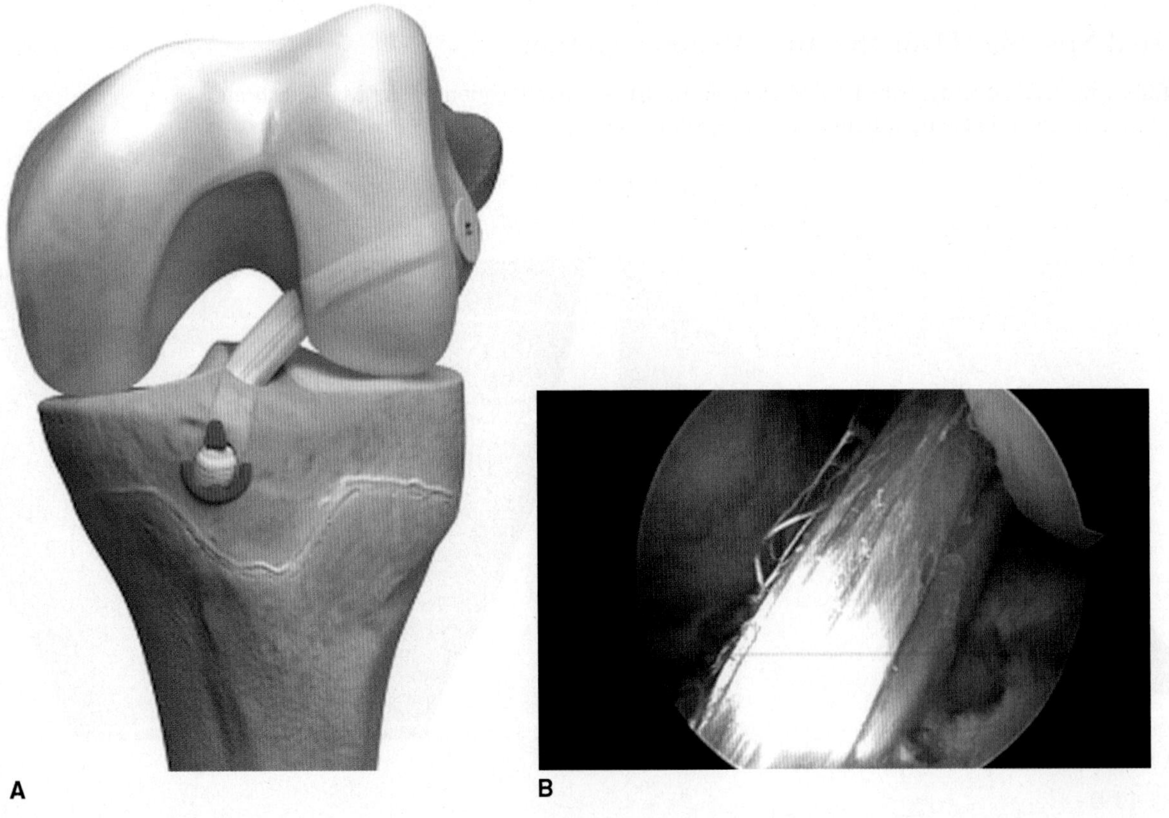

FIGURE 13-10

The final construct (**A**). (Copyright 2013 OrthoPediatrics Corp., with permission.) Arthroscopic view of the graft after fixation (**B**).

Diagnostic Arthroscopy and Notch Preparation

A diagnostic arthroscopy is then performed using standard anteromedial and anterolateral portals. The remaining ACL remnant and fat pad are resected. A small notchplasty is performed, and soft tissue is cleared from the over-the-top position of the lateral femoral condyle, taking care to avoid injury to the perichondrial ring, which is in close proximity.

Graft Passage and Fixation

A second incision is made at the medial border of the patellar tendon, starting at the joint line and extending 4 cm distally. Dissection is carried down to the periosteum. A curved clamp is placed under the intermeniscal ligament, followed by a rasp to make a groove in the proximal tibial epiphysis. Fluoroscopy is used to identify the anterior tibial physis to avoid damaging it during rasping. To pass the graft into the knee, a full-length clamp or tendon passer is inserted into the anteromedial portal to the over-the-top position and out the lateral capsule. The iliotibial band graft is then pulled into the knee. The clamp is then passed under the intermeniscal ligament and used to deliver the graft into the medial incision. The graft is placed under tension, with the knee in 90 degrees of flexion and 15 degrees of external rotation, and sutured to the lateral femoral condyle at the insertion of the lateral intermuscular septum (Fig. 13-11A,B). Following this, the periosteum of the tibia is incised distal to the physis, and a trough is made in the metaphysis. The graft is then seated into the groove in the tibial epiphyses, placed under tension, and sutured to the periosteum of the metaphysis with the knee in 20 degrees of flexion. The residual defect in the iliotibial band is closed to prevent herniation of the vastus lateralis muscle. The lateral patella reticulum is left open to avoid excessive pressure on the lateral facet of the patella. The wounds are closed in a standard fashion.

Transphyseal Reconstruction

The setup of the room, graft harvesting, diagnostic arthroscopy, and notch preparation are the same as described for the all-epiphyseal technique; however, C-arm is not needed for the procedure.

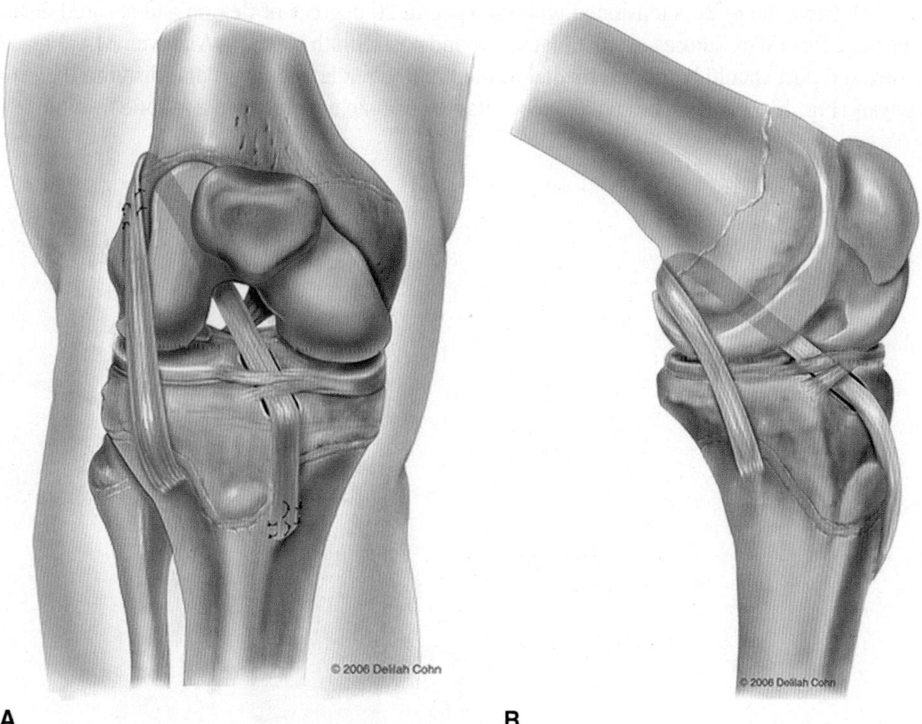

FIGURE 13-11

Anteroposterior (**A**) and oblique (**B**) views of the over-the-top reconstruction after the graft has been passed over the lateral femoral condyle, through the knee, under the intermeniscal ligament, and into the groove in the proximal tibia. (Copyright 2006 Delilah R. Cohn, CMI. Reprinted with permission.)

Femoral and Tibial Tunnel Placement

The tibial drill guide (Acufex-Smith Nephew, Andover, MA) is set to a 55-degree angle, and the tip is inserted through the anteromedial portal. The tip of the guide is placed at the anatomic insertion of the ACL on the tibia with the guide oriented so that the guide pin enters the anteromedial aspect of the tibia at a 65- to 70-degree angle in the coronal plane. Verticalizing the guide in this manner minimizes the cross-sectional area of damage to the physis during reaming. The guide wire is then placed and overreamed with an appropriately sized cannulated reamer selected based on graft size.

After drilling the tibial tunnel, the knee is placed at 90 degrees of flexion. An over-the-top femoral guide that leaves 2 mm of posterior wall is inserted through the tibial tunnel and positioned at the 10:30 position in a left knee or the 1:30 position in a right knee. The 2.7-mm guide pin is advanced into the offset guide and through the lateral femoral condyle until it penetrates through the lateral femoral cortex. A cannulated acorn reamer that matches the diameter of the graft is drilled to a depth of 30 to 35 mm in the femur. The depth of the femoral tunnel should be 10 mm greater than the length of graft desired in the tunnel to allow for rotation of the Endobutton. The 4.5-mm Endobutton reamer is then placed over the guide wire and drilled out the lateral femoral cortex. The femoral hole is chamfered to minimize graft fraying. The Endobutton depth gauge is used to measure the length of the femoral tunnel.

An Endobutton-CL (Smith Nephew, Andover, MA) that leaves 20 to 25 mm of graft within the femoral tunnel is selected. A no. 5 Ethibond suture is passed through one of the outside holes of the Endobutton, and a no. 2 Ethibond suture is passed through the other outside hole. The hamstrings are then passed through the Endobutton-CL to create a quadrupled graft. A 2.7-mm passing pin is inserted up through the tibial and femoral holes, piercing the quadriceps and skin proximally. Both strands of the no. 5 and no. 2 suture in the Endobutton are inserted through the eyelet of the passing pin, and the pin is pulled proximally out of the femur to pass the sutures through the knee (Fig. 13-12). The Endobutton and graft are advanced into the femoral socket by pulling the no. 5 suture. Once the Endobutton is outside the lateral femoral cortex, the no. 2 suture is pulled to rotate the Endobutton (Fig. 13-13). The graft is then pulled distally to firmly seat the Endobutton on the outside of the femoral cortex. Then the no. 2 and no. 5 sutures in the Endobutton are removed, and the knee is cycled to remove any remaining creep from the construct.

The graft is then checked for impingement on the intercondylar notch with the knee in extension (Fig. 13-14). Next, the graft is tensioned with the knee in 20 degrees of flexion and secured distally by tying the no. 2 FiberWire sutures over a tibial screw and post (Smith Nephew, Andover, MA; Fig. 13-15). The screw and post should be placed medial to the tibial tubercle apophysis and distal to the proximal tibial physis (Fig. 13-16A,B). The subcutaneous tissue and skin are closed in a routine fashion.

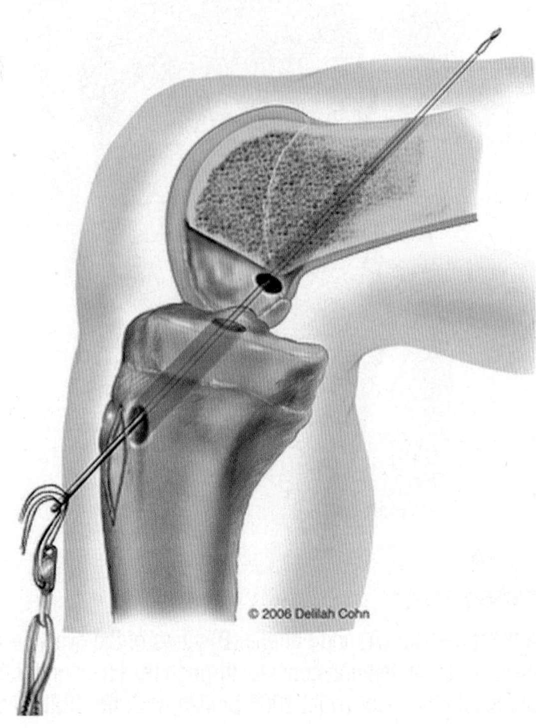

FIGURE 13-12

The passing pin is placed through the tibial and femoral tunnels and pulled proximally to pass the sutures. (Copyright 2006 Delilah R. Cohn, CMI. Reprinted with permission.)

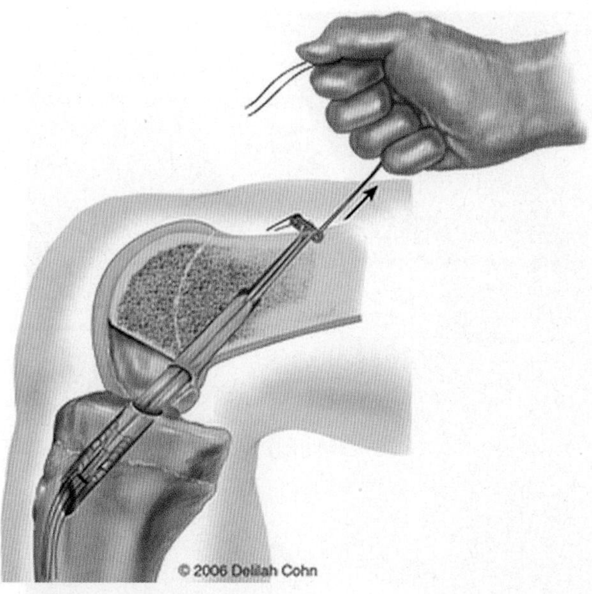

FIGURE 13-13

The graft is pulled into the femoral socked by pulling the no. 5 suture. The Endobutton is flipped by pulling the no. 2 suture. (Copyright 2006 Delilah R. Cohn, CMI. Reprinted with permission.)

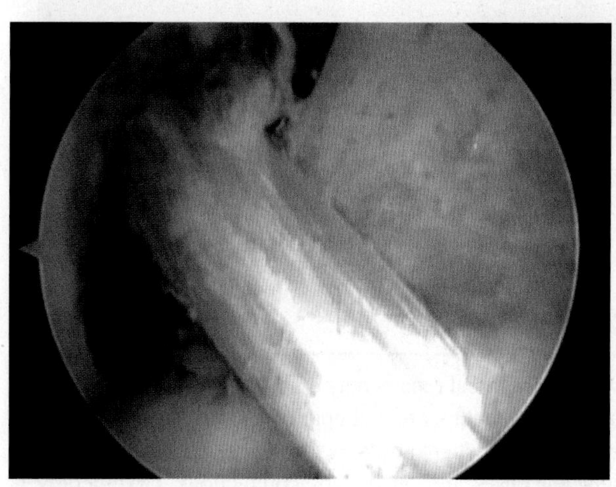

FIGURE 13-14

Arthroscopic view of the graft.

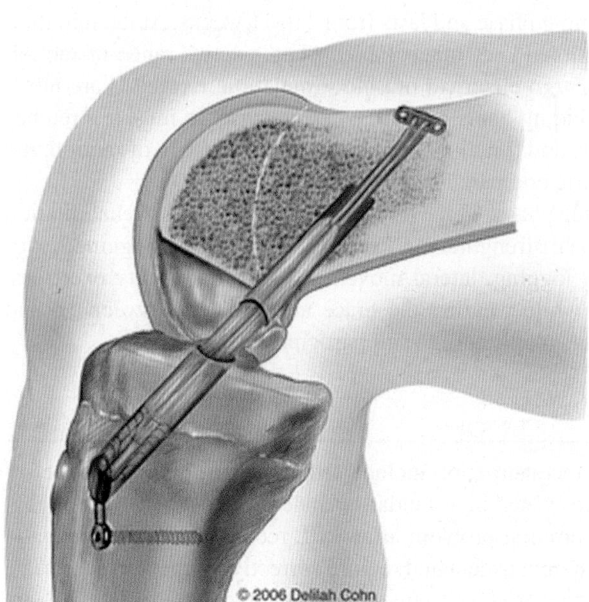

FIGURE 13-15

The graft is pulled distally to lock the Endobutton on the femoral cortex, and the hamstring graft is tied distally over a tibial screw and post. (Copyright 2006 Delilah R. Cohn, CMI. Reprinted with permission.)

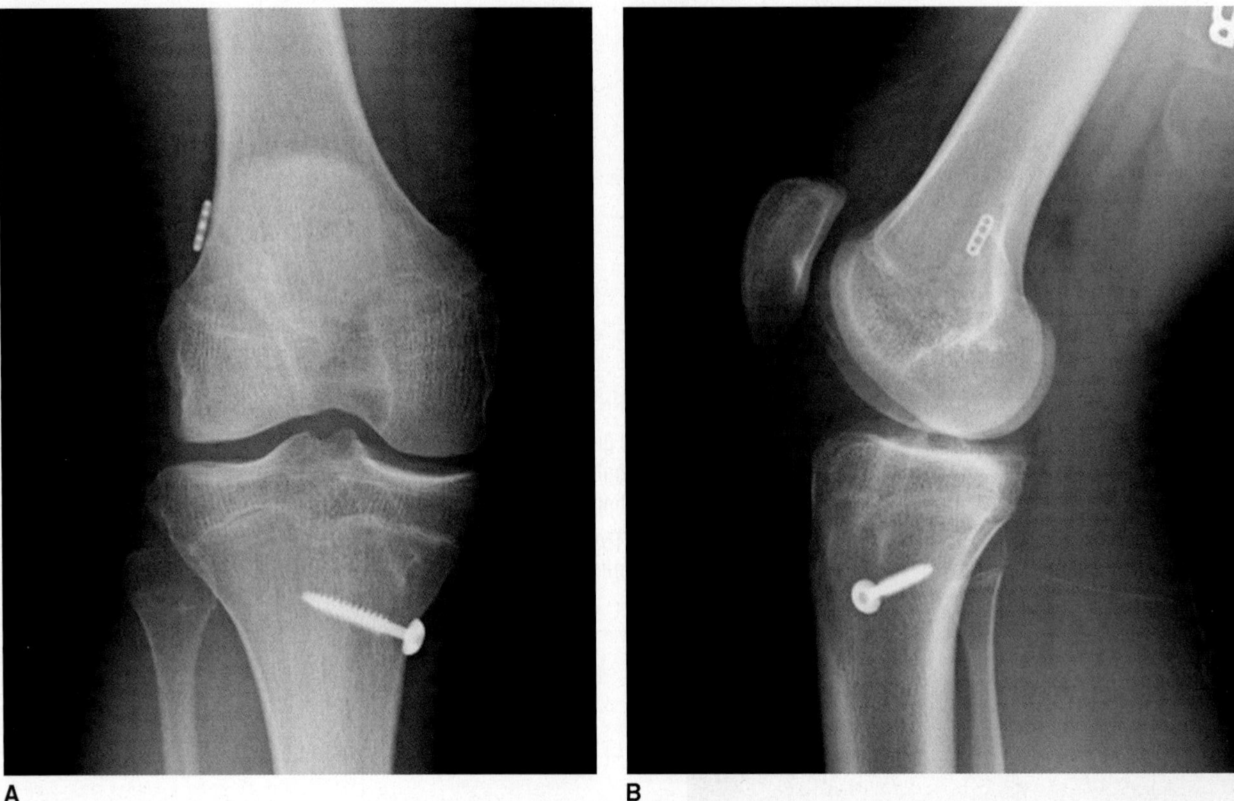

FIGURE 13-16

AP (**A**) and lateral (**B**) radiographs of the knee 2 years after transphyseal ACL reconstruction in a patient with a bone age of 14 years at the time of surgery.

POSTOPERATIVE MANAGEMENT

For all-epiphyseal reconstructions, patients without meniscal repairs may ambulate with crutches and are partial weightbearing for 4 weeks. Postoperative rehabilitation after all-epiphyseal and transphyseal ACL reconstruction has three phases. Phase I begins when the patient awakens from surgery and lasts 2 weeks. The patient is encouraged to perform straight leg raises and quadriceps contractions. Cryotherapy is applied for 5 to 10 minutes each hour. On postoperative day 1, hamstring stretches in a prone position, and range-of-motion exercises are initiated. The goal after 1 week is to have 0 to 90 degrees range of motion.

Phase II of rehabilitation is the strengthening phase and lasts from 2 to 11 weeks. At the initiation of this phase, patients are fitted with a functional knee brace. Patients begin active range-of-motion exercises, do patellar mobilization, and undergo electrical muscle stimulation. Exercises are introduced in order of increasing difficulty, including hamstring stretches, quadriceps muscle stretches and strengthening, proprioception exercises, and functional strengthening. For range of motion, the goal is for the operative knee to be symmetric compared to the normal knee by week 6.

The final phase of rehab is the normalization phase, which lasts from 12 to 20 weeks. Rehabilitation activities during this phase include functional strengthening exercises, straight line jogging, plyometric exercises, sports cord exercises for jogging, lateral movement, and foot agility exercises. Functional activities (full-speed running) while wearing the brace are initiated between 16 and 20 weeks. At postoperative week 32, patients may return to full participation in sports.

COMPLICATIONS

General complications reported with ACL reconstruction include arthrofibrosis, hemorrhagic effusion, and infection. These complications are treated in a standard manner.

Iatrogenic growth disturbance is an uncommon problem after ACL reconstruction in skeletally immature patients, but may cause significant impairment and require corrective surgery. Appropriate risk stratification based on skeletal maturity and subsequent surgical technique selection are paramount in avoiding this complication. Each reconstruction technique carries specific risks for growth disturbance that should be avoided.

For transphyseal ACL reconstruction, both clinical and basic science studies have demonstrated a risk of iatrogenic leg length deficit (LLD) or angular deformity with transphyseal drilling. Consequently, we only recommend this technique in patients who are nearing skeletal maturity and have minimal growth remaining. If transphyseal ACL reconstruction is selected, tunnels should be drilled perpendicular to the physes with the smallest possible reamer to minimize physeal damage and risk of growth deformity. We also recommend using soft tissue autografts to decrease the chance of a physeal bone bridge forming through the drill tunnels. Hardware used for graft fixation in transphyseal ACL reconstruction should always be placed outside and away from the physis to prevent encroachment on and subsequent damage or tethering to the growth plate (Fig. 13-16A,B).

Transphyseal and over-the-top reconstruction rely on extraphyseal graft fixation on the metaphysis on both the tibia and femur. Consequently, graft overtensioning should be avoided in these techniques because it can theoretically create compressive forces on the physis that inhibit longitudinal growth via the Hueter-Volkmann principle. Rasping the femoral over-the-top position and posterior notchplasty should also be avoided in these techniques to prevent damage to the perichondrial ring.

For all-epiphyseal reconstruction, guidewire placement in close proximity to the physis may result in physeal damage during reaming. Consequently, intraoperative fluoroscopy is necessary for guidewire placement that allows both safe reaming relative to the physis and anatomic graft positioning.

Graft rupture is an uncommon complication that can occur from reinjury of the knee. Treatment type depends on the skeletally maturity of the patient. For patients with significant knee growth remaining, we recommend revision all-epiphyseal reconstruction using hamstring autograft from the contralateral knee. Care must be taken to not encroach upon the growth plates when removing residual graft tissues from the tunnels. If previous tunnels are in close proximity to the growth plate on MRI, and there is concern for growth disturbance, the Micheli technique can be utilized to prevent physeal injury. For patients nearing skeletal maturity, revision all-epiphyseal or transphyseal reconstruction with contralateral hamstring autograft can be performed.

CASE EXAMPLE

The following case is an 8-year and 2-month-old male who sustained a right knee injury during an all-terrain vehicle accident (Fig. 13-17A–I). At the time of the injury, the patient was 4′ 6″ tall and weighed 65 pounds. His examination revealed positive Lachman and pivot shift tests. MRI demonstrated a complete midsubstance tear of the ACL (Fig. 13-17A) and a vertical longitudinal tear of the lateral meniscus (Fig. 13-17B). Posteroanterior left hand and wrist radiographs were compared to the Greulich and Pyle atlas and were consistent with a skeletal age of 8 years old (Fig. 13-17C). Given the substantial knee growth remaining in this patient, we performed an all-epiphyseal ACL reconstruction with hamstring autograft to avoid the possibility of growth deformity (Fig. 13-17D,E). An inside-out lateral meniscus repair was also performed at the time of arthroscopy (Fig. 13-17F,G). Nine months out from surgery, he had normal motion and negative Lachman and pivot shift tests and was cleared for sports participation (Fig. 13 17H,I).

PEARLS AND PITFALLS

All-Epiphyseal

The setup for all-epiphyseal and transphyseal reconstruction is important. The patient should be positioned on the operating table with the leg in an arthroscopic leg holder so that the physis may be clearly visualized in both the AP and lateral planes prior to the initiation of surgery.

The drill holes for both the all-epiphyseal and transepiphyseal reconstruction should be as small as possible to minimize the area of damage to the physis in the transphyseal reconstruction and minimize the chance of damaging the physis in the all-epiphyseal reconstruction. The technique used to place a suture in the tendon ends influences the drill hole size. The free ends of the tendons are always larger due to the no. 2 FiberWire sutures placed in the tendon ends. To minimize the diameter of the tendon construct, we recommend placing a locking whipstitch as the first suture pass followed four Bunnell passes up and back the tendon, and the last pass is also a locking whipstitch. The locking whipstitch functions to prevent the suture from pulling out of the tendon ends, and the Bunnell-type stitch minimizes the bulk of the suture in the tendon ends.

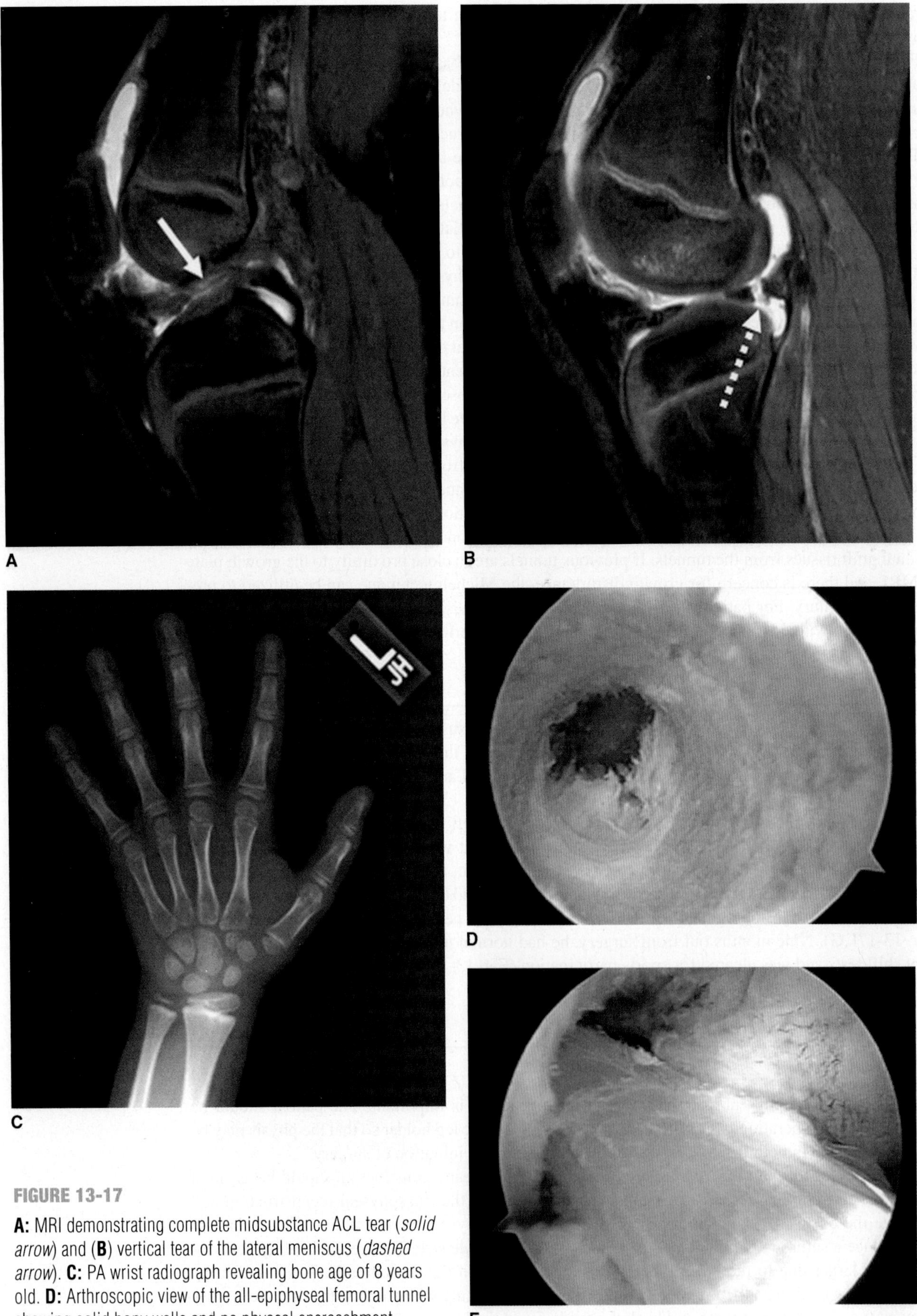

FIGURE 13-17

A: MRI demonstrating complete midsubstance ACL tear (*solid arrow*) and (**B**) vertical tear of the lateral meniscus (*dashed arrow*). **C:** PA wrist radiograph revealing bone age of 8 years old. **D:** Arthroscopic view of the all-epiphyseal femoral tunnel showing solid bony walls and no physeal encroachment.

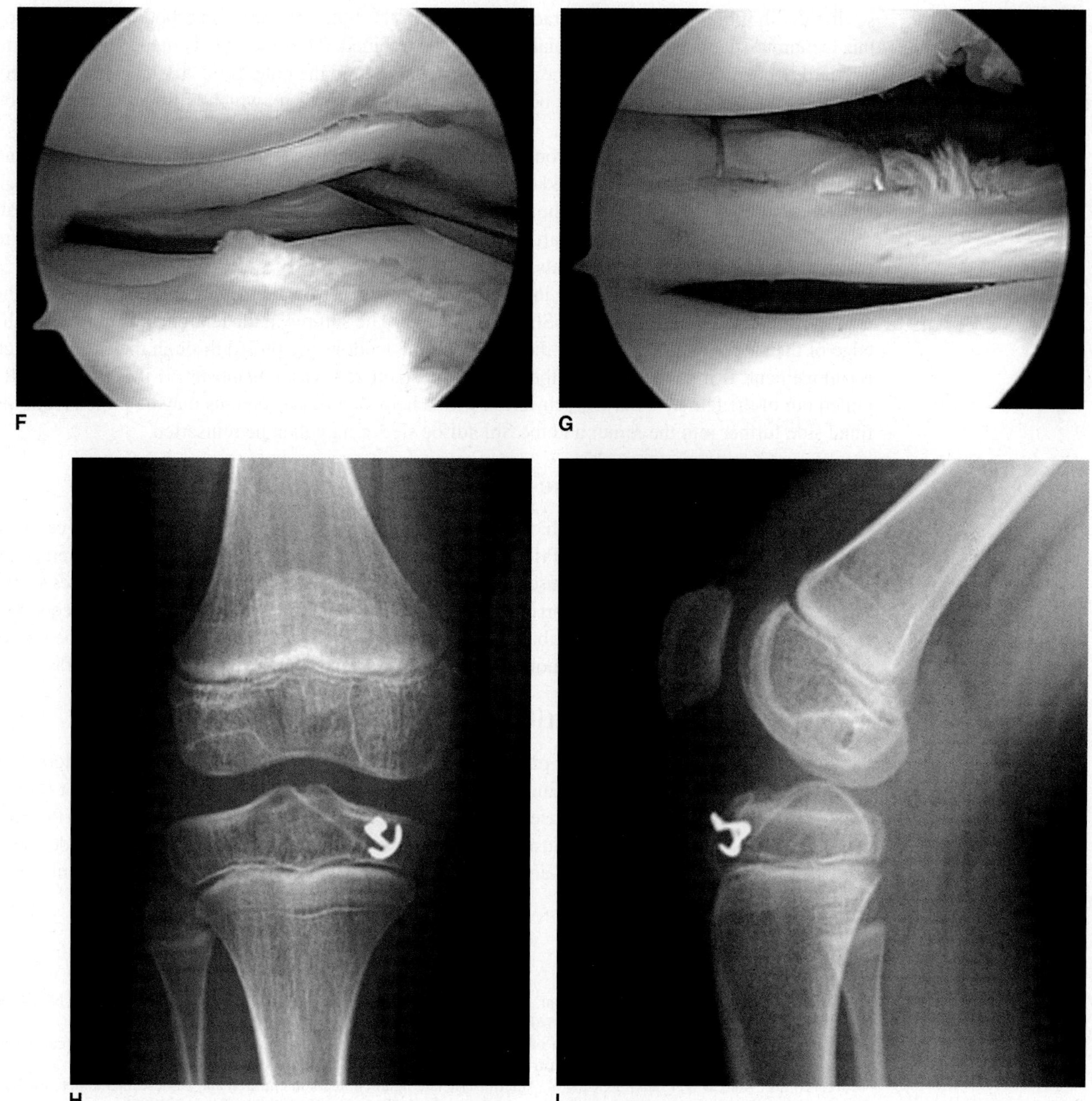

FIGURE 13-17 (*Continued*)

E: Arthroscopic view of the anatomic ACL graft. **F:** Arthroscopic picture of the lateral meniscus tear and (**G**) subsequent inside-out repair. **H:** AP and (**I**) Lateral radiographs of the knee 9 months after reconstruction.

When removing the debris from the intercondylar notch, it is important to clearly identify the insertion site of the ACL on the femur, if possible. Consequently, a minimal notchplasty consisting of primarily soft tissue removal is performed so that the anatomy including the resident's ridge and remaining ACL fibers can be visualized.

During the all-epiphyseal reconstruction, it is important to avoid the insertion sites of the fibular collateral ligament and popliteus tendon on the lateral side of the femur. We have performed pediatric cadaveric dissections, which have demonstrated that these structures may be avoided by elevating the hand holding the guide 30 to 40 degrees from parallel, so that the drill hole is made from anterolateral to posteromedial, entering the joint at the anatomic insertion site of the ACL.

When inserting the counterboard reamer, it is possible for the sharp edges of the reamer to damage the iliotibial tract. Consequently, the lateral skin incision should be approximately 2 cm long, so that the iliotibial tract can be retracted away from the flutes on the counterboard reamer. Using this technique, damage to the iliotibial tract will be avoided. After the hole is made with the counterboard reamer, carefully remove the soft tissue from around the hole. If this tissue is not removed, it may become trapped between the bone and the ShieldLoc sleeve, which will reduce the fixation of the ShieldLoc sleeve in bone.

We prefer to place a fiber tape through the graft passer and pull it through the femoral tunnel and out the tibial tunnel. Then the doubled tendons are passed through the fiber tape and shuttled through the femur and out the tibia. Using the fiber tape to pass, the graft spreads the pressure on the graft over a larger area and minimizes graft damage, should a substantial amount of force be required to pull the graft through the tight tunnels.

After the Armor Link implant is inserted, it is important to watch the ShieldLoc sleeve as the tendons are pulled back through the ShieldLoc sleeve. The sutures in the tendon ends may catch the edge of the sleeve and pull it out of the femur. As the tendons are pulled through the sleeve, watch for movement. If it starts to move, then it may be stabilized with a hemostat. If it is inadvertently pulled out of the femur, it may be reinserted with a hemostat or the tendons may be pulled from the tibial side further into the femur and the ShieldLoc sleeve may then be reinserted.

Physeal Sparing "Over-the-top" Reconstruction

Avoid rasping on the femoral side, which may damage the perichondrial ring of La Croix and cause an iatrogenic valgus flexion deformity. Prior to passing the iliotibial band through the posterolateral capsule, the full-length clamp should be used to dilate the hole in the capsule so that the graft passes easily.

The lateral incision is relatively short compared to the length of the iliotibial band graft. Consequently, it may be difficult to repair the iliotibial band proximally. We have found a Deaver or appendiceal retractor and a long vascular needle holder to be useful for repairing the proximal iliotibial tract.

Transphyseal Reconstruction

The Endobutton continuous loop is pulled through the femur using the sutures in the Endobutton. Occasionally, it is possible for the Endobutton to become lodged within the tunnel and not flipped outside the femoral cortex. In this case, the graft may feel secure when pulling distally, but the construct may fail postoperatively because the Endobutton is not properly seated on the outside of the cortex. We recommend use of the C-arm to confirm the position of the Endobutton on the outside of the femoral cortex in every case.

REFERENCES

1. Dodwell ER, LaMont LE, Green DW, et al. 20 years of pediatric anterior cruciate ligament reconstruction in New York state. *Am J Sports Med.* 2014. doi:10.1177/0363546513518412.
2. Anderson AF, Anderson CN. Correlation of meniscal and articular cartilage injuries in children and adolescents with timing of anterior cruciate ligament reconstruction. *Am J Sports Med.* 2014. doi:10.1177/0363546514559912.
3. Ramski DE, Kanj WW, Franklin CC, et al. Anterior cruciate ligament tears in children and adolescents: a meta-analysis of nonoperative versus operative treatment. *Am J Sports Med.* 2013. doi:10.1177/0363546513510889.
4. Anderson AF. Transepiphyseal replacement of the anterior cruciate ligament in skeletally immature patients a preliminary report. *J Bone Joint Surg Am.* 2003;85(7):1255–1263.
5. Green WT, Anderson M. Experiences with epiphyseal arrest in correcting discrepancies in length of the lower extremities in infantile paralysis a method of predicting the effect. *J Bone Joint Surg Am.* 1947;29(3):659–678.
6. Micheli LJ, Rask B, Gerberg L. Anterior cruciate ligament reconstruction in patients who are prepubescent. *Clinical Orthopaedics and Related Research.* 1999;(364):40–47.
7. Kocher MS, Garg S, Micheli LJ. Physeal sparing reconstruction of the anterior cruciate ligament in skeletally immature prepubescent children and adolescents. *J Bone Joint Surg Am.* 2005;87(11):2371–2379.

14 ACL Reconstruction Using BPTB

Robert A. Arciero and Justin Shu Yang

PATIENT SELECTION

Several items are important in the history when considering a patellar tendon autograft for anterior cruciate ligament (ACL) reconstruction. An advantage of this graft is that it is similar in length to the ACL. Bony attachments at each end of the graft permit bone-to-bone healing, which many surgeons believe that it provides the strongest method of healing. For the general population, age is an important determining factor in choosing an autograft. We generally recommend autograft in patients under the age of 40 in the primary setting. For athletes, we prefer autograft due to the higher activity level. We take into account the participation level, sport, position, and future careers in determining the specific autograft type. The ideal candidate for a patellar tendon graft is a young high-demand athlete without any preexisting anterior knee pain, does not require kneeling, and have normal patellar height.

The primary disadvantage of the patellar tendon graft is an increased incidence (upward of 30%) of anterior knee pain postoperatively. Preexisting anterior knee pain can predispose patients to have the same, if not worse, problem postoperatively. Further, preexisting symptomatic patellofemoral arthritis is a relative contraindication. Classically, baseball and softball catchers who kneel constantly on their knees will often complain of pain at the donor site after surgery. Other sports may have positions that put direct pressure on the anterior knee that may not be as intuitive, such as a volleyball player who dives or a rower that canoes. Professions such as carpentry, construction, carpet laying, plumbing, and electricians are also at an increased risk of developing anterior knee pain. Also, by removing the middle third of the patellar tendon, it is weakened and the patient is put at risk for patellar tendon rupture as well as patella fracture. A history of patellar tendon rupture or fracture of the patella would be a contraindication to using patellar tendon autograft. The other issue is a residual ossicle in the distal portion of the graft from Osgood-Schlatter disease. There is some debate whether the presence of this ossicle is a contraindication to use of the patellar tendon autograft. We believe this should be individualized and certainly, extremely large ossicles may preclude the use of this graft. We also do not use a patellar tendon graft in patients with open physis and tanner stage less than 3. Finally, a patient with patellar baja on radiograph and exam may be a contraindication if the tendon length is shorter than 3 cm, although we rarely have found this to be the case.

PREOPERATIVE PLANNING

After a careful history noting all the factors mentioned above, a physical examination is performed. We believe it is important to take a history and physical prior to viewing any imaging as it may bias the surgeon. The patient's skin status is an often overlooked portion of the physical exam but important in considering a patellar tendon graft. Patients that have abrasions, small lacerations, psoriatic lesions and inflamed bursa directly over the patellar tendon should be counseled as wound complications may occur. If the patient hyperextends or have generalized soft tissue laxity, we would favor a patellar tendon graft over a hamstring graft. A careful examination of collateral ligaments and the posterior cruciate ligament (PCL) is performed to rule out any concomitant injury.

Weight-bearing radiographs are then obtained. Our standard views include weight-bearing anterior-posterior, Rosenberg, lateral, and merchant views. If there is any suspicion of malalignment or varus thrust on the physical exam, then bilateral weight-bearing full hip to ankle views are needed.

SURGICAL PROCEDURE

After induction of anesthesia, an examination is performed to confirm the diagnosis of an ACL tear. The knee is then positioned in a leg holder; standard prep and drape are applied. A longitudinal incision is made 1 cm medial to midline from the inferior pole of the patella to the tibial tubercle (Fig. 14-1).

The incision is carried down to the level of the paratenon; skin flaps are raised medially and laterally. After the paratenon is completely exposed, it is divided longitudinally and reflected on either side (Fig. 14-2). A scissor can be used to spread above and below the paratenon to detach any adhesions (Fig. 14-3). After the patellar tendon is exposed, the central third of the patellar tendon is identified. The graft is typically 10 to 11 mm in width. Using a blade, the tendon is divided up to the patella and down to the tubercle (Fig. 14-4). Care should be taken to maintain the 10 to 11 m width as there is a tendency to make the graft narrower distally.

Attention is turned first to the tibial plug harvest. A 10-mm by 25-mm plug outline is delineated on the tibial tubercle using a knife or Bovie cautery. Using a microsagittal ½-in saw introduced perpendicular to the bone, and cut approximately 10 mm deep (Fig. 14-5). A horizontal bone cut with the saw behind the patellar tendon is often needed to free the tibial plug. On the patellar side, a similar 10-mm by 20-mm plug is outlined (Fig. 14-6). The saw is introduced at a 45-degree angle and the tip of the plug is rounded by curving the saw (Figs. 14-7 and 14-8). Osteotome is used to gently free up both plugs. We do not recommend using a mallet on the patella as this may fracture the bone plug. We would prefer to almost entirely remove the patellar plug of the graft using the oscillating saw by beveling the cuts. After both bone plugs are freed, the graft is detached from adhesions to the fat pad using a knife taking care to cut away from the tendon.

The graft is prepared on the back table first by removing any excess fat from the tendon (Fig. 14-9). Using a crimper and a rongeur, the bone plugs are made into 10 mm in diameter (Fig. 14-10). The total length of the tendon is calculated. Ideally, the patellar tendon is 30 to 50 mm in length with bone plugs that are 20 to 25 mm in length. The total length of the graft should not exceed 100 mm; if this is the case, the bone plugs should be shortened. The patellar bone plug is used in the tibia and the tubercle bone plug is used in the femur. We prefer to place the tibial bone portion of the graft into the femoral socket as there is a natural step-off between the bone and tendon insertion on the tibial end. This protects the soft tissue during interference screw placement (Fig. 14-11). One stitch is put through the femoral plug, and three ultra-high-strength sutures are put through the tibial plug along with a stitch through the tendon. This is pretensioned at 10 N on the back table and wrapped in antibiotic-soaked sponge (Fig. 14-12).

After a diagnostic arthroscopy and any relevant meniscal work are performed, the notch is debrided free of any remnant ACL tissue through a medial portal that can normally be made inside the tendon harvest incision. The tibial and femoral ACL attachments are preserved. An accessory low anterior medial portal is made using an 18-gauge needle to set up this portal (Figs. 14-13 and 14-14). The over-the-top position is identified on the femur and a microfracture awl is used to make a small hole at the center of the femoral footprint (Fig. 14-15). The top of the leg holder is removed and the knee is hyperflexed to 120 degrees. A 7-mm over-the-top guide is introduced through the accessory portal and a guide pin is placed at the previously made hole (Fig. 14-16). The guide pin should exit the femur laterally through the skin anterior and superior to the lateral epicondyle (Fig. 14-17). This avoids the potential for posterior wall blowout.

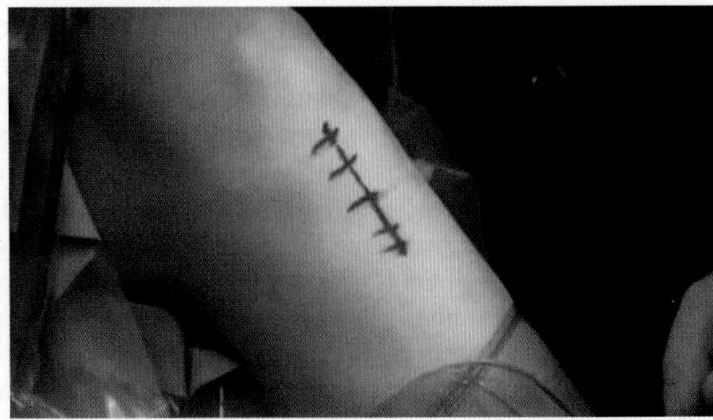

FIGURE 14-1

Longitudinal incision is made 1 cm medial to midline from the inferior pole of the patella to the tibial tubercle.

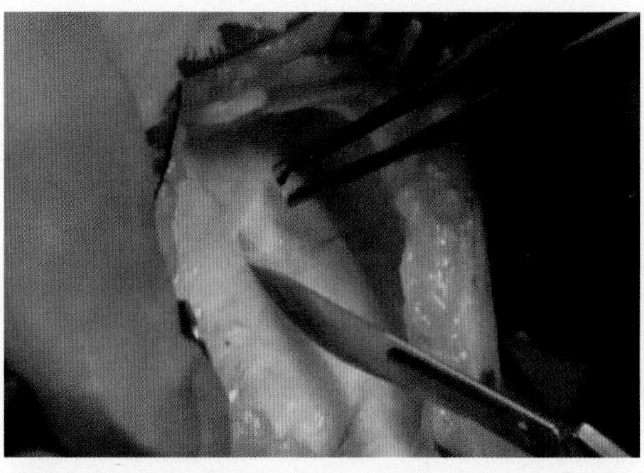

FIGURE 14-2

Paratenon is divided longitudinally.

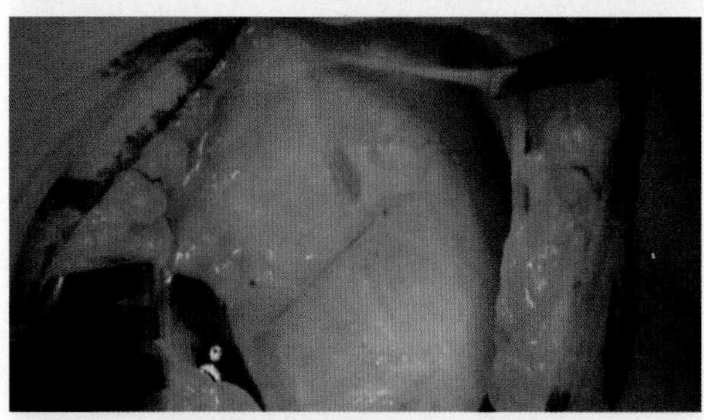

FIGURE 14-3

Paratenon is elevated and retracted.

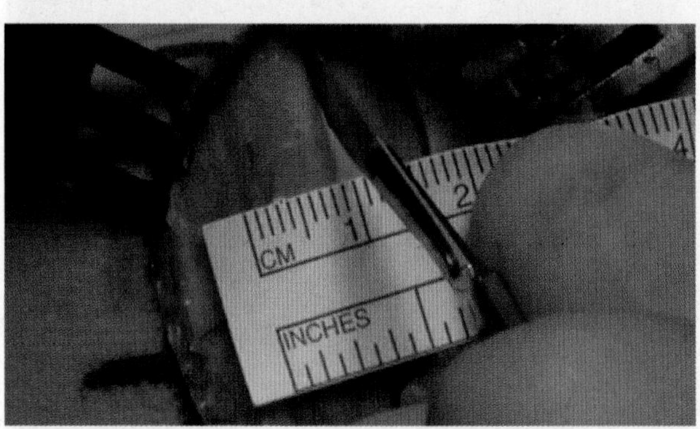

FIGURE 14-4

The middle one-third of the patellar tendon is split longitudinally at a distance 10 to 11 mm wide.

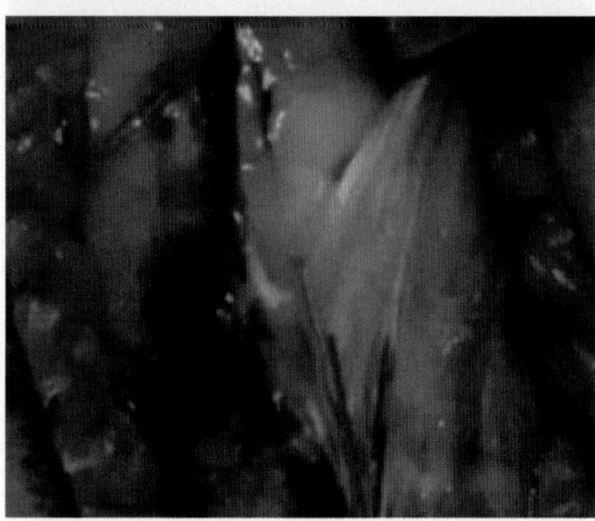

FIGURE 14-5

Tibial bone plug harvest.

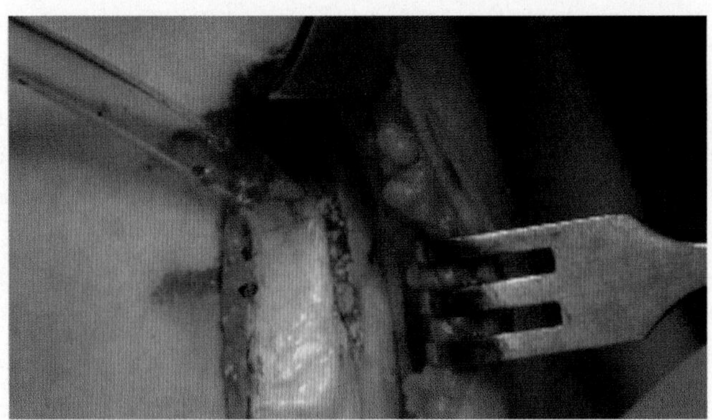

FIGURE 14-6
Patellar bone plug outlined.

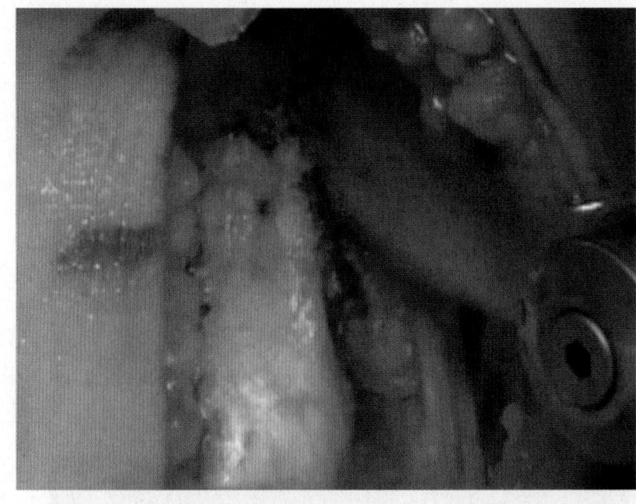

FIGURE 14-7
Beveling the saw 45 degrees for patellar plug harvest.

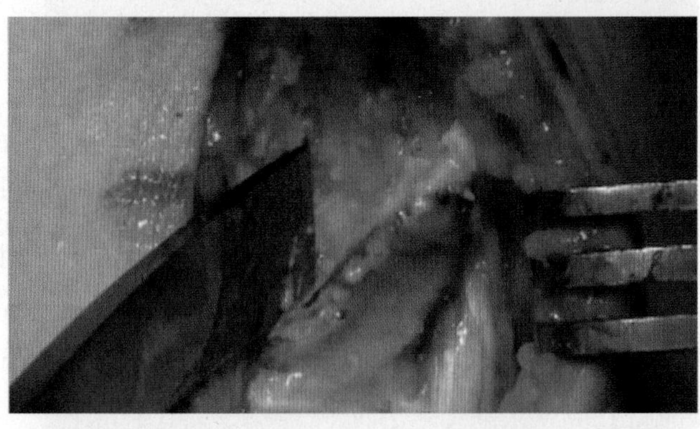

FIGURE 14-8
Small osteotome is used to free the bone plug.

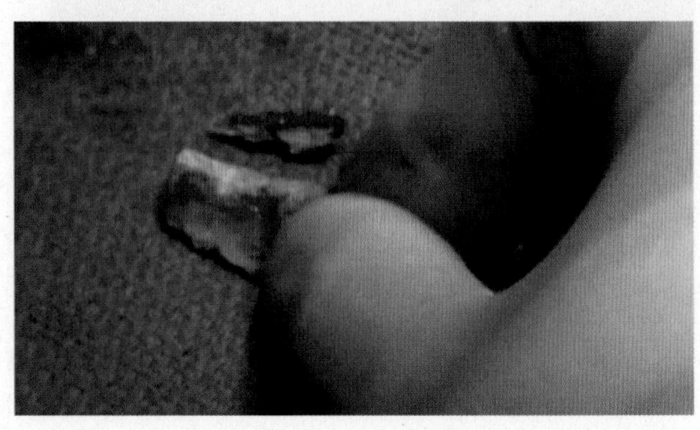

FIGURE 14-9
Bone plugs are cut down to a smaller size.

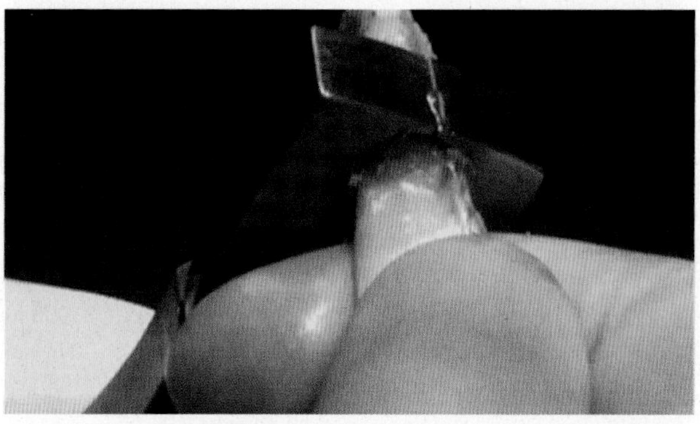

FIGURE 14-10

Bone crimper can be used to make the plugs round.

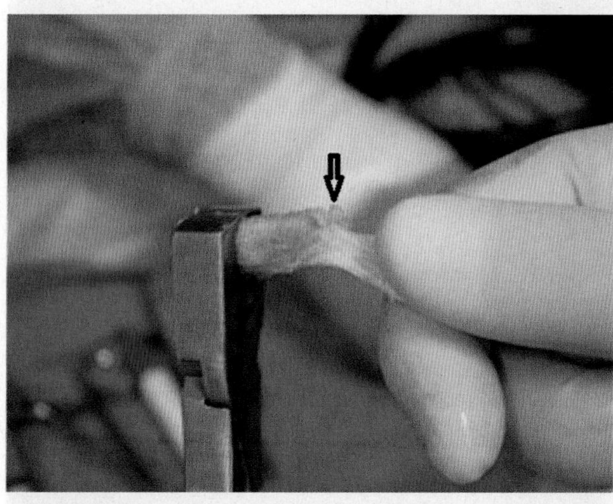

FIGURE 14-11

Arrow points to the bone behind the patellar tendon on the tibial harvest that can protect the graft during interference screw fixation.

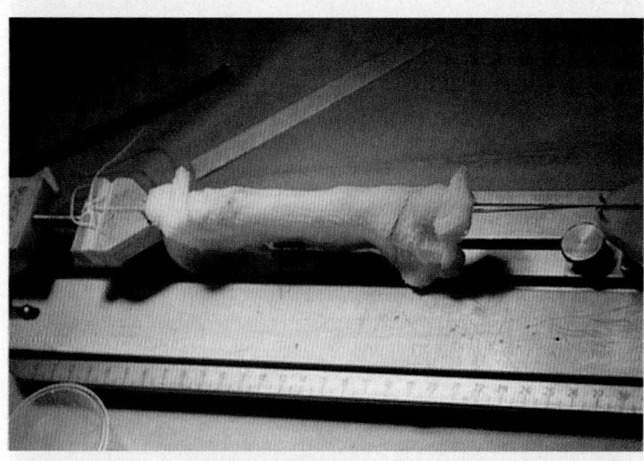

FIGURE 14-12

The graft is wrapped in an antibiotic- and saline-soaked sponge.

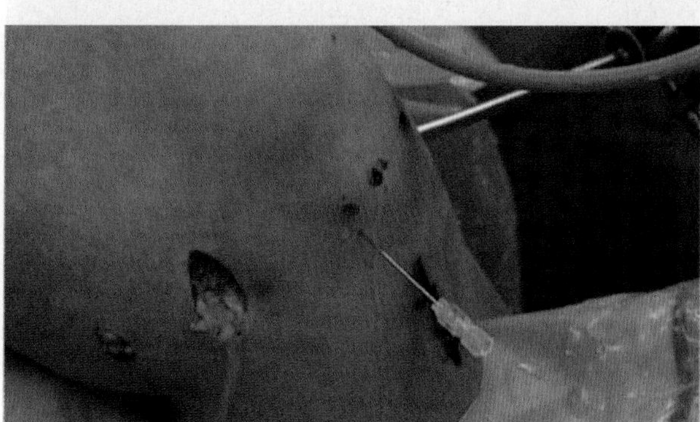

FIGURE 14-13

An accessory low anterior medial portal is made using an 18-gauge needle to confirm location.

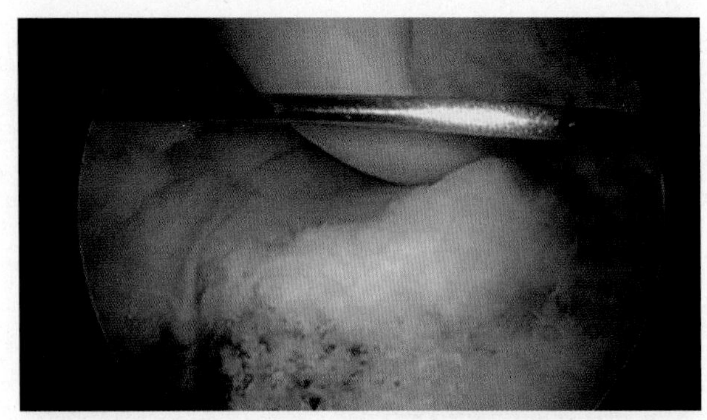

FIGURE 14-14

An accessory low anterior medial portal is made using an 18-gauge needle to confirm location.

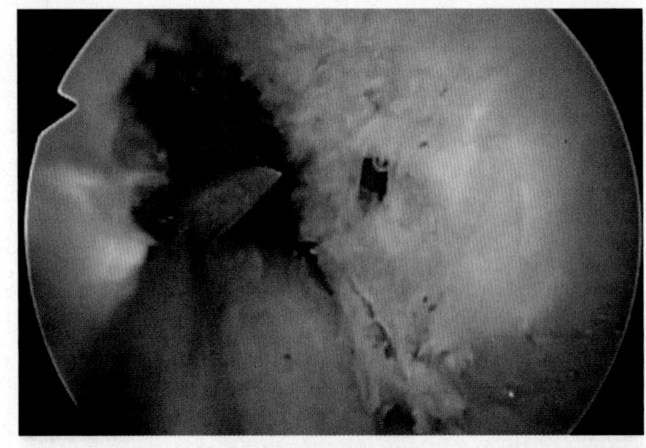

FIGURE 14-15

A microfracture awl is used to make a small hole at the center of the femoral footprint.

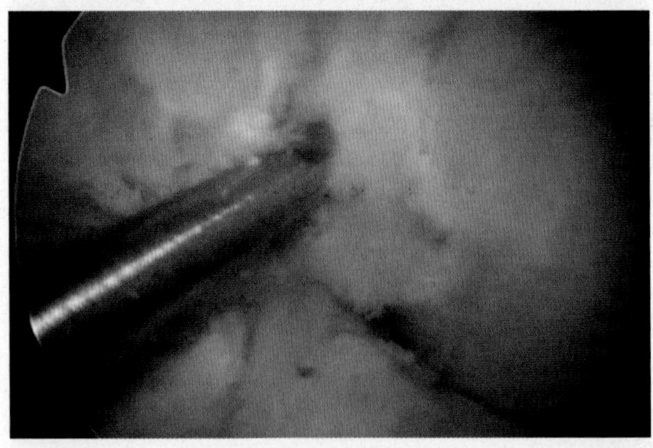

FIGURE 14-16

A guide pin is placed at the previously made hole.

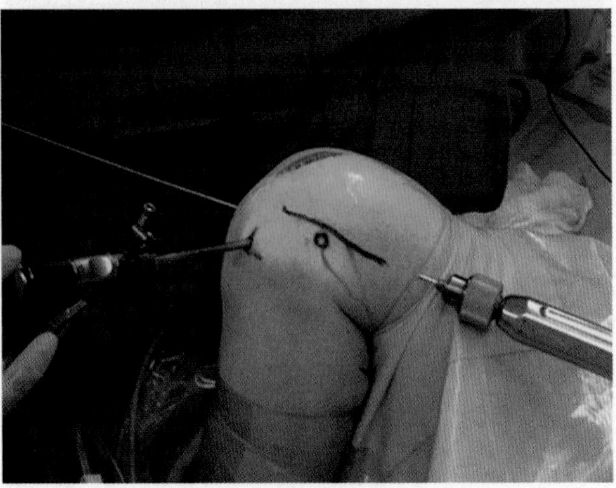

FIGURE 14-17

The guide pin should exit the femur laterally through the skin anterior and superior to the lateral epicondyle.

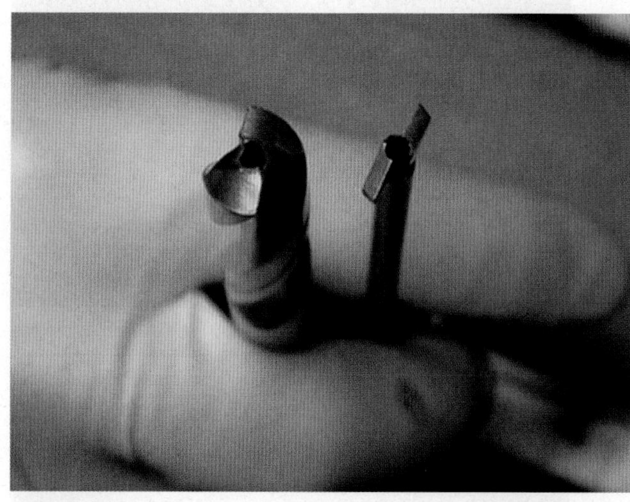

FIGURE 14-18

A low-profile reamer is used on the femur, and a full conical reamer is used on the tibia.

A 10-mm low-profile reamer is then used to make a 10 mm × 25 mm hole (Fig. 14-18). Care should be taken while reaming to make sure the posterior wall is intact. Excess bone debris is cleaned from the tunnel using a disassembled shaver (the sleeve of a spinal needle also works well). A notcher is used to make a notch anteriorly in the femoral tunnel for future interference screw placement. A suture loop is introduced using the guide pin and pulled through the femoral tunnel (Fig. 14-19).

For the standard length graft, the tibial guide angle is set to 55 degrees. However, in longer grafts, the angle will need to be increased accordingly. The formula n + 7 is often used where n is the length of the patellar tendon. The tibial guide is introduced into the knee through the medial portal. The guide is placed in the middle of the tibial footprint medially-laterally and at the level of the posterior border of the anterior lateral meniscus anteriorly-posteriorly (Figs. 14-20 and 14-21). A guide pin is drilled and a 10-mm full conical reamer is used to make the tibial tunnel. Bone reamings are collected for future donor site grafting (Fig. 14-22). Excess soft tissue is removed at the apertures of the tunnel using rongeur and shaver. The suture looped from the femoral tunnel is passed through the tibial tunnel.

The graft is brought from the back table and pulled through the tibial tunnel using the suture loop (Fig. 14-23). The femoral plug is docked into the femoral tunnel with the bone plug facing anteriorly (Fig. 14-24). The guidewire for the interference screw is then introduced anterior to the bone plug using the previously notched hole; a large guidewire is recommended to avoid wire bending (Fig. 14-25). A 7 mm × 20 mm metal interference screw is then secured in place while pulling tension on the femoral plug (Fig. 14-26). The knee is then cycled multiple times making sure the graft tightens in extension. The knee is placed in 10 degrees of flexion, and a postwasher plate is implanted just distal to the tibial tunnel (Fig. 14-27). The two sutures through the tibial plug and the

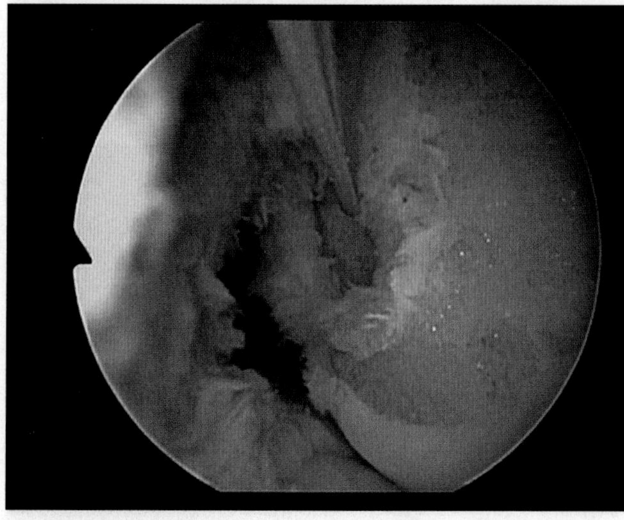

FIGURE 14-19

A suture loop is introduced using the guide pin and pulled through the femoral tunnel.

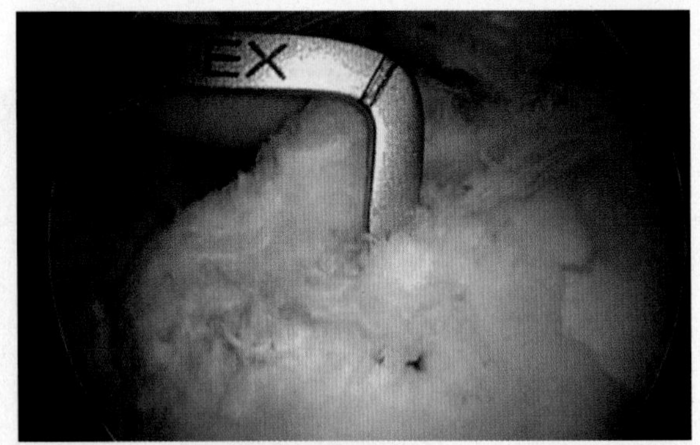

FIGURE 14-20

The guide is placed in the middle of the tibial footprint medially-laterally and at the level of the posterior border of the anterior lateral meniscus anteriorly-posteriorly.

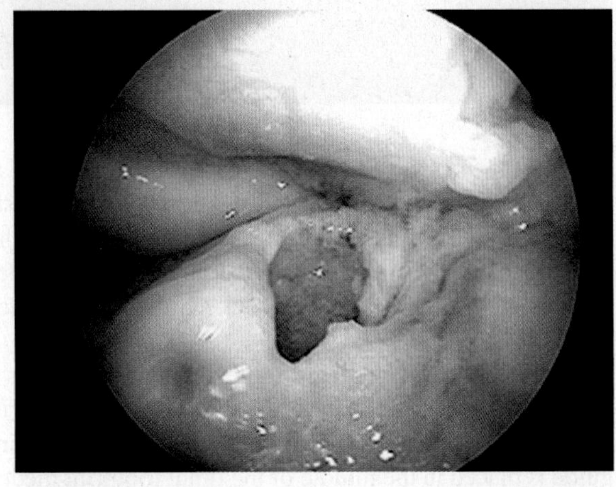

FIGURE 14-21

A 10-mm drill hole is made using the full conical reamer.

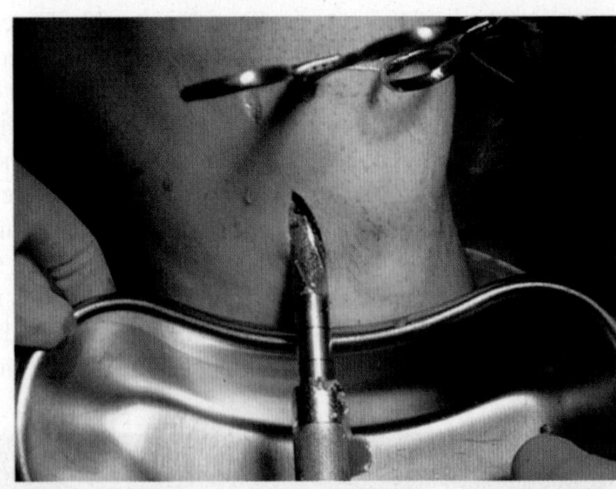

FIGURE 14-22

Bone reamings is collected in a kidney basin for later grafting.

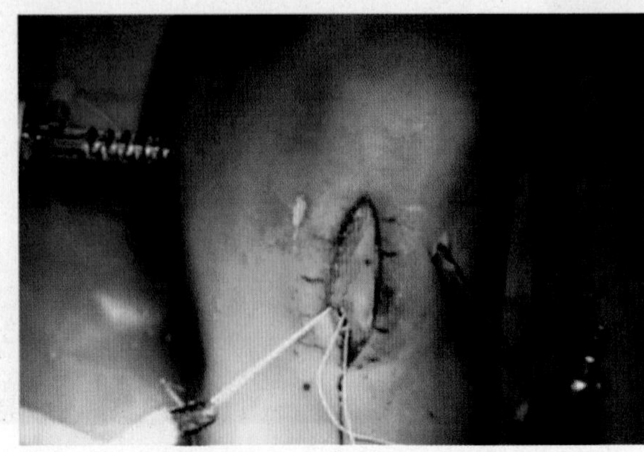

FIGURE 14-23

The graft is brought from the back table and pulled through the tibial tunnel using the suture loop.

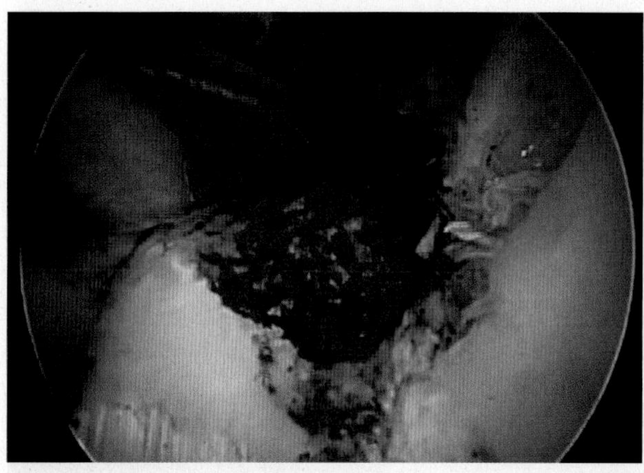

FIGURE 14-24

The femoral plug is docked into the femoral tunnel with the bone plug facing anteriorly. *Blue* markings can be made at the anterior plug face to ensure this is visualized.

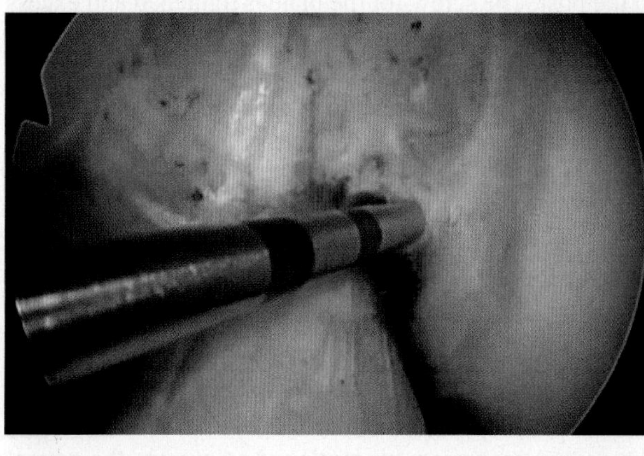

FIGURE 14-25

Large guidewire for the interference screw is introduced anterior to the bone plug.

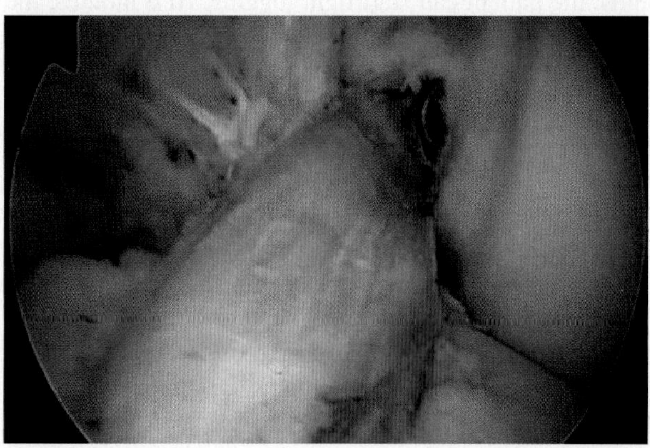

FIGURE 14-26

A metal interference screw is then secured in place while pulling tension on the femoral plug.

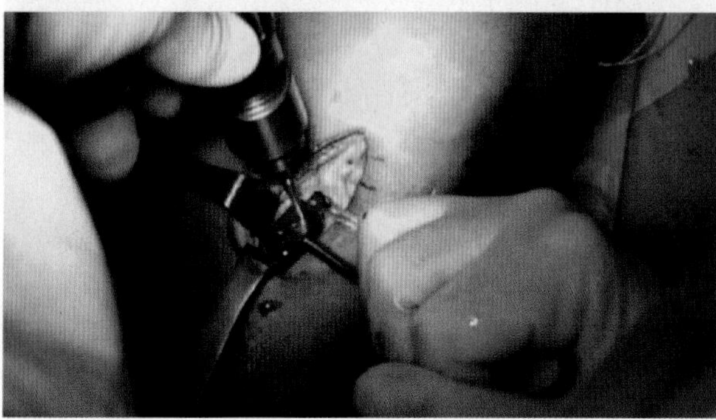

FIGURE 14-27

The tibial plug sutures are tied to a postwasher plate with the knee in 10 degrees of flexion.

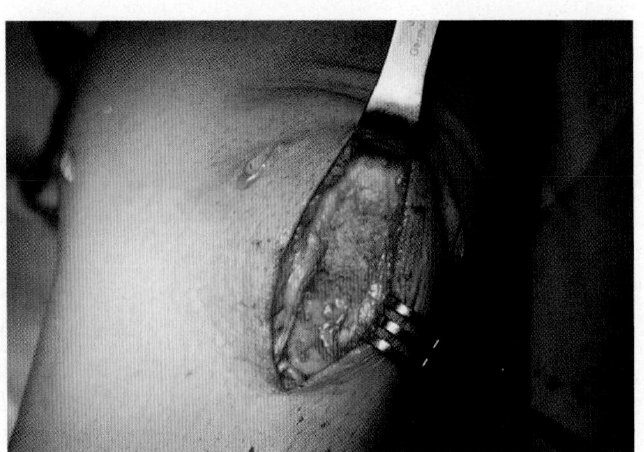

FIGURE 14-28

The excess bone reamings are first grafted into the patellar donor site and then the tibial donor site.

one suture through the tendon is tied around the post. The screw for the plate is tightened and excess suture is cut. The graft is examined through the scope to make sure it is free of impingement and the femoral plug has not moved.

The excess bone reamings are first grafted into the patellar donor site and then the tibial donor site (Fig. 14-28). The paratenon is closed using 0 Vicryl suture (Fig. 14-29). The skin is closed using 2-0 and 3-0 Monocryl suture. Sterile dressing is applied along with an ice pack. The patient is put into a hinged knee brace locked in extension.

POSTOPERATIVE MANAGEMENT

The patient will be partial or full weight bearing based on if any meniscal repair was performed. We recommend the patient do isometric quad sets and ankle pumps immediately. Therapy starts after the first week with passive and active range of motion. The patient remains in a brace locked in extension for 1 week, and then, we unlock the brace and progress with motion. At 6 weeks, the patient should have regained the preoperative motion and can be started on quad strengthening; the brace can be discontinued at this point. At 3 months, the patient can start light jogging. At 6 months, the patient can start sport-specific drills, cutting and jumping. Return to play ideally is at 9 months but can be earlier based on the patient's rehab.

COMPLICATIONS TO AVOID

Bone plug harvest can be tricky especially on the patellar side. We make sure the longitudinal bone cuts on either side of the patellar plug are deep enough with the saw and only use the osteotome to gently pry the plug from the patella. We never use a mallet for fear of propagating a fracture. We also never use the osteotome on the horizontal cut of the patella or tibia as it may break the plug in two.

Metallic screw advances have decreased the risk of cutting the tendon as the interference screw is advanced into the femoral tunnel. We chose to use the tubercle bone plug as the femoral graft due to the retropatellar bone that comes with the tubercle plug (Fig. 14-11). This piece of bone acts as

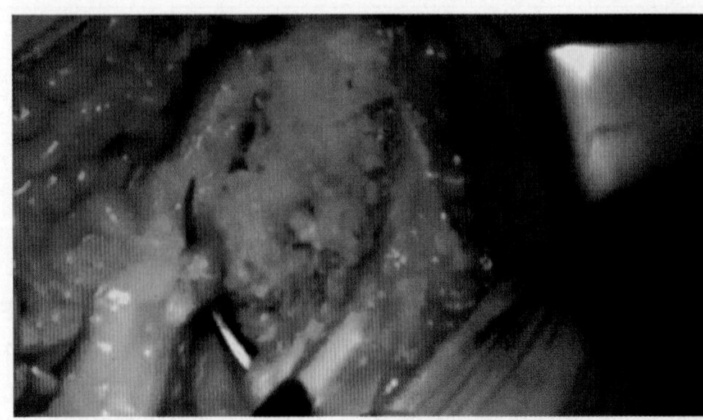

FIGURE 14-29

The paratenon is closed using 0 Vicryl suture.

a protector to the patellar tendon from the cutting effect of the metal screw. Alternatively, a plastic sleeve can be used to protect the tendon from being cut by the screw.

Posterior wall blowout can be an issue when reaming the femoral tunnel. Using a 7-mm over-the-top guide with a 10-mm bone plug will theoretically leave a 2-mm posterior wall if the guide is used correctly. We suggest using a 70-degree scope to visualize the over-the-top position if there's any doubt. If a posterior wall blowout is encountered, then a suspensory fixation device can be used to fix the graft to the lateral femoral cortex. Alternatively, a second lateral incision can be made and a screw postwasher can be placed in the femur with the sutures from the bony portion of the autograft tied around this device.

Anatomic tunnel placement is critical to the success of any ACL surgery. We recommend using the low anterior medial accessory portal to get to the anatomic femoral insertion of the ACL. A low-profile reamer is needed to protect the medial femoral condyle as the reamer is passed into the joint. We typically do this under direct visualization with the scope with the reamer free from the power assembly under manual control.

RECOMMENDED READINGS

Bradley JP, Klimkiewicz JJ, Rytel MJ, et al. Anterior cruciate ligament injuries in the National Football League: epidemiology and current treatment trends among team physicians. *Arthroscopy.* 2002;18(5):502–509.

Duffee A, Magnussen RA, Pedroza AD, et al. Transtibial ACL femoral tunnel preparation increases odds of repeat ipsilateral knee surgery. *J Bone Joint Surg Am.* 2013;95(22):2035–2042.

Jackson DW, Grood ES, Goldstein JD, et al. A comparison of patellar tendon autograft and allograft used for anterior cruciate ligament reconstruction in the goat model. *Am J Sports Med.* 1993;21(2):176–185.

Kaeding CC, Aros B, Wright RW, et al. Allograft versus autograft anterior cruciate ligament reconstruction: predictors of failure from a MOON prospective longitudinal cohort. *Sports Health.* 2011;3(1):73–81.

Mohtadi NG, Chan DS, Dainty KN, et al. Patellar tendon versus hamstring tendon autograft for anterior cruciate ligament rupture in adults. *Cochrane Database Syst Rev.* 2011;9:CD005960.

Moller E, Weidenhielm L, Werner S. Outcome and knee-related quality of life after anterior cruciate ligament reconstruction: a long-term follow-up. *Knee Surg Sports Traumatol Arthrosc.* 2009;17:786–794.

Reinhardt KR, Hetsroni I, Marx RG. Graft selection for anterior cruciate ligament reconstruction: a level I systematic review comparing failure rates and functional outcomes. *Orthop Clin North Am.* 2010;41:249–262.

Tomita F, Yasuda K, Mikami S, et al. Comparisons of intraosseous graft healing between the doubled flexor tendon graft and the bone-patellar tendon bone graft in anterior cruciate ligament reconstruction. *Arthroscopy.* 2001;17:461–476.

15 Anatomic Single-Bundle Hamstring ACL Reconstruction

Charles H. Brown Jr and James Robinson

INTRODUCTION

A tear of the anterior cruciate ligament (ACL) is usually sustained in athletic activities involving cutting, pivoting, changing directions, deceleration, and landing from a jump. In the United States, the incidence of ACL tears in the general population has been reported to be 3.8 per 10,000 individuals (1). A complete tear of the ACL often results in rotational instability of the knee, which can lead to meniscal tears, articular cartilage damage, and the early onset of osteoarthritis (2,3). Following an ACL tear, many patients elect to undergo ACL reconstruction to return to athletic activities that involve running, jumping, deceleration, changing directions, and pivoting. In the United States, the incidence of ACL reconstruction has been reported to be 45 per 100,000 capita (4). In the year 2006, it was reported that approximately 130,000 ACL reconstructions were performed in the United States (5).

The success of ACL reconstruction is influenced by many factors such as the initial tensile properties of the ACL graft tissue, ACL graft placement, initial fixation of the ACL graft, healing of the ACL graft tissue within the bone tunnels, and biological remodeling of the ACL graft tissue. Due to its high initial tensile strength and stiffness, ability to be rigidly fixed to bone, and rapid bone-to-bone healing at the ACL graft fixation sites, the central-third bone-patellar tendon-bone (BPTB) autograft is considered by many surgeons to be the "gold standard" for ACL reconstruction. Clinical studies have shown that ACL reconstructions performed using a BPTB autograft result in predictable success in restoring anterior tibial translation and eliminating the pivot shift phenomena (6–10). However, harvest of a BPTB autograft is associated with a higher incidence of donor site problems such as anterior knee pain, kneeling pain, quadriceps muscle weakness, and extensor mechanism dysfunction (6–10). Due to decreased harvest site morbidity, a lower incidence of harvest site complications, and improvements in soft tissue graft fixation techniques that have resulted in equivalent objective stability to that of BPTB autograft reconstructions, hamstring tendon autografts have become an increasingly popular graft choice for ACL reconstruction. In a survey of international knee surgeons conducted at the 2011 American Academy of Orthopaedic Surgeons (AAOS) and the European Federation of National Associations of Orthopaedics and Traumatology (EFORT) meetings, 66% of the respondents reported using hamstring tendon autografts as their first choice for ACL reconstructions (11). Hamstring tendon autograft was the most common graft choice (58%) of members of the Magellan Society, a group of greater than 150 sports knee surgeons from four continents (12). In a 2016 survey of members of the ACL Study Group, 48% of the respondents reported that hamstring tendon autografts were their first graft of choice for primary ACL reconstructions. This chapter discusses the following: indications for using hamstring tendon autografts, how to safely harvest hamstring tendon grafts; how to prepare a 4-strand, 5-strand, or 6-strand hamstring ACL autograft; and the surgical technique for performing an anatomic single-bundle hamstring ACL reconstruction and a tissue-preserving ACL augmentation technique.

INDICATIONS AND CONTRAINDICATIONS

Hamstring tendon autografts can generally be used in any patient with an acute or chronic ACL tear. Due to the lower incidence of anterior knee pain and kneeling pain and less interference with kneeling and crawling, hamstring tendon grafts are preferred for patients whose occupation, lifestyle, or religion requires kneeling, crawling, or squatting. Hamstring tendon grafts are also preferred in patients with a history of anterior knee pain, patellar instability, extensor mechanism dysfunction, or previous extensor mechanism trauma such as a patellar fracture or a quadriceps or patellar tendon rupture. The only absolute contraindication for using hamstring tendon autografts for an ACL reconstruction is previous harvest of the hamstring tendons. If the surgeon wishes to avoid using a BPTB or quadriceps tendon autograft in the situation of previous ipsilateral hamstring tendon harvest, the hamstring tendons can be harvested from the contralateral leg.

There are a number of situations where the use of hamstring tendons may be inadvisable and an alternative graft choice considered. Previous open surgery on the medial side of the knee may change the normal anatomical relationships of the medial hamstring tendons, and postoperative scarring may alter the normal tissue planes, potentially making harvest of the hamstring tendons difficult and unpredictable. Harvest of the hamstring tendons has been shown to result in loss of flexion and internal tibial rotation strength at high flexion angles (13). Hamstring tendon ACL grafts should be avoided in athletes that require maximum hamstring strength at high flexion angles such as wrestlers, sprinting athletes, gymnasts, ice and rock climbers, and athletes who must back pedal while playing their sport. In patients with excessive hyperextension and generalized ligamentous laxity, BPTB autografts seem to function better in restoring anterior and rotational stability (14). Finally, an alternative graft source may be considered in patients with a history of chronic hamstring muscle strains.

PREOPERATIVE PLANNING

Patients undergoing ACL reconstruction should have a detailed history taken. The history should include details of the initial injury and subsequent episodes of instability and their treatment. The diagnosis of a torn ACL is confirmed clinically with the Lachman and pivot shift tests. Patients who give a history consistent with an ACL injury and on clinical examination are found to have a lower-grade Lachman, and pivot shift test may have a partial ACL tear. Similar to a patient with a complete ACL tear, symptomatic patients with a partial ACL tear should be considered for ACL reconstruction. Preoperative radiographs of the involved knee should be taken to look for associated bony injuries and joint space narrowing and to determine skeletal maturity. Recommended views include an anteroposterior (AP) radiograph of the involved knee and standing AP and posteroanterior (PA) 45 degree flexion views of both knees. A true lateral radiograph of the injured knee in maximum extension is useful for preoperative planning of the sagittal position of the ACL tibial tunnel. Merchant's views of both knees are helpful in assessing patellar alignment and tilt. A full-length standing AP, hip-to-ankle radiograph of both lower extremities is indicated in patients with joint space narrowing or malalignment of the lower extremities. Although not needed in most cases to diagnose an ACL tear, magnetic resonance imaging (MRI) is useful in assessing concomitant meniscal injuries, damage to the articular cartilage, and collateral ligament injuries. An MRI scan with images taken in the oblique sagittal and coronal planes can also be helpful for diagnosing partial ACL tears.

THE CONCEPT OF ANATOMIC ACL RECONSTRUCTION

The technique of ACL reconstruction has evolved from a transtibial surgical technique in which the objectives were "isometric" femoral tunnel placement and avoidance of intercondylar roof and PCL impingement, toward an anatomic surgical technique that attempts to reproduce the anatomy of the patient's native ACL (15–17). This change occurred because it was recognized that the technique of transtibial drilling often placed the ACL tibial tunnel in the posterior part of the native ACL tibial attachment site and the ACL femoral tunnel onto or in the roof of the intercondylar notch (18). These resulting tunnel positions often produced a nonanatomic vertical ACL graft in both the sagittal and coronal planes (18,19). Although a vertical ACL graft is potentially able to resist anterior tibial translation, it is poorly aligned to resist the coupled motions of anterior tibial translation and internal tibial rotation that occur during the pivot shift phenomena. As a result, a patient with a vertical ACL graft would often have a negative Lachman test, with a firm endpoint, but a positive pivot shift test and continued complaints of instability (19). Recognition of the limitations of transtibial drilling has led to a reevaluation of ACL surgical technique and ACL tunnel placement (15–17).

The concept of anatomic ACL reconstruction was developed to improve postoperative rotational stability and knee kinematics (15–17). An anatomic ACL reconstruction refers to an ACL reconstruction in which the ACL femoral and tibial bone tunnels are positioned within the native ACL femoral and tibial attachment sites. It has been proven biomechanically and clinically that placing the bone tunnels of the ACL reconstruction within the native ACL attachment sites better restores rotational stability and knee kinematics compared to a nonanatomic ACL reconstruction (20,21). The constraints of transtibial drilling, which often placed the ACL bone tunnels outside of the native ACL attachment sites, have led to a move toward independent drilling techniques, such as medial portal and outside-in drilling. Independent drilling techniques allow the surgeon to consistently place the ACL tibial and femoral ACL bone tunnels within the native ACL attachment sites (15–18).

THREE-PORTAL TECHNIQUE FOR ANATOMIC ACL RECONSTRUCTION

ACL reconstruction has traditionally been performed using 2 arthroscopic portals, the anterolateral (AL) and the anteromedial (AM) portals. In the 2-portal technique, the AL portal is used as the arthroscopic viewing portal and the ACL femoral tunnel is drilled through the AM portal. However, this approach has several limitations. First of all, the lateral wall of the intercondylar notch when viewed through the AL portal results in a tangential view of the ACL femoral attachment site. Viewing the ACL femoral attachment site tangentially can potentially compromise the surgeon's ability to accurately place the ACL femoral tunnel within the native ACL femoral attachment site. Secondly, drilling the ACL femoral tunnel through the AM portal can result in a shorter ACL femoral tunnel, limiting the length of ACL graft that can be inserted into the ACL femoral tunnel when a cortical suspensory fixation device is used for femoral fixation.

Anatomic ACL reconstruction is facilitated by using 3 arthroscopic portals (16,17,22–24). In the 3-portal technique, the AL and AM portals are used as viewing portals, and the ACL femoral tunnel is drilled through a low accessory anteromedial (AAM) portal. There are several advantages of the 3-portal technique compared to the traditional 2-portal approach. The 3-portal technique allows the surgeon to interchange the working and viewing portals according to the specific task that is being performed. In the 3-portal technique, the lateral wall of the intercondylar notch can be viewed orthogonally through the AM portal while the AAM portal is used as a working portal for instrumentation. This approach allows the surgeon to look and work in the same direction, making it easier to achieve more accurate and consistent placement of the ACL femoral tunnel within the native ACL femoral attachment site (Fig. 15-1). Viewing the lateral wall of the intercondylar notch through the AM portal also eliminates the need to perform a notchplasty for visualization purposes. Drilling the ACL femoral tunnel through the AAM portal increases the obliquity of the ACL femoral tunnel relative to the lateral wall of the intercondylar notch, resulting in a longer ACL femoral tunnel and a more elliptical

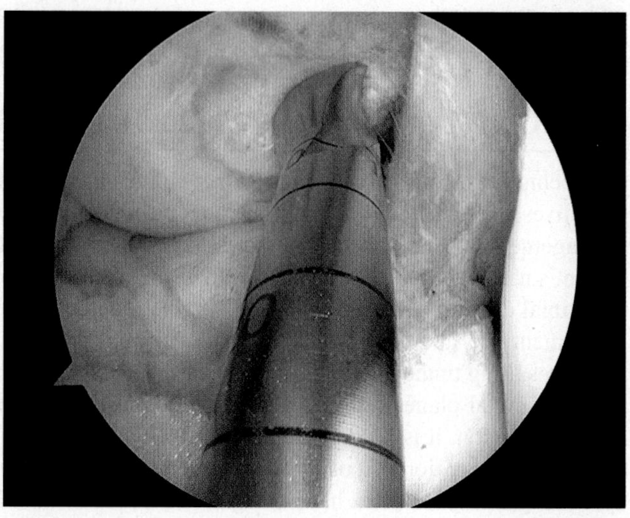

FIGURE 15-1

Anteromedial portal view of the ACL femoral attachment site in hyperflexion. Viewing the lateral wall of the intercondylar notch with the arthroscope in the anteromedial portal affords a more orthrogonal view of the ACL femoral attachment. This approach allows the surgeon to look and work in the same direction, making it possible to see if the drill bit will safely pass the medial femoral condyle and see exactly where in the ACL femoral attachment site the ACL femoral tunnel will be created.

shape to the ACL femoral tunnel aperture (25,26). An elliptically shaped ACL femoral tunnel aperture has the advantage of covering more of the native ACL femoral attachment site compared to a circular femoral tunnel (26). Another advantage of the 3-portal technique is that the lateral wall of the intercondylar notch can be viewed through the AM portal and an ACL ruler (Smith & Nephew Advanced Surgical Devices, Andover, MA) can be inserted through the AL portal and positioned along the lateral wall of the intercondylar notch. An angled microfracture awl can then be inserted into the notch through the AAM portal, and positions along the lateral wall of intercondylar notch can be accurately measured and marked (24,27). Finally, when drilling the ACL femoral tunnel with the knee in hyperflexion, a motorized shaver blade can be inserted into the intercondylar notch through the AL portal and areas of the fat pad restricting visualization can be resected and bony debris created during drilling of the ACL femoral tunnel can be suctioned out of the knee joint. These steps help improve visualization in the intercondylar notch while drilling the ACL femoral tunnel.

Surgeons making the transition from transtibial to medial portal drilling may experience some unique issues and challenges not normally encountered with transtibial drilling. The medial portal technique requires that the knee be flexed to 120 degrees or greater when a rigid guide pin and drill bit are used to drill the ACL femoral tunnel. Hyperflexion of the knee is necessary for the following reasons: to avoid the femoral guide pin exiting the lateral soft tissue of the thigh too posteriorly, placing the peroneal nerve at risk, to avoid a "blow-out" of the posterior femoral cortex, and to insure adequate length of the ACL femoral tunnel. Compared to working at the more familiar 90 degrees of flexion, working with the knee in hyperflexion can potentially compromise joint distention and arthroscopic visualization, and the unfamiliar orientation of the lateral wall of the notch can result in spatial disorientation. Other challenges that the surgeon may encounter while drilling the ACL femoral tunnel through a medial portal in hyperflexion include difficulty passing the cannulated endoscopic drill bit over the guide pin into the knee joint as a result of the medial portal tightening with hyperflexion; the drill bit may drag the fat pad into the notch, further limiting visualization; and difficulty advancing the endoscopic drill bit over the guide pin into the knee joint due to a bend or kink in the guide pin. However, with attention to details, all of these potential issues and challenges can be overcome. Drilling the ACL femoral tunnel through a medial portal is the most frequently used surgical technique by surgeons around the world. In a survey of international knee surgeons, 68% of the respondents drilled their ACL femoral tunnel using a medial portal (11). Medial portal drilling of the ACL femoral tunnel was used by 64% of the members of the Magellan Society (12). In a 2016 survey of members of the ACL Study Group, 66% of the respondents reported that they drilled the ACL femoral tunnel through the medial portal.

Three-Portal Technique: Indications and Contraindications

The 3-portal technique as described in this chapter is versatile and can be used when performing an ACL reconstruction with any graft type and most ACL femoral fixation devices. The 3-portal technique may be used for any primary, revision, single- or double-bundle ACL reconstruction. The technique is particularly useful in cases where only one of the two ACL bundles is torn or where there is a large remnant of the native ACL present. In these situations, an augmentation or tissue-preserving procedure may be performed. Augmentation and tissue-preserving procedures cannot be performed using a transtibial or an all-inside technique. When used in revision ACL surgery, the 3-portal technique usually allows a new anatomic ACL femoral tunnel to be drilled away from a previous nonanatomic transtibial femoral tunnel. This may eliminate the need to remove the original ACL femoral fixation hardware and can bypass a malpositioned or enlarged ACL femoral tunnel, thereby avoiding the need for a two-stage revision and bone grafting of the original femoral tunnel. The only contraindication to drilling the ACL femoral tunnel through an AM or AAM portal using a rigid guide pin and drill bit is the inability to flex the knee to at least 120 degrees. This limitation may be encountered in some obese patients, in which case consideration should be given to drilling the ACL femoral tunnel using an outside-in technique or using a flexible guide pin and flexible reamers.

SURGICAL TECHNIQUE

Examination under Anesthesia

The patient is positioned supine on the operating room table, time out is called, and the patient's identity, operative site, and planned surgical procedure are confirmed. The patient is given 1 g of a first-generation cephalosporin intravenously at least 30 minutes prior to the skin incision being made. The operation can be performed under general or regional anesthesia or a peripheral nerve block. An adductor canal nerve block minimizes quadriceps muscle weakness and reduces the risks of falls in the postoperative period and is preferred over a femoral nerve block. A comprehensive ligament examination of both knees is performed under anesthesia. In the situation of a ++ or +++ Lachman test and a Grade II or III pivot shift test and/or an MRI demonstrating a complete tear of both bundles of the ACL, the hamstring tendons are harvested before performing a diagnostic arthroscopy. However, when examination reveals a lower-grade Lachman and pivot shift test, the nature of the ACL tear is confirmed by performing a diagnostic arthroscopy prior to harvesting the hamstring tendons. In the situation of a one-bundle ACL tear, the surgeon may elect to perform an augmentation technique rather than completely resecting the torn ACL and performing a traditional single-bundle ACL reconstruction.

Surgical Preparation and Patient Positioning

A padded pneumatic tourniquet is placed high on the thigh of the operative leg. The tourniquet is rarely inflated during the procedure as adequate joint distention, and visualization can usually be achieved using an infusion pump. If intraoperative fluoroscopy is planned during the procedure, a lead gonad shield is placed over the pelvis or scrotum to protect the patient from radiation exposure. When drilling the ACL femoral tunnel through the AAM portal, it is important to have the ability to achieve full, unrestricted knee flexion during the procedure. The requirement that the knee be flexed to greater than 120 degrees when drilling the ACL femoral tunnel may be difficult to achieve when using a circumferential leg holder and the foot of the operating room table is flexed down. Keeping the operating room table flat and using a padded thigh post and two padded L-shaped foot supports to stabilize the lower extremity allow full unrestricted flexion of the knee during the procedure (24). Using two foot supports allows the knee to be maintained at the two most commonly needed flexion angles during the procedure, 70 to 90 degrees and greater than 120 degrees, eliminating the need for an assistant to hold the leg. Although it is possible to tape sandbags or rolled blankets to the operating table to maintain the knee at these flexion angles, using L-shaped foot supports that can be moved along the side rail of the operating room table allows the surgeon to adjust the knee flexion angle during the procedure.

The first padded L-shaped foot support is placed and attached to the side rail near the end of the operating table. The patient's foot is placed on this support and the patient's torso moved down the operating room table until the knee is flexed to 90 degrees. The patient's foot is placed on this support during harvest of the ACL graft and preparation of the intercondylar notch and while drilling the ACL tibial tunnel. Next, a padded thigh post and a padded hip positioner are fixed to the side rail of the operating room table at the level of the tourniquet. The padded hip positioner stabilizes the patient's pelvis on the operating table and prevents the pelvis from sliding on the operating table when valgus stress is applied to the knee to open the medial compartment. The padded thigh post prevents the hip from abducting and the leg from externally rotating during the procedure. This post also acts as a fulcrum and allows valgus stress to be applied to the knee to distract and open up the medial compartment when performing surgery on the medial meniscus. The knee is placed into extension, and a second padded L-shaped support is placed just proximal to the popliteal fossa. It is important to avoid placing this support under the popliteal fossa as this may result in compression of the popliteal vessels. The proximal support should also not be placed under the proximal tibia as this will apply an anterior force to the tibia and sublux the tibia anteriorly during tensioning and final fixation of the ACL graft. The knee is hyperflexed and the height of the proximal L-shaped foot support adjusted so that the patient's foot can be placed under the horizontal limb of the support, resulting in the knee being maintained in hyperflexion. The knee is placed back into extension and positioned on the two L-shaped supports. The relative height of the two L-shaped supports can be adjusted such that the knee can be maintained at a known flexion angle during tensioning and fixation of the ACL graft (Fig. 15-2). The skin is prepared with a chlorhexidine or iodine soap solution, followed by an alcohol-based skin prep solution. Sterile draping of the operative extremity is performed using impervious arthroscopic drapes. Standard arthroscopic equipment is required: a 30-degree arthroscope, an HD digital video camera, a high-resolution video monitor, an image capture unit, a high-intensity arthroscopic light source, a motorized shaver, a radiofrequency (RF) wand, and an infusion pump.

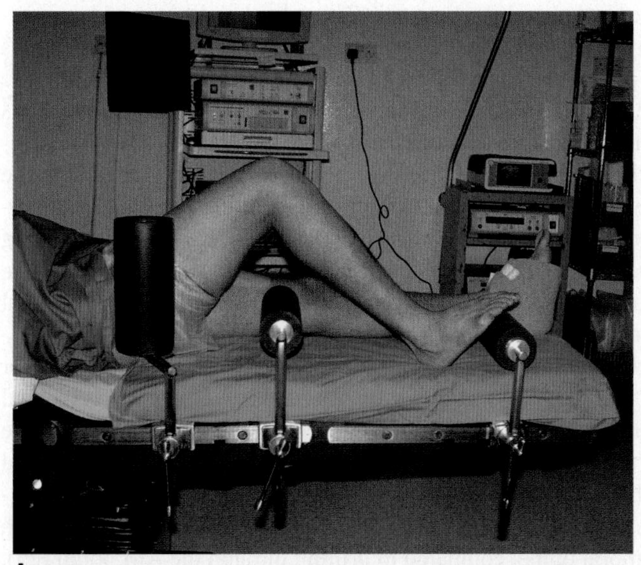
A

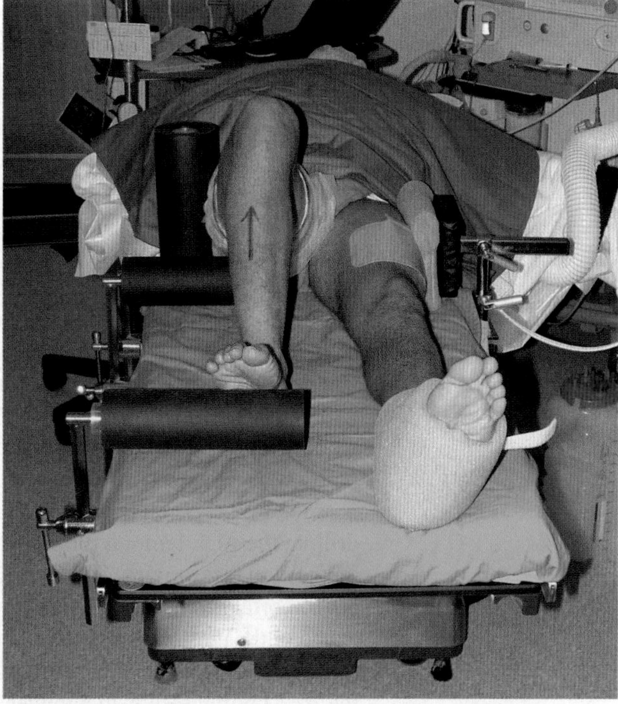
B

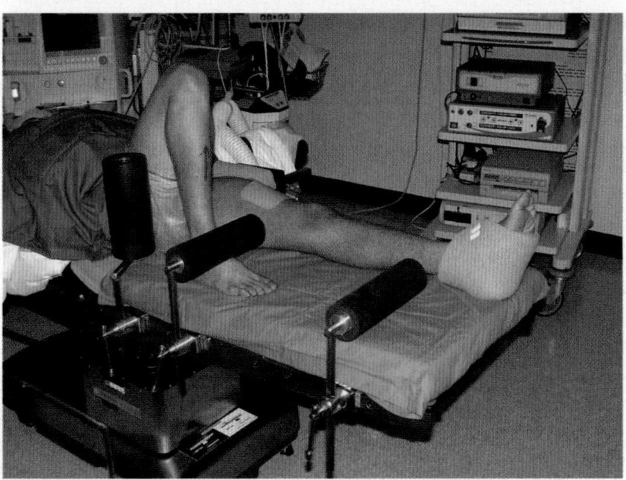
C

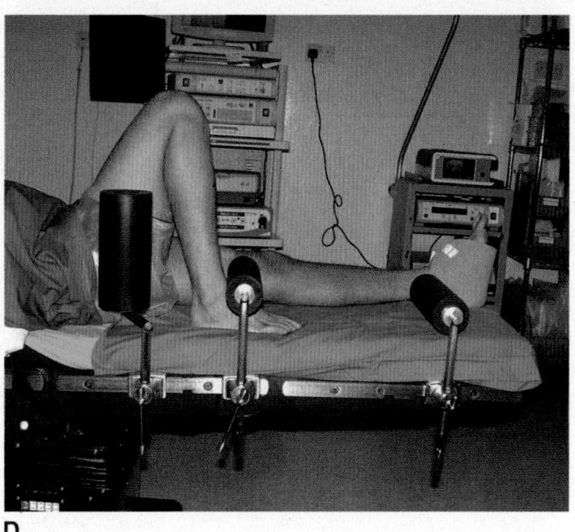
D

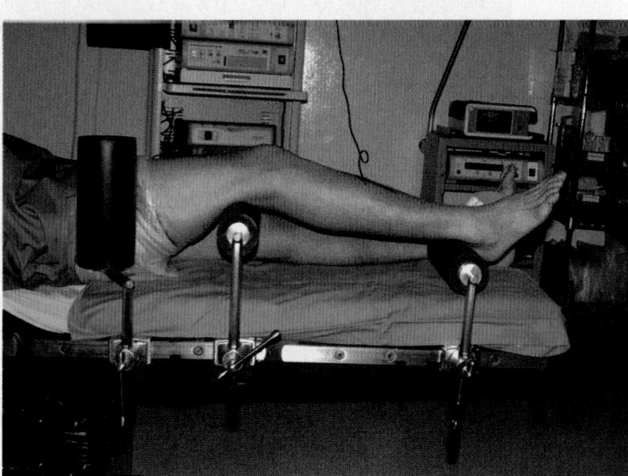
E

FIGURE 15-2

Patient positioning. **A, B:** Patient's pelvis and torso are stabilized on the operating room table by a padded lateral hip positioner and padded thigh post. The L-shaped foot support is secured to the side rail of the operating room table near the end of the table.The patient's foot is placed on this support, maintaining the knee at 70 to 90 degrees of flexion. **C, D:** A second L-shaped foot support is used to maintain the knee in hyperflexion during drilling of the ACL femoral tunnel. **E:** The height of the proximal and distal foot supports can be adjusted such that the knee can be maintained at a known flexion angle (usually 20 degrees) during tensioning and fixation of the ACL graft.

Arthroscopic Portals

Proper placement of the arthroscopic portals is critical to the success of the procedure. With the knee at 90 degrees of flexion, the medial, lateral, superior, and inferior borders of the patella, the medial and lateral borders of the patellar tendon, the tibial tubercle, and the medial and lateral joint lines are marked on the skin with a sterile surgical marking pen. These landmarks are used as references for placing the arthroscopic portals and the skin incision for harvest of the hamstring tendons (Fig. 15-3). The vertical AL portal is placed at the height of the inferior pole of the patella, as close as possible to the lateral border of the patellar tendon. Placing the AL portal at this height positions the arthroscope above the fat pad, minimizing the amount of fat pad resection required for visualization when working in the intercondylar notch. The vertical AM portal is positioned medial to the medial border of the patellar tendon, slightly higher than the inferior pole of the patella. It is important that the AM portal be placed high above the medial joint line; otherwise, instrument crowding will occur when the AM portal is used as the viewing portal and the low AAM portal is used as the working portal. The preliminary location for the AM portal is marked on the skin. However, the final position of the AM portal is made under direct arthroscopic visualization.

A low AAM portal is used as a working portal to insert instrumentation into the knee joint and for drilling the ACL femoral tunnel. The preliminary location for the transverse AAM portal is marked on the skin just proximal to the medial joint line. Similar to the AM portal, the final position for the AAM portal is created under direct arthroscopic visualization. Proper placement of the AAM portal is one of the most critical aspects of the technique. The location of the AAM portal is the major factor determining the length of the ACL femoral tunnel (25). Drilling the ACL femoral tunnel through the AAM portal results in a longer femoral tunnel compared to drilling through the AM portal (25). Using an AAM portal also allows the surgeon to view the lateral wall of the intercondylar notch through the AM portal while drilling the ACL femoral tunnel through the AAM. Thus, the surgeon can look and work in the same direction (see Fig. 15-1). The AAM portal is created under direct vision as low as possible, just above the anterior horn of the medial meniscus. A transverse incision is used for the AAM portal as this allows for adjustments of the femoral guide pin in the medial-lateral direction. The arthroscopic portal sites are infiltrated with a local anesthetic with epinephrine using a 25-gauge needle.

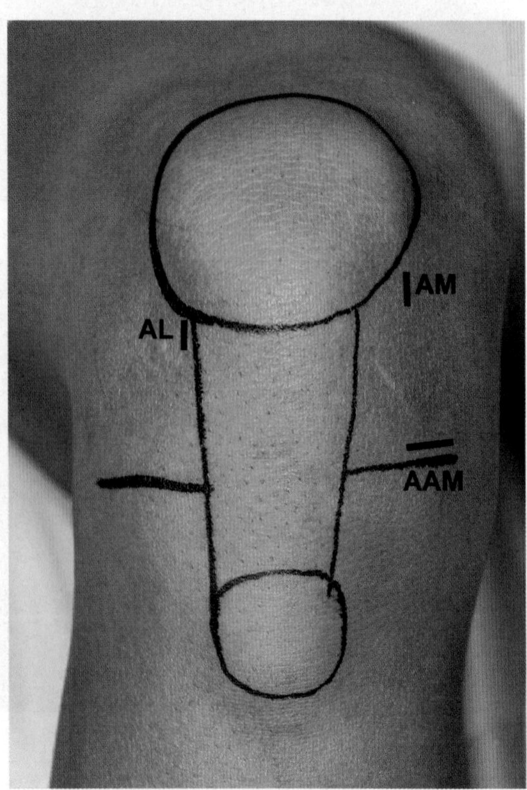

FIGURE 15-3

Surface landmarks and arthroscopic portals. Anterolateral (AL) portal, high anteromedial (AM) portal, low accessory anteromedial (AAM) portal.

Hamstring Tendon Graft Harvest

Unlike the harvest of a BPTB or quadriceps tendon autograft, harvesting the hamstring tendons is essentially a closed, blind procedure that involves introducing a tendon stripper through a small distal skin incision. For many surgeons, harvesting the hamstring tendon is often the most stressful part of the procedure. Although in general there is less surgical morbidity when harvesting hamstring tendon grafts compared to the harvest of a BPTB autograft, complications can occur (28). Surgeons unfamiliar with harvesting hamstring tendons are encouraged to review articles describing the anatomy of the pes anserinus (29–32). Hamstring tendon grafts can be harvested using a vertical, horizontal, or oblique skin incision (Fig. 15-4). Advantages of the horizontal or oblique skin incision are they allow better proximal exposure of the hamstring tendons and run parallel to Langer's lines, resulting in a more cosmetic scar. Additionally, harvesting the hamstring tendons using a horizontal or oblique skin incision has been shown to result in a lower incidence of injury to the infrapatellar branch of the saphenous nerve and a smaller area and lower incidence of sensory disturbance compared to a vertical incision. The major disadvantage of the horizontal or oblique incision is that these incisions are not extensile and if premature amputation of a tendon should occur, an additional skin incision is required to harvest a BPTB autograft. A vertical incision has the advantages of providing good exposure of the tibial attachment of the two tendons and it is extensile allowing harvest of a BPTB autograft using the same incision should it become necessary.

In the average-size patient, the superior border of the pes anserinus is located approximately 1 fingerbreadth below the tibial tubercle or 3 fingerbreadths below the medial joint line. The proximal edge of the vertical skin incision is placed at the level of the gracilis tendon and approximately 2 cm medial to the crest of the tibia. The skin incision is typically 2.5 to 3 cm long. The hamstring tendons

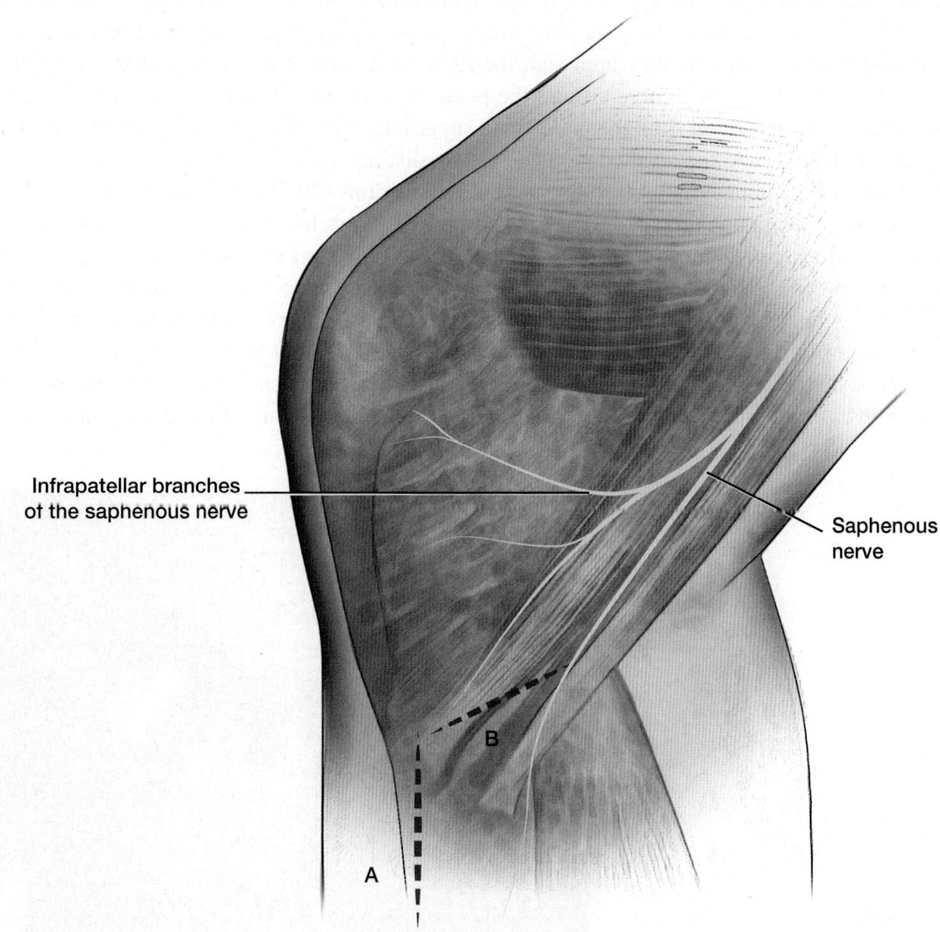

FIGURE 15-4
A vertical (*A*) or oblique/horizontal (*B*) skin incision may be used to harvest the hamstring tendons.

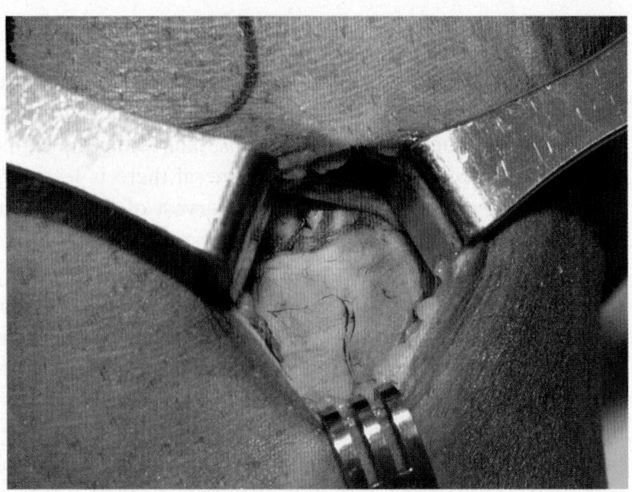

FIGURE 15-5

The sartorius fascia overlying the pes anserinus is exposed by blunt dissection.

are routinely harvested without inflating the tourniquet. Using a 25-gauge needle, the skin incision is infiltrated with a local anesthetic with epinephrine. The skin is incised with a #15 knife blade and two sharp Senn retractors are used to lift the skin and subcutaneous fat away from the sartorius fascia (layer 1). The sartorius fascia (layer 1) is exposed by bluntly dissecting the subcutaneous fat off the fascia with a small sponge (Fig. 15-5). This step minimizes bleeding and injury to branches of the infrapatellar nerve. The upper border of the pes anserinus is usually marked by a small leash of vessels that run on the sartorius fascia. These vessels should be coagulated to prevent bleeding when the fascia is divided. The gracilis and semitendinosus tendons lie deep to the sartorius fascia and can be rolled against the underlying tibia with a curved clamp (Fig. 15-6). The two tendons join together and become flatter as they approach the tibia, so it is often easier to identify and palpate them more posteriorly as they curve around the posteromedial corner of the tibia. In this location, the two tendons are separated from the underlying superficial medial collateral ligament (sMCL) by the pes anserine bursa and they can be palpated as two distinct, round structures.

An "inside-out" technique is used to harvest the two tendons (29,31). This approach provides an excellent view of the internal aspect of the two tendons and allows for identification of any associated anatomic variations, anomalous tendon attachments to the tibia, and accessory bands (31). The two tendons lie between the sartorius fascia (layer 1) and the sMCL (layer 2) so the sartorius fascia must be divided to gain access to them. The sartorius fascia is incised a few millimeters proximal to the superior border of the gracilis tendon. This incision can be made either bluntly using a curved clamp (Fig. 15-7) or sharply using a #15 knife blade. Care must be taken when dividing the sartorius fascia using a knife to avoid injury to the underlying sMCL. Blunt entry through the sartorius fascia is less

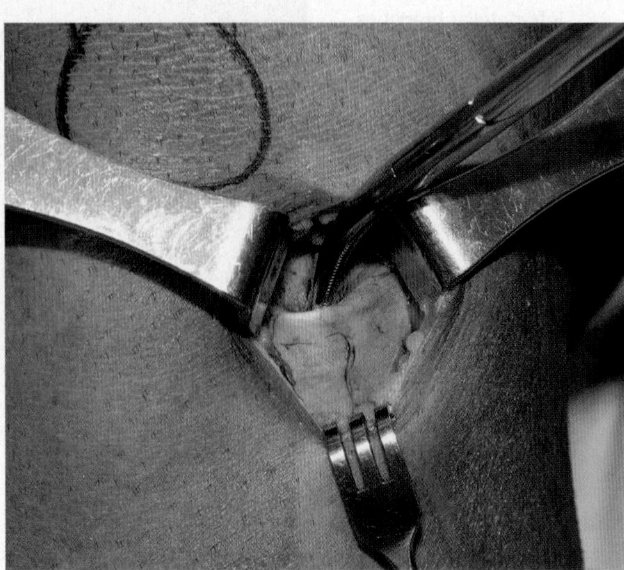

FIGURE 15-6

A curved clamp is used to identify the upper border of the gracilis tendon, which lies deep to the sartorius fascia.

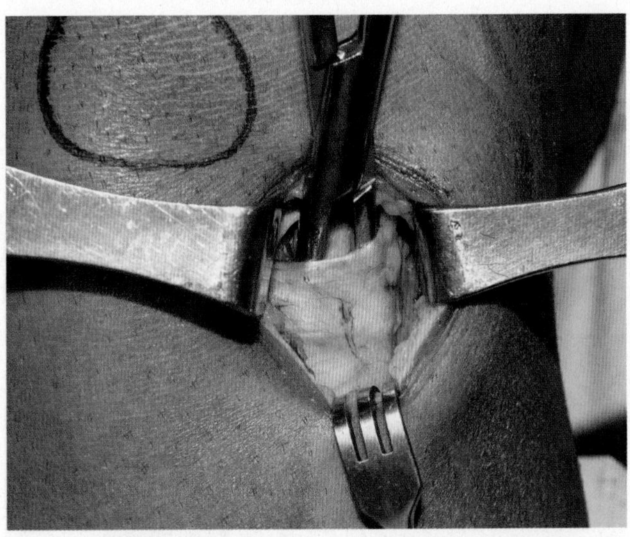

FIGURE 15-7

The sartorius fascia is opened just proximal to the superior border of the gracilis tendon using a curved clamp.

likely to injure the underlying sMCL. After dividing the sartorius fascia, the shiny parallel fibers of the underlying sMCL can be seen and identified. The sMCL is further protected from injury by grasping the divided sartorius fascia with an Allis clamp and lifting the sartorius fascia away from the underlying sMCL and tibia. The incision through the sartorius fascia is extended back to the posteromedial border of the tibia using Metzenbaum scissors. To prevent injury to the saphenous nerve, it is important to avoid extending the incision and dissecting posterior to the posteromedial corner of the tibia.

The vertical limb of an L-shaped incision is made, 1 cm medial to the crest of the tibia with a #15 knife blade. This incision cuts across the conjoined insertion of the gracilis and semitendinosus tendons, detaching them from the tibia. The superior corner of the sartorius fascia flap is grasped with an Allis clamp and the insertion of the two tendons sharply dissected off the medial surface of the tibia. During this step, it is possible for the sMCL to be erroneously dissected off the tibia if the two tendons are not clearly identified and separated from the underlying sMCL. Blunt dissection with the index finger is used to free the "web-like" fascial bands that run from the undersurface of the two tendons to the sMCL and tibia. Release of these bands allows the sartorius fascial flap containing the two tendons to be retracted further away from the underlying sMCL and tibia, improving the proximal exposure of the two tendons.

Soft tissue on the internal surface of the two tendons is removed using blunt dissection with a small sponge and Metzenbaum scissors. It is important to identify a clear distinction between the gracilis and semitendinosus tendons prior to harvesting the tendons (Fig. 15-8). The tip of a right-angle–type clamp is used to individually separate the two tendons from the undersurface of

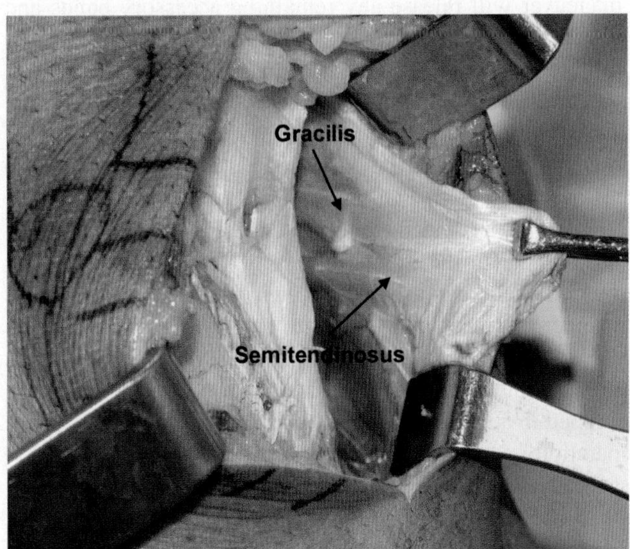

FIGURE 15-8

The sartorius fascia is retracted medially. This step exposes the under surface of the sartorius fascia, providing a clear view of the gracilis and semitendinosus tendons.

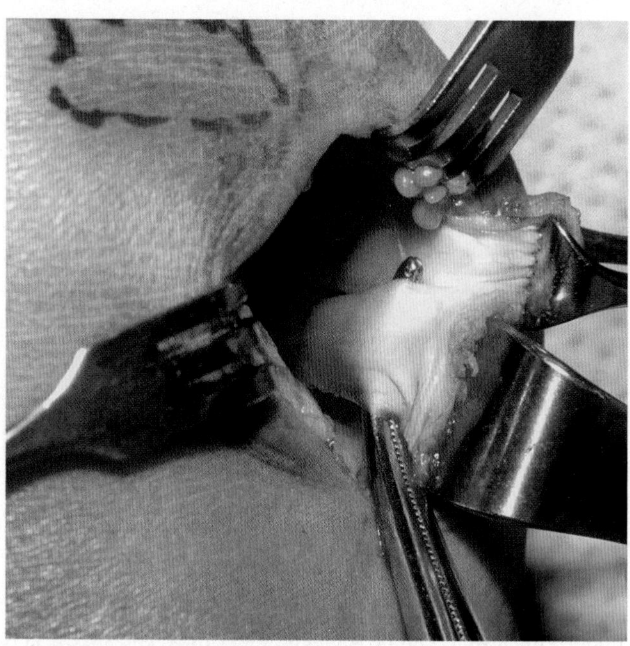

FIGURE 15-9

A right-angle clamp is used to separate the tendons from the undersurface of the sartorius fascia.

the sartorius fascia (Fig. 15-9). The gracilis tendon is then hooked with the right-angle clamp, and using firm traction, the tendon is bluntly peeled off the sartorius fascia. This technique leaves the sartorius fascial flap intact for later closure. The distal end of the gracilis tendon is grasped with a wide Allis-Adair forceps (Symmetry Surgical, Antioch, TN). The sartorius fascia is retracted medially with an Army-Navy–type retractor and the gracilis tendon is dissected off the undersurface of the sartorius fascia using Metzenbaum scissors. The accessory bands running from the gracilis to the semitendinosus tendon are released with Metzenbaum scissors and blunt finger dissection along the inferior border of the gracilis tendon. The saphenous nerve exits the adductor canal and crosses over the superior border of the gracilis at the posteromedial border of the knee as it travels to become subcutaneous (28,29,32) (Fig. 15-10). Scissor dissection along the superior border of the gracilis tendon should be avoided as this can injure the saphenous nerve. The distal end of the gracilis tendon is whipstitched with five to seven throws of a running baseball-style suture using a #2 FiberWire suture (Arthrex, Naples, FL). It is important to use a high-strength suture material such as FiberWire as this allows the connecting knots used in tripling the tendons to be tied with maximum tension. Polyester suture material may break during the process of tripling the tendons. The tendons are harvested by placing the knee at 90 degrees. Pagnani et al. (32) suggest placing the knee in the figure-four position to decrease risk of injury to the saphenous nerve. The sartorius fascia is retracted medially with an Army-Navy– or Langenbeck-type retractor and firm traction applied to the gracilis tendon using the whipstitch. In most instances this maneuver will release any remaining accessory bands and allow additional distal excursion of the tendon. Any remaining proximal accessory bands should be released using blunt finger dissection until the muscle belly of the gracilis tendon can be palpated. Complete release of the accessory bands can be verified by the absence of skin dimpling on the posterior aspect of the thigh when traction is applied to the gracilis tendon.

Depending on the surgeon's preference, the tendons can be harvested with a closed or slotted tendon stripper or a Tendon Harvester (Linvatec, Largo, FL). Traction is applied to the gracilis tendon using the whipstitch and the tendon stripper advanced along the tendon using a slow, steady, push-pull sliding motion up into the thigh aiming for the ischial tuberosity. If the tendon stripper fails to advance smoothly, it is best to stop, remove it, and use further blunt finger dissection to free the area of obstruction. As the tendon stripper advances into the thigh, contraction of the gracilis muscle confirms that the musculotendinous junction has been reached. The tendon is released from its muscle belly by slowing pulling the tendon out of the incision keeping the tendon stripper in place. The gracilis tendon is carefully wrapped in a moist laparotomy pad, placed in a marked graft pan and passed to the back table for preparation.

A similar technique is used to harvest the semitendinosus tendon. When harvesting the semitendinosus tendon, it may be advantageous to use a larger 7.4-mm diameter closed tendon stripper (Smith & Nephew Advanced Surgical Devices, Andover, MA). There are more extensive and thicker

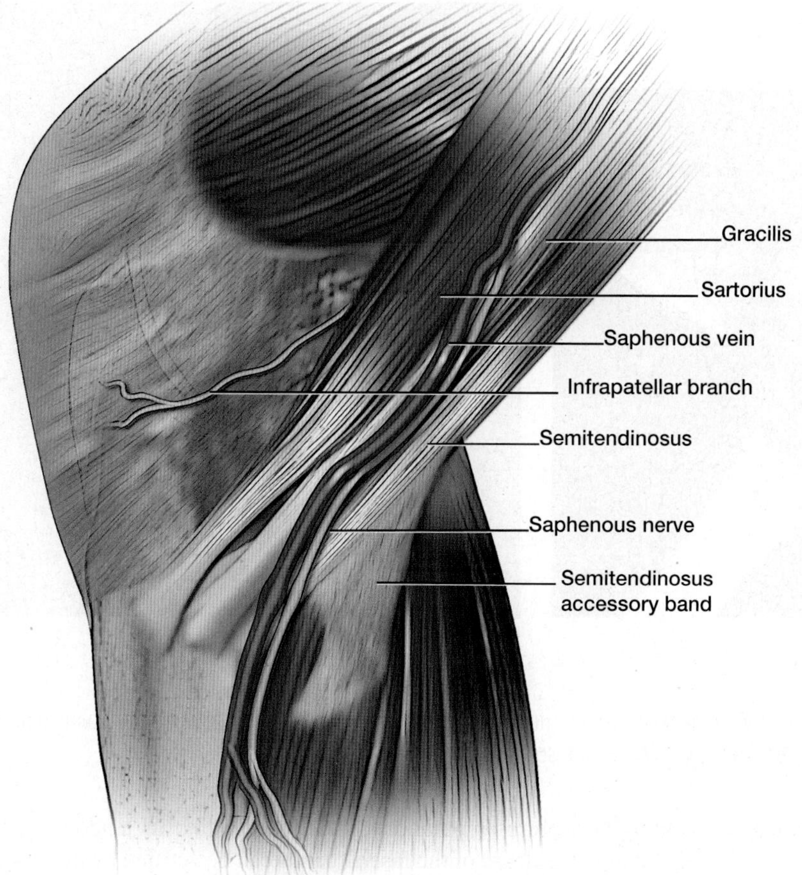

FIGURE 15-10

Drawing illustrating the anatomic relationships on the medial side of the knee. Note the relationship of the saphenous nerve to the superior border of the gracilis tendon and the fascial connection from the inferior border of the semitendinosus tendon to the medial head of the gastrocnemius muscle.

accessory tendon insertions and fascial bands that course from the inferior border of the semitendinosus to the tibia and the medial head of the gastrocnemius (28–30,33–35). The most consistent fascial band lies approximately 5 to 9 cm from the tibial insertion of the semitendinosus tendon and runs between the inferior border of the semitendinosus tendon and the medial head of the gastrocnemius muscle (Fig. 15-11). Recognizing these accessory insertions and fascial bands and releasing

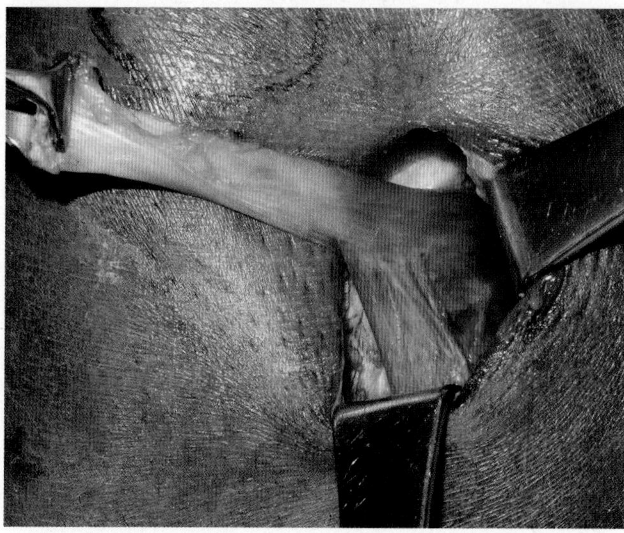

FIGURE 15-11

Retraction of the semitendinosus tendon demonstrating the fascial band running between inferior border of the semitendinosus and the medial head of the gastrocnemius muscle.

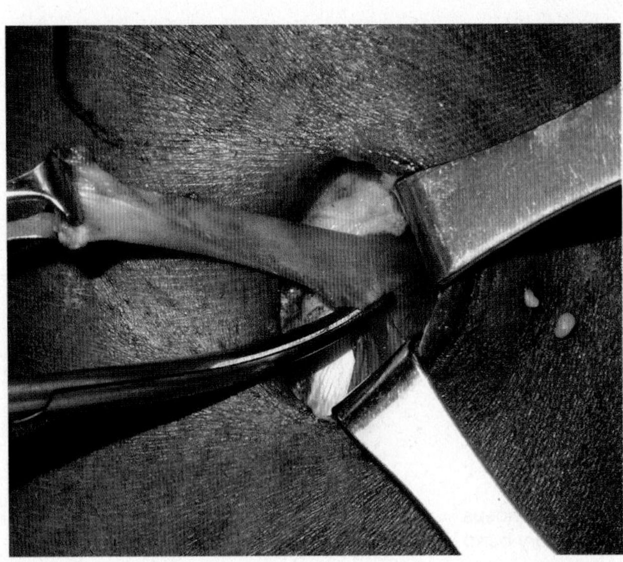
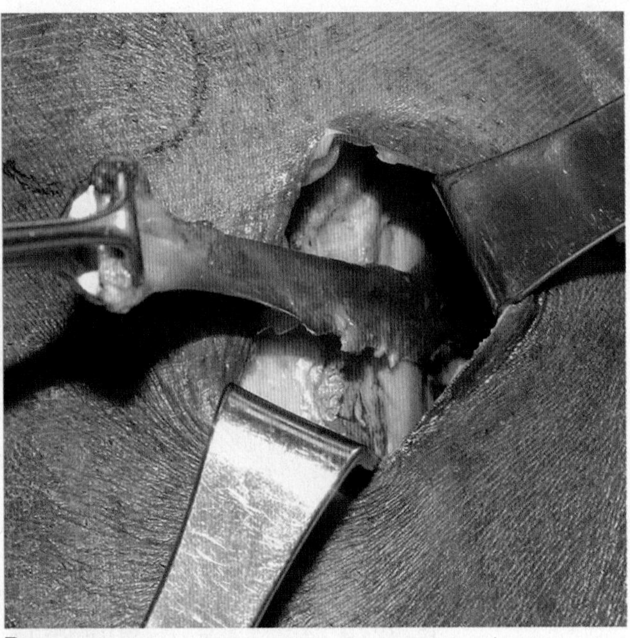

A B

FIGURE 15-12

A: Curved Metzenbaum scissors are used to divide the fascial band running from the inferior border of the semitendinosus tendon to the medial head of the gastrocnemius muscle. **B:** This step releases the semitendinosus tendon.

them is critical to avoiding premature amputation of the semitendinosus tendon and harvest of a short graft (Fig. 15-12). Complete release of the fascial bands can be verified by the absence of bowing of the tendon and puckering of the medial head of the gastrocnemius when traction is applied to the semitendinosus tendon. Proximally in the thigh, approximately 12 to 15 cm proximal to the tibial insertion of the semitendinosus tendon, the semitendinosus tendon is suspended from the inferior surface of the semimembranosus tendon by a fascial sling or thickening (29,32). Premature amputation of the semitendinosus tendon can occur if the tendon stripper takes an aberrant path outside the fascial sling (Fig. 15-13). If excessive resistance is encountered while attempting to advance the tendon stripper up into the thigh, it is tempting to pull harder on the semitendinosus tendon and apply more force to the tendon stripper to get it to advance. However, this may tighten the fascial sling, making passage of the tendon stripper even more difficult. Decreasing tension on the semitendinosus tendon and gently "navigating" the stripper so that it passes inside the fascial sling will often result in the stripper advancing. If the tendon stripper does not pass easily beyond the 12 to 15 cm mark, it should be removed and blunt finger dissection performed to release the area of resistance. A successful graft harvest typically results in graft lengths of 22 to 28 cm for the gracilis and 24 to 32 cm for the semitendinosus tendon. The harvested semitendinosus tendon is wrapped in a separate moist laparotomy pad and placed in the marked graft pan.

Hamstring Tendon Graft Preparation

Single-bundle hamstring anterior cruciate ligament (ACL) reconstruction is most commonly performed using a doubled gracilis and doubled semitendinosus, 4-strand hamstring tendon autograft. The initial tensile strength of a 4-strand hamstring tendon graft increases linearly with the cross-sectional area of the graft. Since the diameter of the gracilis and semitendinosus tendons is variable from patient-to-patient, there is concern amongst knee surgeons that hamstring ACL reconstructions performed using smaller diameter hamstring tendon grafts may have inadequate initial tensile strength. A systematic review demonstrated a 6.8 times greater relative risk for failure of hamstring ACL reconstructions performed with hamstring tendon graft diameters less than 8 mm (36). Thus, it is important to achieve a minimum hamstring tendon ACL graft diameter of 8 mm. This goal may be achieved using a conventional doubled gracilis and semitendinosus 4-strand graft in some patients, but in others, this objective may require adding additional hamstring tendon graft stands. There is significant variation in the diameter and length of hamstring tendons from patient to patient and among different nationalities. In the local population of the Gulf States, the average diameter of a 4-strand hamstring

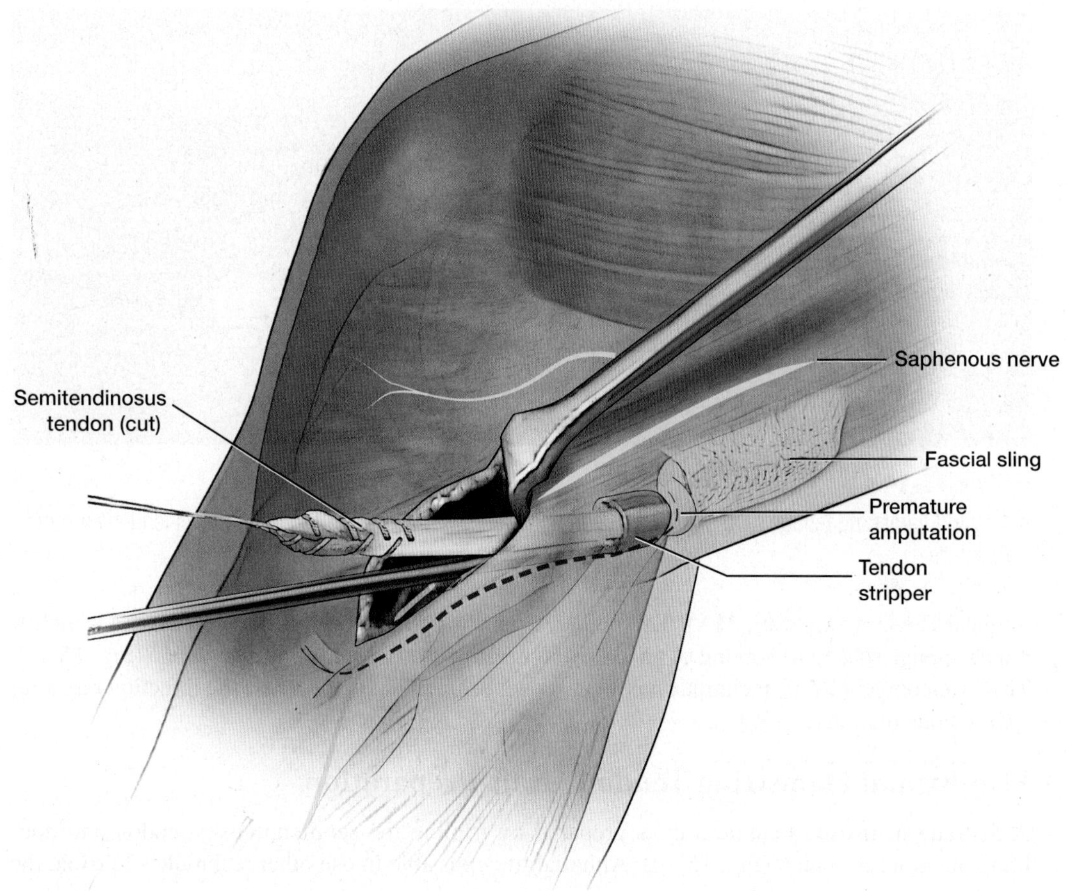

FIGURE 15-13

Passage of the tendon stripper outside of the fascial sling beneath the semimembranous muscle may result in premature amputation of the semitendinosus tendon graft.

tendon graft is 7 to 7.5 mm, so in most situations preparation of a 5- or 6-strand hamstring tendon graft is required to achieve a graft with a minimum 8 mm diameter. Preparation of the hamstring tendons is facilitated by use of a graft preparation board (Graftmaster III, Smith & Nephew Advanced Surgical Devices, Andover, MA). Residual muscle fiber on the proximal end of both tendons is removed using blunt dissection with a metal ruler, a large curette or a Cushing-type periosteal elevator.

Four-Strand Hamstring Tendon Graft Preparation

The semitendinosus and gracilis tendons are looped around a #2 or #5 polyester suture and the resulting 4-stranded graft sized using sizing block or sizing tubes. If the diameter of the 4-stranded graft is greater than or equal to 8 mm, then a 4-strand graft can be used. The two tendons are cut to equal length and the proximal end of each tendon is tubularized with a running, baseball-style whipstitch using a #2 FiberWire suture. The FiberWire sutures on each end of the tendons are pretensioned with a "cinching" motion to remove slack from the whipstitches. The two tendon grafts are looped around a #5 polyester suture creating a 4-stranded graft (Fig. 15-14). The diameter of the 4-stranded graft is measured to the nearest 0.5 mm using a sizing block or sizing tubes. The 4-strand graft is looped around an ENDOBUTTON Tensioning Post (Smith & Nephew Advanced Surgical Devices, MA), and the whipstitches from the gracilis and semitendinosus tendon on each side of the 4-stranded graft are tied together at a distance of 12 to 15 cm from the end of the two tendons. This step creates a suture loop on each side of the graft. The two suture loops are attached to opposite ends of a graft tensioning device (Smith & Nephew Advanced Surgical Devices, MA) during final tensioning and fixation of the graft. It is important to not suture the 4-graft strands together, as this will prevent the 4 strands from sliding and being equally tensioned at the time of graft fixation. The 4-strand hamstring tendon graft is pretensioned to 10 pounds for the remainder of the procedure on the graft preparation board using a suture vise with tensiometer (Smith & Nephew Advanced

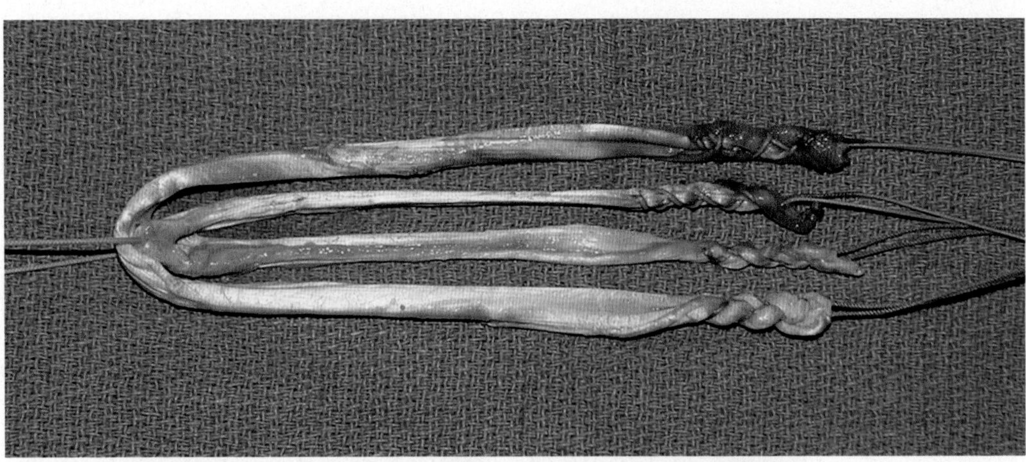

FIGURE 15-14

A 4-strand hamstring tendon ACL graft is created by looping the gracilis and semitendinosus tendons around a #5 suture.

Surgical Devices, Andover, MA). The prepared hamstring tendon graft is wrapped in a 4 inch × 4 inch sponge soaked in 500 mg of vancomycin mixed with 100 mL of normal saline (Fig. 15-15). This "vancomycin wrap" technique has been shown to significantly decrease the infection rate after ACL reconstruction (37–39).

Five-Strand Hamstring Tendon Graft Preparation

A 5-strand hamstring tendon graft is prepared by tripling the semitendinosus tendon and doubling the gracilis tendon (Fig. 15-16). Although it is possible to use other techniques to triple the

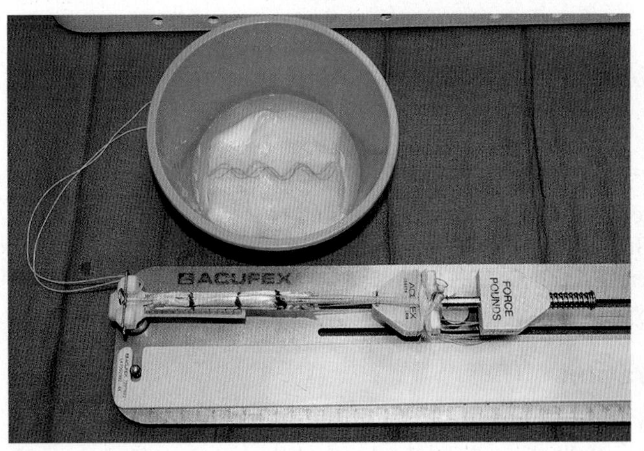

A

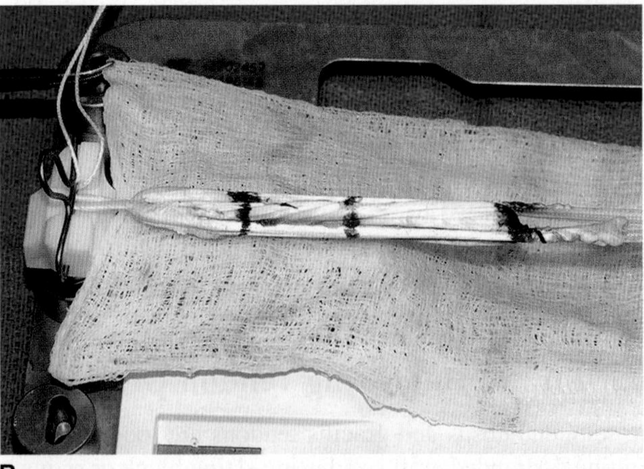

B

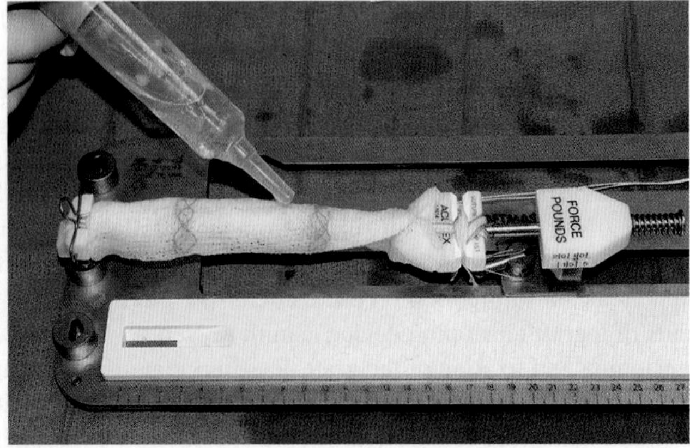

C

FIGURE 15-15

"Vancomycin wrap" technique. **A:** A 4″ × 4″ in sponge is soaked in a solution of 500 mg of vancomycin mixed with 100 mL of normal saline. **B, C:** The soaked sponge is wrapped around the prepared hamstring tendon ACL graft and the graft is kept moist with the remaining vancomycin solution.

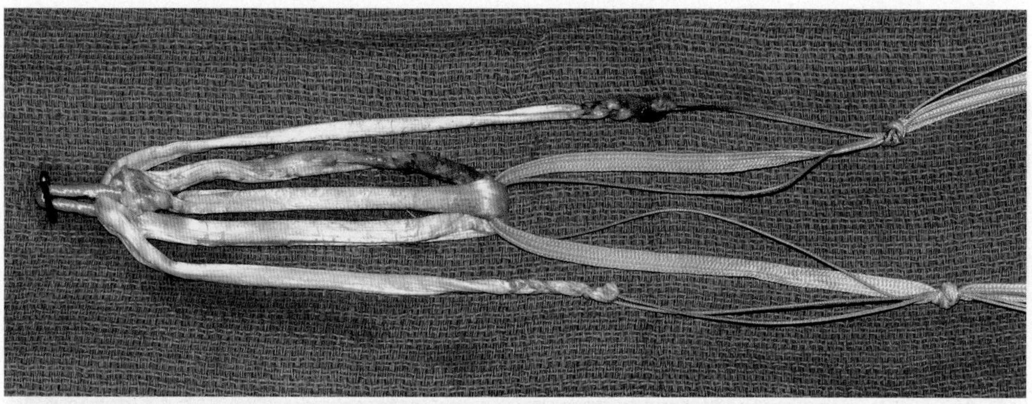

FIGURE 15-16

A 5-strand hamstring tendon ACL graft is prepared by tripling the semitendinosus tendon graft and doubling the gracilis tendon graft.

semitendinosus tendon, one of the advantages of the technique described below is that the whipstitch sutures on each end of the graft are stress shielded by the looped part of the semitendinosus graft. A minimum length of 24 to 25 cm is required to triple the semitendinosus tendon. A semitendinosus tendon in this length range will produce an 8 cm long graft after tripling. An 8 cm tripled semitendinosus graft will allow 20 to 25 mm of tendon graft to be inserted into the ACL femoral tunnel, 25 to 30 mm across the joint for the intra-articular length of the ACL, and 25 to 30 mm of tendon graft in the ACL tibial tunnel. The proximal ends of the gracilis and semitendinosus tendons are whipstitched with a #2 FiberWire suture (Arthrex, Naples, FL). It is important to use a high-strength suture as this allows the connecting knots used to tie the ends of the semitendinosus tendon to the polyester loop of the ENDOBUTTON CL ULTRA implant and the Dacron tape to be tied firmly. Polyester sutures may break during this process. A minimum of five whipstitch throws in the proximal end of each tendon is usually required to achieve adequate strength and security. Thinner tendons will require more suture throws. Slack in the whipstitches is removed ,and the ends of the hamstring tendon grafts are compressed by applying tension to the FiberWire sutures at both ends of the tendon in a direction parallel to the tendon using a back and forth "cinching" motion. This is a very important step as the ends of the two tendons will compress, shortening the total length of the tendon by approximately 5 to 10 mm. Cinching the FiberWire sutures also removes slack from the suture-tendon construct.

A 15-mm ENDOBUTTON CL ULTRA implant (Smith & Nephew Advanced Surgical Devices, Andover, MA) is most commonly used for femoral fixation of the ACL graft. Drilling the ACL femoral tunnel through the AAM portal typically results in a femoral tunnel length of 35 to 45 mm. When used in ACL femoral tunnels of this length, a 15-mm ENDOBUTTON CL ULTRA implant will allow 20 to 30 mm of tendon graft to be inserted into the ACL femoral tunnel. A 15-mm ENDOBUTTON CL ULTRA implant is inserted into the ENDOBUTTON Holder (Smith & Nephew Advanced Surgical Devices, Andover, MA) and the #2 FiberWire sutures from the proximal end of the semitendinosus tendon are tied to the polyester loop of the ENDOBUTTON implant (Fig. 15-17). The knots should be tied as tightly as possible. It is important that the proximal and not the distal end of the semitendinosus tendon be tied to the polyester loop of the ENDOBUTTON CL ULTRA implant. Tying the proximal end of semitendinosus tendon to the ENDOBUTTON CL ULTRA implant will typically produce a 5-strand graft that is 0.5 to 1 mm larger on the tibial end of the ACL graft. Since the native ACL tibial attachment site is larger than the native ACL femoral attachment site, an ACL graft with a larger diameter on the tibial end will increase the percentage of the native ACL tibial attachment site that is restored.

Using a tapered free needle, the FiberWire sutures from the distal end of the semitendinosus tendon are passed 5 mm apart through the midpoint of a 5-mm Dacron tape, creating a horizontal mattress suture (Fig. 15-18). The FiberWire sutures are tied tightly against the Dacron tape. This step connects the distal end of the semitendinosus tendon to the Dacron tape. Although it is possible to create a 5-stranded hamstring tendon graft without using Dacron tape, the Dacron tape improves the seating of the middle strand of the tripled semitendinosus graft in the axilla of the looped part of the graft, and allows all three graft strands to be equally tensioned (Fig. 15-19). This allows more uniform tension to be applied to all 3-graft strands.

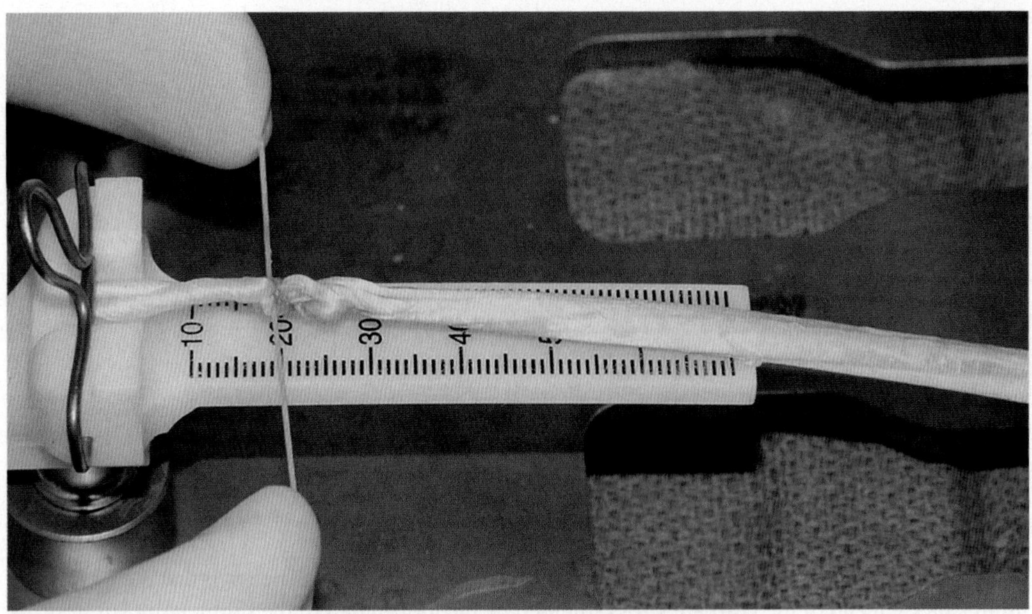

A

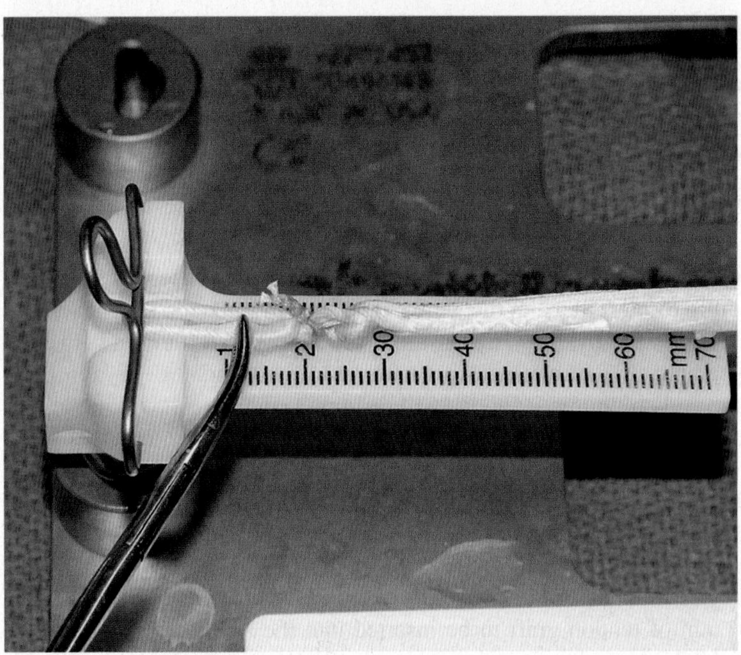

B

FIGURE 15-17

A: The FiberWire sutures used to whipstitch the proximal end of the semitendinosus tendon are tied to the polyester loop of the ENDOBUTTON CL implant. **B:** This step connects the proximal end of the semitendinosus graft to the polyester loop of the ENDOBUTTON implant.

The semitendinosus tendon is tripled by passing both ends of the Dacron tape and FiberWire sutures through the polyester loop of the ENDOBUTTON implant (Fig. 15-20). This step creates a loop of semitendinosus tendon on the opposite end of the graft. The ends of the Dacron tape and FiberWire sutures are separated and one end of the Dacron tape and one of the FiberWire sutures are passed on each side of the loop of semitendinosus tendon. This step results in the looped part of the semitendinosus tendon being straddled on both sides by the Dacron tape and one FiberWire suture. Tension is applied to both ends of the Dacron tape and the FiberWire sutures, docking the distal end of the semitendinosus tendon into the axilla of the looped part of the semitendinosus tendon, in

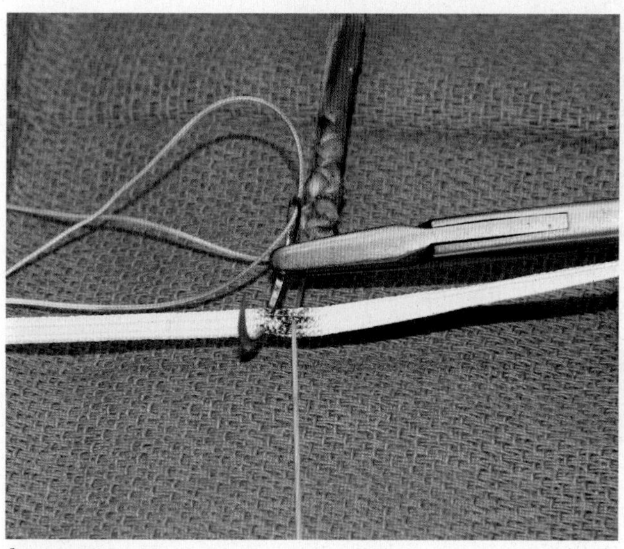
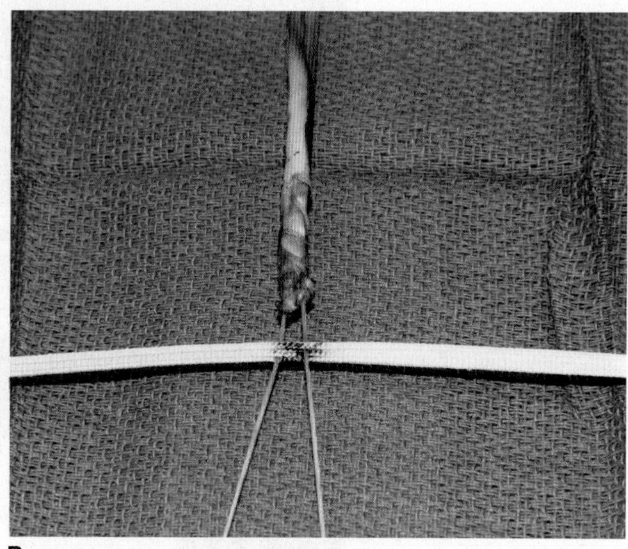

A B

FIGURE 15-18

A, B: The FiberWire sutures from the distal end of the semitendinosus graft are passed through the 5 mm Dacron tape using a tapered free needle, creating a horizontal mattress suture.

the process creating a tripled semitendinosus tendon graft. Tension is applied to the Dacron tape and the FiberWire sutures. This step aligns and locks the distal end of the semitendinosus tendon inside the looped part of the semitendinosus tendon and equally tensions all 3 strands of the tripled semitendinosus tendon graft (Fig. 15-21).

The gracilis tendon is then passed through the polyester loop of the ENDOBUTTON implant and the ends of the gracilis tendon are adjusted so they are equal in length. This will create a 5-strand hamstring tendon graft (Fig. 15-22). The two FiberWire sutures from the same end of the gracilis and one FiberWire suture and Dacron tape from the same side of the semitendinosus graft are tied together 12 to 15 cm from the end of the graft using a single throw. The Dacron tape and FiberWire sutures on the opposite side of the graft are marked with a surgical marker at the same length as the previously tied knot on the other side of the graft. The Dacron tape and the FiberWire suture are tied together at the marked location. This step will create two equal-length suture/tape loops on each side of the 5-strand graft (Fig. 15-23). The suture loops are connected to a graft tensioning device at the time of final graft fixation, equally tensioning all 5-graft strands. It is important to not suture

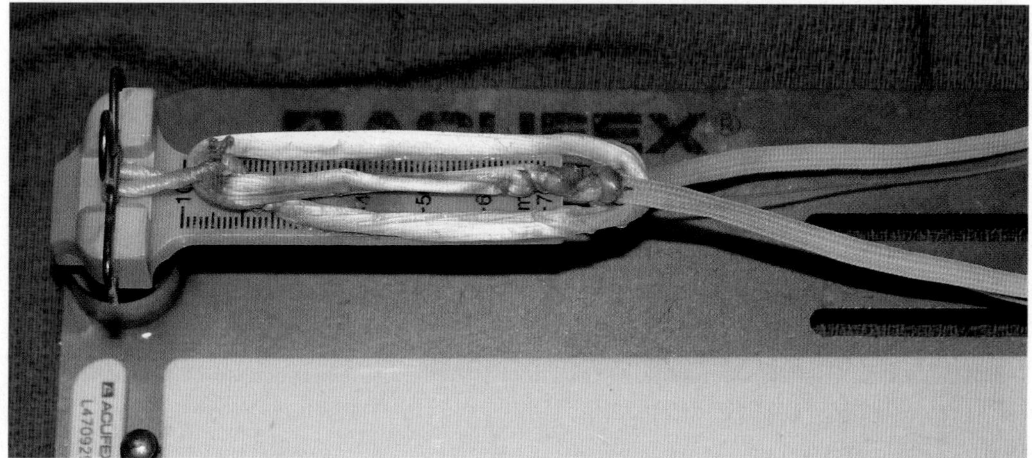

FIGURE 15-19

The use of Dacron tape improves the seating of the middle strand of the tripled semitendinosus graft in the axilla of the looped part of the graft and allows even tension to be applied to all three strands of the tripled graft.

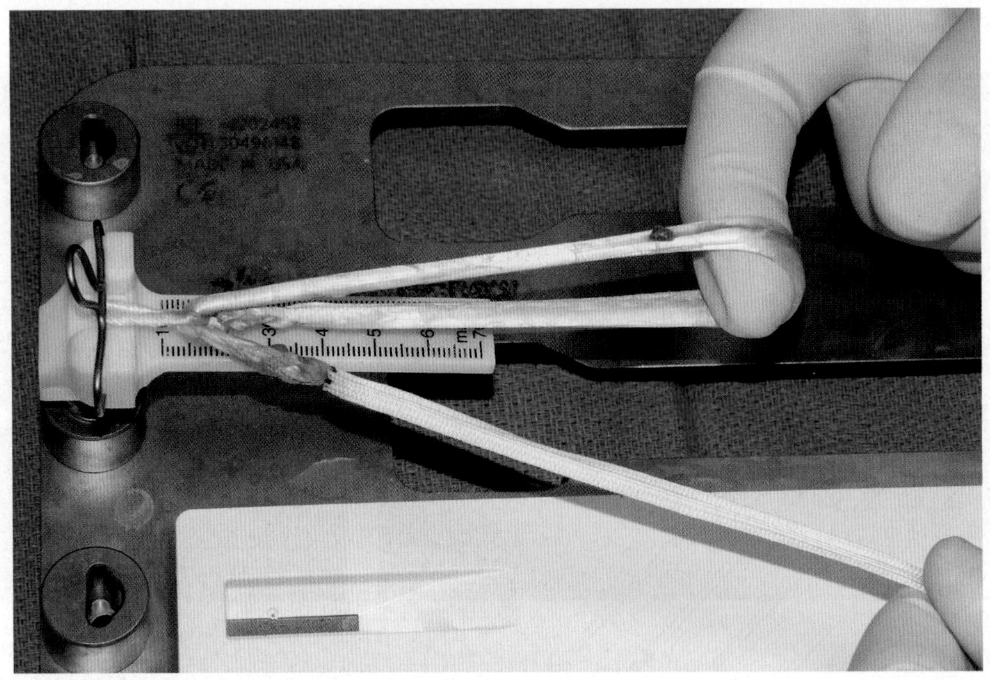

FIGURE 15-20

Both ends of the Dacron tape and FiberWire sutures are passed through the polyester loop of the ENDOBUTTON implant. This step creates a loop of semitendinosus graft on the opposite end of the construct.

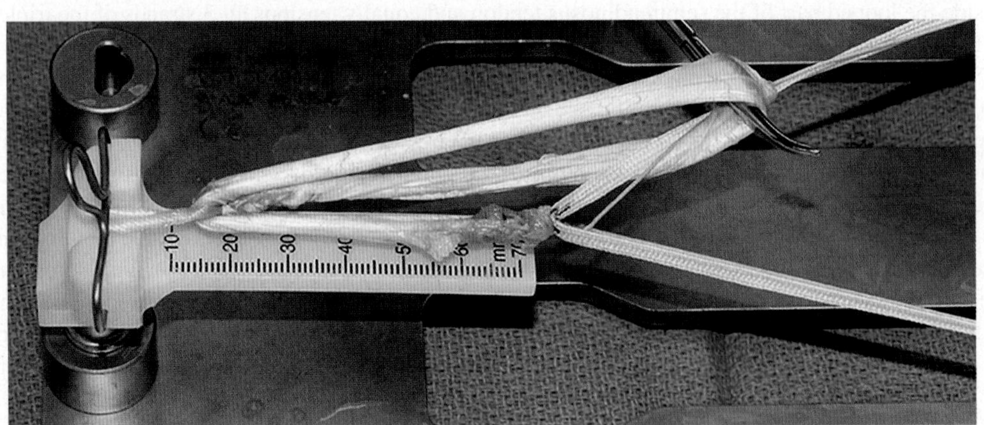

A

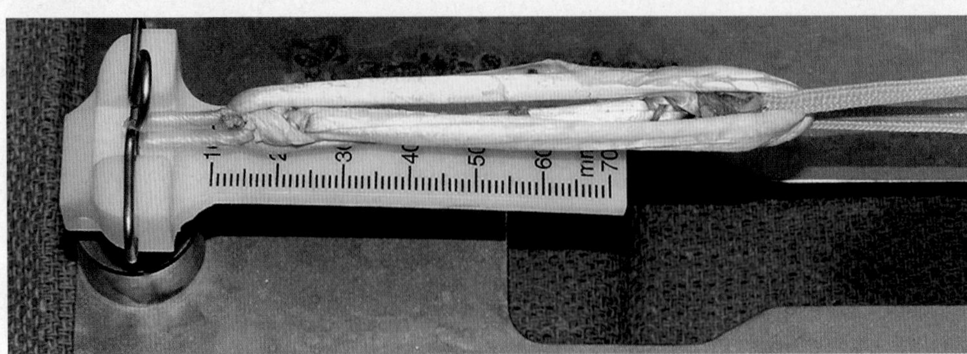

B

FIGURE 15-21

A: The ends of the Dacron tape and FiberWire sutures are separated and one end of the Dacron tape and one of the FiberWire sutures are passed on each side of the loop of semitendinosus tendon. **B:** Both ends of the tape and the sutures are tensioned, seating the middle strand of the semitendinosus tendon in the axilla of the looped end, creating a tripled semitendinosus graft.

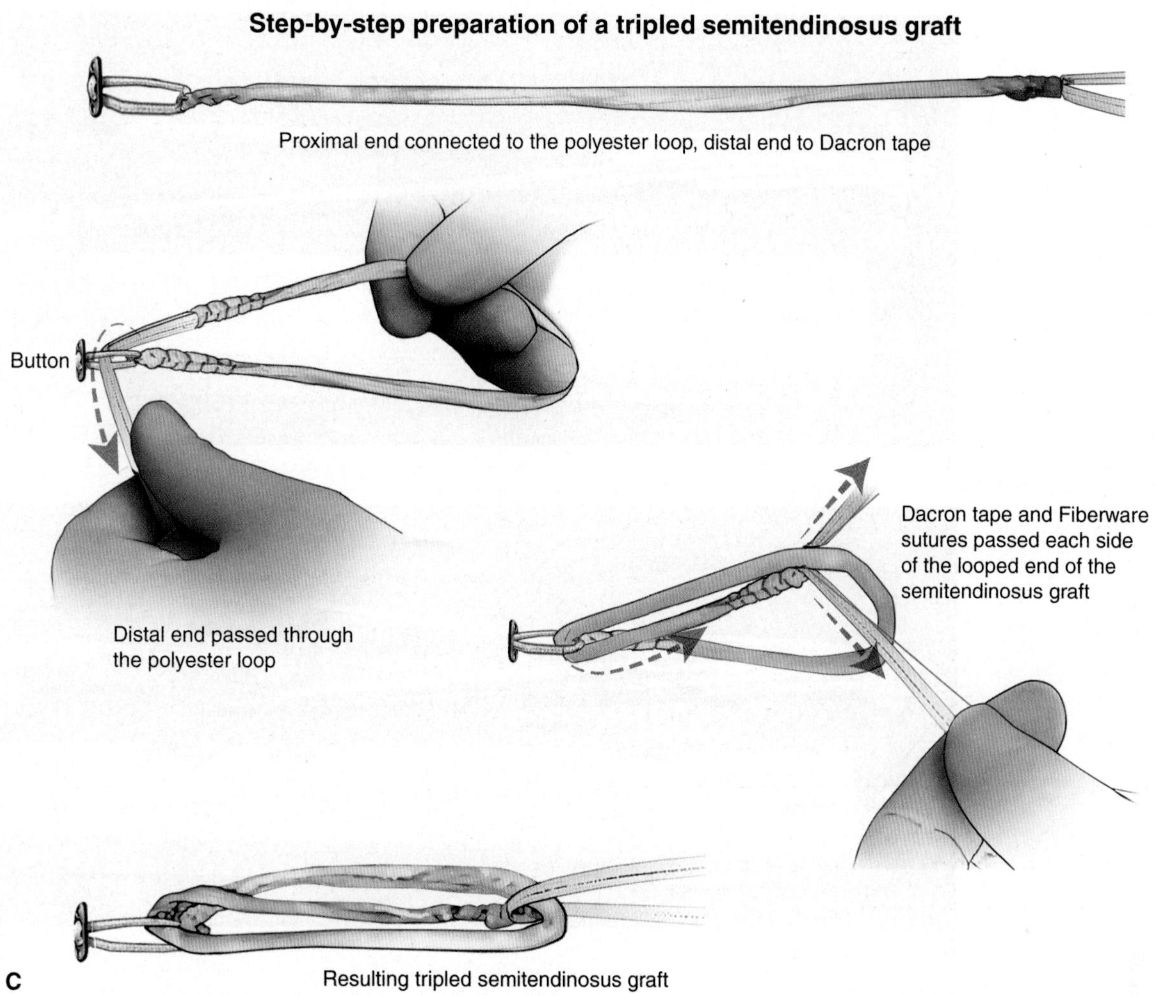

Step-by-step preparation of a tripled semitendinosus graft

Proximal end connected to the polyester loop, distal end to Dacron tape

Button

Dacron tape and Fiberware sutures passed each side of the looped end of the semitendinosus graft

Distal end passed through the polyester loop

C

Resulting tripled semitendinosus graft

FIGURE 15-21 (*Continued*)

C: Drawing illustrating the steps used to create a tripled semitendinosus graft.

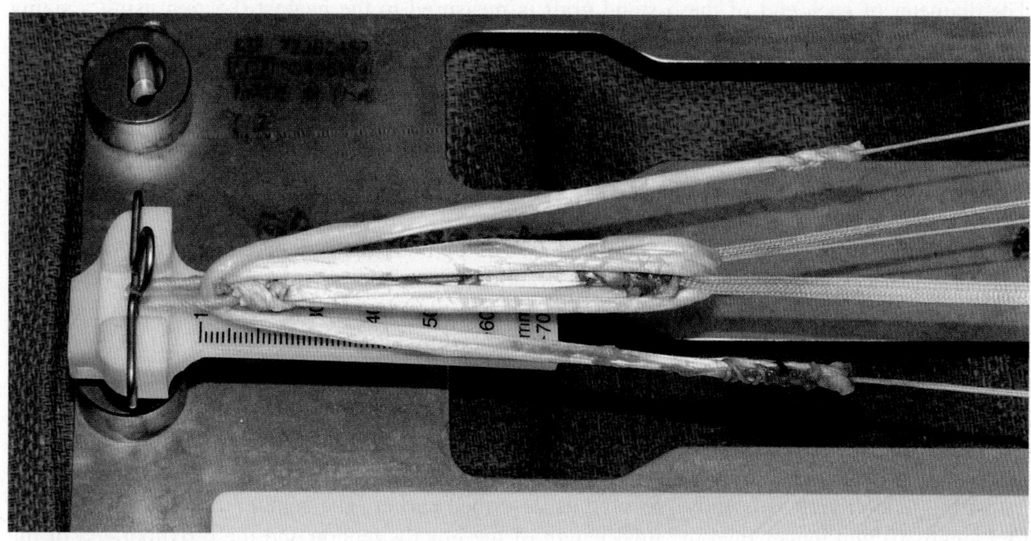

FIGURE 15-22

The gracilis tendon is doubled by passing the ends through the polyester loop of the ENDOBUTTON implant, creating a 5-strand hamstring tendon graft.

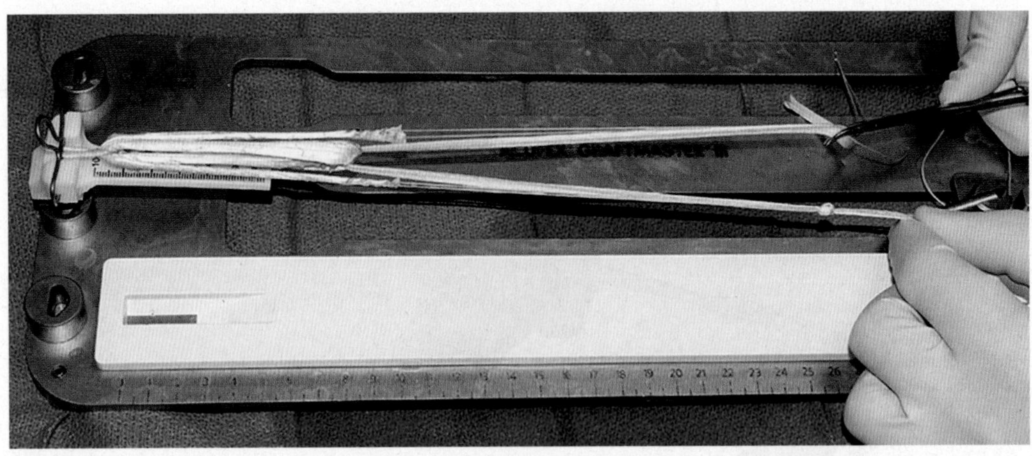

A

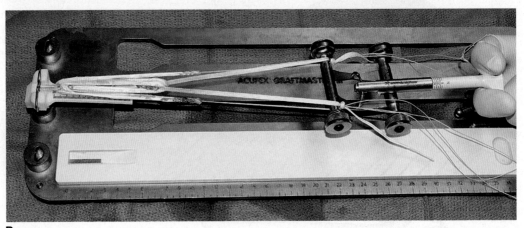

B

FIGURE 15-23

A: The Dacron tape and the FiberWire sutures are tied together on each side of the 5-strand graft, creating two equal-length suture/tape loops. **B:** The suture loops can be connected to a graft tensioning device at the time of final graft fixation, equally tensioning all 5-graft strands.

the graft strands together, as this will not allow the 5-graft strands to slide and be equally tensioned. The diameter of each end of the 5-stand graft is measured to the nearest 0.5 mm using a sizing block. The ENDOBUTTON CL ULTRA implant is placed back in the ENDOBUTTON Holder and the 5-strand graft is pretensioned to 10 to 15 pounds using a suture vise with tensiometer (Smith & Nephew Advanced Surgical Devices, Andover, MA) and the graft wrapped with a surgical sponge soaked in a vancomycin saline solution as described previously.

6-Strand Hamstring Tendon Graft Preparation

A 6-strand hamstring tendon graft is prepared by tripling both the semitendinosus and gracilis tendons (Fig. 15-24). The proximal end of the gracilis tendon is whipstitched with a #2 FiberWire suture. Slack in the FiberWire whipstitch sutures is removed and the tendon compressed by applying tension to the sutures using a "cinching" motion. The length of the gracilis tendon is then measured. The minimum length for tripling the gracilis tendon is around 23 cm. Tendon lengths less than 23 cm will result in less than 20 mm of tendon graft being inserted into the ACL femoral tunnel and less than 30 mm of graft in the tibial tunnel when a 15 mm ENDOBUTTON CL implant is used and the ACL femoral tunnel length is 40 mm. If the gracilis tendon is less than 23 cm, a 5-strand hamstring tendon graft is usually prepared as described earlier. The semitendinosus tendon is cut to a length 10 mm longer than the final length of the gracilis tendon and the proximal end of the semitendinosus tendon whipstitched with a #2 FiberWire suture. The two tendons will end up being the same length as the semitendinosus tendon will typically shorten by 10 mm after the ends of the graft have been compressed and slack removed from the whipstitches.

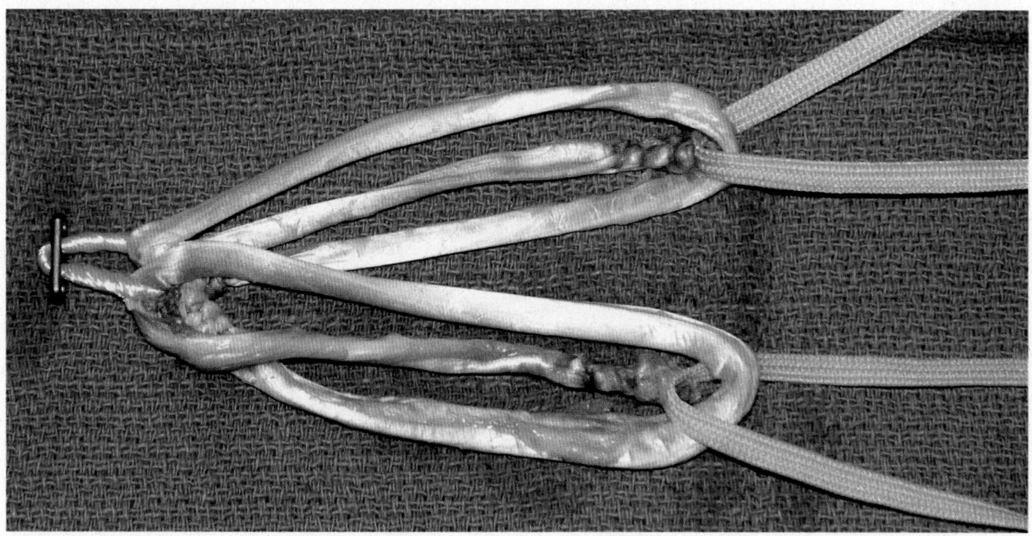

FIGURE 15-24
The gracilis and semitendinosus tendon are both individually tripled, creating a 6-strand hamstring tendon ACL graft.

A 15-mm ENDOBUTTON CL ULTRA implant is placed in the ENDOBUTTON Holder and the proximal ends of both tendons are individually tied to the polyester loop using the FiberWire sutures. After tying each tendon to the polyester loop, one suture from the semitendinosus tendon is tied to one FiberWire suture from the gracilis tendon. This step is repeated for the remaining two FiberWire sutures. This step locks the two tendons together and provides additional strength and security to the construct. The gracilis and semitendinosus tendon grafts are individually tripled as previously described for a 5-strand graft. The distal end of each tendon is passed through the polyester loop of the ENDOBUTTON CL ULTRA implant from inside the axilla of the two tendons to an outside direction. Passing the tendons in this direction will bury the connecting knot inside the tendons, decreasing the bulk of the femoral end of the graft. The tripled gracilis and semitendinosus grafts are combined to create a 6-strand graft (Fig. 15-25). A loop of Dacron tape is created by tying the Dacron tape together with a single throw, 12 to 15 cm from the end of the semitendinosus graft. The tape on the gracilis tendon is marked and tied together at the same length as the knot on the semitendinosus tendon. These steps create two equal-length tape loops. The FiberWire sutures on each tendon are left untied. If required, the FiberWires sutures can be tied around a screw/washer or small staple to provide supplemental tibial fixation. Equal tension is applied to the 6-graft strands by looping the two tape loops around the arms of a graft tension device at the time of final tensioning and graft fixation (Fig. 15-26). The diameter of each end of the 6-strand graft is measured to the nearest 0.5 using a sizing block. The 6-strand graft is pretensioned to 10 to 15 pounds using a suture vise with tensiometer and wrapped with a 4″ × 4″ sponge soaked in a vancomycin saline solution as previously described.

Tibial Tunnel Length

The final step after preparing either a 5- or 6-strand hamstring tendon graft involves estimating the femoral and tibial tunnel lengths necessary to avoid a graft-tunnel mismatch. A sterile surgical marking pen is used to mark the femoral end of the graft at the estimated femoral tunnel length (e.g., 40 mm) from the ENDOBUTTON implant. From the first mark, a second mark is made on the hamstring tendon graft at the estimated intra-articular length of the ACL (25 mm for patients in the Gulf States, 28 to 30 mm for Western populations). Thus, for the average size Western patient, the first mark would lie at 40 mm (femoral tunnel length) from the ENDOBUTTON implant, and the second mark at 70 mm (femoral tunnel length + intra-articular length of the ACL). The length of hamstring tendon graft that lies beyond the 70-mm mark represents the amount of tendon graft that will be inserted in the ACL tibial tunnel (Fig. 15-27). Typically, this length is in the 30 to 35 mm range, in which case a 40-mm length tibial tunnel would be drilled. An extra #5 polyester suture is passed through the end hole of the ENDOBUTTON CL ULTRA implant containing the white passing suture. This provides an additional traction suture minimizing the possibility of suture breakage when passing the hamstring tendon graft.

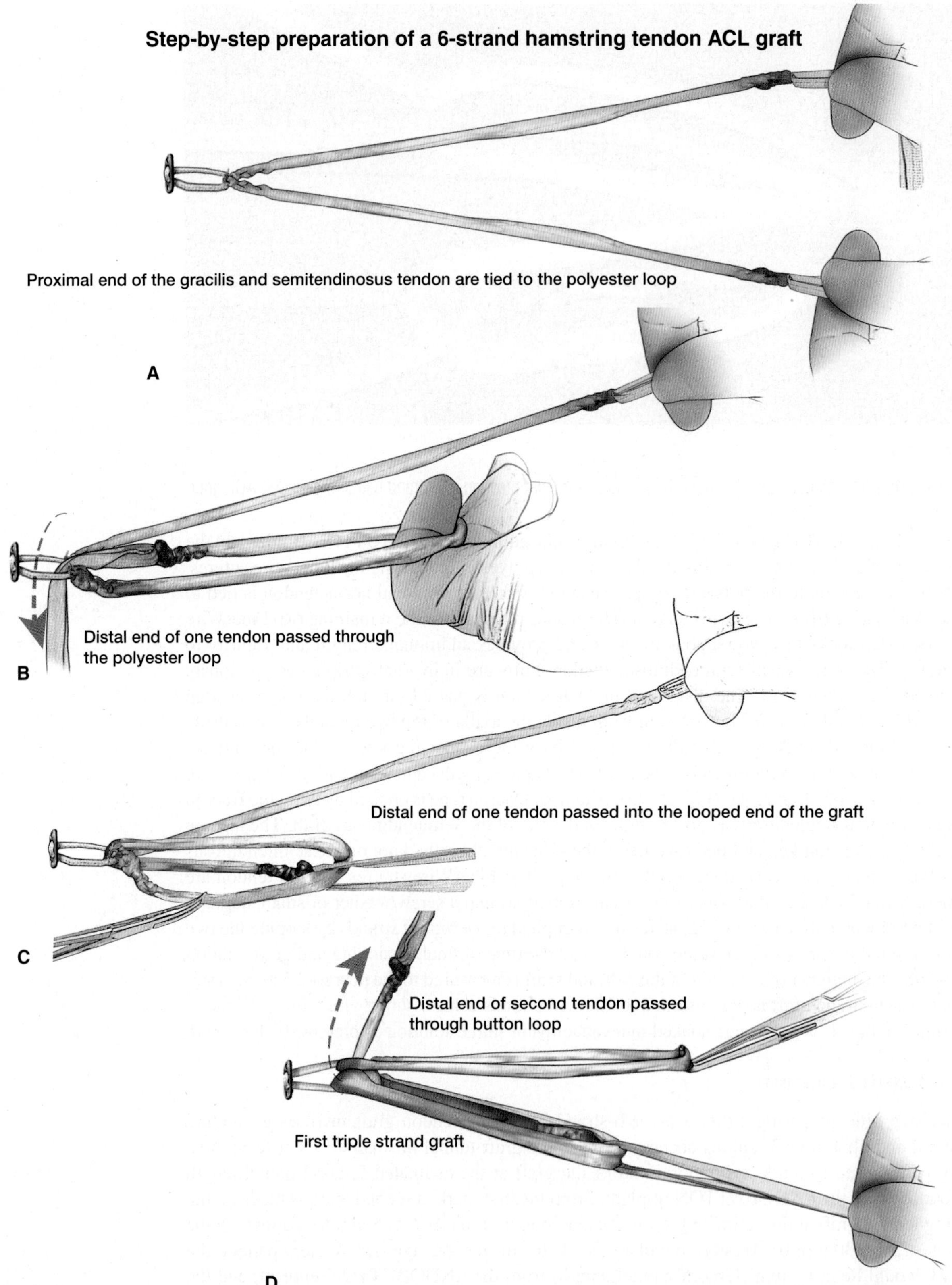
Step-by-step preparation of a 6-strand hamstring tendon ACL graft
Proximal end of the gracilis and semitendinosus tendon are tied to the polyester loop
A
Distal end of one tendon passed through
the polyester loop
B
Distal end of one tendon passed into the looped end of the graft
C
Distal end of second tendon passed
through button loop
First triple strand graft
D

FIGURE 15-25

Step-by-step preparation of 6-strand hamstring tendon ACL graft. **A:** The FiberWire sutures from the proximal end of both the gracilis and semitendinosus tendons are tied to the polyester loop of the ENDOBUTTON CL implant. **B:** The distal end of one tendon graft is passed through the ENDOBUTTON CL polyester loop. The tendon graft is passed from inside the axilla of the tendons, exiting in an outside direction. **C:** The ends of the Dacron tape and FiberWire sutures are separated and one end of the Dacron tape and one of the FiberWire sutures are passed on each side of the loop of the tendon, creating the first tripled tendon graft. **D:** The distal end of the second tendon is passed through the ENDOBUTTON CL polyester loop in an inside-out direction.

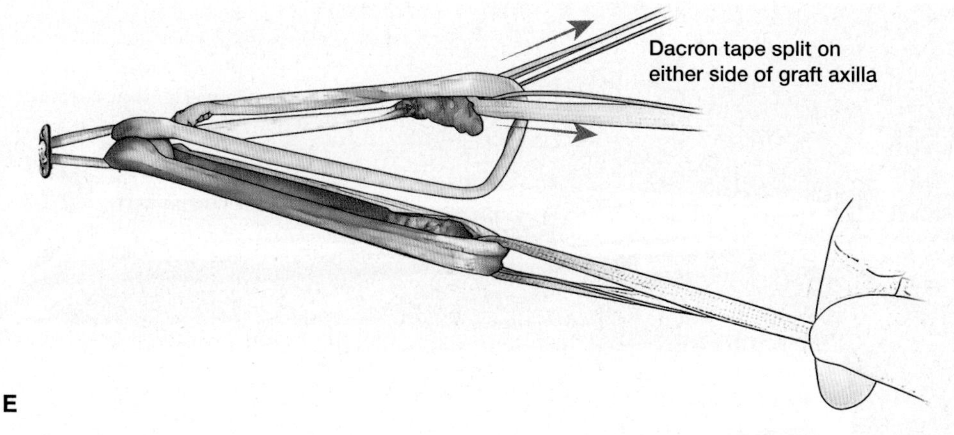

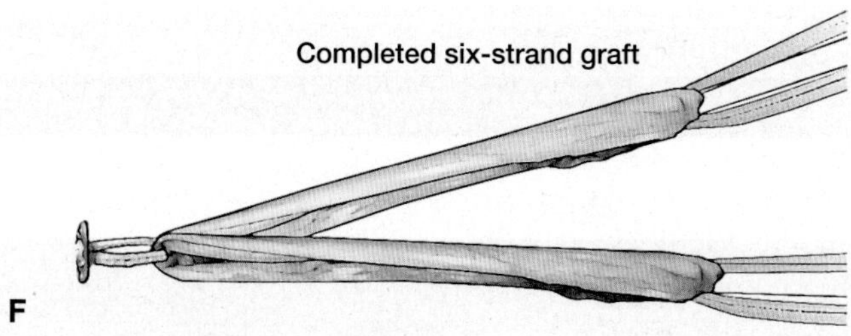

FIGURE 15-25 *(Continued)*
E: The ends of the Dacron tape and FiberWire sutures are separated and one end of the Dacron tape and one of the FiberWire sutures are passed on each side of the loop of the second tendon graft, creating the second tripled tendon graft. **F:** The final 6-strand hamstring tendon ACL graft construct, consisting of tripled semitendinosus and gracilis tendon grafts.

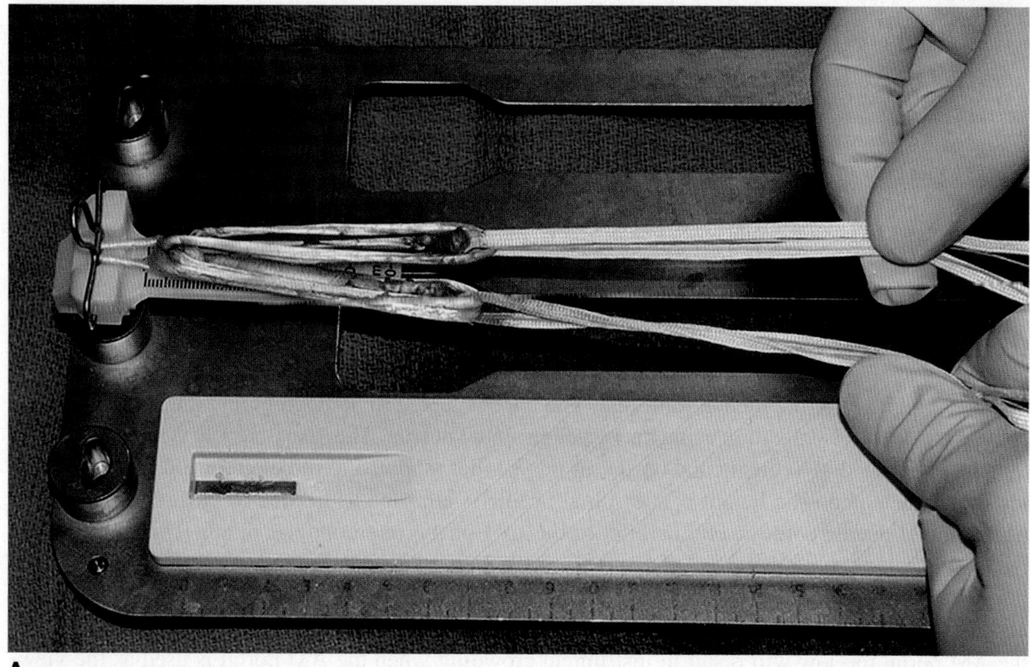

A

FIGURE 15-26
A, B: The ends of the Dacron tapes from the tripled gracilis and semitendinosus tendons are tied together to create two equal-length tape loops allowing equal tension to be applied to the 6 tendon strands.

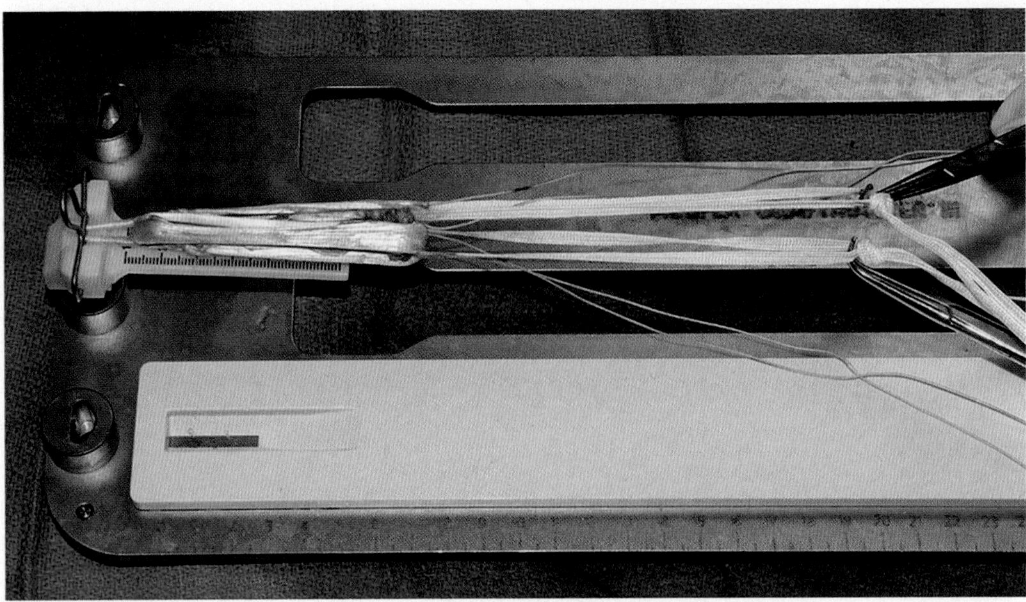

B

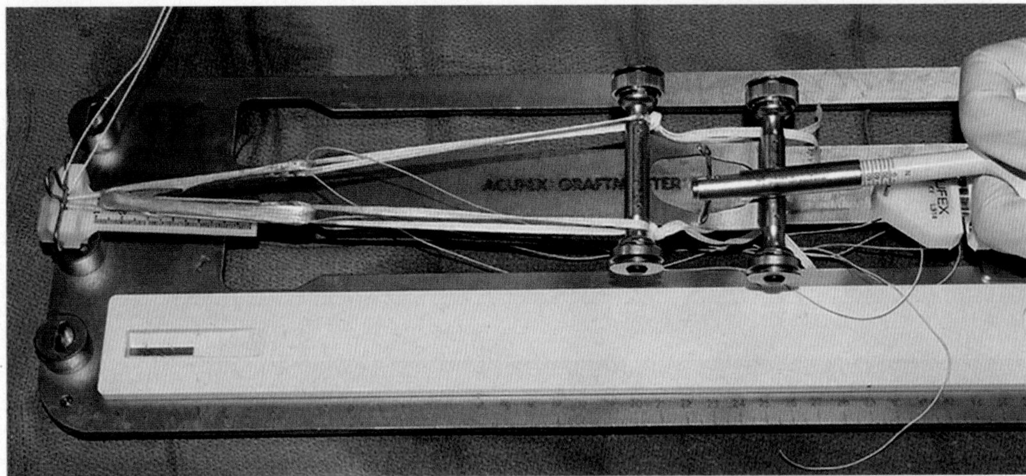

C

FIGURE 15-26 ***(Continued)***
C: A spring loaded tensioning device may be used to apply equal tension to the 6-strand graft.

Arthroscopy

A 30-degree arthroscope is inserted into the knee joint through the AL portal and a diagnostic arthroscopy performed. It is important for the ease and success of the procedure that the AM portal be placed high above the medial joint line. The knee is flexed to 90 degrees and the AM portal created under direct visualization using an 18-gauge spinal needle. The spinal needle is introduced into the knee joint medial to the medial border of the patellar tendon and directed toward the roof of the intercondylar notch. The height of the spinal needle is adjusted as needed to ensure that the shaft of the spinal needle comes to lie parallel to the roof of the intercondylar notch. This step usually results in the external position of the spinal needle being located slightly more proximal than the inferior pole of the patella and higher than the AL portal. Placing the spinal needle at this height ensures adequate spatial separation between the viewing AM and the working AAM portals. Placing the AM portal too low will result in instrument crowding when the AM portal is used as the viewing portal and the AAM portal is used as a working portal. A low AM portal will also result in the arthroscope passing through the fat pad and the fat pad being dragged into the field of view by the tip of the arthroscope limiting visualization in the intercondylar notch when the knee is hyperflexed. Due to the curvature of the medial border of the patellar, moving the spinal needle position more medially will allow the AM portal to be created higher above the medial joint line. Once the correct

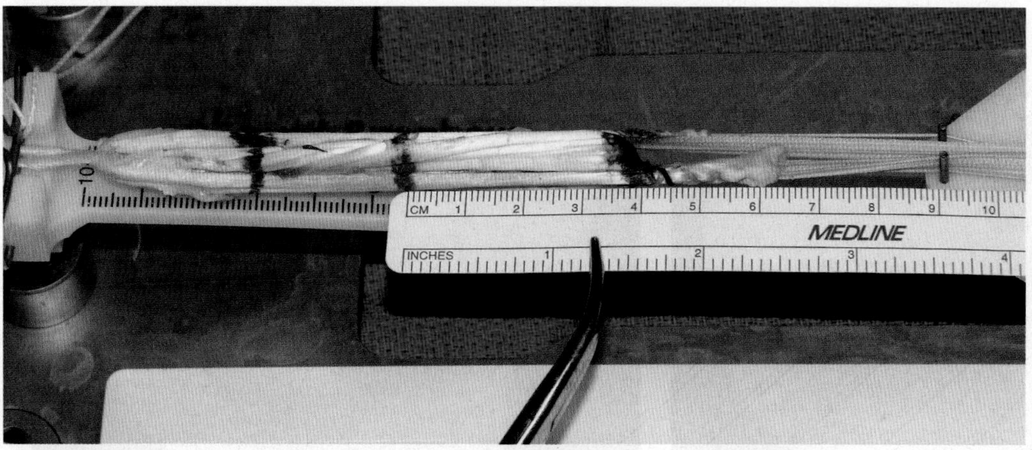

FIGURE 15-27

The hamstring ACL graft is marked at the estimated femoral tunnel length, 40 mm (first mark on the left), and at the estimated intra-articular length of the ACL, 25 mm in this case (middle mark). The distance from the estimated intra-articular length of the ACL to the end of the tendon graft (third mark) represents the amount of graft in the tibial tunnel. The drilled tibial tunnel length should be greater than this distance to avoid a graft-tunnel mismatch.

position for the AM portal is determined, a vertical incision is created using a #11 knife blade. The AM portal is used primarily as a working portal when performing diagnostic arthroscopy and chondral and meniscal surgery and as a viewing portal for the ACL femoral and tibial attachment sites. A motorized 4.5-mm shaver blade is inserted through the working AM portal and the ligamentum mucosum resected. This step releases the fat pad, exposing the intercondylar notch. Instrumentation is inserted through the working AM portal and a diagnostic arthroscopy and any necessary meniscal or chondral procedures performed.

Accessory Anteromedial Portal

Proper placement of the AAM portal is critical to the success of the procedure, since it is the most important factor determining the length of the ACL femoral tunnel (24,25). Positioning the AAM portal more medially results in a more perpendicular orientation of the drill bit with respect to the lateral wall of the notch, producing a shorter femoral tunnel with a more circular-shaped tunnel aperture. However, placing the AAM portal too far medially can result in iatrogenic damage to the medial femoral condyle when passing a cannulated endoscopic drill bit through the AAM portal into the intercondylar notch. Moving the AAM portal more laterally, toward the medial border of the patellar tendon, orients the drill bit more obliquely with respect to the lateral wall of the notch, producing a longer femoral tunnel length with a more elliptically shaped tunnel aperture (Fig. 15-28). An elliptically shaped femoral tunnel aperture is the preferred shape for hamstring tendon grafts since this geometry restores a greater percentage of the native ACL femoral attachment site.

The AAM portal is created under direct vision using an 18-gauge spinal needle. The fat pad above the anterior horn of the medial meniscus and in front of the medial femoral condyle should be removed to allow visualization to correctly place the AAM portal. During this step care should be taken to avoid injury to the anterior horn of the medial meniscus and the intermeniscal ligament. The arthroscope is rotated medially to visualize the spinal needle entering the knee joint just above the anterior horn of the medial meniscus. The spinal needle should be directed toward the center of the ACL femoral attachment site and should be seen to easily pass by the medial femoral condyle. The arthroscope is rotated medially to determine if the spinal needle is positioned too close to the medial femoral condyle and the position adjusted accordingly. The skin and fat is incised transversely with a #11 knife blade along the upper aspect of the spinal needle under direct vision. Sliding the knife blade along the superior border of the spinal needle protects the anterior horn of the medial meniscus from iatrogenic injury. A transverse skin incision is recommended for this portal as this allows adjustments in the medial-lateral position of the femoral guide pin to be made and is less likely to result in injury to the anterior horn of the medial meniscus. Instrument passage through the AAM portal can be eased by dilating the portal in line with the skin incision using the tips of Metzenbaum scissors or a curved clamp.

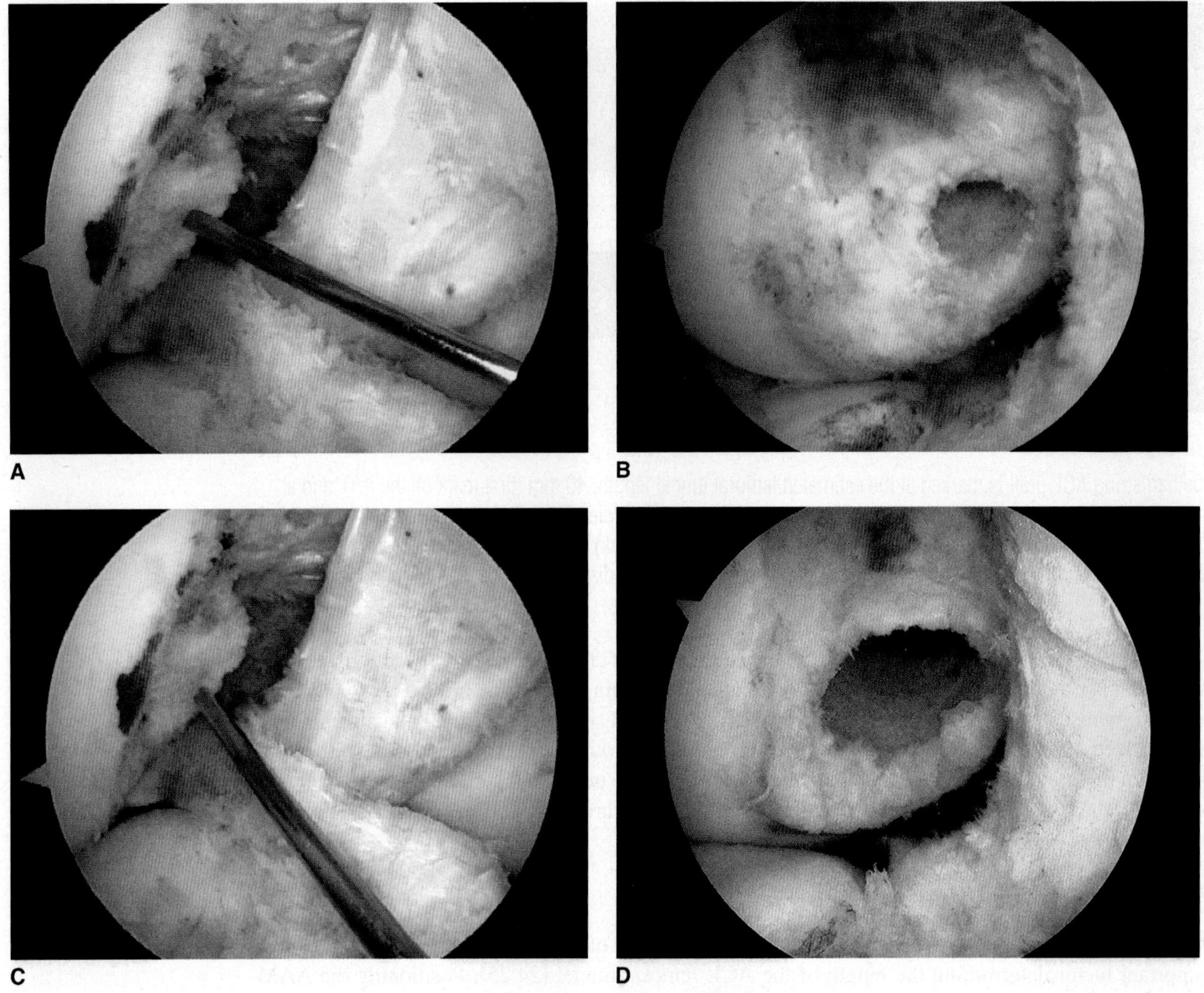

FIGURE 15-28

The effect of accessory anteromedial (AAM) portal position on femoral tunnel length and femoral tunnel aperture shape. **A, B:** A more medially placed AAM portal orients the femoral guide pin/drill more orthogonally to the lateral wall of the intercondylar notch, producing a more circular tunnel aperture and a shorter ACL femoral tunnel. **C, D:** Moving the AAM portal more laterally, closer to the patellar tendon, orients the femoral guide pin/drill more tangentially to the lateral wall of the intercondylar notch, producing a more elliptically shaped tunnel aperture and a longer femoral tunnel.

Intercondylar Notch Preparation

A motorized shaver blade is inserted through the working AM portal and any fat pad limiting view of the ACL tibial attachment site and intercondylar notch is removed. Resection of the fat pad should be limited to that which is necessary for visualization. It is important to carefully inspect and classify the ACL tear pattern. ACL tears can be classified according to the location of the tear, proximal, midsubstance, or distal, complete (two-bundle tear) versus partial (one-bundle tear of the AM or PL bundle). This information may affect the surgical approach. In cases where only a one-bundle tear of the ACL is found or where ACL remnants are found connecting the tibia to the femur, the intact bundle or remnant ACL fibers may be preserved and a single-bundle augmentation or tissue-preserving procedure performed as opposed to resecting the intact fibers of the ACL and performing a complete ACL reconstruction. Preserving native ACL tissue may have some potential biomechanical, vascular, biological and proprioceptive advantages (40).

In cases of a complete tear of both ACL bundles, the torn ACL fibers in the midsubstance are resected using a basket punch and motorized shaver blade. It is important to preserve some of the native ACL fibers at the femoral and tibial attachment sites to aid with later placement of the

ACL femoral and tibial bone tunnels. In chronic cases with narrow notch or notch osteophytes, the distance from the lateral border of the PCL to the lateral wall of the intercondylar notch can be measured with an ACL ruler to ensure that there is adequate space for the ACL replacement graft. In the case of large-diameter ACL grafts or small notch widths, a limited wallplasty may be required. However, the wallplasty should be performed after the ACL femoral tunnel is drilled to avoid removing the native ACL fibers and the underlying bony landmarks, which are valuable aids in achieving anatomic tunnel placement. If a wallplasty is required, bone is only removed at the shallow (distal) part of the notch. It is important to avoid removing bone in the area of the ACL attachment site as this will lateralize the ACL femoral tunnel, changing the axis of the ACL graft.

Anatomic ACL Femoral Tunnel Placement

Although there is an ongoing debate about the optimal position for the ACL femoral tunnel, it is widely accepted that when performing an anatomic ACL reconstruction, the ACL femoral tunnel should be placed within the native ACL femoral attachment site (16,17,21). When performing an ACL reconstruction, anatomic placement of the ACL femoral tunnel is best achieved by first identifying the center of the native ACL femoral attachment site. Using the center of the native attachment site as a defined anatomic reference point, the surgeon may choose to alter the position of the ACL femoral tunnel within the ACL femoral attachment site based on different philosophies (41,42). Placing the center of the ACL femoral tunnel at the center of the native ACL femoral attachment site is favored by many surgeons based on biomechanical and gait analysis studies demonstrating that a single-bundle ACL graft positioned at the center of the native ACL femoral and tibial attachment sites best controls anterior tibial translation and tibial rotation during a simulated pivot shift test and more closely restores kinematics to that of the normal knee compared with other ACL graft placements within the native ACL femoral attachment site (20,21,43,44). Moving the center of the femoral tunnel away from the center of the native ACL femoral attachment site toward the center of the AM bundle attachment site results in an ACL graft that has smaller length changes (isometric) and experiences lower and relatively constant in situ graft forces (41,44,45). Lower ACL graft forces may theoretically reduce the risk of graft rerupture compared to a centrally placed ACL graft (41,45). However, moving the femoral tunnel toward the center of the AM bundle attachment site results in a more vertical ACL graft that is not as well aligned as a centrally placed graft to control the pivot shift phenomena (19,20). Moving the center of the femoral tunnel toward the area of the PL bundle attachment site will result in larger graft length changes and higher in situ graft forces as the knee is extended (20,41,45). Although this femoral tunnel position results in a more horizontal ACL graft orientation that is better aligned to control the pivot shift, higher in situ graft forces and greater ligament strain may theoretically increase the risk of graft rerupture (20,41,44). At the present time, there are no clinical studies documenting the superiority of one anatomic femoral tunnel location versus another.

Center of the ACL Femoral Attachment Site

To find the center of the ACL femoral attachment site, the knee is positioned at 90 degrees of flexion. This is the most reproducible position to visualize the lateral wall of the intercondylar notch and orients the ACL femoral attachment site in the reference position most commonly used in anatomical studies of the ACL femoral attachment site. The ACL femoral attachment site is viewed through the AM portal as this provides an orthogonal view of the lateral wall of the notch compared to the more tangential view when viewing through the AL portal (Fig. 15-29). Viewing the lateral wall of the notch and ACL femoral attachment site through the AM portal improves the accuracy of ACL femoral tunnel placement in both the shallow-deep (distal-proximal) and high-low (anterior-posterior) directions and eliminates the need to perform a routine notchplasty for visualization purposes. Performing an initial notchplasty or using a curette, motorized shaver blade or burr to remove soft tissue and bone along the lateral wall of the notch should be avoided in order to preserve the bony and soft tissue ACL landmarks. An improved view of the ACL femoral attachment site can be achieved by maintaining the knee at 90 degrees of flexion and placing the leg in the figure-four position. This maneuver distracts the lateral compartment and lifts the lateral femoral condyle away from the lateral meniscus, allowing better visualization of the low (posterior) part of the ACL femoral attachment site and the area of insertion of the indirect fibers (fan-like extension fibers) (Fig. 15-30).

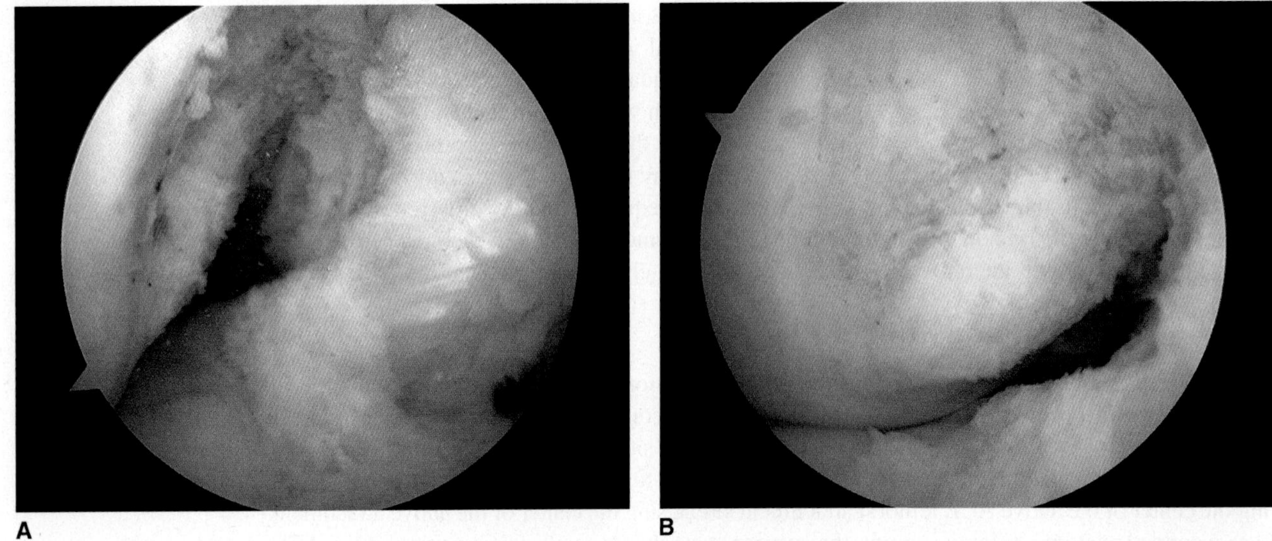

FIGURE 15-29

(A) The view through the AM portal provides an orthogonal view of the lateral wall of the notch compared to the more tangential view through the AL portal **(B)**. Viewing through the AM portal allows more accurate ACL femoral tunnel placement.

Although the clock-face reference is often used to specify the location of the ACL femoral tunnel, this reference method has several limitations (Fig. 15-31). First of all, it ignores the depth of the intercondylar notch. Secondly, there is no agreed-upon reference position for the 3 and 9 o'clock locations. Finally, the clock-face reference does not rely on any known anatomic ACL landmarks and cannot be used when viewing the lateral wall of the intercondylar notch through the AM portal. Finding the center of the ACL femoral attachment site is most reliably achieved using one or all of the following methods: when present directly referencing from the native ACL femoral footprint, referencing from the bony ACL ridges, measuring along the lateral wall of the intercondylar notch with an ACL ruler, and using intraoperative fluoroscopy (24).

In most situations, there are remnant fibers of the native ACL present and these fibers can be used to locate the center of the ACL femoral attachment site. With the arthroscope in the AM portal, an RF wand is inserted through the AAM portal and the borders of the native ACL footprint marked. It is possible to estimate the center location of the ACL femoral footprint. However, the parallax that occurs with the use of a 30-degree arthroscope tends to result in estimating a center position that is shallower than the actual true position. The true center position is more accurately located by choosing a location that is 1 to 2 mm deeper than the visually estimated position. The center of the ACL femoral attachment site can be located with greater accuracy by using an ACL ruler to measure the length of the patients' native ACL footprint.

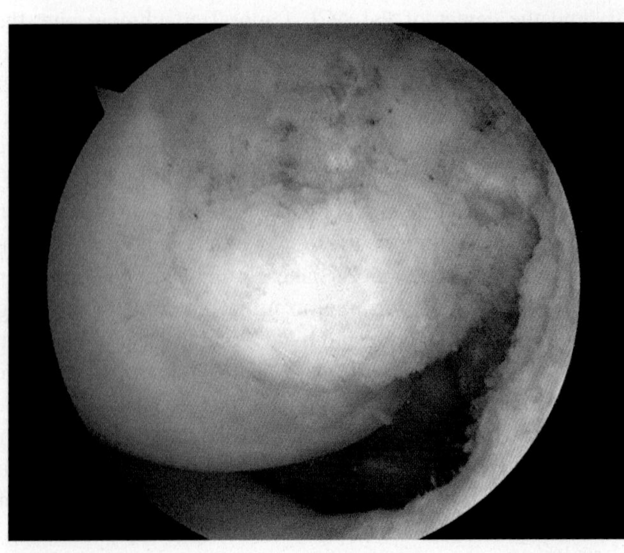

FIGURE 15-30

Viewing the ACL femoral attachment site through the AM portal with knee in the figure-of-four position distracts the lateral compartment, providing a better view of the low (posterior) part of the ACL femoral attachment site. This helps avoid placing the ACL femoral tunnel too low (posterior).

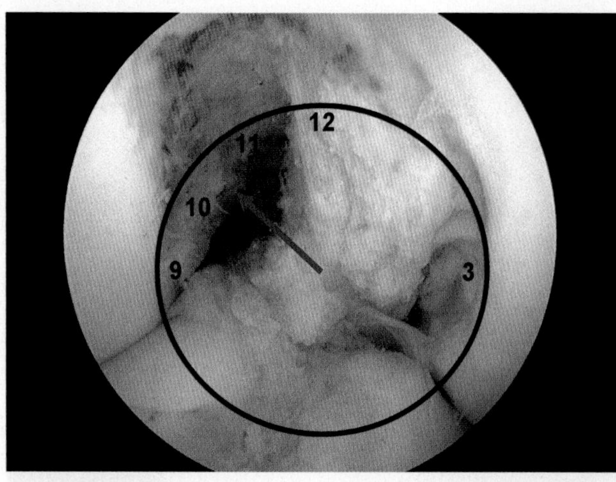

FIGURE 15-31

Placing the ACL femoral tunnel using a "clock-face" reference has several limitations and can result in nonanatomic tunnel placement.

The ACL ruler is bent at a 45-degree angle at the 24-mm mark and inserted into the intercondylar notch through the AL portal. Dilating the AL portal and fat pad with the tips of Metzenbaum scissors or a small clamp is often necessary to ease passage into the knee joint. The ACL ruler is orientated to lie flat against the lower third of the lateral wall of the notch, parallel to the long axis of the native ACL footprint. For the ruler to lie parallel to the long axis of the native ACL femoral attachment site, it is often necessary to flex the knee beyond 90 degrees. The length of the femoral footprint is measured from the deep (proximal) border of the footprint (zero position) to the shallow (distal) margin along its long axis. Using the measured length of the footprint, the center position (50% of the measured footprint length) is calculated and marked by inserting a 45-degree microfracture awl through the AAM portal (Fig. 15-32). Using this measurement technique, it is possible for the surgeon to individualize placement of the ACL femoral tunnel. Choosing a tunnel location that is less than 50% of the measured femoral footprint length will position the femoral tunnel deeper in the ACL femoral attachment site, resulting in a tunnel that covers more of the AM part of the ACL femoral attachment site. Choosing a tunnel location that is greater than 50% of the measured femoral footprint length will position the tunnel shallower in the notch, resulting in more coverage of the PL part of the attachment site. The height of the ACL femoral footprint can be measured by inserting the ACL ruler through the AAM

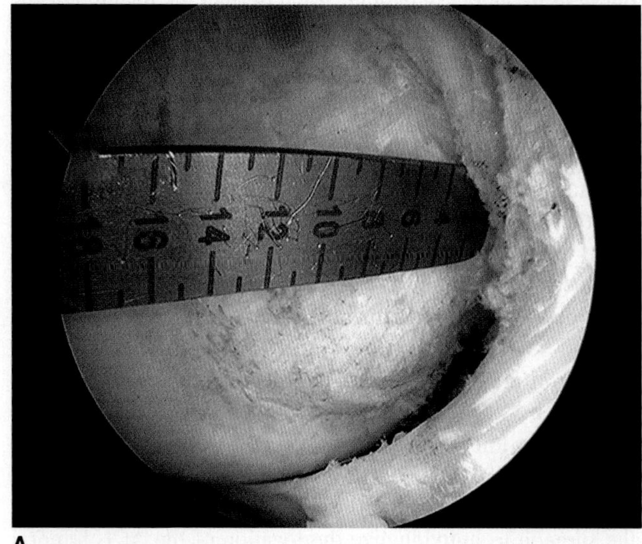

A

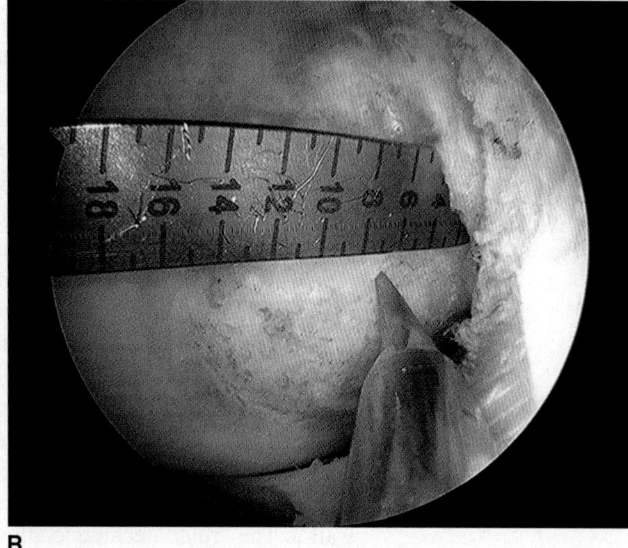

B

FIGURE 15-32

Measuring the center of the ACL femoral attachment site. The ACL femoral attachment site is viewed through the anteromedial portal. **A:** An ACL ruler is inserted into the intercondylar notch through the AL portal and oriented to lie flat against the lower third of the lateral wall of the notch, parallel to the long axis of the native ACL footprint. The length of the native ACL footprint measures 14 mm in this case. **B:** A 45-degree angled microfracture awl is inserted through the AAM portal and is used to mark the center position of the ACL femoral attachment length (50% of the measured length of the ACL footprint), 7 mm in this case.

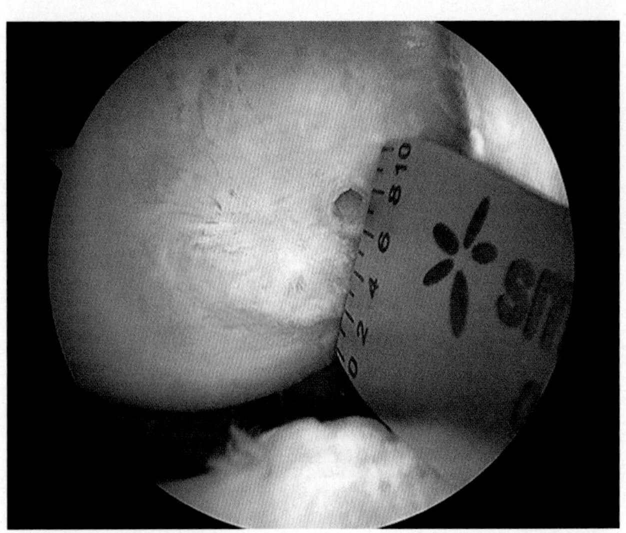

FIGURE 15-33

The height of the ACL femoral footprint can be measured using an ACL ruler inserted through the AAM portal.

portal (Fig. 15-33). This measurement can be used to determine the high-low position of the ACL femoral tunnel. Locating the center of the ACL femoral tunnel equidistant between the lateral intercondylar ridge and the inferior articular cartilage border may position the tunnel too low in the femoral attachment site, covering more of the region where the indirect fibers of the ACL insert (41,42). Moving the center of the femoral tunnel higher, toward the lateral intercondylar ridge, will position the center of the ACL tunnel in the area where the direct fibers of the ACL insert. Biomechanical studies have demonstrated that the direct fibers contribute more to resisting anterior tibial translation and a simulated pivot shift test than the indirect fibers (46).

When fibers of the native ACL are absent, as is often the case in chronic ACL tears and in revision cases, the bony ACL ridges can be used to find the center of the femoral attachment site. The lateral intercondylar ridge ("resident's ridge") is visible in 88% to 100% of chronic ACL-deficient knees and is an important bony landmark as it marks the superior (anterior) border of the ACL. Approximately 50% of the time, it is possible to identify a second bony ridge, the lateral bifurcate ridge, which separates the ACL femoral attachment site into the anteromedial (AM) and posterolateral (PL) bundle attachment sites. It is important to remember that because the cross-sectional area of the PL and AM bundles may be variable from patient to patient, when present the location of the lateral bifurcate ridge does not necessarily represent the true center of the ACL femoral attachment site. Anatomic studies have shown that the center of the ACL femoral attachment site is approximately 1.7 mm deep (proximal) to the lateral bifurcate ridge (47).

With the knee positioned at 90 degrees of flexion, a 90-degree RF wand is inserted through the working AAM portal. The lateral intercondylar ridge is most easily identified by dissecting from the low (posterior) part of the ACL femoral attachment site and working in a high (anterior) direction. A distinct step off will be encountered as the RF wand contacts the lateral intercondylar ridge. The lateral intercondylar ridge is used as a bony reference for the high-low position of the ACL femoral tunnel. The lateral bifurcate ridge if present can be identified as a shelf or prominence perpendicular to the intercondylar ridge in the mid part of the ACL femoral attachment site. The center of the ACL femoral attachment site has been reported to be 8.6 mm superior to the inferior articular cartilage margin and approximately 1.7 mm deep to the bifurcate ridge (47). A 45-degree microfracture awl is inserted through the AAM portal and the center of the attachment site marked (Fig. 15-34).

Using an ACL ruler to measure along the lower third of the lateral wall of the intercondylar notch from the proximal articular cartilage border to the distal articular cartilage border is especially useful in chronic and revision cases where soft tissue and bony landmarks are often absent ("naked lateral wall"). The "ruler" technique allows the surgeon to individualize the location of the ACL femoral tunnel based on the specific anatomy of the patient (24,27). This technique allows for "a la carte" or patient-specific surgery to be performed versus a "one size fits all" approach associated with the use of offset femoral aimers. The ACL ruler is bent at a 45-degree angle at the 24-mm mark and inserted into the notch through the AL portal. Using the AM portal as the viewing portal, the ACL ruler is oriented to lie flat against the lower third of the lateral wall of the notch. Inserting the ACL ruler through the AL portal allows a microfracture awl to be inserted through the working AAM portal, making it

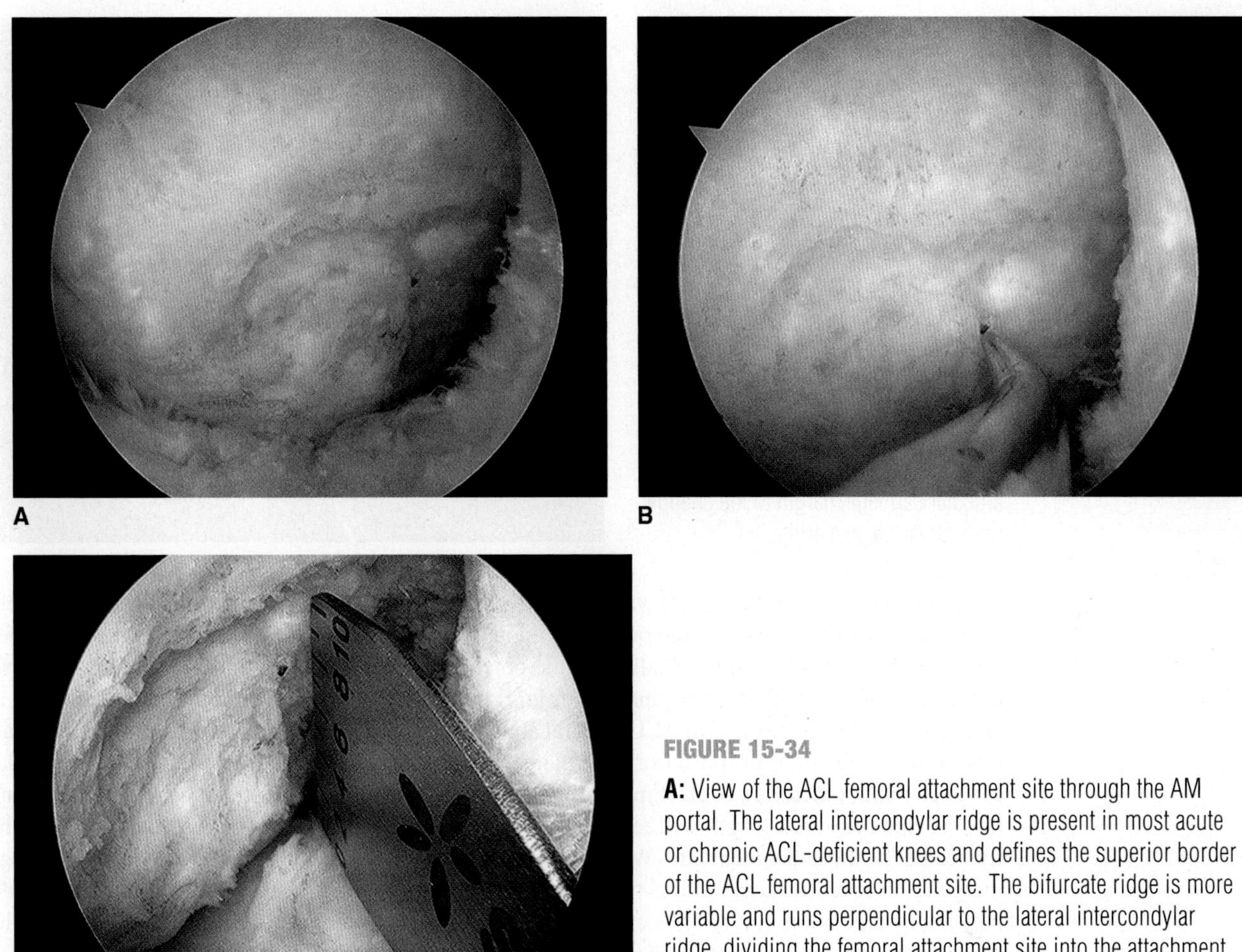

FIGURE 15-34

A: View of the ACL femoral attachment site through the AM portal. The lateral intercondylar ridge is present in most acute or chronic ACL-deficient knees and defines the superior border of the ACL femoral attachment site. The bifurcate ridge is more variable and runs perpendicular to the lateral intercondylar ridge, dividing the femoral attachment site into the attachment areas for the anteromedial and posterolateral bundle fibers. Anatomical studies have shown that on average, the center of the attachment is 1.7 mm deep to the bifurcate ridge **(B)** and 8.6 mm superior to the inferior articular cartilage margin **(C)**.

possible to simultaneously measure and mark positions along the lateral wall of the notch. The lower edge of the ACL ruler is positioned along the lower third of the lateral wall of the intercondylar notch or the lateral intercondylar ridge if it is visible. Slide the ruler along the lateral wall of the notch until the tip is positioned at the deep (proximal) margin of the articular cartilage. This point represents the starting or zero reference position for the ruler. Note that this position is different than the commonly referenced "over-the-top" position that lies higher and deeper in the notch. To insure that the ACL ruler is placed at the correct starting position, it is important to remove soft tissue along the deep (proximal) margin of the lateral femoral condylar until the proximal articular cartilage border is clearly visible. Placing the knee in the figure-four position often helps with visualizing the proximal articular cartilage border. To mark the starting point for the ruler, a 45-degree microfracture awl can be inserted through the AAM portal and the tip of the awl placed at the proximal articular cartilage border. Slide the ACL ruler along the lateral wall of the notch until the end of the ruler contacts the tip of the microfracture awl. This step will align the ruler at the correct starting point. With the knee at 90 degrees of flexion, the lateral wall of the notch is measured from the deep (proximal) articular cartilage margin to the shallow (distal) articular cartilage margin. Bird et al. (27) have shown that 50% of the measured distance from the proximal articular cartilage margin to the shallow articular cartilage margin is a close approximation to the midbundle position of the ACL femoral attachment (Fig. 15-35). In some knees, the height of the AL portal above the lateral joint line may make it difficult to correctly align the ACL ruler along the lower third of the lateral wall of the notch. This limitation can often be overcome by placing the knee in the figure-four position. If this maneuver is unsuccessful, bend the blade of the ruler in the opposite direction and insert the ruler into the notch through the AAM portal. The lower position of the AAM portal will allow the ruler to be positioned

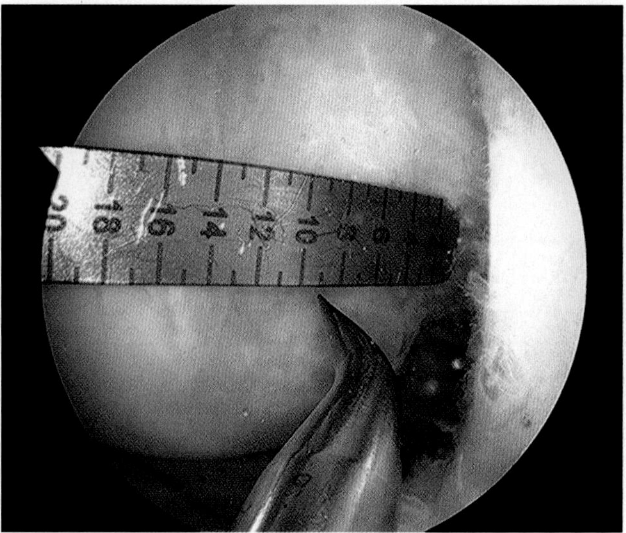

FIGURE 15-35

The "ruler" technique estimates the midbundle position of the ACL femoral attachment site as being 50% of the measured distance from the proximal articular cartilage margin to the shallow articular cartilage margin.

along the lower third of the lateral wall of the notch. The most common error when using the "ruler" technique is failing to position the ruler deep enough in the notch. This will result in the ACL femoral tunnel being positioned too shallow in the notch. An ACL graft positioned at this location will experience larger length changes and higher graft forces in extension. It is important to note that at 90 degrees of flexion, the native ACL femoral attachment site does not extend completely to the shallow (distal) or the inferior (posterior) articular cartilage margins. Measuring to the shallow articular cartilage margin therefore overestimates the true length of the ACL femoral attachment site. Using 50% of this measured length will result in the calculated center position being shallower than the true center of the attachment site. When measuring from the deep to the shallow articular cartilage margin, it is better to choose a final tunnel position that is 1 to 2 mm deeper than the calculated 50% position or a position that is 45% of the proximal-distal measurement. This will avoid having the ACL femoral tunnel being positioned too shallow in the ACL femoral attachment site.

Intraoperative fluoroscopy is the most accurate and reproducible method to position the bone tunnels for an ACL reconstruction (24,42,48–50). ACL tunnel placement using fluoroscopy does not depend on visualizing soft tissue or bony landmarks so this method is applicable in all situations. Fluoroscopy is especially valuable in chronic ACL ruptures where there may be no remnants of the native ACL present and in revision cases where the bony morphology of the ACL femoral attachment site has been altered or destroyed by prior notchplasty and/or malposition of the previous ACL femoral bone tunnel. Fluoroscopy is also extremely valuable when performing an augmentation technique for a single-bundle ACL tear or a remnant-preserving procedure. In these situations, identification of the bony ACL ridges is not feasible as exposure of the lateral wall of the notch would require removal of intact ACL fibers. The "ruler" method is also not applicable in this situation since the intact bundle or remnant tissue prevents accurate alignment of the ACL ruler along the lateral wall of the notch. Using fluoroscopy, the location of the ACL femoral tunnel can be easily determined without relying on soft tissue or bony landmarks.

The knee is positioned at 90 degrees of flexion and the lateral wall of the intercondylar notch is viewed through the AM portal. A 45-degree microfracture awl is passed into the intercondylar notch through the AAM portal and the tip of the awl is positioned along the lateral wall of the intercondylar notch at the proposed location for the center of the ACL femoral tunnel. When present and identified, anatomic landmarks such as the native ACL footprint and the ACL bony ridges can be used as references to help position the tip of the awl. A sterile-draped digital C-arm is used to take a true lateral radiograph of the knee. A true lateral radiograph is one where the inferior (posterior) and deep (proximal) borders of the medial and lateral femoral condyles overlap. Due to the size difference between the medial and lateral femoral condyles, it is often difficult to achieve a perfect overlap of the shallow (distal) borders of both condyles. However, this is not essential to obtain reliable information. A lateral C-arm image of the knee is taken and the initial position of the tip of the microfracture awl evaluated. The microfracture awl should be rotated so that the tip is clearly visible on the C-arm image. The location of the tip of the microfracture awl can be compared to a preoperatively planned ideal ACL femoral tunnel position or alternatively compared to data from published radiographic anatomic studies of the native ACL femoral attachment site. Any difference between the planned or desired femoral tunnel position and the achieved position can be corrected by adjusting the position of the tip of the microfracture awl under fluoroscopic guidance.

The grid system described by Bernard et al. (51) is used to plot the location of ACL femoral tunnel. This rectangular grid is applied to the lateral femoral condyle and allows any position along the inner wall of the lateral femoral condyle to be measured in the shallow-deep (distal-proximal) direction (x-axis) and the high-low (anterior-posterior) direction (y-axis). This method is easy to use and has been shown to be independent of the knee size, shape, and the distance between the x-ray tube and the patient (51). This measurement method is versatile and can be plotted on plain lateral knee radiographs, lateral C-arm images and CT images. Intra-and interobserver reliability of ACL femoral tunnel measurements on lateral CT images using the Bernard-Hertel grid has been found to be reliable (48). The Bernard-Hertel grid is drawn on a lateral knee radiographic image in the following way:

1. Draw a tangent to the roof of the intercondylar notch (Blumensaat's line).
2. Draw two lines perpendicular to the first line, one at the intersection of the tangent line with the shallow (distal) border of the lateral femoral condyle and the other with the intersection of the tangent line and the deep (proximal) border of the lateral femoral condyle. The lateral femoral condyle can be identified by an indentation at the distal margin (Grant's notch) and the fact that the medial femoral condyle extends more distally.
3. Draw another line parallel to Blumensaat's line and tangent to the inferior (posterior) border of the lateral femoral condyle.

Measurements of the ACL femoral tunnel position are made as percentages along Blumensaat's line (t), which represents the maximum sagittal diameter of the lateral femoral condyle, and line (h), which represents the maximum intercondylar notch height (Fig. 15-36).

The Bernard-Hertel grid method has been used to measure the location of the center of the PL and AM bundles in human cadaveric specimens (48,51–66). Using data from these published studies, a weighted average position for the center of the PL and AM bundles can be calculated (Table 15-1). Although the position of the center of the ACL femoral attachment site was directly measured in only a few of the studies, it is possible to perform a linear extrapolation of the location of the center position by assuming that the center of the ACL femoral attachment site lies halfway between the center of the PL and AM bundle attachment sites. The calculation for the extrapolated weighted average for the center of the ACL femoral attachment site across all the included studies reveals that the center of the ACL femoral attachment site is located at a point which is 28% along Blumensaat's line and 34% along the height of the intercondylar notch (Fig. 15-37). The weighted average location for the center of the PL and AM bundles and the extrapolated center of the ACL femoral attachment site can

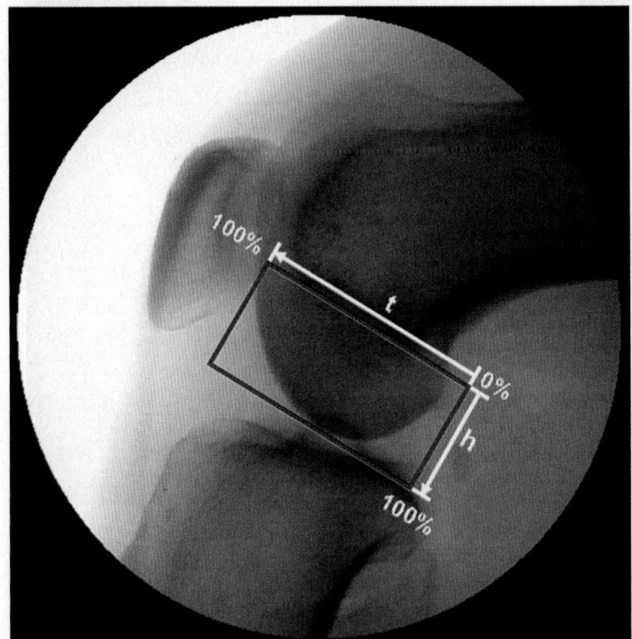

FIGURE 15-36

ACL femoral tunnel positions are plotted on the lateral C-arm image using the Bernard-Hertel grid. Measurements are made as percentages along Blumensaat's line (t) and the height of the intercondylar notch (h).

TABLE 15-1 Radiographic Measurements of the ACL Femoral Attachment Site

Author	*N*	AMB Depth (%)	PLB Depth (%)	Average Center Depth (%)	AMB Height (%)	PLB Height (%)	Average Center Height (%)
Bernard et al. (1997) (51)	10			24.8			28.5
Luites (2000) (64)	29	21.0	26.6	23.5	19.2	42.2	32.3
Musahl et al. (2003) (52)	8			27			28
Yamamoto et al. (2004) (53)	10	25	29	27	16	42	29
Columbet et al. (2006) (54)	7	26.4	32.3	29.4	25.3	47.6	36.5
Zantop et al. (2008) (55)	20	18.5	29.3	23.9	22.3	53.6	38.0
Tsukada et al. (2008) (56)	36	25.9	34.8	30.4	17.8	42.1	30.0
Lorenz et al. (2009) (57)	12	21	27	24	22	45	34
Forsythe et al. (2010) (58)	8	21.7	35.1	28.4	33.2	55.3	44.3
Iriuchishima et al. (2010) (59)	15	15	32	23.5	26	52	39
Pietrini et al. (2011) (60)	12	21.6	28.9	25.3	14.6	42.3	28.5
Moloney et al. (2013) (48)	20			33.7			32.0
Abreu-e-Silva et al. (2015) (61)	8			30.0			35.3
Lee et al. (2015) (62)	15	33.5	38.3	35.9	27.6	55.1	41.4
Luites and Verdonschot (2015) (64)	12	23.2	25.2	24.9	15.1	38.1	31.9
Davis et al. (2016) (65)	12	27.1	39.3	32.9	24.1	49.3	36.6
Weighted average	**234**	**23.2**	**31.4**	**27.8**	**21.1**	**46.3**	**33.7**

AMB, anteromedial bundle; PLB, posterolateral bundle.

be plotted on a preoperative lateral radiograph or a C-arm image and these images can be used as a reference to guide placement of the ACL femoral tunnel during surgery. Some authors have criticized using averaged data from radiographic anatomical studies to guide placement of the ACL bone tunnels in an individual patient (64). An individualized anatomic ACL reconstruction is best performed by identifying the native ACL footprint or bony anatomic ACL landmarks in each patient. However, this approach also has limitations since the native ACL footprint and anatomic bony landmarks may not always be present or be correctly identified by the surgeon. The goal of using intraoperative fluoroscopy is not necessarily to place the ACL bone tunnels in the same location in every patient, but rather to avoid unintended tunnel placements or unrecognized deviation in tunnel placements that might lead to failure of the ACL reconstruction.

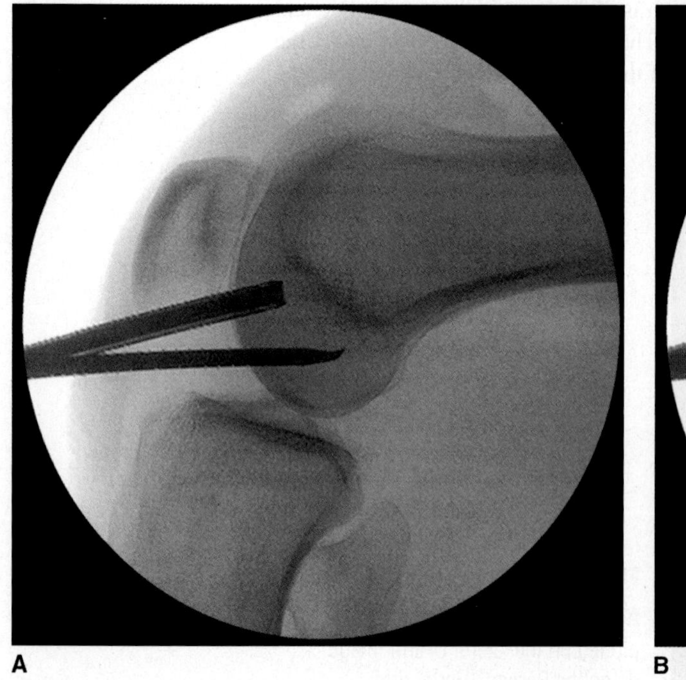

A

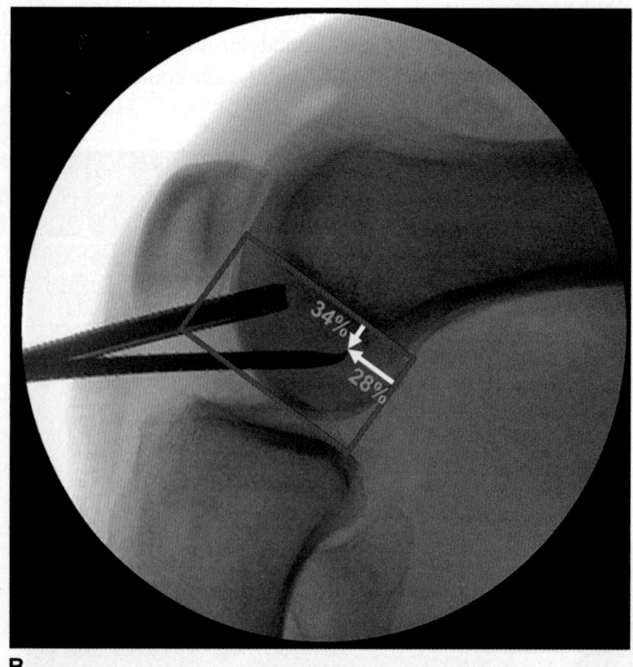

B

FIGURE 15-37

A: Intraoperative fluoroscopy image. The tip of the angled microfracture awl is positioned at the location of the center of the proposed ACL femoral tunnel. **B:** The tip of the microfracture awl is located at 28% along Blumensaat's line and 34% along the height of the intercondylar notch, which represents the center of the ACL femoral attachment site based on the weighted average of radiographic measurements.

Using any or all of the above methods eliminates the need to use the clock-face reference, an offset femoral aimer, and referencing from the "over-the-top" position to determine the location for the ACL femoral tunnel. ACL femoral offset aimers place the femoral guide pin a set number of millimeters from the over-the-top position and thus can lead to nonanatomic placement of the ACL femoral tunnel in some patients. The above methods allow the surgeon to individualize the placement of the ACL femoral tunnel using established anatomic and radiographic landmarks.

DRILLING THE ACL FEMORAL TUNNEL

The AM portal is used as the viewing portal and a 45-degree microfracture awl is inserted through the working AAM portal and a pilot hole is created at the chosen ACL femoral tunnel position. The knee is slowly flexed to greater than 120 degrees while keeping the microfracture awl in place in the pilot hole. The knee is stabilized in hyperflexion by placing the foot of the operative leg under the most proximal foot support. Positioning the knee in hyperflexion causes the ACL femoral attachment site to rotate, providing an excellent view of the low and deep aspects of the ACL femoral attachment site. Hyperflexion of the knee will often result in a loss of joint distention due to external compression of the joint capsule by the soft tissues of the thigh. This may cause bleeding and encroachment of the fat pad into the notch, which can comprise visualization during this critical part of the procedure. One solution to maintaining visualization is to increase the infusion pump pressure to 120 mm Hg. The pump pressure is decreased back to the normal setting after drilling the ACL femoral tunnel and the knee is extended back to 90 degrees. If the fat pad limits visualization, limited resection of the fat pad should be performed using a motorized shaver blade inserted through the AAM portal.

The microfracture awl is removed from the knee and a 0-degree offset femoral aimer inserted through the AAM portal and positioned at the previously created pilot hole. The offset femoral aimer is used only to pass the guide pin through the skin portal and fat pad and for directing the femoral guide pin, and it is not used to reference from the over-the-top position. A drill-tip graduated passing pin is passed through the 0-degree offset femoral aimer into the pilot hole and the guide pin tapped into the bone using a small mallet (Fig. 15-38). Avoid using power to initially drill the guide pin into the bone as this will cause the guide pin to skive out of the pilot hole. With the tip of the drill-tip guide pin in the pilot hole, the handle of the 0-degree offset aimer is slowly moved in a lateral direction and the guide pin tapped further into the bone until the drill-tip part of the pin is fully buried. This maneuver increases the obliquity of the guide pin relative to the lateral wall of the notch, resulting in a longer femoral tunnel length and also produces a more elliptically shaped femoral tunnel aperture. An elliptically shaped bone tunnel covers more of the ACL femoral attachment site and more closely reproduces the anatomy of the native ACL femoral attachment site versus a circular-shaped femoral tunnel. Guide pin breakage may occur if an attempt is made to simultaneously drill and change the angle of the guide pin. To prevent guide pin breakage, insure that the drill-tip portion of the guide pin is fully inserted into the bone before using power to drill the pin through the lateral femoral condyle. The drill-tip graduated passing pin is slowly drilled through the lateral femoral condyle until the resistance of the lateral femoral cortex is encountered. Note the depth mark on the passing pin at the lateral wall of the notch at the point of maximum resistance and cortical break through. This

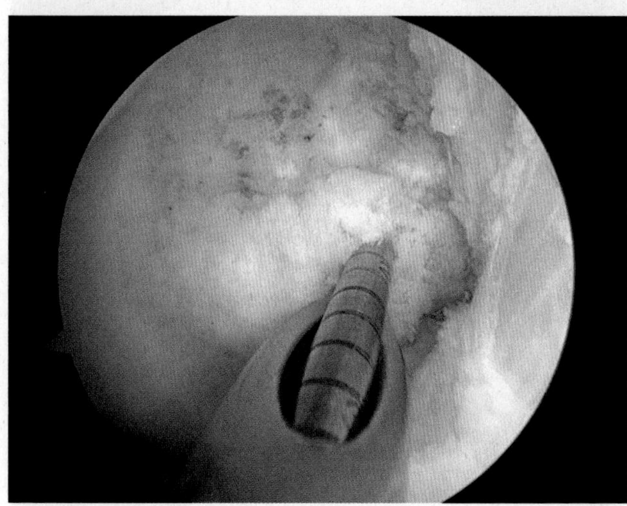

FIGURE 15-38

Anteromedial portal view of the ACL femoral attachment site with the knee in hyperflexion. A drill-tip graduated passing pin is passed through a 0-degree offset femoral aimer into a pilot hole created at the location of the center of the ACL femoral. The offset aimer is not used to locate the ACL femoral tunnel position but rather to direct the drill-tip passing pin through the AAM portal and to increase the obliquity of the guide pin relative to the lateral wall of the notch. The later step increases the length of the femoral tunnel.

distance will provide a good estimate of the ACL femoral tunnel length. Using the above technique, the femoral tunnel length should average 40 mm with a range from 35 to 45 mm. If the resulting ACL femoral tunnel length is less than desired, it is possible to increase the tunnel length by reversing the guide pin back to the entry point into the bone and redirecting the guide pin by moving the offset aimer more laterally and increasing the knee flexion angle. These maneuvers will redirect the guide pin more proximally up the femoral shaft, producing a longer femoral tunnel length.

A 4.5-mm ENDOBUTTON drill bit (Smith & Nephew Advanced Surgical Devices, Andover, MA) is used to drill a 4.5-mm femoral tunnel through the lateral femoral cortex. Visualization can be improved while drilling the ACL femoral tunnel by inserting a motorized shaver blade through the AL portal and suctioning bony debris from the notch. The shaver blade can also be used to resect parts of the fat pad restricting passage of the drill bit or obstructing visualization in the notch. The length of the ACL femoral tunnel may again be estimated using the measurement scale on the ENDOBUTTON drill bit at the time of cortical break through. The femoral socket is drilled with a low-profile single-fluted endoscopic drill bit the same size as the measured diameter of the femoral end of the hamstring tendon graft (Fig. 15-39). Single-fluted drill bits are easier to pass through the AAM portal and are less likely to cause injury to the medial femoral condyle or meniscus. For the ENDOBUTTON CL ULTRA implant, the minimum depth of the ACL femoral socket must equal the amount of ACL graft to be inserted into the ACL femoral socket plus an additional distance of 6 mm to allow the ENDOBUTTON implant to pass out of the femoral tunnel and flip on the lateral femoral cortex. Assuming a femoral tunnel length of 40 mm and a 15-mm ENDOBUTTON CL ULTRA implant, the femoral socket must be drilled at least 25 mm + 6 mm = 31 mm. In practice, these calculations can be eliminated by drilling the ACL femoral socket up to but not through the lateral femoral cortex. The endoscopic drill bit is removed from the knee joint and a full-length number 2 or 5 polyester passing suture threaded through the eyelet of the passing pin. The free ends of the passing suture are pulled out through the lateral soft tissues of the thigh, leaving the loop of the suture in the femoral socket. An ENDOBUTTON depth probe (Smith & Nephew Advanced Surgical Devices, Andover, MA) is inserted through the AAM portal and used to measure the true length of the femoral tunnel. The tunnel edges at the entrance of the femoral socket are beveled with an ACL chamfer rasp to minimize graft abrasion. In chronic cases with notch osteophytes or in patients with small notches, a limited wallplasty at the shallow border of the notch is performed using a small curved compound gouge, curette, and/or a motorized shaver blade and burr (Fig. 15-40).

Preparation of the ACL Tibial Attachment Site

The direct insertion of the ACL fibers at the tibial attachment site has recently been reported to be C-shaped rather than oval shaped (67). The direct tibial insertion of the ACL runs just anterior to the medial tibial tubercle (spine) and curves to the anterior aspect of the anterior root attachment of the lateral meniscus. The posterior border of the direct tibial insertion of the ACL lies just anterior to a bony ridge connecting the medial and lateral tubercles (intercondylar eminence). The tibial

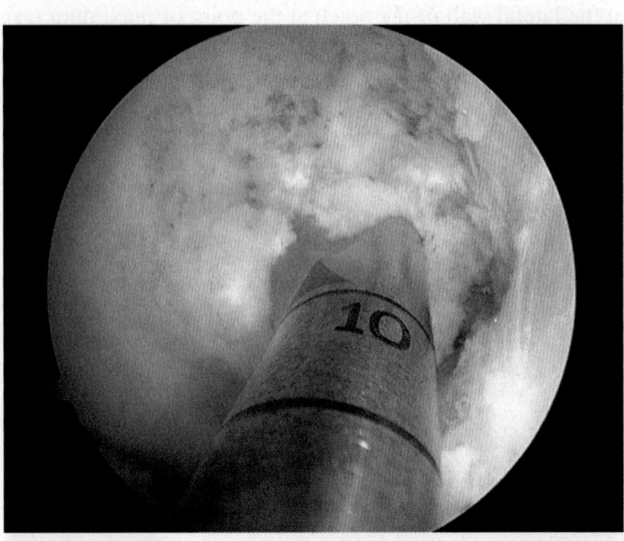

FIGURE 15-39

AM portal view of the ACL femoral attachment site in hyperflexion. Drilling the femoral tunnel with a single-fluted drill. Viewing the ACL femoral attachment site through the AM portal allows the surgeon to see exactly what part of the ACL footprint will be covered by the femoral tunnel.

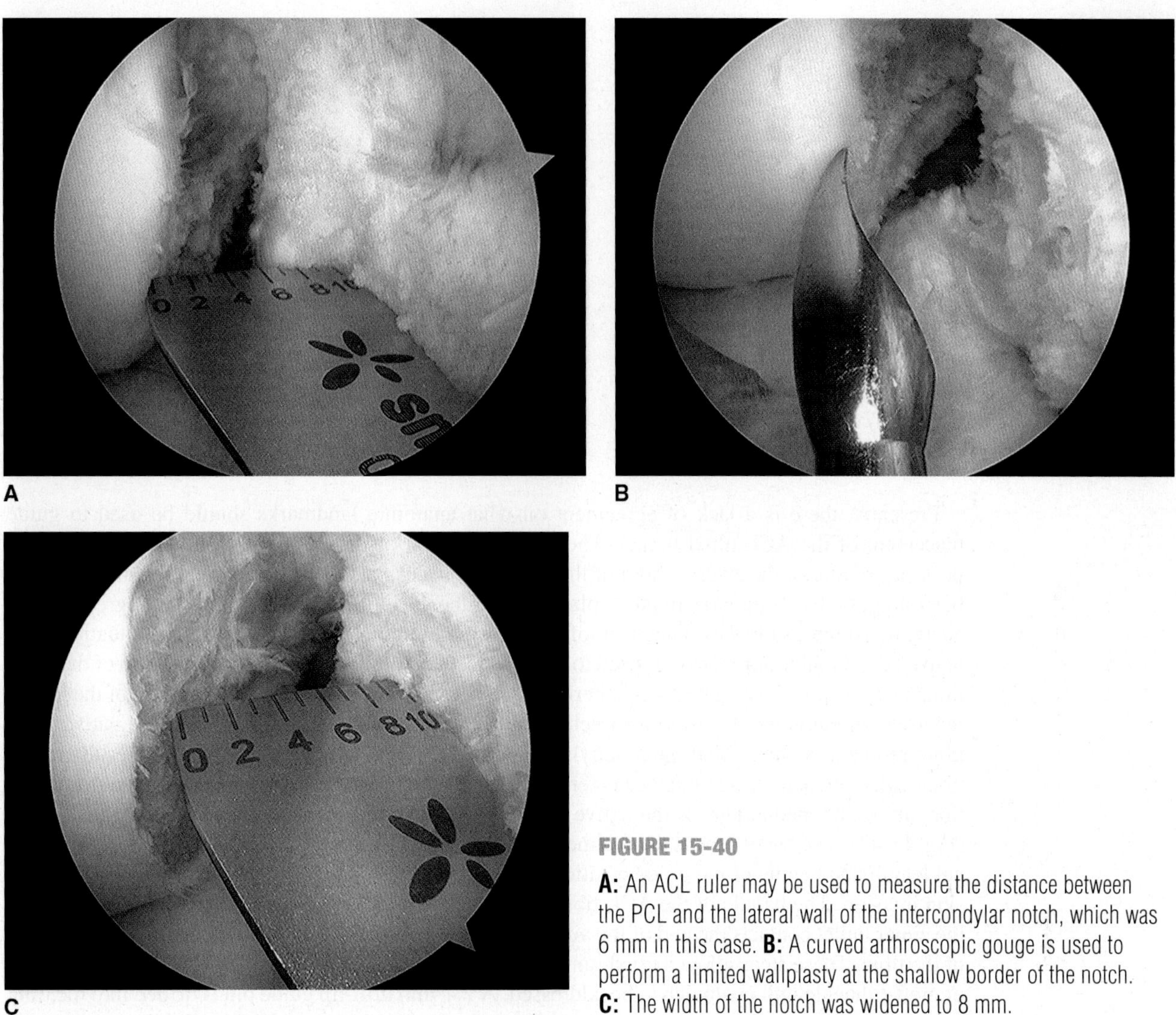

FIGURE 15-40

A: An ACL ruler may be used to measure the distance between the PCL and the lateral wall of the intercondylar notch, which was 6 mm in this case. **B:** A curved arthroscopic gouge is used to perform a limited wallplasty at the shallow border of the notch. **C:** The width of the notch was widened to 8 mm.

attachment of the ACL does not insert directly on the medial or lateral tibial tubercles. The medial border of the ACL tibial attachment site is defined by a bony ridge, the medial intercondylar ridge of the tibia, which extends anteriorly from the medial tubercle. The lateral border blends with the anterior horn of the lateral meniscus (Fig. 15-41). The length and width of the ACL tibial attachment site can be measured by inserting an ACL ruler through the AAM portal. Attachment site lengths greater than 14 mm are best restored with 5- or 6-strand hamstring tendon grafts.

Drilling the Tibial Tunnel

The tibial tunnel is drilled with the knee at 50 to 70 of flexion. This position improves visualization of the anterior aspect of the ACL tibial attachment site. In the traditional approach for drilling the ACL tibial tunnel, the AL portal is used as the viewing portal and the ACL tibial aimer is inserted into the knee joint through the AM portal. When the AL portal is used as the viewing portal, the arthroscope is positioned lateral to the ACL tibial attachment site, resulting in an oblique view. Using the AM portal as the viewing portal positions the arthroscope directly over the ACL tibial attachment site, resulting in an orthogonal view. This approach allows for more accurate assessment of the tibial guide pin position within the ACL tibial attachment site in both the anterior-posterior and medial-lateral directions. When the AM portal is used as the viewing portal, the ACL tibial aimer can be inserted into the knee joint through the AAM portal. This results in the arm of the ACL tibial aimer being oriented parallel to the medial tibial plateau, making it easier to drill longer tibial tunnels. The ACL tibial aimer is set at a 55-degree angle and the tip of the aimer is inserted through the working AAM portal into the knee joint.

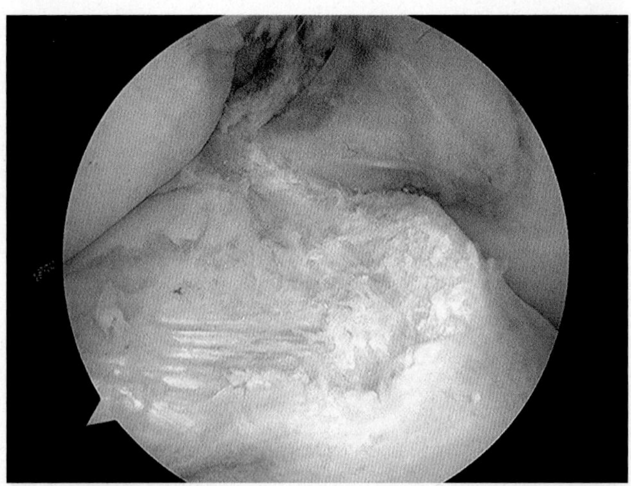

FIGURE 15-41

Arthroscopic view of the "C-shaped" ACL tibial attachment site in a right knee. The ACL fibers are densest along the medial intercondylar ridge of the tibia. Note the intimate relationship with the anterior lateral meniscus root attachment. Drilling the ACL tibial tunnel too laterally may result in iatrogenic injury to this structure.

Presently, there is a lack of agreement on what anatomic landmarks should be used to guide placement of the ACL tibial tunnel. The anterior margin of the PCL, the medial tibial spine, the posterior border of the anterior horn of the lateral meniscus, and the intermeniscal ligament have all been suggested as landmarks to guide placement of the ACL tibial tunnel. The lack of agreement on anatomic landmarks makes placement of the ACL tibial tunnel challenging. In most situations, the native ACL tibial footprint can be used to guide placement of the tibial guide pin. The tip of the ACL tibial aimer is positioned 2 to 3 mm anterior to the posterior margin of the anterior horn of the lateral meniscus in the anterior-posterior direction and 2 mm lateral to medial border of the native ACL tibial remnant or the medial intercondylar ridge of the tibia. This location typically results in the tibial guide pin being placed in the center of the tibial attachment site in the anterior-posterior direction and in the medial part of the native ACL tibial attachment site in the medial-lateral direction (Fig. 15-42). The bullet for the tibial aimer is marked with a surgical marker at the desired tibial tunnel length and handle of the guide positioned in the center of the vertical hamstring tendon harvest skin incision. The handle of the ACL tibial aimer is raised or lowered until the marked position on the aimer bullet contacts the end of the aimer handle when the bullet is flush with the anterior cortex of the tibia. These steps allow a tibial tunnel of a known length to be drilled, thus allowing the issue of graft-tunnel length mismatch to be addressed. A 2.4-mm drill-tip guide pin is drilled into the tibia until the resistance of the aimer tip is encountered. Avoid drilling the tibial guide pin completely into the knee joint as this will result in the guide pin hitting the tip of the aimer and deflecting away

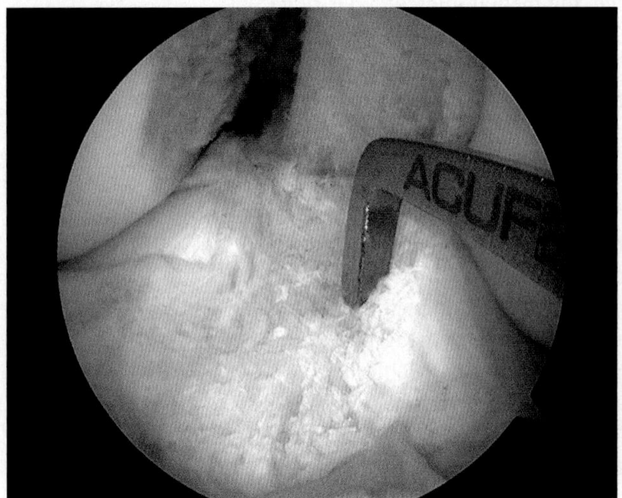

A

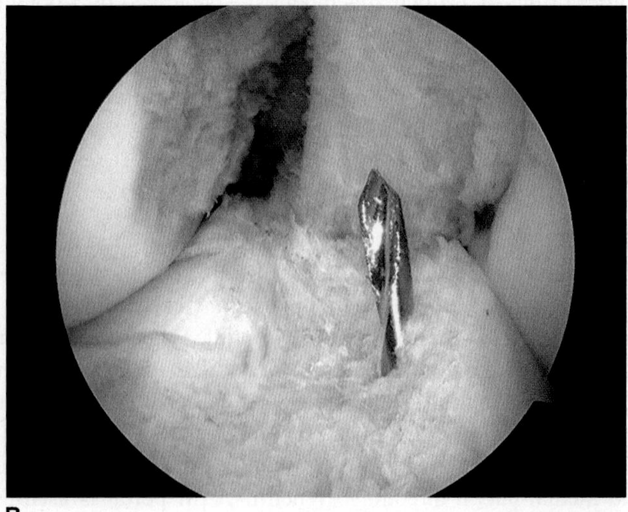

B

FIGURE 15-42

A: View through the AM portal. The tip of the tibial aimer is positioned as medially as possible and 2 to 3 mm anterior to the posterior margin of the anterior horn of the lateral meniscus and slightly medial to the medial intercondylar ridge of the tibia. **B:** Resulting tibial guide pin position.

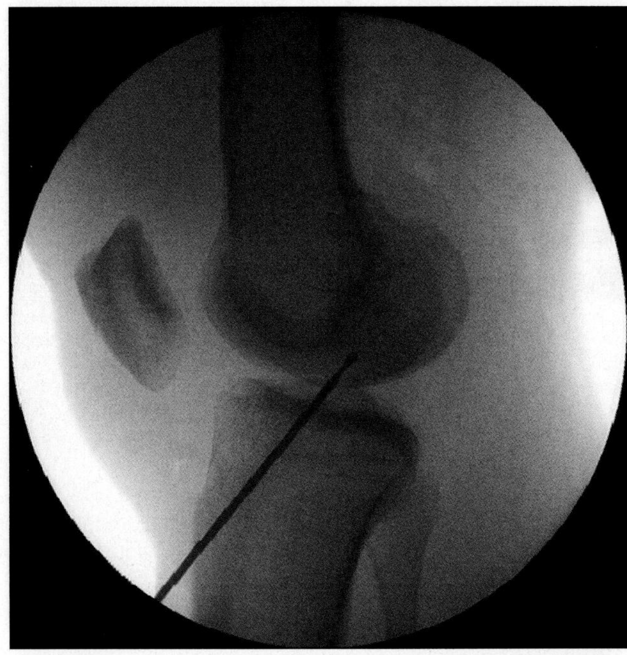

FIGURE 15-43

Lateral c-arm image. The posterior borders of the medial and lateral tibial condyles are overlapping and the concave medial joint line is clearly seen. The tibial guide pin is located parallel and posterior to Blumensaat's line (impingement free tibial tunnel).

from its intended target. Instead, remove the tibial aimer from the joint and use a small mallet to tap the guide pin until it is visible in the joint.

Fluoroscopy is the most accurate way to assessment placement of the tibial guide pin position (68). The location of the tibial guide pin in the sagittal plane is determined by taking a lateral C-arm image of the knee in maximum extension or 90 degrees of flexion as described earlier for the ACL femoral tunnel. One advantage of evaluating the tibial guide pin position in maximum extension is that the guide pin position can be accessed for roof impingement by checking the relationship of the guide pin to Blumensaat's line. The knee is extended and held in maximum extension and a lateral image of the knee is obtained (Fig. 15-43). The goal is to obtain a lateral view of the tibia with the posterior borders of the medial and lateral tibial condyles overlapping. Internally or externally rotating the knee will adjust the overlap of the posterior borders of the medial and lateral tibial and femoral condyles, while abducting and adducting the knee affects the overlap of the medial and lateral joint lines and the proximal borders of the medial and lateral tibial condyles. Although one should aim to obtain a perfect image with complete overlap of the posterior borders of the tibial condyles, small amounts of malrotation can be accepted. An alternative method for checking the position of the tibial guide pin is to insert the tip of the ACL tibial aimer at the desired location in the ACL tibial attachment site and to take a lateral C-arm image with the knee at 90 degrees of flexion (Fig. 15-44). An advantage of this method is that the tip of the ACL tibial aimer can be adjusted under fluoroscopic control until the desired sagittal position of the ACL tibial tunnel is achieved. Once the desired position is achieved, the guide pin is then drilled into position. This method eliminates the possibility of drilling an errant tibial guide pin and having to reposition it. However, a disadvantage of this method is that the relationship of the guide pin to Blumensaat's line cannot be established with the knee at 90 degrees of flexion. If this information is desired, then the knee will need to be placed in maximum extension and a new lateral C-arm image taken. It is possible to use intraoperative fluoroscopy to check the medial-lateral position of the tibial guide pin. However, this will require rotating the C-arm to take an anterior-posterior image of the knee. In our experience, the medial-lateral position of the tibial guide pin can be reliably assessed arthroscopically.

The position of the tibial guide pin is measured using the method of Amis and Jakob (69). In this method, a line is drawn from the highest point of the anterior aspect of the medial tibial joint line to the highest point of the posterior aspect of the medial tibial joint line. The medial joint line is identified by the fact that the medial tibial condyle is concave. The Amis-Jakob line is drawn from the anterior aspect of the tibia to the posterior corner of the widest part of the medial tibial condyle parallel to the previously placed line marking the medial joint line. The posterior aspect of the medial tibial condyle is indentified by the fact that the posterior contour is squared off, while the posteror aspect of the lateral

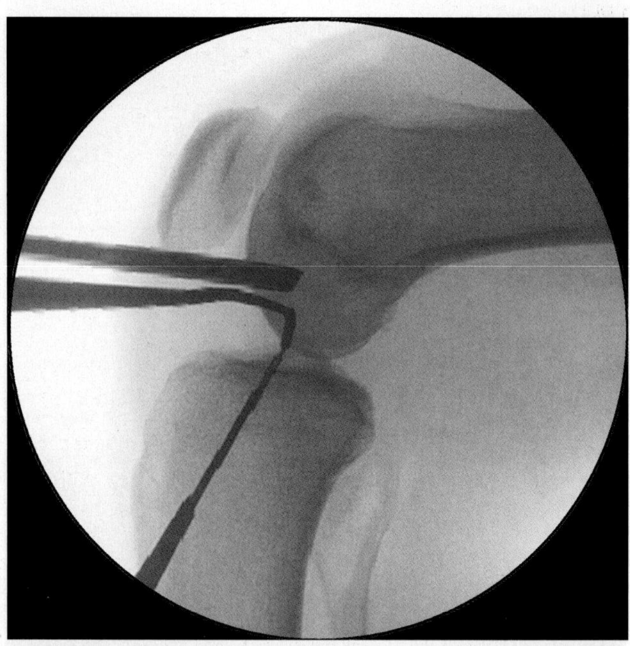

FIGURE 15-44

Lateral fluoroscopy image of the tibial aimer and guide pin, taken with the knee at 90 degrees of flexion, demonstrating correct guide pin placement.

tibial condyle has a downward slope. The anterior tibial cortex represents 0% and the posterior tibial cortex 100% of the sagittal width of the tibia. The tibial guide pin position is calculated by dropping an orthogonal line from the point where the tibial guide pin crosses the medial joint line onto the Amis-Jakob line. The distance from the anterior tibial cortex (0%) to the orthogonal projection onto the Amis-Jakob line is represented as a percentage of the total length of the Amis-Jakob. The goal is to place the tibial guide pin in the center of the ACL tibial insertion site (Fig. 15-45). The location of the centers of the AM and PL bundles and the center of the ACL tibial attachment site has been measured using the Amis-Jakob line and the anterior-posterior diameter of the tibia on cadavers, on patients undergoing surgery, and on the normal population using radiographs, CT, and MRI (66,70–74) (Table 15-2). The weighted average position of the center of the ACL tibial attachment site based on published x-ray studies that used the Amis-Jakob line as the measurement method is 40% (Table 15-3).

It is possible to "fine-tune" the final tibial tunnel position by incrementally increasing the diameter of the tibial tunnel and drilling eccentrically. A clamp is inserted through the AL portal and the tip of the guide pin grasped. A preliminary tibial tunnel is drilled with a small diameter drill bit such as a 5-mm fully fluted cannulated drill bit. The guide pin is repositioned

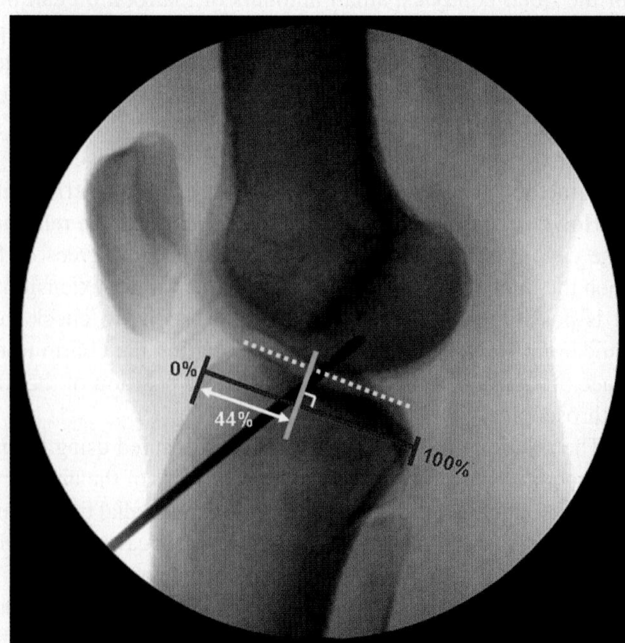

FIGURE 15-45

The position of the tibial guide pin can be measured as a percentage distance along Amis and Jacob's line (drawn parallel to the medial joint surface at the widest part of the tibia on a true lateral radiograph).

TABLE 15-2 Radiographic Measurements of the ACL Tibial Attachment Site

Author	Methods	N	Evaluation Method	Average AMB Center	Average PLB Center	Average ACL Center
Staubli et al. (1994) (70)	Cadaver	10	AP width tibia			41.2%
	Cryosection	5				43.3%
	MRI (male)	23				44.1%
	MRI (female)	12				43.7%
Musahl et al. (2003) (52)	Cadaver: radiograph	8	AP width tibia			46.2%
	Cadaver: CT scan	8	AP width tibia			45.4%
Columbet et al. (2006) (54)	Cadaver: radiograph	7	Amis-Jakob line	36%	52%	
Zantop et al. (2008) (55)	Cadaver: radiograph	20	Amis-Jakob line	30%	44%	
Doi et al. (2009) (71)	Cadaver: radiograph	31	Amis-Jakob line	34.6%	38.4%	
Lorenz et al. (2009) (57)	Cadaver: CT scan	12	AP width tibia	41%	52%	
Forsythe et al. (2010) (58)	Cadaver: CT scan	8	AP width tibia	25%	46.4%	
Iriuchishima et al. (2010) (59)	Cadaver: radiograph	15	AP width tibia	31%	50%	
Frank et al. (2010) (72)	Normal population: MRI	100	AP width tibia			46%
Kasten et al. (68) (2010)	Surgery: C-arm	67	Amis-Jakob line	35%	48%	41%
Pietrini et al. (2011) (60)	Cadaver: radiograph	12	Amis-Jakob line	36.3%	51.0%	
Scheffel et al. (2012) (73)	Normal population: MRI	138	AP width tibia			44.1%
Lee et al. (2015) (62)	Cadaver: dissection	8	AP width tibia	37.6%	43.8%	
	Cadaver: radiograph			36.3%	43.4%	
	Cadaver: CT scan			36.7%	42.2%	
Abreu-e-Silva et al. (2015) (61)	Cadaver: CT scan	8	AP width tibia			40.5%
Parkinson et al. (2015) (74)	Normal population: MRI	76	Amis-Jakob line			39%
	Normal population: CT	26				38%

eccentrically in the desired direction within the drilled tunnel using the clamp and the tunnel sequentially drilled by 1-mm increments using fully fluted cannulated drill bits up to the desired size of the tunnel (Fig. 15-46). An ACL rasp is used to smooth the edges of the tunnel to minimize abrasion and soft tissue is cleared from around the tunnel using a motorized shaver blade.

Graft Passage

An arthroscopic probe or grasper is used to retrieve the suture loop that was left in the ACL femoral tunnel and the suture is pulled out of the tibial tunnel. The passing and flipping sutures on the ENDOBUTTON implant are passed through the suture loop and pulled out through the lateral thigh. Traction is applied to the ENDOBUTTON passing sutures and the hamstring tendon graft is pulled into the knee joint and then into the femoral socket. The graft is pulled into the femoral socket until the mark placed at the femoral tunnel length is advanced into the femoral socket. The ENDOBUTTON CL ULTRA implant is anchored on the lateral femoral cortex using the flipping suture attached to the implant. The flipping suture is pulled in a proximal direction parallel to the femoral tunnel and the ENDOBUTTON will be felt to flip against the lateral femoral cortex. Successful deployment of the ENDOBUTTON can be verified by the simultaneously pulling on the passing and flipping sutures and feeling the ENDOBUTTON "seesaw" against the lateral femoral cortex. If any doubt exists about successful deployment of the ENDOBUTTON, intraoperative fluoroscopy or an x-ray can be used to confirm the position of the ENDOBUTTON implant.

TABLE 15-3 Radiographic Measurements of the ACL Tibial Attachment Site using the Amis-Jakob Line

Author	Methods	N	Evaluation Method	Average AMB Center	Average PLB Center	Average ACL Center
Columbet et al. (2006) (54)	Cadaver: radiograph	7	Amis-Jakob line	36%	52%	44%
Zantop et al. (2008) (55)	Cadaver: radiograph	20	Amis-Jakob line	30%	44%	37%
Doi et al. (2009) (71)	Cadaver: radiograph	31	Amis-Jakob line	34.6%	38.4%	36.5%
Kasten et al. (2010) (68)	Surgery: C-arm	67	Amis-Jakob line	35%	48%	41.5%
Pietrini et al. (2011) (60)	Cadaver: radiograph	12	Amis-Jakob line	36.3%	51.0%	43.6%
Weighted average		**137**		**34.3%**	**45.7%**	**40.2%**

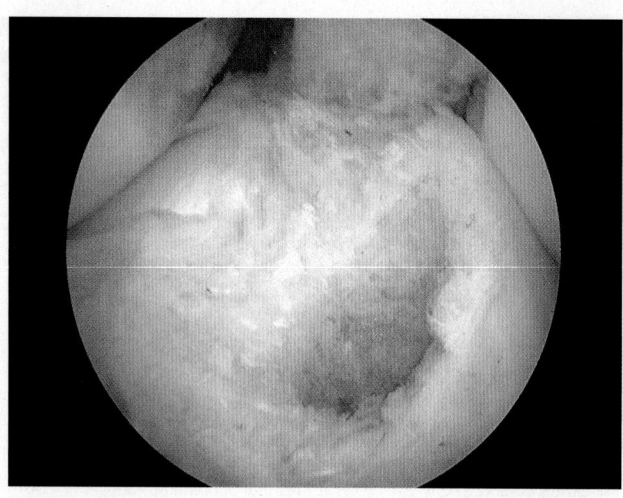

FIGURE 15-46

Final position of the ACL tibial tunnel. Eccentric drilling results in an elliptically shaped tibial tunnel. The medial edge of the tunnel is positioned as far medially as possible within the native ACL tibial attachment site. This avoids injury to the attachment of the anterior horn of the lateral meniscus.

Graft Tensioning and Fixation

The Dacron tape/suture loops from opposite ends of the hamstring tendon graft are looped around the arms of a graft tensioning device (Smith & Nephew Advanced Surgical Devices, Andover, MA). The spring-loaded connecting handle is used to apply a preload of 80 to 100 N to the graft. The knee is cycled from 0 to 90 degrees with an 80- to 100-N preload for a minimum of 30 cycles. Applying a preload and cycling the knee are important steps as they insure that the ENDOBUTTON implant sits flush on the lateral femoral cortex. In addition, preloading the graft and cycling the knee allows stress relaxation of the polyester continuous loop, the tendon whipstitches, and the hamstring tendon graft. At the present time, the optimal graft tension and knee flexion angle for a single-bundle ACL reconstruction are unknown. The usual graft excursion pattern for a femoral tunnel positioned near the center of the ACL attachment site results in the ACL graft tightening (pulling into the tibial tunnel) during the last 30 degrees of extension. In this situation, the graft is fixed at 20 degrees of flexion with a posterior force applied to the anterior tibia to hold the tibia in a reduced position.

The tibial end of the graft is fixed with a plastic or resorbable 30-mm–length tapered interference screw such as a GTS-tapered screw (Smith & Nephew Advanced Surgical Devices, Andover, MA). This screw comes in two sizes, 7 to 9 mm × 30 mm and 8 to 10 mm × 30 mm. The 7- to 9-mm screw is typically used for 8.5 mm or smaller diameter grafts and the 8 to 10 screws for grafts greater than 8.5 mm. The knee is extended and rested on the two L-shaped foot supports that can be adjusted at the beginning of the operation to maintain the knee in 20 degrees of flexion. The hamstring tendon graft is tensioned at 60 N for a 4- or 5-strand hamstring tendon graft and 70 to 80 N for 6-strand hamstring tendon grafts. The guide wire is inserted posterior to the hamstring tendon graft and parallel to the long axis of the tibial tunnel. While maintaining the desired tension on the ACL graft using the graft tensioning device (Fig. 15-47), the tibia is held in a reduced position by applying a posteriorly directed force to the proximal tibia and the GTS-tapered screw is screwed into the tibial tunnel

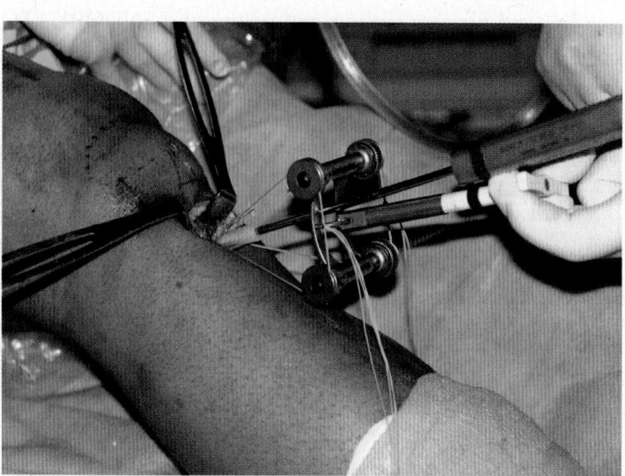

FIGURE 15-47

Tibial interference screw insertion. Tension on the ACL graft is maintained with the aid of a graft tensioning device.

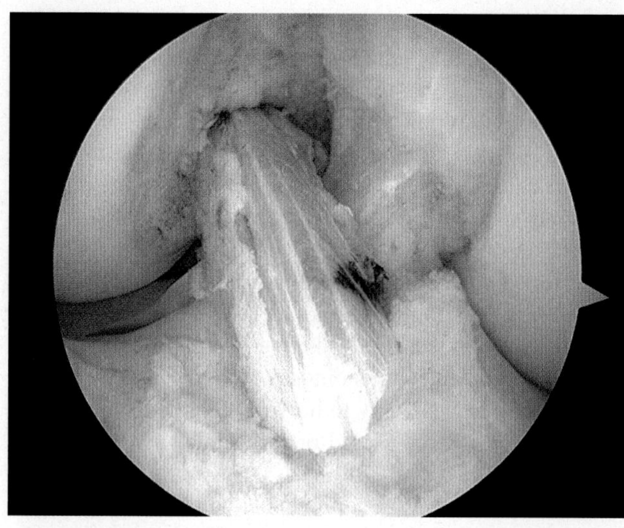

FIGURE 15-48

Anteromedial portal view with the knee in the figure-four position. The hamstring ACL graft can be seen to be positioned in the anatomic footprint of the native ACL.

until the end of the screw is buried just below the cortex. If the surgeon feels that there is inadequate screw insertion torque during insertion of the interference screw, supplemental tibial fixation using a small barbed staple or tying the graft sutures around an AO screw and washer may be considered. The stability and range of motion of the knee are checked. It is important to verify that the patient has full range of motion and the pivot shift test is negative. The arthroscope is inserted back into the joint to document the absence of wall or roof impingement (Fig. 15-48).

Closure

The arthroscope sheath is inserted back into the knee joint through the AL portal and a Hemovac drainage tube inserted through the sheath into the suprapatellar pouch. A second Hemovac drain is inserted under the sartorius fascia up into the hamstring harvest site. The L-shaped flap of sartorius fascia is sutured back to the crest of the tibia and over the MCL with a 0 absorbable suture. The subcutaneous tissue is closed in layers with a 2-0 undyed absorbable suture. The arthroscopic portals are closed with a 3-0 nylon suture. A running subcuticular suture produces a cosmetic closure. A single 4″ × 8″ gauze pad is placed over the hamstring tendon harvest incision and the arthroscopic portals, followed by a cotton compression dressing. A thigh-length TED stocking is applied to the leg followed by an extension splint.

AUGMENTATION AND REMNANT-PRESERVING TECHNIQUE

Augmentation of a single-bundle ACL tear or preservation of remnant ACL tissue is performed using similar principles and surgical technique as described for a single-bundle ACL reconstruction. However, these procedures are more technically demanding due to the following reasons:

- Visualization in the intercondylar notch is restricted due to the intact ACL fibers.
- Anatomic bone tunnel placement is more difficult due to the inability to reference from soft tissue and bony landmarks.
- Special care must be taken to protect and preserve the intact ACL fibers.

Indications for an augmentation or remnant-preserving procedure include a one-bundle AM or PL bundle tear and complete ACL tears with tissue remnants, which maintain an intact bridge of tissue between the tibia and lateral wall of the notch or the tibia and the PCL. Augmentation and remnant preservation have several potential advantages: preservation of remnant tissue that contains mechanoreceptors may enhance proprioceptive function of the knee, remnant tissue may aid healing of the ACL graft, and the intact bundle or remnant tissue may contribute to biomechanical stability of the knee (40).

Diagnostic arthroscopy is performed prior to hamstring tendon graft harvest when there is suspicion of a partial ACL tear based on the presence of a low-grade Lachman and pivot shift test or MRI findings. The low-grade clinical laxity tests are the result of either a tear of one of the ACL bundles and the remaining bundle is intact or stretched or both bundles are torn and the ruptured ACL fibers have become adherent and scarred to the PCL or the wall or roof of the intercondylar notch. Careful probing of the torn ACL fibers is necessary to determine which of the above possibilities exist. It is important to keep in mind that even in the situation of a one-bundle ACL tear, the remaining intact bundle or remnant fibers are unlikely to have normal biomechanical function. Therefore, the surgeon should not compromise placement of the ACL bone tunnels for the sack of preserving tissue that may ultimately contribute little biomechanical stability. If there is any doubt about the integrity or quality of the remaining bundle or remnant tissue or there is difficulty achieving anatomic bone tunnel placement, it is advisable to revert to the approach described earlier for a complete ACL tear.

The ideal hamstring tendon graft diameter for an augmentation or remnant-preserving procedure is 8 to 9 mm. Grafts in this size range are easier to pass through or adjacent to the intact bundle or remnant tissue. In addition, bone tunnels in this size range are less likely to injure the intact bundle or remnant tissue. In many cases, a tripled or quadrupled semitendinosus tendon graft can achieve a graft diameter in this size range. However, it may be necessary to harvest the gracilis tendon and construct a 4-, 5-, or 6-strand hamstring tendon graft if the tripled or quadrupled semitendinosus tendon graft is less than 8 mm.

Visualization while working in the notch is more limited due to the intact bundle or remnant tissue, and therefore, care needs to be taken to avoid injury to the intact bundle or remnant tissue when using a motorized shaver or an RF wand. Preparation of the intercondylar notch is performed as previously described for a single-bundle ACL reconstruction. When drilling the ACL femoral tunnel, the AM portal is used as the viewing portal and the AAM portal as the working portal. With a one-bundle tear, the center of the attachment site of the torn bundle is marked with a microfracture awl or RF wand. It is important to remember that in a one-bundle tear, the intact bundle is unlikely to have normal biomechanical function (40). Therefore, the goal of the procedure is not simply to replace the torn bundle, but rather, to augment the partially functioning intact bundle with a biomechanically functioning ACL graft. When performing an augmentation technique for a one-bundle tear, the femoral bone tunnel should not be placed exactly at the center of the torn bundle but rather it should be placed at a location that will also partially restore the attachment site of the intact bundle. According to Kazusa et al. (40), one-quarter of the new bone tunnel should lie in the attachment site area of the intact bundle. In the situation of a complete ACL tear with an intact remnant, the remnant is left untouched and the native ACL femoral attachment site is prepared using a motorized shaver and RF wand as previously described for a single-bundle ACL reconstruction. The remnant ACL fibers usually adhere to the lateral border of the PCL or along the roof or lateral wall of the notch. In either case, these intact ACL fibers are nonanatomic and will not provide normal biomechanical function. In this situation, the recommendations for anatomic single-bundle femoral tunnel placement as described earlier should be followed.

When trying to preserve intact ACL fibers, femoral tunnel placement strategies such as referencing from the native footprint; the shallow, deep, and inferior cartilage borders; and the bony ACL ridges or using an ACL ruler are all impractical as the intact fibers limit access to these landmarks (Fig. 15-49). Intraoperative fluoroscopy is the most accurate and reliable method to insure that the bone tunnels are placed at the desired position. ACL bone tunnel placement using fluoroscopy does

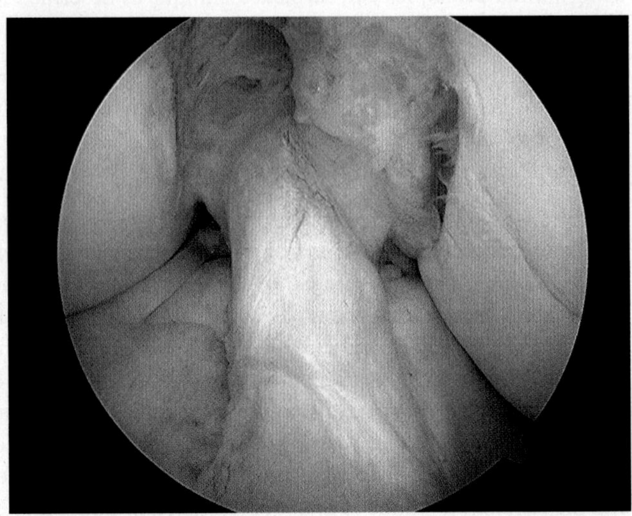

FIGURE 15-49

AM portal view. The intact ACL remnant obscures the usual landmarks used for placement of the ACL femoral tunnel.

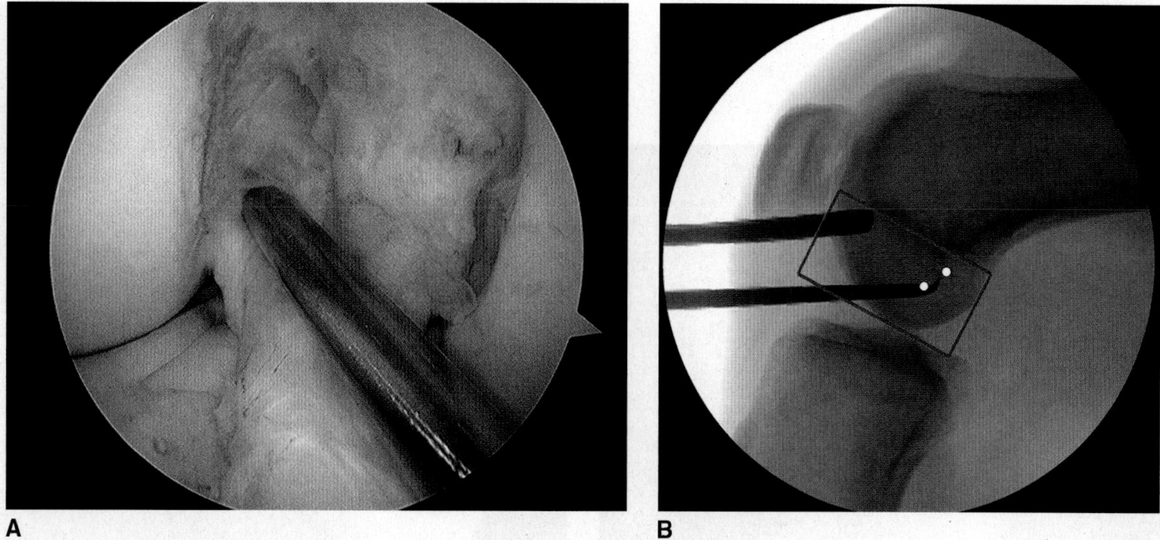

FIGURE 15-50

A: AM portal view. The tip of an angled microfracture awl is placed at the proposed ACL femoral tunnel position. **B:** The position of the microfracture awl is determined using fluoroscopy. In this case, a position between the center of the AM and PL bundles (*white circles*) has been selected.

not rely on referencing off of soft tissue or bony landmarks, and this method can be used in the presence of an intact bundle or intact remnant fibers. While viewing the ACL femoral attachment site through the AM portal, a 45-degree microfracture awl is inserted into the intercondylar notch through the working AAM portal. The tip of the microfracture awl is placed at the chosen ACL femoral tunnel location and a true lateral fluoroscopic image taken. The awl position is analyzed (Fig. 15-50) using the Bernard-Hertel grid and data from published anatomical studies (51–66) (Table 15-1). The awl location can be repositioned under fluoroscopic guidance until the desired ACL femoral tunnel position is achieved. Once identified, a pilot hole is created at the desired ACL femoral tunnel location using the microfracture awl. The femoral tunnel is drilled as previously described for an anatomic single-bundle ACL reconstruction. To minimize trauma to the intact ACL fibers, it is helpful to use low-profile single-fluted endoscopic reamers or smooth tunnel dilators when drilling the ACL femoral tunnel. A #2 or #5 polyester passing suture is passed out through the lateral thigh and the looped end of the suture left at the entrance of the femoral tunnel. This suture will be retrieved and used to pass the ACL graft after the tibial tunnel is drilled.

The tibial tunnel is drilled using the AM or AL portal as the viewing portal and the ACL tibial aimer is introduced into the knee through the AAM portal. To ease instrument passage, the AAM portal is dilated using the tips of Metzenbaum scissors. A #15 knife blade on a long handle is inserted into the knee joint through the AAM portal and a longitudinal slit is made in the tibial remnant. The slit is made in the middle of the tibial remnant for a PL bundle augmentation or a remnant-preserving procedure. This will allow the tibial guide pin to be positioned in the center of the ACL tibial attachment site. For an AM bundle augmentation, the slit should be made in the anterior and medial part of the tibial remnant. This will allow the tibial guide pin to be positioned in area of the AM bundle tibial attachment site. An ACL tibial guide is inserted into the knee joint through the AAM portal and the tip of the aimer passed through the slit in the tibial remnant and positioned on the bone at the desired location in the tibial attachment site. It is helpful to use an elbow ACL tibial aimer as this will allow the tip of the guide pin to be visualized. The length of the tibial tunnel is adjusted as previously described for a single-bundle ACL reconstruction, and a 2.4-mm drill-tip guide pin is drilled into the joint until it can be felt to contact the aimer tip. The ACL tibial aimer is removed from the joint and a small curved clamp is inserted through the AAM portal and used to spread the slit in the intact ACL fibers open. The guide pin is tapped into the tibia using a small mallet until the tip of the guide pin can be seen to pass through the slit and exit into the ACL tibial attachment site. Proper placement of the tibial guide pin is confirmed by taking a true lateral C-arm image (Fig. 15-51). The tip of the tibial guide pin is grasped with curved clamp and the tibial tunnel drilled with a small diameter drill bit such as a 4.5-mm ENDOBUTTON

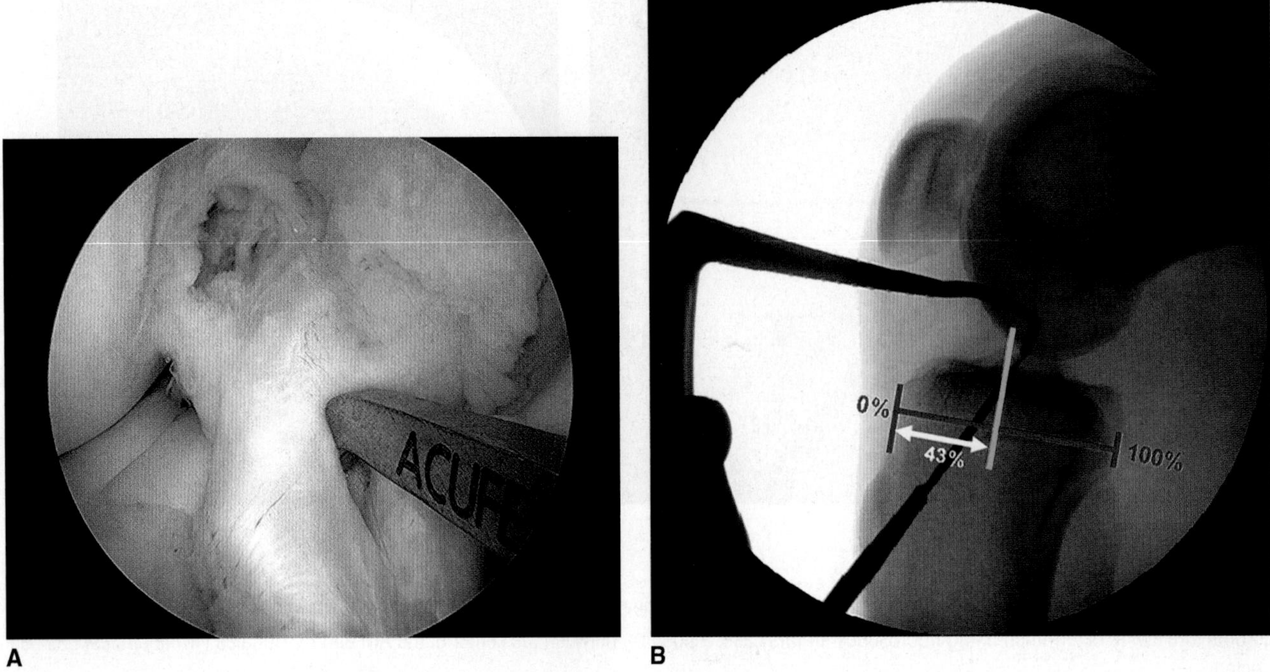

FIGURE 15-51

A: The tip of the ACL tibial aimer is placed in the ACL tibial attachment site through the slit in the tibial remnant. **B:** The position of the ACL tip aimer and guide pin is confirmed using fluoroscopy and the Amis and Jacob's line.

drill bit. The drill bit is advanced under power until the cortex is felt. The cortex is penetrated by drilling by hand. These steps will minimize trauma to the intact ACL fibers. The tibial tunnel is eccentrically drilled with fully fluted cannulated drills or dilators. To ease graft passage, the final diameter of the tibial tunnel should be 0.5 mm larger than the measured diameter of the tibial end of the hamstring tendon graft.

Graft passage depends on the type of ACL tear. When the PL bundle is torn, the hamstring tendon augmentation graft should be passed through the slit in the tibial remnant, posterior to the intact AMB fibers. This will position the augmentation graft in the correct anatomical position, which is the posterior to intact AM bundle fibers. Passing the PL bundle augmentation graft anterior to the intact AM bundle positions the augmentation graft incorrectly and could lead to notch impingement. To pass the ACL graft posterior to the AM bundle, an arthroscopic probe is passed through the AAM portal and the passing suture retrieved and "parked" next to the tibial remnant. The probe is then advance up the tibial tunnel and the passing suture retrieved and passed out of the ACL tibial tunnel. When only the AM bundle is torn, the hamstring tendon augmentation graft should be passed anterior to the intact PL bundle. This will position the hamstring tendon augmentation graft in the correct anatomical position. The passing suture in the femoral tunnel is passed anterior to the PL bundle and retrieved out of the tibial tunnel using a probe or arthroscopic grasper. This step will result in the augmentation graft being positioned anterior and medial to the intact PL bundle fibers. For cases of 2-bundle ACL tears with an intact remnant, the ACL hamstring tendon graft is passed through the slit in the center of the tibial remnant fibers. This places the augmentation graft in the central region of the ACL femoral attachment site and in the center of the tibial attachment site, which is the anatomically correct position. To avoid overstuffing the intercondylar notch, a 2.4-mm drilled-tip guide pin is manually passed down the center of the ACL remnant and the tip of the pin tapped into the roof of the intercondylar notch. This step anchors the guide pin and avoids having to reposition the pin during reaming of the tibial tunnel. An endoscopic cannulated drill bit is drilled by hand up the remnant. This step creates a path through the remnant for the hamstring tendon graft. An arthroscopic grasper is passed through the remnant and used to retrieve the passing suture left in the femoral tunnel. The augmentation graft is passed through the center of the tibial remnant into the femoral tunnel (Fig. 15-52). Graft fixation is performed as previously described for a single-bundle reconstruction.

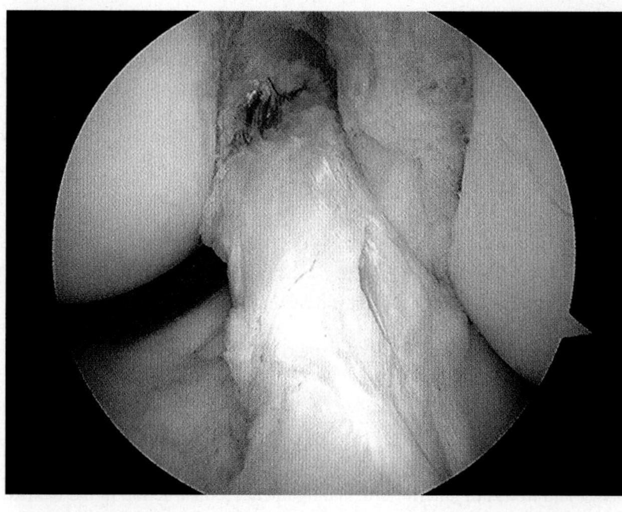

FIGURE 15-52

Final arthroscopic view of the ACL reconstruction. The preserved ACL remnant can be seen enveloping the graft.

POSTOPERATIVE MANAGEMENT

The Hemovac drains are removed at the time the patient is discharged. Due to the slower bone tunnel healing of soft tissue grafts and the fact that our patient population has a normal varus morphotype and increased tibial slope, anatomic factors that are known to increase loading of the ACL graft, we use a rehabilitation program that minimizes cyclic loading and anterior shear forces on the ACL graft during the early healing period. Important aspects of our rehabilitation program include:

- Immediate full passive extension
- Full unrestricted ROM
- No bike, elliptical, or StairMaster exercises during the first 6 weeks to reduce cyclic loading of the ACL graft fixation sites
- Use of a knee extension splint for 4 weeks to further reduce cyclic loading and anterior shear ACL graft forces during walking
- Partial weight bearing (25% body weight) for the first 2 weeks, 50% body weight, weeks 2 to 3, 75% body weight, weeks 3 to 4, full weight bearing end of week 4
- No leg extension exercises using a knee extension machine until 4 months
- No cutting/pivoting sports activities until 6 months
- Unrestricted return to sport no earlier than 9 months

SUMMARY

- Due to the lower incidence of donor site morbidity, hamstring tendon autografts are now the most common graft choice for primary ACL reconstruction worldwide.
- A 5- or 6-strand hamstring tendon graft may be necessary to ensure a minimum graft diameter of 8 mm.
- Due to the limitations of transtibial drilling, medial portal drilling is now the most common surgical technique used to perform an ACL reconstruction.
- A 3-portal surgical technique facilitates anatomic ACL reconstruction as it allows interchange of the portals as both viewing and working portals.
- Arthroscopic viewing through the AM portal improves visualization of the ACL femoral attachment site and allows more accurate assessment of ACL femoral tunnel placement.
- Anatomic ACL femoral tunnel placement is facilitated by using one or all of the following strategies: referencing the native ACL femoral footprint, referencing the ACL ridges, measuring with an ACL ruler, or using intraoperative fluoroscopy.
- Drilling through a low AAM portal achieves acceptable femoral tunnel lengths and allows consistent placement of the ACL femoral tunnel within the native ACL femoral attachment site.
- The ACL tibial attachment site is best visualized through the AM portal with the knee at 50 to 70 degrees of flexion. This improves accuracy of guide pin positioning in both the anterior-posterior and medial-lateral directions.

- In cases of one-bundle AM or PL tears and complete ACL tears with remnants that maintain an intact bridge of tissue between the tibia and femur, a tissue-preserving, ACL augmentation procedure may be undertaken. Preservation of native tissue may enhance knee proprioception, aid healing of the ACL graft, and contribute to knee stability.
- A rehabilitation program that avoids early postoperative cyclic loading of the ACL graft is advantageous to hamstring graft healing within the bone tunnels.

REFERENCES

1. Miyasaka KC, Daniel DM, Stone ML, et al. The incidence of knee ligament injuries in the general population. *Am J Knee Surg.* 1991;4:43–48.
2. Parat A, Roos EM, Roos H. High prevalence of osteoarthritis 14 years after an anterior cruciate ligament tear in male soccer players: a study of radiographic and patient relevant outcomes. *Ann Rheum Dis.* 2004;63:269–273.
3. Lohmander LS, Englund PM, Dahl LL, et al. The long-term consequences of anterior cruciate ligament and meniscus injuries. *Am J Sports Med.* 2007;35:1756–1769.
4. Buller LT, Best MJ, Baraga MG, et al. Trends in anterior cruciate ligament reconstruction in the United States. *Orthop J Sports Med.* 2015;3:1–8.
5. Mall NA, Chalmers PN, Moric M, et al. Incidence and trends of anterior cruciate ligament reconstruction in the United States. *Am J Sports Med.* 2014;42:2363–2370.
6. Salmon LJ, Russell VJ, Refshauge K, et al. Long-term outcome of endoscopic anterior cruciate ligament reconstruction with patellar tendon autograft. Minimum 13-year review. *Am J Sports Med.* 2006;34:721–732.
7. Biau DJ, Tournoux C, Katsahian S, et al. Bone-patellar tendon-bone autografts versus hamstring autografts for reconstruction of anterior cruciate ligament: meta-analysis. *Br Med J.* 2006;332(7548):995–1001.
8. Chahal J, Lee A, Heard W, et al. A retrospective review of anterior cruciate reconstruction using patellar tendon: 25 years of experience. *Orthop J Sports Med.* 2013;1(3):2325967113501789.
9. Mohtadi NGH, Chan DS, Dainty KN, et al. Patellar tendon versus hamstring tendon autograft for anterior cruciate ligament rupture in adults. *Cochrane Database Syst Rev.* 2011;18:287–293. Review.
10. Thompson SM, Salmon LJ, Waller A, et al. Twenty-year outcomes of a longitudinal prospective evaluation of isolated endoscopic anterior cruciate ligament reconstruction with patellar tendon or hamstring tendon autograft. *Am J Sports Med.* 2015;43(9):2164–2174.
11. Chechik O, Amar E, Khashan M, et al. An international survey on anterior cruciate ligament reconstruction practices. *Int Orthop.* 2013;37:201–206.
12. Lee YHD, Kuroda R, Chan KM. Anterior cruciate ligament reconstruction: a 2015 global perspective of the Magellan Society. *Asia Pac J Sports Med Arthrosc Rehab Technol.* 2015;2:122–128.
13. Ardern CL, Webster KE. Knee flexor strength recovery following hamstring tendon harvest for anterior cruciate ligament reconstruction: a systematic review. *Orthop Rev.* 2009;1:e12.
14. Kim, S-J, Kumar P, Kim S-H. Anterior cruciate ligament reconstruction in patients with generalized joint laxity. *Clin Orthop Surg.* 2010;2:130–139.
15. Getgood A, Spalding T. The evolution of anatomic anterior cruciate ligament reconstruction. *Open Orthop J.* 2012;6:287–294.
16. Martins CAQ, Kropf EJ, Shen W, et al. The concept of anatomic anterior cruciate ligament reconstruction. *Oper Tech Sports Med.* 2012;20:7–18.
17. Irarrazaval S, Kurosaka M, Cohen M, et al. Anterior cruciate ligament reconstruction. *J ISAKOS.* 2016;1:38–52.
18. Kopf S, Forsythe B, Wong AK, et al. Transtibial ACL reconstruction technique fails to position drill tunnels anatomically in vivo 3D CT study. *Knee Surg Sports Traumatol Arthrosc.* 2012;20:2200–2207.
19. Lee MC, Seong SC, Lee S, et al. Vertical femoral tunnel placement results in rotational knee laxity after anterior cruciate ligament reconstruction. *Arthroscopy.* 2007;23:771–778.
20. Kato Y, Ingham SJM, Kramer S, et al. Effect of tunnel position for anatomic single-bundle ACL reconstruction on knee biomechanics in a porcine model. *Knee Surg Sports Traumatol Arthrosc.* 2010;18:2–10.
21. Abebe ES, Utturkar GM, Taylor DC, et al. The effects of femoral graft placement on in vivo knee biomechanics after anterior cruciate ligament reconstruction. *J Biomech.* 2014;47:96–101.
22. Cohen SB, Fu FH. Three-portal technique for anterior cruciate ligament reconstruction: use of a central medial portal. *Arthroscopy.* 2007;23:325.e1–325.e4.
23. Araujo PH, van Eck CF, Macalena JA, et al. Advances in the three-portal technique for single- or double-bundle ACL reconstruction. *Knee Surg Sports Traumatol Arthrosc.* 2011;19:1239–1242.
24. Brown CH, Spalding T, Robb C. Medial portal technique for single-bundle anatomical anterior cruciate (ACL) reconstruction. *Int Orthop.* 2013;37:253–269.
25. Erdem M, Gulabi D, Asil K, et al. Far medial versus anteromedial portal drilling of the femoral tunnel in ACL reconstruction: a computed tomographic analysis. *Arch Orthop Trauma Surg.* 2015;135:539–554.
26. Hensler D, Working Z, Illingworth K, et al. Medial portal drilling: effects on the femoral tunnel aperture morphology during anterior cruciate ligament reconstruction. *J Bone Joint Surg Am.* 2011;93:2063–2071.
27. Bird J, Carmont M, Dhillon M, et al. Validation of a new technique to determine mid-bundle femoral tunnel position in anterior cruciate ligament reconstruction using 3-D computed tomography analysis. *Arthroscopy.* 2011;27: 1259–1267.
28. Wittstein JR, Wilson JB, Moorman CT. Complications related to hamstring tendon harvest. *Oper Tech Sports Med.* 2006;14:15–19.
29. Brown CH, Sklar JH. Endoscopic anterior cruciate ligament reconstruction using doubled gracilis and semitendinosus tendons and endobutton femoral fixation. *Oper Tech Sports Med.* 1999;7:201–213.
30. Charalambous CP, Kwaees TA. Anatomical considerations in hamstring tendon harvesting for anterior cruciate ligament reconstruction. *Muscles Ligaments Tendons J.* 2012;2:253–257.
31. Levy M, Prud'homme J. Anatomic variations of the pes anserinus: a cadaveric study. *Orthopedics.* 1993;16: 601–606.

32. Pagnani MJ, Warner JJ, O'Brien SJ, et al. Anatomic considerations in harvesting the semitendinosus and gracilis tendons and a technique of harvest. *Am J Sports Med.* 1993;21:565–571.
33. Caudal-Couto JJ, Deehan DJ. The accessory bands of the gracilis and semitendinosus: an anatomical study. *Knee.* 2003;10:325–328.
34. Tuncay I, Kucuker H, Uzun I, et al. The fascial band from semitendinosus to gastrocnemius: the critical point of hamstring harvesting. *Acta Orthop.* 2007;78:361–363.
35. Reina N, Abbo O, Gomez-Brouchet A, et al. Anatomy of the bands of the hamstring tendon: how can we improve harvest quality. *Knee.* 2013;20:90–95.
36. Conte EJ, Hyatt AE, Gatt CJ, et al. Hamstring autograft size can be predicted and is a potential risk factor of anterior cruciate ligament failure. *Arthroscopy.* 2014;30:882–890.
37. Vertullo CJ, Quick M, Jones A, et al. A surgical technique using presoaked vancomycin hamstring grafts to decrease the risk of infection after anterior cruciate ligament reconstruction. *Arthroscopy.* 2012;28:337–342.
38. Pérez-Prieto D, Torres-Claramunt R, Gelber PE, et al. Autograft soaking in vancomycin reduces the risk of infection after anterior cruciate ligament reconstruction. *Knee Surg Sports Traumatol Arthrosc.* 2015;24:2724–2728.
39. Phegan M, Grayson JE, Vertullo CJ. No infections in 1300 anterior cruciate ligament reconstructions with vancomycin pre-soaking of hamstring grafts. *Knee Surg Sports Traumatol Arthrosc.* 2016;24:2729–2735.
40. Kazusa H, Nakamae A, Ochi M. Augmentation technique for anterior cruciate ligament injury. *Clin Sports Med.* 2013;32:127–140.
41. Pearle AD, McAllister D, Howell SM. Rationale for strategic graft placement in anterior cruciate ligament reconstruction: I.D.E.A.L. femoral tunnel position. *Am J Orthop.* 2015;44:253–258.
42. Dhawan A, Gallo RA, Lynch SA. Anatomic tunnel placement in anterior cruciate ligament reconstruction. *J Am Acad Orthop Surg.* 2016;24:443–454.
43. Budny J, Fox J, Rauh M, et al. Emerging trends in anterior cruciate ligament reconstruction. *J Knee Surg.* 2017;30(1):63–69.
44. Harms SP, Noyes FR, Grood ES, et al. Anatomic single-graft anterior cruciate ligament reconstruction restores rotational stability: a robotic study in cadaveric knees. *Arthroscopy.* 2015;31(10):1981–1990.
45. Araujo PH, Asai S, Pinto M, et al. ACL graft position affects in situ force following ACL reconstruction. *J Bone Joint Surg Am.* 2015;97:1767–1773.
46. Nawabi DH, Tucker S, Schafer KA, et al. ACL fibers near the lateral intercondylar ridge are the most load bearing during stability examinations and isometric through passive flexion. *Am J Sports Med.* 2016;44(10):2563–2571.
47. Ziegler CG, Pietrini SD, Westerhaus BD, et al. Arthroscopically pertinent landmarks for tunnel positioning in single-bundle and double-bundle anterior cruciate ligament reconstructions. *Am J Sports Med.* 2011;39:743–752.
48. Moloney G, Araujo P, Rabuck S, et al. Use of a fluoroscopic overlay to assist arthroscopic anterior cruciate ligament reconstruction. *Am J Sports Med.* 2013;41:1794–1800.
49. Sven S, Maurice B, Hoeher J, et al. Variability of tunnel positioning in fluoroscopic-assisted ACL reconstruction. *Knee Surg Sports Traumatol Arthrosc.* 2015;23:2269–2277.
50. Inderhaug E, Larsen A, Waaler PA, et al. The effect of intraoperative fluoroscopy on the accuracy of femoral tunnel placement in single-bundle anatomic ACL reconstruction. *Knee Surg Sports Traumatol Arthrosc.* 2015. doi: 10.1007/s00167-015-3858-3.
51. Bernard M, Hertel P, Hornung H, et al. Femoral insertion of the ACL. Radiographic quadrant method. *Am J Knee Surg.* 1997;10:14–22.
52. Musahl V, Burkart A, Debski RE, et al. Anterior cruciate ligament tunnel placement: comparison of insertion site anatomy with the guidelines of a computer-assisted surgical system. *Arthroscopy.* 2003;19:154–160.
53. Yamamoto Y, Hsu WH, Woo SL, et al. Knee stability and graft function after anterior cruciate ligament reconstruction: a comparison of a lateral and an anatomical femoral tunnel placement. *Am J Sports Med.* 2004;32:1825–1832.
54. Columbet P, Robinson J, Christel P, et al. Morphology of anterior cruciate ligament attachments for anatomic reconstruction: a cadaveric dissection and radiographic study. *Arthroscopy.* 2006;22:984–992.
55. Zantop T, Wellman M, Fu FH, et al. Tunnel positioning of anteromedial and posterolateral bundles in anatomic anterior cruciate ligament reconstruction. Anatomic and radiographic findings. *Am J Sports Med.* 2008;36:65–72.
56. Tsukada H, Ishibashi Y, Tsuda E, et al. Anatomical analysis of the anterior cruciate ligament femoral and tibial footprints. *J Orthop Sci.* 2008;13:122–129.
57. Lorenz S, Elser F, Mitterer M, et al. Radiographic evaluation of the insertion sites of the 2 functional bundles of the anterior cruciate ligament using 3-dimensional computed tomography. *Am J Sports Med.* 2009;37:2368–2376.
58. Forsythe B, Kopf S, Wong AK, et al. The location of femoral and tibial tunnels in anatomic double-bundle anterior cruciate ligament reconstruction analyzed by three-dimensional computed tomography models. *J Bone Joint Surg Am.* 2010;92-A:1418–1429.
59. Iriuchishima T, Ingham SJM, Tajima G, et al. Evaluation of the tunnel placement in the anatomical double-bundle ACL reconstruction: a cadaver study. *Knee Surg Sports Traumatol Arthrosc.* 2010;18:1226–1231.
60. Pietrini SD, Ziegler CG, Anderson CJ, et al. Radiographic landmarks for tunnel positioning in double-bundle ACL reconstructions. *Knee Surg Sports Traumatol Arthrosc.* 2011;19:792–800.
61. Abreu-e-Silva GM, Oliveira MHGCN, Maranhao GS, et al. Three-dimensional computed tomography evaluation of anterior cruciate ligament reconstruction footprint for anatomic single-bundle reconstruction. *Knee Surg Sports Traumatol Arthrosc.* 2015;23:770–776.
62. Lee JK, Lee S, Seong SC, et al. Anatomy of the anterior cruciate ligament insertion sites: comparison of plain radiography and three-dimensional computed tomographic imaging to anatomic dissection. *Knee Surg Sports Traumatol Arthrosc.* 2015;23:2297–2305.
63. Sullivan JP, Cook S, Gao Y, et al. Radiographic anatomy of the native anterior cruciate ligament: a systematic review. *HSS J.* 2015;11:154–165.
64. Luites WH, Verdonschot N. Radiographic positions of femoral ACL, AM and PL centres: accuracy of guideline based on the lateral quadrant method. *Knee Surg Sports Traumatol Arthrosc.* 2015. doi:10.1007/s00167-015-3681-x.
65. Davis AD, Manaqibwala MI, Brown CH, et al. Height and depth guidelines for anatomic femoral tunnels in anterior cruciate reconstruction. *Arthroscopy.* 2016;32:1098–1105.
66. Parkar AP, Adriaensen M, Vinfeld S, et al. The anatomic centers of the femoral and tibial insertions of the anterior cruciate ligament. A systematic review of imaging and cadaveric studies reporting normal center location. *Am J Sports Med.* 2017 (in press).

67. Siebold R, Schuhmaker P, Fernandez F, et al. Flat midsubstance of the anterior cruciate ligament with tibial "c"-shaped insertion site. *Knee Surg Sports Traumatol Arthrosc.* 2015;23:3136–3142.
68. Kasten P, Szczodry M, Irrgang J, et al. What is the role of intra-operative fluoroscopic measurement to determine tibial tunnel placement in anatomical anterior cruciate ligament reconstruction. *Knee Surg Sports Traumatol Arthrosc.* 2010;18:1169–1175.
69. Amis A, Jakob R. Anterior cruciate ligament graft positioning, tensioning and twisting. *Knee Surg Sports Traumatol Arthrosc.* 1998;6(Suppl 1):S2–S12.
70. Staubli HU, Rauschning W. Tibial attachment area of the anterior cruciate ligament in the extended knee position. Anatomy and cryosections in vitro complemented by magnetic resonance arthrography in vivo. *Knee Surg Sports Traumatol Arthrosc.* 1994;2:138–146.
71. Doi M, Takahashi M, Abe M, et al. Lateral radiographic study of the tibial insertions of the anteromedial and posterolateral bundles of human anterior cruciate ligament. *Knee Surg Sport Traumatol Arthrosc.* 2009;17:347–351.
72. Frank RM, Seroyer ST, Lewis PB, et al. MRI analysis of tibial position of the anterior cruciate ligament. *Knee Surg Sports Traumatol Arthrosc.* 2010;18:1607–1611.
73. Scheffel PT, Henninger HB, Burks RT. Relationship of the intercondylar roof and the tibial footprint of the ACL. Implications for ACL reconstruction. *Am J Sports Med.* 2012;41:396–401.
74. Parkinson B, Gogna R, Robb C, et al. Anatomic ACL reconstruction: the normal central tibia footprint position and a standardized technique for measuring tibial tunnel location on 3D CT. *Knee Surg Sports Traumatol Arthrosc.* 2015. doi:10.1007/s00167-015-3683-8.

16 ACL Reconstruction Using Quadriceps Tendon Autograft

John W. Xerogeanes and Harris S. Slone

INDICATION

There are many variables to consider when selecting a graft choice for anterior cruciate ligament (ACL) reconstruction. The advantages and disadvantages to each graft must be considered in addition to patient-specific factors, in order to achieve optimal outcomes. The quadriceps tendon is a versatile graft, which can be used for primary or revision reconstruction. It is an excellent choice for anatomic, transtibial, all-inside, or all-epiphyseal techniques, and the anatomy of the quadriceps makes it amenable to either single-bundle or double-bundle reconstruction. Additionally, the quadriceps tendon graft can be harvested with or without a patellar bone block based on surgeon preference, although we used all soft tissue grafts exclusively for our quadriceps tendon autograft ACL reconstructions.

Despite excellent clinical outcomes, biomechanical properties, and low donor site morbidity, quadriceps tendon autograft is still relatively infrequently used compared to alternative graft options. We believe that this is largely due to surgeon unfamiliarity with the technique and anatomy. Most quadriceps tendon harvests have historically been performed through larger incisions, and cosmetic concerns may have also limited its utility. Recently, minimally invasive harvest techniques and instrumentation have allowed for easy and reproducible graft harvest through a small incision.

The vast majority of patients who require ACL reconstruction are good candidates for quadriceps tendon autograft reconstruction. We have transitioned to soft tissue–only quadriceps tendon reconstruction for nearly all patients where a soft tissue autograft reconstruction is indicated. We have found quadriceps tendon autografts to be most useful in patients where anterior knee pain and/or kneeling pain is unacceptable due to professional or recreational demands. There is little variability with regard to quadriceps tendon graft diameter when compared to hamstring autografts, and the thickness of the graft can be evaluated preoperatively.

CONTRAINDICATIONS

In patients where ACL reconstruction is indicated, contraindications to quadriceps tendon ACL reconstruction are few. While we require most all patients requiring ACL reconstruction to obtain full extension preoperatively, it is especially important for those who are undergoing quadriceps tendon reconstruction as the intra-articular volume of graft tends to be larger (and more anatomic) than bone-tendon-bone reconstructions. Specific relative contraindications include:

- Prior quadriceps tendon injury or preexisting quadriceps tendonitis
- Prior quadriceps tendon surgery or parapatellar approach to the knee
- Untreated coagulopathy
- Large cystic or cavitary lesions in the revision setting

PREOPERATIVE PREPARATION

When evaluating a patient for suspected ACL tear, one should always start with a detailed history and physical examination. Assessing patients' functional demands, activity level, and expectations following surgery allows the surgeon to choose the most appropriate graft after a diagnosis has been established.

Restoration of preoperative knee motion, especially extension, is essential prior to any ACL reconstruction, unless a bucket-handle meniscus tear or comparable injury limits motion. Comparison to the contralateral side should serve as reference for normal motion.

Once the decision has been made to perform a quadriceps tendon autograft ACL reconstruction, the MRI can be evaluated to assess quadriceps tendon thickness. The quadriceps tendon is measured midsagittal from anterior to posterior, 3 cm above the proximal pole of the patella (Fig. 16-1). In general, we prefer partial-thickness quadriceps tendon harvest; however, full-thickness grafts can be harvested in patients with thinner tendons (≤6 mm). We have found no increased morbidity when harvesting full-thickness grafts as long as the capsular rent is closed or approximated.

TECHNIQUE

In this chapter, we describe our minimally invasive harvest technique, which has evolved with newer instrumentation. Some surgeons prefer a larger incision and more "open" technique, but we have found our minimally invasive technique to be reproducible, easy, and more cosmetic. Patients tend to not like larger incisions over the quadriceps tendon, as the scar is readily visible when they are sitting.

Positioning

After successful general anesthetic, examination under anesthesia is performed and findings recorded. A tourniquet is applied to the operative thigh. We prefer positioning the operative leg in a circumferential leg holder with the foot of the bed dropped and the contralateral side in a lithotomy positioner with bony prominences well padded. Alternatively, the bed can be left flat with an arthroscopic post, and the knee can be flexed over the side of the bed. The operative extremity is then prepped and draped. An Esmarch bandage is used to exsanguinate the leg and the tourniquet is inflated.

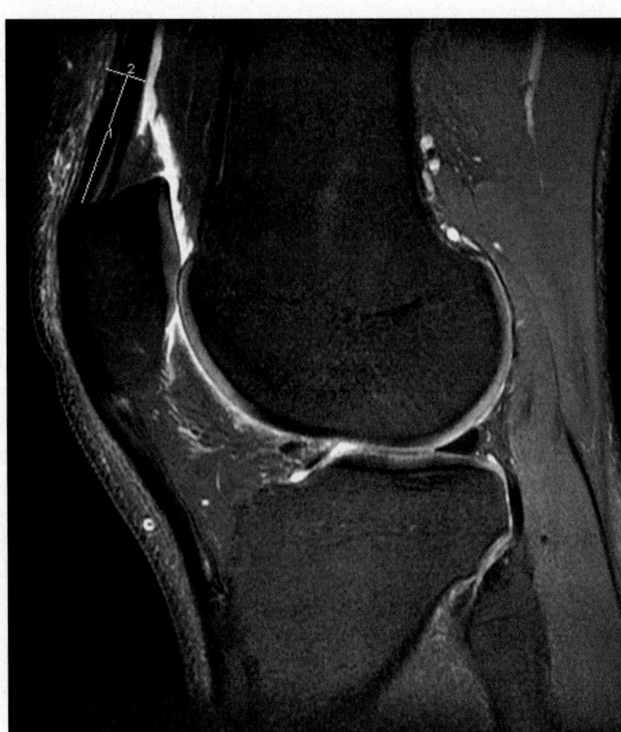

FIGURE 16-1

The thickness of the quadriceps tendon is measured preoperatively on the sagittal MRI, 3 cm above the proximal pole of the patella.

Graft Harvest

We generally start with graft harvest, although it can be performed before or after diagnostic arthroscopy. If diagnostic arthroscopy is performed first, it is helpful to completely drain the knee of fluid prior to graft harvest. This limits capsular distention and pressure on the deep surface of the quadriceps tendon, making capsular violation less likely.

With the knee flexed to 90 degrees, the proximal pole of the patella, medial patellar border, lateral patellar border, and vastus medialis obliquus (VMO) are marked. It is important to distinguish the lateral trochlear ridge from the superior pole of the patella, which can be difficult at 90 degrees of flexion. Gentle flexion and extension of the knee helps to distinguish between the mobile patella and the immobile lateral trochlear ridge. The incision site is marked with a 1.5- to 2-cm longitudinal mark made extending just from the lateral to the midline of the proximal pole of the patella proximally in line with the femur. A second mark is made between 7 and 7.5 cm (depending on planned graft length) from the proximal pole of the patella (Fig. 16-2).

Local anesthetic with epinephrine is infiltrated into the subcutaneous tissue deep to the previously marked incision site. This helps to define tissue layers during later dissection. A 15-blade scalpel is used to make the incision. It is critical to widely ellipse the subcutaneous fat and paratenon to allow for visualization (Fig. 16-3). A Ray-Tec sponge over a key elevator is used to sweep away tissue on the anterior surface of the quadriceps tendon and patella. Soft tissue should be removed at least 7 cm proximal to the incision. An Army-Navy retractor is placed into the proximal apex of the incision, and the arthroscope (fluid off, looking down toward the tendon) is placed in the wound. The VMO, proximal aspect of the rectus, and vastus lateralis are identified (Fig. 16-4). When the proximal rectus tendon is identified, the arthroscope is turned so the light is shining through the skin on the anterior thigh, and this point is marked (Fig. 16-5). If any crossing vessels are seen, they should be coagulated with the radiofrequency device or Bovie electrocautery.

The Arthrex (Naples, FL) minimally invasive double-blade harvest knife is designed to cut a predetermined width and depth based on surgeon preference. We generally use a 10-mm wide by 7-mm deep blade for most adult patients. The design of the blade allows for a "push" or "pull" cutting technique; we recommend using a push technique as cutting seems to be easier in this direction. The knife handle has markings that allow for appropriate length of incision based on the superior pole of the patella. The knife carefully is placed into the wound incising in line with the proximal pole of the patella and the previously placed mark of transillumination, indicating the direction of the rectus

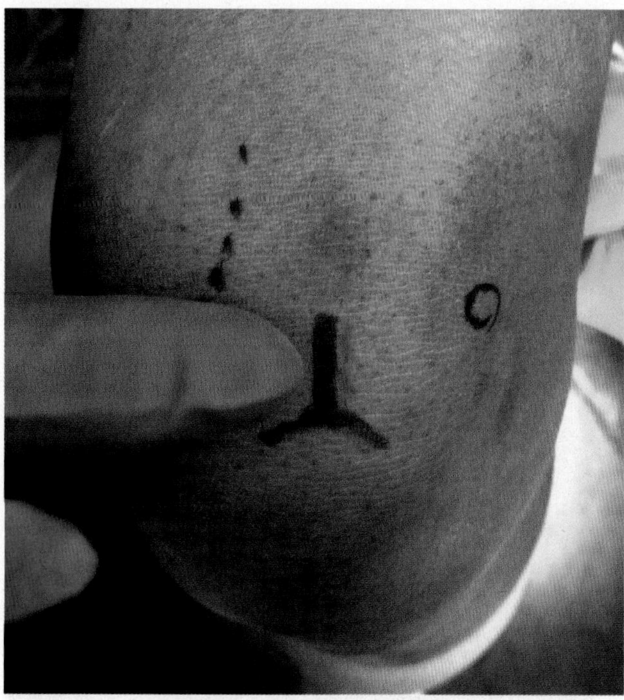

FIGURE 16-2

Preoperative marking of bony and soft tissue landmarks.

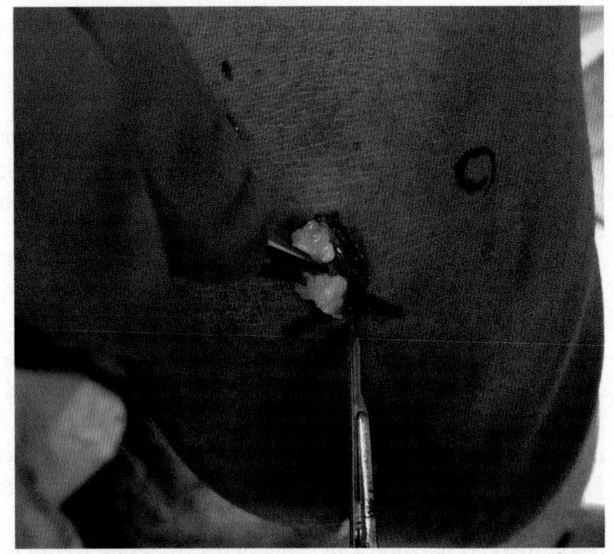

FIGURE 16-3

Subcutaneous fat is widely excised to facilitate visualization through a small incision.

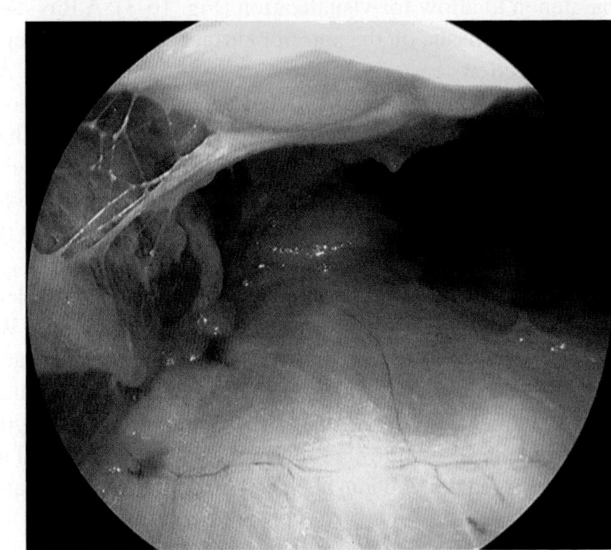

FIGURE 16-4

The arthroscope is used to visualize the quadriceps tendon, vastus medialis, vastus lateralis, and distal rectus femoris musculotendinous junction.

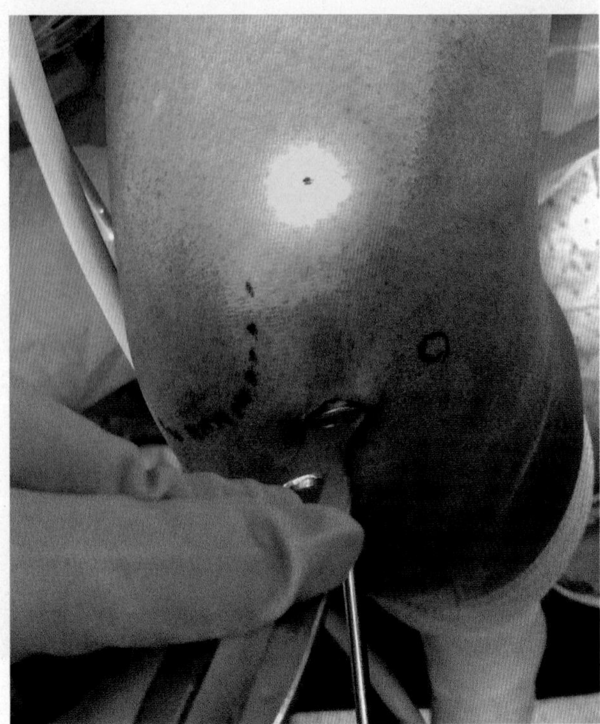

FIGURE 16-5

A mark is made on the anterior skin at the point of maximum transillumination, which identifies the trajectory of the quadriceps tendon and distal rectus muscle.

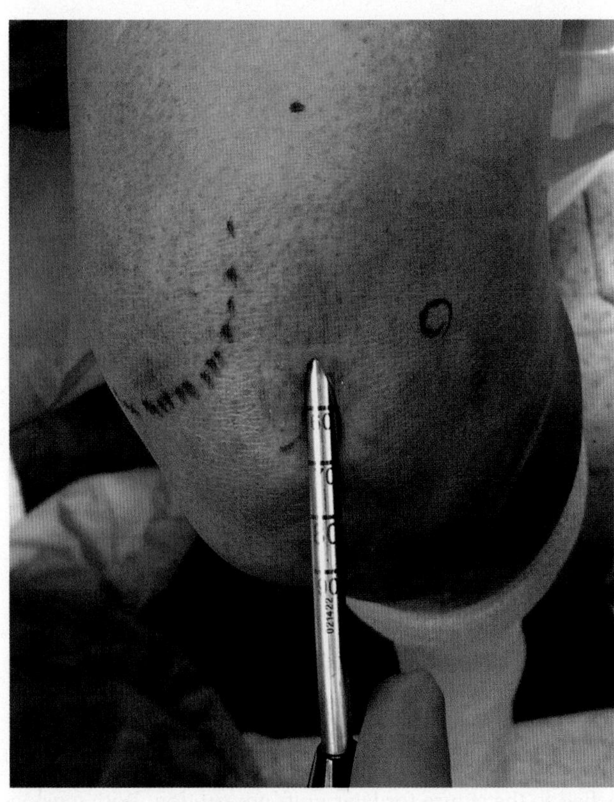

FIGURE 16-6

The harvest knife is used to incise the tendon longitudinally, starting at the proximal pole of the patella, extending toward the previously placed mark on the skin overlying the distal musculotendinous junction of the rectus femoris.

femoris (Fig. 16-6). The longitudinal incisions are extended down to the patella with a 15 blade. The tendon is then dissected off the proximal pole of the patella, connecting the two longitudinal incisions. The depth of the dissection can be determined based on the depth of the longitudinal incisions from the double-blade knife. If fat is encountered, avoid deeper dissection or risk capsular violation (Fig. 16-7A,B). An Allis clamp is used to lift the central soft tissue quadriceps graft anteriorly, and Metzenbaum scissors are used to continue proximal dissection. It is important to taper the distal end of the graft slightly, as additional 1 mm of girth will be added with suture. Once 3 cm of graft has been elevated, an Arthrex (Naples, FL) FiberLoop suture is placed about 2 cm proximal from the

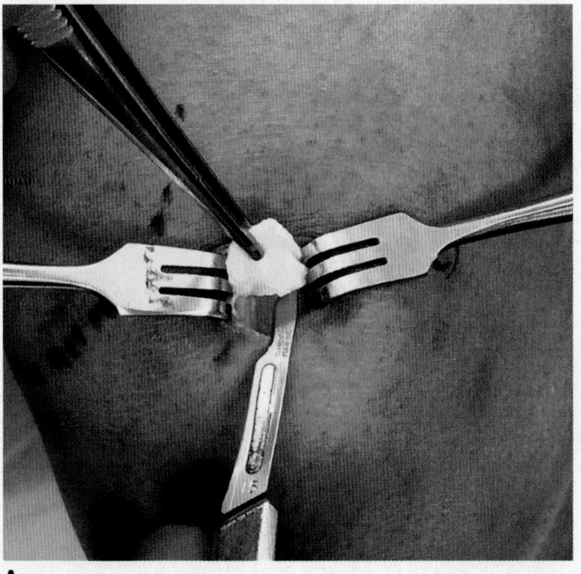

A

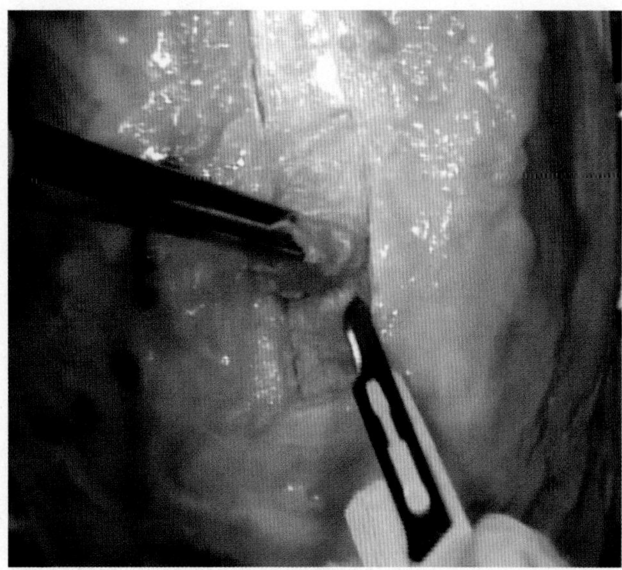

B

FIGURE 16-7

A, B: A scalpel is used to dissect the tendon of the proximal pole of the patella.

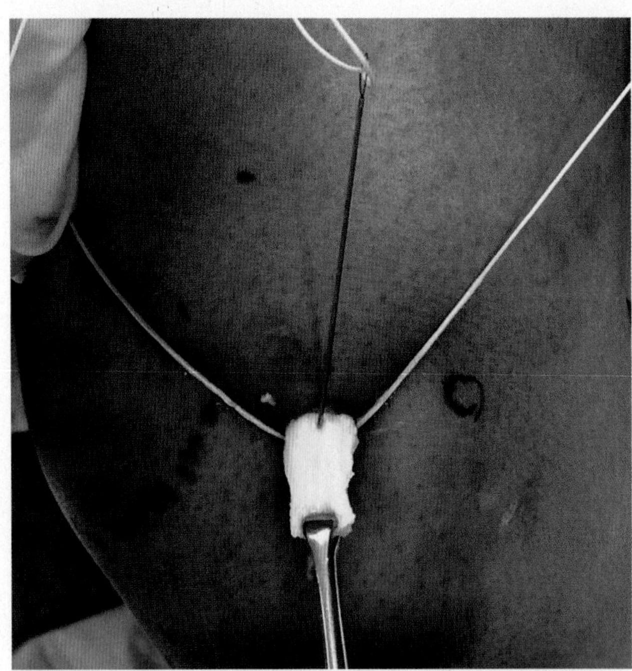

FIGURE 16-8
Looped suture is used to whipstitch the tendon.

end of the graft (Fig. 16-8). Four suture throws are placed from proximal to distal, and the last suture is "locked" by entering the tendon proximal to the last throw and exiting the central portion of the tendon (Fig. 16-9). The needle is left attached to the suture for later graft preparation. With tension on the sutures, dissection is carried further proximally with Metzenbaum scissors. Assistants can aid in visualization with Senn retractors. Once 5 to 6 cm of graft has been elevated, the Arthrex (Naples, FL) Quadriceps Tendon stripper/cutter is used to strip the tendon proximally, with firm tension on the placed sutures. It is important to note that this tendon stripper is used differently than a hamstring tendon stripper, since only a portion of the tendon is being harvested. Markings on the shaft of the stripper/cutter allow the surgeon to identify graft length. We cut the graft at 7 cm, which gives 2 cm

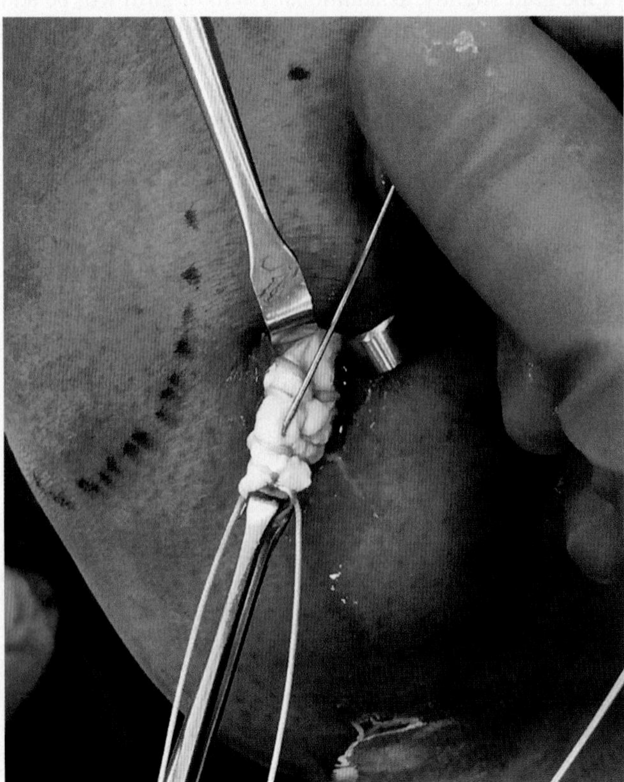

FIGURE 16-9
The last throw is "locked" by passing the suture behind the previously placed stitch, which then exits the central portion of the tendon.

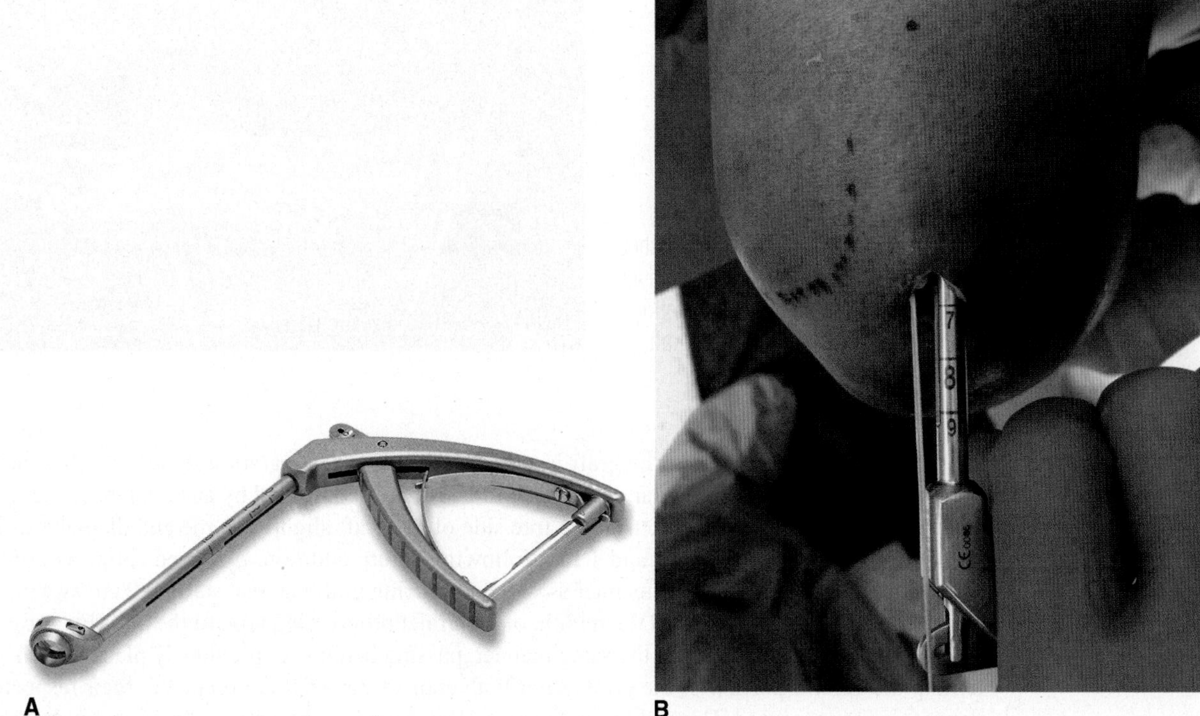

FIGURE 16-10

A: The stripper/cutter device is used to mobilize the tendon proximally. **B:** The graft length can be estimated off the markings on the stripper/cutter handle. Firm tension on the sutures facilitates stripping and then cutting of the graft.

or more of graft in both the femoral and tibial tunnels. Harvesting grafts greater than 8 cm can lead to an increased incidence of both bleeding and cosmetic deformity. Once the desired graft length has been obtained, the handle of the stripper/cutter is squeezed while tension is applied to the sutures, cutting the graft proximally (Fig. 16-10A,B). The graft is then removed from the wound and taken to the back table for preparation.

The arthroscope (fluid off, looking down toward the tendon) is the placed back into the wound and partial-thickness harvest can be confirmed. If full-thickness rents or capsular violation is identified, they are closed with 0 Vicryl. The tendon edges of the harvest site are injected with 0.25% Marcaine for postoperative pain relief. A strip of gel-foam is placed in the harvest site. Subcutaneous layer is closed with 2-0 Vicryl, and the skin is closed with 3-0 Monocryl (Fig. 16-11). Remember when using an arthroscopy pump, check the tenseness of the thigh periodically during the case to ensure no significant fluid extravasation is occurring.

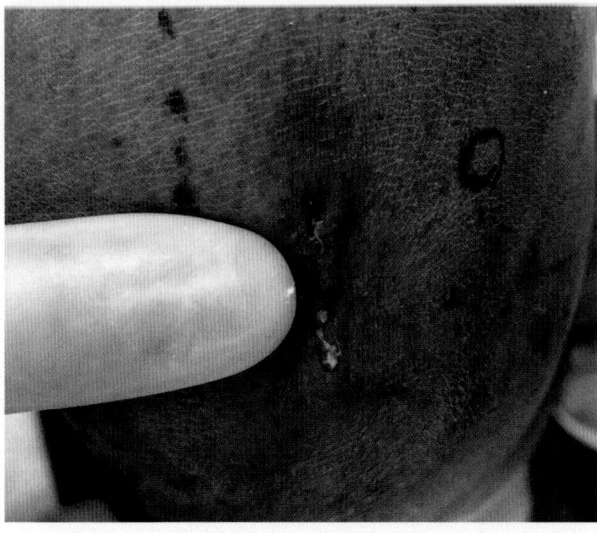

FIGURE 16-11

The graft is harvested through a small cosmetic incision.

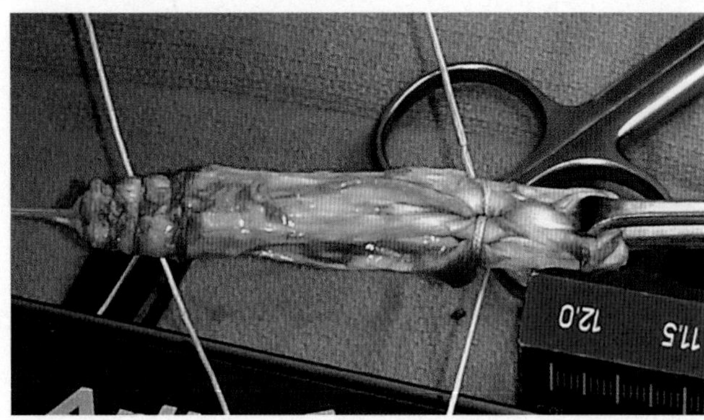

FIGURE 16-12

Graft preparation is performed. Both ends of the graft have been whipstitched with looped sutures. The needles are left in place on the suture if button fixation is to be used on that side of the graft.

Graft Preparation

The previously sutured end of the graft is secured to the graft preparation stand. An Aliss clamp is placed on the free multilaminar end of the graft, which is controlled by an assistant to facilitate graft preparation. It is critical to trim the free side of the graft slightly, as the end diameter of the graft will increase between 0.5 and 1 mm following suture addition. A looped suture is used to whipstitch the graft in the same manner as was done during graft harvest, starting 2 cm away from the end of the graft (i.e., toward the middle of the graft) progressing toward the end (Fig. 16-12). The last suture is also locked in the same manner, passing behind the previously placed stitch and exiting the central portion of the graft. After both ends of the graft are prepared, their respective diameters are measured. Depending on the size of each end of the graft, a decision can be made as to which end will be used for the femoral or tibial tunnels. One must keep in mind that the side selected for the femoral tunnel will have its diameter increased 0.5 mm after the attachment of the femoral fixation device.

We prefer adjustable loop suspensory fixation for the femoral side, which provides the opportunity for graft adjustment on the femoral side after the graft is passed. The previously placed FiberLoop (with attached needle) is passed through the loop of the Arthrex TightRope RT (Naples, FL). The needle is then passed through the central portion of the graft exiting the surface of the graft 5 mm away from the graft end (Fig. 16-13). Three or four subsequent whipstitches are placed in the graft proceeding centrally. The needle is then cut from the suture, and the two limbs of suture are wrapped around the graft in opposite directions from each other and tied. The ends of sutures can be passed through the needle, and the knot can be shuttled into the midsubstance of the tendon, before suture tails are cut on the opposite side of the tendon.

The tibial side can be fixed with a variety of methods, including suspensory fixation with a button or tie-over-post screw. If a suspensory button is used for the tibial side, it is attached to the graft in the same manner as the femoral side. The final diameter of each graft ends are then measured.

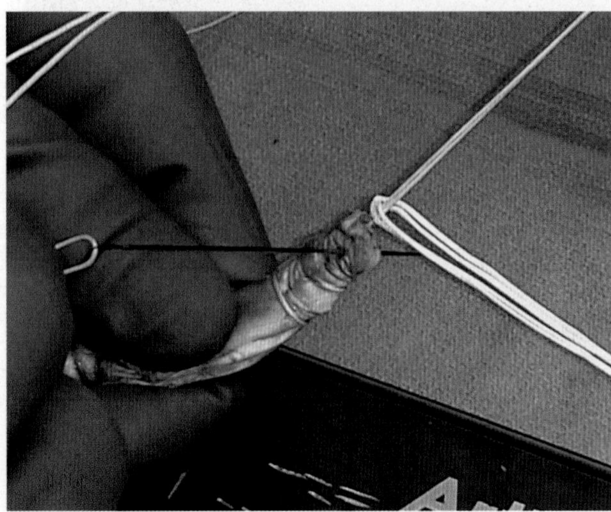

FIGURE 16-13

The adjustable loop button is attached to the graft.

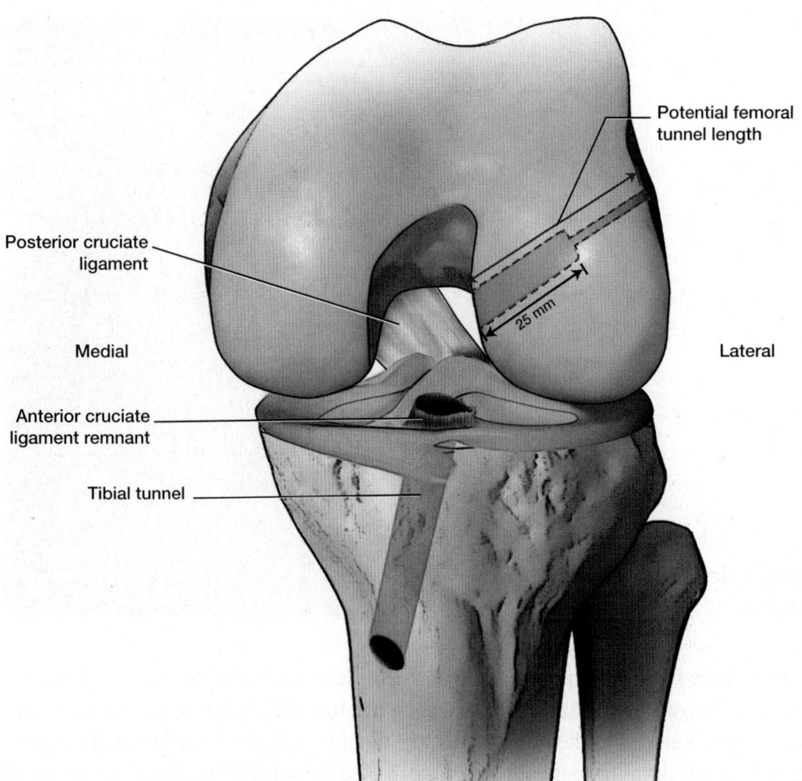

FIGURE 16-14

The femoral intraosseous distance or potential femoral tunnel length is measured with a spade-tipped pin. A femoral socket is drilled to 25 mm.

ACL Reconstruction

We use three arthroscopic portals: the standard anterior lateral (AL) portal, a low anterior medial (AM) portal placed just medial to the patellar tendon, and an accessory far medial (FM) portal. When identifying the correct placement of the femoral tunnel, we look through the AM portal with the arthroscope. In the acute setting, there is often sufficient soft tissue left on the wall, which can help identify the center of the footprint. We drill anatomic tunnels centered on the bifurcate ridge in the center of the ACL femoral origin. No matter which femoral drilling technique a surgeon utilizes, it is vital to accurately measure the distance from the ACL footprint to the lateral femoral cortex or "potential femoral tunnel length." We prefer to do this with a spade-tipped eyelet pin with measurement marking. The potential tunnel length is normally between 30 and 40 mm with an AM portal technique. In general, no more than a 25-mm tunnel is needed with a 7-cm graft (Fig. 16-14). A looped suture is placed in the femoral tunnel for later graft passage. The adjustable loop button is shortened to the length of the potential femoral tunnel +5 mm (Fig. 16-15A,B).

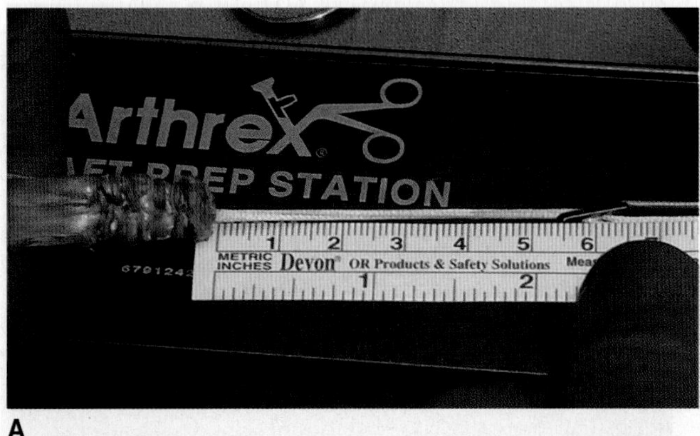

A

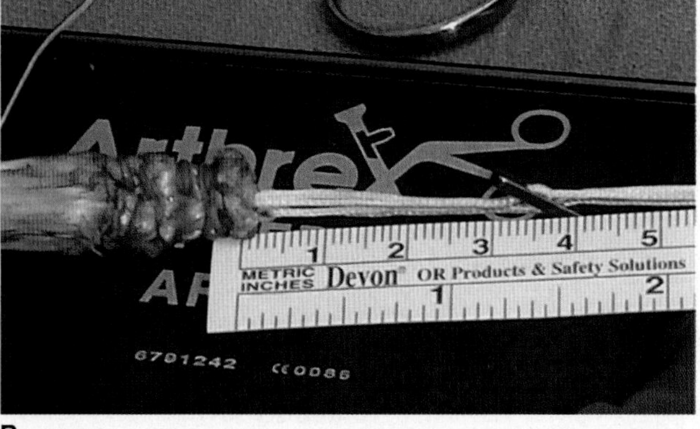

B

FIGURE 16-15

A, B: The adjustable loop is shortened to 5 mm greater than the potential femoral tunnel length.

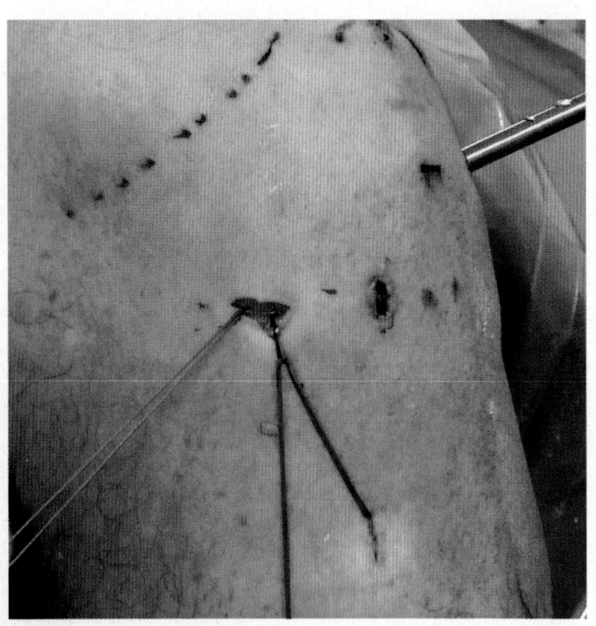

FIGURE 16-16

Passing sutures are controlled with a hemostat to prevent inadvertent removal of the suture.

The arthroscope is then switched to the AL portal and the tibial side is marked in the center of the tibial footprint. When present, we leave a small stump of tibial footprint to aid in anatomic graft placement. The mark is approximately 2 mm anterior to the posterior aspect of anterior horn of the lateral meniscus. Either a full length or blind socket tibial tunnel can be drilled, based on surgeon preference. If a blind socket is preferred, we generally prepare 25 mm of tunnel with the Arthrex Flip Cutter (Naples, FL) to allow for adequate graft tensioning. A looped suture is placed in the tibial tunnel for later graft passage.

Graft Passage

We prefer graft passage through the FM portal. Passing the graft through the FM is not only easier but also provides flexibility to place the larger diameter end on the femoral side without enlarging the tibial tunnel, which may be helpful in revision settings.

Opening the FM portal with a large hemostat facilitates easy suture and graft passage. A grasper is used to retrieve passing sutures from both the femoral and tibial side out the FM portal. Care must be taken to ensure no soft tissue suture bridge is created. A hemostat is used to clamp the tibial passing suture out of the way (Fig. 16-16).

The passing suture is used to shuttle the sutures from the femoral TightRope RT (Arthrex, Naples, FL) out through the lateral thigh. The graft is then pulled through the FM portal until the proximal end of the graft reaches the aperture of the femoral tunnel (Fig. 16-17). If the potential femoral tunnel measurement and the loop shortening were done correctly, the button should be deployed on the lateral aspect of femoral cortex and not outside of the IT band. Deployment can be confirmed by

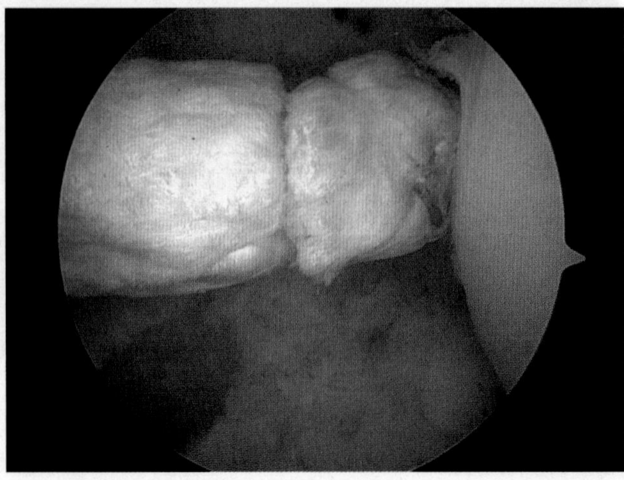

FIGURE 16-17

The graft is pulled into the notch until the end of the graft reaches the aperture of the femoral tunnel.

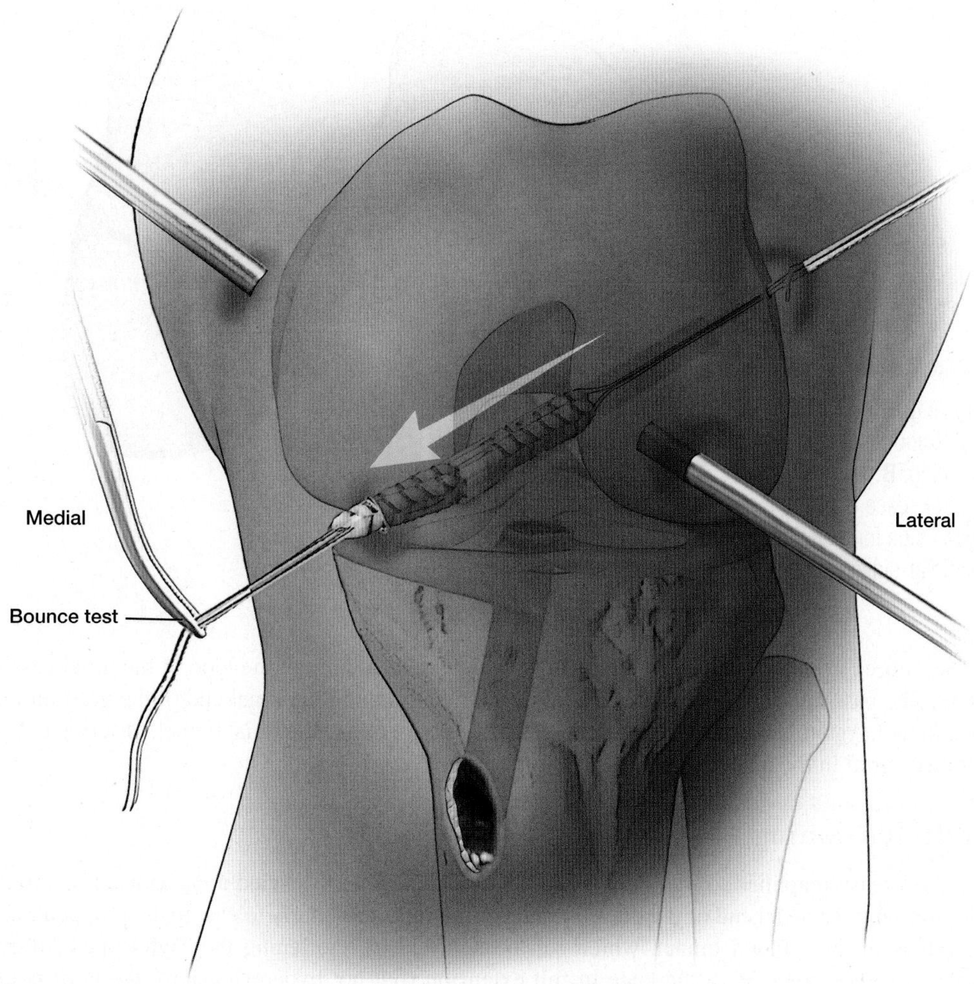

FIGURE 16-18

The "bounce test" is used to confirm the button has successfully been deployed on the femoral side.

performing the "TightRope" maneuver. To perform this maneuver, the femoral sutures are grasped in one hand, and the tibial in the other hand. The button is pulled a 1 to 2 mm off of the femoral cortex, and then, tension is quickly placed on the tibial sutures. The surgeon should feel a firm end point as the button reaches the femoral cortical bone (Fig. 16-18). Once the femoral button is successfully deployed, the adjustable loop is shortened until 20 mm of graft enters the femoral tunnel (i.e., when no suture is seen on the femoral side) (Fig. 16-19). Approximately 5 mm of space is left in the femoral socket for final tightening after tibial-sided fixation (Fig. 16-20).

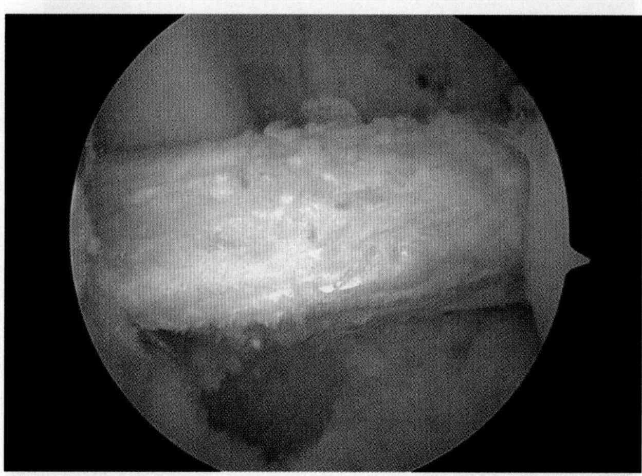

FIGURE 16-19

About 2 cm of graft is pulled into the femoral tunnel by tightening the adjustable loop.

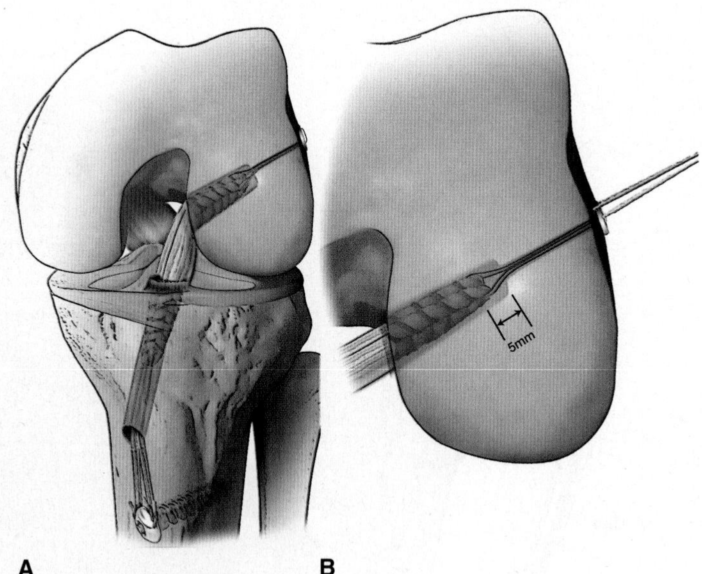

FIGURE 16-20

A: Final graft in place following tibial fixation and final femoral tightening. **B:** Approximately 5 mm of space is left on the femoral side for final tightening after tibial-sided fixation.

The sutures from the distal end of the graft are then placed through the loop of the tibial passing suture. The passing suture is then pulled out of the tibia bringing the tibial end of the graft into the tibial tunnel. Again, the suture from graft preparation should be in the tibial tunnel, ensuring at least 20 mm of graft in the tunnel.

Graft Tensioning

With firm tension applied to the tibial fixation sutures, the knee is cycled approximately 20 times. Prior to fixing the distal end of the graft, we again look intra-articularly to ensure the proper amount of graft is in the femoral tunnel, which can be adjusted by shortening the TightRope (Arthrex, Naples, FL) construct. With the knee in full extension (but not hyperextension), the graft is tensioned and the tibial side secured. If a screw is used, we prefer the Arthrex (Naples, FL) low-profile flat-headed screw, which does not require a washer. Alternatively, the tibial side can be fixed with an adjustable loop cortical button as previously noted. The adjustable loop is then maximally shortened while maintaining the knee in extension. A Lachman maneuver and final arthroscopic evaluation are then performed to confirm appropriate graft tension (Fig. 16-21A,B).

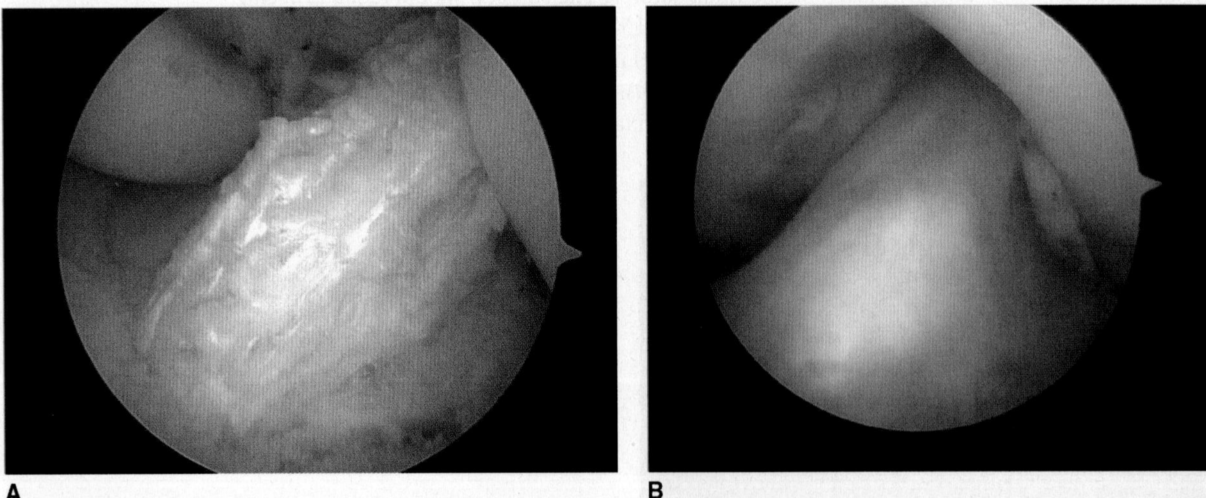

FIGURE 16-21

A: Graft following immediate reconstruction. **B:** Graft appearance following second-look arthroscopy.

PEARLS AND PITFALLS

- If arthroscopy is performed prior to graft harvest, ensure all fluid is drained from the knee to minimize capsular distention on the deep surface of the quadriceps tendon.
- It is critical to adequately excise the subcutaneous fat and overlying paratenon following skin incision to allow for adequate visualization following incision for graft harvest.
- Any crossing vessels identified with the arthroscope prior to graft harvest should be coagulated.
- A layer of fat lies deep to the quadriceps tendon as it attaches to the patella; if fat is encountered, avoid deeper dissection or risk capsular violation.
- The ends of the graft should be trimmed prior to suture addition, as the graft diameter will increase by 0.5 to 1 mm following suture addition.
- Passing the graft from the FM portal allows the surgeon to customize tunnel diameter on both the femoral and tibial sides.
- Ensure that FM portal is large enough to ensure easy graft passage and cleared of fat and soft tissue so that passing sutures do not get tangled or caught.
- Shorten femoral tightrope so it is just 5 mm longer than femoral length measurement so that it is not pulled through the IT band.
- Cycle knee 20 times and look at graft position in femoral tunnel to ensure the proper amount of graft remains in the tunnel.
- Graft tensioning should be performed in full extension, but not hyperextension.
- Always check the operative thigh prior to discharging the patient from the recovery room to ensure no potential compartment syndrome.

POSTOPERATIVE MANAGEMENT

Postoperatively, we treat our quadriceps tendon autograft ACL reconstructions similar to alternative graft options. We do not routinely use a brace, except with meniscal repair or coexisting extra-articular ligamentous injury. Extension (prone hangs, forced extension) is emphasized in the immediate postoperative period. Patients are instructed to use crutches with minimal weight bearing for their first 3 to 4 days, which coincides with their first postoperative visit. At that point, they began full weight bearing with crutches for 2 weeks. They are then transitioned off crutches when they can walk without a limp.

COMPLICATIONS

One complication specific to quadriceps tendon graft harvest includes harvest site hematoma. This condition presents with swelling directly under the harvest site wound and must be differentiated from intra-articular hematoma. Wound hematomas can be from damage to a crossing vessel overlying the quadriceps tendon, inadvertent muscle damage, or intra-articular bleeding, which may escape through a full-thickness rent. Although uncommon, this can be a source of severe pain within 2 to 3 days of surgery. Once identified, this should be evacuated immediately. We have seen no long-term sequelae of harvest site hematoma following evacuation. Most of these complications happened early in the development of this technique, although they can still occur. Since we have started to identify and coagulate any crossing vessels, placed gel-foam in the harvest site, and limited graft harvest length to less than 8 cm, we have observed fewer problems with postoperative hematoma.

Although extremely rare, we have diagnosed one impending thigh compartment syndrome following quadriceps tendon harvest in the postanesthesia care unit. This was immediately evacuated, explored, and found to emanate from a proximal muscle arteriole. This complication occurred early in our quadriceps harvest experience and was secondary to harvesting a graft greater than 8 cm in length going into the rectus femoris muscle.

We have seen one postoperative deformity with proximal retraction of the rectus femoris muscle belly. Despite the deformity, the patient reported no functional deficit and had an otherwise normal recovery. Rates of other complications such as reruptures and arthrofibrosis are similar to alternative autografts and will be discussed in more detail below.

RESULTS

Over the past 4 years, the senior author has performed over 400 primary ACL and revision reconstructions using the quadriceps tendon. This is the senior author's primary graft choice for all patients under 25 years old and all elite collegiate and professional athletes. All of the patients have been prospectively followed. We have not had early clinical failures (less than 3 months), or significant changes in KT-1000 values from 6 weeks to 3 months, suggesting our preferred method of fixation is sufficient. We have had no significant changes in KT-1000 from 6 weeks to 6 months. Our overall failure rate from the first 200 reconstructions stands at 5.2% with over 2-year follow-up. As expected, patients between 15 and 20 years old had higher rates of graft failure (8.2%) compared to patients over 20 (2.8%). Overall rate of arthrofibrosis (loss of extension) requiring intervention was 6.2% with the majority being in patients under 20 years old. Initially, we did not recognize the importance of tensioning the graft in full extension and emphasizing early postoperative full extension and believe this may have contributed to higher early rates of extension loss. If the patient does not achieve full extension within 6 weeks of surgery, the odds of them having a cyclops-type lesion are very high. Patients who did not achieve full extension by 3 months underwent an arthroscopy, and all were found to have a cyclops lesion and all achieved full or near-full extension after the procedure.

RECOMMENDED READINGS

Geib TM, Shelton WR, Phelps RA, et al. Anterior cruciate ligament reconstruction using quadriceps tendon autograft: intermediate-term outcome. *Arthroscopy.* 2009;25(12):1408–1414. Available at http://doi.org/10.1016/j.arthro.2009.06.004

Lund B, Nielsen T, Faunø P, et al. Is quadriceps tendon a better graft choice than patellar tendon? A prospective randomized study. *Arthroscopy.* 2014;30(5):593–598. Available at http://doi.org/10.1016/j.arthro.2014.01.012

Slone HS, Romine SE, Premkumar A, et al. Quadriceps tendon autograft for anterior cruciate ligament reconstruction: a comprehensive review of current literature and systematic review of clinical results. *Arthroscopy.* 2015;31(3):541–554. Available at http://doi.org/10.1016/j.arthro.2014.11.010

17 Anatomic Anterior Cruciate Ligament Double-Bundle Reconstruction

Garth Nyambi Walker, Daniel Guenther, Chad Griffith, and Freddie H. Fu

INDICATIONS/CONTRAINDICATIONS

Rupture of the anterior cruciate ligament (ACL) is one of the most common injuries worldwide. Traditional ACL reconstruction/repair techniques have been sufficient in providing anteroposterior (AP) tibiofemoral stability. However, current techniques such as anatomic single-bundle (SB) and double-bundle (DB) reconstruction have been shown to restore both AP and rotational stability more effectively. Indications for ACL reconstruction, either SB or DB, are patients desiring to return to cutting and pivoting activities or symptomatic instability despite nonoperative management. Additionally, concomitant meniscal injury is a relative indication for surgical repair especially in younger patients. While it is theorized that chronic knee instability from ACL deficiency may lead to early-onset osteoarthritis, this outcome has never been proven by literature. Ultimately, the decision of whether or not to undergo ACL reconstruction is a combined decision between surgeon and patient based on lifestyle choices and objective evaluation. Contraindications for DB ACL reconstruction include tibial insertion size less than 14 mm, open physes, severe arthritic changes (grade 3 or greater), and multiligamentous injuries. Relative contraindications include narrow notch and severe bone bruising over the lateral femoral condyle.

DOUBLE-BUNDLE CONCEPT

Anatomy studies have well documented that the ACL consists of the anteromedial (AM) and posterolateral (PL) bundles. While biomechanical studies have demonstrated improved rotational stability with DB reconstruction, this has not been demonstrated in vivo. Understanding the DB concept is more important than the decision between performing an SB or DB reconstruction. Paramount to the DB concept is an understanding of the bony morphology and native footprints of the ACL, as improper tunnel placement can cause increased graft rupture rates, persistent rotational instability, or loss of extension. Another key feature of the DB concept is the ability to distinguish between partial, complete SB, and complete DB tears both preoperatively and intraoperatively so that treatment can be individualized with either an SB augmentation or complete reconstruction. Finally, it is important to take measures both on the preoperative MRI and intraoperatively to ensure that the patient's knee is large enough to accommodate a DB reconstruction. Tibial insertion size greater than 18 mm is large enough to undergo DB graft placement, whereas a tibial insertion size less than 14 mm is too small. A footprint size of 14 to 18 mm is controversial whether it is large enough to accommodate a DB reconstruction without excessive risk of tunnel coalescence. The notch morphology is also important to assess with a notch width less than 14 mm being too small to accommodate the DB reconstruction.

PREOPERATIVE PLANNING

Preoperative planning includes a detailed history, physical exam, preoperative clearance, x-rays (Fig. 17-1), and MRI (Fig. 17-2).

Physical exam should include a range of motion (ROM) exam, Lachman exam, anterior drawer test, and pivot shift test as well as a thorough examination assessing for concomitant ligamentous injuries. Often, patients will have concomitant medial collateral ligament (MCL) injuries, which can be found on valgus stress test at 0 and 20 degrees of knee flexion. It is important to discern whether these are femoral or tibial-sided injuries since femoral-sided injuries have a high rate of healing with nonoperative management. In addition, valgus gapping in extension is indicative of a higher-grade injury. It is also important to assess for concomitant posterolateral corner (PLC) injuries with a varus stress test at 0 and 20 degrees of knee flexion, Dial test, PL drawer test, and external rotation recurvatum test as an undiagnosed PLC injury increases the risk of ACL graft failure.

Patients must gain full ROM and resolution of any swelling prior to surgery. On average, regaining full ROM takes 2 to 4 weeks from the time of injury. Surgery should also be delayed if a concomitant MCL injury is discovered to allow time for the MCL injury to heal without surgical intervention.

Preoperative measurements of tibial insertion size, quadriceps tendon thickness, and patella tendon thickness can be obtained from the MRI to assist in preparation for DB indication and graft choice (Fig. 17-3).

SURGERY

After induction, an examination under anesthesia (EUA) is performed on both the involved and uninvolved knee including Lachman exam, pivot shift test, anterior drawer, posterior drawer, dial test, and varus and valgus stress test in 0 and 20 degrees of knee flexion. A Lachman exam of 1B or 2A in the absence of a clunk on pivot shift test can be indicative of an SB tear. In this case, consideration for arthroscopic examination of the ACL prior to autograft harvest should be considered. In this way,

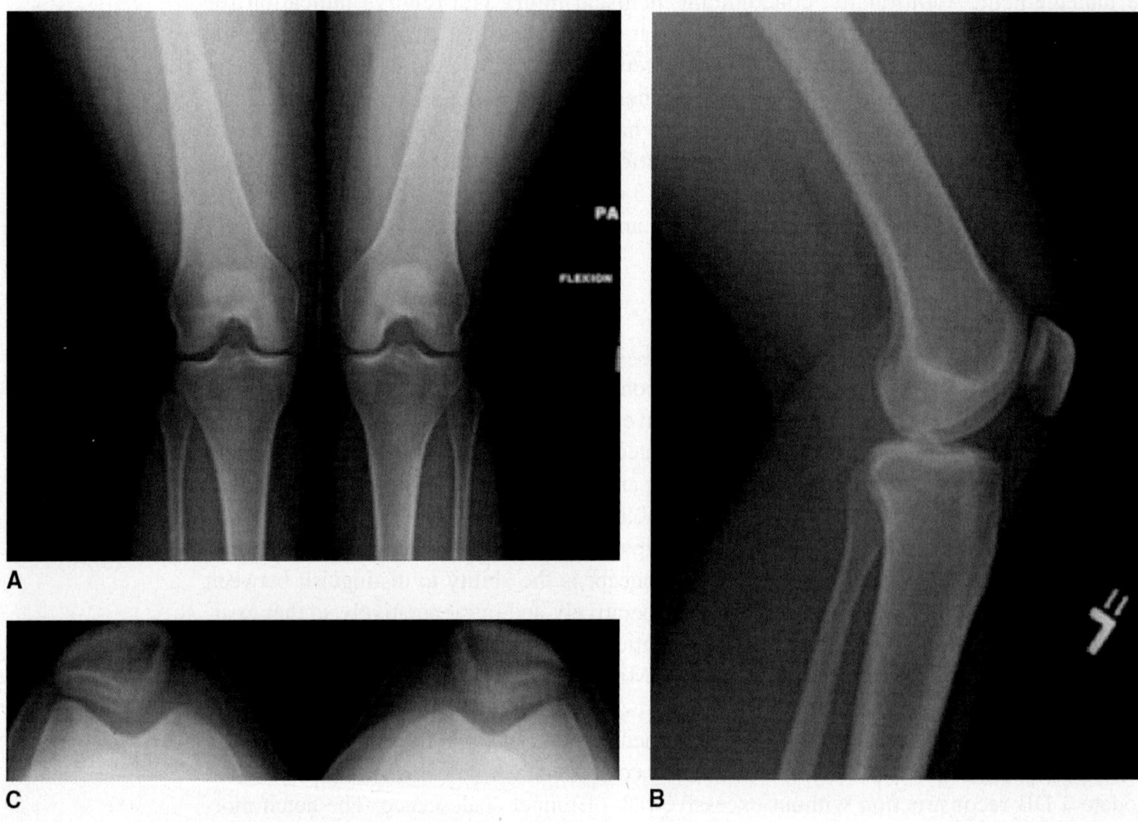

FIGURE 17-1

Anteroposterior (**A**), lateral (**B**), and Merchant (**C**) views of radiographs are taken at the patient's initial visit. Possible injuries, like fractures and osteoarthritis, and the alignment of the lower extremity, are examined.

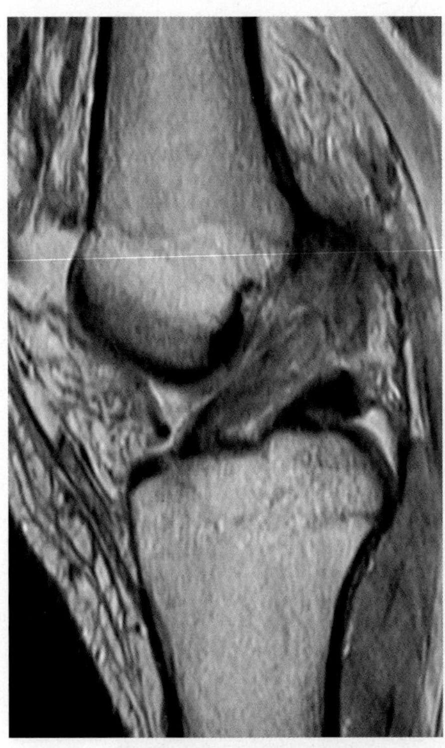

FIGURE 17-2
A sagittal view of MRI confirms a torn ACL.

if an SB tear is found on arthroscopy and augmentation is planned, then the morbidity from harvesting a bone block or both hamstring tendons can be avoided.

Patients are positioned supine with the foot of the table dropped and the operative leg secured in a circumferential leg holder (Fig. 17-4). This position is the preference of the senior author of this chapter and multiple positioning methods can be used.

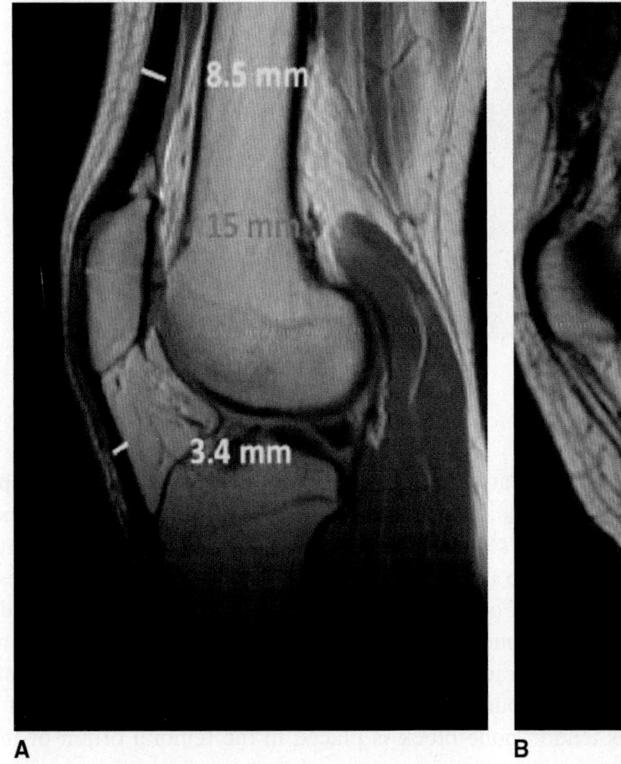

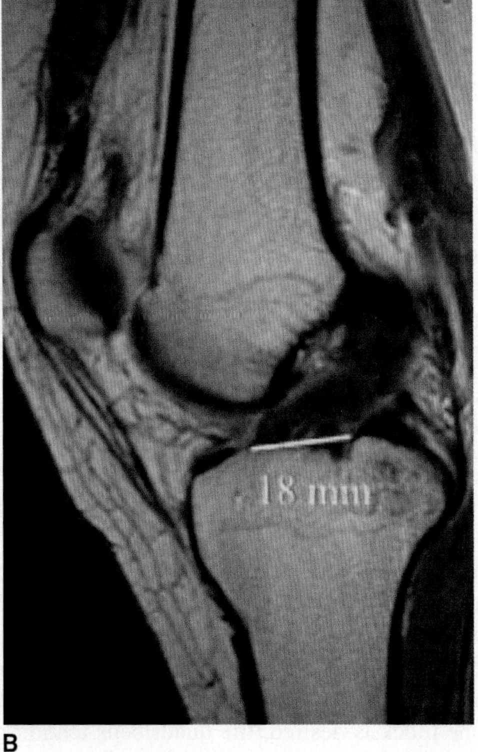

A B

FIGURE 17-3
MRI measurements of quad tendon and patella tendon thickness (**A**) as well as ACL tibial insertion site length (**B**).

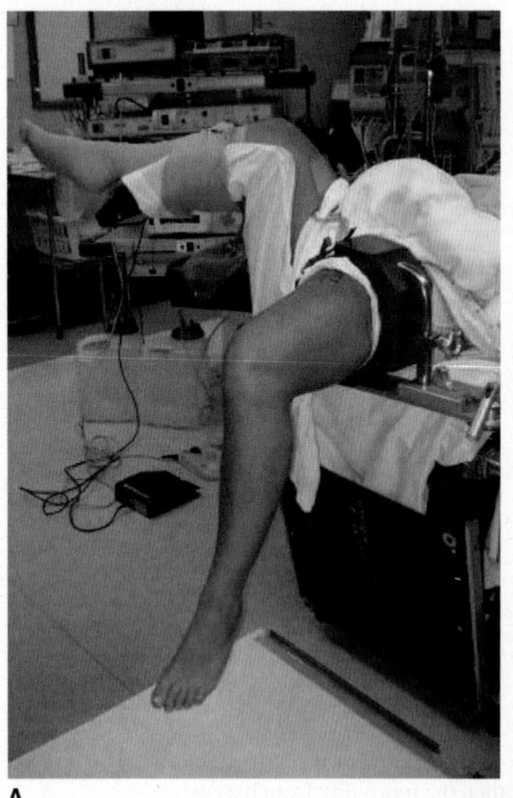

A

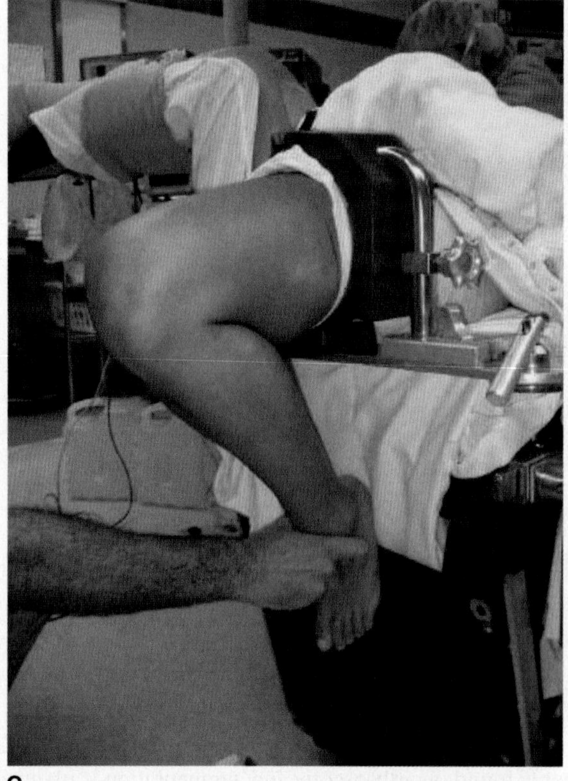

C

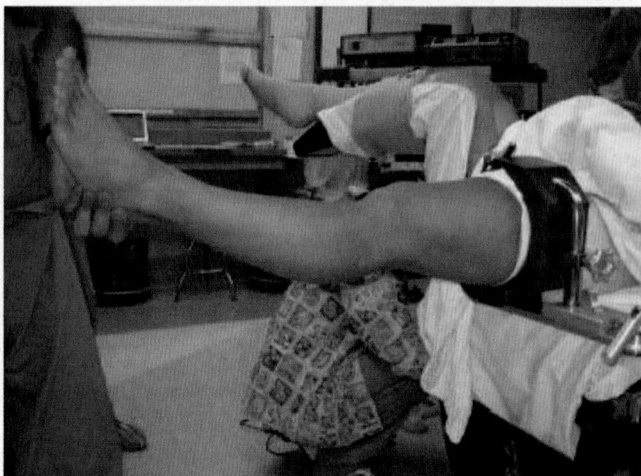

B

FIGURE 17-4

A knee holder is used to keep the surgery knee stable during the surgery (**A**). It also allows a good range of motion, both extension (**B**) and flexion (**C**), during the surgery.

Graft Selection

Preoperative MRI is used to assess potential graft choices. Minimum thicknesses for quadriceps tendon and patellar tendon are 7 and 5 mm, respectively. Autografts are preferred for patients less than 35 years of age, while allografts are often selected for patients greater than 40 years of age. However, all patients are consented for possible allograft use in case graft augmentation is necessary due to insufficient size of the autograft. For DB reconstruction, autograft options include hamstring or quad tendon (with or without a bone block). Hamstring autografts use the semitendinosus graft doubled for the AM bundle and gracilis graft tripled for PL. If inadequate autograft size based on coverage for tibial insertion is found, an allograft can be used to supplement. If a bone block is desired, the quadriceps tendon bone block is placed in the femoral origin of the ACL and the tendon is separated between the rectus femoris and vastus intermedius portions. These two portions of the tendon are used for the tibial insertions of the AM and PL bundles.

Allograft tissue has the advantage of predetermined size prior to incision as well as possibility of prep before incision for efficiency. However, drawbacks include delayed vascularization, potential

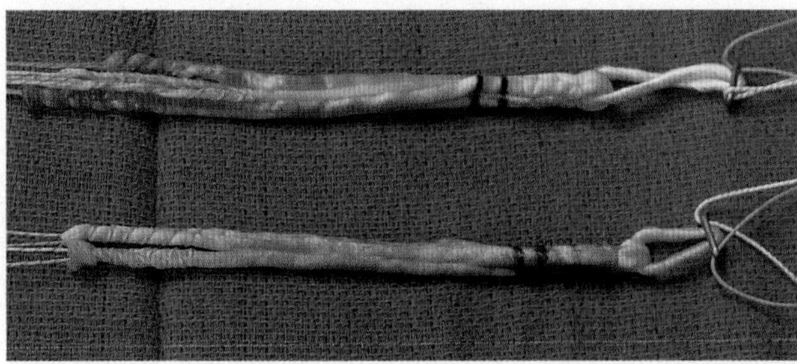

FIGURE 17-5

The graft is prepared on a back table by an assistant surgeon. The length of the femoral tunnels is measured, and the length of the grafts is adjusted accordingly.

reaction or disease transmission, increased cost, or lack of availability/variable supply. Allograft is not recommended in younger patients (less than 35 years old) involved in high-risk sports who have suitable autograft options.

Graft Preparation

Discussion of a closed-loop suspensory fixation will be discussed in this chapter; however, the authors acknowledge that multiple fixation systems are viable. For soft tissue grafts, the ends of both tendons are whipstitched with no. 2 braided nonabsorbable sutures. The tendons are then placed through the closed loop of the suspensory devices and folded in half (Fig. 17-5). The grafts are then placed on 15 pounds. of tension until they are ready to be passed into the knee to remove any creep from the graft construct. The femoral portion of the graft is marked at the appropriate depth at which the button will be able to exit the tunnel and flip into position.

Portal Placement and Diagnostic Arthroscopy

Appropriate portal placement is critical in performing thorough diagnostic arthroscopy and for accurate tunnel placement drilling. The senior author recommends three portals to ensure optimal visualization of the appropriate anatomic landmarks and an unobstructed access to the femoral insertion site for tunnel drilling (Fig. 17-6). The first portal is created superior to the inferior pole of the patella directly alongside the lateral border of the patella. This high lateral portal (LP) gives a good overview of ACL anatomy within the notch. Subsequently, AM and accessory anteromedial (AAM) portals are created under direct visualization of an 18-gauge spinal needle. The AM portal is

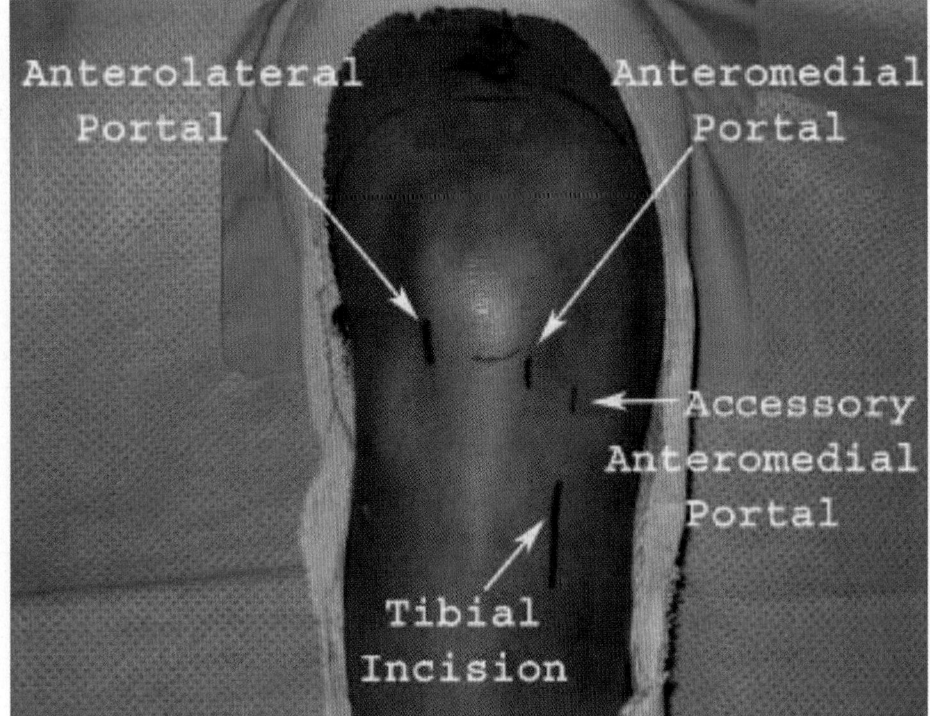

FIGURE 17-6

Standard anterolateral and anteromedial portal are used. In addition, an accessory anteromedial portal is used to provide better view of the lateral wall of the femoral notch. Tibial incision is made at the medial aspect of the tibia, and it is anterior to the tibial attachment of MCL.

placed such that the spinal needle is directly in line with the fibers of the ACL. This portal is either adjacent to the medial edge of the patella tendon or transtendinous. The AM portal has many uses including direct visualization of the ACL insertion sites and use in measuring the ACL dimensions. Medially above the joint line, the AAM portal is created with a direct trajectory of the spinal needle to the ACL femoral origin. The AAM portal should be slightly proximal to the AM portal and should provide adequate space from the medial femoral condyle cartilage for passage of instruments to avoid iatrogenic cartilage injury when the reamer is passed over the guidewire. The AAM portal is used for drilling the femoral tunnels and for best viewing of the AP profile of the medial wall of the lateral femoral condyle. All three compartments of the knee are examined in diagnostic arthroscopy to evaluate for associated injuries to cartilage or menisci and pathology addressed as indicated.

Reconstruction Method Decision-Making

The ACL rupture pattern is thoroughly evaluated. The ACL stump is cut to evaluate the insertion sites of both the AM and PL bundles of the ACL (Fig. 17-7). Before preparation of the medial wall of the LFC,

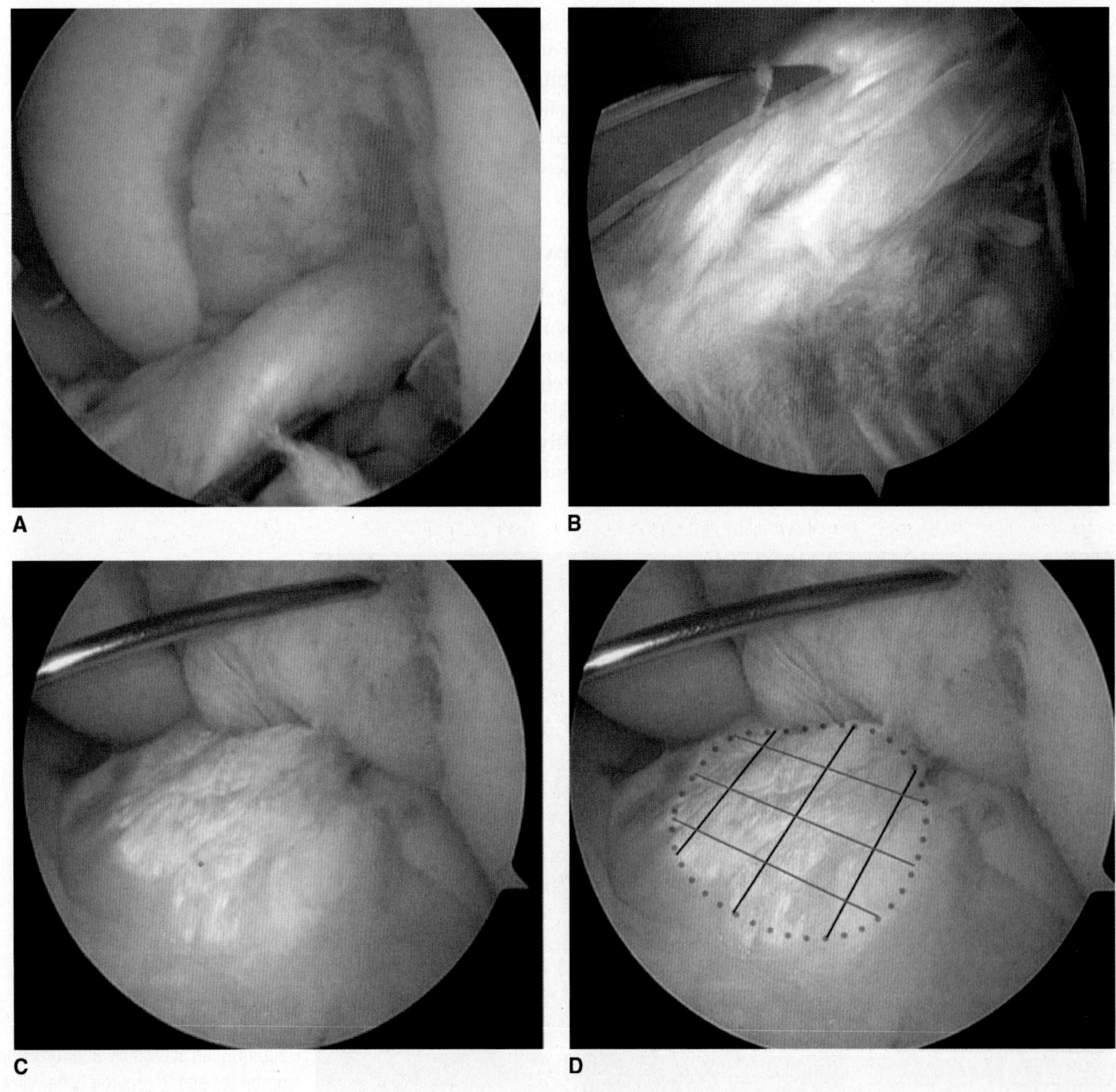

FIGURE 17-7

The ACL remnant is evaluated (**A**). Then, the stump is cut (**B**) to visualize the tibial insertion site (**C**). Measurements can be taken to determine length, width, and area (**D**).

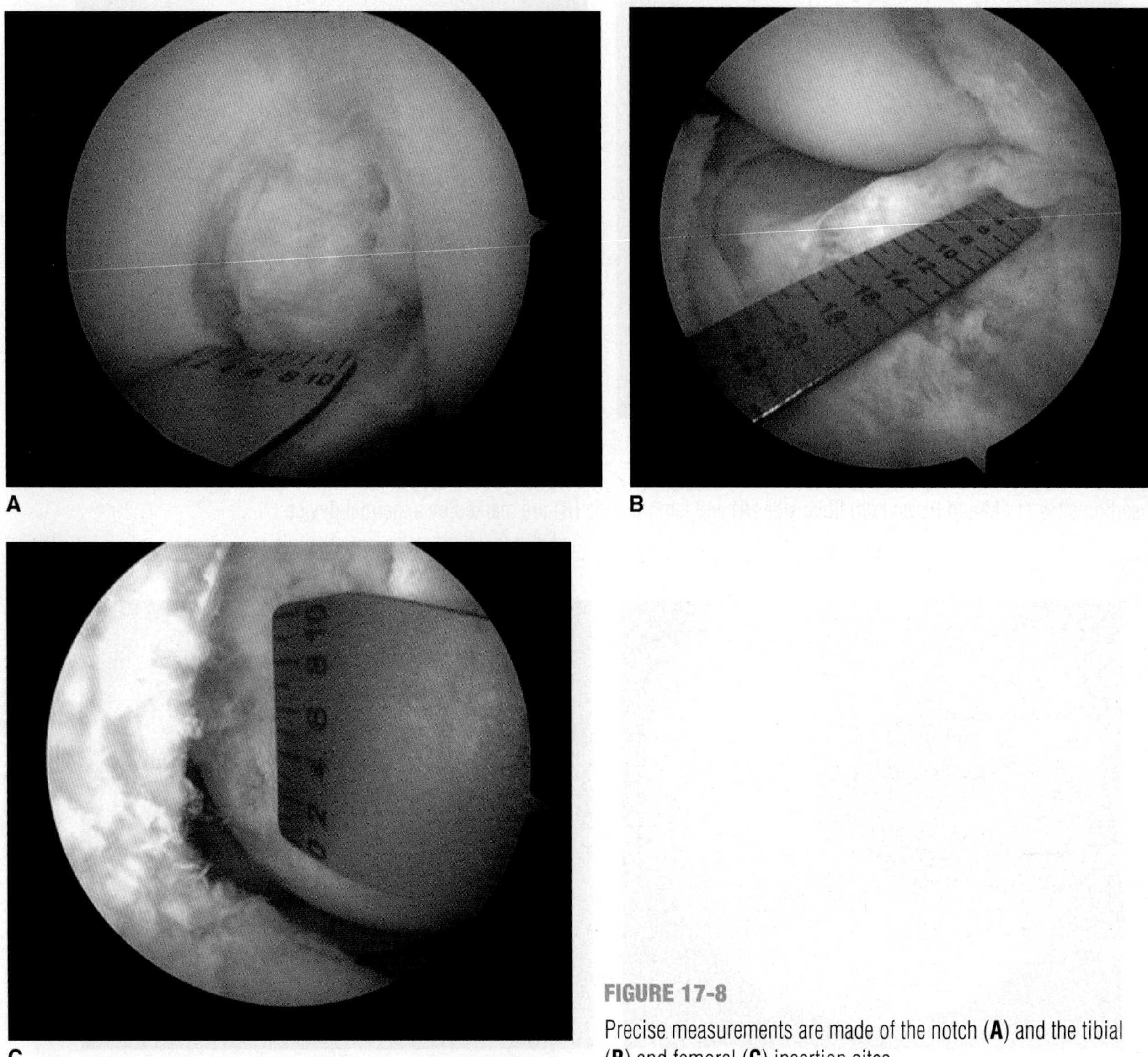

FIGURE 17-8

Precise measurements are made of the notch (**A**) and the tibial (**B**) and femoral (**C**) insertion sites.

soft tissue at the origin is carefully probed and the outline of the origin is preserved with the aid of an arthroscopic shaver and radiofrequency thermal ablator. The lateral intercondylar ridge and the bifurcate ridge are used to determine the native femoral insertion site. The LP is used to evaluate the tibial insertion, and appreciation of the entire footprint for both bundles is critical to placement of the tunnels. When remnant tissue is present, the surgeon may carefully dissect the tissue to get a good overview of the entire footprint. It is also important to note that for chronic cases where visualization of the footprint is difficult, the posterior margin of the anterior horn of the lateral meniscus marks the center of the tibial footprint in the AP direction. Precise measurements are made during this portion of the case as well (Fig. 17-8).

Tunnel Placement and Drilling

Once the femoral origin and tibial insertion site positions and dimensions are appreciated, the next step is to mark the center of the planned tunnels (Fig. 17-9) and then to perform drilling (Fig. 17-10). The tunnel size will vary between patients based on the footprint size and graft size, but, typically, the AM tunnel is 7 to 8 mm and the PL tunnel is 5 to 7 mm. The tunnel diameters should be 1 to 2 mm smaller than the native bundle sizes to allow for an adequate bone bridge between the two tunnels on both the tibial and femoral sides.

The femoral PL tunnel is created first. If a quadriceps tendon bone block has been harvested with the plan of inserting the bone block into the femoral condyle, then the femoral tunnel should be

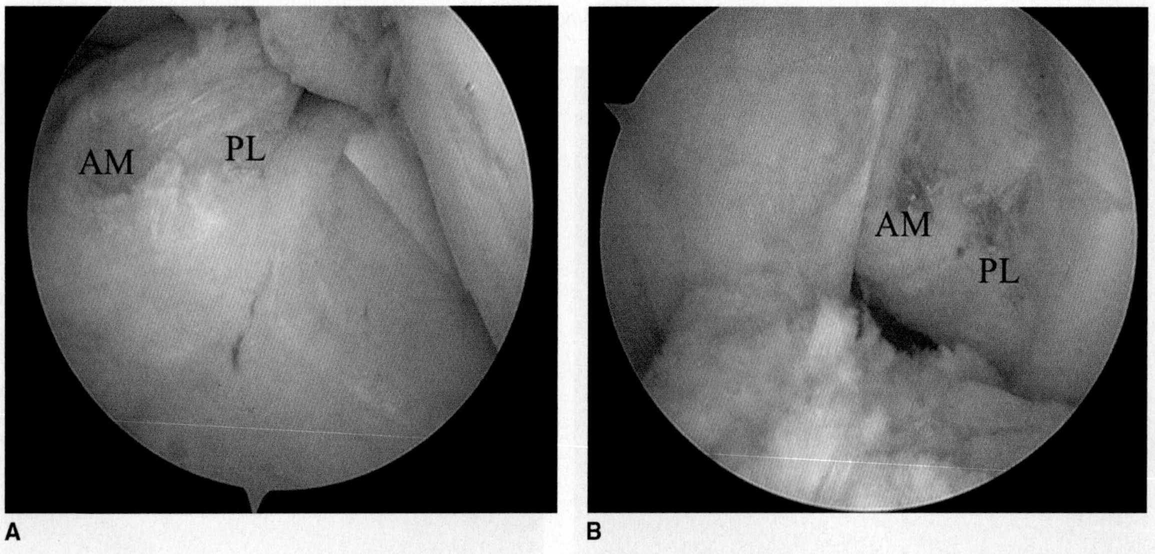

FIGURE 17-9

The insertion sites of AM and PL on both tibial side (**A**) and femoral side (**B**) are marked by a thermal device.

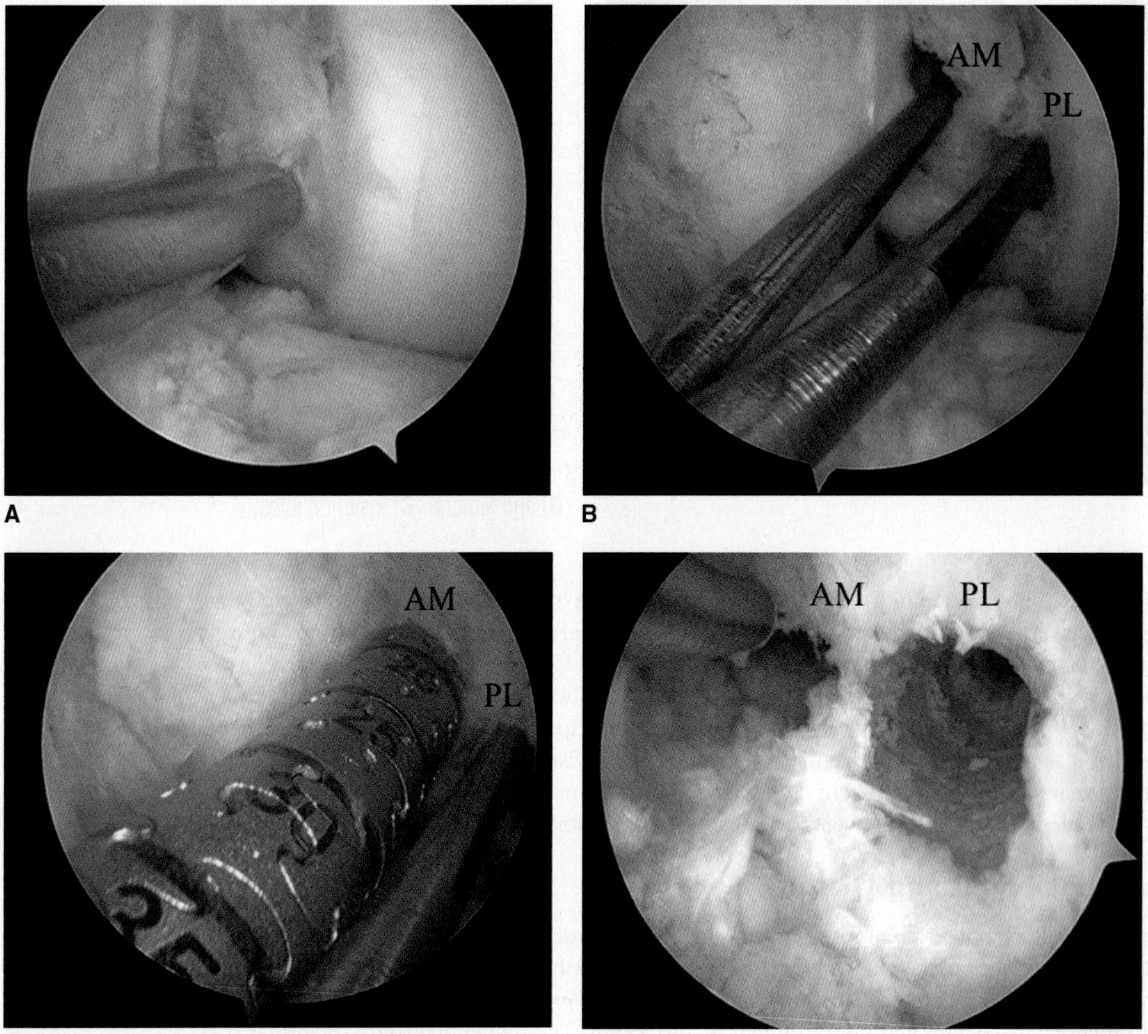

AM

PL

A

B

AM

PL

AM

PL

C

D

FIGURE 17-10

A Steadman awl is used to mark the desired femoral AM and PL positions for guide pins and to make it easier for the guide pins to stick to the chosen spot (**A**). Subsequently, guide pins are used (**B**), followed by a flexible drill (**C**). After using an EndoButton drill, the finished femoral tunnels are shown (**D**).

drilled in an SB manner. The senior author recommends drilling through the AAM portal with the knee in a hyperflexed position to best access the anatomic footprint. The senior author does acknowledge that other techniques such as outside-in drilling are also plausible as long as tunnels are placed into the centers of the AM and PL bundles with a 1- to 2-mm bone bridge between the tunnels.

If a soft tissue graft is planned, then with the arthroscope in the AM portal, a microfracture awl is used to make a pilot hole in the center of the PL bundle. A flexible guidewire is then placed into the center of the PL bundle footprint. A straight guidewire can also be used. The knee is then hyperflexed and the pin advanced through the lateral femoral cortex and skin. The length of the femoral tunnel should then be determined using a multitude of proprietary systems. Ideally, the length of the tunnel should be in the 30 to 40 mm range as the goal is to create a socket of at least 27 mm such that 20 mm of the graft can be present within the tunnel and an additional 7 mm to allow for the button to flip. If the tunnel is of insufficient length, the most likely cause is a lack of hyperflexion during drilling. If a straight pin is used, it is important to keep the knee in a hyperflexed position to avoid bending the pin. The cannulated reamer is advanced over the guidewire, taking care not to damage the articular cartilage of the medial femoral condyle as the reamer is introduced into the joint. A socket of at least 27 mm is created as stated above. As the socket is created, it is important not to drill through the lateral cortex. If the lateral cortex is perforated, then an extended or revision button will be necessary for suspensory fixation. The smaller proprietary drill is then used to perforate the lateral cortex for passage of fixation device later on the femoral side. A suture is then passed through the eyelet on the guidewire for future graft passage.

The next step is to create the tibial tunnels (Fig. 17-11). This step is the same whether two femoral tunnels were created or a single femoral tunnel was created for a quadriceps tendon bone block. A vertical 3- to 4-cm incision is made over the proximal portion of the AM tibia 2 cm below the joint line and 1 to 2 cm medial to the tibial tubercle. The incision site is roughly the same incision as was used for hamstring autograft harvest. The arthroscope is then placed in the LP and an ACL tip guide set at 55 degrees is introduced through the AM or AAM portal to the marked center of the PL bundle (Fig. 17-12). The tip guidewire is then advanced to the center of the PL bundle. The ACL tip guide is then changed 45 degrees and the tip is placed in the center of the AM bundle. A second guidewire is advanced to the center of the AM bundle. The starting point for the second guidewire needs to be at least 10 mm away from the PL bundle guidewire, although 15 mm is preferred. The knee is brought in figure of four positions to achieve a better view on the anatomic landmarks (Fig. 17-13).

With both guidewires in place, the knee is brought into full extension to evaluate impingement with the roof of the notch. The distance between the guidewires is also scrutinized to ensure that there is enough distance between the wires to accommodate both tunnels and a 1- to 2-mm bone bridge. Both tibial tunnels are then drilled using cannulated barrel reamers approximately 1 to 2 mm smaller than planned final diameter of the tunnel and sequentially dilated by hand in 0.5-mm increments up to the final desired size (Fig. 17-14). Care must be used in this step to prevent tunnel convergence, which is why this step is done by hand.

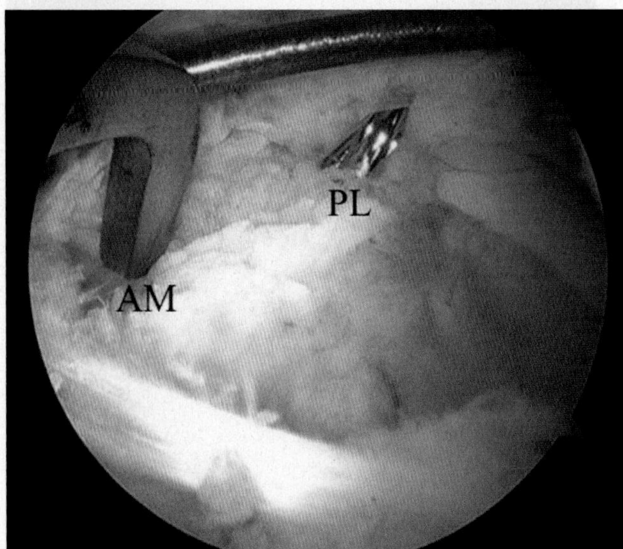

FIGURE 17-11

The tibial insertion sites of AM and PL bundles are shown. The aiming elbow is used to guide the direction of the guide pin.

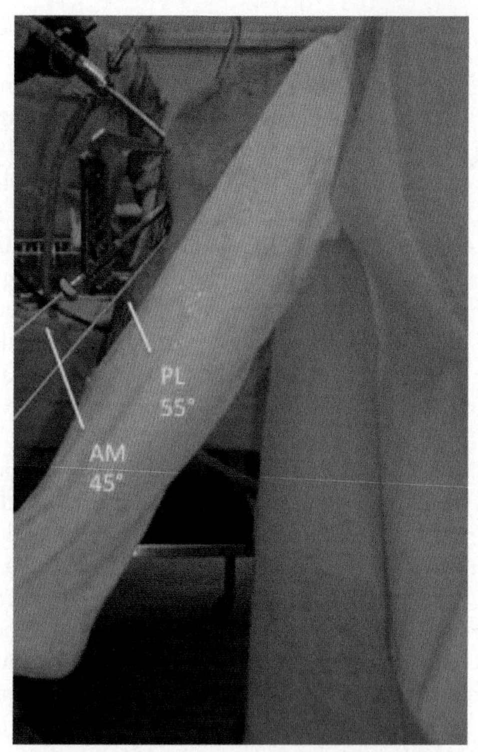

FIGURE 17-12

The AM and PL guide pins are inserted at 45 and 55 degrees, respectively.

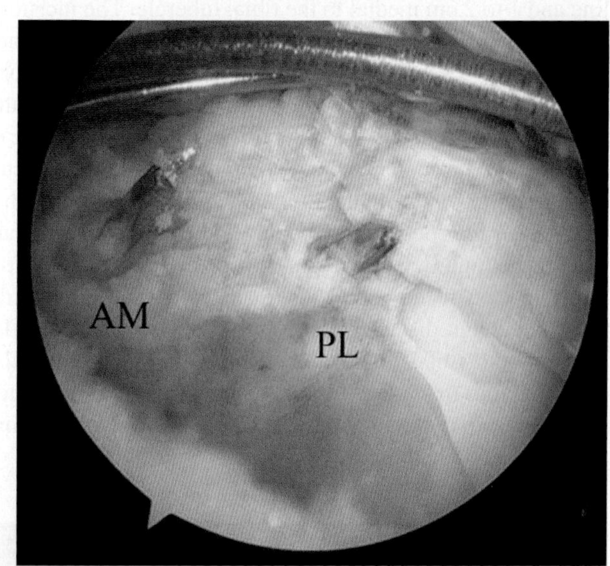

FIGURE 17-13

The knee is brought in figure of four position to achieve a better view on the anatomic landmarks.

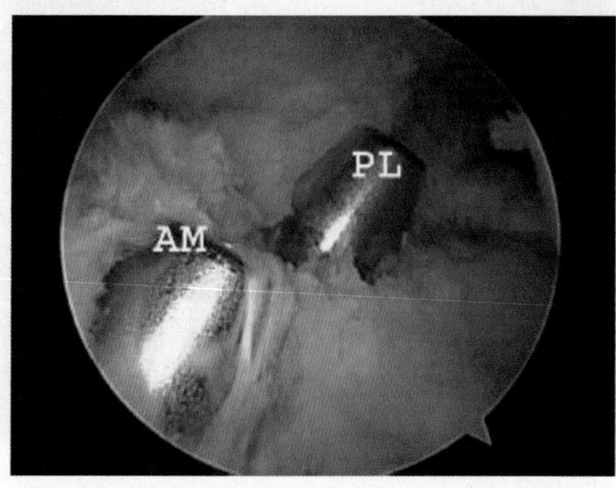

FIGURE 17-14

Dilators are used to enlarge the tibial tunnels.

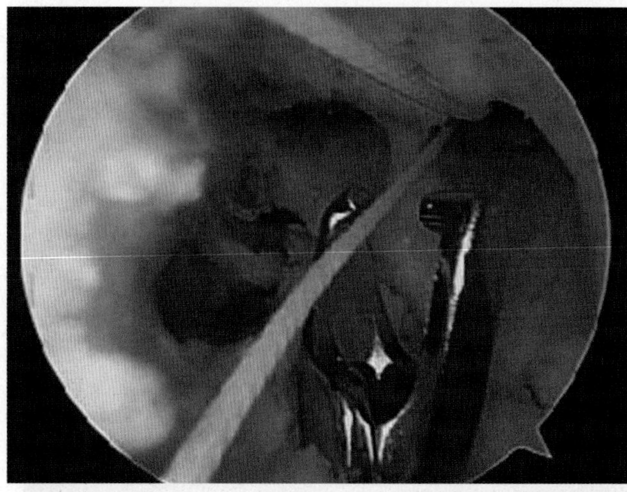

FIGURE 17-15

The looped suture is visualized and retrieved with an arthroscopic suture grasper through the PL tibial tunnel.

Similar to the PL femoral tunnel, the femoral AM tunnel center is identified with the arthroscope viewing from the AM portal and the microfracture awl is used to make the pilot hole through the AAM portal. The femoral AM tunnel guidewire placement and reaming may take place through three sites (via accessory medial portal; transtibially through the PL tibial tunnel, transtibially through the AM tibial tunnel). However, true anatomic placement can be found through the accessory medial portal, which will nearly always produce the desired starting point. Drilling the femoral AM tunnel through the PL tibial tunnel increases the risk of creating a high femoral tunnel. Whichever option is chosen, the most important factors are anatomic, divergent tunnels that maximize tunnel length. After choosing a drilling method, the guidewire placement, socket reaming, perforation of the lateral cortex with the smaller proprietary drill, and suture passage are performed in the same manner as the PL femoral tunnel.

Graft Passage, Tensioning, and Fixation

The looped sutures within the femoral tunnels are retrieved out of their respective tibial tunnels (Fig. 17-15). Different colored sutures are used to aid identification of tunnels and grafts as a supplement to direct visualization (Fig. 17-16).

If a quadriceps bone block has been used, passing sutures need to be inserted through the AAM portal and the tibial tunnels. The sutures from both tibial tunnels and the femoral tunnel should be retrieved out the AAM portal at the same time to avoid a soft tissue bridge. The quadriceps bone block is then inserted through the AAM portal and pulled into the femoral tunnel until its suspensory fixation device is engaged on the lateral cortex. Then, the PL bundle is reduced into its tibial tunnel followed by the AM bundle.

For soft tissue grafts, it is important to note the orientation of the passing sutures. The PL suture must sit posterior to the AM bundle suture. The PL bundle graft is passed through its tibial and femoral tunnels until its suspensory fixation device is secured on the femoral side. The AM bundle graft is then passed in a symmetric manner (Fig. 17-17).

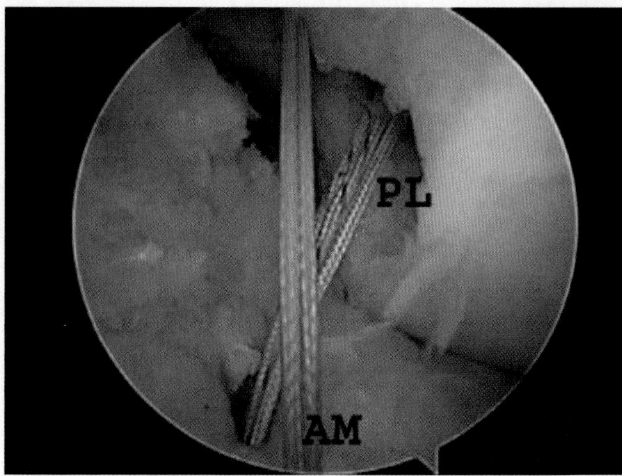

FIGURE 17-16

When in flexion, the AM and PL graft sutures show a crossing pattern, which is also true in intact ACL.

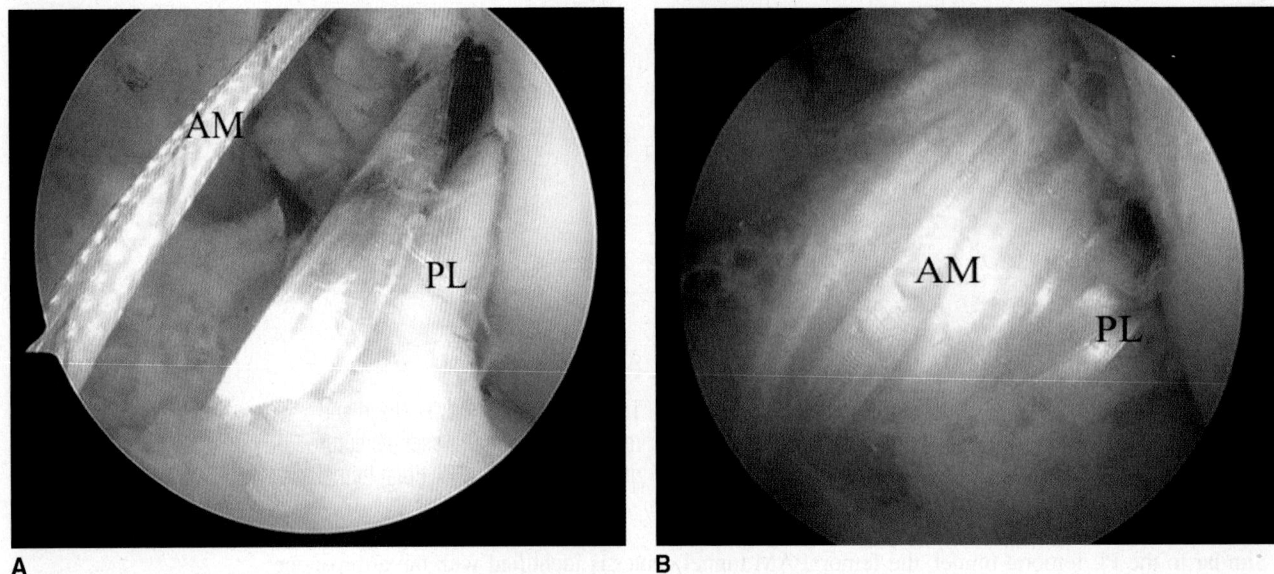

FIGURE 17-17

The grafts with the incorporated fibrin clot are passed (**A**). An EndoButton fixation is used to fix on the femoral side. The grafts will be pulled through (**B**) and the EndoButton will be flipped on the femoral cortex.

Fluoroscopic evaluation is performed with a mini C-arm to confirm engagement of the suspensory fixation devices on the lateral femoral cortex. Holding tension on both grafts, the knee is brought into full extension to ensure that no notch impingement is present. The knee is then cycled 15 to 20 times making sure to bring the knee into full extension with each cycle.

The tibial fixation of the PL bundle is performed at 0 degrees of knee flexion and the AM bundle fixation is secured at 20 to 30 degrees of knee flexion. The leg is placed on an adjustable-height Mayo stand for stability during tibial fixation. The senior author prefers tibial fixation interference screws but acknowledges that multiple fixation options exist. The interference screw size is usually line-to-line with the tunnel diameter but may need to be upsized if there is poor screw purchase. Final arthroscopic inspection is performed to evaluate graft position, ensure absence of impingement at full extension, and probe graft to confirm adequate tension. This final inspection of the graft analyzes the femoral origin and tibial insertion sites and is done from all three portals for the best overview. A Lachman exam is also performed to confirm that there is no residual laxity. If laxity is present, then the tibial side may need to be retightened. If a "pop" is felt during testing, then careful evaluation of the femoral fixation should be done with fluoroscopy. Following closure, a hinged knee brace locked in extension is applied.

PEARLS AND PITFALLS

- A high lateral portal is crucial in order to avoid poorly desired visualization from the fat pad.
- Optimal placement of the accessory medial portal under direct visualization above the meniscus is recommended to allow clearance from medial femoral condyle for drilling is critical to avoid iatrogenic injury.
- Be prepare to supplement a graft that is too small with adequate allograft in order to provide sufficient coverage of the tibial insertion site.
- Maintain appropriate bone bridge between tunnels.
- Mark the PL bundle graft with ink in order to maintain appropriate orientation of AM and PL bundle relationship during graft passage and graft fixation.
- Use bony and soft tissue landmarks in order to best estimate AM and PL bundle insertion site for less than ideal anatomy.

POSTOPERATIVE MANAGEMENT

Patients are expected to return 1 to 2 weeks after surgery where post-op x-rays are obtained (Fig. 17-18). Postoperative management of rehabilitation is separated into five stages. In order to

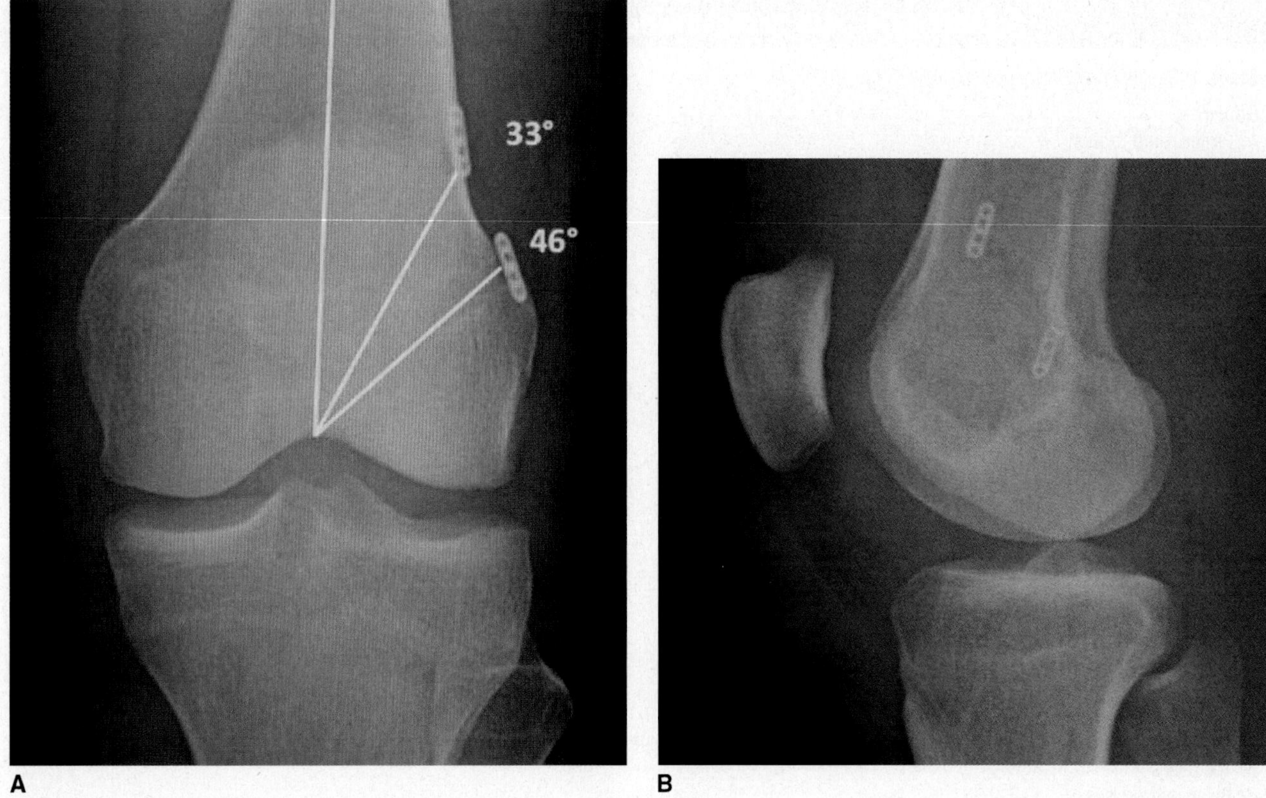

FIGURE 17-18

Anteroposterior **(A)** and lateral **(B)** views of radiographs are taken after the surgery to check the position of hardwares. Femoral tunnel angle greater than 33 degrees indicates potential anatomic placement of graft.

progress to each stage, certain milestones must be met. Stage 1 begins immediately postoperatively where the goal is to protect graft fixation, control inflammation, achieve full extension and ROM, and educate the patient. The goal is to obtain full ROM by 4 to 6 weeks postoperatively. If patients are struggling to regain their ROM, then they need closer observation with the possibility of a manipulation under anesthesia between 8 and 12 weeks post-op if they fail to regain motion. Manipulations after 12 weeks have a higher risk of fracture. Once patients have gained all of their ROM, between weeks 4 and 16, they may progress to strengthening, gait training, and endurance exercises. This focuses on stationary bike, leg press, fast walking on a treadmill, double and single leg squats, and lunges. In order to progress to stage 2, the patient must be able to walk 15 minutes without any symptoms, perform 10 single leg squats to 45 degrees of flexion without loss of balance, and be at least 4 months postoperative. Stage 2 is the introduction of running and lasts between 4 and 6 months postoperatively. Continual work on strengthening and proprioception is necessary in this stage. In order to advance to stage 3, the patient must be able to jog greater than 2 miles without any difficulty and perform a leg press at greater than 85% to their contralateral side. Stage 3 begins around 6 to 8 months postoperatively. It involves light agility including lateral shuffling, forward/backward shuttle runs, carioca, and ladder drills. To advance to stage 4, they must be able to perform leg press at 90% of their contralateral side, 10 consecutive single leg squats to 60 degrees of knee flexion without loss of balance or significant trunk shift, and demonstrate no compensatory mechanisms during deceleration and agility drills. Stage 4 begins around 7 to 9 months and is the start of jumping. Jumping starts straight up and down with observation for the knee falling into any type of functional valgus position. Once the patient has mastered up and down jumping with good mechanics, they may progress to forward, side, and box jumps. When patients have mastered all jumping without compensatory mechanisms and continue to have good core, pelvifemoral, and quad strength, they may progress to stage 5 no earlier than 9 months postoperatively. Stage 5 involves a gradual progression to single leg hops, sprinting activities, pivoting, and cutting activities. Finally, a return to sport participation test can be administered to clear for full activity. At all points, quadriceps strengthening and neuromuscular control are emphasized (Table 17-1). However, we recommend MRI evaluation of graft healing before the patient returns to high activity levels (Fig. 17-19).

TABLE 17-1 ACL Reconstruction and Rehabilitation Protocol

Stage 1: Begins immediately postoperatively through ~6 wk

Goals:
1. Protect graft fixation
2. Minimize effects of immobilization
3. Control inflammation
4. Full extension and flexion range of motion
5. Educate patient on rehabilitation progression

Therapeutic exercises:
1. Heel slides
2. Quadriceps sets
3. Patellar immobilization
4. Non–weight-bearing gastro/soleus stretches, begin hamstring stretches at 4 wk
5. Straight leg raises in all planes with brace in full extension until quadriceps strength is sufficient to prevent extension lag
6. Quadriceps isometrics at 60 and 90 degrees

Stage 2: Begins immediately 6 wk postoperatively and extends to ~8 wk

Goals:
1. Restore normal gait
2. Maintain full extension, progress flexion range of motion
3. Protect graft fixation

Therapeutic exercise
1. Wall slides 0–45 degrees
2. Four-way hip machine
3. Stationary bike
4. Closed-chain terminal extension with resistance tubing or weight machine
5. Toe raises
6. Balance exercises
7. Hamstring curls
8. Aquatic therapy with emphasis on normalization of gait
9. Continue hamstring stretches, progress to weight-bearing gastro/soleus stretches.

Stage 3: Begins ~8 wk and extends through ~6 mo

Goals:
1. Full range of motion
2. Improve strength, endurance, and proprioception of the lower extremity to prepare for functional activities

Therapeutic exercises:
1. Continue flexibility exercises as appropriate for patient.
2. StairMaster (begin with short steps, avoid hyperextension)
3. NordicTrack
4. Advanced closed-chain strengthening (one-leg squats, leg press 0–50 degrees, step-ups, etc.)
5. Progress proprioception activities (slide board, use of ball with balance activities, etc.)
6. Progress aquatic therapy to include pool running, swimming (no breaststroke)

Stage 4: Begins ~6 mo and extends through ~9 mo

Goals:
1. Progress strength, power, proprioception to prepare for return to functional activities

Therapeutic exercises:
1. Continue to progress flexibility and strengthening program
2. Initiate plyometric program as appropriate for patient's functional goals
3. Functional progression including, but not limited to, walk/jog progression, forward/backward running at 1/2, 3/4, full speed, cutting, crossover, carioca, etc.
4. Initiate sport-specific drills as appropriate for patient

Stage 5: Begins ~9 mo postoperatively

Goals:
1. Safe return to athletics
2. Maintenance of strength, endurance, proprioception
3. Patient education with regard to any possible limitations

Therapeutic exercises:
1. Gradual return to sports participation
2. Maintenance program for strength and endurance

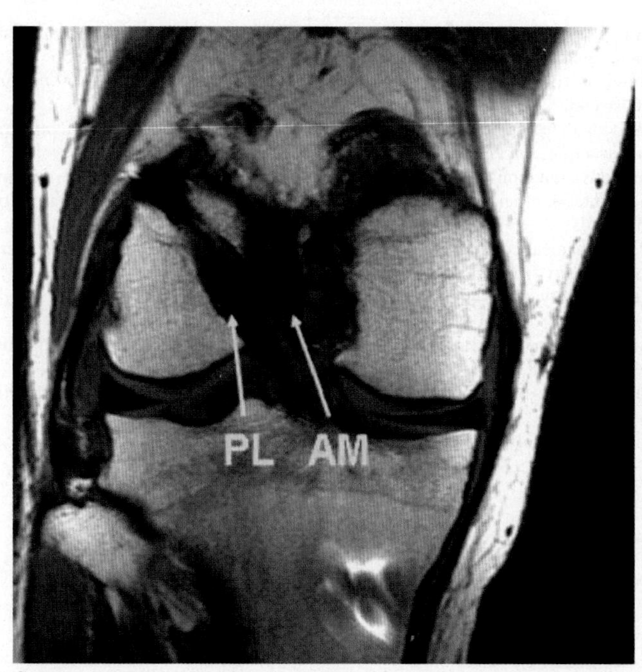

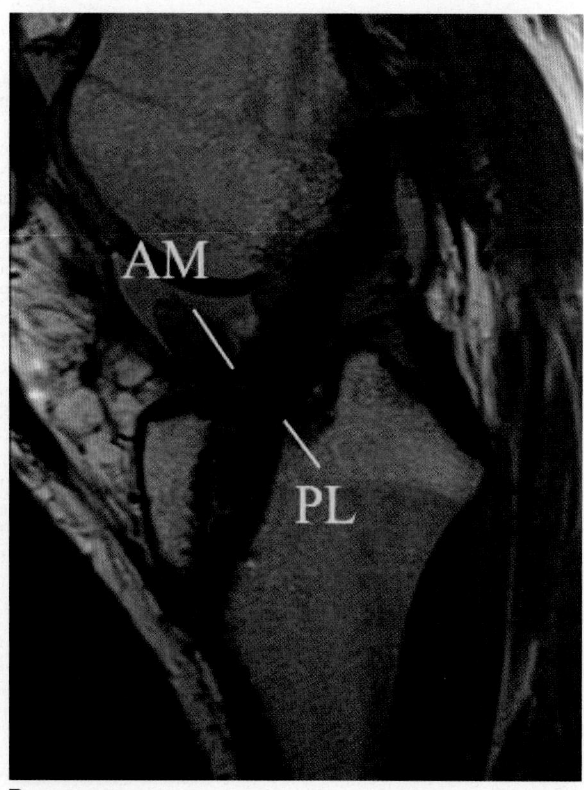

FIGURE 17-19

Coronal (**A**) and sagittal (**B**) views of MRI show the AM and PL grafts.

COMPLICATIONS

When considering DB reconstruction, it is important to address potential complications. General complications after knee surgery include hemarthrosis, effusions, and wound infection, which are treated according to the common postoperative procedures. Tunnel widening and sclerosis, tibial and femoral fractures, and notch or posterior cruciate ligament impingement following ACL reconstruction are known to occur in an SD reconstruction but can also occur during anatomic ACL DB reconstruction. When performing the tibial incision, the infrapatellar branch of the saphenous nerve can be damaged, leaving a small numb area along the anterolateral aspect of the knee and, rarely, a painful neuroma. Additionally, loss of motion and arthrofibrosis can occur secondary to poor preoperative ROM and tunnel placement or cyclops lesion. Lastly, high portal placement can disrupt proper visualization of the ACL.

RESULTS

Comparison of anatomic and DB and SB reconstruction has been documented in literature, but the need for more prospective and randomized control trials still exists. A randomized prospective study involving 281 patients compared ACL reconstruction using anatomic DB, anatomic SB, and nonanatomic SB techniques. Statistically significant differences were found between the groups with anterior tibial translation of 1.2, 1.6, and 2 mm for anatomic DB, anatomic SB, and nonanatomic SB techniques, respectively. This study suggests that anatomic DB reconstruction was superior to anatomic and nonanatomic SB reconstructions. Pivot shift supported the superiority of DB and anatomic reconstruction in that the percentage of patients who had scores of 0 for pivot shift were 93.1% for anatomic DB, 66.7% for anatomic SB, and 41.7% for nonanatomic SB. There were no differences in subjective IKDC scores between the groups. A follow-up study was completed where SB and DB results were compared using an individualized technique dependent on intraoperative measurements of ACL insertion sizes. No difference was found between anatomic DB reconstruction and anatomic SB reconstruction suggesting that individualizing patients by ACL anatomy can produce superior results to nonanatomic ACL reconstruction.

RECOMMENDED READINGS

Casagranda BU, Maxwell NJ, Kavanagh EC, et al. Normal appearance and complications of double-bundle and selective-bundle anterior cruciate ligament reconstructions using optimal MRI techniques. *AJR Am J Roentgenol.* 2009;192(5):1407–1415.

Chu CR, Williams AA, West RV, et al. Quantitative magnetic resonance imaging UTE-T2* mapping of cartilage and meniscus healing after anatomic anterior cruciate ligament reconstruction. *Am J Sports Med.* 2014;42(8):1847–1856.

Fu FH, van Eck CF, Tashman S, et al. Anatomic anterior cruciate ligament reconstruction: a changing paradigm. *Knee Surg Sports Traumatol Arthrosc.* 2015;23(3):640–648.

Hussein M, van Eck CF, Cretnik A, et al. Individualized anterior cruciate ligament surgery: a prospective study comparing anatomic single- and double-bundle reconstruction. *Am J Sports Med.* 2012;40(8):1781–1788.

Hussein M, van Eck CF, Cretnik A, et al. Prospective randomized clinical evaluation of conventional single-bundle, anatomic single-bundle, and anatomic double-bundle anterior cruciate ligament reconstruction: 281 cases with 3- to 5-year follow-up. *Am J Sports Med.* 2012;40(3):512–520.

Kato Y, Maeyama A, Lertwanich P, et al. Biomechanical comparison of different graft positions for single-bundle anterior cruciate ligament reconstruction. *Knee Surg Sports Traumatol Arthrosc.* 2013;21(4):816–823.

Kopf S, Pombo MW, Szczodry M, et al. Size variability of the human anterior cruciate ligament insertion sites. *Am J Sports Med.* 2011;39(1):108–113.

Tashman S, Collon D, Anderson K, et al. Abnormal rotational knee motion during running after anterior cruciate ligament reconstruction. *Am J Sports Med.* 2004;32(4):975–983.

Van Eck CF, Lesniak BP, Schreiber VM, et al. Anatomic single- and double-bundle anterior cruciate ligament reconstruction flowchart. *Arthroscopy.* 2010;26(2):258–268.

Yagi M, Wong EK, Kanamori A, et al. Biomechanical analysis of an anatomic anterior cruciate ligament reconstruction. *Am J Sports Med.* 2002;30(5):660–666.

18 Revision ACL Reconstruction

Adam V. Metzler and Darren L. Johnson

INDICATIONS

Anterior cruciate ligament reconstructions (ACLRs) have become one of the most commonly performed procedures by orthopedic surgeons. The number of ACL reconstructions has risen over the past few decades and is estimated to be around 250,000 per year. As the number of ACL reconstructions continues to increase, so will the number of revisions. Evidence has shown that the number one cause for ACL failure is technical error with tunnel placement. Biomechanical studies have shown that accessory medial portal drilling techniques and outside-in techniques more accurately reproduce the anatomic femoral footprint. We believe this should not only be implemented for primary ACLRs but also in the revision setting. When a surgeon is faced with a revision, ACLR numerous challenges are faced including the following: (a) removing the hardware implanted during the primary surgery, (b) avoiding previously drilled tunnels and managing tunnel osteolysis, (c) selecting the appropriate graft type for the patient, and (d) managing postoperative rehabilitation and patient expectations after surgery.

Contraindications to revision ACL reconstruction:

1. Revision ACL reconstruction in the setting of arthritis
2. Revision ACL reconstruction for pain alone
3. Revision ACL at the same time as a stiffness operation

Evaluation

A thorough preoperative evaluation is imperative when presented with patient with a prior ACLR. It is vital to determine the cause of graft failure and determine what the patient's expectations for a revision ACLR are. Both the surgeon and the patient should have realistic expectation for revision ACLR, as it has been shown that success rates of revision ACLR do not match that of primary ACLR. For many patients, revision surgery may be considered a "salvage" procedure. For some patient, simply returning to activities of daily living without instability could be considered a success. Return to sports or high-level activities may not always be possible and should be stressed pre-op.

History

The initial evaluation must include a careful history that addresses the nature of the primary injury and procedure, postoperative regimen, ability to return to activity, and timing of recurrent instability. The surgeon must have the operative notes from the primary surgery and ideally the intraoperative images to help guide the revision surgery. Information regarding the original graft, fixation type and manufacturer, and status of the menisci and articular cartilage is extremely important in preoperative planning. Symptoms of pain and instability must be clearly differentiated as the treatment and prognosis may significantly differ. Did the patient ever have a period of stability and return to level 1 sports after the index ACL procedure? Typically, patients with symptomatic instability and objective findings of patholaxity have the highest potential for successful outcome after revision ACLR.

Physical Exam

Physical exam of the extremity must be comprehensive. It must include all objective and subjective tests to qualify and quantify the amount of patholaxity present as well as concomitant pathology that will affect the revision surgery. These include evaluation of the ACL, menisci, PLC, and PMC. You must have the patient walk in your office hallway to not miss any gait abnormalities.

- The "best test" is the exam under anesthesia (EUA) and provides the most accurate indications of pathology compared to the in-office evaluation.

Radiographic Evaluation

- High-quality preoperative x-rays should be obtained, including standing AP, PA 45, lateral, and sunrise views. Alignment films must also be done to rule out mechanical axis issues. One must measure and compare the posterior slope of the tibia compared to the uninvolved knee. An increased posterior slope in a varus failed ACL knee may often be "cured" with an HTO that decreases the tibial slope. Degenerative changes should be noted and discussed with the patient, as many revision ACLR patients have degenerative pathology. Preoperative x-rays should be used to evaluate hardware used, tunnel position, and expansion. Previously placed metal screws do not always need to be removed depending on their location. If the previously placed metallic screws do not interfere with revision tunnel location, then the screws should be left to prevent bone void defects. If hardware removal is necessary, a complete set of implant drivers and screw removal instruments must be on hand.
- Tunnels should be assessed for osteolysis and bone loss. Excessively posterior femoral tunnels from the original procedure may have caused back wall blowout. When the tunnel exceeds 15 mm, we recommend staged bone grafting and returning in 6 months for revision ACL after the bone graft has incorporated.
- MRI and 3-D CT scan may be useful tools to fully evaluate tunnel osteolysis and tunnel position. MRI is more useful in determining integrity of the graft, chondral and meniscal pathology, but has limited use when metallic screws are present due to metallic artifact.

Graft Selection

There is no single optimal graft option for revision ACLR, and each patient should be individualized in regard to graft choice. Studies have shown no significant difference in allograft and autograft use in the revision setting. Our preferred graft choice in the under 25 years old athletically active is autograft tissue, especially patellar tendon autograft. However, in those less active and lower-demand patients, allograft tissue remains an excellent option. We prefer the use of autogenous tissue particularly if the previous surgeon used allogenic tissue. Factors such as previous graft used, tunnel placement and enlargement, presence of patellofemoral symptoms, existing skin incision, other surgical procedures planned as part of the revision, and patient preference should all be taken into account when making this decision. Allograft tissue offers several advantages that are relevant in the revision setting. Lack of donor site morbidity, decreased operative time, and smaller incision are all beneficial to the patient. For the surgeon, variable graft sizes, ability to create larger bone plugs, and increased tissue availability provide improved surgical flexibility. BPTB and Achilles tendon grafts are the most commonly used allograft in the revision setting; however, slower graft incorporation and the risk of disease transmission still are concerns. Return to level 1 sports should be delayed until at least 9 to 12 months if allograft tissue is used.

TECHNIQUE

Equipment Needed

The surgeon must have all necessary equipment ready at the time of surgery. There should be no questions what implants were used for the primary surgery and any special equipment needed for their possible removal.

Patient Positioning

The patient's operative leg is placed in the Acufex (Smith & Nephew, Andover, MA) leg holder, and the nonoperative leg is placed in a well-leg holder. The operative leg or femur should be parallel to the floor when placed in the leg holder (Fig. 18-1). A high and tight anterolateral portal, a low and

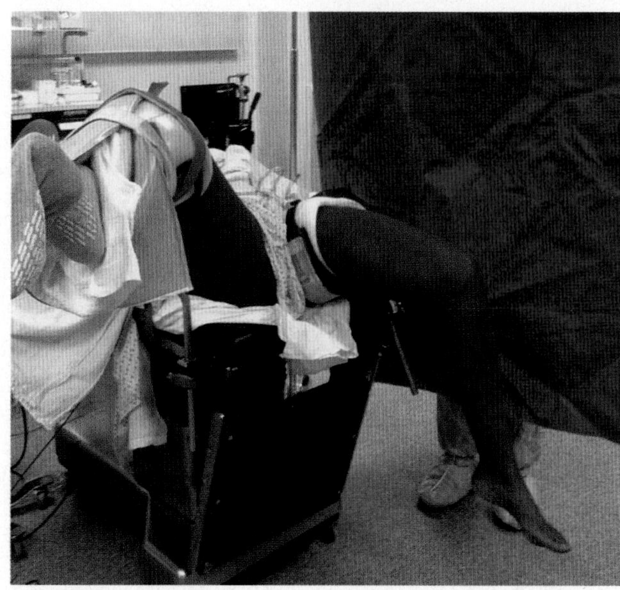

FIGURE 18-1

Standard arthroscopic setup for primary or revision ACLR. The left leg is in the arthroscopic leg holder. The nonoperative leg is in the well-leg holder.

tight anteromedial portal, and an accessory anteromedial portal are created (Fig. 18-2). The fat pad is debrided enough to allow full visualization in addition to a limited (3 mm) wall- and notchplasty. Complete visualization of the ACL femoral and tibial footprints is imperative. The scope can alternate between the three portals for better visualization as needed. This setup allows for hyperflexion if needed for accessory medial portal femoral drilling and also allows for complete access to the operative leg for assistants to hold retractors and perform meniscal repairs, etc. This setup also allows for outside-in reaming as well, which will be described below (Fig. 18-3).

Hardware Removal

The decision to remove or retain hardware can be one of the hardest decisions in revision ACLR. Two questions should be asked: (a) Can the hardware be safely removed? (b) Does the hardware need to be removed? In general, hardware should only be removed when it interferes with the planned procedure, but the surgeon should be prepared for hardware removal in all cases. The importance of previous surgical reports and having the appropriate instrumentation available cannot be overemphasized.

Tunnel Placement

Previous tunnel position may also affect revision graft integrity and therefore the ability to perform a single-stage revision. For example, a transtibial primary ACL reconstruction commonly results in a posteriorly placed tibial tunnel and an anterior and superiorly placed femoral tunnel. In this scenario,

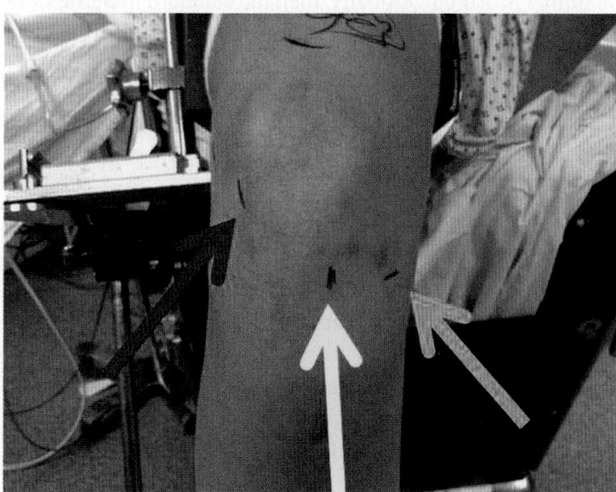

FIGURE 18-2

Portal placement—*red arrow*: "high and tight" anterolateral portal; *yellow arrow*: central medial portal; *blue arrow*: accessory anteromedial portal.

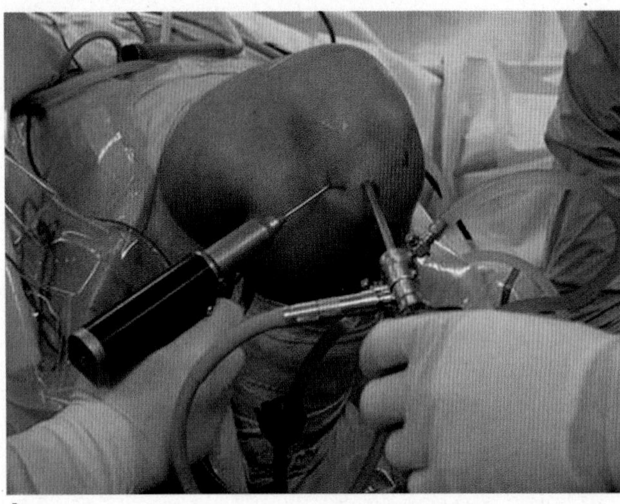

A

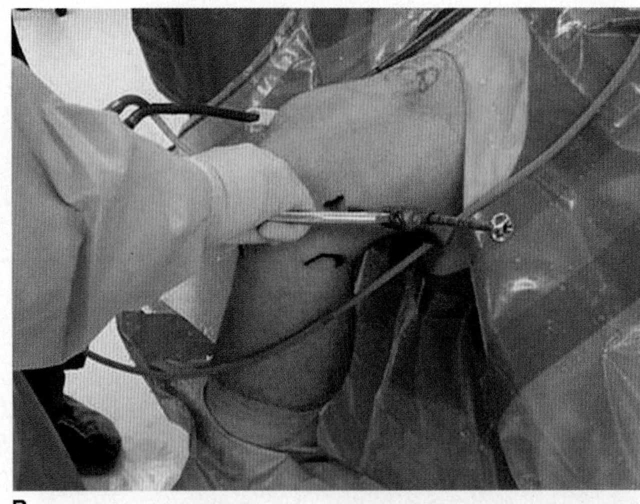

B

FIGURE 18-3

A: Hyperflexion ACL femoral tunnel reaming through accessory anteromedial portal. **B:** Outside-in femoral tunnel Pinpoint guide (Smith and Nephew Endoscopy, Andover, MA).

drilling an anatomic femoral tunnel in native bone is often possible; however, it is more common that the tibial tunnel necessitates bone grafting and staged surgery. Prior tunnel position can be described as anatomically placed (entire tunnel opening is 100% in the native ACL footprint), nonanatomically placed (commonly seen in transtibial femoral tunnel drilling), or partially anatomic (overlapping). The greatest variation in tunnel placement is seen on the femur. When the femoral tunnel is nonanatomically placed, it rarely interferes with the revision tunnel placement and can be ignored, leaving the previous fixation hardware in place. Partially overlapping tunnel placement creates the most difficult scenario because the existing and revision tunnels will create a figure-of-eight tunnel. Often, redirection of the tunnel (diverging from the existing tunnel) can address this on the femur (drilling outside-in on the femur), allowing for adequate fixation of the new graft. In the authors' experience, outside-in femoral tunnel drilling has proven successful in this situation. A revision ACL surgeon must be comfortable with multiple techniques to reproduce anatomic tibial and femoral tunnels.

Outside-In (2-Incision) ACL Revision Reconstruction

The choice of surgical technique should be guided by the preoperative plan, intraoperative findings, and comfort level with the diverse revision methods. Decisions regarding single-incision arthroscopic versus outside-in (2-incision) technique and double-bundle versus single-bundle ACLR must be made after vigilant considerations of all variables. At present, the senior author prefers the outside-in (2-incision) technique for most revision ACLRs and in some instance performs a double-bundle ACLR. In cases where the femoral tunnel is drilled vertically, then the standard hyperflexion/accessory anteromedial portal drilling technique is used for femoral tunnel revision drilling. The technique described below will discuss the outside-in (2-incision) technique.

TECHNIQUE

Bone Grafting

Before the start of the case, the surgeon should determine whether or not bone grafting needs to be performed. If significant tunnel osteolysis is noted on pre-op x-rays, CT scan, etc., then bone grafting and staging are performed. The bone grafting technique is discussed below.

Bone grafting case example:

Figure 18-4 shows significant femoral and mild tibial tunnel osteolysis after failed ACLR with a previous hamstring autograft. The femoral tunnel osteolysis measured 17 mm (Fig. 18-5), and the tibia tunnel osteolysis measured 14 mm (Fig. 18-6). Due to significant tunnel widening, a staged

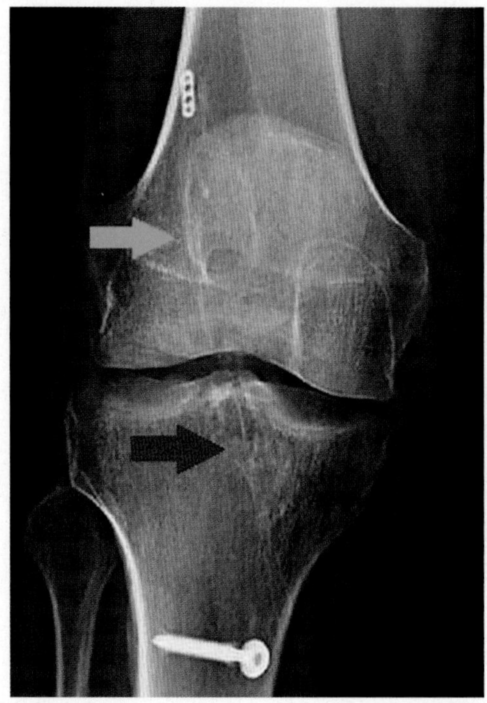

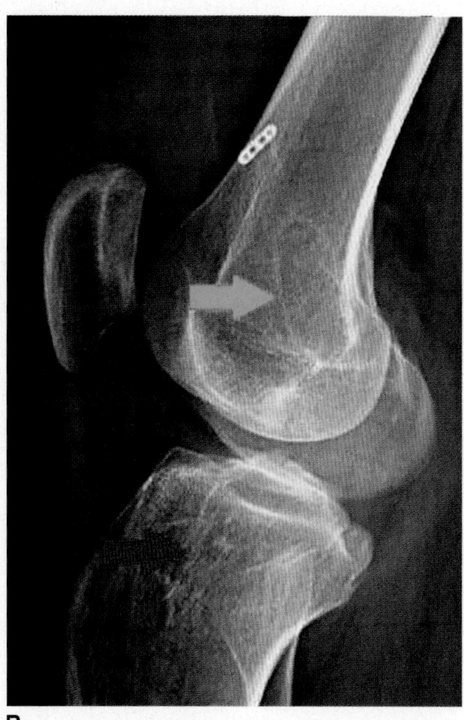

A B

FIGURE 18-4

Femoral and mild tibial tunnel osteolysis after failed ACLR with a previous hamstring autograph. **A:** AP radiograph. **B:** Lateral radiograph. *Green arrows* show the femoral tunnel, and *red arrows* show the tibial tunnel.

revision involving bone grafting of the femoral and tibial tunnels with femoral head allograft was recommended. Intraoperatively, the ACL retear was confirmed (Fig. 18-7A), the femoral tunnel was prepared with curettes, and a shaver until bleeding bone was exposed (Fig. 18-7B). The femoral tunnel was measured and filled with an allograft dowel that was subsequently tamped in place (Fig. 18-7C). The tibial tunnel was prepared with reamers, curettes, and a shaver. Bleeding bone was visualized, and the tunnel was also filled with an allograft dowel (Fig. 18-7D). Figure 18-8 shows the radiographs after bone grafting. The patient underwent a staged revision ACLR 6 months later to allow for integration of the allograft dowel into the patient's bone.

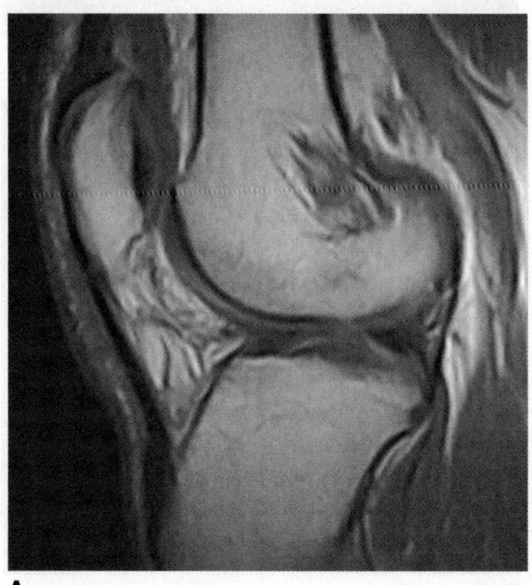

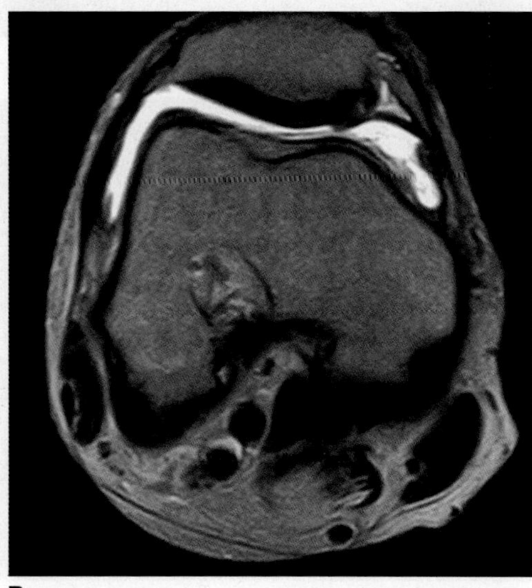

A B

FIGURE 18-5

A: Sagittal MRI showing femoral tunnel osteolysis. **B:** Axial image showing femoral tunnel osteolysis.

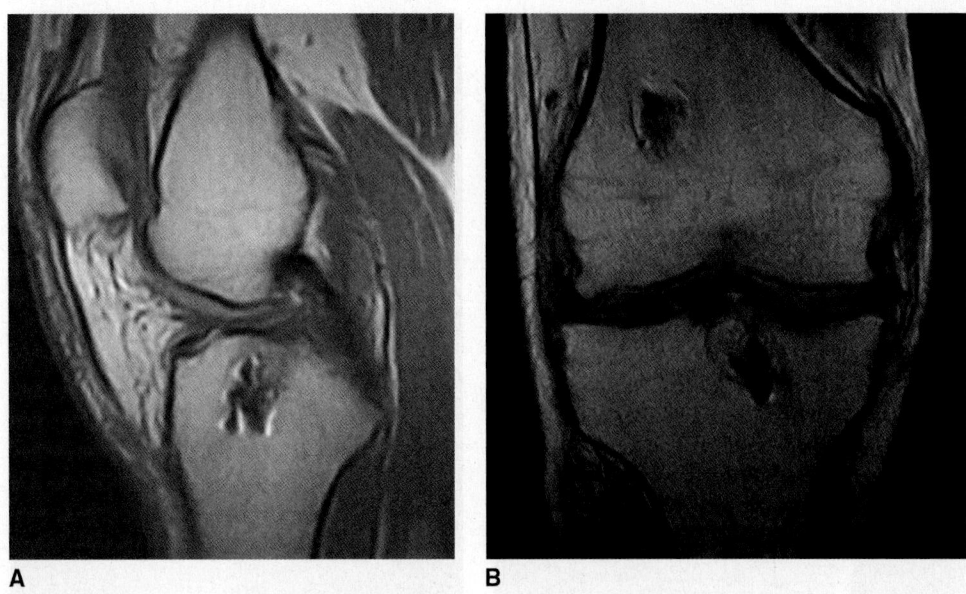

FIGURE 18-6

A: Sagittal MRI showing tibial tunnel osteolysis. **B:** Coronal MRI showing tunnel osteolysis.

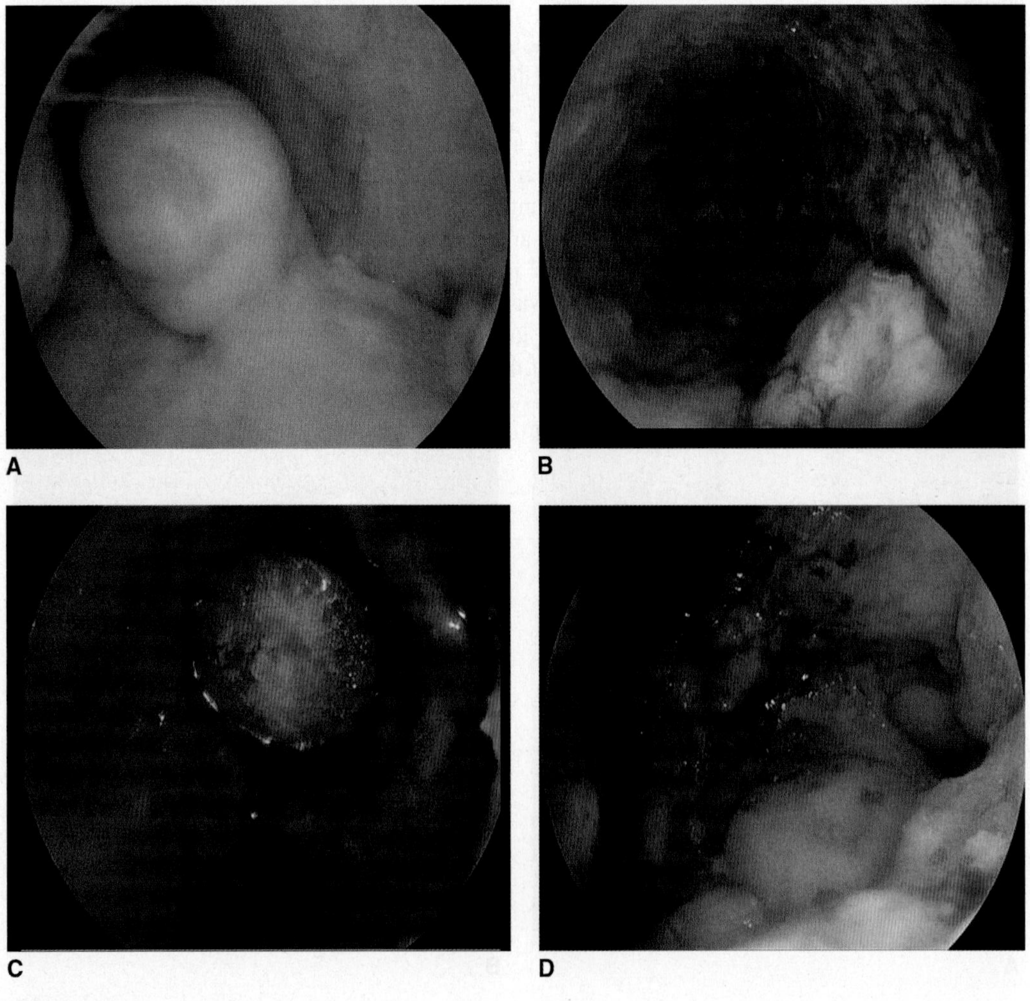

FIGURE 18-7

A: Torn ACL. **B:** Tunnel debrided with circumferential bone in the tunnel. **C:** Bone dowel placed in the femur. **D:** Bone dowel in place on the tibia.

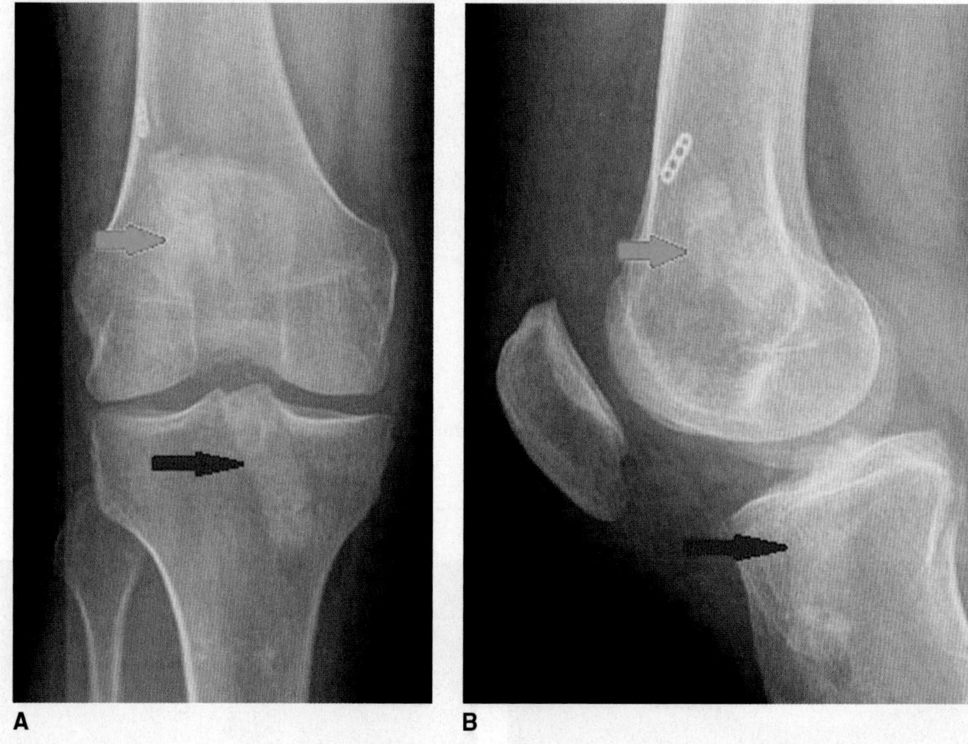

FIGURE 18-8

Post-op radiographs after bone grating. *Green arrows* show femoral dowel, and *red arrows* show the tibial tunnel dowels. **A:** AP radiograph. **B:** Lateral radiograph.

Outside-In Technique (2-Incision)

Once adequate visualization has been obtained with the previously described portals placed (Fig. 18-2), a full diagnostic evaluation of the knee is performed. A full evaluation of the cartilage and meniscus must be performed. The menisci should be repaired if possible due to their importance as secondary stabilizers. If there is a medial or lateral drive-through sign, this would indicate significant MCL/POL or PLC laxity and should be addressed concomitantly at the time of revision ACLR. The previous ACL graft should be debrided, and critical arthroscopic analysis of the tunnels should be done. Once all of the above has been addressed, the appropriate Acufex Pinpoint guide (Smith & Nephew) size is chosen, with options ranging from 6 to 10 mm. The scope is placed in the central medial portal, and the outside-in Pinpoint guide is placed through the anterolateral portal (Fig. 18-9). The intra-articular portion of the guide is placed on the anatomic position on the medial aspect of the lateral femoral condyle (Fig. 18-10A). Next, the trochar is placed through the handle to mark the skin incision laterally (Fig. 18-9). The starting point for the drill in general is anterior and proximal to the lateral epicondyle, except for use in skeletally immature patients. In these patients, the entrance point must be distal to the femoral physis, which is directly above the epicondyle or femoral attachment of the fibular collateral ligament. Care must be taken to maintain the intra-articular portion of the guide in the anatomic position.

The trochar is removed once the skin is marked, and a 2- to 3-cm skin incision is made in line with the iliotibial band. Skin retractors are placed, the trochar is reinserted, the IT band is incised in line with its fibers, and the trochar is advanced through the guide handle abutting the lateral femoral condyle (Fig. 18-11). While the guide is held firmly in place, a Beath pin is slowly advanced through the trochar and visualized with the scope, passing a few millimeters into the intercondylar notch (Fig. 18-10A). The guide is removed, and retractors are placed deep to the iliotibial band on each side of the Beath pin to prevent the reamer from injuring the iliotibial band (Fig. 18-11). The Beath pin is grabbed with a pituitary grabber via the low anteromedial portal. The appropriately sized, fully fluted reamer is drilled in an outside-in manner while an assistant holds the Beath pin to prevent advancement. The pin and reamer are removed, the tunnel is debrided, and a plug is placed into the tunnel to prevent fluid extravasation (Fig. 18-10A–C). One can clearly see fibers of the original ACL circumscribing the outside-in tunnel indication anatomic femoral tunnel ACL placement. As described above, drilling outside-in allows for a new virgin tunnel to be drilled with tunnel convergence at the notch.

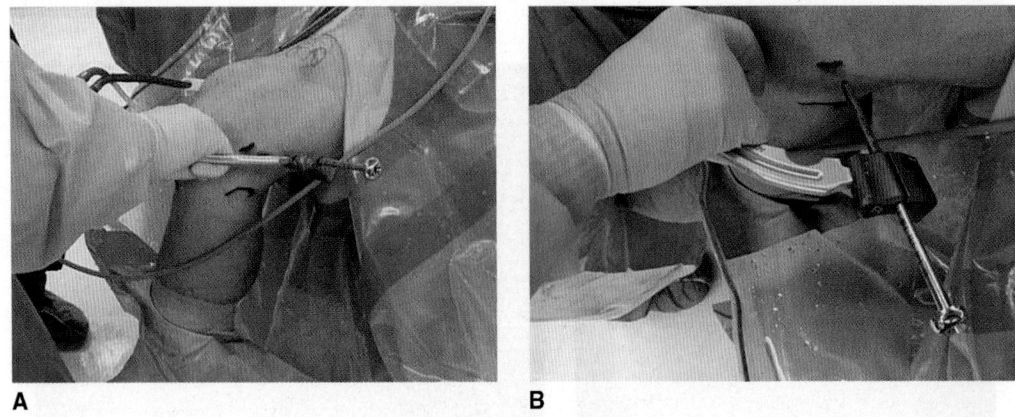

FIGURE 18-9

Outside-in femoral tunnel Pinpoint guide (Smith and Nephew Endoscopy, Andover, MA). The guide is placed through the lateral portal.

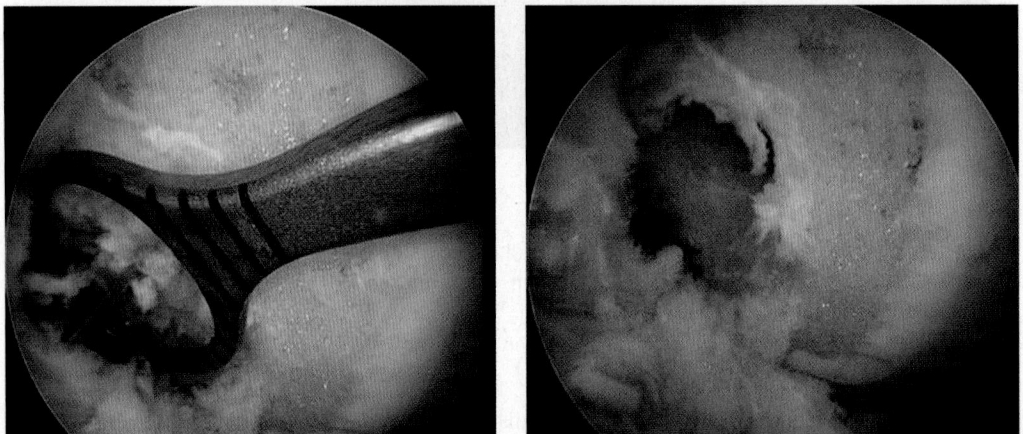

A B

C D

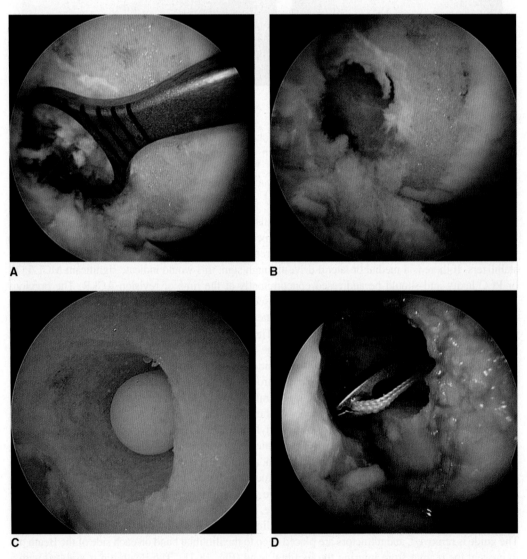

FIGURE 18-10

Intraoperative arthroscopic images as viewed through the anteromedial portal. **A:** Pinpoint guide (Smith and Nephew, Andover, MA) placed in anatomic ACL footprint with Beath pin advanced into the femoral notch. **B:** Anatomic placement of femoral tunnel via Pinpoint guide. The femoral tunnel is completely within the anatomic ACL footprint as fibers can be seen circumferentially around the drilled tunnel. **C:** Bone plug placed to prevent fluid extravasation from outside-in. **D:** Passing suture shuttled through the femoral tunnel for graft passage.

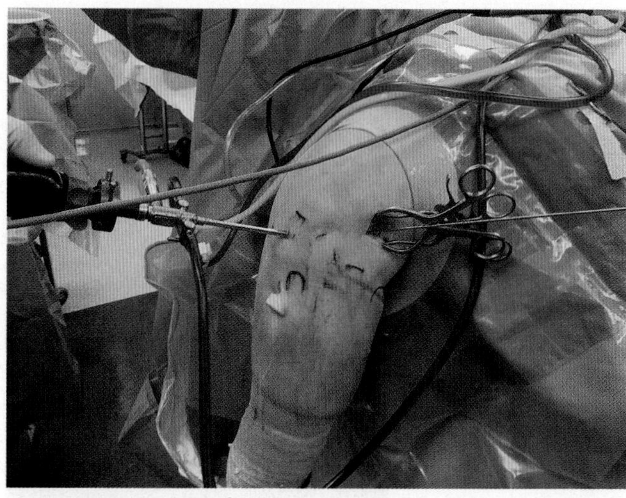

FIGURE 18-11

Retractors are placed under the IT band, and the trochar is advanced through the guide handle abutting the lateral femoral condyle. The Beath pin is advanced. The Pinpoint guide was used for placement (Smith and Nephew, Andover, MA).

The tibial tunnel is drilled in a standard fashion. If the previously used screw can be avoided, then the screw is left in place. In some cases, the screw is removed, and the tunnel is rereamed to allow for good bleeding bone. In addition, in some cases, if biocomposite screws were used in the original case, then they are drilled through. It is important to start reaming with small reamers and progress up in size as previously placed screws can cause deflection of the reamers and cause nonanatomic tunnels. One should dock the guide pin in the femoral bone before using your reamers on the tibia. This prevents the reamers for migrating to softer bone in the tibial metaphysis. To pass the graft, a passing suture is looped and grabbed with a pituitary grabber. The passing suture is placed in a retrograde fashion through the lateral femoral condyle and passed off to another grabber through the drilled tibial tunnel. The graft can then be pulled into appropriate position. If a BTB graft is chosen, then the bone plug is fixed on the femoral side with a metal or a bio-screw placed from outside-in. The guidewire is placed in a retrograde manner, and the bone plug must be directly observed to prevent aberrant screw placement. The tibial side is fixed with a metal or a bio-screw in standard fashion (Fig. 18-12).

If a hamstring tendon graft is used, the graft is passed in a similar manner; however, a 10-mm EndoButton (Smith & Nephew) with an Xtendobutton (Smith & Nephew) attachment is used for femoral fixation. A biocomposite crew and a staple or a screw with a spiked washer are used for tibial fixation (Fig. 18-13).

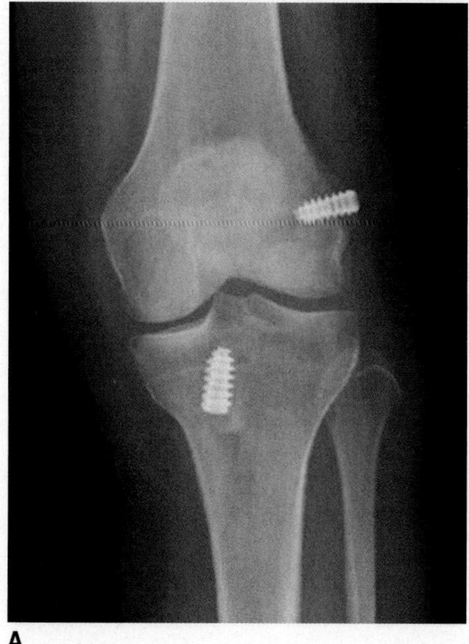

A

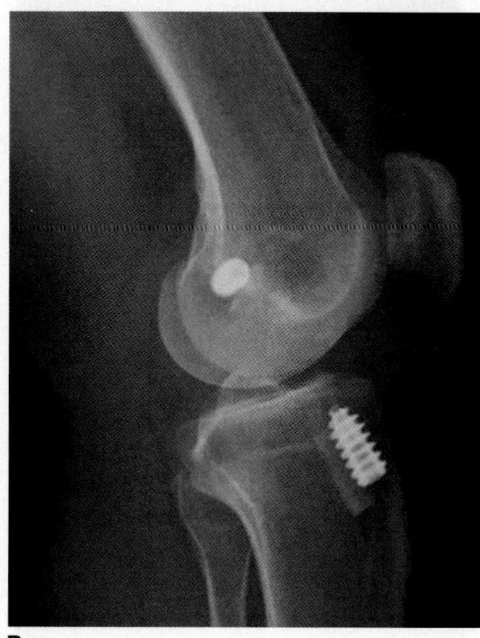

B

FIGURE 18-12

AP and lateral radiograph showing metal screw placement for outside-in femoral tunnel reaming.

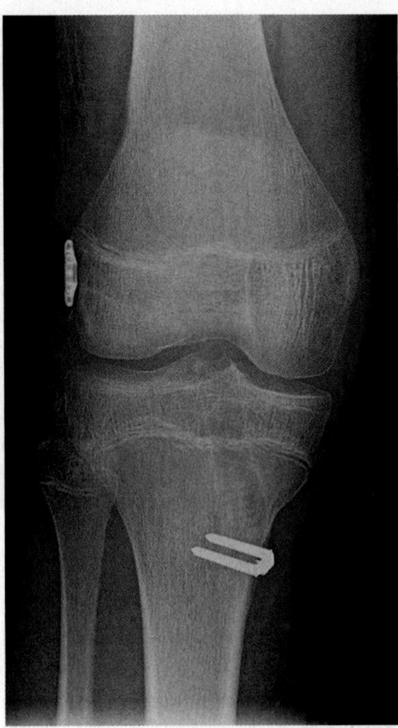

FIGURE 18-13

AP radiograph after hamstring ACL reconstruction in skeletally immature patient with outside-in reaming to avoid the femoral physis with Xtendobutton (Smith & Nephew) attachment used for femoral fixation. A biocomposite screw and a staple or a screw with a spiked washer are used for tibial fixation.

CASE EXAMPLE

Figure 14-17 shows the case example of a patient with a previous ACL reconstruction with a quadrupled hamstring allograft via a flexible reaming system from an accessory medial portal. A plastic screw and sheath were used for femoral interference fixation, and a biocomposite screw was used for tibial interference fixation. The patient was an active 42-year-old karate instructor. He retore his ACL 5 years after his index procedure. His preoperative exam showed a positive Lachman with normal mechanical axis and no collateral or rotational pathology on knee exam. Figures 18-14 and 18-15

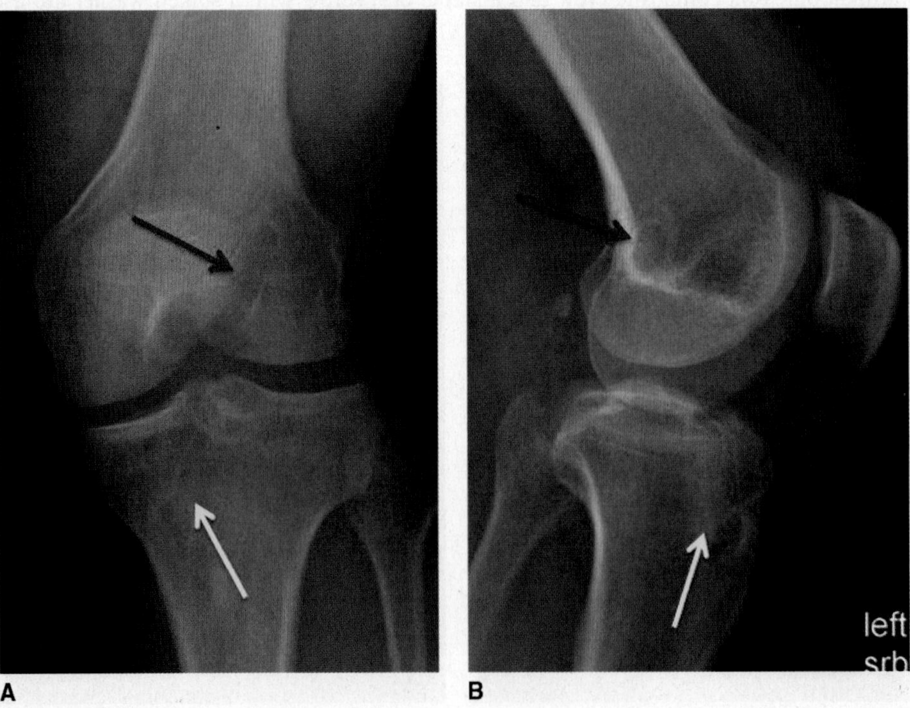

FIGURE 18-14

Case example. AP **(A)** and lateral **(B)** radiographs of failed hamstring allograft with minimal tunnel osteolysis. *Yellow arrows* indicate the tibial tunnel, and *red arrows* indicate the femoral tunnel.

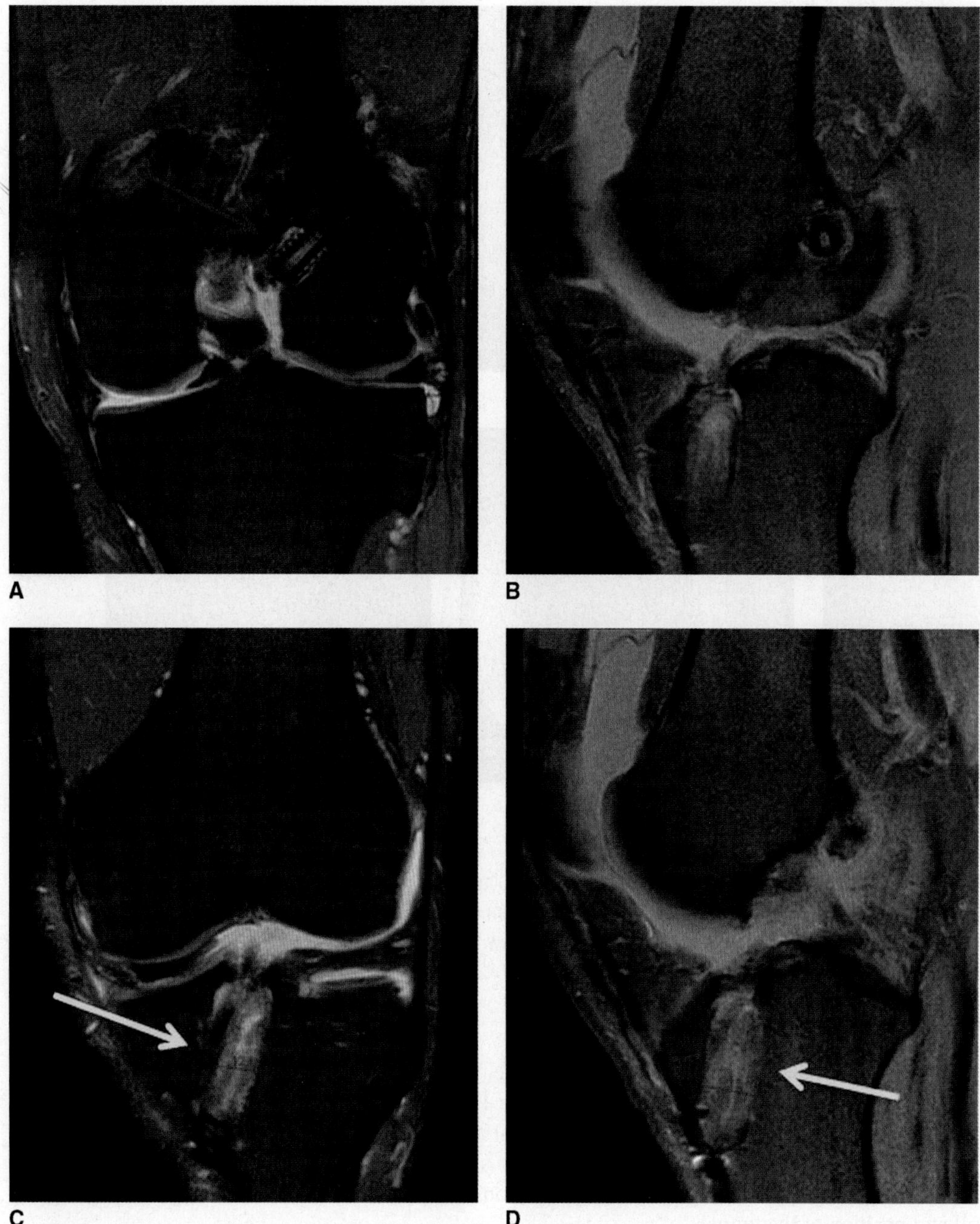

FIGURE 18-15

Case example. **A:** Coronal MRI showing peak screw in the femoral socket. Femoral tunnel osteolysis was 12.2 mm. **B:** Sagittal MRI, *red arrow* indicates peak screw with femoral tunnel osteolysis of 12.2 mm. **C:** Coronal MRI, *yellow arrow* shows tunnel osteolysis of 12.4 mm. **D:** Sagittal MRI, *yellow arrow* shows tibial tunnel.

show the preoperative x-rays and MRI. The femoral tunnel osteolysis was 12.2 mm, and the tibial tunnel osteolysis was 12.4 mm. He was revised with a bone tendon bone allograft to allow bone fixation in the tunnels. Due to the high and posterior placement of the previously placed femoral tunnel and screw, it was left in place and a new inferior, and more anatomic tunnel was drilled (Fig. 18-16B–D). The previous tibial tunnel was reused and was sequentially reamed up to allow for circumferential fresh bone in the tunnel. Figure 18-16A shows the torn ACL. Figure 18-16B shows the high and posterior placed previous femoral tunnel in a nonanatomic location (*yellow arrow*). Figure 18-16C shows the ACL Pinpoint guide being placed in the anatomic position of the ACL inferior to the plastic screw. Figure 18-16D shows the bone plug in place to prevent fluid extravasation. The tunnel is below the lateral intercondylar ridge and is appropriately placed in the anterior to posterior plane on the lateral femoral condyle. Figure 18-16E shows that fresh virgin bone (*blue arrow*) was able to

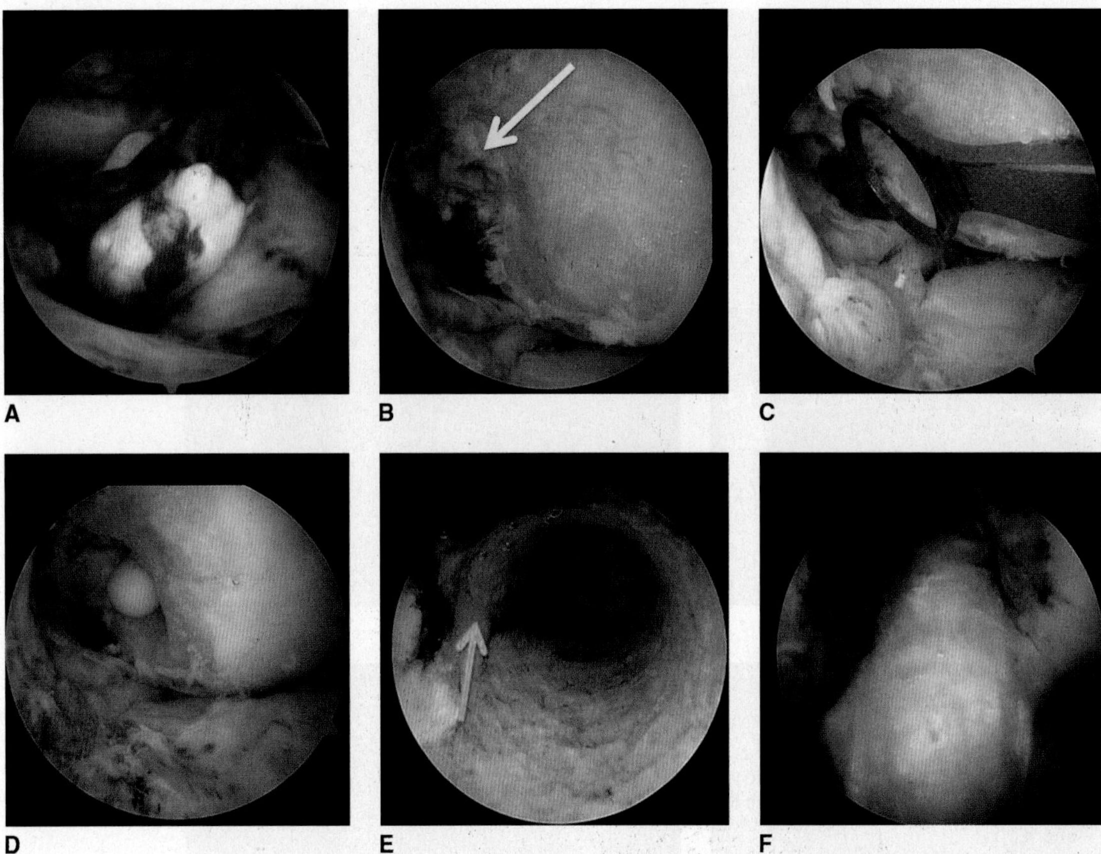

FIGURE 18-16

Case example. **A:** Torn ACL. **B:** *Yellow arrow* shows a peak screw in a nonanatomic location (too high and too posterior). **C:** ACL femoral Pinpoint guide placed at the anatomic footprint of the ACL. **D:** Tunnel was reamed from outside-in, and a bone plug was placed. **E:** View from the accessory medial portal shows "virgin" bone circumferentially around the new femoral tunnel. *Blue arrow* shows bone between the previous femoral socket and the new tunnel. **F:** Bone-tendon-bone allograft in place.

be obtained with the outside-in drilling technique, with the previous plastic screw and blue sheath just off the edge of left side of the picture. Figure 18-16F shows the BTB allograft in position after fixation with biocomposite screws on the femoral and tibial side. A spiked washer and screw were used to tie the tibial bone block sutures over for supplemental fixation on the tibia. Figure 18-17 shows the postoperative x-rays. The x-rays demonstrate a new femoral tunnel trajectory and good fill and position of the tunnels.

PEARLS

1. If the previously placed metallic or plastic screws do not interfere with revision tunnel location, then the screws should be left to prevent bone void defects.
2. Bone graft and stage if tunnel widening is greater than 15 mm.
3. Before revision surgery, the previous operative report must be available for preoperative planning.
4. Secondary stabilizer pathology must be addressed to prevent ACL graft retear.
5. When reaming through biocomposite screws, sequentially ream up starting with smaller reamers (must dock the guide pin into femur first) to prevent deflection of the reamer and nonanatomic tunnels.
6. Drill outside-in on the femur; this almost universally allows one to avoid the previous tunnel and guarantees the revision surgery virgin bone. It also allows for fixation of the graft at the lateral cortex of the distal femur.

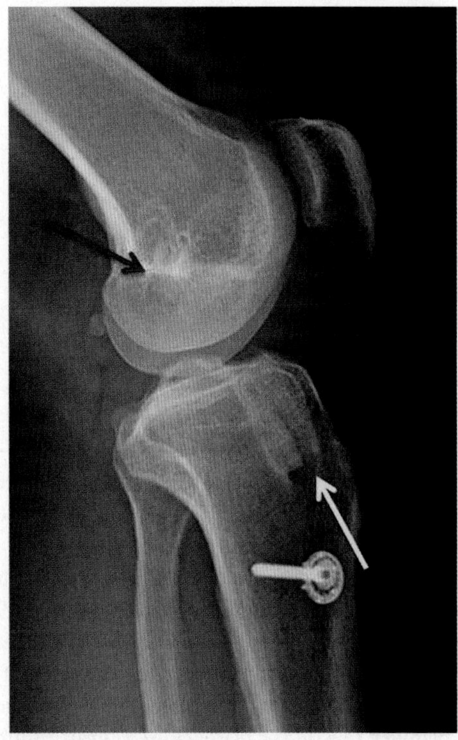

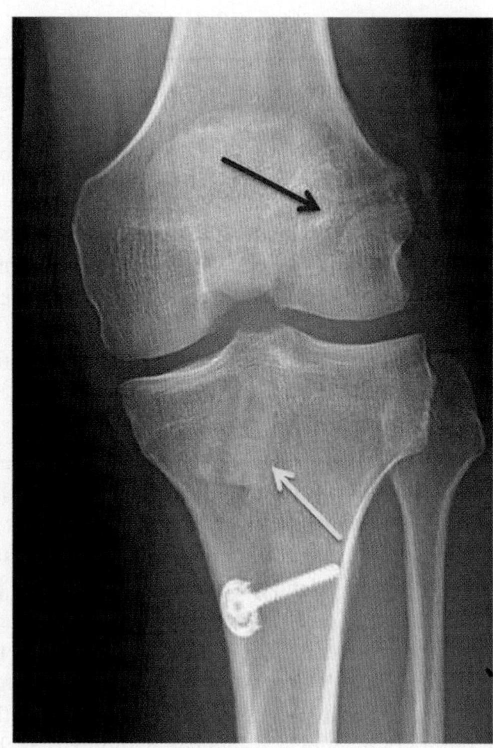

A B

FIGURE 18-17

A, B: Case example: AP and lateral radiographs showing bone tendon bone graft in place in the femoral tunnel (*red arrow*) and tibial tunnel (*yellow arrow*). Fixation was performed with biocomposite screws on the femoral and tibial side. A spiked washer and screw were used to tie the tibial bone block sutures over for supplemental fixation on the tibia.

PITFALLS

1. Anterior placement of the femoral tunnel in the notch should be avoided, and the back wall must be visualized with appropriate soft tissue debridement.
2. The femoral insertion of the lateral collateral ligament can also be injured when drilling with any outside-in guide. The guide must be placed anterior and proximal to the LCL insertion.
3. If the guide is placed too inferior with knee at 90 degrees, this could risk a Hoffa fracture.
4. Avoid intra-articular advancement of the Beath pin and associated cartilage injury by grabbing the Beath pin with a pituitary grabber in the notch.

POSTOPERATIVE MANAGEMENT

We place all of our patients in a telescoping brace locked in full extension for one month when ambulating and weight bearing as tolerated. The patient's brace can be unlocked for sleep at night and is removed when the patient is seated and immediate full range of motion (ROM) is started post-operative day (POD) 1. Formal physical therapy is started in 3 to 5 days from the index procedure. At 1 month, the telescoping brace is shortened and unlocked. At 2 months, the patient is fitted with a standard off the shelf knee sleeve. Functional ACL braces are used for patient returning to contact sports such as football and hockey for the first year from the reconstruction. Patients are advised to start immediate full ROM POD 1 with quad sets and straight leg raises initiated. Around 1 month, mini squats, wall slides, and mini squats are started, and bicycle is added. The patient in general is advised not to jog for 4 months with no running for 5 months. Sports-specific drill is initiated around 6 months, and return to sports after a revision is advised between 9 and 12 months, depending on quadriceps function. The rehabilitation protocol is adjusted depending on associated meniscal, cartilage, or alignment procedures performed.

COMPLICATIONS

This is an abbreviated list of the many complications that can occur with revision ACLR.

1. Arthrofibrosis
2. Graft rerupture
3. Inability to return to play
4. Lateral collateral ligament femoral insertion disruption, from outside-in reaming
5. Poor graft fixation (if done in single stage and not bone grafted or if tunnels converge)
6. Lateral femoral condyle fracture (from multiple drill tunnels)
7. Chronic pain
8. Broken hardware or inability to remove previously placed hardware

CONCLUSION

As the number of primary ACLRs increase, so will the number of revisions. Failure of an ACL can be attributed to numerous factors. Loss of motion, chronic pain, and recurrent laxity are all reason for patient to present to the surgeon's office dissatisfied with their primary reconstruction. It is imperative to understand the exact reason why the primary ACLR failed to ensure a successful outcome for the revision ACLR. Return to play after revision ACLR is noted to be approximately 60%. Many of these patients will not be able to return to their previous level of play. The greatest concern is that greater than 50% of patients have early radiographic findings of degenerative changes as early as 5 years after primary ACL surgery. We believe that the use of nonanatomic principles combined with failure to recognize associated patholaxity is the primary reason for primary ACL graft failure. The outside-in technique allows for a predictable method for revision ACLR. By adhering to anatomic reconstruction principles and addressing missed injuries to the secondary stabilizers should restore knee kinematics to as normal as possible and therefore improve overall outcomes. The senior author currently uses the outside-in technique on the majority of his revision ACLRs.

RECOMMENDED READINGS

Johnson DL, Harner CD, Maday MG, et al. Revision anterior cruciate ligament surgery. In: Fu FH, Harner CD, Vince KG, eds. *Knee Surgery*. Baltimore: Lippincott Williams & Wilkins; 1994;1:877–895.

Maday MG, Harner CD, Fu FH. Revision ACL surgery: evaluation and treatment. In: Feagin JA, ed. *The Crucial Ligaments*. New York: Churchill-Livingston; 1994:711–723.

Fu FH, Jordan SS. The lateral intercondylar ridge—a key to anatomic anterior cruciate ligament reconstruction. *J Bone Joint Surg Am.* 2007;89(10):2103–2104.

Piefer JW, Pflugner TR, Hwang MD, et al. Anterior cruciate ligament femoral footprint anatomy: systematic review of the 21st century literature. *Arthroscopy.* 2012;28(6):872–881.

Hwang MD, Piefer JW, Lubowitz JH. Anterior cruciate ligament tibial footprint anatomy: systematic review of the 21st century literature. *Arthroscopy.* 2012;28(5):728–734.

Gadikota HR, Sim JA, Hosseini A, et al. The relationship between femoral tunnels created by the transtibial, anteromedial portal, and outside-in techniques and the anterior cruciate ligament footprint. *Am J Sports Med.* 2012;40(4):882–888.

Marchant BG, Noyes FR, Barber-Westin SD, et al. Prevalence of nonanatomical graft placement in a series of failed anterior cruciate ligament reconstructions. *Am J Sports Med.* 2010;38(10):1987–1996.

Duffee A, Magnussen RA, Pedroza AD, et al. Transtibial ACL femoral tunnel preparation increases odds of repeat ipsilateral knee surgery. *J Bone Joint Surg Am.* 2013;95(22):2035–2042.

Magnussen RA, Lawrence JT, West RL, et al. Graft size and patient age are predictors of early revision after anterior cruciate ligament reconstruction with hamstring autograft. *Arthroscopy.* 2012;28(4):526–531.

Mariscalco MW, Flanigan DC, Mitchell J, et al. The influence of hamstring autograft size on patient-reported outcomes and risk of revision after anterior cruciate ligament reconstruction: a Multicenter Orthopaedic Outcomes Network (MOON) Cohort Study. *Arthroscopy.* 2013;29(12):1948–1953.

The MARS Group. Descriptive epidemiology of the Multicenter ACL Revision Study (MARS) cohort. *Am J Sports Med.* 2010;38(10):1979–1986.

Grossman MG, El Attrache NS, Shields CL, et al. Revision anterior cruciate ligament reconstruction: three to nine year follow-up. *Arthroscopy.* 2005;21:418–423.

Johnson DL, Coen MJ. Revision ACL surgery: etiology, indications, techniques, and results. *Am J Knee Surg.* 1995; 8:155–167.

19 Anterior Cruciate Ligament Reconstruction with Extra-articular Reconstruction

Philippe Neyret, Daniel C. Wascher, Olivier Reynaud, and German Jose Filippi

INTRODUCTION

Instability of the anterior cruciate ligament (ACL)-deficient knee has been described for over 100 years. In the 1970s, the term "pivot shift" was first used by Galway to describe the complex rotational and translational instability that occurs in ACL-deficient knees. At that time, diagnostic physical exam tests were described to elicit the increased anterior translation and internal rotation that occur during this phenomenon. As early as 1967, a variety of extra-articular procedures were developed to attempt to restore anterolateral stability to the ACL-deficient knee. Unfortunately, only half of patients had good or excellent results with an isolated extra-articular tenodesis as these procedures did not restore normal anterior stability to the knee. Combined intra- and extra-articular ACL reconstructions were frequently utilized during the 1980s; good to excellent results were reported in 80% to 90% of patients. However, concerns about postoperative stiffness and degenerative changes developing in the lateral tibiofemoral compartment as well as the development of arthroscopic techniques for intra-articular ACL reconstruction led most surgeons to abandon extra-articular procedures in the 1990s. However, a few centers continued to perform combined intra- and extra-articular reconstructions with encouraging results.

There is a population of patients who continue to experience instability and a demonstrable pivot shift despite having an intact intra-articular ACL reconstruction. Double-bundle ACL (DB-ACL) reconstruction techniques were developed to address the rotational instability in these patients. Other surgeons began revisiting the addition of an extra-articular procedure to address this rotatory instability. Two in vivo studies have compared single-bundle ACL (SB-ACL) reconstruction with extra-articular tenodesis to double-bundle ACL reconstruction. One study showed the DB-ACL technique better controlled the pivot shift phenomenon, whereas the other study showed the SB-ACL with extra-articular tenodesis was more effective in reducing the internal rotation of the tibia at 30 degrees of flexion.

In the past 5 years, there has been an improvement in the understanding of the complex anatomy of the lateral capsule. The anterolateral ligament (ALL) is a thickening of the lateral capsule that is tensioned with internal rotation at 30 degrees of flexion. Its fibers originate off the femur 5 mm posterior and proximal to the fibular collateral ligament (FCL) (Fig. 19-1). The tibial attachment of the ALL is located posterior to Gerdy tubercle. Biomechanical and clinical data have shown that the Segond fracture is an avulsion of the tibial attachment of the ALL. The ALL has a mean maximum load of 175 N. The ALL is clearly injured in many patients with ACL tears. Reconstruction of the ALL, in combination with an intra-articular ACL reconstruction, may improve rotational stability in ACL-deficient knees.

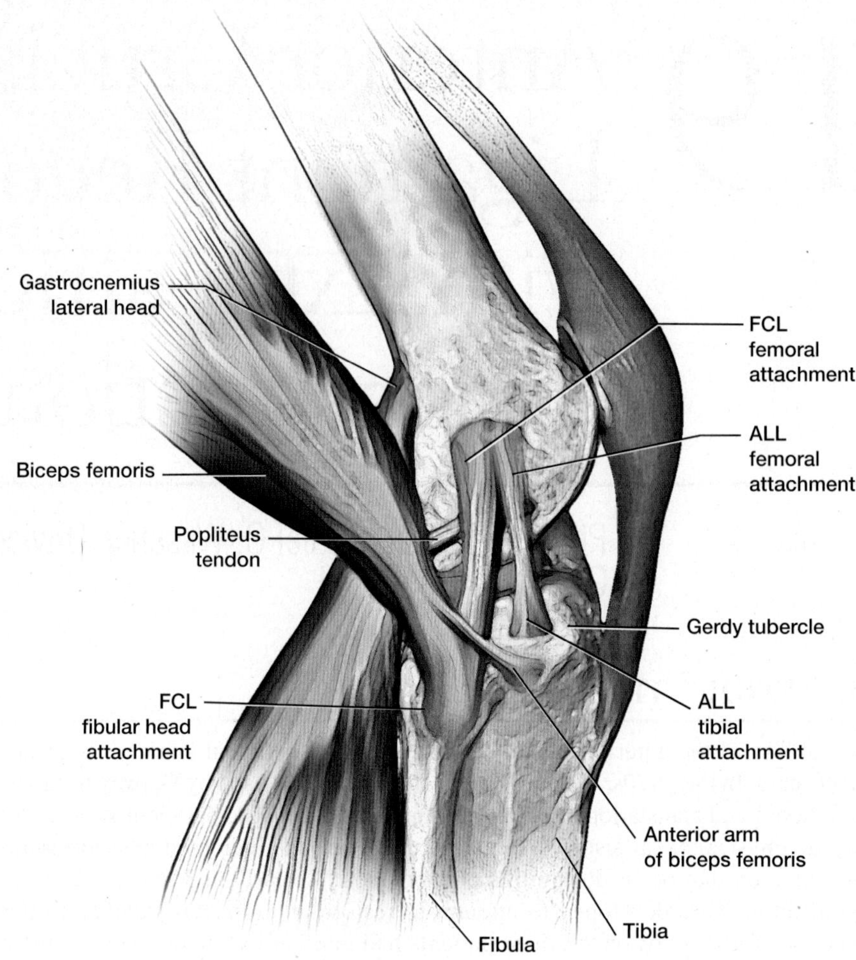

FIGURE 19-1

Representation of the anatomy of the anterolateral ligament. Note the tibial attachment just posterior to Gerdy tubercle and the femoral attachment between the insertions of the FCL and the lateral gastrocnemius tendon.

SURGICAL INDICATIONS

We have several indications for adding an extra-articular tenodesis to an intra-articular ACL reconstruction. In general, our philosophy is to perform the procedure in cases where the expected failure rate is increased. Our primary indication for an extra-articular tenodesis is a 3+ pivot shift on physical examination. In these patients, an intra-articular graft alone may not completely control excessive anterior tibial translation and internal rotation in the lateral compartment. These are generally patients with chronic ACL deficiency. It is unusual for us to perform an extra-articular reconstruction in the acute setting. Similarly, patients with generalized hyperlaxity are treated with the combined procedure. We also consider extra-articular augmentation in patients who plan to return to collision sports. The additional constraint may help protect these knees from the high loads seen in these sports and may decrease the rerupture rate. We also consider an extra-articular tenodesis in patients less than 20 years of age. It has been shown that these patients are at an increased risk of rerupture of an isolated intra-articular graft. Finally, we perform this procedure in cases of revision ACL surgery. Objective laxity is greater in patients with failed ACL reconstructions, especially those that have undergone concomitant medial meniscectomies, and the addition of an extra-articular tenodesis has improved the results of revision ACL surgery in some studies.

SURGICAL CONTRAINDICATIONS

The addition of an extra-articular reconstruction is contraindicated in ACL-deficient patients that have an associated posterolateral corner injury. In this situation, the lateral augmentation may fix the tibia in a posterolaterally subluxed position. We also do not perform an extra-articular reconstruction in skeletally immature patients because of the risk of injury to the femoral physis. Older studies have shown increased risk of lateral tibiofemoral degeneration after an isolated extra-articular reconstruction. This may have been a result of overtensioning of the graft leading to overconstraint of the lateral compartment or may have been related to the 4 to 6 weeks of postoperative immobilization that was standard at that time. We have not seen lateral tibiofemoral arthritis in our extra-articular patients where the lateral meniscus was intact.

PREOPERATIVE PLANNING

Physical examination remains the most important factor in deciding when to add an extra-articular procedure to an intra-articular ACL reconstruction. The examiner must be skilled in performing both the Lachman test to assess anterior translation and the pivot shift test to assess rotatory laxity. KT-1000 measurements and anterior tibial stress radiographs can help quantify global anterior laxity, but a measurement of the translation of the individual tibiofemoral compartments would be more useful to identify patients who would benefit from an extra-articular procedure. Several research techniques, including computer-assisted measurements, are being developed to quantitate the rotatory laxity of the knee, but these are not yet widely available. Radiographs should be obtained in all patients with suspected knee injuries. The presence of a Segond fracture confirms that there has been injury to the ALL. Unfortunately, magnetic resonance imaging (MRI) has not been shown to be useful to identify an injured ALL and does not help the surgeon in the decision of when to add an extra-articular procedure. In cases of revision ACL surgery, old operative reports should be obtained to know what grafts will be available and what instrumentation might be required to remove previously placed hardware.

SURGICAL TECHNIQUE

Two different surgical approaches can be utilized. One option is to use an extended anterior incision that will allow access to both the patellar tendon and the iliotibial band (Fig. 19-2A). Alternatively, two incisions can be used: an anteromedial one for harvesting the patellar tendon and a lateral incision for the extra-articular procedure (Fig. 19-2B). Subcutaneous skin flaps are raised, and a central 10-mm strip of patellar tendon is harvested. The patellar bone block is 9 mm × 25 mm to allow for easy graft passage, while the 25-mm long tibial bone block is harvested as a trapezoid being 10 mm wide at the tendon insertion and fanning out to 12 mm distally. A passing stitch of no. 2 reinforced nonabsorbable suture is placed through a small drill hole in each bone block. The patella tendon graft is then placed in a moist saline sponge until ready for passage.

Next, the lateral skin flap is dissected subcutaneously to expose the iliotibial band and Gerdy tubercle. A distally based strip of iliotibial band 10 mm wide and 70 to 100 mm long is harvested

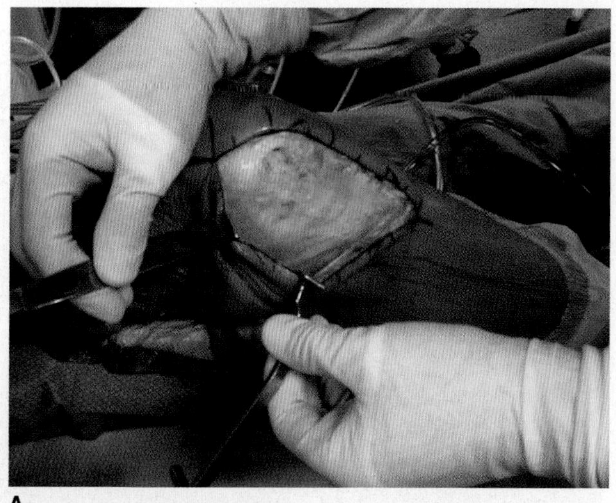

A

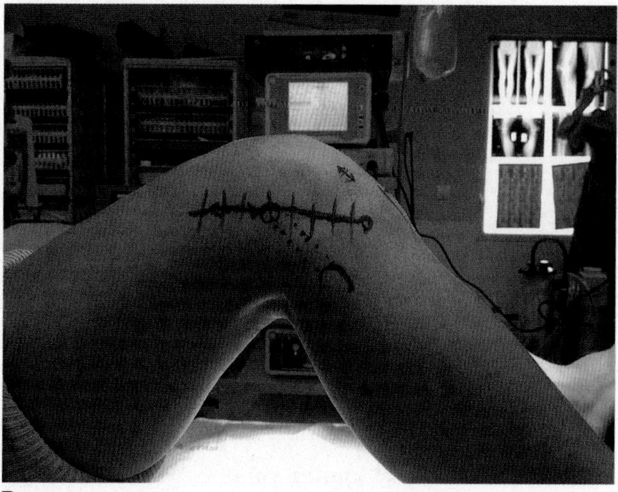

B

FIGURE 19-2

A: Extended anterior incision. **B:** Lateral incision.

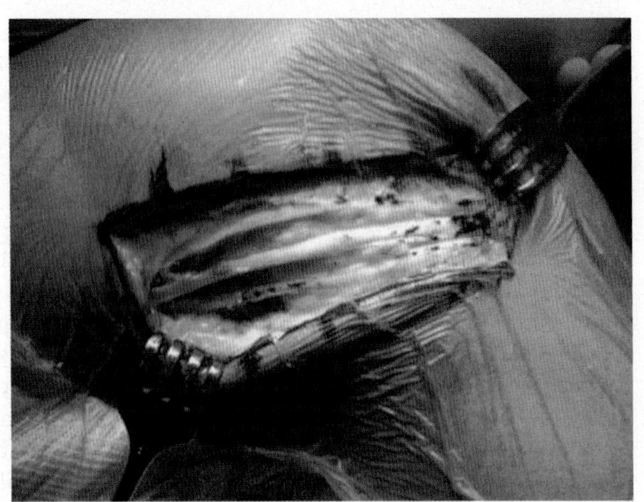

FIGURE 19-3

Harvesting of the iliotibial band. The IT band is left attached distally, and a 10-mm wide strip, 70 to 100 mm in length, is harvested.

using a scalpel and scissors (Fig. 19-3). A whipstitch of no. 2 suture is placed in the proximal end of the graft. Next, the surgeon should identify the fibular collateral ligament and its attachment on the femur. Dissection is carried out so that a clamp can be passed underneath the ligament (Fig. 19-4).

An arthroscopic evaluation of the knee joint is then undertaken and any associated intra-articular pathology is addressed. The ACL remnant is debrided. A femoral tunnel guide pin is drilled with an outside-in guide starting just 5 mm posterior and proximal to the FCL femoral insertion and exiting inside the knee joint at the center of the ACL femoral attachment (Fig. 19-5A, B). The guide pin is then reamed up to a 10-mm diameter tunnel. Finally, a 9-mm tibial tunnel is created in the center of the ACL tibial footprint using standard technique.

A passing suture is then placed through both tunnels and a second passing stitch placed through the femoral tunnel and exiting out the anteromedial portal. With the patellar bone block leading, the graft is then passed proximal to distal until the tibial bone block is just about to enter the femoral tunnel (Fig. 19-6). The strip of iliotibial band is then passed underneath the FCL and then pulled into the femoral tunnel (Fig. 19-7). With the leg held in 30 degrees of flexion and neutral rotation, tension is applied through the iliotibial band sutures. The tibial bone plug is then press fit into the femoral tunnel with the aid of a bone tamp (Fig. 19-8). This provides secure fixation for both the patellar tendon graft and the extra-articular reconstruction. The leg is then brought out into full extension, and the patellar bone plug is tensioned and secured with a 9-mm tibial interference screw. The split in the iliotibial band is closed with no. 1 absorbable suture, and if necessary, a limited lateral retinacular release is performed to avoid increased pressure on the lateral facet of the patella.

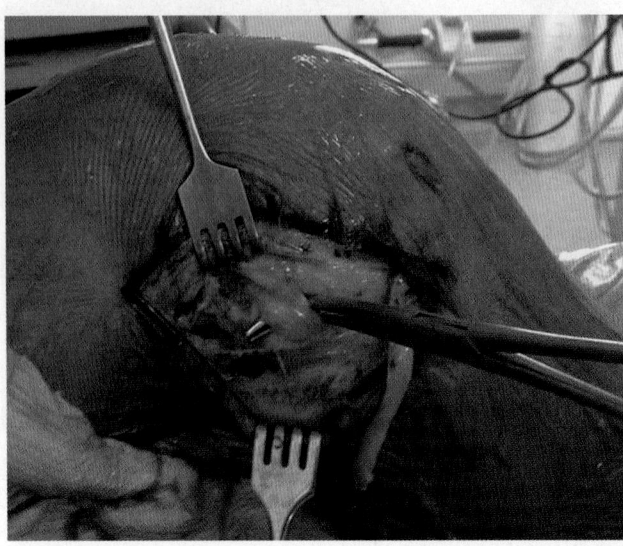

FIGURE 19-4

The FCL is dissected and a right angle clamp passed beneath it to allow for graft passage.

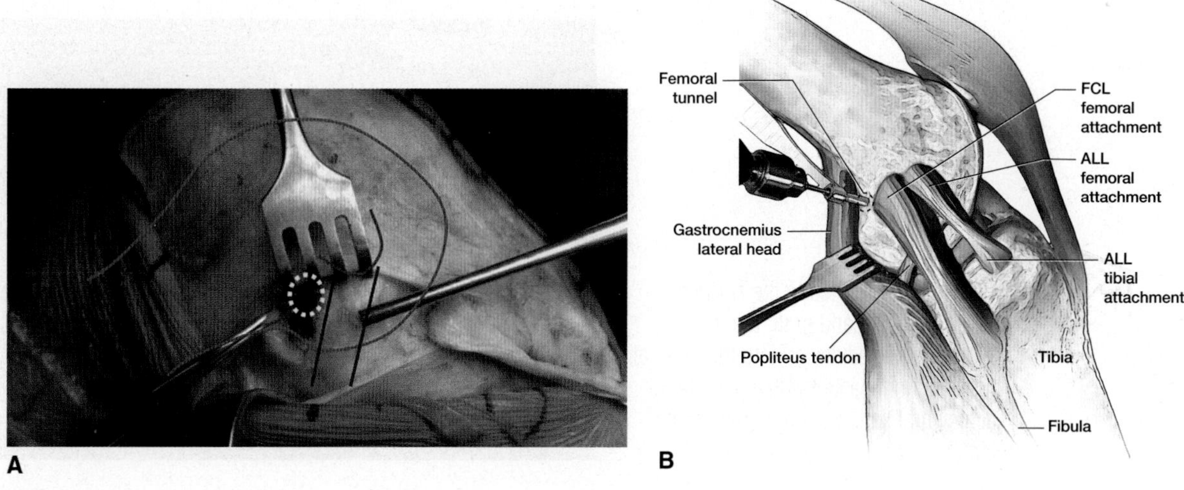

FIGURE 19-5

A: The femoral tunnel starting point is located between the insertions of the FCL and the lateral gastrocnemius tendons. **B:** Schematic representation of the femoral tunnel location.

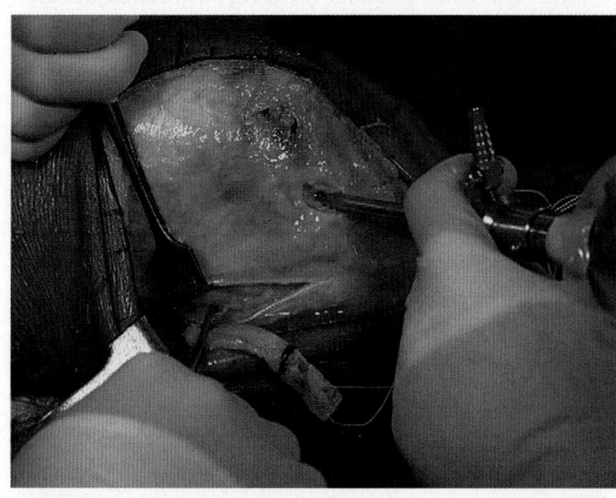

FIGURE 19-6

The ACL graft is passed until the trapezoidal tibial bone block is just about ready to enter the femoral tunnel.

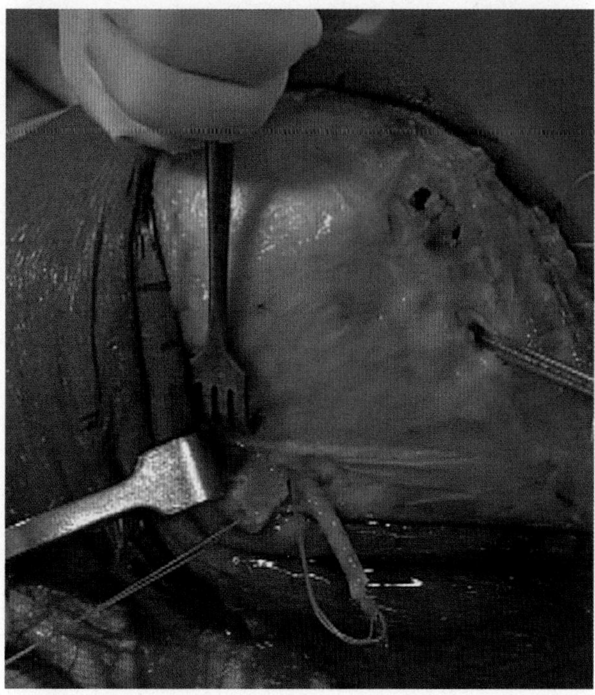

FIGURE 19-7

The IT band graft is then passed into the femoral tunnel, prior to seating the tibial bone block.

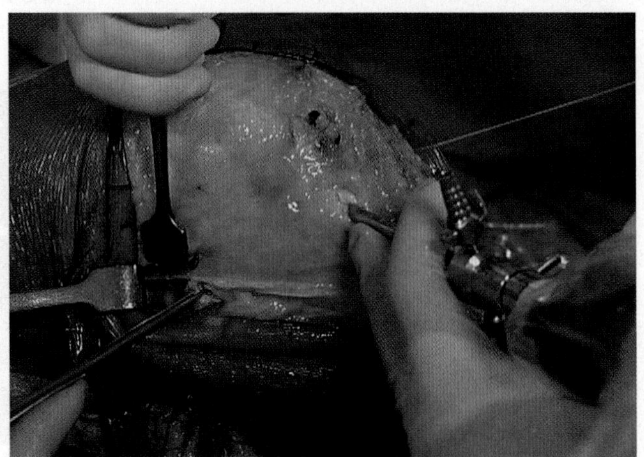

FIGURE 19-8
With tension applied to the sutures holding the IT band graft, the tibial bone block is advanced into the femoral tunnel and impacted with a bone tamp achieving fixation of both graft on the femur.

POSTOPERATIVE MANAGEMENT

Patients who have undergone the combined intra- and extra-articular ACL reconstruction undergo the same rehabilitation protocol as isolated intra-articular ACL reconstruction patients. The knee is immobilized in a hinged brace at 0 degrees for the first 2 weeks while the patient is at rest. The patient is then allowed range of motion as tolerated. Weight bearing is progressed as pain, swelling, and quadriceps strength allows. Full range of motion is expected by 6 weeks. After the first 6 weeks, no brace is required. Closed-chain exercises are emphasized the first 3 months. In patients with isolated ACL reconstructions, assuming normal motion, no effusion, and sufficient strength, running and sports-specific conditioning is allowed at 3 months. In patients with no severe laxity, return to play can be allowed at 6 months because the extra-articular augmentation protects the ACL graft during pivoting activities.

COMPLICATIONS TO AVOID

All complications that can occur with an isolated intra-articular ACL reconstruction can happen with this combined procedure. These include infection, stiffness, errors in tunnel placement, and residual laxity. The extra-articular ACL reconstruction described above should not be performed as an isolated procedure as it will not adequately control anterior tibial translation nor completely restore normal knee kinematics in young, active patients. Care must be taken to avoid overconstraining rotational laxity. We believe that appropriately tensioning the graft and maintaining the knee in neutral rotation during fixation can avoid this complication. Graft placement is also critical. The starting point for the outside-in femoral tunnel is extremely important to reproduce the femoral attachment point of the ALL. The surgeon must also insure that the tibial bone block achieves excellent fixation in the femoral tunnel while being fully seated. Appropriately trimming the graft and trialing with tunnel sizers prior to graft passage can minimize these problems. The closure of the IT band split can overtension the lateral retinaculum, causing lateral patellar facet overload. Performing a lateral retinacular release can help avoid this complication. Finally, pain and lateral tenderness can occur if the extra-articular reconstruction is passed superficial to the FCL. Making sure the graft passes beneath the FCL will avoid this complication.

ILLUSTRATIVE CASE

A 26-year-old man presented with a reinjury to his right knee. He had undergone ACL reconstruction of that knee 18 months previously, using bone-patellar tendon-bone autograft. After an appropriate rehabilitation period, he had returned to full activity, including recreational soccer. Three weeks prior to presentation, he had reinjured the knee with a twisting episode in a soccer match. Physical examination showed a 2+ Lachman and a 3+ pivot shift. Radiographs showed good positioning

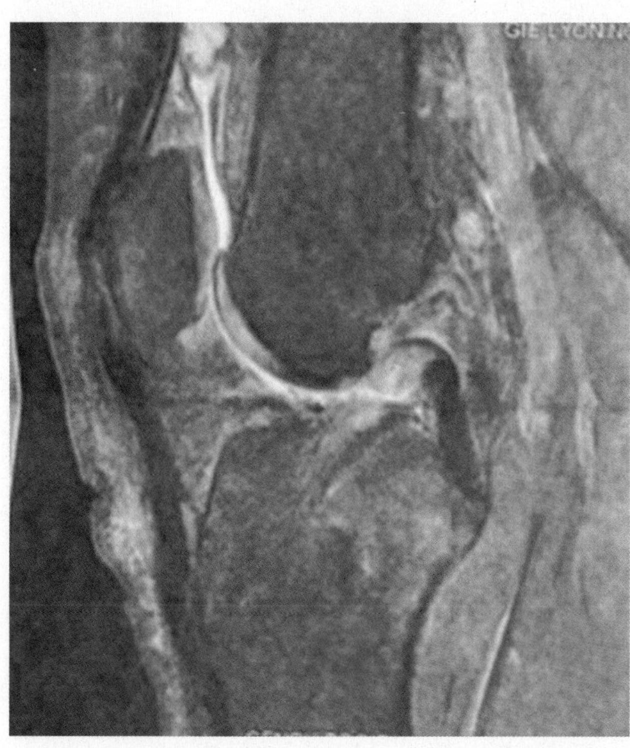

FIGURE 19-9
MRI scan showing traumatic ACL graft rupture 18 months after an ipsilateral patellar tendon graft ACL reconstruction.

of the previous tunnels. An MRI scan showed rupture of the ACL graft (Fig. 19-9). The patient underwent a combined intra- and extra-articular ACL reconstruction. The contralateral patellar tendon was used for the intra-articular graft, and a strip of iliotibial band was used for the extra-articular tenodesis as outlined above. A postoperative CT scan (Fig. 19-10) showed good positioning of the femoral tunnel. He went through our standard gradual rehabilitation program and returned to full activities at 10 months.

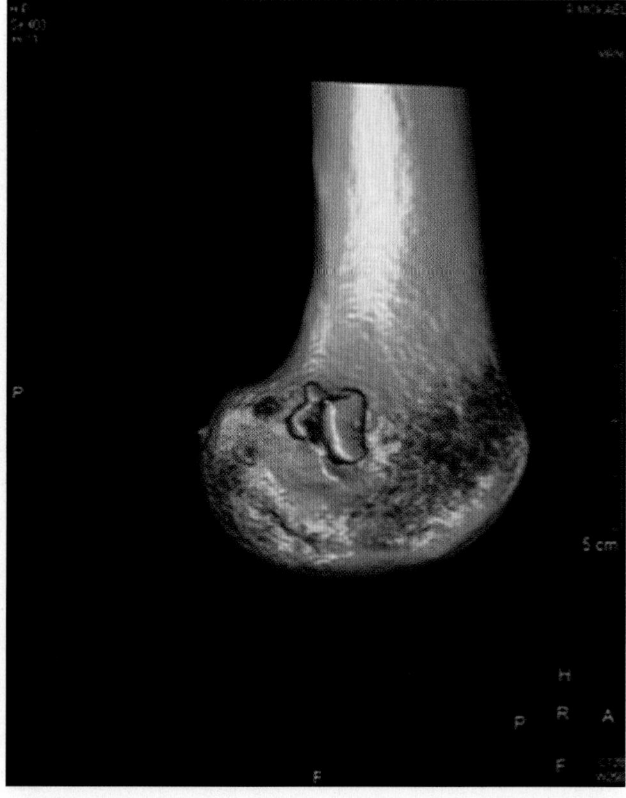

FIGURE 19-10
Postoperative CT scan showing the position of the femoral tunnel and the tibial bone block secured in the tunnel.

RECOMMENDED READINGS

Colombet P. Knee laxity control in revision anterior cruciate ligament reconstruction versus anterior cruciate ligament reconstruction and lateral tenodesis: clinical assessment using computer-assisted navigation. *Am J Sports Med.* 2011;39(6):1248–1254.

Claes S, Vereecke E, Maes M, et al. Anatomy of the anterolateral ligament of the knee. *J Anat.* 2013;223(4):321–328.

Dodds AL, Gupte CM, Neyret P, et al. Extra-articular techniques in anterior cruciate ligament reconstruction: a literature review. *J Bone Joint Surg Br.* 2011;93:1440–1448.

Dodds AL, Halewood C, Gupte CM, et al. The antero-lateral ligament: anatomy, length changes and association with the Segond fracture. *Bone Joint J.* 2014;96-B(3):325–331.

Duthon VB, Magnussen RA, Servien E, et al. ACL reconstruction and extra-articular tenodesis. *Clin Sports Med.* 2013;32(1):141–153.

Kennedy MI, Claes S, Fuso FAF, et al. The anterolateral ligament: an anatomic, radiographic, and biomechanical analysis. *Am J Sports Med.* 2015;43(7):1606–1615.

Lemaire M, Combelles F. Plastic repair with fascia lata for old tears of the anterior cruciate ligament (author's transl). *Rev Chir Orthop Reparatrice Appar Mot.* 1980;66:523–525 [in French].

Marcacci M, Zaffagnini S, Giordano G, et al. Anterior cruciate ligament reconstruction associated with extra-articular tenodesis: a prospective clinical and radiographic evaluation with 10- to 13-year follow-up. *Am J Sports Med.* 2009;37(4):707–714.

Pernin J, Verdonk P, Si Selmi TA, et al. Long-term follow-up of 24.5 years after intra-articular anterior cruciate ligament reconstruction with lateral extra-articular augmentation. *Am J Sports Med.* 2010;38(6):1094–1102.

Sonnery-Cottet B, Thaunat M, Freychet B, et al. Outcome of a combined anterior cruciate ligament and anterolateral ligament reconstruction technique with a minimum 2-year follow-up. *Am J Sports Med.* 2015;43(7):1598–1605.

Trojani C, Beaufils P, Burdin G, et al. Revision ACL reconstruction: influence of a lateral tenodesis. *Knee Surg Sports Traumatol Arthrosc.* 2012;20:1565–1570.

Vincent JP, Magnussen RA, Gezmez F, et al. The anterolateral ligament of the human knee: an anatomic and histologic study. *Knee Surg Sports Traumatol Arthrosc.* 2012;20(1):147–152.

Zaffagnini S, Signorelli C, Lopomo N, et al. Anatomic double-bundle and over-the-top single-bundle with additional extra-articular tenodesis: an in vivo quantitative assessment of knee laxity in two different ACL reconstructions. *Knee Surg Sports Traumatol Arthrosc.* 2012;20:153–159.

20 Single-Bundle Transtibial Posterior Cruciate Ligament Reconstruction

Gregory C. Fanelli

INDICATIONS AND CONTRAINDICATIONS

Posterior cruciate ligament (PCL) injuries in my practice rarely occur as an isolated knee ligament injury. The PCL injuries are most often combined with at least one other knee ligament injury. The reasons for PCL reconstruction surgical failure most commonly are failure to address associated ligament instabilities, failure to address lower extremity malalignment, and incorrect tunnel placement. Identifying the multiple planes of instability in these complex knee ligament injuries is essential for successful treatment of the PCL injured knee. The PCL disruption will lead to increased posterior laxity at 90 degrees of knee flexion. Recognition and correction of the medial and/or lateral side instability is the key to successful posterior and anterior cruciate ligament (ACL) surgery.

There are three different types of instability patterns that I have observed in medial and lateral side knee injuries. These are, type A (axial rotation instability only), type B (axial rotation instability combined with varus and/or valgus laxity with a firm end point), and type C (axial rotation instability combined with varus and/or valgus laxity with little or no end point). In my experience, the axial rotation instability (type A) medial or lateral side is most frequently overlooked. It is also critical to understand that combined medial and lateral side instability of different types occurs with bicruciate and unicruciate multiple ligament knee injuries. Examples include PCL, ACL, lateral side type C, and medial side type A, or PCL, medial side type B, and lateral side type A instability patterns.

A combination of careful clinical examination, radiographs, and MRI studies aids in determining the correct diagnosis of multiple ligament knee injuries. Knee examination under anesthesia combined with fluoroscopy, stress radiography, and diagnostic arthroscopy also contributes to accurately diagnose the multiple planes of instability. My indications for surgical treatment of acute PCL injuries include insertion site avulsions, a decrease in tibial step of 8 mm or greater, and PCL tears combined with other structural injuries. Our indications for surgical treatment of chronic PCL injuries are when an isolated PCL tear becomes symptomatic or when progressive functional instability develops. Contraindications include poor skin condition, uncorrected bony malalignment, severe degenerative joint disease, and medical conditions preventing surgical intervention. The purpose of this chapter is to describe the arthroscopic transtibial tunnel PCL reconstruction surgical technique.

PREOPERATIVE PLANNING

Posterior cruciate ligament–based reconstruction procedures are routinely performed in an outpatient setting unless specific circumstances indicate the necessity of an inpatient environment. The same experienced surgical teams are assembled for these complex surgical procedures. Experienced and familiar teams provide for a smoother operation, shorter surgical times, enhanced patient care, and a greater probability of success in these difficult surgical procedures. Preoperative and postoperative prophylactic antibiotics are routinely used in these complex and time-consuming surgical procedures to decrease the probability of infection.

My preferred graft for the PCL reconstruction is the Achilles tendon allograft for single-bundle PCL reconstructions and Achilles tendon (anterolateral bundle) and tibialis anterior (posteromedial bundle) allografts for double-bundle PCL reconstructions. The allograft tissue used is from the same tissue bank with the same methods of tissue procurement and preservation that provide a consistent graft of high quality. It is very important for the surgeon to "know the tissue bank" and to obtain high-quality allograft tissue that will maximize the probability of surgical success.

POSTERIOR CRUCIATE LIGAMENT RECONSTRUCTION SURGICAL PROCEDURE

The principles of PCL reconstruction are to identify and treat all pathology, accurately place tunnels to produce anatomic graft insertion sites, and utilize strong graft material, mechanical graft tensioning, secure graft fixation, and a deliberate postoperative rehabilitation program.

The patient is placed on the operating room table in the supine position, and after satisfactory induction of anesthesia, the operative and nonoperative lower extremities are carefully examined. A tourniquet is applied to the upper thigh of the operative extremity but is not routinely inflated, and that extremity is prepped and draped in a sterile fashion. The well leg is supported by the fully extended operating room table that also supports the surgical leg during medial and lateral side surgery. A lateral post is used to control the surgical extremity. An arthroscopic leg holder is not used. Preoperative and postoperative antibiotics are given, and antibiotics are routinely used to help prevent infection in these time-consuming, difficult, and complex cases. Allograft tissue is prepared prior to bringing the patient into the operating room to minimize general anesthesia time for the patient. Autograft tissue is harvested prior to beginning the arthroscopic portion of the procedure. The Biomet Sports Medicine PCL/ACL System (Biomet Sports Medicine, Warsaw, IN) are the surgical instruments used for this surgical procedure. Intraoperative radiography and C-arm image intensifier are not routinely used for this surgical procedure.

The arthroscopic instruments are inserted with the inflow through the superolateral patellar portal. Instrumentation and visualization are positioned through inferomedial and inferolateral patellar portals and can be interchanged as necessary. Additional portals are established as necessary. Exploration of the joint consists of evaluation of the patellofemoral joint, the medial and lateral compartments, medial and lateral menisci, and the intercondylar notch. The residual stumps of the PCLs are debrided; however, the posterior (and ACL when applicable) anatomic insertion sites are preserved to serve as tunnel reference points. The notchplasty for the ACL portion of the procedure in combined PCL/ACL reconstruction cases is performed at this time.

An extracapsular extra-articular posteromedial safety incision is made by creating an incision approximately 1.5 to 2 cm long starting at the posteromedial border of the tibia approximately 1 in below the level of the joint line and extending distally (Figs. 20-1 and 20-2). Dissection is carried down to the crural fascia, which is incised longitudinally. An interval is developed between the medial head of the gastrocnemius muscle and the nerves and vessels posterior to the surgeon's finger and the capsule of the knee joint anterior to the surgeon's finger. The posteromedial safety incision enables the surgeon to protect the neurovascular structures, confirm the accuracy of the PCL tibial tunnel, and facilitate the flow of the surgical procedure. The neurovascular structures of the popliteal fossa are in close proximity to the posterior capsule of the knee joint and are at risk during transtibial PCL reconstruction. The posteromedial safety incision is very important for the protection of these structures.

The curved over-the-top PCL instruments (Biomet Sports Medicine, Warsaw, IN) are used to sequentially lyse adhesions in the posterior aspect of the knee and elevate the capsule from the posterior tibial ridge. This will allow accurate placement of the PCL/ACL drill guide, and correct placement of the tibial tunnel (Fig. 20-3).

The arm of the PCL/ACL guide (Biomet Sports Medicine, Warsaw, IN) is inserted through the inferior medial patellar portal (Fig. 20-4). The tip of the guide is positioned at the inferior lateral aspect of the PCL anatomic insertion site. This is below the tibial ridge posterior and in the lateral aspect of the PCL anatomic insertion site. The bullet portion of the guide contacts the anteromedial surface of the proximal tibia at a point midway between the posteromedial border of the tibia and the tibial crest anterior at or just below the level of the tibial tubercle. This will provide an angle of graft orientation such that the graft will turn two very smooth 45 degree angles on the posterior aspect of

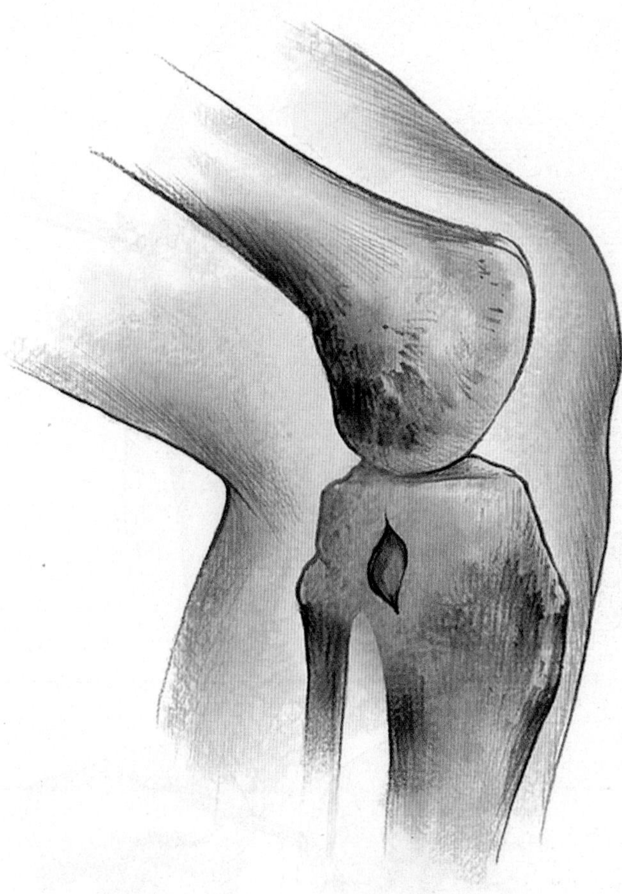

FIGURE 20-1

Posteromedial extra-articular extracapsular safety incision. (From Fanelli GC. *Rationale and surgical technique for PCL and multiple knee ligament reconstruction.* 3rd ed. Warsaw, IN: Biomet Sports Medicine; 2012, with permission.)

the tibia (Figs. 20-5 and 20-6). The tip of the guide, in the posterior aspect of the tibia, is confirmed with the surgeon's finger through the extracapsular extra-articular posteromedial safety incision. Intraoperative AP and lateral x-ray may also be used; however, I do not routinely use intraoperative x-ray. When the PCL/ACL guide is positioned in the desired area, a blunt spade-tipped guide wire is drilled from anterior to posterior. The surgeon's finger confirms the position of the guide wire through the posterior medial safety incision.

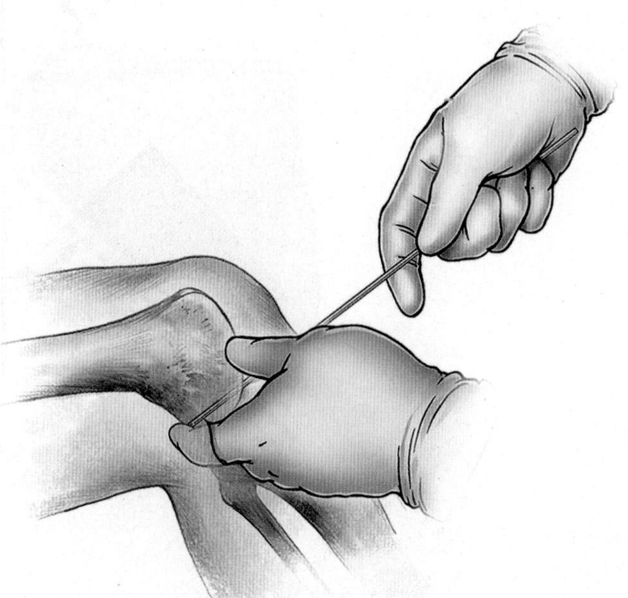

FIGURE 20-2

The surgeon is able to palpate the posterior aspect of the tibia through the extracapsular extra-articular posteromedial safety incision. This enables the surgeon to accurately position guide wires, create the tibial tunnel, and protect the neurovascular structures. (From Fanelli GC. *Rationale and surgical technique for PCL and multiple knee ligament reconstruction.* 3rd ed. Warsaw, IN: Biomet Sports Medicine; 2012, with permission.)

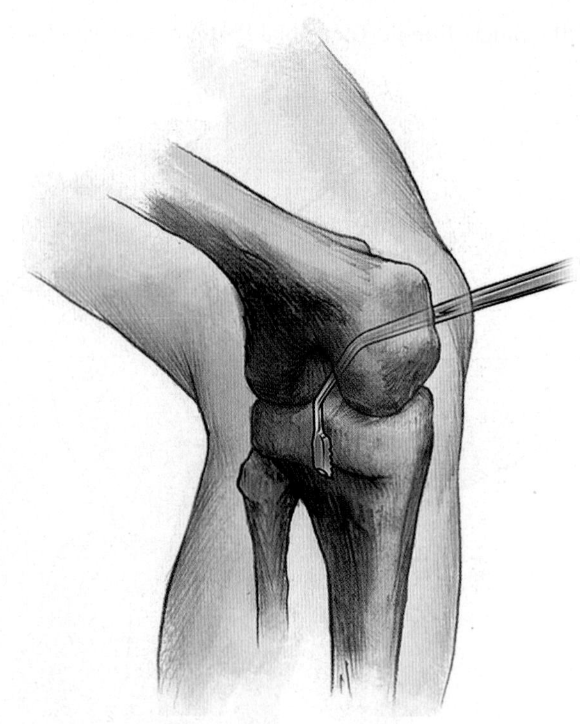

FIGURE 20-3

Posterior capsular elevation. (From Fanelli GC. *Rationale and surgical technique for PCL and multiple knee ligament reconstruction.* 3rd ed. Warsaw, IN: Biomet Sports Medicine; 2012.)

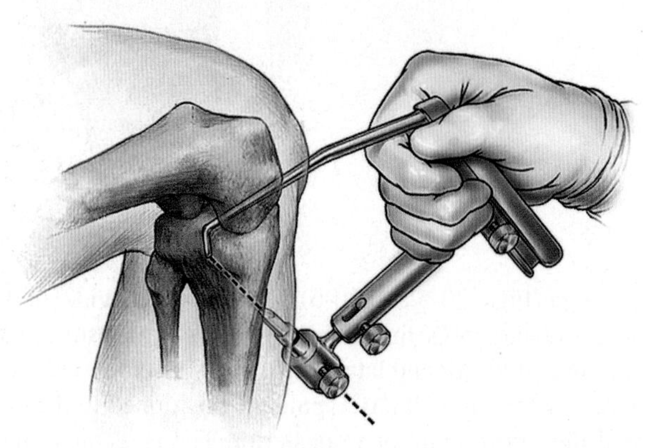

FIGURE 20-4

PCL-ACL drill guide positioned to place guide wire in preparation for creation of the Transtibial PCL tibial tunnel. (From Fanelli GC. *Rationale and surgical technique for PCL and multiple knee ligament reconstruction.* 3rd ed. Warsaw, IN: Biomet Sports Medicine; 2012.)

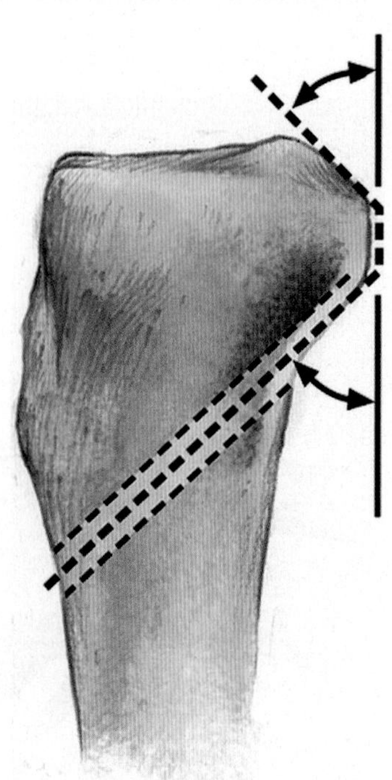

FIGURE 20-5

Drawing demonstrating the desired turning angles the PCL graft will make after the creation of the tibial tunnel. (From Fanelli GC. *Rationale and surgical technique for PCL and multiple knee ligament reconstruction.* 3rd ed. Warsaw, IN: Biomet Sports Medicine; 2012.)

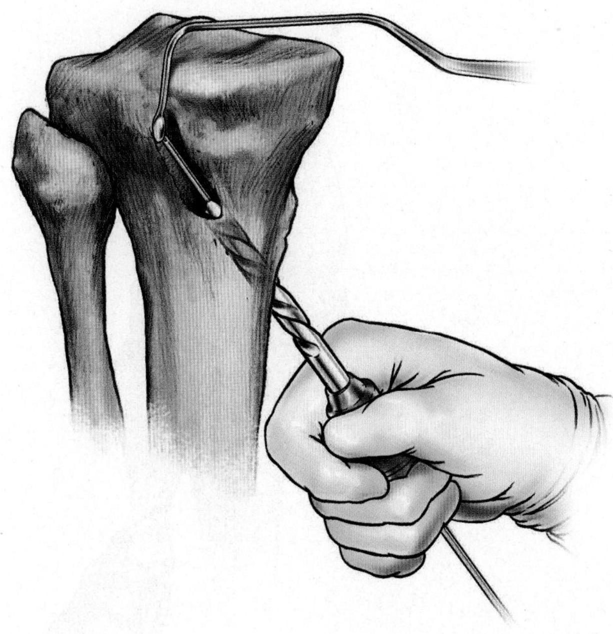

FIGURE 20-6

Final PCL tibial tunnel reaming by hand for an additional margin of safety. Note the trough created on the posterior aspect of the tibia that is similar to the tibial inlay PCL reconstruction surgical technique. This trough creation minimizes stress in the graft and provides a biomechanical advantage for graft positioning and function. (From Fanelli GC. *Rationale and surgical technique for PCL and multiple knee ligament reconstruction.* 3rd ed. Warsaw, IN: Biomet Sports Medicine; 2012.)

The appropriately sized standard cannulated reamer is used to create the tibial tunnel. The surgeon's finger through the extracapsular extra-articular posteromedial incision is monitoring the position of the guide wire. When the drill is engaged in bone, the guide wire is reversed, blunt end pointing posterior, for additional patient safety. The drill is advanced until it comes to the posterior cortex of the tibia. The chuck is disengaged from the drill, and completion of the tibial tunnel is performed by hand.

The PCL single-bundle or double-bundle femoral tunnels are made from inside out using the double-bundle aimers, or an endoscopic reamer can be used as an aiming device (Biomet Sports Medicine, Warsaw, IN) (Figs. 20-7 to 20-10). The appropriately sized double-bundle aimer or endoscopic reamer is inserted through a low anterior lateral patellar arthroscopic portal to create the PCL anterior lateral

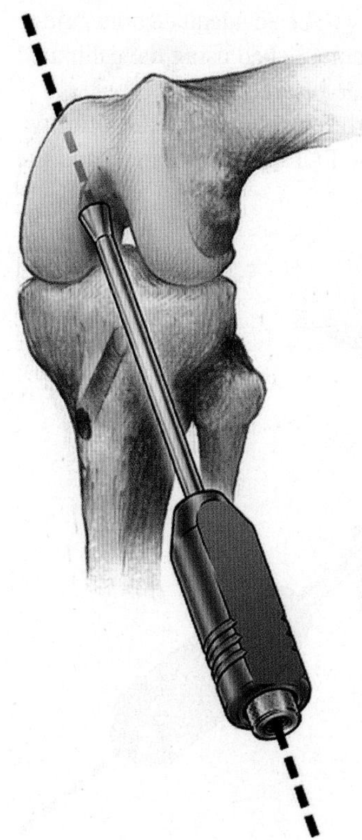

FIGURE 20-7

Double-bundle aimer positioned to drill a guide wire for creation of the PCL anterolateral bundle tunnel. (From Fanelli GC. *Rationale and surgical technique for PCL and multiple knee ligament reconstruction.* 3rd ed. Warsaw, IN: Biomet Sports Medicine; 2012.)

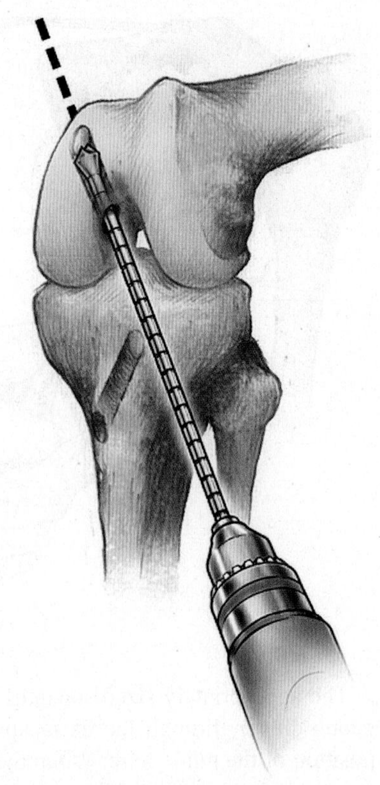

FIGURE 20-8

Endoscopic acorn reamer is used to create the PCL anterolateral bundle femoral tunnel through the low anterolateral patellar portal. (From Fanelli GC. *Rationale and surgical technique for PCL and multiple knee ligament reconstruction.* 3rd ed. Warsaw, IN: Biomet Sports Medicine; 2012.)

bundle femoral tunnel with the surgical knee in 90 to 110 degrees of knee flexion. The double-bundle aimer or endoscopic reamer is positioned directly on the footprint of the femoral anterior lateral bundle PCL insertion site. The appropriately sized guide wire is drilled through the aimer or endoscopic reamer, through the bone, and out a small skin incision. Care is taken to prevent any compromise of the articular surface. The double-bundle aimer is removed, and the endoscopic reamer is used to drill the anterior lateral PCL femoral tunnel from inside to outside. When the surgeon chooses to perform a double-bundle double femoral tunnel PCL reconstruction, the same process is repeated for the posterior medial bundle of the PCL. Care must be taken to ensure that there will be an adequate bone bridge (~5 mm) between the two femoral tunnels prior to drilling. This is accomplished using the calibrated probe and direct arthroscopic visualization of the PCL femoral anatomic insertion sites.

My preferred surgical technique of PCL femoral tunnel creation from inside to outside is for two reasons. There is a greater distance and margin of safety between the PCL femoral tunnels and the

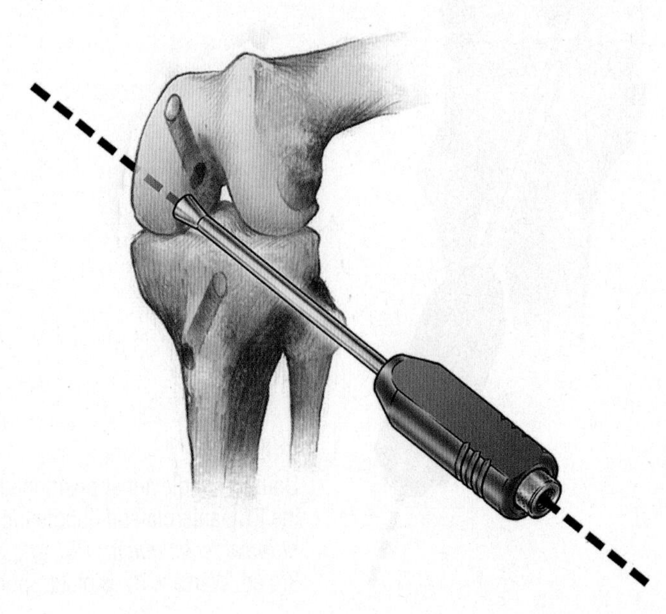

FIGURE 20-9

Double-bundle aimer positioned to drill a guide wire for creation of the PCL posteromedial bundle femoral tunnel through the low anterolateral patellar portal. (From Fanelli GC. *Rationale and surgical technique for PCL and multiple knee ligament reconstruction.* 3rd ed. Warsaw, IN: Biomet Sports Medicine; 2012.)

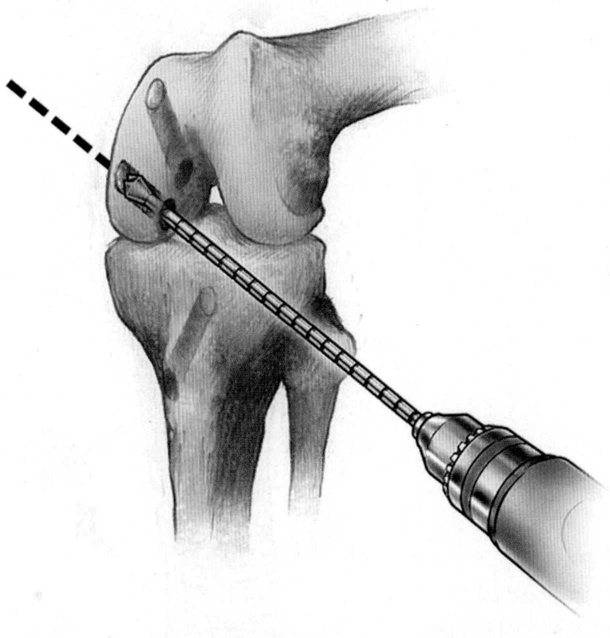

FIGURE 20-10

Endoscopic acorn reamer is used to create the PCL posteromedial bundle femoral tunnel. A 5-mm bone bridge is maintained between tunnels. (From Fanelli GC. *Rationale and surgical technique for PCL and multiple knee ligament reconstruction.* 3rd ed. Warsaw, IN: Biomet Sports Medicine; 2012.)

medial femoral condyle articular surface using the inside to outside method. Additionally, a more accurate placement of the PCL femoral tunnels is possible, in my opinion, because I can place the double-bundle aimer or endoscopic reamer on the anatomic foot print of the anterior lateral or posterior medial PCL insertion site under direct visualization.

A Magellan suture retriever (Biomet Sports Medicine, Warsaw, IN) is introduced through the tibial tunnel into the joint and retrieved through the femoral tunnel (Fig. 20-11). The traction sutures of the graft material are attached to the loop of the Magellan suture retriever, and the graft is pulled into position. The graft material is secured on the femoral side using a bioabsorbable interference screw for primary aperture opening fixation and a polyethylene ligament fixation button for backup fixation.

The cyclic dynamic method of graft tensioning using the Biomet graft tensioning boot is used to tension the posterior and ACL grafts (Fig. 20-12). Tension is placed on the PCL graft distally using the

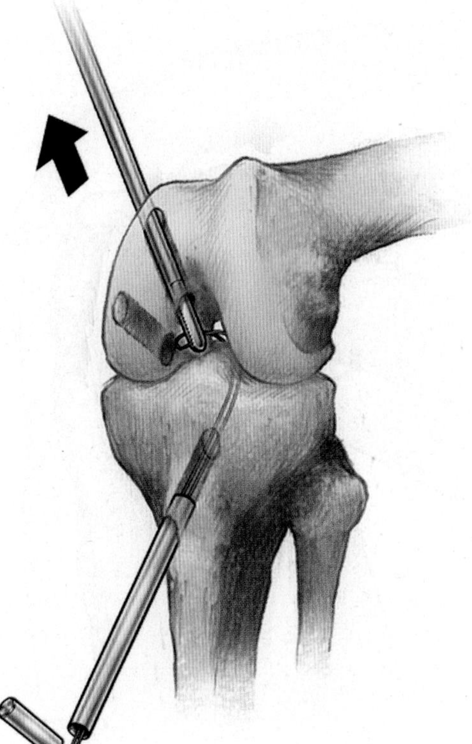

FIGURE 20-11

Magellan suture-passing device. (From Fanelli GC. *Rationale and surgical technique for PCL and multiple knee ligament reconstruction.* 3rd ed. Warsaw, IN: Biomet Sports Medicine; 2012.)

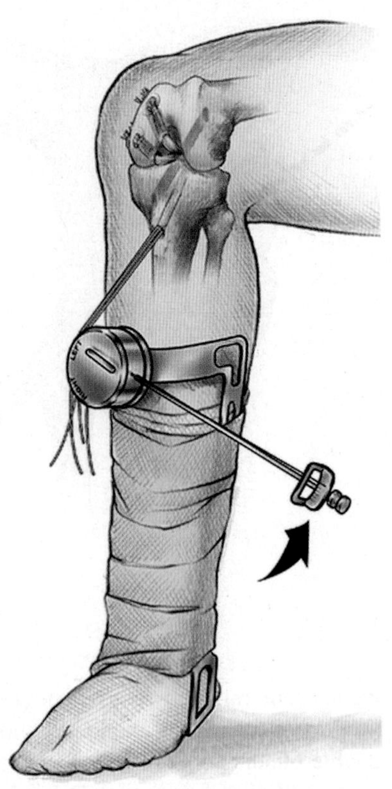

FIGURE 20-12

Knee ligament graft-tensioning boot is used to tension the PCL graft. This mechanical tensioning device uses a ratcheted torque wrench device to assist the surgeon during graft tensioning. (From Fanelli GC. *Rationale and surgical technique for PCL and multiple knee ligament reconstruction.* 3rd ed. Warsaw, IN: Biomet Sports Medicine; 2012.)

Biomet graft-tensioning boot (Biomet Sports Medicine, Warsaw, IN). Tension is gradually applied with the knee in zero degrees of flexion (full extension) reducing the tibia on the femur. This restores the anatomic tibial step off. The knee is cycled through a full range of motion multiple times to allow pre-tensioning and settling of the graft. The process is repeated until there is no further change in the torque setting on the graft tensioner. The knee is placed in 70 to 90 degrees of flexion, and fixation is achieved on the tibial side of the PCL graft with a bioabsorbable interference screw, and backup fixation with a bicortical screw and spiked ligament washer or polyethylene ligament fixation button (Fig. 20-13).

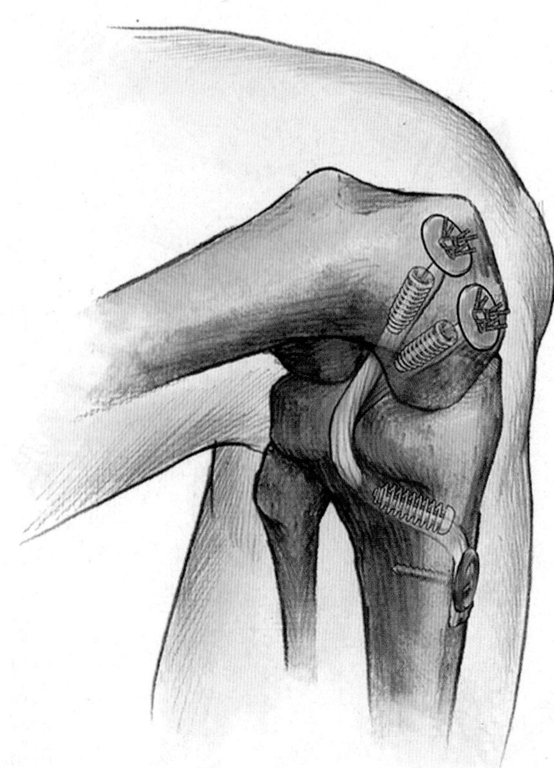

FIGURE 20-13

PCL final graft fixation using primary and backup fixation. (From Fanelli GC. *Rationale and surgical technique for PCL and multiple knee ligament reconstruction.* 3rd ed. Warsaw, IN: Biomet Sports Medicine; 2012.)

POSTOPERATIVE REHABILITATION

The knee is maintained in full extension for 3 to 5 weeks non–weight-bearing. Progressive range of motion occurs during postoperative weeks 3 to 5 through 10. Progressive weightbearing occurs at the beginning of postoperative weeks 3 through 5. Progressive closed kinetic chain strength training, proprioceptive training, and continued motion exercises are initiated very slowly beginning at postoperative week 12. The long leg range of motion brace is discontinued after the tenth week. Return to sports and heavy labor occurs after the ninth to twelfth postoperative month when sufficient strength, range of motion, and proprioceptive skills have returned. It is very important to carefully observe these complex knee ligament injury patients and get a feel for the "personality of the knee." The surgeon may need to make adjustments and individualize the postoperative rehabilitation program as necessary. Careful and gentle range of motion under general anesthesia is a very useful tool in the treatment of these complex cases and is utilized as necessary.

COMPLICATIONS TO AVOID

The posteromedial safety incision protects the neurovascular structures, confirms the accuracy of the PCL tibial tunnel placement, and enhances the flow of the surgical procedure. We have found it very important to use primary and backup fixation. During cruciate ligament reconstruction, primary aperture fixation is achieved with bioabsorbable interference screws, and backup fixation is performed with a screw and spiked ligament washer and ligament fixation buttons. Secure fixation is critical to the success of this surgical procedure. Mechanical tensioning of the PCL at zero degrees of knee flexion (full extension), and restoration of the normal anatomic tibial step-off at 70 to 90 degrees of flexion, and fixation of the PCL graft at 70 to 90 degrees of knee flexion have provided the most reproducible method of establishing the neutral point of the tibiofemoral relationship in our experience. Full range of motion is confirmed on the operating table to assure the knee is not "captured" by the reconstruction.

AUTHOR'S RESULTS

The author's experience over the past 26 years has revealed the following important points regarding PCL and multiple knee ligament (MLK) reconstruction. Allograft and autograft tissue are both successful in both the acute and chronic setting for PCL and MLK reconstruction with no statistically significant difference in KT 1000, stress x-rays, and knee ligament rating scales. Mechanical graft tensioning using the Biomet mechanical graft tensioning boot (Biomet Sports Medicine, Warsaw, IN) produced an 87% to 92% normal posterior drawer compared to a 46% normal posterior drawer in PCL reconstruction without the tensioning boot. Single- and double-bundle PCL reconstructions are both successful with no statistically significant difference in the acute and chronic setting when evaluated with KT 1000, stress radiography, and return to preinjury level of function. Long-term postoperative results of 18 to 22 years reveal a 23% to 30% incidence of degenerative joint disease in PCL and MLK reconstruction patients even when stability is retained when evaluated by physical examination, KT 1000, and stress radiography. Transtibial PCL reconstruction is effective in restoring stability and return to function in patients 18 years of age and younger in PCL and MLK reconstruction with no physeal growth arrest or resultant angular deformity in this population of patients. Restoration of posterolateral and posteromedial stability is essential to achieve stability in these complex knee ligament injuries.

ILLUSTRATIVE CASE

The patient is a 17-year-old competitive gymnast who had a missed landing during a gymnastics event injuring her left knee. At the time of injury, the patient had a hyperextension and varus force applied to her knee with the right foot planted firmly on the ground. The patient developed immediate pain and swelling and was unable to continue participation in the athletic competition. The patient's initial presentation upon reporting to the emergency department included a right knee effusion with posterior and lateral right knee pain. Neurovascular status of the involved right lower extremity was intact, and the skin was intact. There was anterior posterior and varus laxity with guarding by the patient. The patient was referred to me for evaluation and treatment of the knee injury.

Initial evaluation of this patient in our clinic revealed nearly symmetrical range of motion of both knees with minimal effusion of the injured left knee. The neurovascular examination of the involved left lower extremity was symmetrical to the normal right lower extremity, and the skin was intact on both legs. Physical examination comparing the injured left knee to the normal right knee revealed negative tibial step-offs with the proximal tibia dropped back posterior to the distal femur with the knee at 90 degrees of knee flexion, a grade three posterior drawer test, positive posterior lateral drawer test, and varus laxity at 30 and 0 degrees of knee flexion with 10 mm of increased lateral joint line opening compared to the normal knee, but with a firm end point. The dial test was positive at both 30 and 90 degrees of knee flexion, and the posteromedial drawer test was negative. The knee was stable to valgus stress throughout the flexion-extension arc, and the Lachman and pivot shift tests were negative. The hyperextension external rotation recurvatum and heel lift off tests were symmetrical. The extensor mechanism was stable.

Plain radiographs demonstrated symmetrical positioning of the tibiofemoral and patellofemoral joints compared to the patient's normal knee. Stress radiography at 90 degrees of knee flexion with a posterior directed force applied to the proximal tibial comparing the injured left knee to the normal right knee revealed 12 mm more posterior tibial displacement of the injured knee. MRI study of the left knee revealed a medial femoral condyle bone bruise, complete PCL tear, and disruption of the posterolateral structures of the knee.

The diagnosis in this case is an acute PCL tear combined with posterolateral instability type B in a 17-year-old competitive athlete. The plan was to proceed with reconstruction of the PCL, primary repair of the posterolateral structures, and posterolateral reconstruction at approximately 3 to 4 weeks postinjury. Preoperatively, the patient achieved full range of motion of the injured knee. There was a complete disruption of the PCL, and PCL reconstruction was performed using the single-bundle arthroscopically assisted transtibial tunnel technique using an Achilles tendon allograft to reconstruct the anterolateral bundle of the PCL (Fig. 20-14). The injury complex on the lateral side of the knee consisted of femoral insertion site avulsion of the fibular collateral ligament and popliteus tendon and attenuation of the midlateral and posterolateral capsule. Primary repair of fibular collateral ligament and popliteus tendon injuries was performed combined with a posterolateral capsular shift procedure and a posterolateral reconstruction using a fibular head based figure of eight posterolateral reconstruction technique (Fig. 20-15). Postoperatively, the surgical knee was immobilized in a long leg brace locked in full extension and was non–weight-bearing with crutches. Prophylactic preoperative and postoperative antibiotics were utilized. Progressive weightbearing and range of knee motion were gradually initiated according to our postoperative rehabilitation program.

Ten years postoperatively, the patient's range of motion is 0 to 135 degrees on the surgical left knee and 0 to 150 degrees on the uninvolved right knee. The posterior drawer is negative, posteromedial and posterolateral drawer tests are negative, and the dial test is symmetrical at 30 and 90 degrees of knee flexion. The Lachman test is negative, the pivot shift test is negative, and the surgical knee is stable to varus and valgus stress throughout the flexion extension arc. The hyperextension external rotation recurvatum and heel lift off tests are symmetrical compared to the normal knee.

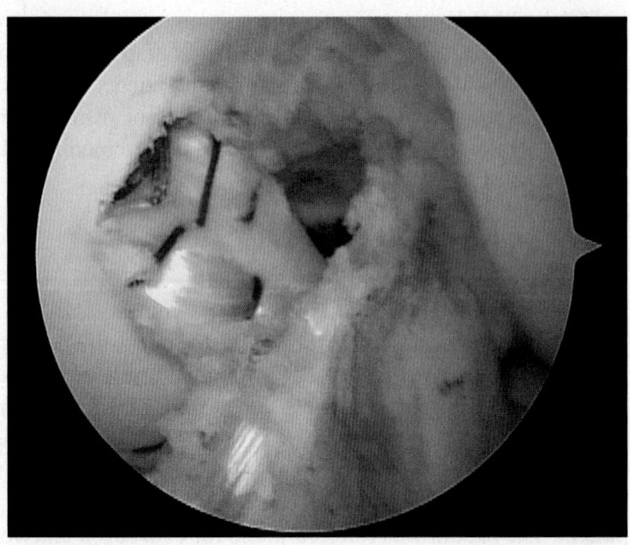

FIGURE 20-14

There was a complete disruption of the PCL, and PCL reconstruction was performed using the single-bundle arthroscopically assisted transtibial tunnel technique using an Achilles tendon allograft to reconstruct the anterolateral bundle of the PCL.

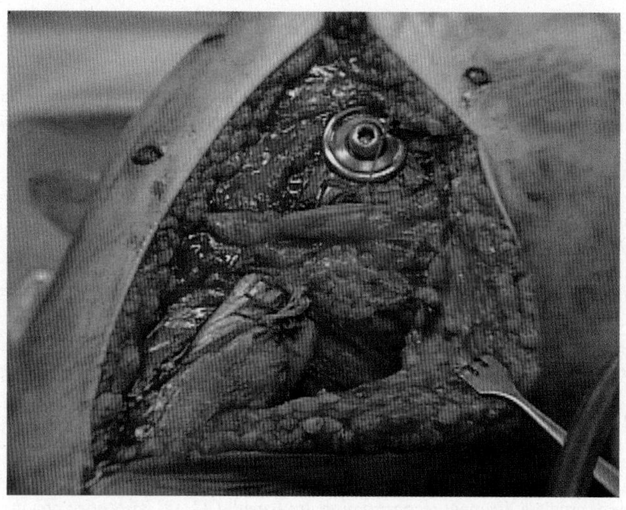

FIGURE 20-15

The injury complex on the lateral side of the knee consisted of femoral insertion site avulsion of the fibular collateral ligament and popliteus tendon and attenuation of the midlateral and posterolateral capsule. Primary repair of fibular collateral ligament and popliteus tendon injuries was performed combined with a posterolateral capsular shift procedure and a posterolateral reconstruction using a fibular head based figure-of-8 posterolateral reconstruction technique.

Side-to-side difference on KT 1000 measurements on the PCL screen, corrected posterior, and corrected anterior measurements are 3.5, 2.0, and −2.0 mm, respectively. Side-to-side difference on the KT 1000 anterior displacement measurement at 30 degrees of knee flexion is 1.0 mm. The Hospital for Special Surgery, Lysholm, and Tegner knee ligament rating scale scores are 94/100, 94/100, and 5. Five-year postoperative stress x-rays at 90 degrees of knee flexion using the Telos device comparing the surgical to the knee normal knee reveal a 0.5-mm side-to-side difference.

PEARLS AND PITFALLS

- The posteromedial safety incision protects the neurovascular structures, confirms the accuracy of the PCL tibial tunnel placement, and enhances the flow of the surgical procedure.
- We have found it very important to use primary and backup fixation. During cruciate ligament reconstruction, primary aperture fixation is achieved with bioabsorbable interference screws, and backup fixation is performed with a screw and spiked ligament washer and ligament fixation buttons. Secure fixation is critical to the success of this surgical procedure.
- Mechanical tensioning of the PCL at 0 degrees of knee flexion (full extension), restoration of the normal anatomic tibial step-off at 70 to 90 degrees of flexion, and fixation of the PCL graft at 70 to 90 degrees of knee flexion have provided the most reproducible method of establishing the neutral point of the tibiofemoral relationship in our experience. Full range of motion is confirmed on the operating table to assure the knee is not "captured" by the reconstruction.
- Recognition and correction of the medial and/or lateral side instability is the key to successful posterior and ACL surgery.

SUMMARY

The goals leading to successful PCL reconstruction surgery include identification and treatment of associated pathology such as posterolateral instability, posteromedial instability, and lower extremity malalignment. The use of strong graft material, properly placed tunnels to as closely as possible approximate the PCL insertion sites, and minimization of graft bending also enhance the probability of PCL reconstruction success. In addition, mechanical graft tensioning, primary and backup PCL graft fixation, and the appropriate postoperative rehabilitation program are also necessary ingredients for PCL reconstruction success. Both single-bundle and double-bundle PCL reconstruction surgical techniques are successful when evaluated with stress radiography, KT 1000 arthrometer measurements, and knee ligament rating scales. Indications for double-bundle PCL reconstruction as of this writing include severe hyperextension of the knee and revision PCL reconstruction. Our 2- to 18-year postsurgical results in combined PCL, ACL, and medial and lateral side knee injuries (global laxity) revealed very successful PCL reconstruction using the arthroscopic transtibial tunnel surgical technique.

RECOMMENDED READINGS

Edson CJ, Fanelli GC. Postoperative rehabilitation of the multiple ligament injured knee. In: Fanelli GC, ed. *The multiple ligament injured knee. A practical guide to management.* 2nd ed. New York: Springer-Verlag; 2013:437–442.

Edson CJ, Fanelli GC, Beck JD. Postoperative rehabilitation of the posterior cruciate ligament. *Sports Med Arthrosc Rev.* 2010;18(4):275–279.

Edson CJ, Fanelli GC, Beck JD. Rehabilitation after multiple ligament reconstruction of the knee. *Sports Med Arthrosc Rev.* 2011;19(2):162–166.

Fanelli GC. PCL injuries in trauma patients. *Arthroscopy.* 1993;9:291–294.

Fanelli GC. *Rationale and surgical technique for PCL and multiple knee ligament reconstruction.* 3rd ed. Warsaw, IN: Biomet Sports Medicine; 2012.

Fanelli GC, ed. *The multiple ligament injured knee. A practical guide to management.* 2nd ed. New York: Springer-Verlag; 2013.

Fanelli GC. Surgical treatment of combined PCL ACL medial and lateral side injuries (global laxity): acute and chronic. In: Fanelli GC, ed. *The multiple ligament injured knee. A practical guide to management.* 2nd ed. New York: Springer-Verlag; 2013:281–301.

Fanelli GC. Mechanical graft tensioning in multiple ligament knee surgery. In: Fanelli GC, ed. *The multiple ligament injured knee. A practical guide to management.* 2nd ed. New York: Springer-Verlag; 2013:323–330.

Fanelli GC. Arthroscopic transtibial tunnel posterior cruciate ligament reconstruction. In: Fanelli GC, ed. *Posterior cruciate ligament injuries. A practical guide to management.* 2nd ed. New York: Springer; 2015:111–122.

Fanelli GC. Mechanical graft tensioning in posterior cruciate ligament reconstruction. In: Fanelli GC, ed. *Posterior cruciate ligament injuries. A practical guide to management.* 2nd ed. New York: Springer; 2015:263–270.

Fanelli GC. Fibular head based posterolateral reconstruction of the knee: surgical technique and outcomes. *J Knee Surg.* 2015;28(6):455–463.

Fanelli GC. Fibular head based posterolateral reconstruction. *Oper Tech Sports Med.* 2015;23(4):321–330.

Fanelli GC. Selected case studies in posterior cruciate ligament reconstruction. In: Fanelli GC, ed. *Posterior cruciate ligament injuries. A practical guide to management.* 2nd ed. New York: Springer; 2015:349–358.

Fanelli GC, ed. *Posterior cruciate ligament injuries: a practical guide to management.* 2nd ed. New York: Springer; 2015.

Fanelli GC, Edson CJ. PCL injuries in trauma patients. Part II. *Arthroscopy.* 1995;11:526–529.

Fanelli GC, Edson CJ. Arthroscopically assisted combined ACL/PCL reconstruction: 2–10 year follow-up. *Arthroscopy.* 2002;18(7):703–714.

Fanelli GC, Edson CJ. Combined posterior cruciate ligament—posterolateral reconstruction with Achilles tendon allograft and biceps femoris tendon tenodesis: 2–10 year follow-up. *Arthroscopy.* 2004;20(4):339–345.

Fanelli GC, Edson CJ. Surgical treatment of combined PCL, ACL, medial, and lateral side injuries (global laxity): surgical technique and 2 to 18 year results. *J Knee Surg.* 2012;25(4):307–316.

Fanelli GC, Fanelli DG. Management of chronic combined posterior cruciate ligament and posteromedial instability of the knee. *Sports Med Arthrosc Rev.* 2015;23(2):96–103.

Fanelli GC, Fanelli DG. Fibular head based posterolateral reconstruction of the knee combined with capsular shift procedure. *Sports Med Arthrosc Rev.* 2015;23(1):33–43.

Fanelli GC, Fanelli DG. Knee dislocations in patients 18 years of age and younger. Surgical technique and outcomes. *J Knee Surg.* 2016;29(4):269–277.

Fanelli GC, Feldmann DD. Management of combined anterior cruciate ligament/posterior cruciate ligament/posterolateral complex injuries of the knee. *Oper Tech Sports Med.* 1999;7(3):143–149.

Fanelli GC, Harris JD. Surgical treatment of acute medial collateral ligament and posteromedial corner injuries of the knee. *Sports Med Arthrosc Rev.* 2006;14(2):78–83.

Fanelli GC, Harris JD. Late MCL (medial collateral ligament) reconstruction. *Tech Knee Surg.* 2007;6(2):99–105.

Fanelli GC, Beck JD, Edson CJ. Arthroscopic trans tibial double bundle PCL reconstruction. *J Knee Surg.* 2010;23(2):89–94.

Fanelli GC, Beck JD, Edson CJ. Single compared to double bundle PCL reconstruction using allograft tissue. *J Knee Surg.* 2012;25(1):59–64.

Fanelli GC, Edson CJ, Orcutt DR, et al. Treatment of combined ACL, PCL, medial lateral side injuries of the knee. *J Knee Surg.* 2005;28(3):240–248.

Fanelli GC, Giannotti BF, Edson CJ. The posterior cruciate ligament: arthroscopic evaluation and treatment. Current concepts review. *Arthroscopy.* 1994;10(6):673–688.

Fanelli GC, Sousa P, Edson CJ. Long term follow-up of surgically treated knee dislocations: stability restored, but arthritis is common. *Clin Orthop Relat Res.* 2014;472(9):2712–2717.

LaPrade RF. Arthroscopic evaluation of the lateral compartment of knees with grade 3 posterolateral knee complex injuries. *Am J Sports Med.* 1997;25(5):596–602.

Noyes FR, Barber-Westin SD. Posterior cruciate ligament revision reconstruction. Part 1. Causes of surgical failure in 52 consecutive operations. *Am J Sports Med.* 2005;33(5):646–654.

21 Inlay Posterior Cruciate Ligament Reconstruction

Dean Wang, Edward C. Cheung, Nirav B. Joshi, and David R. McAllister

In recent years, posterior cruciate ligament (PCL) injury has received increased attention as the biomechanical function of the PCL, and the natural history of chronic insufficiency have become better elucidated. Although many patients may clinically tolerate a PCL-deficient knee, recent studies have described altered loads and kinematics during functional activities (1–3). The natural history of chronic PCL deficiency is not well established but can involve premature degeneration of articular cartilage in the medial and patellofemoral compartments in addition to an increased risk for injury to the meniscus and posterolateral structures (2,4–6). Although the available literature is limited, the outcomes of isolated PCL reconstruction are generally good, with patient-reported outcomes greatly improved from preoperative level of function (7–9). However, return to preinjury activity level is less predictable, and current techniques do not seem to reliably restore normal laxity and prevent degenerative arthritis (9,10).

Current surgical treatment options for PCL reconstruction include transtibial and tibial inlay techniques with single- or double-bundle reconstruction. Using the transtibial technique, the graft must make an acute turn as it passes from the tibial tunnel into the knee joint. This "killer" turn has been implicated as a potential cause of graft attenuation and eventual graft failure (11). Additionally, the acute angle of the graft as it enters the notch in the transtibial tunnel can make tensioning more difficult. To address these concerns, the tibial inlay technique was developed to avoid the "killer" turn by direct fixation of the graft at the PCL tibial attachment site (12). We believe that the tibial inlay technique leads to better biomechanical stability, and it is our preferred method for PCL reconstruction. In this chapter, we present our operative technique for single-bundle tibial inlay PCL reconstruction using an Achilles tendon allograft.

INDICATIONS/CONTRAINDICATIONS

Indications

Treatment decisions for PCL injuries should be made on the basis of symptoms, grade of the injury, associated injuries, and activity level of the patient. As with any orthopedic condition, operative intervention should only be chosen if it results in improved outcomes compared to nonoperative management. Because good outcomes have been reported with nonoperative treatment for isolated PCL injuries, the indications for surgical treatment remain controversial among orthopedic surgeons. Proponents of nonoperative treatment argue that most patients can clinically tolerate a PCL-deficient knee, while others argue that diminishing results may be seen in the long term (13).

Level I evidence does not currently exist to support strong recommendations on the management of PCL injuries. We generally reserve operative treatment for chronic isolated grade III PCL injuries with symptoms of pain or instability when an adequate course of conservative treatment has failed. Additionally, we usually recommend operative treatment for acute and chronic combined ligamentous injuries involving the PCL.

Contraindications

- Acute, isolated grade I or II PCL injuries
- Isolated PCL injury in a patient who has not undergone a formal physical therapy program focused on quadriceps strengthening

- Acute knee dislocation with vascular injury resulting in limb compromise
- Flexion contracture greater than 10 degrees or extension contracture greater than 30 degrees
- Complex regional pain syndrome

PREOPERATIVE PLANNING

History

A thorough history of the patient's complaints and the mechanism of injury can help in identifying PCL injuries and distinguishing them from other knee derangements. Often, the patient has sustained a traumatic injury or a sports-related injury (14). In a high-energy trauma such as a motor vehicle accident, patients typically report an inability to bear weight, instability, and decreased knee range of motion. The classic "dashboard" injury pattern results from a posteriorly directed force on the anterior aspect of the proximal tibia with the knee in a flexed position. Associated capsuloligamentous injury should be suspected in these patients due to the possibility of a transient knee dislocation.

In athletics, the typical mechanism of isolated PCL injury is a direct blow to the anterior tibia or a fall onto the knee with the foot in a plantarflexed position (Fig. 21-1). In contrast to acute ACL injuries, patients seldom report feeling or hearing a "pop" and may be able to continue play. Isolated PCL injuries may have more subtle presentations, with patients reporting stiffness, swelling, and pain located in the back of the knee or pain with deep knee flexion. In chronic isolated PCL injuries, complaints of anterior knee pain, difficulty ascending stairs, and instability are typical (15).

Physical Examination

Physical examination should begin with assessment of the patient's gait and overall limb alignment. Varus alignment, external rotation recurvatum, and varus thrust during the stance phase of gait may be present in patients with chronic posterolateral corner (PLC) injury with or without PCL injury. An effusion is usually present after an acute injury. A complete neurovascular examination of the lower extremity should be performed on all patients with suspected ligamentous injuries.

The integrity of the PCL is most accurately assessed with the posterior drawer test. With the patient lying supine and the knee flexed to 90 degrees, a posteriorly directed force is placed on the proximal tibia. In a PCL-deficient knee, the tibia may be posteriorly subluxed; therefore, an anteriorly directed force is usually needed to reduce the tibia to neutral position before applying the

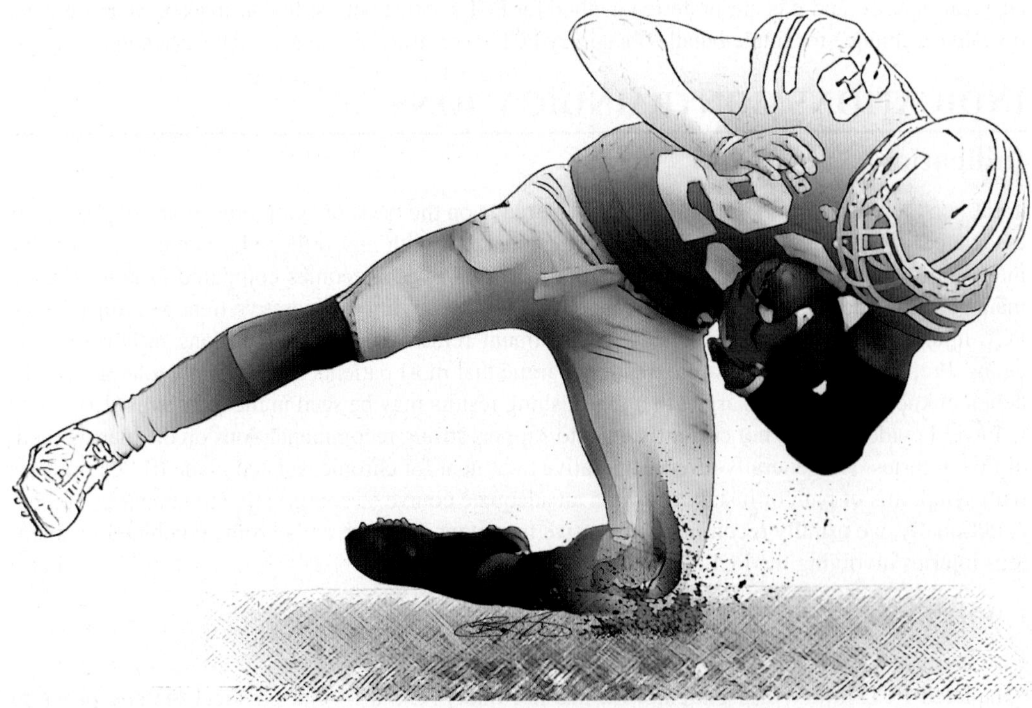

FIGURE 21-1

Mechanism of isolated PCL injury by falling on a flexed knee with the foot in a plantarflexed position.

posteriorly directed force. In cases of isolated PCL tears, posterior tibial translation is decreased with internal rotation of the tibia as a result of tightening of the superficial medial collateral ligament and posterior oblique ligament, which act as secondary restraints to posterior tibial translation. Grading of PCL injuries is based on the amount of posterior tibial translation during the posterior drawer test. Grade 1 injuries are defined as those with 0 to 5 mm of increased posterior tibial translation compared to the contralateral knee. Grade 2 injuries are defined as those with 6 to 10 mm of increased posterior tibial translation. Grade 3 injuries are defined as those with more than 10 mm of increased posterior tibial translation. The presence or lack of a firm end point should also be noted. PCL insufficiency can also be graded based on the position of the medial tibial plateau relative to the medial femoral condyle during the posterior drawer test. In grade 1 injuries, the plateau remains anterior to the medial femoral condyle. In grade 2 injuries, the plateau is flush with the medial femoral condyle. In grade 3 injuries, the plateau displaces posterior to the medial femoral condyle.

The quadriceps active test can aid in the diagnosis of complete PCL tears. With this test, the patient lies supine and the knee is flexed to 90 degrees. While the examiner stabilizes the foot, the patient is asked to contract the quadriceps isometrically. In a complete PCL tear, the posteriorly subluxed tibia will dynamically reduce during quadriceps contraction.

Combined PCL and PLC injuries can be diagnosed with the "dial" test or external rotation test. This test is performed with the patient positioned prone or supine. An external rotation force is applied to both feet with the knees at 30 degrees and then 90 degrees of flexion. More than a 10-degree side-to-side difference is considered abnormal. Increased external rotation at 30 degrees but not at 90 degrees indicates an isolated PLC injury, while increased external rotation at both 30 and 90 degrees suggests a combined PCL and PLC injury. The examiner should also evaluate for varus laxity.

Imaging

Plain radiographs of the knee should be obtained, including bilateral standing anteroposterior, 45-degree flexion weightbearing posteroanterior, Merchant patellar, and lateral views of the affected extremity. These views allow for assessment of fractures, preexisting arthritis, and tibial slope. Any posterior tibial subluxation, avulsion fractures, and tibial plateau fractures should be ascertained. Medial Segond fractures indicate a medial capsular avulsion that may be associated with a peripheral meniscus tear. Medial or patellofemoral compartment arthritic changes may be indicative of the chronicity of the PCL injury. If coronal malalignment is suspected, full-length hip-to-ankle films are helpful in determining overall limb alignment.

Magnetic resonance imaging (MRI) is the imaging modality of choice to confirm the presence of an acute PCL tear (Fig. 21-2) and any associated ligamentous or cartilage injury. On T1- and T2-weighted sagittal MRI images, the normal PCL appears dark in nature and is curvilinear in appearance. With an acute PCL injury, the MRI will reveal increased signal within the PCL or a

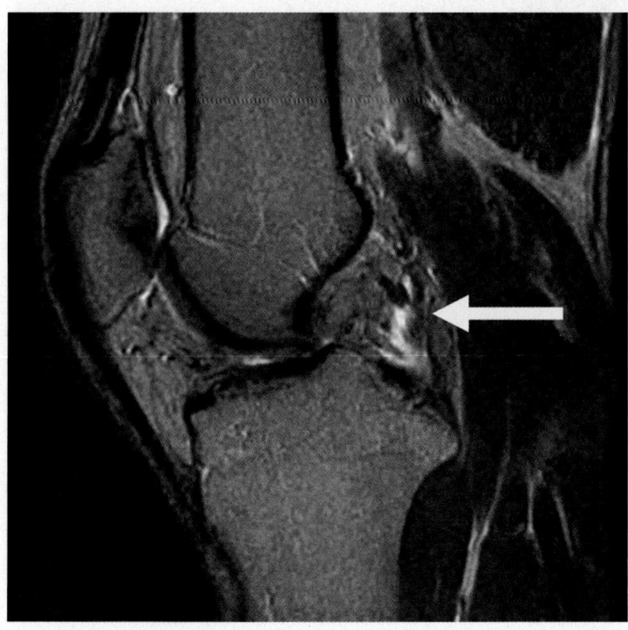

FIGURE 21-2

MRI demonstrating a disrupted PCL (*white arrow*).

disrupted PCL. In contrast, chronic PCL tears can heal and assume a curvilinear appearance on MRI. Thus, MRI is less sensitive in the diagnosis of chronic PCL tears.

SURGICAL TECHNIQUE

Equipment

- 30- and 70-degree arthroscopes with full arthroscopy setup
- PCL femoral drill guide
- 18-Gauge wire loop
- Oscillating saw, osteotomes, rongeur, burr
- 6.5-mm partially threaded cancellous screw, 35 mm in length, with washer

Graft Options

Multiple options are available for graft tissue, and no study has conclusively demonstrated a superior graft. Bone-patellar tendon-bone (BTB), hamstring, and quadriceps tendons are common autograft sources. BTB grafts have the advantage of bone-to-bone healing on both sides of the graft. Harvest and subsequent weakening of the quadriceps tendon are a concern due to its function as a dynamic restraint to posterior tibial translation. Use of allograft tissue has the advantages of avoiding donor site morbidity, reducing operative time, and offering improved graft diameter and tissue bulk. We use an Achilles tendon allograft for most of our PCL reconstructions because of its size, strength, and versatility.

Graft Preparation

The bone plug of the Achilles allograft is fashioned 22 mm in length and 13 mm in width on the cortical surface using an oscillating saw and rongeur. The side cuts are tapered inward so that the cancellous surface is 10 mm in width, forming a trapezoidal shape. The bone plug is predrilled and tapped for a 6.5-mm cancellous screw. This is achieved by drilling the bone plug with a 4.5-mm drill from the cancellous to soft tissue/cortical surface to prevent wrapping of the soft tissue over the drill bit. The drill hole should be angled slightly distal to account for the posterior slope of the tibia and avoid penetration of the screw into the joint during tibial fixation. The drill hole is tapped with a 6.5-mm tap. A partially threaded 6.5-mm cancellous screw, approximately 35 mm in length, and a metal washer are placed into the bone plug from the cortical surface to the cancellous surface (Fig. 21-3A). The screw is placed so that the tip is 5 mm past the cancellous surface to facilitate later tibial fixation.

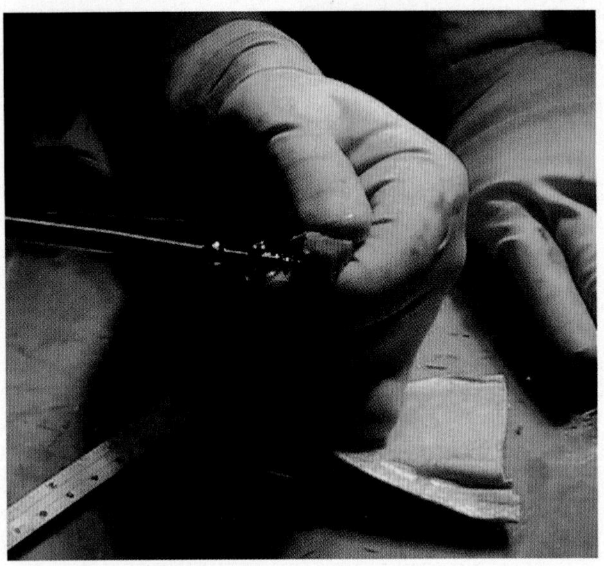

A

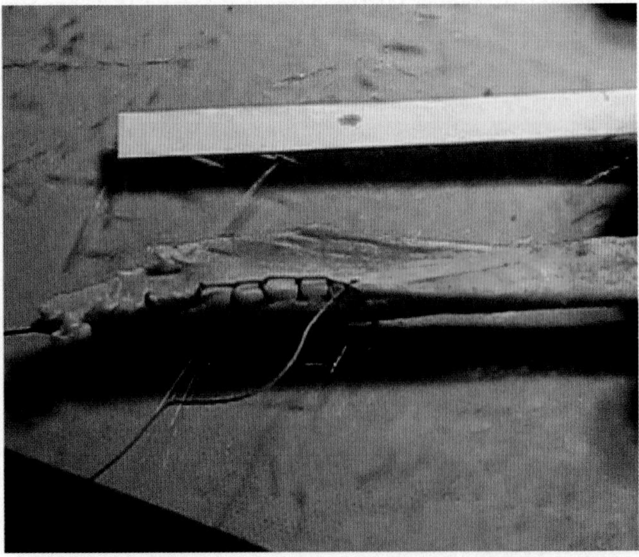

B

FIGURE 21-3

Preparation of Achilles tendon allograft with placement of a **(A)** 6.5-mm cancellous screw into the bone plug and **(B)** running locking stitch suture in the tendon.

The soft tissue portion of the Achilles is sized for a 10-mm bone tunnel to allow for passage and fixation in the femoral tunnel. A running locking stitch is placed along approximately 30 mm of tendon using a No. 2 braided polyester suture (Fig. 21-3B). Any excess soft tissue that will interfere with smooth passage of the graft is trimmed. The graft is now ready for implantation.

Arthroscopy/Femoral Tunnel

The patient is first positioned supine on the operative table for a diagnostic arthroscopy. We recommend that the patient be intubated to protect the airway during position changes. A complete examination under anesthesia is performed prior to placement of a tourniquet. It is very important to evaluate for both PCL and associated capsuloligamentous injuries at this time. A thigh tourniquet is then placed but not inflated. To maintain sterility of the drapes during position changes, we prep and drape the patient in the lateral decubitus position midway between the supine and prone positions used for the procedure. The patient is then rotated back to the supine position after draping is complete. A routine diagnostic arthroscopy is performed, and any meniscal or chondral injuries are treated at the same time. The ACL may appear lax because of posterior tibial subluxation and should tighten with an applied anterior drawer. The PCL is then examined, and often, the ligament is lax or stretched out rather than frankly torn (Fig. 21-4).

Once incompetence of the PCL has been confirmed, the residual PCL tissue is removed with hand-operated punches and a shaver. If the meniscofemoral ligaments of Humphrey and Wrisberg are intact, they should be preserved if possible. The native footprint is saved as a guide for femoral tunnel placement. Previous studies have demonstrated that the anterolateral (AL) bundle is the most important component of the PCL because it has a higher cross-sectional area and is stronger than the posteromedial bundle (16). Thus, we attempt to restore the AL bundle of the PCL by placing the tunnel in the distal and anterior portion of the native footprint (Fig. 21-5). A curette is used to score the desired femoral tunnel site.

The femoral tunnel is drilled from outside-in through a small medial arthrotomy. A medial incision is made through the skin and then through the medial retinaculum along the anteromedial aspect of the patella. An outside-in arthroscopic guide is used to establish the tunnel position. The outer edge of the femoral tunnel should be 5 to 6 mm away from the articular margin of the medial femoral condyle (Fig. 21-6). A femoral guide pin is placed. The femoral tunnel is then created with a cannulated drill, typically 10 mm in width, over the guide pin. The edges are chamfered and smothered with a rasp. An 18-gauge wire loop is then passed through the femoral tunnel from the outside and directed into the posterior notch to be retrieved later for graft passage.

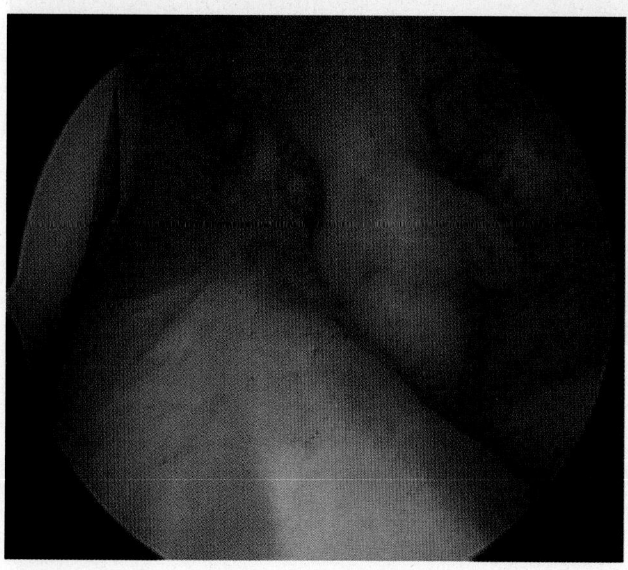

A

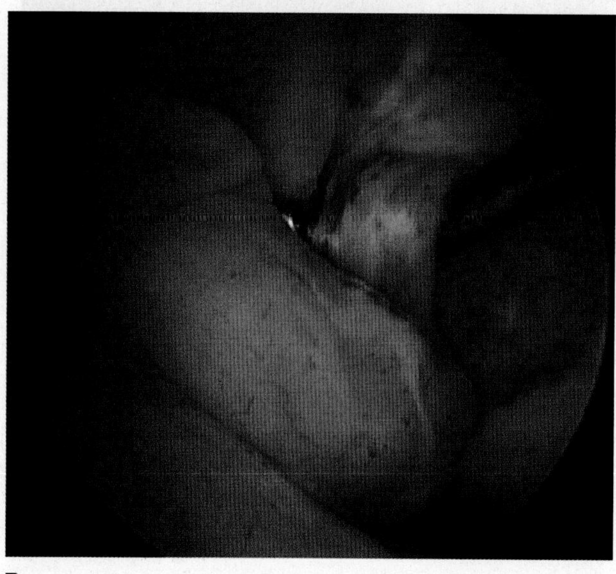

B

FIGURE 21-4

Arthroscopic views of the **(A)** notch and **(B)** probed posterior cruciate ligament, demonstrating a tear. Often, the ligament is lax or stretched out rather than frankly torn.

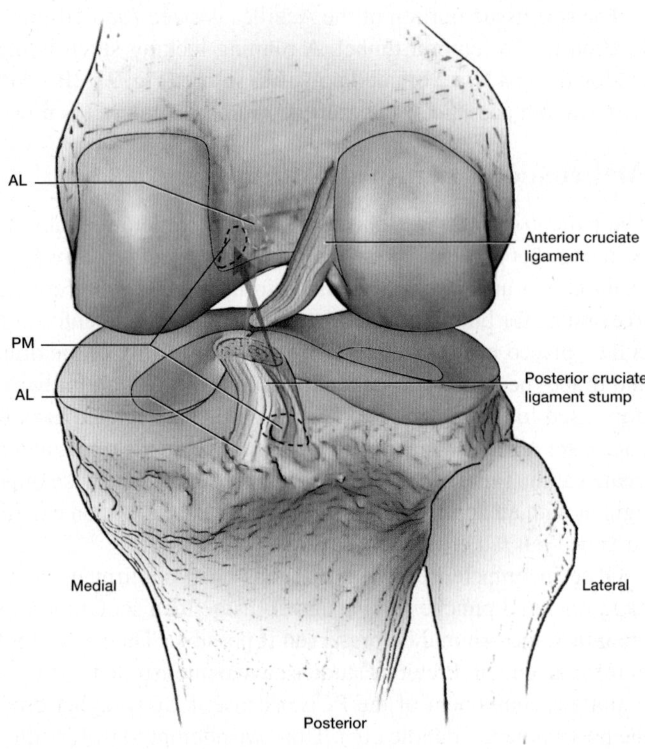

FIGURE 21-5

Femoral and tibial insertions sites of the anterolateral (AL) and posteromedial (PM) bundles of the posterior cruciate ligament.

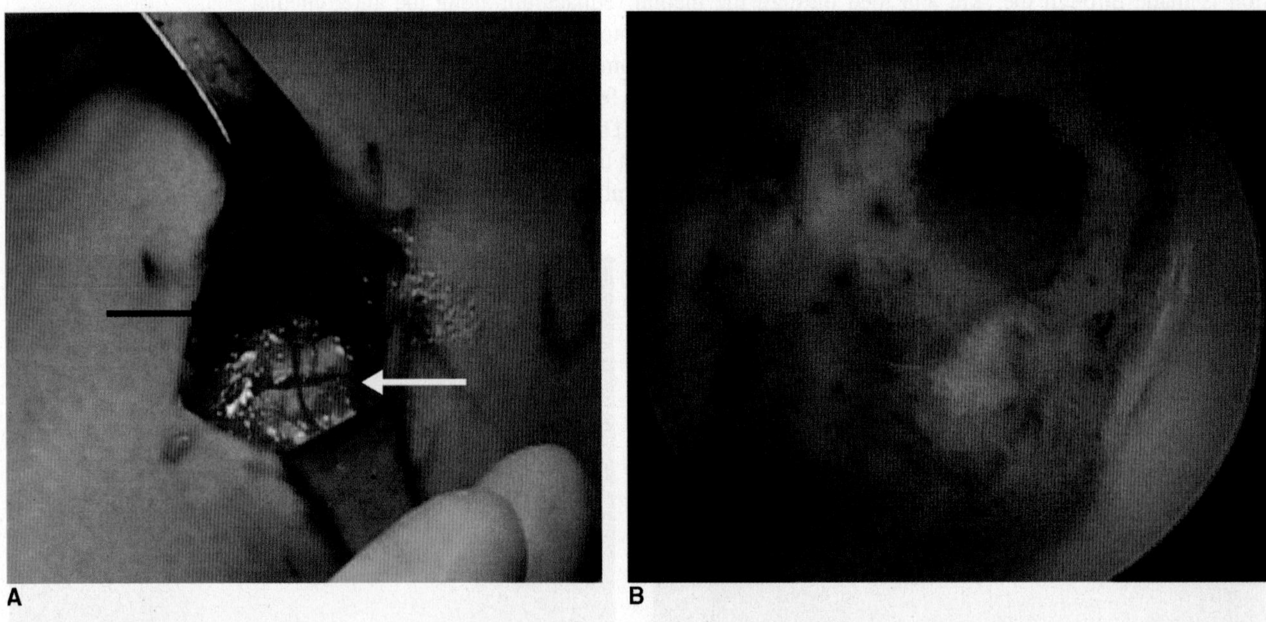

FIGURE 21-6

A: An "X" (*white arrow*) marks the starting point for outside-in drilling of the femoral tunnel. The edge of the tunnel should be 5 to 6 mm away from the articular margin of the medial femoral condyle (*black arrow*). **B:** An arthroscopic view of the femoral tunnel created in the footprint of the native anterolateral bundle.

Tibial Inlay

The patient is sterilely rotated into the prone position for the tibial inlay portion of the case. The extremity is exsanguinated and the tourniquet inflated. The posteromedial exposure to the tibia, as described by Burks and Schaffer (17), is performed (Fig. 21-7). A curvilinear incision is made traversing horizontally across the medial half of the popliteal crease and extending down over the medial head of the gastrocnemius. Dissection is carried down to the investing fascial layer. The medial sural cutaneous nerve can be vulnerable near the midline but typically perforates the fascia distal to the horizontal limb of the incision. The fascia is incised over the medial gastrocnemius, and the interval between the medial gastrocnemius and semimembranosus tendon is developed with blunt dissection (Fig. 21-8). If necessary, the fascia over the proximal popliteus muscle may be incised to allow for retraction of the muscle. The medial head of the gastrocnemius is retracted laterally with a blunt-tipped retractor, protecting the neurovascular bundle. At this point, the posterior proximal tibia and posterior femoral condyles are palpated and a vertical capsulotomy is made, exposing the posterior notch and tibial attachment of the native PCL. The knee may be slightly flexed and the tibia externally rotated to facilitate additional exposure.

The tibial insertion site is then prepared for placement of the graft. Typically, two prominent processes are found on the medial and lateral borders of the PCL insertion site and can be palpated. Using osteotomes, a cortical window containing the insertion site and remnant PCL is removed. A trapezoid-shaped bony trough corresponding to the bone plug previously prepared is created using both osteotomes and a burr (Fig. 21-9). The bone plug of the graft is then placed into the recipient site and secured with the 6.5-mm cancellous screw and washer. It is not necessary to predrill the cancellous tibial bone. The sutures in the tendinous portion of the graft are then shuttled through the femoral tunnel using the previously placed wire loop. After the sutures are passed, the capsule

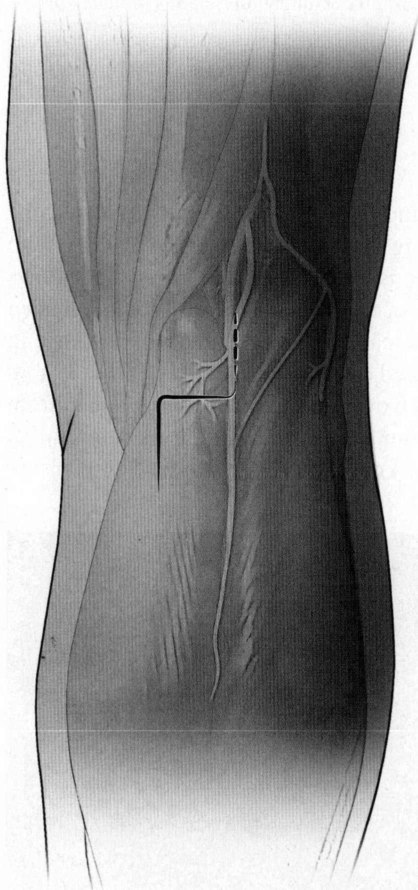

FIGURE 21-7
Modified Burks posteromedial approach to the tibia.

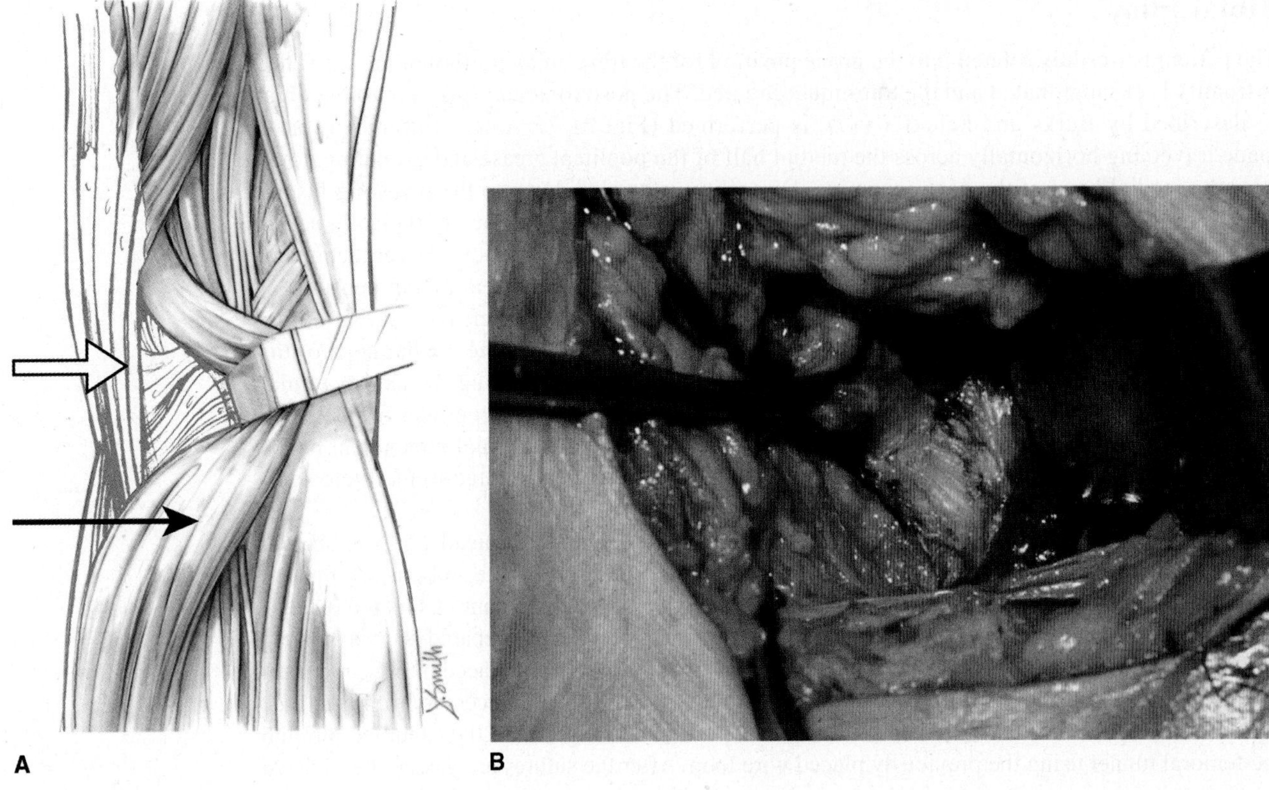

FIGURE 21-8

Drawing **(A)** and photograph **(B)** of the interval between the medial gastrocnemius (*black arrow*) and semimembranosus (*white arrow*).

is repaired. The tourniquet is deflated, and hemostasis is achieved. The wound is irrigated and closed in layers.

Graft Tensioning

After wound closure, the patient is returned to the supine position in a sterile fashion. The arthroscope is placed back into the knee and the graft is confirmed entering the femoral tunnel (Fig. 21-10). With manual tension applied to the graft via the sutures, the knee is cycled several times, which allows the surgeon to evaluate knee range of motion and isometry of the graft. The graft should lengthen slightly as the knee is moved into full extension. Tension is reapplied to the graft with the knee in 70 to 90 degrees of flexion and an anterior drawer force placed on the proximal tibia. A 9 × 25-mm soft tissue interference screw is placed over a guide wire to fix the graft in the femoral tunnel from outside-in. A staple is then placed over the soft tissue portion of the graft on the medial femoral condyle to augment fixation (Fig. 21-11). After fixation, the knee is flexed and extended to ensure

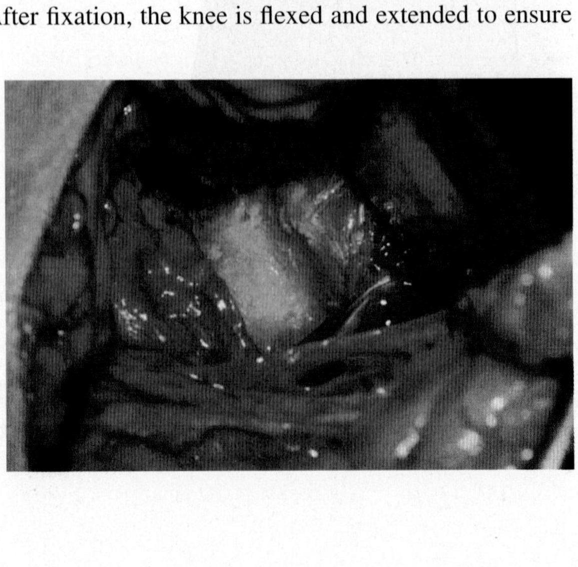

FIGURE 21-9

Bony trough created in the posterior tibia for inlay of the graft.

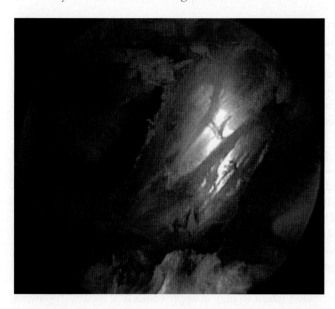

FIGURE 21-10
An arthroscopic view of the completed posterior cruciate ligament reconstruction.

an adequate range of motion. A gentle posterior drawer at 90 degrees can be performed, and the anterior tibial step-off should be restored. The medial wound is irrigated and closed in layers, and the arthroscopic incisions are closed in standard fashion.

PEARLS AND PITFALLS

- When drilling the femoral tunnel using the outside-in technique, place the drill guide as far anterior as possible without violating the articular cartilage of the medial femoral condyle. This will optimize the trajectory of the femoral tunnel to minimize graft bending.
- It is usually necessary to divide a portion of the proximal aspect of the popliteus muscle to gain good exposure of the posterior tibia.

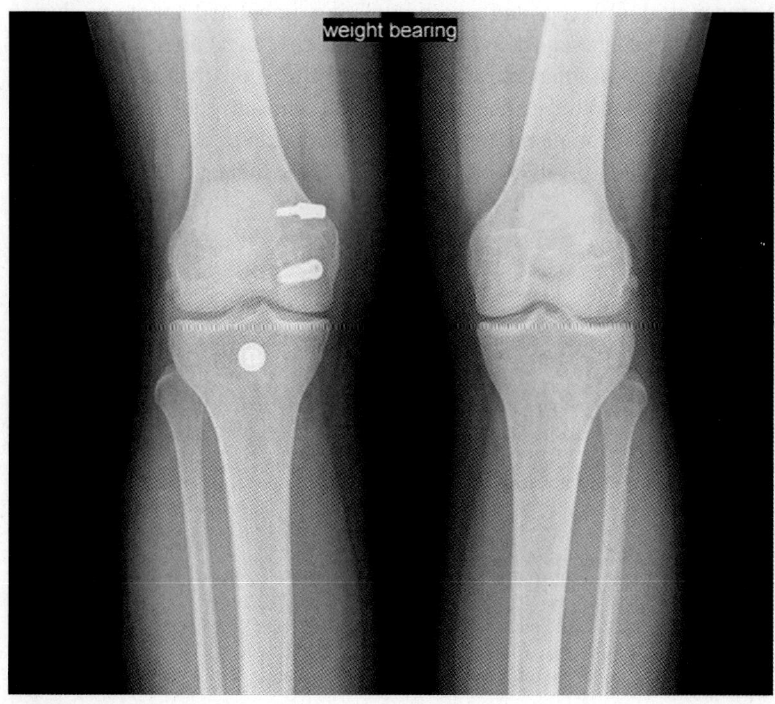

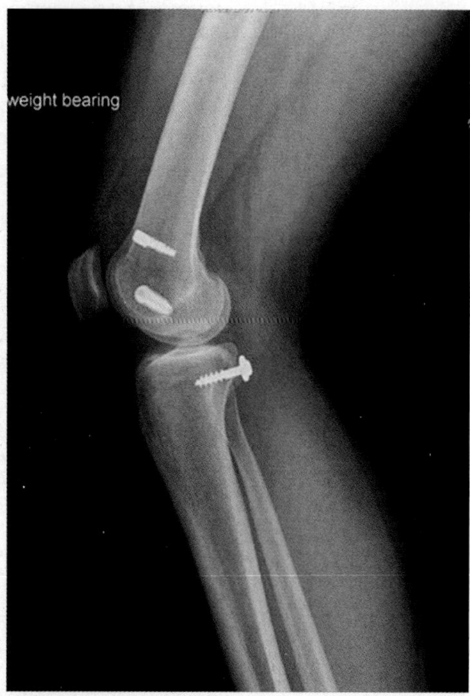

A B

FIGURE 21-11
Anteroposterior **(A)** and lateral **(B)** radiographs of the knee after completion of single-bundle posterior cruciate ligament reconstruction.

- When placing the 6.5-mm screw in the tibia, it is helpful to angle slightly distal to avoid penetrating the articular cartilage of the tibial plateau.
- If an ACL reconstruction is performed in conjunction with a PCL reconstruction, direct the 6.5-mm screw slightly lateral to avoid the ACL tibial tunnel.
- After drilling the femoral tunnel, an 18-gauge wire loop can be placed in the femoral tunnel and pushed up against the posterior capsule. This can be used to shuttle the sutures and graft into the femoral tunnel after the graft has been secured via the posterior approach.

POSTOPERATIVE MANAGEMENT

In the immediate postoperative period, the knee is immobilized in full extension with no weightbearing. At 3 weeks, passive range of motion is initiated from 0 to 70 degrees of knee flexion. Partial weightbearing is permitted. The patient is started on isometric exercises and quadriceps strengthening while minimizing hamstring activation. At 6 weeks, weightbearing is advanced to as tolerated with no limit on knee flexion. The patient is started on isotonic quadriceps strength exercises. Hamstring and quadriceps cocontraction exercises are permitted at 3 months postoperatively. Unopposed hamstring exercises are avoided for 4 months postoperatively. Agility drills and sports-specific activities follow, with an anticipated return to play at approximately 9 months following surgery.

COMPLICATIONS TO AVOID

There are several complications that are associated with the specific nature of the inlay technique. In a series of 41 patients, Cooper and Stewart (18) reported three cases of postoperative posterior hematoma formation after posteromedial exposure. As a result, the authors routinely ligate the inferior medial geniculate vessels and use a drain for 2 days after surgery. Bone plug fracture is possible during fixation. To prevent this complication, caution should be taken to avoid overtightening the screw on the inlayed bone plug. Additionally, the bone plug should rest in an inlay slot (not onlay) on the tibia, which minimizes the formation of stress risers. If the patient's bone density is poor, a longer screw that captures the anterior cortex of the tibia can be used to improve fixation strength (18).

Vascular injury during PCL reconstruction is rare but is a known complication, especially in the setting of prior surgery. Nemani et al. (19) reported a case involving a popliteal venotomy during PCL reconstruction. In this case, the patient had previously received a popliteal artery bypass graft after suffering a knee dislocation with vascular injury. During the PCL reconstruction, an anomalous branch of the popliteal vein was found to be adherent to the PCL remnant, and a venotomy was noted after debridement. The authors recommend considering a preoperative vascular workup in a patient with possible aberrant vascular anatomy when performing these higher-risk procedures.

REFERENCES

1. Logan M, Williams A, Lavelle J, et al. The effect of posterior cruciate ligament deficiency on knee kinematics. *Am J Sports Med.* 2004;32:1915–1922.
2. Skyhar MJ, Warren RF, Ortiz GJ, et al. The effects of sectioning of the posterior cruciate ligament and the posterolateral complex on the articular contact pressures within the knee. *J Bone Joint Surg Am.* 1993;75:694–699.
3. Van de Velde SK, Bingham JT, Gill TJ, et al. Analysis of tibiofemoral cartilage deformation in the posterior cruciate ligament-deficient knee. *J Bone Joint Surg Am.* 2009;91:167–175.
4. Dejour H, Walch G, Peyrot J, et al. [The natural history of rupture of the posterior cruciate ligament]. *Rev Chir Orthop Reparatrice Appar Mot.* 1988;74:35–43.
5. Kozanek M, Fu EC, Van de Velde SK, et al. Posterolateral structures of the knee in posterior cruciate ligament deficiency. *Am J Sports Med.* 2009;37:534–541.
6. Strobel MJ, Weiler A, Schulz MS, et al. Arthroscopic evaluation of articular cartilage lesions in posterior-cruciate-ligament-deficient knees. *Arthroscopy.* 2003;19:262–268.
7. Hermans S, Corten K, Bellemans J. Long-term results of isolated anterolateral bundle reconstructions of the posterior cruciate ligament: a 6- to 12-year follow-up study. *Am J Sports Med.* 2009;37:1499–1507.
8. Jackson WF, van der Tempel WM, Salmon LJ, et al. Endoscopically-assisted single-bundle posterior cruciate ligament reconstruction: results at minimum ten-year follow-up. *J Bone Joint Surg Br.* 2008;90:1328–1333.
9. Voos JE, Mauro CS, Wente T, et al. Posterior cruciate ligament: anatomy, biomechanics, and outcomes. *Am J Sports Med.* 2012;40:222–231.
10. Kim YM, Lee CA, Matava MJ. Clinical results of arthroscopic single-bundle transtibial posterior cruciate ligament reconstruction: a systematic review. *Am J Sports Med.* 2011;39:425–434.
11. Markolf KL, Zemanovic JR, McAllister DR. Cyclic loading of posterior cruciate ligament replacements fixed with tibial tunnel and tibial inlay methods. *J Bone Joint Surg Am.* 2002;84-A:518–524.

12. Jakob RP, Ruegsegger M. [Therapy of posterior and posterolateral knee instability]. *Orthopade.* 1993;22:405–413.
13. Boynton MD, Tietjens BR. Long-term follow-up of the untreated isolated posterior cruciate ligament-deficient knee. *Am J Sports Med.* 1996;24:306–310.
14. Schulz MS, Russe K, Weiler A, et al. Epidemiology of posterior cruciate ligament injuries. *Arch Orthop Trauma Surg.* 2003;123:186–191.
15. Margheritini F, Mariani PP. Diagnostic evaluation of posterior cruciate ligament injuries. *Knee Surg Sports Traumatol Arthrosc.* 2003;11:282–288.
16. Markolf KL, Feeley BT, Tejwani SG, et al. Changes in knee laxity and ligament force after sectioning the posteromedial bundle of the posterior cruciate ligament. *Arthroscopy.* 2006;22:1100–1106.
17. Burks RT, Schaffer JJ. A simplified approach to the tibial attachment of the posterior cruciate ligament. *Clin Orthop Relat Res.* 1990:216–219.
18. Cooper DE, Stewart D. Posterior cruciate ligament reconstruction using single-bundle patella tendon graft with tibial inlay fixation: 2- to 10-year follow-up. *Am J Sports Med.* 2004;32:346–360.
19. Nemani VM, Frank RM, Reinhardt KR, et al. Popliteal venotomy during posterior cruciate ligament reconstruction in the setting of a popliteal artery bypass graft. *Arthroscopy.* 2012;28:294–299.

RECOMMENDED READINGS

Cooper DE, Stewart D. Posterior cruciate ligament reconstruction using single-bundle patella tendon graft with tibial inlay fixation: 2- to 10-year follow-up. *Am J Sports Med.* 2004;32(2):346–360.

Jung YB, Tae SK, Jung HJ, et al. Replacement of the torn posterior cruciate ligament with a mid-third patellar tendon graft with use of a modified tibial inlay method. *J Bone Joint Surg Am.* 2004;86-A(9):1878–1883.

Markolf KL, Feeley BT, Jackson SR, et al. Where should the femoral tunnel of a posterior cruciate ligament reconstruction be placed to best restore anteroposterior laxity and ligament forces? *Am J Sports Med.* 2006;34(4):604–611.

Markolf KL, Zemanovic JR, McAllister DR. Cyclic loading of posterior cruciate ligament replacements fixed with tibial tunnel and tibial inlay methods. *J Bone Joint Surg Am.* 2002;84-A(4):518–524.

Montgomery SR, Johnson JS, McAllister DR, et al. Surgical management of PCL injuries: indications, techniques, and outcomes. *Curr Rev Musculoskelet Med.* 2013;6(2):115–123.

Panchal HB, Sekiya JK. Open tibial inlay versus arthroscopic transtibial posterior cruciate ligament reconstructions. *Arthroscopy.* 2011;27(9):1289–1295.

22 Double-Bundle Posterior Cruciate Ligament Reconstruction

Craig R. Bottoni

INDICATIONS/CONTRAINDICATIONS

The posterior cruciate ligament (PCL), the primary restraint to posterior tibial translation, is reportedly disrupted in 5% to 20% of all knee ligament injuries (1–6). Multiligamentous injuries of the knee that include the PCL often fare better with operative reconstruction. However, the treatment of isolated PCL injuries is controversial. The "isolated" PCL rupture, although rare, typically occurs during sporting events by a direct blow to the proximal tibia, by a fall onto a flexed knee, or with knee hyperflexion or hyperextension. Unfortunately, operative reconstructions of PCL injuries have not obtained the equivalent success as that of anterior cruciate ligament (ACL) reconstructions. Isolated PCL injuries (grades I and II) can be treated nonoperatively with protected weightbearing and rehabilitation focused on quadriceps strengthening. However, some studies have demonstrated degenerative changes and poor objective outcomes associated with conservative treatment of PCL injuries (7–9).

The indication for acute reconstruction or, if feasible, repair of an isolated PCL tear would be for a bony avulsion of the PCL, which can occur off of the tibia or femoral attachment. Operative indication for an isolated PCL tear would be persistent symptomatic instability (grade II or III) despite 4 to 6 months of rehabilitation. Although some authors have suggested that athletes can function at high levels without a PCL (7,8,10,11), it is the author's experience that isolated PCL injuries in active duty service members who cannot return to the obligatory physical demands of their job may require an operative reconstruction.

Better understanding of the anatomy and biomechanics of the PCL has led to an increased interest in arthroscopic techniques to reconstruct the PCL. The PCL is an intra-articular but extrasynovial structure. Anatomic studies have delineated definitive bundles of the PCL with different tensioning characteristics based upon the degree of knee function. The average length of the PCL is 38 mm, and its average width is 13 mm. The PCL can be anatomically separated into the anterolateral (AL) and posteromedial (PM) bundles named for their footprint on the femur and tibia, respectively (Fig. 22-1). The larger AL bundle has increased tension in knee flexion, whereas the PM bundle becomes tighter in extension. In addition, the smaller meniscofemoral ligaments also contribute to the overall strength of the PCL. The timing of PCL reconstruction is controversial, but an acute or early reconstruction is generally accepted for open injuries, bony avulsions, and in conjunction with operative treatment of combined ligamentous injuries, especially a posterolateral corner injury.

Although there are no absolute contraindications to a PCL reconstruction, there are relative contraindications. Some surgeons would delay or forgo a PCL reconstruction in the setting of a traumatic knee arthrotomy with ligament rupture. Others would not reconstruct the PCL in a multiligamentous knee injury, instead choosing to reconstruct the ACL, medial, and/or lateral sides. However, the reconstruction of the PCL and ACL reestablishes the central pivot of the knee, and anatomic reconstruction of all ruptured ligaments is recommended by many surgeons (12–18). One recently cited anatomic abnormality, which may increase the risk of vascular injury, is a proximal takeoff of the anterior tibial artery from the main popliteal artery (19). When this occurs, the anterior tibial artery descends anterior to the popliteus muscle, closely adherent to the posterior capsule, putting it at risk during tibial tunnel

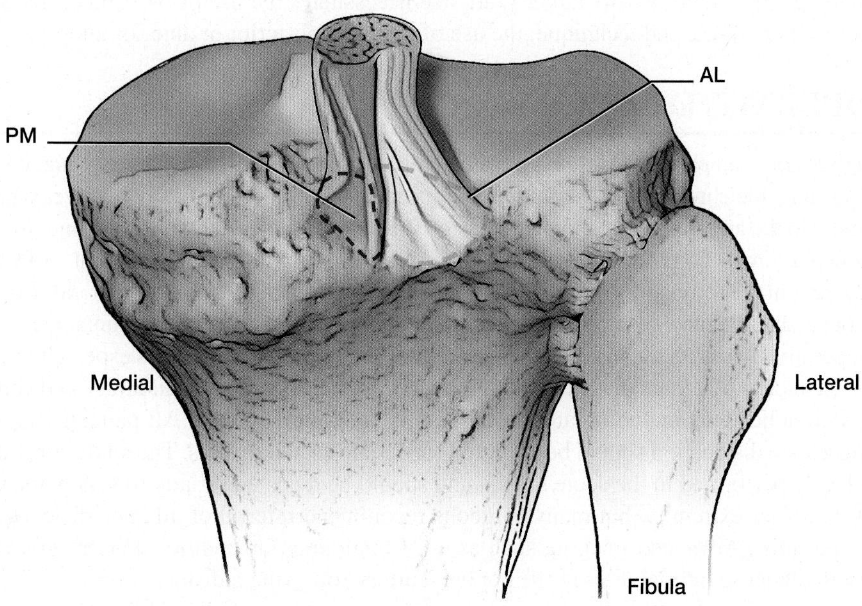

FIGURE 22-1

This drawing depicts the anatomical insertion sites of the anterolateral (AL) and posteromedial (PM) bundles of the posterior cruciate ligament (PCL).

drilling. An axial view at the level of the joint on preoperative magnetic resonance image (MRI) should always be reviewed to ascertain whether this anomaly is present (Fig. 22-2).

There have been a large number of PCL reconstruction techniques published, including single and double bundle, arthroscopically assisted, all-inside arthroscopic, and open inlay. Multiple techniques to drill both the tibial and femoral tunnels have also been described, including outside-in, transportal inside-out, and retrograde (15,17,18,20–31). The use of a double-bundle technique was proposed to better recreate the larger size and definitive bundle anatomy of the PCL (17,23,32). When utilizing a single-bundle technique, only the larger AL bundle is reconstructed with femoral and tibial tunnel sizes from 9 to 12 mm depending upon the graft or bone plug sizes. However, the double-bundle technique reconstructs both of the two bundles separately, allows for differential

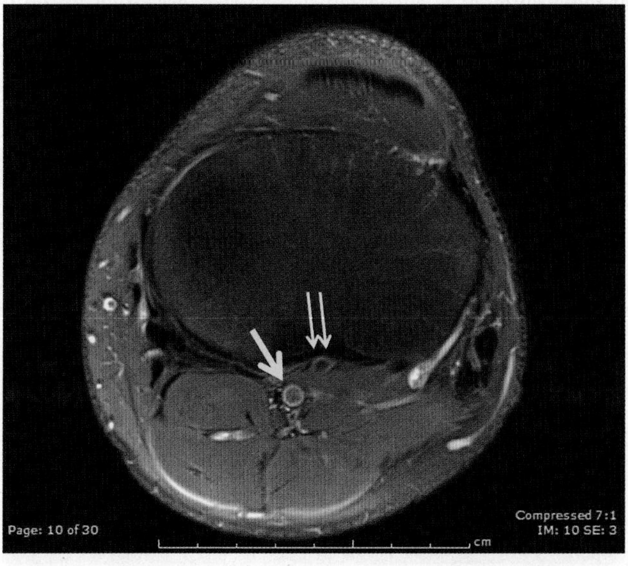

FIGURE 22-2

The MRI, axial view at the level of the proximal tibia, demonstrates the anatomical anomalous position of the anterior tibial artery (*double arrows*), which courses anterior to the popliteus muscle and just behind the posterior capsule. The normal position of the popliteal artery is noted (*arrow*).

tightening, and, theoretically, better recreates the native anatomy. Since the tunnel sizes are typically 6 to 9 mm on both the tibia and femur, the DB technique results in a larger total graft size, which may provide greater stability. The larger graft size necessitates the use of two autografts or, in the case of the author's preferred technique, the use of a tibialis posterior or anterior allograft.

PREOPERATIVE PLANNING

A thorough history and physical examination are obtained preoperatively in a clinic setting. It is important to determine the chronicity of the injury. The mechanism of injury typically involves a history of a direct blow to the anterior leg or a hyperextension injury with subsequent mild swelling. In contrast, the large hemarthrosis commonly seen in an acute ACL injury is not usually present. A PCL injury may also occur in the setting of a knee dislocation with involvement of the posterolateral structures. A spontaneous reduction may occur; therefore, a high index of suspicion must be maintained.

It is imperative to assess the neurovascular status of the injured limb. This is especially important if there is suspicion of a knee dislocation, which has a higher risk of such an injury and can lead to disastrous complications including an above-knee amputation if missed. All patients suspected of sustaining a knee dislocation should be admitted for serial vascular exams. The ankle-brachial index (ABI) is easily performed in the acute setting and should be repeated serially to follow the vascular status of the lower extremity, but many surgeons recommend referral of all knee dislocations to a vascular specialist. Advanced imaging such as a CT angiogram or traditional arteriogram may be necessary to diagnose intimal tears in the popliteal artery following a dislocation.

Initial examination should include an inspection for an effusion followed by assessment of the knee range of motion; however, active motion and an accurate ligament examination may be limited by pain. In the setting of a large hemarthrosis, aspiration of the blood followed by intra-articular injection of a local anesthetic may greatly improve the diagnostic examination as well as provide significant pain relief to the patient with an acutely injured knee. In the chronic setting, a more thorough exam is usually possible. With the knee in a flexed position, palpate for the natural tibial step-off and evaluate the anterior border of the tibial plateau in relation to the femoral condyles. In addition, the presence of a sag sign can be determined. The leg is elevated with the knee flexed approximately 90 degrees to assess for the presence of a "sag" as the tibia is displaced posteriorly in relation to the distal femur. A *quadriceps active test* is assessed by active contraction of the quadriceps and is positive if the sag is eliminated as the tibia is translated anteriorly. A posterior drawer with the knee in 90 degrees of flexion, the most sensitive exam for PCL laxity, is also performed to evaluate the amount of posterior tibial translation (Fig. 22-3). The use of the TELOS device allows for a standardized force applied to the proximal tibia and a quantitative assessment of posterior tibial translation (30,33,34) (Fig. 22-4). This test can be used to compare the injured knee with the normal contralateral knee as well as to assess pre- and postoperative stability.

Plain radiographs of the knee should be obtained to inspect for a ligamentous avulsion or fracture. Posterior tibial subluxation can, at times, be seen on the lateral radiograph. Long-leg cassette films should be obtained if any coronal malalignment is suspected. An MRI is essential not only

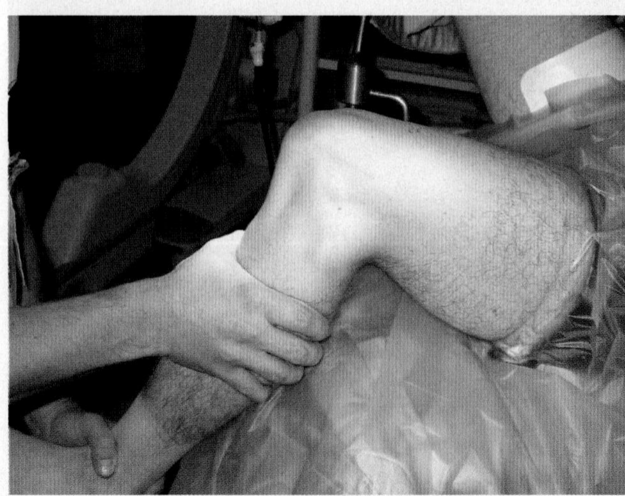

FIGURE 22-3

With the patient's knee at 90 degrees of flexion, the posterior drawer test is the most sensitive examination for PCL laxity.

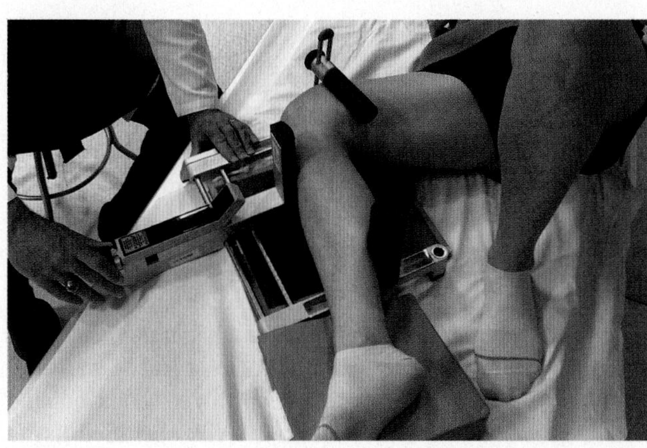

FIGURE 22-4
The TELOS device allows for a quantitative assessment of posterior tibial laxity by applying a standard posteriorly directed force on the proximal tibia.

to confirm a PCL injury but more importantly to assess for any concomitant ligament injuries and chondral or meniscal pathology that may affect the operative plan.

SURGERY

Patient Positioning

The patient is positioned supine with the uninvolved lower extremity secured in a padded well-leg holder that allows flexion of both the hip and knee (Fig. 22-5). This places the contralateral extremity in an abducted and externally rotated position and allows the unencumbered use of the C-arm fluoroscopy unit. The operative extremity is prepared with a standard tourniquet and a hinged lateral thigh post placed proximal to the patella. The hinged post is advantageous because it allows the knee to be fully flexed on the table or to be placed in the "figure four" position, and then, the post can be released through the drapes when no longer required. The operative extremity is allowed to flex off the end of the table. To prevent posterior thigh injury, most notably compartment syndrome, we ensure that the thigh is not in contact with the hard edge of the operative table, and padding is added underneath the distal thigh. The fluoroscopy unit is brought in before draping to ensure adequate visualization of the proximal tibial in a lateral view and the entire knee via an AP view.

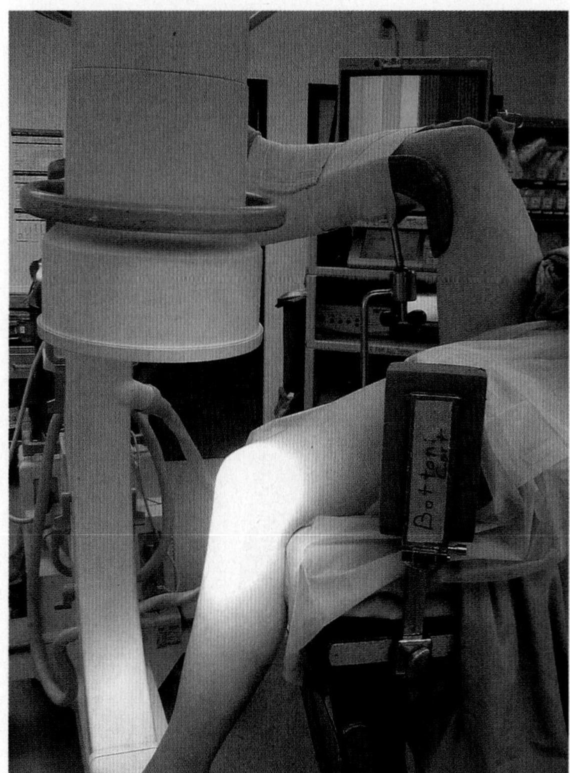

FIGURE 22-5
The patient is positioned with the operative (left) knee flexed over the padded operative table. The fluoroscopy is brought in from the contralateral side prior to draping to ensure adequate visualization of the knee.

Examination Under Anesthesia

Both an examination under anesthesia (EUA) and fluoroscopic joint assessment are recommended to confirm the diagnosis and quantify the amount of joint laxity. Especially during acute reconstructions in multiligamentous knee injuries where the knee examination may be limited due to pain, the EUA and fluoroscopic examinations are invaluable to assess knee laxity and confirm the diagnosis. The lateral view is used to plan the tibial tunnels.

Graft Preparation

A fresh-frozen tibialis posterior tendon allograft is soaked in warm saline and bacitracin antibiotic solution for 20 to 30 minutes prior to its preparation. We prefer grafts that are at least 8 to 9 mm in diameter and a minimum length of 24 cm. We specifically request fresh frozen, nonirradiated allografts in these sizes from an American Association of Tissue Banks (AATB) certified tissue bank. The ends are secured with a locking stitch using a high-strength suture and then secured to a graft tensioning board where the graft is placed under 15 to 20 pounds of tension until insertion (Fig. 22-6). Prior to tensioning, the diameters of the two free ends of the graft are measured with the standard cylindrical guides. This determines the individual AL and PM tunnel diameters. One end of the allograft is typically larger than the other and is clearly marked to properly identify this end upon graft insertion and during arthroscopic passage. Because the allograft ends are passed down through the tibial tunnel, they should be bulletized to allow easier passage through the bony tunnels. Lastly, the graft is marked at its midpoint.

Arthroscopy and Tunnel Preparation

In cases of chronic PCL reconstructions, the extremity is exsanguinated with gravity and the tourniquet inflated. However, in acute reconstructions and multiligamentous injuries, to mitigate the risk of extravasation due to capsular disruption, arthroscopy without a tourniquet may be advisable. Standard arthroscopy portals are used, but a superolateral outflow portal is recommended because a medial incision is required to place the graft through the distal femur. A routine arthroscopic evaluation of the knee is performed and meniscal and/or chondral pathology addressed. In isolated PCL injuries, meniscal tears are not commonly found because the mechanism of injury is typically a straight posteriorly directed force and not rotational as is the case in ACL tears. The PCL is confirmed to be disrupted, but given the interstitial failure of many PCL injuries, the ligament often

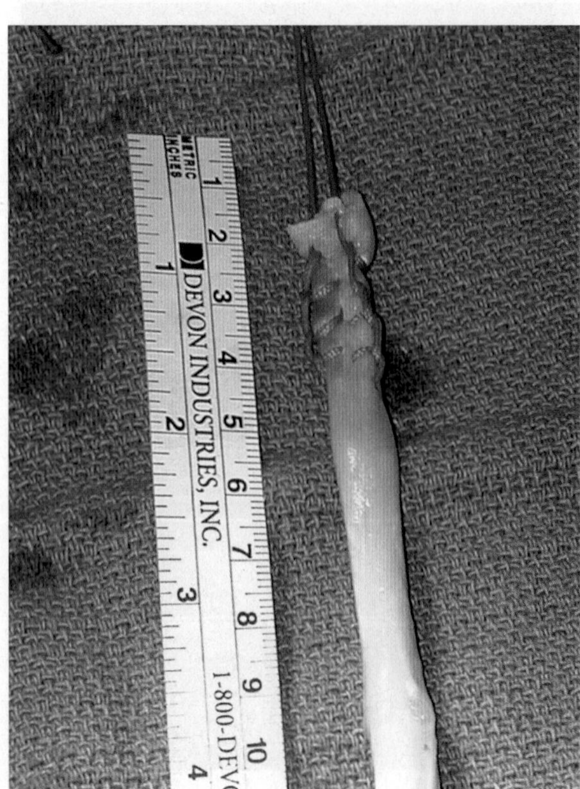

FIGURE 22-6

The allograft is prepared by suturing then sizing both ends and then tensioning the graft prior to its use.

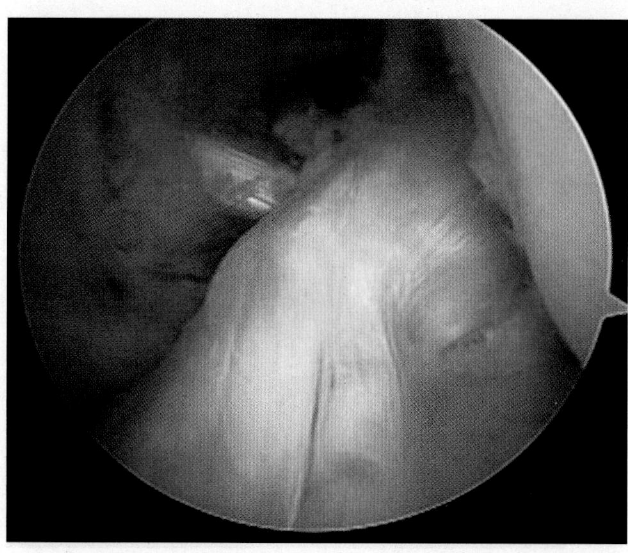

FIGURE 22-7

Arthroscopic view of pseudolaxity of the ACL as is commonly seen with PCL deficiency due to the posteriorly displaced tibia and should not be mistaken for injury or rupture of the ACL.

remains in continuity with its bony insertions. A secondary sign of PCL disruption is ACL pseudolaxity that can be mistaken for an ACL disruption (Fig. 22-7). Because the tibia displaces posteriorly with a PCL injury, the ACL may appear at arthroscopy to be loose. However, with an anterior drawer applied, the ACL becomes taut. In isolated PCL reconstructions, care must be taken to preserve and avoid inadvertent injury to the ACL.

An electrocautery is used to resect the PCL from its femoral origin (Fig. 22-8A). Once released completely, the PM capsule is well visualized. A spinal needle is used to localize the proper trajectory (Fig. 22-8B), and a cannula is inserted into the PM compartment. The PCL is then debrided with the mechanical shaver and electrocautery. To obtain better visualization of the PCL tibial insertion around the ACL, a 70-degree arthroscope is used. Alternatively, the 30-degree arthroscope can be placed through the PM cannula. Good visualization and judicious use of electrocautery are crucial to avoid inadvertent injury to the posterior horns of either the medial or lateral menisci or penetration of the posterior capsule, which increases the risk of neurovascular injury.

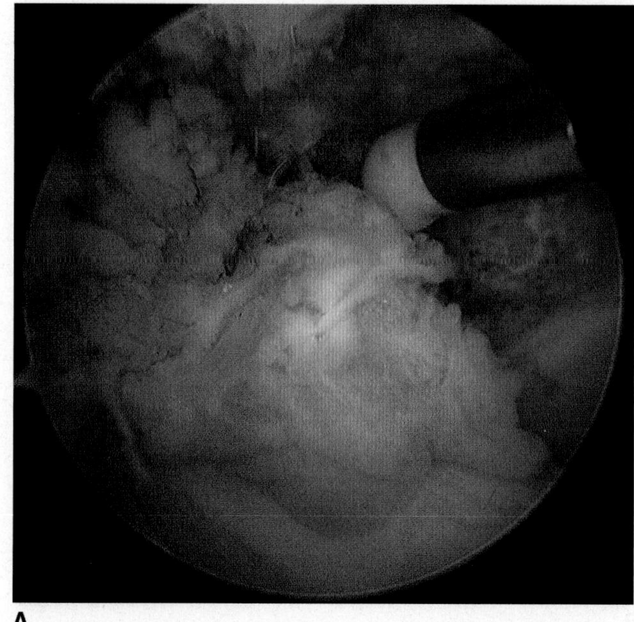

A

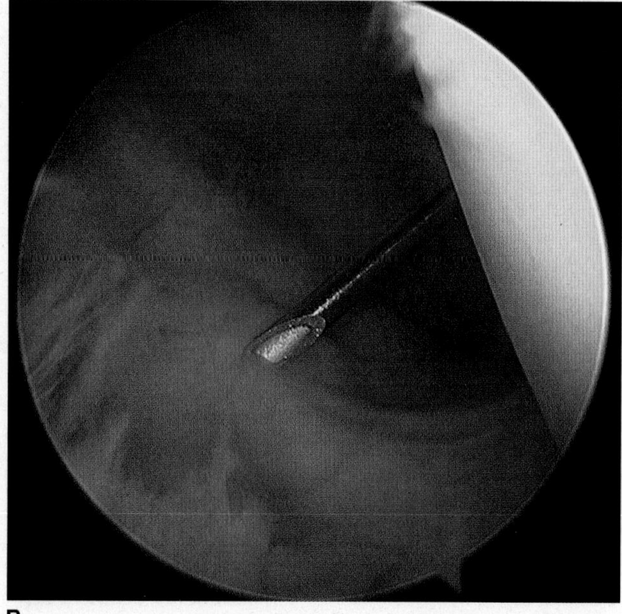

B

FIGURE 22-8

A: Arthroscopic view of right knee. The PCL is resected from its femoral origin while protecting the ACL in an isolated PCL reconstruction. **B:** Once the ligament is completely released from the medial wall, a spinal needle is used to localize the proper trajectory for the posteromedial cannula.

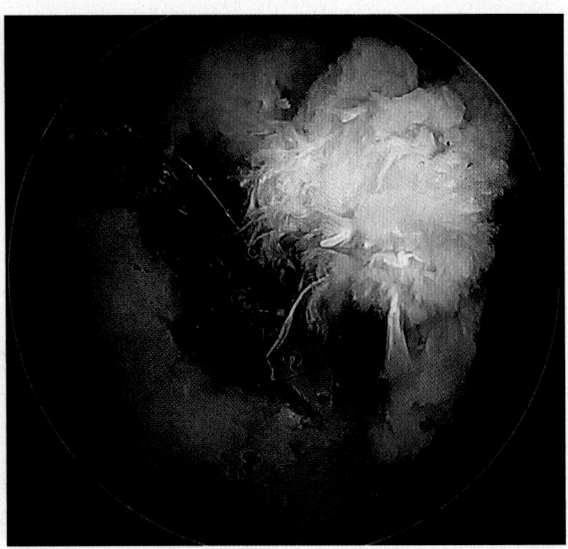

FIGURE 22-9

Arthroscopic view of left knee with 70 degrees arthroscopic, showing tibial footprint with right angle PCL tibial guide.

Tibial Tunnel Preparation

The distal 2 to 3 cm of the PCL is left in continuity and reflected off of its tibial insertion. This allows accurate guide pin placement and retains an additional layer of soft tissue to help prevent inadvertent penetration through the posterior capsule during tunnel drilling. Once the tibial insertion is reflected for 1 to 2 cm down the posterior slope of the tibia, the PCL tibial guide is positioned at the footprint of the PCL tibial insertion (Fig. 22-9).

A 3-cm incision is made over the proximal medial tibia just superior to the pes anserinus. The periosteum is split and reflected to expose the tibia. The fluoroscopy unit is now used, first via an anteroposterior view to confirm proper intra-articular placement of the guide. The guide tip should be positioned slightly lateral to the midline (Fig. 22-10A,B). To avoid unnecessary delay,

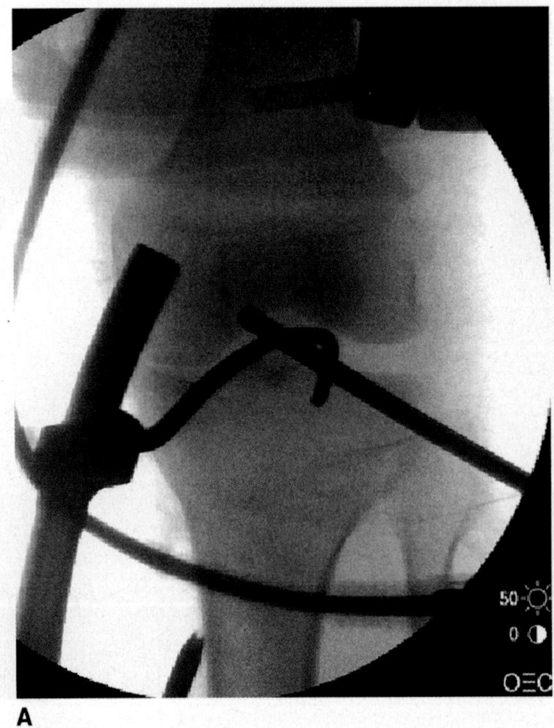

A

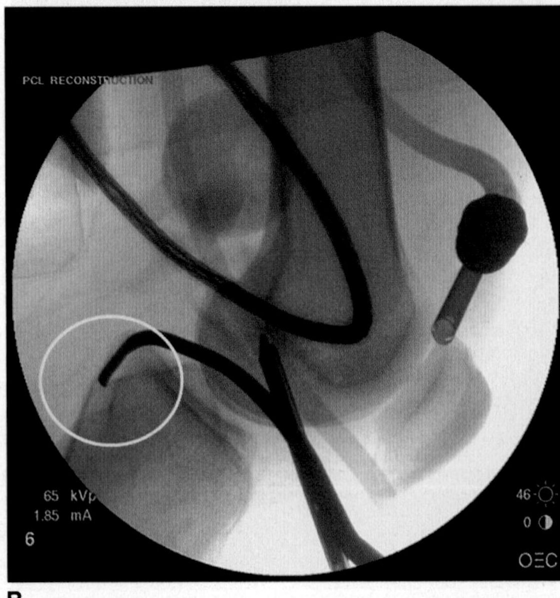

B

FIGURE 22-10

A: Prior to drilling of the tibial tunnel, fluoroscopic views of the knee with the tibial guide in place are obtained. Anteroposterior fluoroscopic view. **B:** Lateral fluoroscopic view of knee demonstrating proper position of tibial guide.

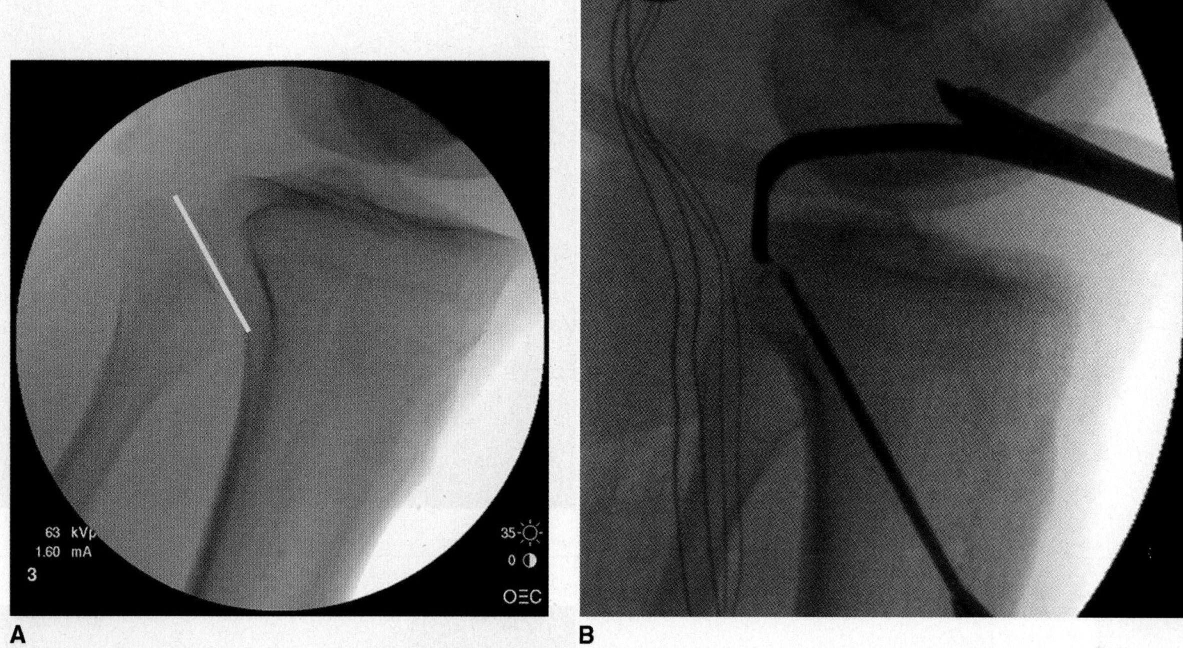

FIGURE 22-11

A: The fluoroscopic view of the proximal tibia demonstrating the alignment of the proximal tibiofibular joint as a guide to drilling the tibial tunnels. **B:** Fluoroscopic image of tibial guide pin being drilled into position.

the arthroscope and tibial guide may remain in the knee joint while obtaining fluoroscopic confirmation. The tibial guide is held firmly in place while the fluoroscopy unit is then rotated to obtain a lateral view of the knee. The tip of the guide should be positioned at the downslope of the posterior tibia approximately 1.5 cm from the articular surface. However, the tibial anatomy is variable and arthroscopic position should be correlated with the fluoroscopic views. The first tibial pin for the AL tibial tunnel is drilled under fluoroscopic guidance and arthroscopic visualization. The starting point should be fairly central and just proximal to the pes tendons to allow for placement of the second guide pin and PM tunnel. When reconstructing both the ACL and PCL, enough space proximally must be preserved to allow the more anterior ACL tunnel as well. On the lateral projection, the tibial pins should be aligned roughly parallel to the proximal tibiofibular joint (Fig. 22-11A). They should exit approximately 1.0 cm distal to the tibial plateau in the native PCL footprint. The tip of the guide pin should be clearly visualized arthroscopically as it emerges from the bone, and live fluoroscopy can be used to prevent inadvertent pin advancement (Fig. 22-11B). Next, the PM guide pin is drilled. The tibial aiming guide for the PM tibial tunnel exit site is situated more distal and medial from that of the AL pin (Fig. 22-12). This position more accurately reproduces the native PCL tibial insertion sites. The starting point should be more proximal and medial on the face of the anterior tibia with at least 2 cm separating the two pins. This will allow a tibial bone bridge over which the sutures from the two bundles will be tied at the end.

A 90-degree curved curette is placed over the pin tip and held securely while drilling the tibial tunnel (Fig. 22-13). Alternatively, a curette may be passed through the PM cannula to secure the pin tip. This step is crucial because as the reamer advances, the pin can become lodged, and as they emerge from the bone, the guide pin tip can be inadvertently pushed out through the back of the capsule risking neurovascular injury. For additional protection, the last few centimeters may be hand-reamed to afford greater control over pin advancement. Once drilled, the tibial tunnel is rasped of all sharp edges. To ensure circumferential bony integrity, the arthroscope can be passed up the tibial tunnel. Disposable bone tunnel plugs are inserted into the tibial tunnel opening to maintain joint distention. Once both tibial tunnels are drilled and rasped, shuttle sutures of different colors are passed up the tibia and parked in the PM cannula until the femoral tunnels are prepared (Fig. 22-14).

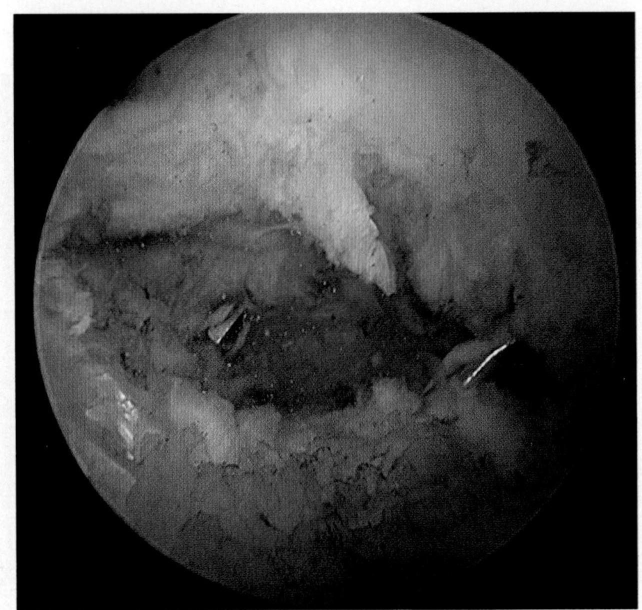

FIGURE 22-12

The two tibial pins arthroscopically visualized from the posteromedial portal.

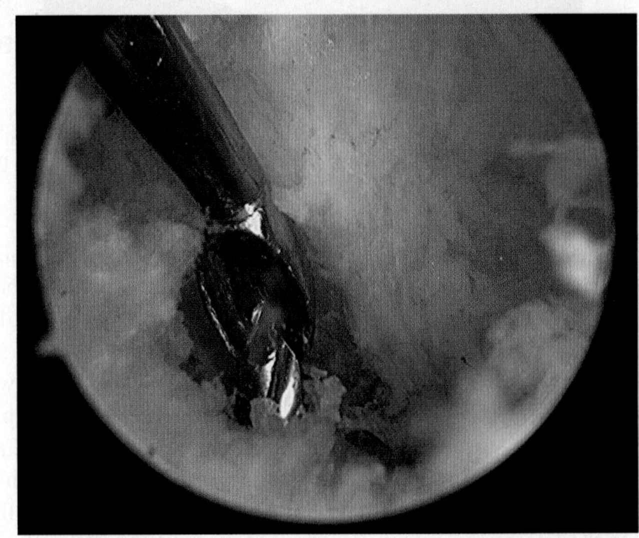

FIGURE 22-13

Arthroscopic view with 90 degrees curette inserted through anteromedial portal to prevent advancement of guide pin during tibial tunnel reaming.

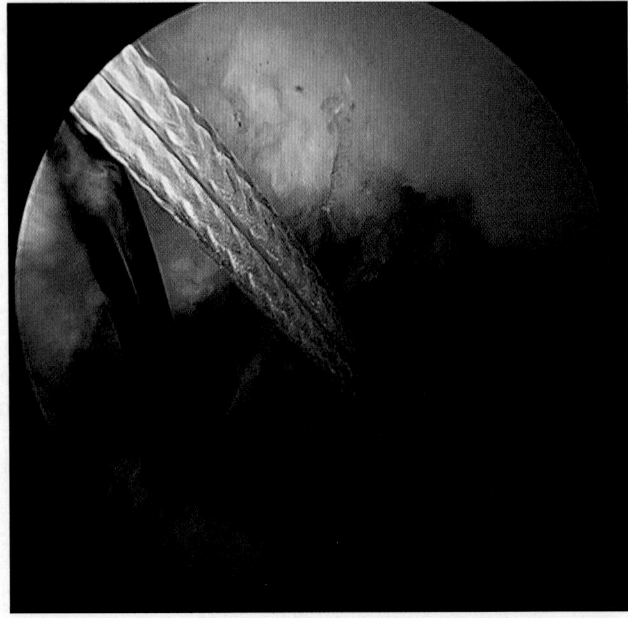

FIGURE 22-14

Arthroscopic view of two shuttle sutures passed up through tibial tunnels into posteromedial cannula.

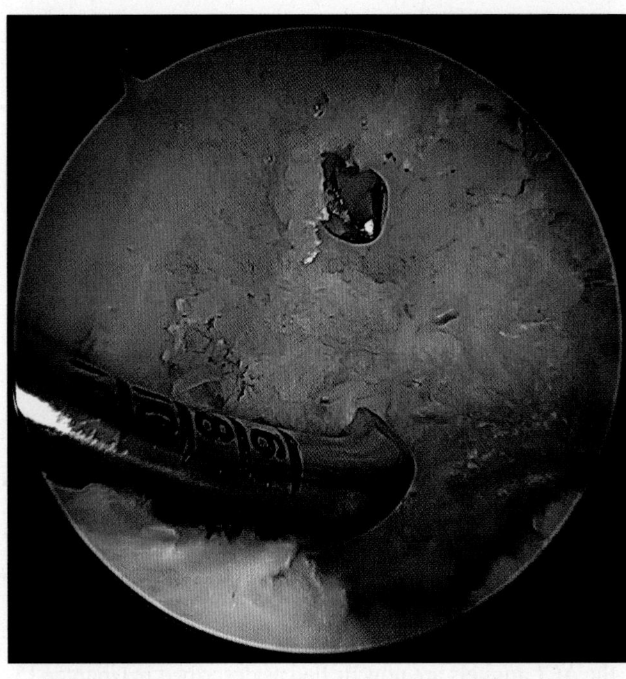

FIGURE 22-15

Arthroscopic view of right knee, medial condyle with AL pin inserted and PCL femoral guide in place to pass PM pin.

Femoral Tunnel Preparation

The 30-degree arthroscope is again used at this point. The two femoral tunnels are created from outside-in using two guide pins. The PCL femoral guide is placed through the anteromedial portal and seated in the 10:30 position (Fig. 22-15) for the AL bundle in the left knee (1:30 for the right knee), and a pin is inserted percutaneously into the joint from just proximal to the medial epicondyle. For the PL bundle, a second pin is passed to emerge at the 9:00 position (3:00 for the right knee) while visualizing the medial side of the notch with the arthroscope from the AL portal. It is imperative when using this technique that these two pins are separated by approximately 2 cm as they enter the cortex of the distal medial femur (Fig. 22-16) allowing a cortical bridge to be maintained when the tunnels are subsequently drilled. To confirm this, your finger should easily fit between the two pins as they enter the bone from the outer cortex. The pins will converge inside the joint, and we have found that maintaining a bony bridge between the two tunnels as they enter the joint facilitates graft passage. Once adequate positioning is confirmed, a skin incision is made between the pins and the vastus medialis is split in line with its fibers. The size of the femoral tunnels has been previously determined by measurement of each limb of the allograft. Typically, one limb is larger, and it is used for the AL bundle. The appropriate-sized reamers (typically 7 to 9 mm) are used to drill these tunnels, and the edges are then rasped with the shaver from within the joint. Additionally, we have found the use of electrocautery to ablate the periosteum around the tunnel entrances while arthroscopically visualizing up the tunnel facilitates subsequent graft and interference screw passage (Fig. 22-17).

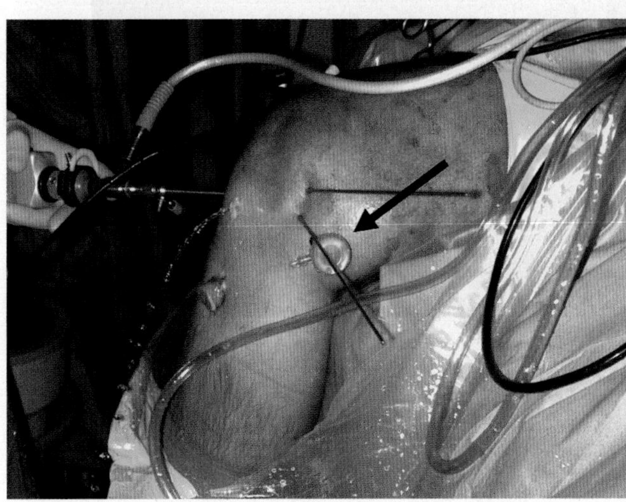

FIGURE 22-16

Intraoperative view of right knee showing two femoral guide pins and posteromedial cannula (*arrow*).

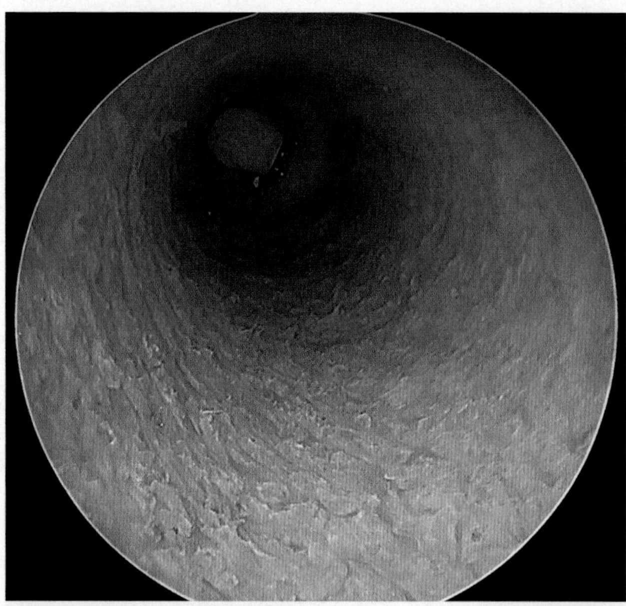

FIGURE 22-17

Arthroscopic view of femoral tunnel demonstrating use of electrocautery to ablate the periosteum at the external aperture to facilitate graft passage.

If the ACL is also to be reconstructed, the ACL tunnels are now drilled as described in Chapter 15. Once all tunnels are prepared, the PCL graft is passed first and secured in the femur, and then, the ACL graft passed and secured in the femur. If medial or lateral reconstructions are needed, the tibial fixation is delayed until after those reconstructions have been performed but not fixated. The PCL is first fixated on the tibia followed by the ACL and then final fixation of the medial and/or lateral sides.

Graft Passage and Fixation

To facilitate passage of both limbs of the allograft, the previously placed shuttle sutures are now retrieved from the PM cannula and passed into the femoral tunnels. It is important to ensure that these sutures are clear of any tangles that may complicate graft passage. These sutures are individually retrieved from the femoral tunnels with an arthroscopic grasper (Fig. 22-18A). The different colored shuttle sutures allow identification of the limbs. The graft is brought to the operative field, and the sutures from the graft are shuttled through the femoral and down the tibial tunnel with the passing sutures (Fig. 22-18B). The graft ends are now passed through the femoral tunnels and down into the tibia. The mark made at the midpoint of the graft facilitates passage of each limb equally;

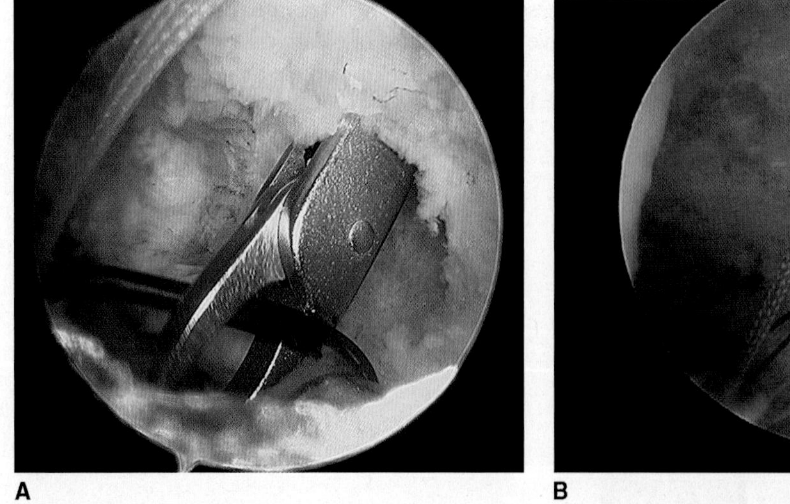

A

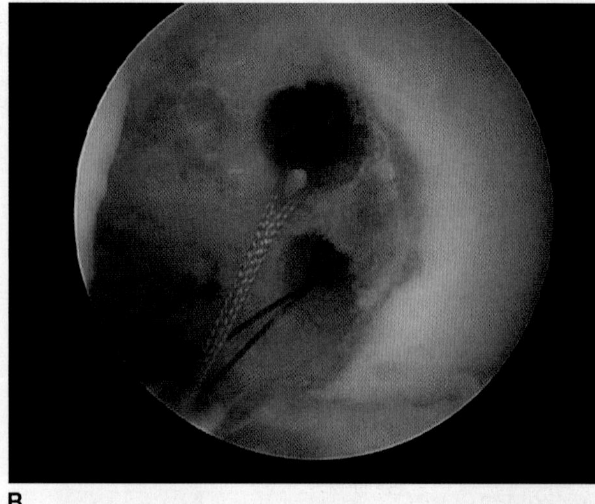

B

FIGURE 22-18

A: Arthroscopic view showing the AL and PM tunnels. An arthroscopic grasper is used to retrieve the sutures from the tibial tunnel. **B:** The shuttle sutures, AL (**green**) and PM (**purple**), are used to pass the sutures from the allograft.

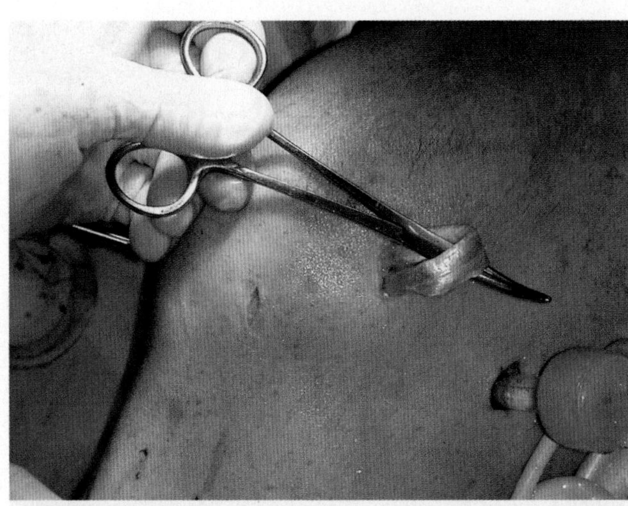

FIGURE 22-19

The intraoperative photo of a right knee, demonstrating passage of the allograft into the femoral tunnels.

however, since the AL limb takes a longer course, the mark should be passed slightly more into the AL femoral tunnel. To facilitate passage and to avoid limb length discrepancy resulting from inadvertently pulling one limb further into the tunnel, a smooth object such as the scope trocar is maintained through the loop of the allograft during passage. Once the graft passage and allograft position are satisfactory, the trocar is slid out allowing the final positioning of the graft (Fig. 22-19).

Femoral Fixation

Once passed, the knee is cycled and the graft secured first in the femoral tunnels. Although the graft passes over the medial bony bridge, to avoid slippage while differentially tightening and to obtain aperture fixation, bioabsorbable interference screws are passed into the femoral tunnels from outside-in. Both guide wires are passed and secured inside the joint while the screws are inserted and tension is maintained on the free ends of the graft (Fig. 22-20). We typically use bioabsorbable interference screws the same size as the diameter of the femoral tunnels and a length of 23 mm. It is important to ensure that these screws are not left proud because any hardware on the medial side can become quite symptomatic.

Tibial Fixation

The knee is again cycled to eliminate any residual graft laxity, and the graft is then differentially tightened on the tibial side. The sutures from the AL bundle are first secured with a bioabsorbable interference screw while the knee is flexed to 70 to 90 degrees and an anterior drawer applied to the proximal tibia.

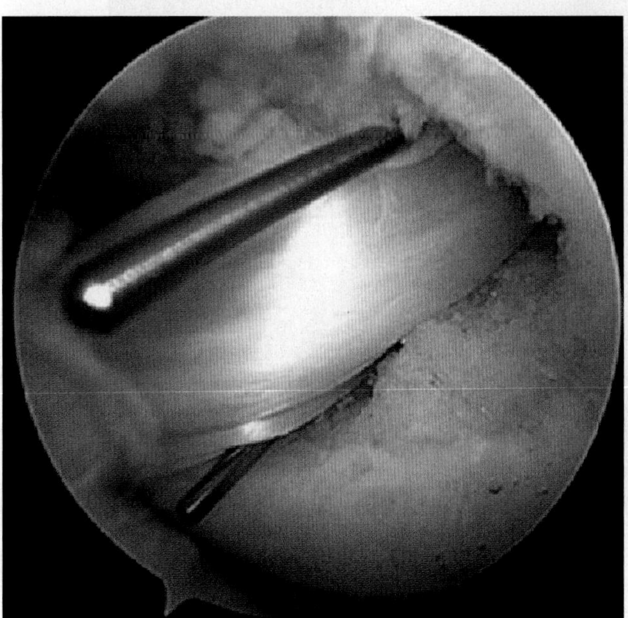

FIGURE 22-20

Arthroscopic view of allograft having been passed into femoral and tibial tunnels. Nitinol guide wires are now used to insert the cannulated bioabsorbable interference screws into the femoral tunnels.

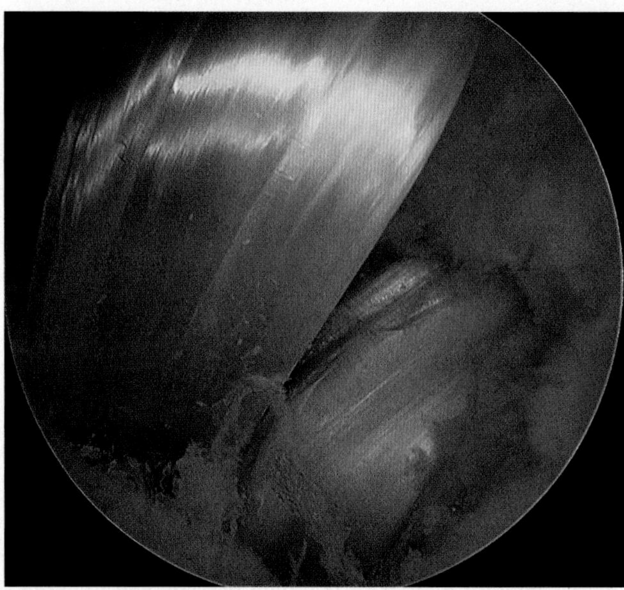

FIGURE 22-21

Arthroscopic view of completed double-bundle PCL reconstruction.

The knee is then extended to 0 to 20 degrees and a second bioabsorbable interference screw is inserted up the PM tunnel securing the allograft while an anterior drawer is again applied and tension maintained on the sutures from the PM bundle. We typically use screws the same diameter as the tibial tunnels but a longer screw (28 mm) is employed than what is used on the femur. For added fixation, the sutures from the PM bundle are now tied to those from the AL over the boney bridge resulting in double fixation on both the femoral and tibial sides (Fig. 22-21). The incisions are closed in standard fashion. A postoperative brace, locked in extension, is applied over a compressive wrap. The incisions, once healed, are typically cosmetically acceptable. As seen in this postoperative radiographs (Fig. 22-22A,B), nonmetallic fixation is used throughout and no prominent hardware is present to cause symptoms.

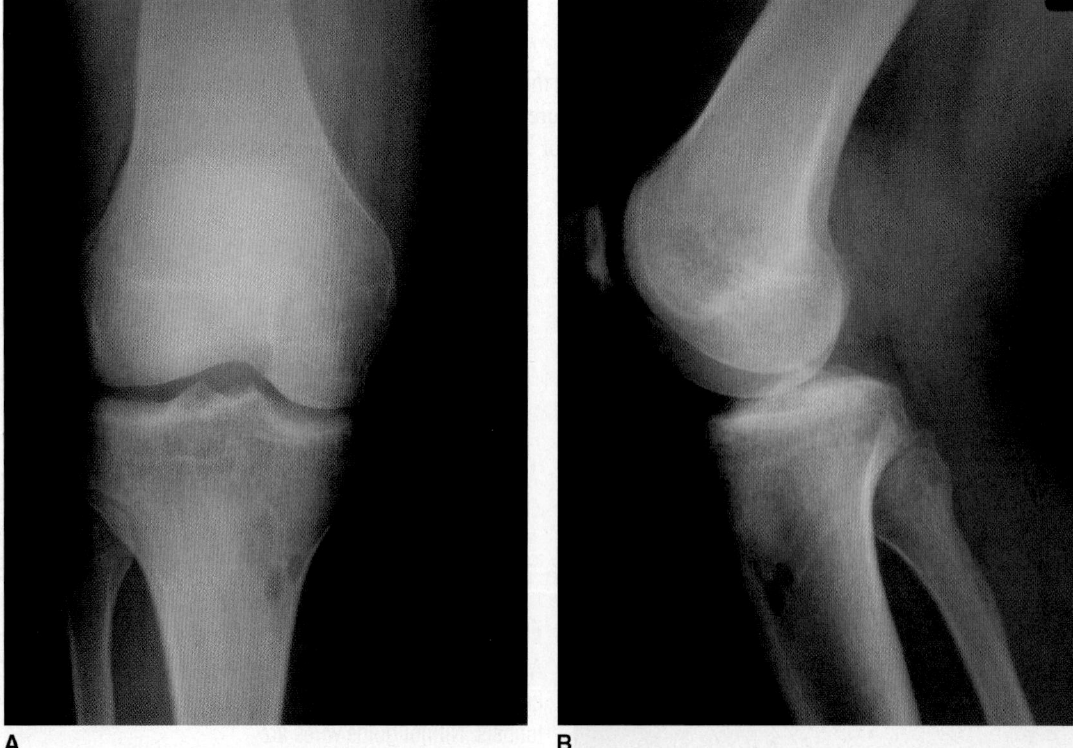

FIGURE 22-22

AP (**A**) and lateral (**B**) postoperative radiographs following PCL reconstruction.

PEARLS AND PITFALLS

- It is important to evaluate for concomitant ligament injuries during preoperative assessment and again during the EUA. Deficiency of other ligaments may lead to early PCL graft failure.
- Visualization of the PCL footprint on the posterior tibia is essential for the success of this technique and to avoid serious complications. This can be tedious, but the surgeon must be careful and patient. Both aggressive debridement and inadequate exposure can lead to neurovascular injury.
- Breach the posterior tibial cortex with the guide pins or reamers in a controlled fashion under direct arthroscopic visualization to avoid overpenetration and potential neurovascular injury.
- A parallel pin guide can be used to make small corrections for placement of the tunnels.
- An arthroscopic switching rod or trocar can be placed within the loop of allograft to facilitate correct limb passage and to avoid inadvertent passage of one limb more than the other.
- Fluid extravasation during arthroscopy is a concern. Limited tourniquet time and decreased pump pressures should be considered. Lower extremity compartments should be monitored throughout the procedure.

POSTOPERATIVE MANAGEMENT

Patients are typically kept overnight for pain management and to monitor their neurovascular status. Postoperative rehabilitation should be very slow. Crutches with touch-toe weightbearing are recommended for the first 6 weeks. The patient's knee is maintained in full extension for the first 2 postoperative weeks and then allowed flexion to 70 degrees for the next 4 to 6 weeks. However, the brace remains locked in extension for ambulation. Quadriceps rehabilitation is emphasized. Progressive weightbearing is allowed at 2 months and the brace is unlocked with restoration of quadriceps control. Full range of motion is allowed at 2 months depending on patient individual progress. Running and sporting activities are allowed after 6 months.

COMPLICATIONS

Complications are rare but can happen. Failure to carefully position the extremity with adequate padding can lead to neuropraxia or compartment syndrome of the posterior thigh. Loss of knee motion, residual laxity, or overt graft failure can result from errors in graft positioning, inadequate fixation, or early motion during the initial postoperative rehabilitation. Injury to the popliteal vessels is an infrequent but very serious complication. With the transtibial technique, great care must be taken to ensure that overpenetration of the posterior tibial cortex does not occur. Fluid extravasation should be avoided. The thigh and calf should be routinely palpated during the case to ensure no compartment syndrome develops from fluid extravasation into the soft tissues.

RESULTS

The plethora of published PCL reconstruction techniques clearly demonstrates the frustration surgeons have had in achieving reproducible results with any single technique. The use of a double-bundle technique has several advantages including the use of a larger graft, the ability to differentially tighten the two bundles, and, theoretically, better recreation of the native PCL anatomy. There are a number of double-bundle techniques described, but the technique described above should be well understood by surgeons who are familiar with arthroscopic ACL reconstructions. Advantages include the use of commonly available equipment, setup, and tunnel drilling. This technique does not require an open posterior approach to the knee, nor does it require any patient position change during the case. There have been several recent publications demonstrating superior results with double-bundle techniques (32,35–38); however, one can cite just as many articles advocating other techniques as well.

Disadvantages of the technique described herein include the need for an exceptionally long and wide allograft that may require special ordering, the difficulty of drilling multiple tunnels, and the challenge of multiple passing sutures. The issue of the "killer turn," a point made by those surgeons advocating the inlay technique, refers to the acute angle the graft passes from the aperture of the tibial tunnel toward the femoral tunnel. This angle can be decreased and any such theoretical disadvantage mitigated by keeping the angle of the tibial tunnels as steep as possible. In summary, for

PCL reconstructions, there are multiple options, each with inherent advantages and disadvantages. The surgeon has to choose a treatment, operative or nonoperative, and if operative, a surgical technique that he or she feels best suits their abilities and their patient's needs.

REFERENCES

1. Bianchi M. Acute tears of the posterior cruciate ligament: clinical study and results of operative treatment in 27 cases. *Am J Sports Med.* 1983;11(5):308–314.
2. DeHaven KE. Diagnosis of acute knee injuries with hemarthrosis. *Am J Sports Med.* 1980;8(1):9–14.
3. DeLee JC, Riley MB, Rockwood CA Jr. Acute straight lateral instability of the knee. *Am J Sports Med.* 1983;11(6):404–411.
4. Lysholm J, Gillquist J. Arthroscopic examination of the posterior cruciate ligament. *J Bone Joint Surg Am.* 1981;63(3):363–366.
5. Rubinstein RA Jr, Shelbourne KD, McCarroll JR, et al. The accuracy of the clinical examination in the setting of posterior cruciate ligament injuries. *Am J Sports Med.* 1994;22(4):550–557.
6. Shelbourne KD, Rubinstein RA Jr. Methodist Sports Medicine Center's experience with acute and chronic isolated posterior cruciate ligament injuries. *Clin Sports Med.* 1994;13(3):531–543.
7. Shelbourne KD, Clark M, Gray T. Minimum 10-year follow-up of patients after an acute, isolated posterior cruciate ligament injury treated nonoperatively. *Am J Sports Med.* 2013;41(7):1526–1533.
8. Keller PM, Shelbourne KD, McCarroll JR, et al. Nonoperatively treated isolated posterior cruciate ligament injuries. *Am J Sports Med.* 1993;21(1):132–136.
9. Song EK, Park HW, Ahn YS, et al. Transtibial versus tibial inlay techniques for posterior cruciate ligament reconstruction: long-term follow-up study. *Am J Sports Med.* 2014;42(12):2964–2971.
10. Shelbourne KD, Muthukaruppan Y. Subjective results of nonoperatively treated, acute, isolated posterior cruciate ligament injuries. *Arthroscopy.* 2005;21(4):457–461.
11. Shelbourne KD, Gray T. Natural history of acute posterior cruciate ligament tears. *J Knee Surg.* 2002;15(2):103–107.
12. Levy BA, Fanelli GC, Miller MD, et al. Advances in posterior cruciate ligament reconstruction. *Instr Course Lect.* 2015;64:543–554.
13. Fanelli GC. Foreword: The posterior cruciate ligament. *J Knee Surg.* 2010;23(2):59.
14. Fanelli GC. Posterior cruciate ligament rehabilitation: how slow should we go? *Arthroscopy.* 2008;24(2):234–235.
15. Fanelli GC, Edson CJ, Reinheimer KN, et al. Posterior cruciate ligament and posterolateral corner reconstruction. *Sports Med Arthrosc.* 2007;15(4):168–175.
16. Fanelli GC, Edson CJ. Arthroscopically assisted combined anterior and posterior cruciate ligament reconstruction in the multiple ligament injured knee: 2- to 10-year follow-up. *Arthroscopy.* 2002;18(7):703–714.
17. Fanelli GC. Treatment of combined anterior cruciate ligament-posterior cruciate ligament-lateral side injuries of the knee. *Clin Sports Med.* 2000;19(3):493–502.
18. Barber FA, Fanelli GC, Matthews LS, et al. The treatment of complete posterior cruciate ligament tears. *Arthroscopy.* 2000;16(7):725–731.
19. Klecker RJ, Winalski CS, Aliabadi P, et al. The aberrant anterior tibial artery: magnetic resonance appearance, prevalence, and surgical implications. *Am J Sports Med.* 2008;36(4):720–727.
20. Kennedy NI, LaPrade RF, Goldsmith MD, et al. Posterior cruciate ligament graft fixation angles, part 1: biomechanical evaluation for anatomic single-bundle reconstruction. *Am J Sports Med.* 2014;42(10):2338–2345.
21. Bait C, Denti M, Prospero E, et al. Posterior cruciate ligament reconstruction with "all-inside" technique: a technical note. *Muscles Ligaments Tendons J.* 2014;4(4):467–470.
22. Spiridonov SI, Slinkard NJ, LaPrade RF. Isolated and combined grade-III posterior cruciate ligament tears treated with double-bundle reconstruction with use of endoscopically placed femoral tunnels and grafts: operative technique and clinical outcomes. *J Bone Joint Surg Am.* 2011;93(19):1773–1780.
23. Fanelli GC, Beck JD, Edson CJ. Current concepts review: the posterior cruciate ligament. *J Knee Surg.* 2010;23(2):61–72.
24. Fanelli GC, Edison CJ, Orcutt DR, et al. Treatment of combined anterior cruciate-posterior cruciate ligament-medial-lateral side knee injuries. *J Knee Surg.* 2005;18(3):240–248.
25. Fanelli GC, Edson CJ. Combined posterior cruciate ligament-posterolateral reconstructions with Achilles tendon allograft and biceps femoris tendon tenodesis: 2- to 10-year follow-up. *Arthroscopy.* 2004;20(4):339–345.
26. Shelbourne KD, Carr DR. Combined anterior and posterior cruciate and medial collateral ligament injury: nonsurgical and delayed surgical treatment. *Instr Course Lect.* 2003;52:413–418.
27. Miller MD, Cooper DE, Fanelli GC, et al. Posterior cruciate ligament: current concepts. *Instr Course Lect.* 2002;51:347–351.
28. Fanelli GC, Giannotti BF, Edson CJ. Arthroscopically assisted combined posterior cruciate ligament/posterior lateral complex reconstruction. *Arthroscopy.* 1996;12(5):521–530.
29. Fanelli GC, Giannotti BF, Edson CJ. Arthroscopically assisted combined anterior and posterior cruciate ligament reconstruction. *Arthroscopy.* 1996;12(1):5–14.
30. Fanelli GC, Edson CJ. Posterior cruciate ligament injuries in trauma patients: part II. *Arthroscopy.* 1995;11(5):526–529.
31. Fanelli GC. Posterior cruciate ligament injuries in trauma patients. *Arthroscopy.* 1993;9(3):291–294.
32. Fanelli GC, Beck JD, Edson CJ. Double bundle posterior cruciate ligament reconstruction: surgical technique and results. *Sports Med Arthrosc.* 2010;18(4):242–248.
33. Jung TM, Reinhardt C, Scheffler SU, et al. Stress radiography to measure posterior cruciate ligament insufficiency: a comparison of five different techniques. *Knee Surg Sports Traumatol Arthrosc.* 2006;14(11):1116–1121.
34. Margheritini F, Mancini L, Mauro CS, et al. Stress radiography for quantifying posterior cruciate ligament deficiency. *Arthroscopy.* 2003;19(7):706–711.
35. Zhao JX, Zhang LH, Mao Z, et al. Outcome of posterior cruciate ligament reconstruction using the single- versus double bundle technique: a meta-analysis. *J Int Med Res.* 2015;43(2):149–160.
36. Li Y, Li J, Wang J, et al. Comparison of single-bundle and double-bundle isolated posterior cruciate ligament reconstruction with allograft: a prospective, randomized study. *Arthroscopy.* 2014;30(6):695–700.
37. Kennedy NI, LaPrade RF, Goldsmith MT, et al. Posterior cruciate ligament graft fixation angles, part 2: biomechanical evaluation for anatomic double-bundle reconstruction. *Am J Sports Med.* 2014;42(10):2346–2355.
38. Tsukada H, Ishibashi Y, Tsuda E, et al. Biomechanical evaluation of an anatomic double-bundle posterior cruciate ligament reconstruction. *Arthroscopy.* 2012;28(2):264–271.

RECOMMENDED READINGS

Ahn JH, Chung YS, Oh I. Arthroscopic posterior cruciate ligament reconstruction using the posterior transseptal portal. *Arthroscopy.* 2003;19(1):101–107.

Fox RJ, Harner CD, Sakane M, et al. Determination of the in situ forces in the human posterior cruciate ligament using robotic technology—a cadaveric study. *Am J Sports Med.* 1998;26(3):395–401.

Giffin JR, Haemmerle MJ, Vogrin TM, et al. Single- versus double-bundle PCL reconstruction: a biomechanical analysis. *J Knee Surg.* 2002;15(2):114–120.

Harner CD, Janaushek MA, Kanamori A, et al. Biomechanical analysis of a double-bundle posterior cruciate ligament reconstruction. *Am J Sports Med.* 2000;28(2):144–151.

LaPrade CM, Civitarese DM, Rasmussen MT, et al. Emerging updates on the posterior cruciate ligament: a review of the current literature. *Am J Sports Med.* 2015;43(5).

Levy BA, Fanelli GC, Miller MD, et al. Advances in posterior cruciate ligament reconstruction. *Instr Course Lect.* 2015;64:543–554.

Margheritini F, Mauro CS, Rihn JA, et al. Biomechanical comparison of tibial inlay versus transtibial techniques for posterior cruciate ligament reconstruction: analysis of knee kinematics and graft in situ forces. *Am J Sports Med.* 2004;32(3):587–593.

Margheritini F, Rihn JA, Mauro CS, et al. Biomechanics of initial tibial fixation in posterior cruciate ligament reconstruction. *Arthroscopy.* 2005;21(10):1164–1171.

Noyes FR, Barber-Westin S. Posterior cruciate ligament replacement with a two-strand quadriceps tendon-patellar bone autograft and a tibial inlay technique. *J Bone Joint Surg Am.* 2005;87(6):1241–1252.

Sekiya JK, Haemmerle MJ, Stabile KJ, et al. Biomechanical analysis of a combined double-bundle posterior cruciate ligament and posterolateral corner knee reconstruction. *Am J Sports Med.* 2005;33(3):360–369.

Sekiya JK, West RV, Ong BC, et al. Clinical outcomes after isolated arthroscopic single-bundle posterior cruciate ligament reconstruction. *Arthroscopy.* 2005;21(9):1042–1050.

Shelbourne KD, Davis TJ, Patel DV. The natural history of acute, isolated, nonoperatively treated posterior cruciate ligament injuries. A prospective study. *Am J Sports Med.* 1999;27:276–283.

Shelbourne KD, Gray T. Natural history of acute posterior cruciate ligament tears. *J Knee Surg.* 2002;15(2):103–107.

Sheps DM, Otto D, Fernhout M. The anatomic characteristics of the tibial insertion of the posterior cruciate ligament. *Arthroscopy.* 2005;21(7):820–825.

Song EK, Park HW, Ahn YS, et al. Transtibial versus tibial inlay techniques for posterior cruciate ligament reconstruction: long-term follow-up study. *Am J Sports Med.* 2014;42(12):2964–2971.

Torg JS, Barton TM, Pavlov H, et al. Natural history of the posterior cruciate ligament-deficient knee. *Clin Orthop Relat Res.* 1989;246:208–216.

Yoon KH, Bae DK, Song SJ, et al. Arthroscopic double-bundle augmentation of posterior cruciate ligament using split Achilles allograft. *Arthroscopy.* 2005;21(12):1436–1442.

23 Surgical Management of Acute Medial-Sided Injuries

Matthew R. Prince, Bruce A. Levy, and Michael J. Stuart

INTRODUCTION

The key structures contributing to valgus and anteromedial rotatory stability to the knee include the superficial medial collateral ligament (sMCL), deep MCL, posterior oblique ligament (POL) and semimembranosus. Injuries to the superficial MCL and its supporting structures constitute the most commonly reported ligamentous injury of the knee (1). The incidence of these injuries has been reported as high as 0.24 per 1,000 per year in the United States (2). Most MCL sprains occur alone without associated meniscal and/or other ligamentous injury (1). The ACL (anterior cruciate ligament), PCL (posterior cruciate ligament), or PLC (posterolateral corner) complex may all be injured in combination with MCL tear, with the overwhelming majority being a combined ACL/MCL injury (3). MCL injuries typically occur during sports activities from a noncontact, valgus and external rotation load or a contact force to the lateral side of the knee creating a valgus moment.

Classification of MCL injuries according to severity of ligament damage are graded as I, II, or III based on asymmetric valgus joint space opening of 2 to 5 mm, 6 to 10 mm, and greater than 10 mm, respectively (4). The vast majority of MCL injuries are managed nonoperatively with excellent results regardless of grade (5,6).

SURGICAL INDICATIONS

There are several knee injury patterns involving the MCL that favor surgical treatment over conservative management. Superior results with operative management have been documented in the setting of multiligament injury, valgus knee alignment, and associated injury to the POL, deep MCL, and semimembranosus tendon (4,7–9). In addition, surgical repair may promote healing for certain cases of distal MCL avulsion with proximal retraction or pes anserine tendon interposition, the so-called Stenar lesion of the knee (10) (Fig. 23-1). Symptomatic valgus patholaxity has been reported with nonoperative management of tibial-based avulsions involving both the superficial and deep MCL (11,12) (Fig. 23-2). These injuries are recognized on MRI from the "wave sign" (a characteristic waving appearance of the superficial MCL) (13) (Fig. 23-3). Although uncommon, a displaced bony MCL avulsion is also an indication for acute repair (14).

The decision to repair or reconstruct the MCL is dependent on the tear location and the quality of the remaining tissue. Stannard et al. have demonstrated inferior results with repair as opposed to reconstruction in the setting of multiligamentous reconstruction and associated medial-side injury (15). However, no differences in clinical results were appreciated when comparing acute repair versus reconstruction in the setting of combined ACL and MCL injuries (16).

Absolute Surgical Indications

- *"Stenar-like" lesion*
- *Bony avulsion*

Relative Surgical Indications

- *Most cases in the setting of multiligament knee injury*

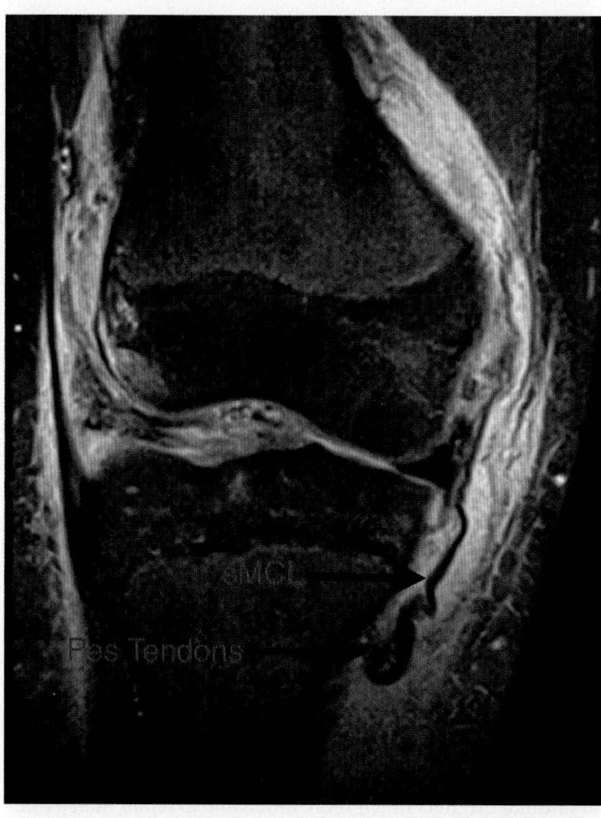

FIGURE 23-1
Distal sMCL avulsion with pes tendon entrapment—"Stenar lesion" of the knee.

- *Selected cases of combined ACL and grade III MCL*
- *Distal tibial avulsion of superficial and deep MCL*
- *Selected cases of valgus knee alignment with grade III MCL*

CONTRAINDICATIONS

Contraindications to acute repair include several preoperative conditions and intraoperative assessment of tissue quality.

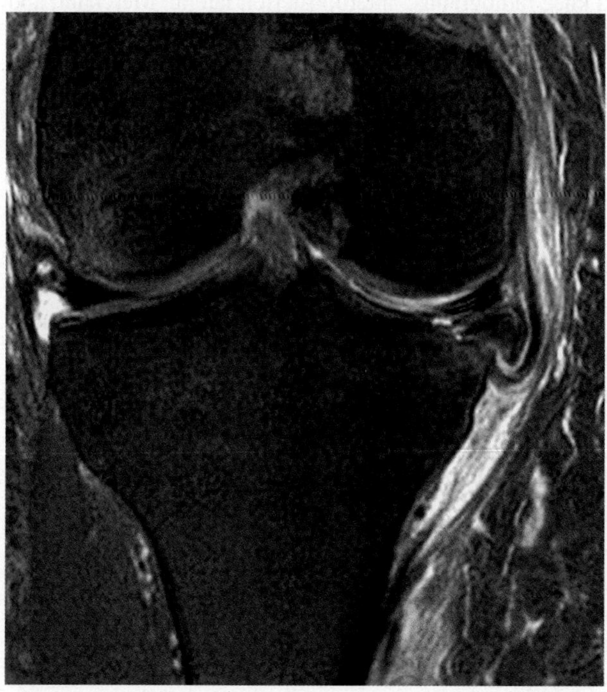

FIGURE 23-2
Distal MCL entrapped in a marginal tibial fracture, demonstrating disruption of both the proximal and distal sMCL tibial insertions along with the meniscotibial insertion of the deep MCL.

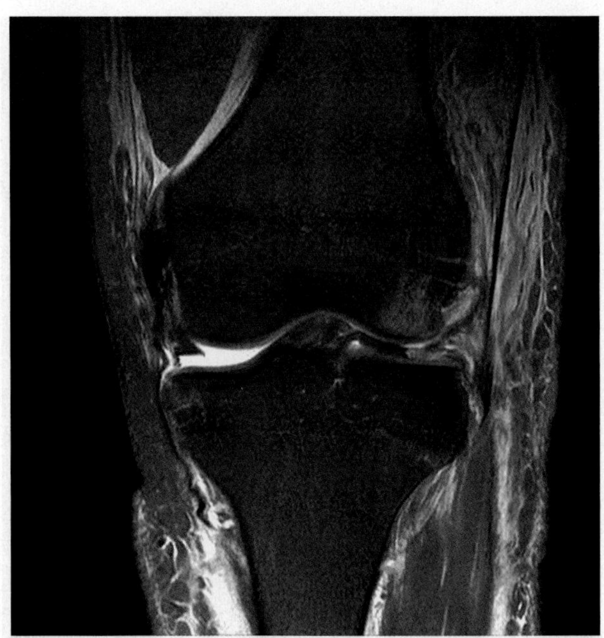

FIGURE 23-3
"Wave sign" with proximal retraction of the sMCL.

Systemic patient assessment may reveal endocrine abnormalities that deserve consideration. Pituitary gland disorders and diabetes mellitus have both been shown to affect MCL healing and repair results (7).

If surgical treatment is undertaken, the location of injury will influence the decision for acute repair versus reconstruction. Tear location at the femoral or tibial origin is much more amenable to repair than a midsubstance rupture. At the time of surgery, tissue quality may be found inadequate to allow repair alone. In this setting, MCL repair can be augmented with a tendon graft or a synthetic internal brace (17,18).

Repair Contraindications

- *Poor tissue quality or extensive tissue damage*
- *Systemic disorders that may inhibit healing*
- *Chronic MCL disruption*

PREOPERATIVE PREPARATION

Preoperative assessment includes standard knee radiographs: anteroposterior, lateral, Merchant, and 30-degree posteroanterior flexion views. A full-length standing, hip to ankle radiograph is recommended if the anteroposterior view reveals excessive valgus malalignment. Magnetic resonance imaging (MRI) is obtained on all patients not only to define the location and extent of the MCL injury but also to evaluate the articular cartilage, menisci, subchondral bone, other ligaments, and joint capsule. Side-to-side comparison using stress imaging with either fluoroscopy or ultrasound is performed before surgery or under anesthesia prior to incision. Stress radiography plays a key role in surgical decision-making for the medial aspect of the knee. Several authors have found that the average physiologic difference in joint space opening between knees under valgus stress should be less than 2.0 mm (19–21). LaPrade et al. found that a side-to-side difference of any greater than 3.2 mm with valgus stress radiography at 20 degrees of knee flexion or greater than 2.0 mm in full extension indicates a grade III MCL injury (21). It is extremely important to maintain identical knee rotation when performing stress radiography to ensure accurate comparison of joint space widening (Fig. 23-4).

Preoperative physical therapy is essential to ensure adequate knee range of motion (ROM), quadriceps activation and resolution of intra-articular effusion.

PATIENT POSITIONING AND SETUP

The patient is placed supine on a radiolucent table. A tourniquet is applied and routinely utilized except in the case of a prior vascular repair or bypass graft. If the medial side surgery is combined with ACL and/or PCL reconstruction, a standard leg holder is used, the foot of the table is dropped, and cruciate ligament surgery is completed first. The foot of the bed is then raised in order to

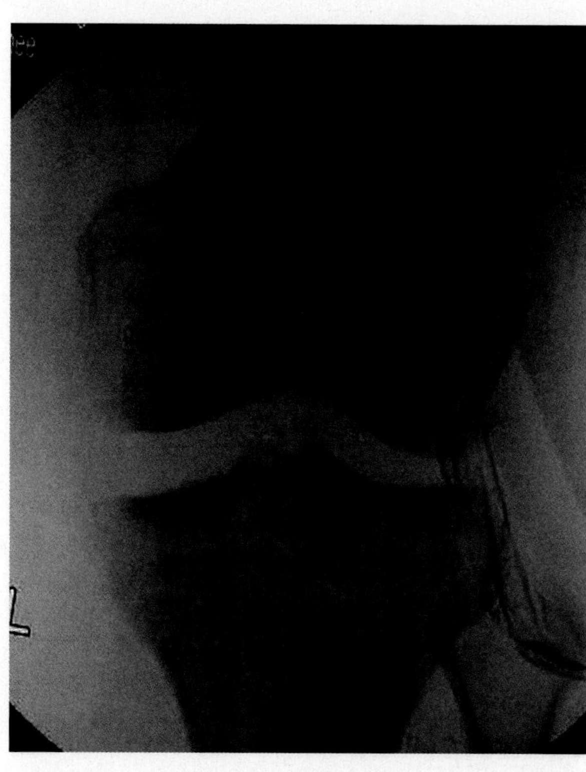

FIGURE 23-4

Valgus stress radiography demonstrating pathologic medial joint space opening.

facilitate MCL repair or reconstruction. Fluoroscopy is positioned on the contralateral side of the injured knee. We typically use a foam riser under the operative leg for a better fluoroscopic view. Recently, we began using a hydrolytic articulated leg holder that allows for secure, intraoperative leg positioning and obviates the need for the standard leg holder or foam riser.

SURGICAL TECHNIQUE

Approach

The initial approach for acute repair of the MCL is influenced by both concomitant injury and location of MCL disruption. Typically, we use an anteromedial, straight skin incision extending from the medial epicondyle to the distal tibial superficial MCL insertion. The incision may be modified if an isolated femoral or tibial avulsion is present.

Tibial-Based Injury

When repairing a tibial-based MCL injury, attention must be paid to both proximal and distal superficial MCL attachments located at 12 and 61 mm from the joint line (on average) (22). In addition, the deep MCL and its medial meniscal attachment should be identified and repaired as necessary. Layer one (sartorius fascia) is identified and incised. The pes anserine tendons are retracted distally exposing the distal MCL insertion site. If the ligament is retracted, proximal dissection is required for identification. A No. 2 nonabsorbable, locking whip stitch is placed at the distal end of the MCL with both free ends exiting on the deep surface of the ligament. Dissection is continued to the joint line in order to assess the proximal insertion and deep MCL integrity.

If disruption of the deep MCL is encountered, suture anchors are placed along the medial tibial plateau rim and passed through the medial meniscus and MCL to reestablish deep MCL (medial meniscotibial ligament) integrity (Fig. 23-5). Two suture anchors are also placed at the proximal superficial MCL insertion site.

A slit is then made in the center of the ligament for placement of a 4.5-mm screw. A 3.2-mm drill bit is used to create a bicortical drill hole at the center of the superficial MCL insertion just anterior to the posterior tibial border. An 18-mm spiked washer and screw are used to secure the ligament at its distal attachment at 20 degrees of knee flexion while applying a varus stress. Fixation is supplemented by tying the locking whipstitch suture around the screw and washer (Fig. 23-6). Finally, the sartorial fascia is repaired, covering the distal fixation (Fig. 23-7).

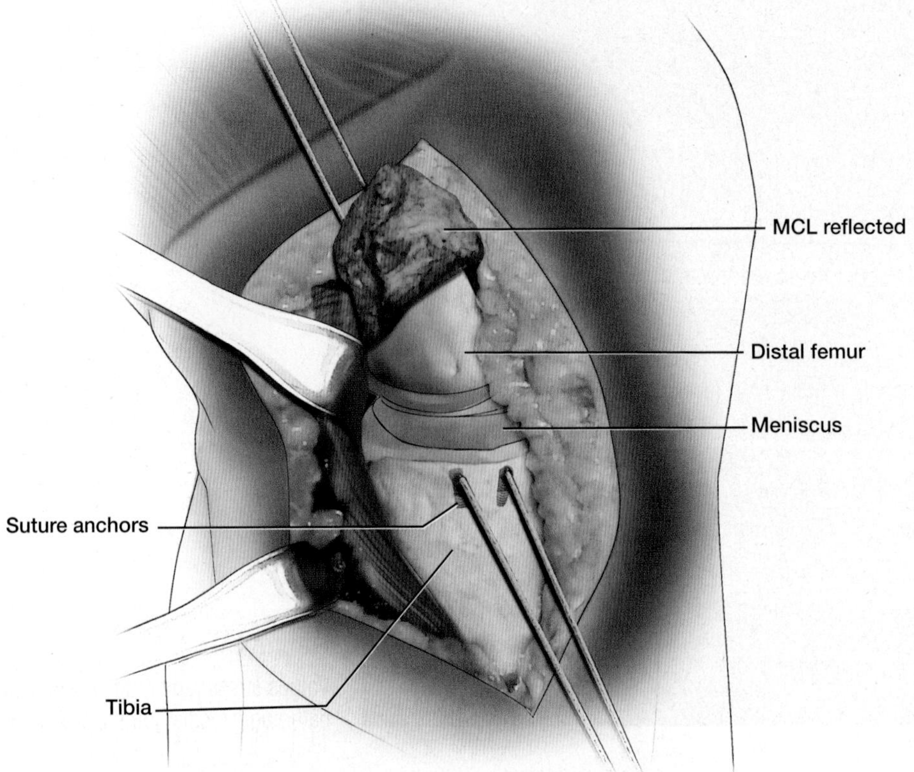

A

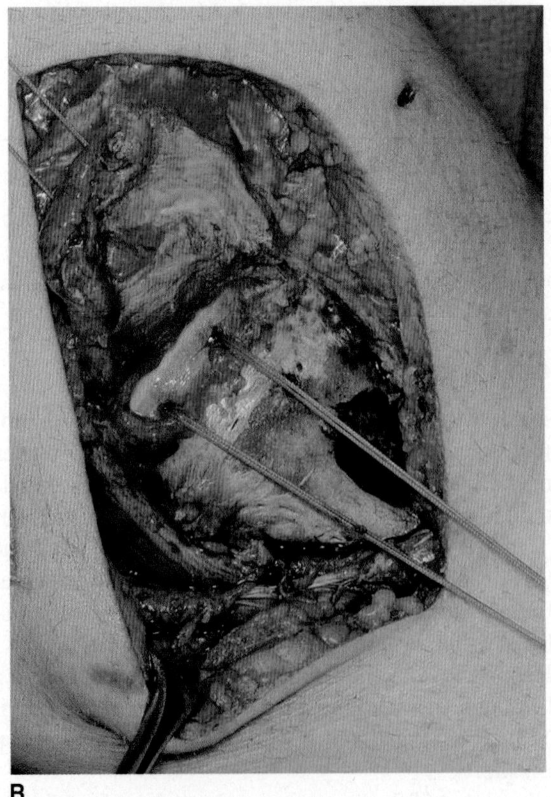

B

FIGURE 23-5

A, B: Tibial suture anchor placement for deep MCL repair.

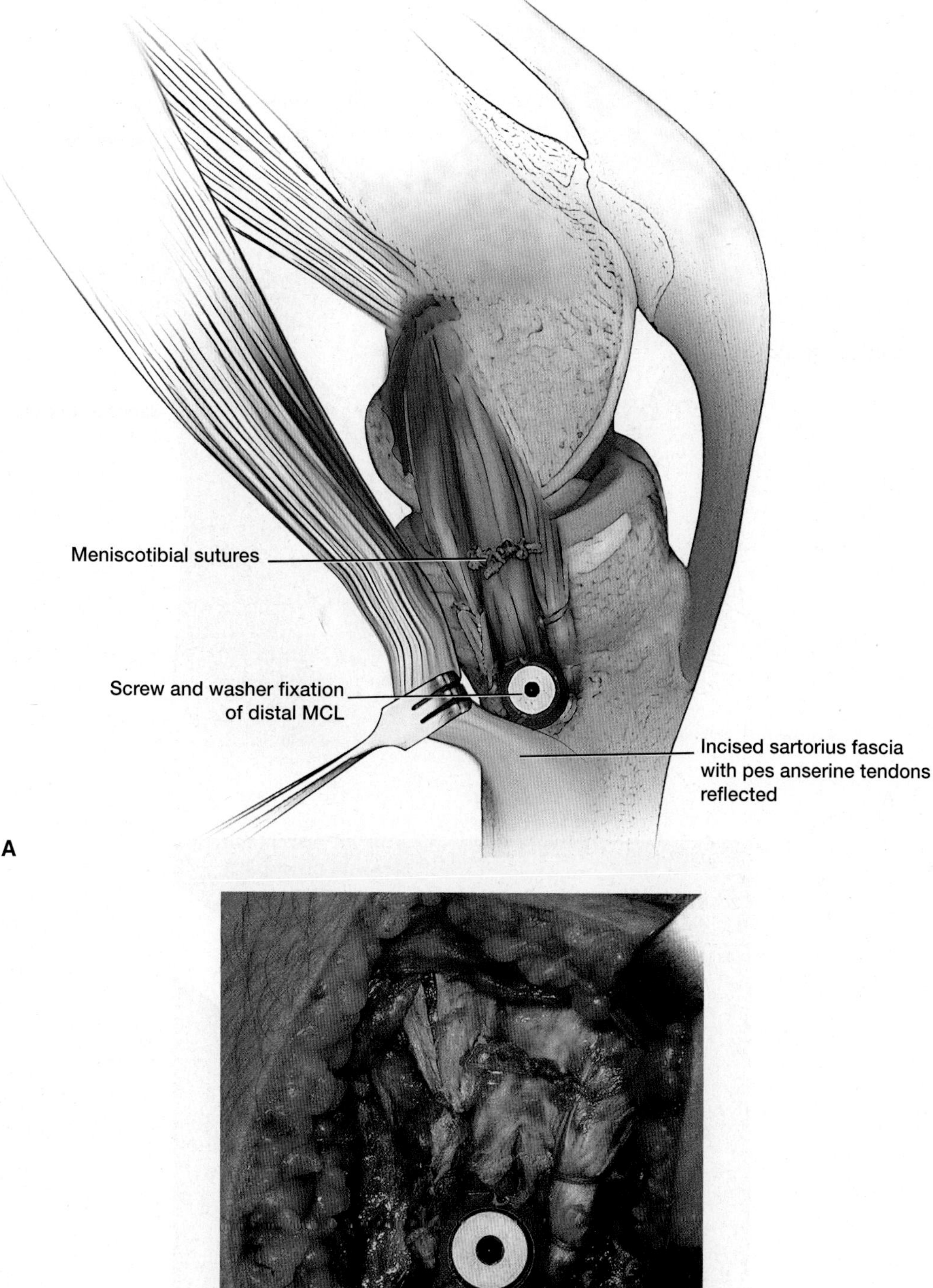

FIGURE 23-6

A, B: Distal insertion of sMCL after screw and washer fixation.

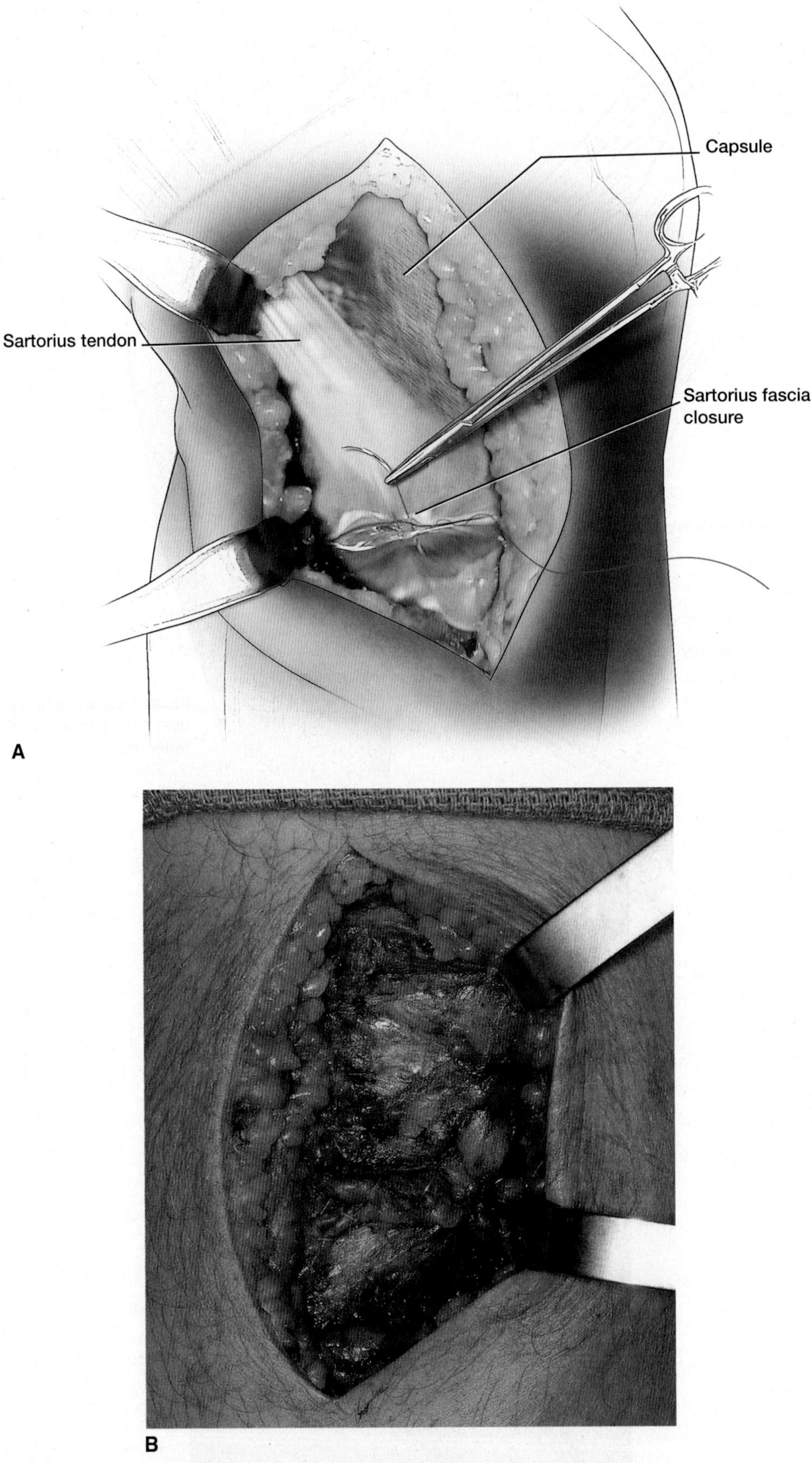

FIGURE 23-7

A, B: Repaired sartorial expansion.

Femoral-Based Injury

If a femoral-based injury to the MCL and posteromedial corner (PMC) is suspected, an incision based over the medial epicondyle is utilized. Fluoroscopy is utilized to locate the sMCL origin about the medial epicondyle. On average, the sMCL insertion is found 3.2 mm proximal and 4.8 mm posterior to the medial epicondyle (23,24). The incision extends down to the crural fascia. The posterior medial corner is explored to assess for damage to the adductor magnus, semimembranosus and medial gastrocnemius tendons, POL, and posteromedial capsule. The tendons are repaired, and suture anchors are placed posterior to the sMCL insertion to recreate the posteromedial capsule and POL attachments. If the PMC is intact but patulous, a longitudinal incision is made posterior to the sMCL margin creating a tissue flap containing the posteromedial capsule and POL. This flap will be advanced and imbricated following sMCL repair. Suture anchors are placed distally on the medial femoral condyle to reestablish the meniscofemoral insertion of the deep MCL. Finally, the ligament washer and suture post technique (same as the distal repair) is employed for the proximal sMCL insertion (Fig. 23-8).

Repair Augmentation

The decision to augment a repair is typically made at the time of surgery. Tissue quality, injury severity, and stability after repair play into this decision. Augmentation is achieved with a tendon graft (autograft or allograft) or a synthetic internal brace. Specifics on preferred reconstruction techniques were discussed in the previous chapter (Fig. 23-9).

Internal bracing is gaining popularity. Lubowitz et al. recently published their technique of internal bracing for medial side ligament repairs (17). Internal bracing utilizes ultra–high-molecular-weight polyethylene/polyester suture tape and knotless bone anchors. Following repair, 4.75-mm knotless suture anchors are used at the sMCL femoral and distal tibial attachment sites. The femoral anchor is loaded with suture tape and placed at the femoral sMCL origin. Tensioning is completed while inserting the second 4.75-mm anchor along the posterior aspect of the distal tibial sMCL insertion site. A high-strength suture through the tibial periosteum just distal to the joint line is tied around the suture tape at the deep MCL insertion.

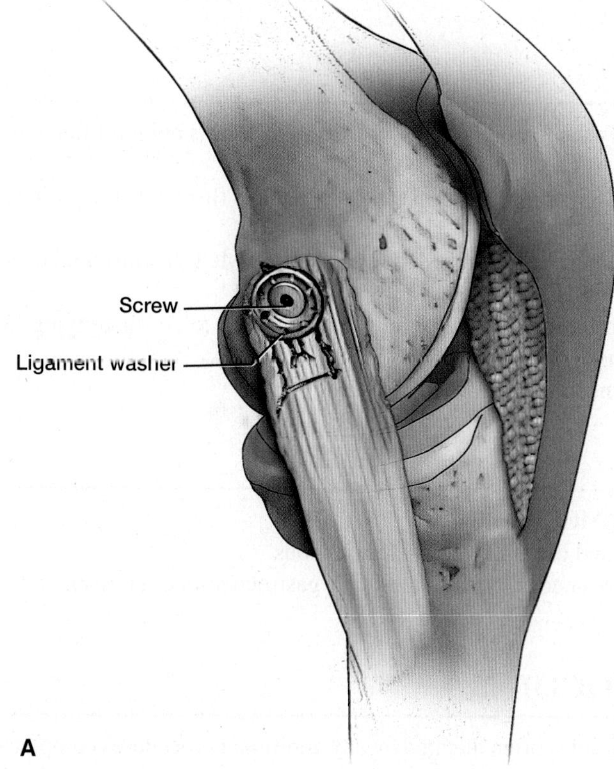

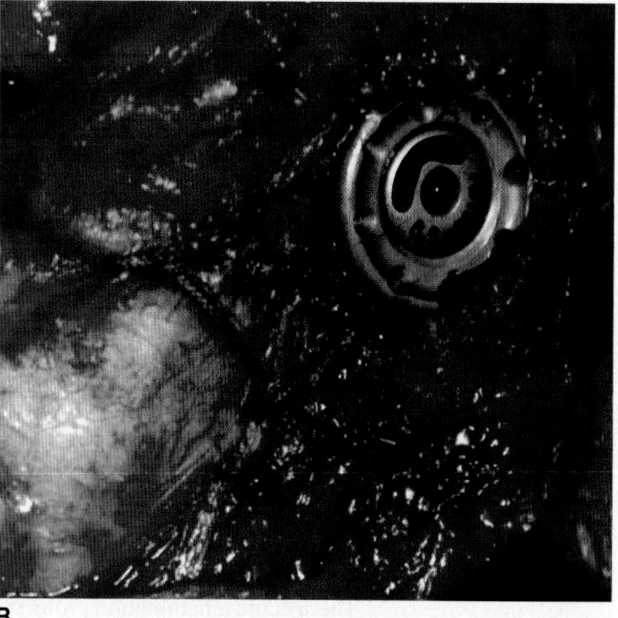

FIGURE 23-8

A, B: Femoral-sided repair with screw and washer, along with suture anchors posteriorly restoring the posteromedial capsule and POL.

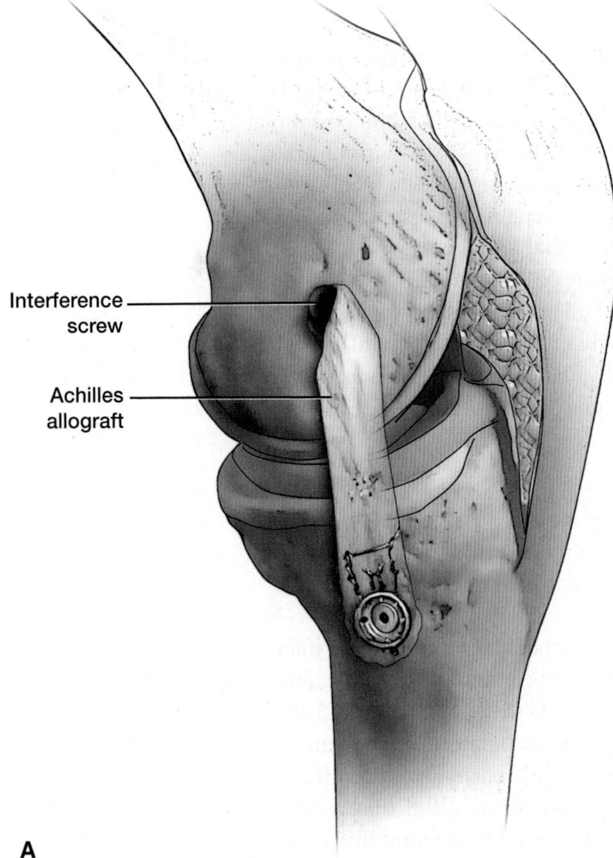

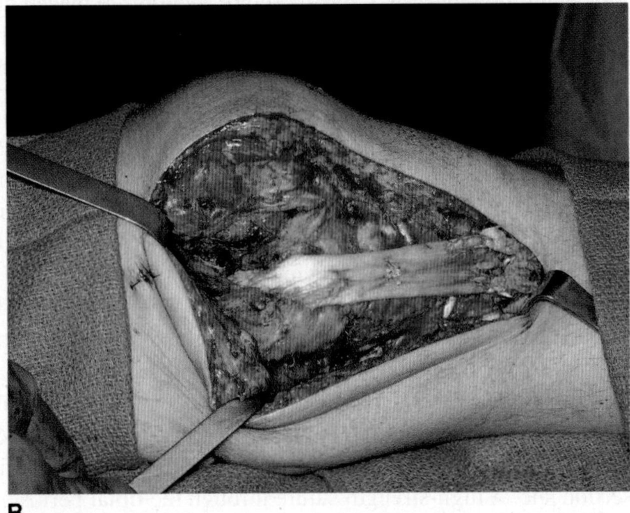

FIGURE 23-9

A, B: Acute MCL-PMC repair with Achilles allograft augmentation.

PEARLS

- Fluoroscopy is very helpful to identify the femoral sMCL insertion site, as this point is often more posterior than expected.
- Position the ligament washer at the distal tibial sMCL insertion so that it is flush with the posterior tibial border.
- Recreate both the proximal tibial attachments of the sMCL and the deep MCL (meniscotibial and meniscofemoral) with suture anchor repair.
- Start and exit the locking whipstitch on the undersurface of the ligament to facilitate tying the suture ends around the screw and washer.
- Tension the repair at 20 degrees of knee flexion with varus stress.

PITFALLS

- Failure to reestablish both deep and sMCL insertions
- Failure to reestablish both proximal and distal tibial sMCL insertions
- Failure to recognize and address associated injuries to the POL, gastrocnemius, semimembranosus, and posteromedial capsule

POSTOPERATIVE PROTOCOL

The specific rehabilitation protocol utilized is often dictated by any additional procedures completed in conjunction with the MCL repair. For the first 6 weeks, a hinged knee brace with a varus mold is worn at all times. When ambulating, the brace is locked in extension, but non–weight-bearing ROM to 90 degrees is allowed in the brace. Progressive weight bearing to tolerance with the brace unlocked is allowed after 6 weeks. By 12 weeks post-op, the patient will get a custom brace with a varus moment and full weight bearing is allowed.

COMPLICATIONS

In general, complications after sMCL repair appear to be minimal. The most commonly reported complication is arthrofibrosis, especially in the setting of multiligamentous injury (25,26). Approach to the medial aspect of the knee can put the saphenous nerve and its cutaneous braches at risk of injury, which can result in anesthesia or neuroma (25,27). Prominent hardware at either the tibia or femoral epicondyle can cause pain, which is commonly resolved with hardware removal.

Complications

- *Arthrofibrosis*
- *Saphenous nerve injury*
- *Irritable hardware*
- *Continued instability*

OUTCOMES

Medial collateral ligament tears are among the most common ligamentous injury of the knee. Fortunately, the vast majority can be managed nonoperatively with functional rehabilitation. There is still considerable controversy over which MCL injuries should be surgically addressed.

Biomechanical studies have demonstrated a significant increase in valgus laxity in dog and rabbit knee models with combined ACL-MCL injuries when the MCL is treated nonsurgically versus repair (28,29). Conversely, a similar animal study has shown that the difference in valgus laxity and tissue quality is only present in the short term, with no difference 1 year after injury (30).

O'Donoghue in the 1950s was the first to publish his case descriptions on acute repair of the MCL and medial supporting structures (31). In 1972, Hughston published his series on 50 athletes after MCL and PMC repair demonstrating excellent stability and return to play (32). Hughston and Eilers were the first to stress the importance of addressing the medial supporting structures in MCL repair to restore knee stability (32).

Clinical series comparing ACL-MCL injured knees undergoing combined ACL reconstruction and MCL repair versus solitary ACL reconstruction have not shown significant differences (33–35). Noyes and Barber-Westin looked at 46 patients with combined ACL-MCL injury with the MCL treated nonsurgically in 12 patients and repaired in 34. While there was no difference in sagittal laxity at 5 years, it should be noted that the surgically treated MCLs had clinically higher-grade medial-sided injuries than did the conservatively treated group. In a randomized prospective study of 47 patients, Halinen et al. found no significant difference between surgical and nonsurgical management of the MCL in ACL-MCL injured knees. In a review of the literature on combined ACL-MCL injuries, Grant et al. (36) concluded that any surgery should be delayed until ROM, quadriceps activation, and swelling have normalized. Furthermore, at the time of ACL reconstruction, persistent valgus laxity should be treated with MCL repair or reconstruction.

There is a dearth of literature to guide the treatment of combined MCL-ACL-PCL injuries. Commonly the MCL is surgically repaired in these injuries, although there is evidence supporting nonoperative treatment. A study by Fanelli et al. (37) demonstrated equal stability in MCL/ACL/PCL injuries treated with 6 weeks of bracing followed by arthroscopic ACL/PCL reconstruction compared to those MCLs treated with primary repair. However, the authors did not report if the clinical outcome scores differed between the two groups.

Repair versus reconstruction of the MCL is also controversial. While the current literature favors reconstruction over repair of the PLC, the literature for medial-sided injuries is less definitive (38,39). Wijdicks et al. (40) published a biomechanical comparison of anatomic repair versus reconstruction of the sMCL in 18 cadaveric knees and found no statistically significant difference in knee kinematics or joint stability.

Kovachevich et al. were unable to find statistically significant different results between repair and reconstruction in their systematic review of the current literature (9). The authors identified inconsistencies in the classification systems, objective outcome scores and levels of evidence, which makes it difficult to judge superiority of either technique (9). Stannard et al. (15) published on a series of 73 knee dislocations with 25 of these undergoing repair of the PMC and 48 treated with PMC reconstruction. The authors found a 20% failure rate in the repair group versus a significantly less failure rate of 4% in the reconstruction group. Recently, Dong et al. (16) reported on 64 patients with a grade III MCL injury and ACL tear with a mean 34-month follow-up. The patients were equally divided between anatomic repair and ligament reconstruction with no clinically significant outcome score difference reported at final follow-up. The authors did report significantly higher postoperative anteromedial rotatory instability in the repair group.

CONCLUSION

In conclusion, initial decision-making when addressing a MCL injury is of paramount importance. The overwhelming majority of MCL injuries are appropriately managed nonoperatively, but it is essential to recognize factors that may favor operative treatment. Concomitant injuries, tear location, and extent of injury all play key roles in decision-making. If surgical management is chosen, the decision to proceed with acute repair, repair with augmentation, or reconstruction is made in combination with both preoperative and intraoperative assessment. With careful selection, acute repair of an MCL-PMC injury can have excellent short- and long-term outcomes.

REFERENCES

1. Wijdicks CA, et al. Injuries to the medial collateral ligament and associated medial structures of the knee. *J Bone Joint Surg Am.* 2010;92(5):1266–1280.
2. Daniel DM, et al. Daniel's knee injuries: ligament and cartilage: structure, function, injury, and repair, 2003:xvii, 636 p. ill. (some col.) 29 cm + 1 CD ROM (4 3/4 in.)]. Available from Publisher description http://www.loc.gov/catdir/enhancements/fy0711/2002035293-d.html
3. Elliott M, Johnson DL. Management of medial-sided knee injuries. *Orthopedics.* 2015;38(3):180–184.
4. Phisitkul P, et al. MCL injuries of the knee: current concepts review. *Iowa Orthop J.* 2006;26:77–90.
5. Petermann J, von Garrel T, Gotzen L. Non-operative treatment of acute medial collateral ligament lesions of the knee joint. *Knee Surg Sports Traumatol Arthrosc.* 1993;1(2):93–96.
6. Holden DL, Eggert AW, Butler JE. The nonoperative treatment of grade I and II medial collateral ligament injuries to the knee. *Am J Sports Med.* 1983;11(5):340–344.
7. Woo SL, Vogrin TM, Abramowitch SD. Healing and repair of ligament injuries in the knee. *J Am Acad Orthop Surg.* 2000;8(6):364–372.
8. Anderson DR, et al. Healing of the medial collateral ligament following a triad injury: a biomechanical and histological study of the knee in rabbits. *J Orthop Res.* 1992;10(4):485–495.
9. Kovachevich R, et al. Operative management of the medial collateral ligament in the multi-ligament injured knee: an evidence-based systematic review. *Knee Surg Sports Traumatol Arthrosc.* 2009;17(7):823–829.
10. Bollier M, Smith PA. Anterior cruciate ligament and medial collateral ligament injuries. *J Knee Surg.* 2014;27(5):359–368.
11. Wilson TC, Satterfield WH, Johnson DL. Medial collateral ligament "tibial" injuries: indication for acute repair. *Orthopedics.* 2004;27(4):389–393.
12. Corten K, et al. Case reports: a Stener-like lesion of the medial collateral ligament of the knee. *Clin Orthop Relat Res.* 2010;468(1):289–293.
13. Taketomi S, et al. Clinical features and injury patterns of medial collateral ligament tibial side avulsions: "wave sign" on magnetic resonance imaging is essential for diagnosis. *Knee.* 2014;21(6):1151–1155.
14. Kuroda R, et al. Avulsion fracture of the posterior oblique ligament associated with acute tear of the medial collateral ligament. *Arthroscopy.* 2003;19(3):E18.
15. Stannard JP, et al. Posteromedial corner injury in knee dislocations. *J Knee Surg.* 2012;25(5):429–434.
16. Dong J, et al. Surgical treatment of acute grade III medial collateral ligament injury combined with anterior cruciate ligament injury: anatomic ligament repair versus triangular ligament reconstruction. *Arthroscopy.* 2015;31(6):1108–1116.
17. Lubowitz JH, MacKay G, Gilmer B. Knee medial collateral ligament and posteromedial corner anatomic repair with internal bracing. *Arthrosc Tech.* 2014;3(4):e505–e508.
18. Court-Brown CM, et al. *Rockwood and Green's Fractures in Adults.* Philadelphia: Wolters Kluwer Health; 2015:1 online resource (xv, 2774 p.).
19. Yoo JC, et al. Measurement and comparison of the difference in normal medial and lateral knee joint opening. *Knee Surg Sports Traumatol Arthrosc.* 2006;14(12):1238–1244.
20. Robinson JR, et al. The role of the medial collateral ligament and posteromedial capsule in controlling knee laxity. *Am J Sports Med.* 2006;34(11):1815–1823.
21. Laprade RF, et al. Correlation of valgus stress radiographs with medial knee ligament injuries: an in vitro biomechanical study. *Am J Sports Med.* 2010;38(2):330–338.
22. LaPrade RF, et al. The anatomy of the medial part of the knee. *J Bone Joint Surg Am.* 2007;89(9):2000–2010.
23. Leiter JR, et al. Accuracy and reliability of determining the isometric point of the knee for multiligament knee reconstruction. *Knee Surg Sports Traumatol Arthrosc.* 2014;22(9):2187–2193.
24. Wijdicks CA, et al. Radiographic identification of the primary medial knee structures. *J Bone Joint Surg Am.* 2009;91(3):521–529.
25. Tibor LM, et al. Management of medial-sided knee injuries, part 2: posteromedial corner. *Am J Sports Med.* 2011;39(6):1332–1340.
26. Klimkiewicz JJ, Petrie RS, Harner CD. Surgical treatment of combined injury to anterior cruciate ligament, posterior cruciate ligament, and medial structures. *Clin Sports Med.* 2000;19(3):479–492, vii.

27. Benjamin Jackson J III, Ferguson CM, Martin DF. Surgical treatment of chronic posteromedial instability using capsular procedures. *Sports Med Arthrosc.* 2006;14(2):91–95.
28. Woo SL, et al. The effects of transection of the anterior cruciate ligament on healing of the medial collateral ligament. A biomechanical study of the knee in dogs. *J Bone Joint Surg Am.* 1990;72(3):382–392.
29. Ohno K, et al. Healing of the medial collateral ligament after a combined medial collateral and anterior cruciate ligament injury and reconstruction of the anterior cruciate ligament: comparison of repair and nonrepair of medial collateral ligament tears in rabbits. *J Orthop Res.* 1995;13(3):442–449.
30. Yamaji T, et al. Medial collateral ligament healing one year after a concurrent medial collateral ligament and anterior cruciate ligament injury: an interdisciplinary study in rabbits. *J Orthop Res.* 1996;14(2):223–227.
31. O'Donoghue DH. Surgical treatment of fresh injuries to the major ligaments of the knee. *J Bone Joint Surg Am.* 1950;32A(4):721–738.
32. Hughston JC, Eilers AF. The role of the posterior oblique ligament in repairs of acute medial (collateral) ligament tears of the knee. *J Bone Joint Surg Am.* 1973;55(5):923–940.
33. Noyes FR, Barber-Westin SD. The treatment of acute combined ruptures of the anterior cruciate and medial ligaments of the knee. *Am J Sports Med.* 1995;23(4):380–389.
34. Halinen J, et al. Operative and nonoperative treatments of medial collateral ligament rupture with early anterior cruciate ligament reconstruction: a prospective randomized study. *Am J Sports Med.* 2006;34(7):1134–1140.
35. Hillard-Sembell D, et al. Combined injuries of the anterior cruciate and medial collateral ligaments of the knee. Effect of treatment on stability and function of the joint. *J Bone Joint Surg Am.* 1996;78(2):169–176.
36. Grant JA, et al. Treatment of combined complete tears of the anterior cruciate and medial collateral ligaments. *Arthroscopy.* 2012;28(1):110–122.
37. Fanelli GC, Giannotti BF, Edson CJ. Arthroscopically assisted combined anterior and posterior cruciate ligament reconstruction. *Arthroscopy.* 1996;12(1):5–14.
38. Levy BA, et al. Repair versus reconstruction of the fibular collateral ligament and posterolateral corner in the multiligament-injured knee. *Am J Sports Med.* 2010;38(4):804–809.
39. Stannard JP, et al. The posterolateral corner of the knee: repair versus reconstruction. *Am J Sports Med.* 2005;33(6):881–888.
40. Wijdicks CA, et al. Superficial medial collateral ligament anatomic augmented repair versus anatomic reconstruction: an in vitro biomechanical analysis. *Am J Sports Med.* 2013;41(12):2858–2866.

24 Reconstruction of the Medial Collateral Ligament of the Knee

Daniel C. Wascher, Gehron Treme, and Heather Menzer

INTRODUCTION

Although injuries to the medial collateral ligament (MCL) of the knee are common, reconstruction of the MCL is only rarely done. The superficial MCL (sMCL) is the primary restraint to valgus loads and is a secondary restraint to rotational loads. Additionally, the posteromedial capsule (PMC) and posterior oblique ligament provide rotational stability and resistance to valgus stress with the knee in extension. The MCL is usually injured by a direct valgus blow to the knee but can also be injured in severe rotational injuries. Nonoperative treatment of isolated tears of the MCL typically results in good stability and allows the athlete to return to full activity. Even in association with cruciate ligament injuries, most partial and complete MCL tears can be successfully treated with nonoperative means. However, there is a small but important subgroup of MCL injuries that will require surgical treatment. A number of MCL reconstruction techniques have been proposed, but only a handful of these have reported clinical outcomes. In this chapter, we present our technique for reconstruction of the MCL of the knee.

SURGICAL INDICATIONS

Several authors have demonstrated that nonoperative treatment of acute, isolated MCL injuries is superior to operative treatment. Treatment of these isolated injuries involves brace protection of the ligament, early range of motion, and gait training, followed by a progressive functional rehabilitation program. Most athletes with acute and isolated injuries can return to play within 6 weeks. Though the majority of isolated MCL injuries heal rapidly with excellent functional results, occasionally these injuries heal with residual valgus laxity. An isolated MCL reconstruction should be considered for those patients who have functional instability with activities.

It is important to recognize MCL injuries that require early surgical treatment in order to achieve good functional results. Early surgical repair is necessary for bony avulsions, MCL tears with tissue incarcerated in the medial compartment, and "Stener-type" lesions where the sMCL has flipped superficial to the pes anserine tendons. If recognized early, these injuries can usually be treated with primary repair of the MCL with good results. Occasionally if there is a mid-substance rupture or if the MCL injury is identified late, poor tissue quality necessitates reconstruction of the MCL.

The most common indication for reconstruction of the MCL involves combined ligament injuries. These include concomitant injuries to the anterior cruciate ligament (ACL), posterior cruciate ligament (PCL), or bicruciate injuries as seen in knee dislocations (Schenck KD III-M or KD IV). The cruciate ligaments function as secondary stabilizers to valgus stress, and cruciate tears can diminish the healing potential of the MCL. Likewise, it has been shown in biomechanical and animal studies that untreated MCL injuries can increase the loads on cruciate ligament grafts and result in residual anteroposterior laxity. Therefore, multiligament knee injuries are the most frequent indication for surgical reconstruction of the MCL. Although some combined injuries will have successful healing of the MCL with bracing and subsequent cruciate ligament reconstruction, occasionally these knees will have persistent valgus instability. Our approach has been to protect the knee in a hinged brace, decrease swelling, and regain range of motion. If 6 weeks later there is persistent 2+ or greater valgus laxity or residual extension laxity, we reconstruct the MCL at the time of cruciate ligament reconstruction. Since all ligaments of the knee have primary and secondary roles in stability, failure to address all pathologic laxity can result in recurrent laxity and a loss of the stability gained with the initial surgery.

SURGICAL CONTRAINDICATIONS

Surgical contraindications to MCL reconstruction are uncommon. Abrasions, cellulitis, and extensive bruising can impede wound healing and increase the risk of infection. Surgery should be delayed until the skin is in good condition. Loss of motion is a relative contraindication to multiple ligament reconstruction. Preoperative stiffness increases the risk of arthrofibrosis from these extensive surgical procedures. In most instances, we prefer to delay surgery and achieve functional range of motion prior to reconstruction. The surgeon must have a high index of suspicion for deep venous thrombosis. Any identified thrombosis should be adequately treated prior to surgical reconstruction. Finally, as most MCL reconstructions also involve cruciate ligament reconstruction(s), these patients face a challenging rehabilitation program. Associated skeletal injuries or closed head trauma necessitates delaying surgery until the patient can participate in a rehabilitation program.

PREOPERATIVE PLANNING

Clinical evaluation begins with a thorough history describing the mechanism of injury, symptoms (pain, swelling, instability), and any previous treatment. A thorough physical exam of the knee is necessary to define the extent of the injury. A hemarthrosis suggests an intra-articular injury (cruciate ligament or fracture). Isolated MCL injuries often present with localized medial swelling and ecchymosis. Tenderness is usually reported over the entire ligament, with maximum focal tenderness over the point of rupture. The grade of injury is based on medial opening with an applied valgus stress at 0 and 30 degrees of flexion compared to uninjured knee. Medial opening of less than 5 mm defines 1+ laxity, 5 to 10 mm indicates 2+ laxity, and 3+ laxity is present if the joint opens more than 10 mm. Valgus laxity in full extension is indicative of posterior oblique ligament (POL) involvement and suggests a combined ligament injury, most commonly injury to the ACL. A careful neurovascular assessment must be documented if a knee dislocation with multiligament injury is suspected. Any abnormality on vascular exam requires further investigation. Knee radiographs should be obtained to evaluate for bony avulsions or lateral tibial plateau fractures. Though not mandatory, stress views comparing to the uninjured limb can be useful to quantify the degree of laxity. Magnetic resonance imaging helps identify the location of the MCL injury, detects "Stener" lesions, and will aid in identifying injuries to articular cartilage, meniscus, or cruciate ligaments. Long leg radiographs are useful in chronic injuries or in patients with marked valgus alignment in which an osteotomy is considered prior to MCL reconstruction.

SURGICAL TECHNIQUE

In order to restore medial stability in the coronal and axial planes we address both the PMC/POL complex as well as the sMCL in our reconstruction. A free hamstring graft is used for the sMCL. A cadaveric study has shown improved biomechanics with a two-stranded graft. The surgeon can utilize a doubled semitendinosus (ST) autograft, both ST and gracilis autografts, or two allograft hamstring tendons. The choice of the graft is frequently affected by the choice of the ACL graft since the two are done together in most situations. The use of allograft tendons provides more graft length, which helps avoid other tibial tunnels in multiligament reconstructions and allows the use of the patient's own hamstrings to reconstruct the ACL. We describe the allograft technique below, but the technique is easily adjusted for use of autograft if the surgeon prefers.

As the length of the sMCL is between 10 and 12 cm, cutting the two hamstring allografts to 16 to 18 cm allows for adequate graft length in the tunnels. Each graft is independently whipstitched at each end with a No. 2 nonabsorbable suture. The grafts are saved on the back table in a damp sponge for later use. With the knee flexed and the hip externally rotated, a curvilinear incision is made along the medial side of the knee from just proximal to the medial epicondyle to the distal aspect of the sMCL. The sartorius fascia is split in line with its fibers and reflected anteriorly and posteriorly to expose the sMCL (Fig. 24-1). This layer blends with the capsule anteriorly, but minimal dissection

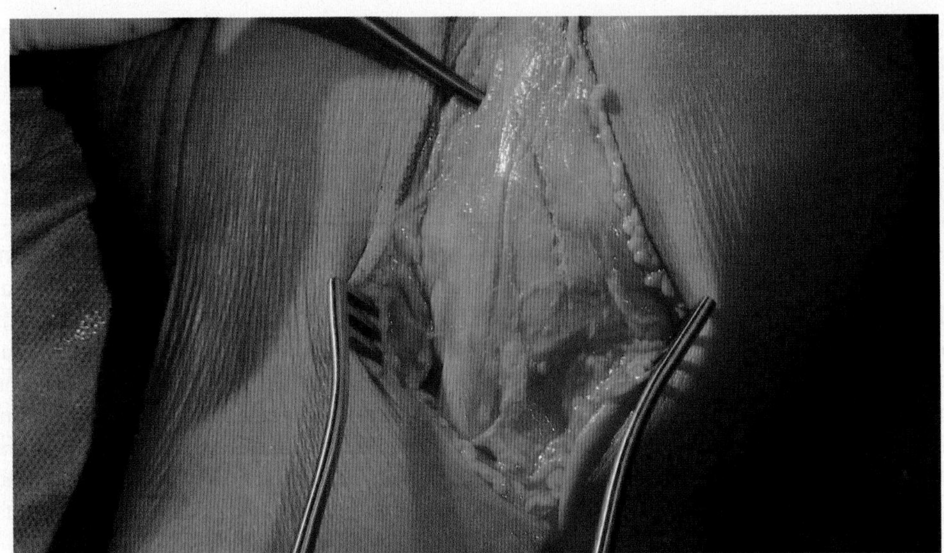

FIGURE 24-1
Exposure of the superficial MCL after splitting the sartorius fascia. The forceps are at the level of the joint line.

is needed in that direction. There is frequent scarring of this layer, and careful dissection is required in order to remain in the proper plane. Remnant fibers of the sMCL are generally readily identifiable and can be used as a landmark for this step.

The PMC complex is identified just posterior to the sMCL at the level of the joint line. This area is readily palpable as a soft spot at the posterior medial corner of the knee joint. A 2- to 3-cm vertical incision is made through the capsule with great care taken to protect the underlying meniscus (Fig. 24-2). The capsule is then repaired with 3 to 4 high-strength No. 2 nonabsorbable sutures in "a pants over vest" technique in which the posterior leaf is advanced over the top of the anterior leaf. All sutures are placed prior to tying, and the knee is then positioned in 15 degrees of flexion for suture tying. Tying sutures in deeper flexion can result in a postoperative contracture or in loss of repair integrity. The repair is then oversewn with another No. 2 suture for reinforcement (Fig. 24-3). With the PMC imbricated, attention is turned to the reconstruction of the sMCL.

The insertion sites of the sMCL are identified on the femur and tibia. The adductor tendon and tubercle, the insertion site for the MPFL, and the medial epicondyle are all palpated to achieve proper

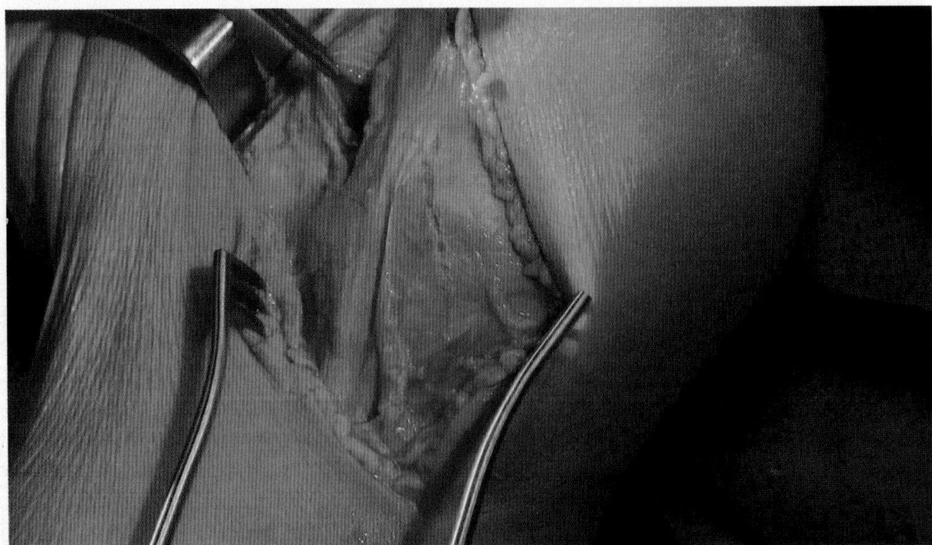

FIGURE 24-2
Opening of the posteromedial capsule.

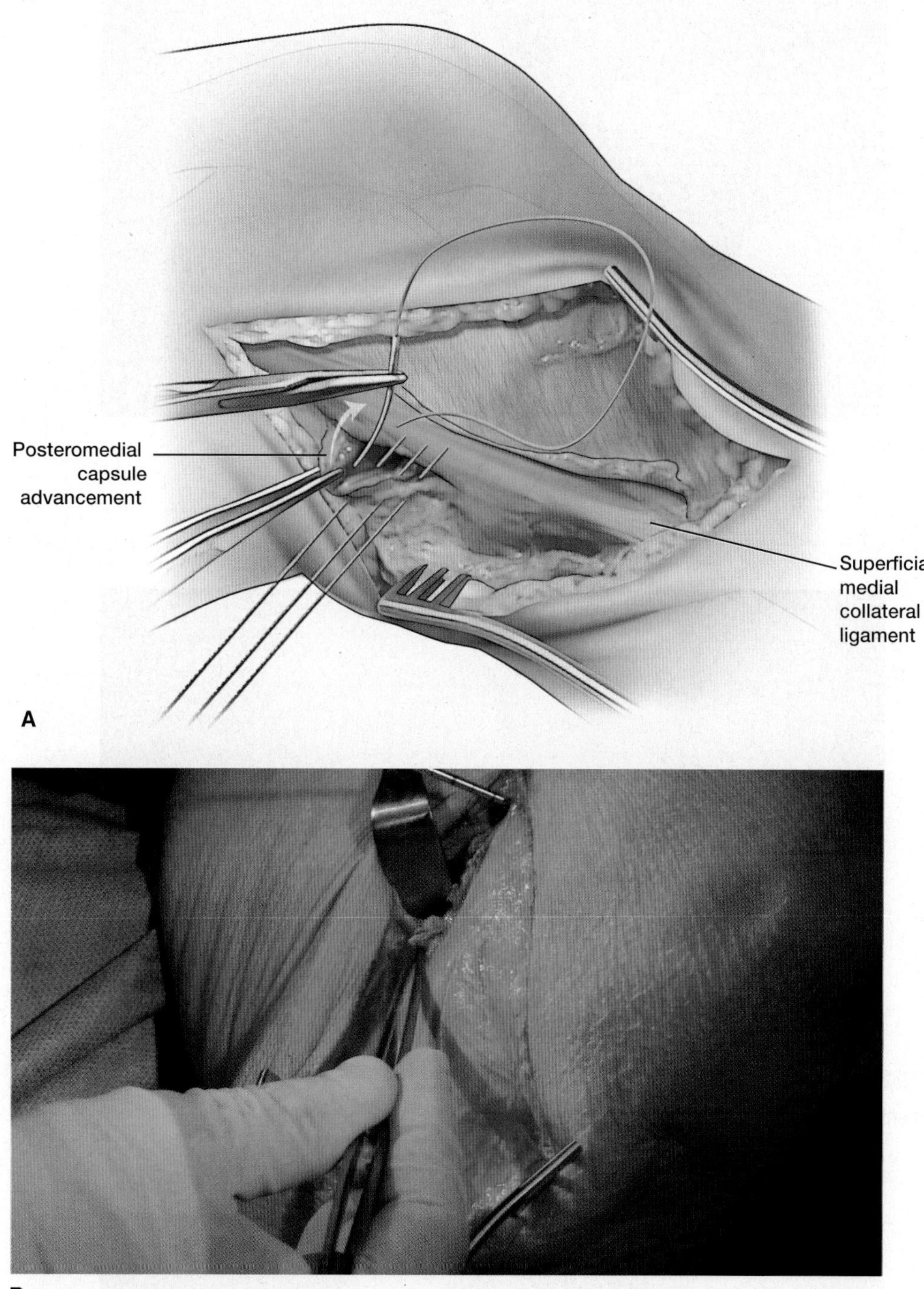

FIGURE 24-3

A, B: Advancement of the posteromedial capsule with No. 2 suture.

orientation. An eyelet guide pin is placed a few mm proximal and posterior to the medial epicondyle and driven through the lateral cortex and out of the lateral skin of the thigh. If the surgeon is having difficulty locating the correct position, fluoroscopy can be helpful. A second eyelet pin is placed in the tibia in the center of the distal one-third of the sMCL. The graft length should be checked in this step in order to place the pin appropriately (Fig. 24-4). Approximately 25 mm of graft will be delivered into the tibia and 30 to 40 mm of graft in the femur, and the tibial pin should be placed in a position that allows the surgeon to achieve both of these criteria (Fig. 24-5). This pin is unicortical and should not be advanced through the lateral cortex of the tibia to minimize the risk of fracture.

Once both pins are placed and location checked against the graft, the pins are overreamed with an 8-mm reamer to, but not through, their respective lateral cortices (Fig. 24-6). Soft tissue should

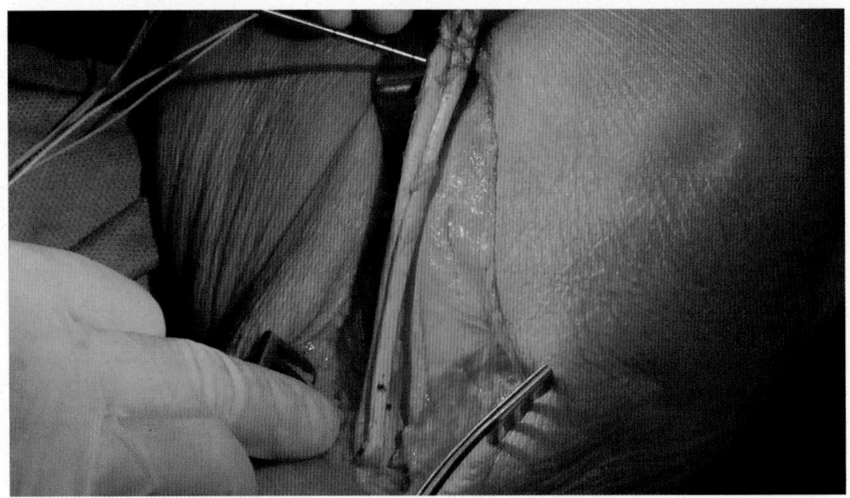

FIGURE 24-4

Measuring graft length prior to placing tibial guide pin.

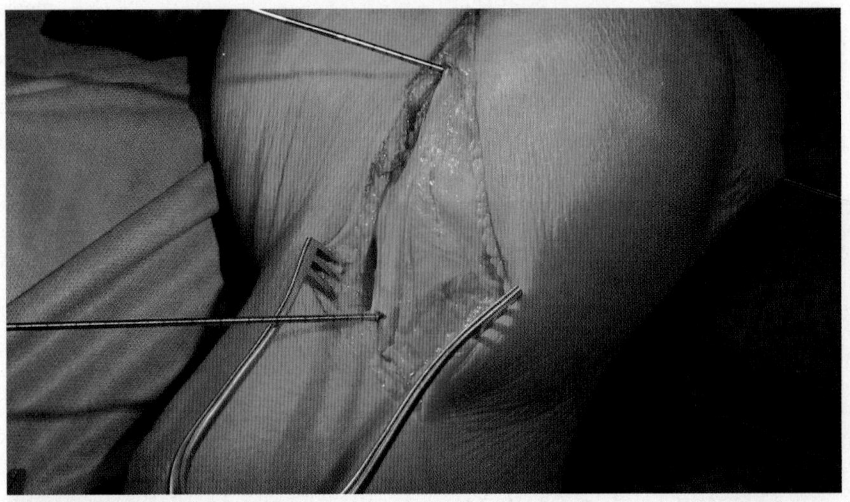

FIGURE 24-5

Placement of femoral and tibial guide pins.

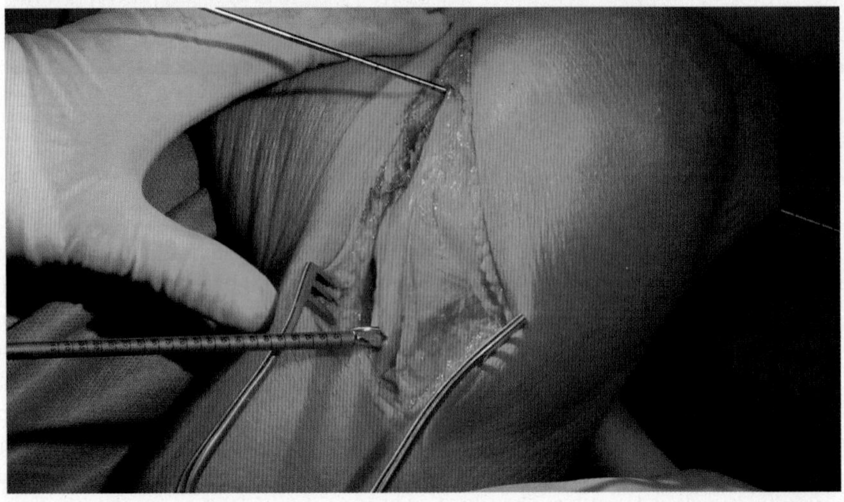

FIGURE 24-6

Reaming of tibial tunnel with 8-mm drill.

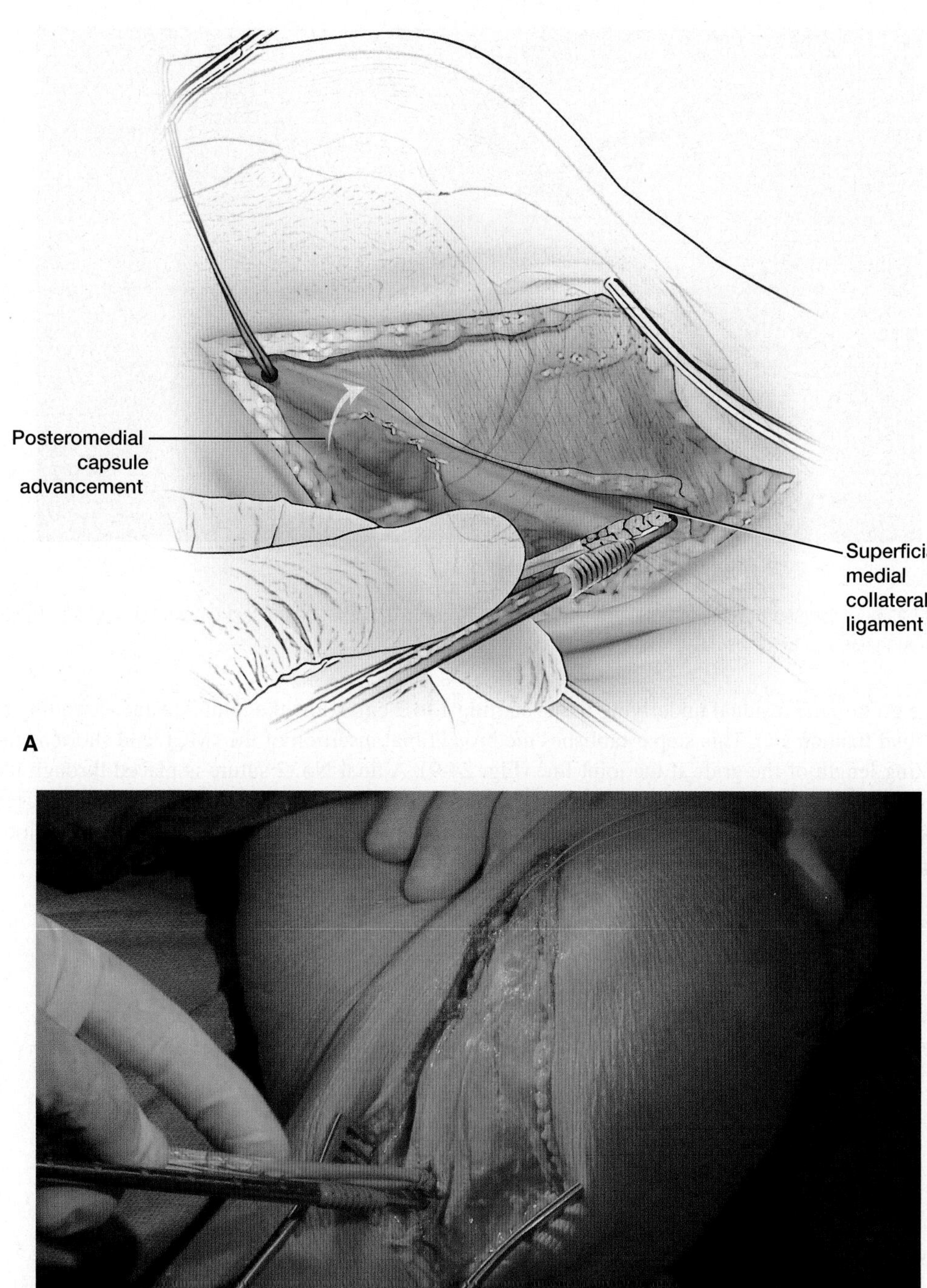

FIGURE 24-7

A, B: Fixation of tibial side of graft with 8 × 23 mm PEEK Bio-Tenodesis screw. Note passing suture exiting femoral tunnel.

be cleaned around the tunnel aperture to improve graft passage, and a passing suture is placed in the femoral tunnel. The free ends of the allograft tendons are then placed into the tibial tunnel using a Bio-Tenodesis driver (Arthrex, Naples, FL) and secured there with an 8 × 23 mm PEEK interference screw (Fig. 24-7). Sutures from the end of the graft are tied to enhance fixation. The graft is then passed into the femoral tunnel and tensioned at 30 degrees of flexion with neutral rotation and a varus stress. Once adequate tension is achieved, the graft is secured with a 9 × 23 mm PEEK interference screw (Fig. 24-8). Final fixation of the MCL reconstruction should be performed after cruciate ligament fixation. Several No. 2 non-absorbable sutures are used to secure the tibial side

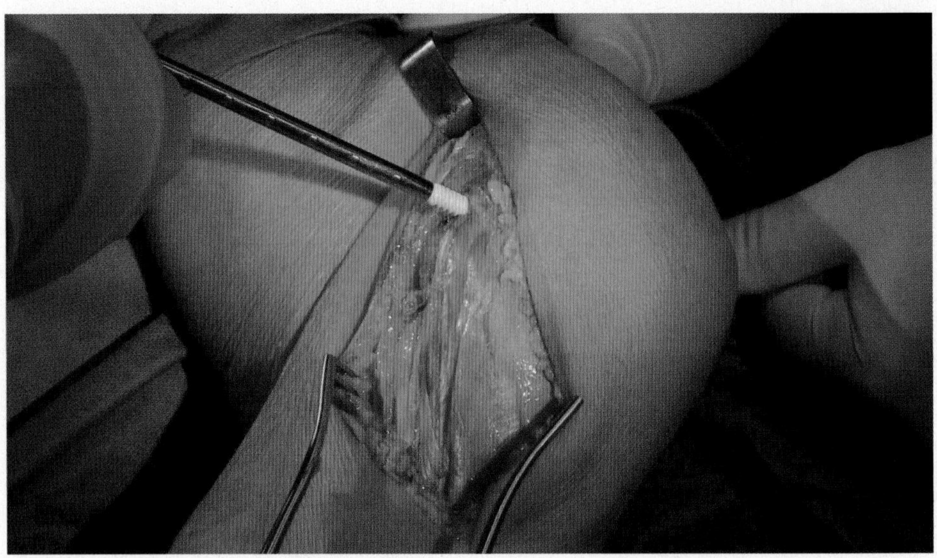

FIGURE 24-8

Graft has been passed into the femoral tunnel, has been tensioned, and is being secured with 9 × 23 mm PEEK Bio-Tenodesis screw.

of the graft to the residual underlying tissue starting 1 to 2 cm below the joint line and extending to the tibial fixation site. This step establishes the broad tibial insertion of the sMCL and shortens the working length of the graft at the joint line (Fig. 24-9). A final No. 2 suture is placed through the native soft tissue and the graft at the femur aperture to backup fixation there. The knee is checked for stability and motion, and closure is performed in a standard manner. The knee is placed in a long hinged brace locked in full extension before leaving the operating room.

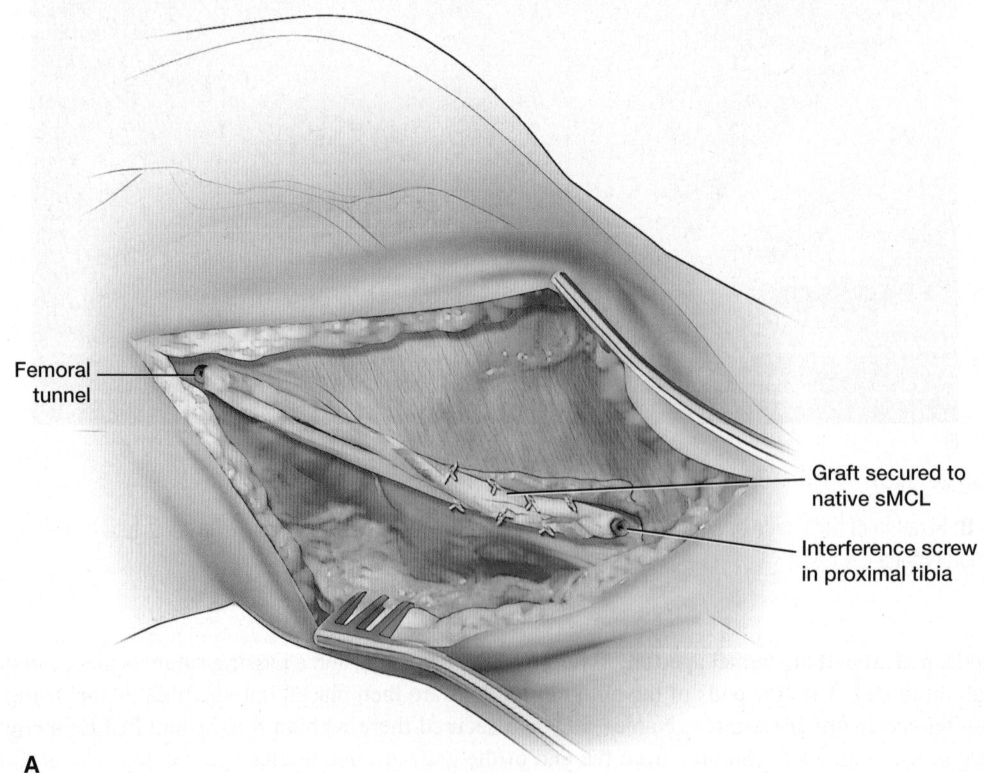

FIGURE 24-9

A, B: Graft has been secured to the native MCL tissue along the entire course of the tibial attachment with No. 2 suture.

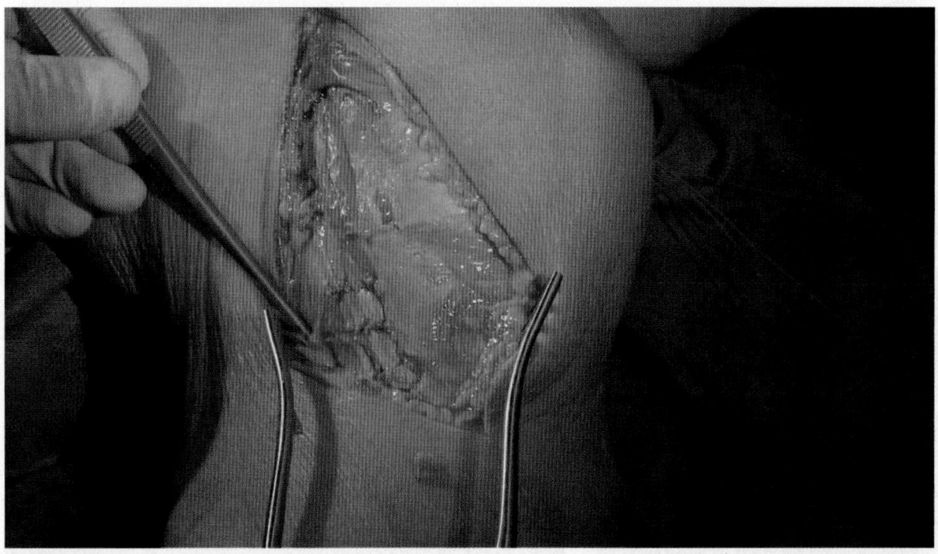

B

FIGURE 24-9 (*Continued*)

POSTOPERATIVE MANAGEMENT

As MCL reconstruction frequently occurs in conjunction with an ACL reconstruction, the postoperative course of this combination will be described here. The patient is discharged from the outpatient surgery center in a long-hinged knee brace locked in extension. They are made 50% weight bearing in the brace with physical therapy to start 2 weeks post operatively. They are placed on 325 mg of aspirin daily as prophylaxis against deep venous thrombosis unless they have additional risk factors that would necessitate more aggressive prevention strategies. The patient is seen at the 2-week post-op mark, sutures are removed, and therapy is started using a standard ACL rehab protocol. Range of motion and weight bearing are advanced to full at this time, and the brace is opened to full motion and left in place for a total of 6 weeks after surgery. Following this protocol, the patient is allowed to run at 3 months post-op and advanced to cutting and sports-specific activities during the second 3 months of recovery. Patients return to sports along the same time course as those with an isolated ACL reconstruction.

COMPLICATIONS TO AVOID

Most of the complications associated with MCL reconstruction are those common to other knee ligament surgery. Residual laxity can arise from improper tunnel placement, inadequate graft tension/fixation, or overly aggressive rehabilitation. Loss of motion can also be a result of improper tunnel placement or an overly cautious rehabilitation program. Symptomatic hardware is common with screw/washer fixation, but we have not seen that problem with interference fixation. Wound healing issues can arise from a postoperative hematoma. The surgeon must obtain meticulous hemostasis and use a drain if there is persistent oozing from the bone tunnels. Prophylactic antibiotics should minimize the risk of wound infection. Deep venous thrombosis prophylaxis should be given until the patient is fully weight bearing. With careful surgical technique and appropriate rehabilitation, most complications can be avoided.

ILLUSTRATIVE CASE

A 17-year-old male presented 10 days after sustaining a valgus injury to his right knee during a high-school football game. He felt a pop, felt his knee give way, and was unable to bear weight on his leg. On physical examination, he had range of motion from 10 to 70 degrees. There was a moderate effusion and soft tissue swelling over the medial side of the knee. There was a 2+ Lachman and 3+ valgus laxity. He was stable to posterior drawer and varus stress. He was point tender over the proximal medial tibia. Radiographs were unremarkable. An MRI scan revealed a complete ACL tear (Fig. 24-10A) and a complete tear of the sMCL at its distal insertion (Fig. 24-10B). He was placed in a long-leg hinged knee brace, kept partial weight bearing, and was begun on gentle range of motion exercises. Four weeks later, he had a mild effusion and full range of motion. On ligament exam, he

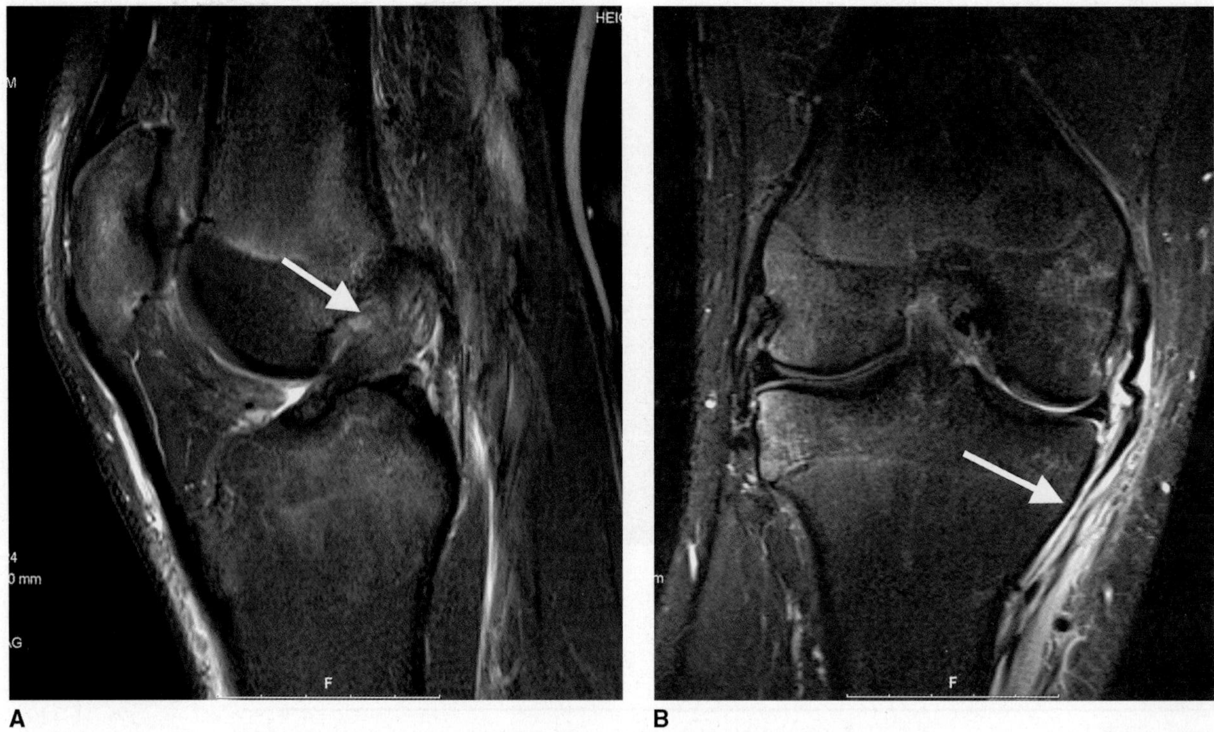

A B

FIGURE 24-10

MRI sagittal **(A)** image showing torn ACL (*arrow*) and coronal **(B)** image showing distal MCL tear (*arrow*).

had a 2+ Lachman and 3+ valgus laxity at 30 degrees of flexion. Six weeks post injury, he underwent surgical treatment. We performed an ACL reconstruction using autogenous bone-tendon-bone and an MCL reconstruction utilizing a doubled semitendinosus autograft using our described technique (Fig. 24-11). He was placed in a hinged knee brace locked in full extension and was made partial

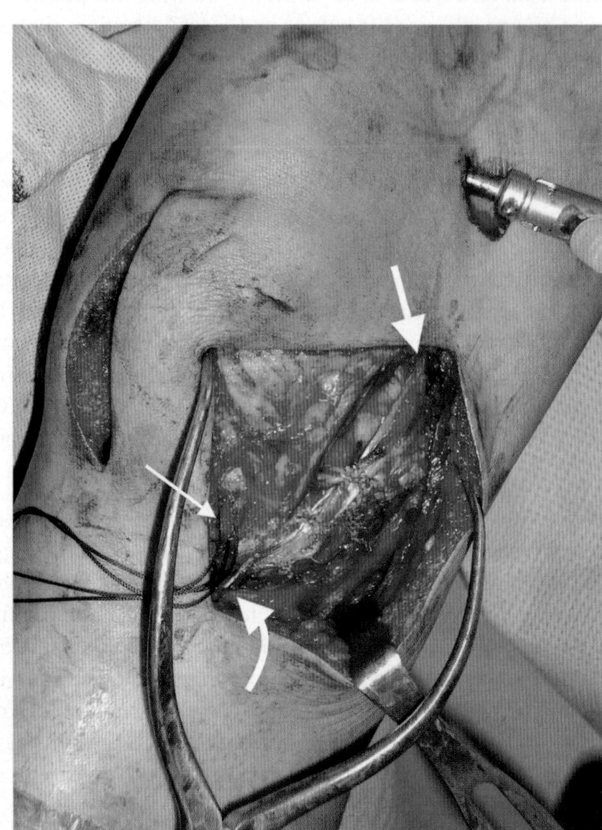

FIGURE 24-11

Intraoperative photograph showing completed MCL reconstruction. Femoral insertion (*large straight arrow*), tibial insertion (*large curved arrow*), and ACL tibial tunnel (*small arrow*).

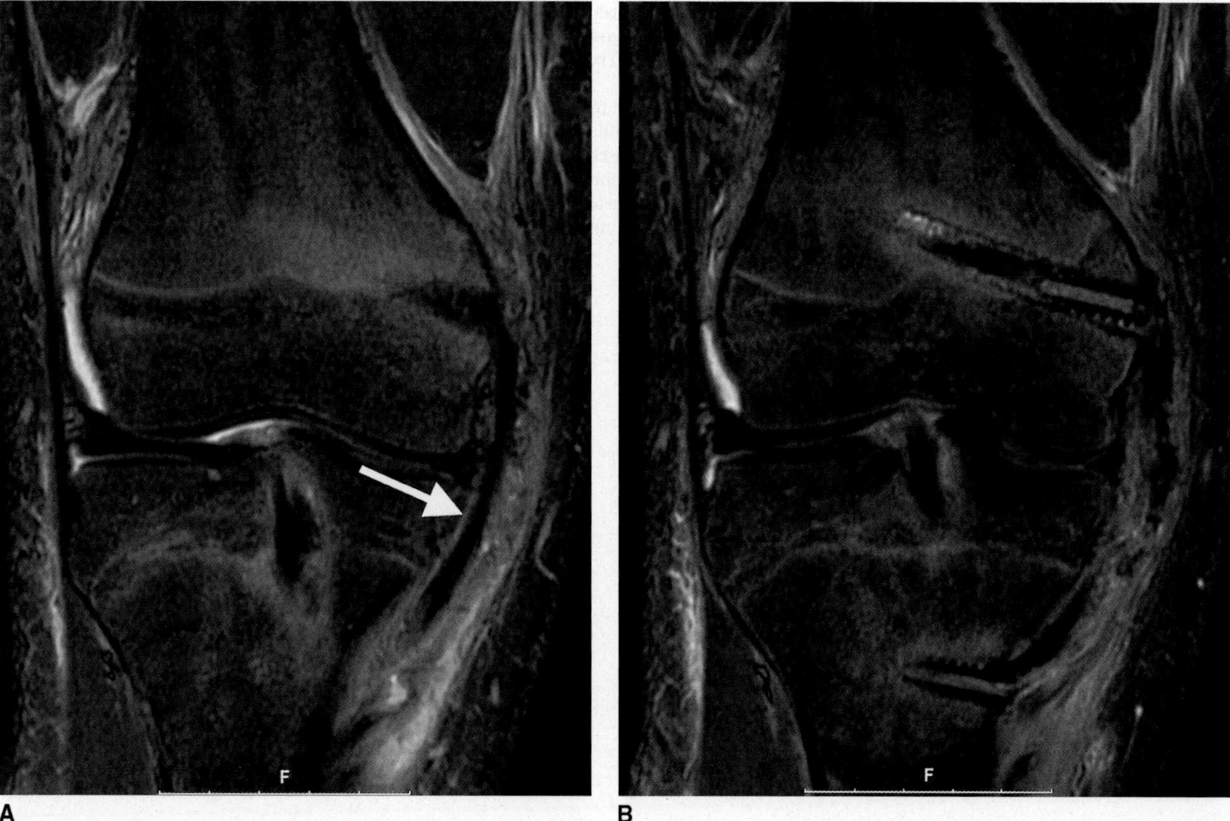

FIGURE 24-12

Postoperative coronal MRI images showing **(A)** intact graft (*arrow*) and **(B)** location of tunnels.

weight bearing. Five days post-op, the patient fell at home. His radiologist mother ordered an MRI scan of his knee, which showed intact grafts (Fig. 24-12). At 2 weeks, the patient was then allowed to increase his knee flexion and weight bearing as tolerated. At 6 weeks post-op, he was fitted with a functional knee brace for activities, and closed chain exercises were initiated. At 4 months, he was begun on a running program. At 6 months, agility drills were started. He had full range of motion and no laxity to Lachman or valgus stress testing.

PEARLS AND PITFALLS

- Examination under anesthesia, stress radiographs, and the amount of medial joint opening at the time of arthroscopy can help determine the need for MCL reconstruction.
- Reconstruct all injured ligaments at the same setting.
- The posteromedial capsular reefing should be tied with the knee in 15 degrees of flexion.
- The old sMCL fibers can be used to help find the femoral insertion site.
- Make sure there is adequate graft length prior to placing the tibial guide pin. As the tibial attachment is broad, the tibial tunnel can be placed slightly more proximally if the graft is short.
- Suture the graft to the old MCL tissue on the proximal tibia to recreate the broad tibial attachment of the sMCL.

RECOMMENDED READINGS

Benjamin Jackson J III, Ferguson CM, Martin DF. Surgical treatment of chronic posteromedial instability using capsular procedures. *Sports Med Arthrosc.* 2006;14(2):91–95.

Bosworth DM. Transplantation of the semitendinosus for repair of laceration of medial collateral ligament of the knee. *J Bone Joint Surg Am.* 1952;34-A(1):196–202.

Feeley BT, Muller MS, Allen AA, et al. Biomechanical comparison of medial collateral ligament reconstructions using computer-assisted navigation. *Am J Sports Med.* 2009;37(6):1123–1130.

Indelicato PA, Hermansdorfer J, Huegel M. Nonoperative management of complete tears of the medial collateral ligament of the knee in intercollegiate football players. *Clin Orthop Relat Res.* 1990;256:174–177.

Kim SJ, Lee DH, Kim TE, et al. Concomitant reconstruction of the medial collateral and posterior oblique ligaments for medial instability of the knee. *J Bone Joint Surg Br.* 2008;90(10):1323–1327.

LaPrade RF, Engebretsen AH, Ly TV, et al. The anatomy of the medial part of the knee. *J Bone Joint Surg Am.* 2007;89(9):2000–2010.

Lind M, Jakobsen BW, Lund B, et al. Anatomical reconstruction of the medial collateral ligament and posteromedial corner of the knee in patients with chronic medial collateral ligament instability. *Am J Sports Med.* 2009;37(6):1116–1122.

Yoshiya S, Kuroda R, Mizuno K, et al. Medial collateral ligament reconstruction using autogenous hamstring tendons: technique and results in initial cases. *Am J Sports Med.* 2005;33(9):1380–1385.

Zhang H, Sun Y, Han X, et al. Simultaneous reconstruction of the anterior cruciate ligament and medial collateral ligament in patients with chronic ACL-MCL lesions: a minimum 2-year follow-up study. *Am J Sports Med.* 2014;42(7):1675–1681.

25 Surgical Management of Acute Lateral Side Injuries

Elad Spitzer, John B. Doyle, Bruce A. Levy, and Robert G. Marx

INTRODUCTION

Injuries to the posterolateral corner (PLC) are uncommon but potentially very problematic for the patient. The most common mechanism of injury for this area of the knee involves a combined hyperextension and varus force that is frequently high energy, although it can also occur from lower-energy athletic injuries (1–3). Because of the force of the injury, other ligament injuries usually occur simultaneously, which makes the diagnosis and surgical reconstruction challenging (4). Associated injuries can include vascular compromise, injury to the common peroneal nerve, and periarticular fracture (5). If surgery is indicated due to a vascular injury or an irreducible knee dislocation, it may be appropriate to repair the lateral side injuries concomitantly. Conversely, acute surgical intervention to treat lateral side injuries may be delayed or not recommended based on the status of the extremity or other patient factors.

PHYSICAL EXAMINATION

Lateral side knee injuries (fibular collateral ligament [FCL] and posterolateral corner [PCL]) injuries are diagnosed according to the history, physical examination, and diagnostic imaging, including standard radiographs and magnetic resonance imaging (MRI). Examination begins with gait assessment, limb alignment, range of motion (ROM), and stability testing. Gait assessment is important to evaluate the presence of a varus thrust, and limb alignment is equally important, especially in the chronic setting to look for varus malalignment. An adductor thrust and varus malalignment are indications for a valgus-producing proximal tibial osteotomy prior to any ligament reconstruction surgery.

The FCL and PLC are evaluated with numerous tests, including varus stress at 0 and 30 degrees of knee flexion, tibial external rotation (Dial test) at 30 and 90 degrees of knee flexion, the posterolateral spin test (6), external rotation (posterolateral) drawer test at 90 degrees, external rotation recurvatum test, and the reverse pivot shift test. The varus stress test is usually graded as I, II, or III, for less than 5 mm, 5 to 10 mm, and greater than 10 mm of opening. The dial test is considered abnormal when side-to-side comparison demonstrates greater than 10 to 15 degrees of external rotation at either 30 or 90 degrees of flexion (7). A positive dial test at 30 degrees of flexion is indicative of an injury to the PLC, whereas a positive dial test at both 30 and 90 degrees is indicative of an injury to both the PLC and the PCL. Measurement error can occur in the dial test due to rotation of the tibia, ankle, or foot, however, and the posterolateral spin test can avoid this error by measuring the posterior lateral rotation at the knee. To examine the amount of posterolateral spin relative to the contralateral side in the posterolateral spin test, the step-off of the lateral tibial plateau from the lateral femoral condyle with the knee flexed at 30 or 90 degrees can be palpated with the thumb. The interrelation between the PCL and PLC also plays out with posterior drawer and external rotation posterior drawer testing. A recent cadaveric study utilizing stress radiography and posterior drawer testing demonstrated a mean posterior translation of 9.8 mm for isolated PCL injuries compared to a mean posterior translation of 19.4 mm for combined PCL/PLC injuries (8). In other words, a grade III posterior drawer (>10 mm) is consistent with a complete injury to both PCL and PLC structures. The external rotation drawer is performed at 90 degrees of knee flexion with the foot in external rotation. Grading is similar to a standard posterior drawer examination, as the examiner feels the amount of posterior translation according to prominence of the anteromedial tibial plateau margin (medial step-off). The external rotation recurvatum test is performed by picking up the great toe of the affected limb in full extension. A positive test is observed when the tibia falls into asymmetric external rotation and recurvatum relative to the femur due to disruption of the PLC, ACL, and PCL.

Laprade has assessed external rotation at 90 degrees and the external rotation recurvatum tests in patients with documented PLC injury (9). He found a positive result for posterolateral external rotation at 90 degrees in 76% (54 of 71 patients) and for external rotation recurvatum in 73% (52 of 71 patients). A positive result on either test was not associated with injury to any specific PLC structure. Hughston found 84% (118 of 140 patients) had positive ER recurvatum, 80% a positive posterolateral drawer, and 72% were positive for both (1). The take-home message from these diagnostic studies is that, while these tests are likely to be positive in patients with PLC injury, they may not be attributed to any one structure nor have their exact sensitivity nor specificity been evaluated in a population of multiligament-injured knees. A positive reverse pivot-shift examination is also indicative of an injury to the PLC. This test is performed starting with the knee in a flexed position, externally rotated foot, and valgus stress. The leg is then brought into an extended position, maintaining valgus load.

IMAGING

Standard anteroposterior (AP) and lateral radiographs are obtained and assessed for fractures, joint space asymmetry, and tibiofemoral subluxation. Often, radiographic findings are very subtle and may include small rim fractures or small bony avulsions, in particular, from the proximal tibia and fibula. A fibular head fracture, sometimes referred to as the arcuate fracture or sign, is pathognomonic for PLC injury (10,11). Although it is difficult to obtain standing radiographs in the acute setting, bilateral standing hip-to-ankle radiographs are routinely obtained in the chronic setting to assess limb alignment.

MRI remains the diagnostic imaging modality of choice. Newer 3-Tesla scans provide high-definition clarity for accurate assessment of injury to the FCL, popliteus muscle and tendon, PFL, posterolateral capsule, and biceps femoris, iliotibial band, and lateral gastrocnemius attachments. MRI is also helpful to identify associated ligamentous, meniscal, and/or chondral injury.

When physical examination findings do not provide sufficient evidence of the degree of injury to the FCL and/or PLC, stress radiography is often helpful. This can be done with routine radiographs or fluoroscopy. Fluoroscopic examination of both knees can be done in the outpatient setting and/or intraoperatively at the time of definitive surgical intervention. LaPrade et al. (12) demonstrated that a varus stress radiograph with a side-to-side difference of less than 2.7 mm was indicative of an isolated injury to the FCL, whereas a side-to-side difference of greater than 4.0 mm was indicative of an injury to both the FCL and PLC.

INDICATIONS FOR SURGICAL INTERVENTION

The indication for reconstruction and/or repair of lateral side injuries depends on the severity of injury to the PLC and the chronicity of the injury. The severity of PLC injuries determines whether nonoperative or operative treatment is recommended. Grade I or grade II PLC injuries with minimal or partial ligament tearing can often be treated nonoperatively with success (5). Grade III (complete tears) PLC injuries, however, are usually associated with uni- or bicruciate injury and have poor results when treated nonoperatively, usually leading to symptomatic instability of the knee (13). Thus, the current treatment recommendation for grade III PLC injuries, which are usually combined with cruciate ligament injuries, is surgical repair and/or reconstruction of all injured structures. If operative treatment is required, the injury pattern and the condition of the injured tissue help determine which type of surgical treatment is recommended.

The chronicity of posterolateral instability also affects the decision to proceed with repair and/or reconstruction. When a PLC injury is diagnosed within the first 2 weeks following injury and the patient's condition and skin around the knee are acceptable for surgery, acute operative intervention may have superior outcomes than late surgery because avulsed tissue can be repaired directly to where it was detached from. As such, early surgical management of all damaged soft tissue structures is generally preferred whenever possible. The advantage of performing the surgery in the first 2 weeks after injury is that the patient's own tissue will be of better quality for repair. However, with acute surgery on a severely injured knee, there is a higher risk of arthrofibrosis, particularly if the patient has not regained motion and/or has severe swelling. Therefore, unless we are able to operate within 2 weeks, we generally prefer to wait for motion to recover to decrease the risk of severe postoperative stiffness and perform delayed PLC reconstruction.

The decision to surgically repair versus surgically reconstruct the PLC remains controversial. Stannard et al. (14) reported results of a level II prospective trial involving repair versus reconstruction of the PLC in 57 knees. Forty-four (77%) of the patients sustained multiligament-injured knees, and minimum follow-up was 24 months. The repair failure rate was 37%, compared with a reconstruction failure rate of 9%. The difference in stability on clinical examination between repairs and reconstructions was significant ($p < 0.05$). Levy et al. (15) reported on the results of patients who underwent repair of the PLC structures in the setting of multiligament knee reconstruction. In this cohort, 28 knees in 28 consecutive patients were evaluated. Group A consisted of 10 acute repairs in 10 patients of the PLC, followed by ACL/PCL reconstructions. Mean follow-up was 34 (range, 24 to 49) months. Group B consisted of 18 reconstructions in 18 patients of the PLC, at the time of ACL/PCL reconstructions. Mean follow-up was 28 (range, 24 to 41) months. Four of the 10 PLC (40%) repairs and 1 of the 18 PLC (6%) reconstructions failed ($p = 0.04$). These findings are similar to those reported by Stannard et al. for the PLC as noted above.

We recommend individualized decision making for each patient taking all factors into account. We recommend thinking of the decision not as whether or not to repair or reconstruct but in terms of repairing with reconstruction when necessary. If we repair early, and the tissue quality is good and we are able to repair all PLC structures anatomically, then repair alone is performed, but this is rarely the case in view of the higher failure rated for isolated repairs.

PREOPERATIVE PLANNING

Posterolateral instability is most commonly associated with multiligament injury, and as such, careful planning of the order and type of ligament reconstruction is of upmost importance. It is also important to assess and document common peroneal nerve function preoperatively. A vertical lateral incision, centered one centimeter anterior to the fibular head is preferred to allow for repair and reconstruction of the PLC as well as for peroneal nerve exposure and neurolysis.

SURGICAL PROCEDURE

In the surgical technique for multiligament injuries described below, the ACL is reconstructed arthroscopically with soft tissue allograft using a single-bundle technique. The PCL is reconstructed arthroscopically using an anterolateral single-bundle, transtibial allograft fixed with interference screws on the femur and tibia with additional backup fixation on the tibia. The PLC technique described below was described by Schechinger et al. (16).

A vertical lateral incision is made one centimeter anterior to the fibular head. Through this incision, the iliotibial band and the biceps femoris muscle complex can be exposed. It is also important to inspect the peroneal nerve, best found proximally, just posterior to the biceps femoris. The peroneal nerve should be isolated and protected with a vessel loop to avoid accidental injury intraoperatively. If the personal nerve is found to be severely injured or scarred, neurolysis should be performed by a surgeon with expertise in nerve surgery.

The iliotibial band is then incised longitudinally and the fibular head is exposed. Subperiosteal dissection is performed on the fibular head anteriorly and posteriorly using a Bovey and small Cobb. Dissection over the lateral aspect of the femur then allows access to the anterior aspect of the popliteal sulcus and the FCL insertion. A K-wire is passed through the anterior one-fifth of the popliteal sulcus using fluoroscopy. A 9-mm reamer is then used to overream the tract to 20 mm in depth. Meanwhile, an Achilles tendon allograft is prepared with a 9 × 20 mm bone plug and 7-mm graft. The tunnel drilled at the popliteal sulcus is filled with the allograft bone plug and fixated with an 8 × 20 mm interference screw.

To create the fibular tunnel, a K-wire is passed under fluoroscopy from the FCL attachment site on the anterolateral fibula to the PFL attachment site on the posteromedial downslope of the fibular styloid. Using a 7-mm reamer, the K-wire is then overreamed to create a hole through which a suture passer can be passed anterior to posterior. Using the previously developed tract, the graft is passed deep to the biceps femoris. The PFL is anatomically reconstructed by passing the graft posterior to anterior through the fibula. The FCL is anatomically reconstructed by looping the graft back over to the insertion of the FCL just proximal and posterior the lateral epicondyle, which is located 18.5 mm proximal and posterior to the popliteus tendon insertion. To make sure that it does not encroach on other reconstructed ligament tunnels, a Beath pin can be passed at the FCL insertion under fluoroscopy. To check the graft for isometry, it is placed in flexion and extension over the Beath pin to a depth of approximately 40 mm.

The Beath pin is used to then pass the graft to the medial side of the knee. The Beath pin and sutures are pulled out from the medial side of the knee, and the graft is tensioned with the leg at approximately 30 degrees of flexion, 10 to 15 degrees of internal rotation, and maximum valgus. To complete the FCL reconstruction, an 8 × 30 mm interference screw is used to secure the graft. A no. 1 Ethibond suture (Ethicon, Somerville, NJ) is used to plicate the capsule in the chronic setting, or anchors can be used to repair capsule to the femur or tibia, as appropriate, in the acute setting. Wounds are then irrigated copiously with saline, and the iliotibial band is closed with no. 1 Ethibond suture. The subcutaneous layers and the skin incision are then both closed to complete the procedure.

PEARLS AND PITFALLS

- Pearls:
  - Place sandbag under buttock or tilt the patient away by tilting the operating room table to make it slightly more vertical, away from the surgeon to facilitate visualization.
  - Perform the procedure with the knee flexed to 90 degrees to minimize tension on the common peroneal nerve.
  - Check for other associated ligament injuries upon presentation and intraoperatively.
  - If surgery within 2 weeks of injury is possible, use MRI to assess for avulsed tissue (FCL, biceps, capsule, etc.) and repair back to bone along with reconstruction.
  - Isolate and protect the peroneal nerve with a vessel loop throughout the procedure.
  - Pass K-wire from the FCL attachment site on the anterolateral fibula to the PFL attachment site on the posteromedial slope of the fibular styloid.
  - Use Beath pin at FCL insertion to ensure that it does not intrude on other reconstructed ligament tunnels.
  - Check graft for isometry in flexion and extension.
  - Tension graft with leg at 30 degrees of flexion 10 to 15 degrees of internal rotation and maximum valgus.
- Pitfalls:
  - Protect nerve throughout the operation.
  - Check for tunnel conversion if concomitant ACL reconstruction is performed.
  - Avoid early or excessive motion, which can lead to repair and/or graft stretch.

POSTOPERATIVE MANAGEMENT

The operated knee should be locked in full extension in a valgus-producing knee brace for the first 4 weeks following surgery. The leg should be nonweight bearing for the first 6 weeks postoperatively. At that point, physical therapy, including range-of-motion exercises and quadriceps training, is recommended with an unlocked brace. By 4 months postoperatively, hamstring exercises can begin. Patients can expect to return to normal activity by 12 months postoperatively, although the time frame varies based on the injury pattern of the multiligament injury, associated injuries, the level of activity, and the patient's progress with rehabilitation.

COMPLICATIONS TO AVOID

- Infected hematoma
- Arthrofibrosis
- Complex regional pain syndrome
- Peroneal nerve injury
- Vascular injury
- Compartment syndrome
- Unaddressed/undiagnosed associated ligament injury

ILLUSTRATIVE CASES

Lateral Side Reconstruction

An 18-year-old football player was tackled in the open field. He had his left foot planted and his knee gave way. He was carried off the field. He was otherwise well. He was referred for consultation 1 month after the injury. There was a large effusion in the left knee and motion from 0 to 130 degrees. The knee was nontender. There was gross AP translation with Lachman test. Medial side was stable but the lateral side opened grossly in full extension and at 30 degrees of flexion. Pedal pulses were normal. Sensation of the deep and superficial peroneal nerve was decreased but clearly present. He could detect light touch. Tibial nerve sensation was normal. Motor function in the distribution of the common peroneal nerve was absent. Tibial nerve motor function was normal.

MRI demonstrated bicruciate disruption and PLC injury (Fig. 25-1). The structures of the posterior lateral corner were torn, including the FCL and popliteus tendon. There was also avulsion of the long head of the biceps and iliotibial band. There were large bone contusions on the anterior medial femoral condyle and tibial plateau. The patient had an EMG, which demonstrated no muscle activation and no nerve function.

The patient underwent bicruciate ligament reconstruction with PLC reconstruction and biceps tendon repair. Achilles tendon allograft was used for both ACL and PCL reconstructions using single-bundle grafts for both, with an arthroscopic, transtibial PCL technique. Extensive and meticulous common peroneal neurolysis was performed because the nerve was extremely scarred to the surrounding tissue. Lateral side reconstruction was performed using the anatomic technique described above with a single Achilles tendon allograft (Figs. 25-2 to 25-4).

The patient was immobilized in full extension for 4 weeks. At 6 months, he began to have an early return of motor function, specifically dorsiflexion. One year after surgery, he had nearly symmetrical dorsiflexion power with only slight weakness and normal peroneal eversion strength. Sensation on the dorsal aspect of the foot was improved, but not quite normal. One year after surgery, he began fielding and batting practice. At 16 months following surgery, he returned to running and sports.

Acute Lateral Side Repair with Reconstruction

A 16-year-old male was seen for consultation following a noncontact varus, hyperextension injury during a football game. On physical exam, he was found to have 10 degrees of asymmetric hyperextension. He had a negative posterior drawer test and a 2+ Lachman with no endpoint. The lateral compartment opened to varus at 30 degrees and also full extension, but slightly less. The patient also had a negative sag and quadriceps active test.

MRI revealed that the patient had ACL and lateral side injury and PLC injury (Figs. 25-5 and 25-6). There was also a proximal avulsion of the FCL and popliteus tendon (Fig. 25-6). During the procedure, the patient had a positive drive-through sign (Fig. 25-7).

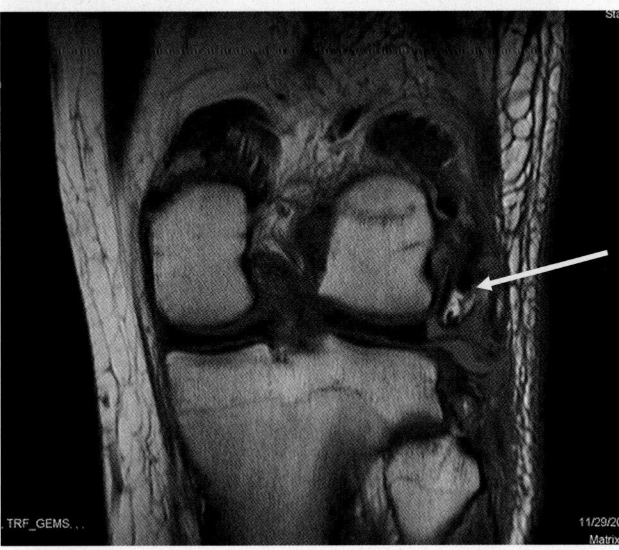

FIGURE 25-1

Bicruciate injury with severe lateral side soft tissue injury (see *arrow*).

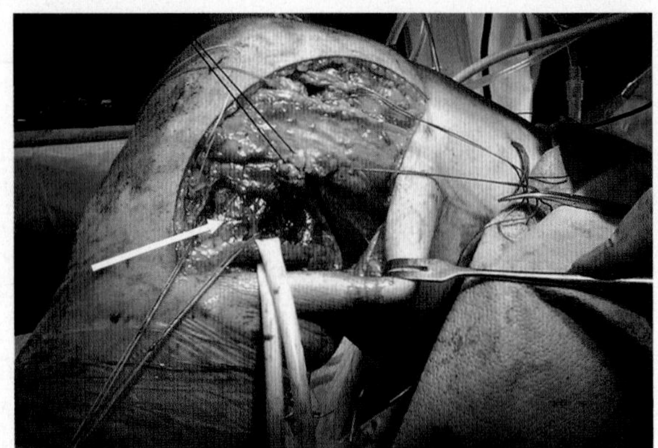

FIGURE 25-2

Intraoperative photo during repair and reconstruction of lateral side with biceps tendon tagged (*black arrow*) and suture in fibula head for graft passage (*white arrow*).

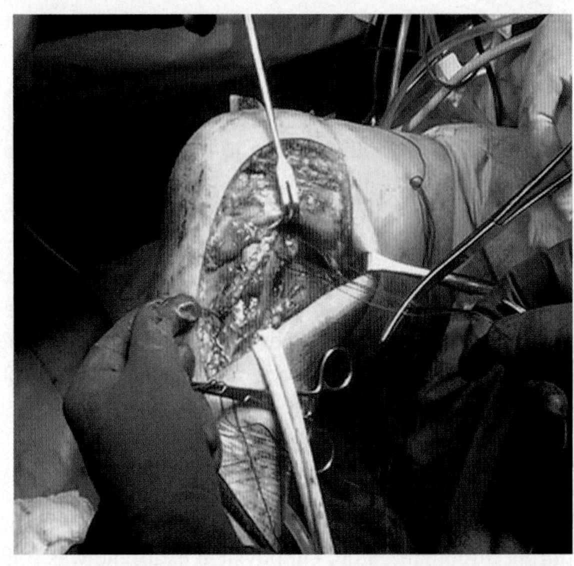

FIGURE 25-3

Graft passed and fixed.

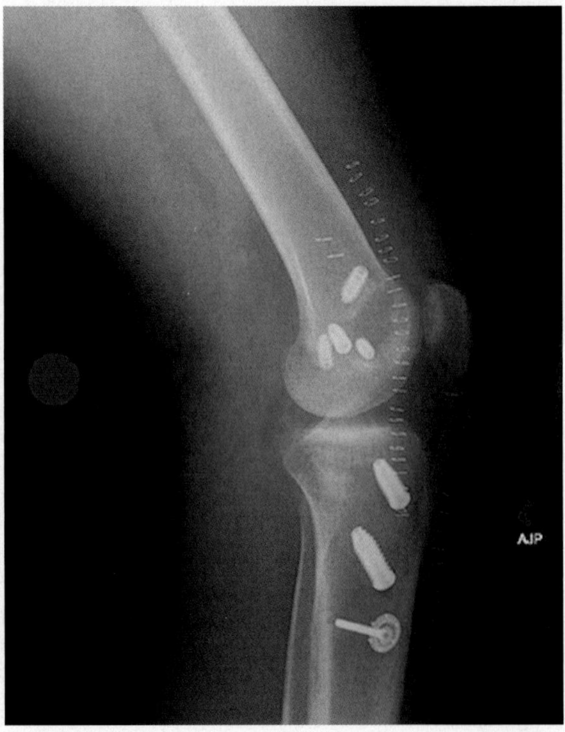

FIGURE 25-4

Postoperative x-ray with fixation in place after ACL reconstruction, PCL reconstruction, and posterolateral repair and reconstruction.

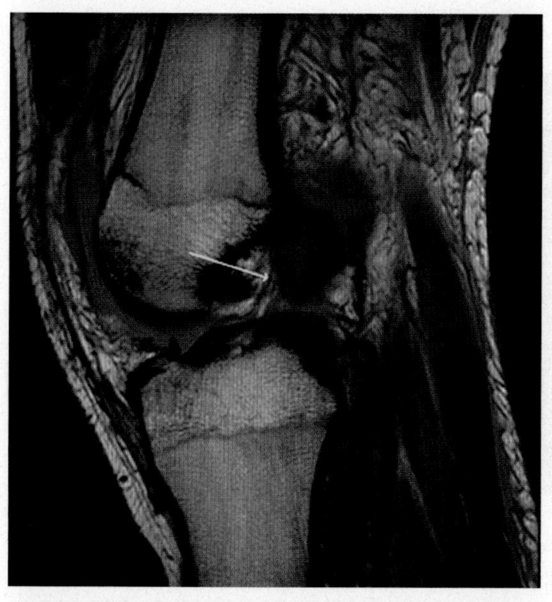

FIGURE 25-5

Bicruciate injury (shown by *arrow*).

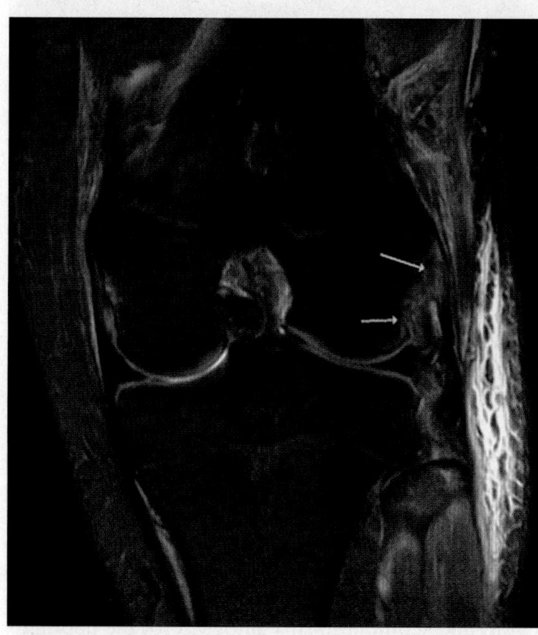

FIGURE 25-6

Proximal avulsion of FCL (indicated by *longer yellow arrow*) and popliteus (indicated by *shorter yellow arrow*).

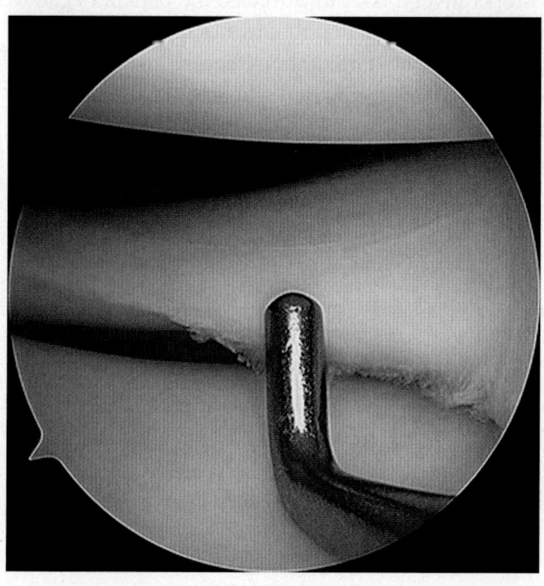

FIGURE 25-7

Drive-through sign lateral compartment.

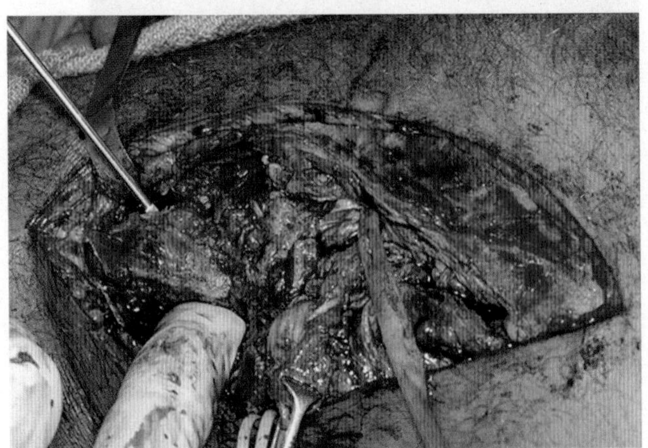

FIGURE 25-8

Drilling fibular tunnel. Repaired all lateral side structures, augmenting with semitendinosus and gracilis autograft.

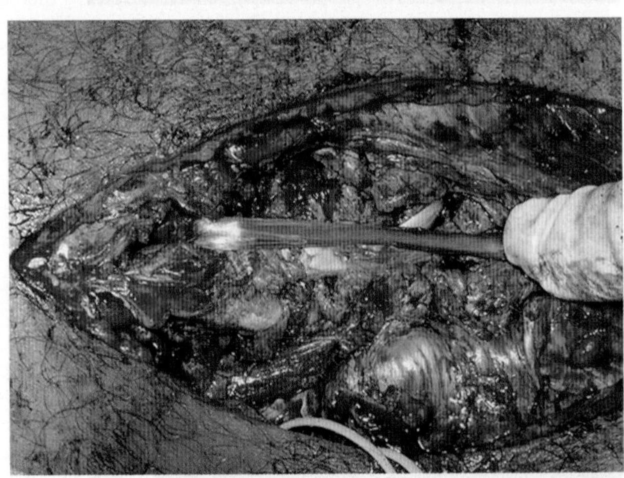

FIGURE 25-9

Graft pulled over top repaired FCL.

The patient underwent ACL reconstruction with a patellar tendon autograft. Other structures including the FCL, popliteofibular ligament, biceps femoris tendon, and popliteus tendon were repaired. The surgeon also performed a lateral meniscal repair and a posterolateral capsule repair. All the repaired structures were further augmented with a two-tailed FCL/PLC reconstruction, utilizing gracilis autograft for the popliteus bypass graft and semitendinosus autograft for the popliteofibular ligament and FCL reconstruction (Figs. 25-8 and 25-9).

The patient was immobilized for 4 weeks postoperatively. At 4 to 6 weeks, the patient began to return to movement with passive motion. The patient then graduated to unrestricted passive, active assisted, and finally active motion. At 3 months, the patient started strengthening his quads with leg press exercises, squats, lunges, and step-ups. At 6 months, he started a hamstring strengthening program with dead lifts, hamstring curls, and single leg bridge curls on an exercise ball. He started progressive running at 6 to 9 months post surgery with plyometrics and agility exercises incorporated at 9 months. Finally, the patient returned to sports 11 months post surgery.

REFERENCES

1. Hughston JC, Jacobson KE. Chronic posterolateral rotator instability of the knee. *J Bone Joint Surg Am.* 1985;67-A:351–359.
2. Baker C, Norwood L, Hughston J. Acute posterolateral rotatory instability of the knee. *J Bone Joint Surg Am.* 1983;65:614–618.
3. Veltri DM, Warren RF. Operative treatment of posterolateral instability of the knee. *Clin Sports Med.* 1994;13:615–627.
4. LaPrade RF, Hamilton CD, Engebretsen L. Treatment of acute and chronic combined anterior cruciate ligament and posterolateral knee injuries. *Sports Med Arthrosc Rev.* 1997;5:91–99.
5. Covey DC. Injuries of the posterolateral corner of the knee. *J Bone Joint Surg Am.* 2001;83A:106–118.
6. Marx RG, Shindle MK, Warren RF. Management of posterior cruciate ligament injuries. *Oper Tech Sports Med.* 2009;17(3):162–166.

7. Bleday RM, Fanelli GC, Giannotti BF, et al. Instrumented measurement of the posterolateral corner. *Arthroscopy.* 1998;14(5):489–494.
8. Sekiya JK, Whiddon DR, Zehms CT, et al. A clinically relevant assessment of posterior cruciate ligament and posterolateral corner injuries. Evaluation of isolated and combined deficiency. *J Bone Joint Surg.* 2008;90(8):1621–1627.
9. LaPrade RF, Terry GC. Injuries to the posterolateral aspect of the knee. Association of anatomic injury patterns with clinical instability. *Am J Sports Med.* 1997;25(4):433–438.
10. Huang GS, Yu JS, Munshi M, et al. Avulsion fracture of the head of the fibula (the "arcuate" sign): MR imaging findings predictive of injuries to the posterolateral ligaments and posterior cruciate ligament. *Am J Roentgenol.* 2003;180(2):381–387.
11. Strub WM. The arcuate sign. *Radiology.* 2007;244(2):620–621.
12. LaPrade RF, Heikes C, Bakker AJ, et al. The reproducibility and repeatability of varus stress radiographs in the assessment of isolated fibular collateral ligament and grade-III posterolateral knee injuries. An in vitro biomechanical study. *J Bone Joint Surg.* 2008;90(10):2069–2076.
13. Pacheco RJ, Ayre CA, Bollen SR. Posterolateral corner injuries of the knee: a serious injury commonly missed. *J Bone Joint Surg Br.* 2011;93-B(2):194–197.
14. Stannard JP, Brown SL, Farris RC, et al. The posterolateral corner of the knee: repair versus reconstruction. *Am J Sports Med.* 2005;33(6):881–888.
15. Levy BA, Dajani KA, Morgan JA, et al. Repair versus reconstruction of the fibular collateral ligament and posterolateral corner in the multiligament-injured knee. *Am J Sports Med.* 2010;38(4):804–809.
16. Schechinger SJ, Levy BA, Dajani KA, et al. Achilles tendon allograft reconstruction of the fibular collateral ligament and posterolateral corner. *Arthroscopy.* 2009;25:232–242.

RECOMMENDED READINGS

LaPrade RF, Johansen S, Agel J, et al. Outcomes of an anatomic posterolateral knee reconstruction. *J Bone Joint Surg Am.* 2010;92:16–22.

LaPrade RF, Johansen S, Wentorf FA, et al. An analysis of an anatomical posterolateral knee reconstruction: an in vitro biomechanical study and development of a surgical technique. *Am J Sports Med.* 2004;32:1405–1414.

Levy BA, Dajani KA, Morgan JA, et al. Repair versus reconstruction of the fibular collateral ligament and posterolateral corner in the multiligament-injured knee. *Am J Sports Med.* 2010;38:804–809.

Peskun CJ, Chahal J, Steinfeld ZY, et al. Risk factors for peroneal nerve injury and recovery in knee dislocation. *Clin Orthop Relat Res.* 2012;470(3):774–778.

Schechinger SJ, Levy BA, Dajani KA, et al. Achilles tendon allograft reconstruction of the fibular collateral ligament and posterolateral corner. *Arthroscopy.* 2009;25:232–242.

Stannard JP, Brown SL, Farris RC, et al. The posterolateral corner of the knee: repair versus reconstruction. *Am J Sports Med.* 2005;33:881–888.

26 Posterolateral Corner Reconstruction with Fibular-Based Tunnel

J. H. James Choi, Eduard Alentorn-Geli, Joseph J. Stuart, and Claude T. Moorman III

INDICATIONS

Injury to the posterolateral corner (PLC) of the knee is a relatively uncommon event with potentially significant long-term adverse sequelae. The mechanism of injury is thought to be a varus, hyperextension force that oftentimes is high energy (1,2). It previously has been referred to as the "dark side of the knee" due to the complexity of the surrounding anatomy and the variability in outcomes from any of a number of reconstruction techniques (3). The PLC is now considered an integral component to maintaining stability of the knee, particularly in the context of rotational, varus, and posterior stresses. Isolated injury to the PLC is a rare occurrence for an infrequently occurring injury pattern, and there almost always is an associated injury to the anterior cruciate ligament, posterior cruciate ligament, or medially based ligaments. Identification of injury to this complex anatomical area is critical as many authors have made note of the increased risk of overall poorer outcomes and higher failure rates of associated ligamentous reconstructions when the PLC remains deficient (1).

Research studies investigating the anatomy of the PLC have identified the critical structures to be the lateral (fibular) collateral ligament (LCL), popliteus tendon, popliteofibular ligament, and the posterolateral capsule (2). Complete disruptions of these structures (grade III injury) or PLC injury resulting in associated laxity in a multiligament-injured knee are candidates for PLC reconstruction (1,4). When injuries are acute and soft tissues are amenable to surgery within the first few weeks following injury, PLC reconstruction is often performed in conjunction with primary repair of damaged structures. For more chronic injuries, reconstruction is generally performed alone as soft tissue planes become scarred and identification of discrete PLC components is difficult if not impossible. The literature demonstrates a broad spectrum of preferences and choices for performing a PLC reconstruction. Autografts are generally reserved for isolated reconstruction of the PLC, while allografts are now almost always used for PLC reconstructions in the multiligament-injured knee as to minimize additional morbidity to the patient.

To date, there remains no gold standard for PLC reconstruction. The fibular-based PLC reconstruction provides a number of advantages to the surgeon. First, it is a technique that is relatively easy to master and reproduce for both acute and chronic injuries. Second, it can be performed with a single-hamstring autograft or allograft tendon. Third, it enables preservation of remaining native tissues of the PLC for either repair or incorporation into the reconstruction. Fourth, it does not require the use of tunnels that are at risk of interfering with other ligament reconstructions in a multiligament-injured knee (5). A cadaver biomechanical study comparing fibular-based reconstruction with combined fibula-tibia–based reconstructions showed no significant differences in varus and external rotation stress at 30 and 90 degrees between the two techniques and also when compared to an intact knee (6). If performed correctly, this fibular-based technique produces a reconstruction that has an anterior limb that reproduces the LCL and a posterior limb that substitutes for the popliteofibular ligament. While this is not a pure anatomical reconstruction, it does provide isometric fixation of the PLC and stability throughout knee range of motion (Table 26-1) (5).

TABLE 26-1 Advantages to Fibular-Based PLC Reconstruction

1. Relatively easy to master and reproduce for both acute and chronic injuries
2. Can be performed with a single-hamstring autograft or allograft tendon
3. Enables preservation of remaining native tissues of the PLC for either repair or incorporation into the reconstruction
4. Does not require the use of tunnels that are at risk of interfering with other ligament reconstructions in a multiligament-injured knee

CONTRAINDICATIONS

Contraindications to PLC reconstruction surgery are few and consistent with other knee ligament reconstructive procedures. These include those patients who are not able to tolerate the surgical procedure secondary to other medical conditions and patients who are not able to comply with postoperative rehabilitation instructions (2). Patients with neurovascular injuries should be delayed until their neurovascular injuries can be stabilized and fully evaluated and any patient with an active infection of the knee or surrounding soft tissues due to trauma of injury or otherwise should be delayed until the infection is cleared. Individuals with preexisting, advanced osteoarthritis in the injured knee may wish to consider knee arthroplasty options that might provide greater long-term benefit to the patient.

PREOPERATIVE PREPARATION

Since PLC injuries rarely occur in isolation, these patients must be thoroughly evaluated for other injuries. In the acute setting, particularly in the setting of a tibiofemoral dislocation, the patient must have a careful evaluation of neurovascular status that may include serial physical examination, ankle-brachial index measurement, and possibly including computed tomography (CT) or traditional angiography if clinical concern warrants additional evaluation. Documentation of motor and sensory function, particularly for the peroneal nerve, is important to establish a functional baseline (7). Once the orthopedic surgeon is assured that there are no further evolving neurovascular concerns, a detailed functional examination of the knee should be performed. Physical examination specifically targeted for the PLC should include varus stress at 0/30 degrees (LCL) and dial testing external rotation of the tibia on the femur at 30/90 degrees (popliteofibular ligament, popliteus tendon, capsule). Absence of the cord-like LCL on palpation with the knee flexed and the hip in external rotation raises concern of LCL disruption. Varus laxity at 0 and/or 90 degrees raises suspicion of cruciate ligament injury, while a finding of exaggerated posterior drawer sign (>2+) should also raise suspicion of PLC injury. A reverse pivot shift may be used by some clinicians but has been reported to have a high false-positive rate that may be upward of 35%. Inspection of the lateral knee in the acute setting may reveal ecchymosis, edema, and tenderness in the area of the PLC that may not be present in more chronic cases. Chronic injury patients may describe a sensation of frequent instability that occurs with relatively low levels of activity as well as pain in the posterolateral aspect of the knee. Some patients may be able to reproduce the sensation or even demonstrate instability with the knee at 90 degrees and contracture of the biceps femoris (8,9). Patients may significantly guard on exam while awake, thus necessitating the examination under anesthesia prior to any planned surgery. In addition to physical examination for PLC injury, evaluation of tibiofibular instability should be evaluated. A finding of tibiofibular instability does not preclude a fibular-based PLC reconstruction but also must be stabilized. Imaging for evaluation of PLC injury should include standard knee radiographs in addition to magnetic resonance imaging (MRI) without contrast. There are limited indications for use of CT for PLC injury evaluation.

Preoperatively, the patient should attempt to regain as much knee range of motion as possible, oftentimes through the assistance of physical therapy in a "prehab" program. Similar to other major knee surgeries, preoperative counseling of the patient regarding the extended postoperative rehabilitative course, expected postoperative pain, and limitations may aid in guiding patient expectations and assist them in understanding the complexities surrounding recovery from surgery. Depending on facility, it may be advantageous to discuss the case and required equipment needs with the operating room (OR) staff and supplier vendors in advance so that necessary equipment is available and OR staff are prepared to assist in an efficient manner.

TECHNIQUE

Fibular-based reconstruction of the PLC is performed with the patient positioned in the supine position. At this institution, the patient usually has regional catheters placed for femoral and sciatic blocks and is sedated during the procedure. Examination under anesthesia is first performed to confirm clinical diagnosis of PLC injury and results documented. A standard tourniquet is placed high on the thigh and a lateral post attached to the operating table at the level of the tourniquet. A prescrub of the operative extremity is completed with chlorhexidine and alcohol then the extremity is sterilely prepped with chlorhexidine and draped in a usual manner.

A diagnostic arthroscopy of the knee is performed prior to reconstruction in both acute and chronic PLC injury cases to evaluate intra-articular structures with particular attention paid to the popliteus and lateral meniscus. If separation of the lateral femoral condyle from the lateral tibial plateau exceeds 10 mm at the midpoint of the lateral compartment with a varus stress, this provides confirmation of PLC incompetence, and a knee arthroscopic "drive-through sign" will be present as seen in Figure 26-1 (10,11). If there is a cruciate ligament injury requiring repair and/or reconstruction, this is typically performed after the diagnostic arthroscopy and prior to PLC reconstruction.

In preparation for PLC reconstruction, either an autograft or allograft semitendinosus tendon is utilized, and a minimum graft length of 25 cm is typically necessary. The ends of the graft are prepared on a back table using any of a number of techniques to secure sutures for passing the graft, securing the graft with suture over 3 cm of each end as shown in Figure 26-2.

For the PLC reconstruction, a slightly curved longitudinal incision line is marked on the lateral aspect of the knee that is centered on the lateral epicondyle at its proximal end and at the midpoint between Gerdy tubercle and the fibular head at its distal end; this will measure approximately 12 cm as seen in Figure 26-3. If other surgeries are performed in conjunction with PLC reconstruction, a 7-cm skin bridge is recommended for other associated incisions. Incision is then made and full-thickness flaps are created down to the iliotibial (IT) band, shown in Figure 26-4. Attention is then directed to identifying the peroneal nerve that is running posterior to the biceps femoris proximally. The nerve is carefully dissected free of any scar tissue and protected throughout the remainder of the PLC reconstruction as seen in Figure 26-5. If the injury is acute and anatomical structures are

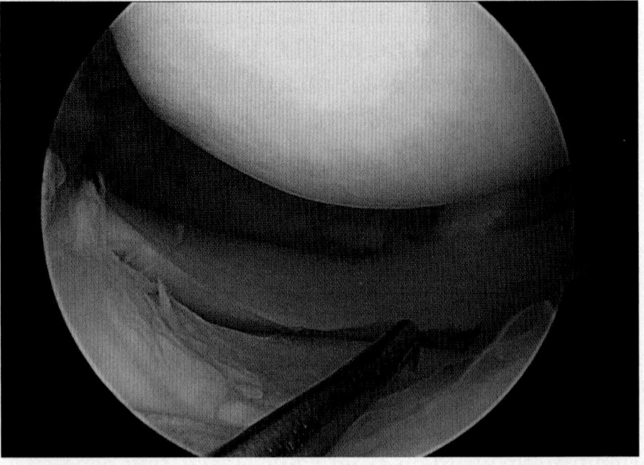

FIGURE 26-1
Arthroscopic "drive-through" sign. (Copyright JHJ Choi.)

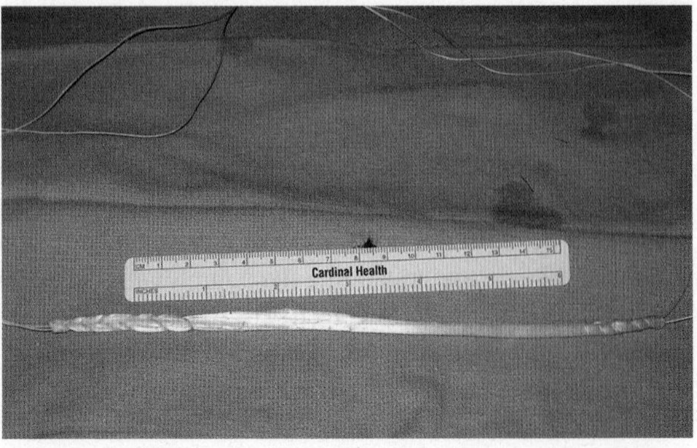

FIGURE 26-2
Graft preparation. (Copyright JHJ Choi.)

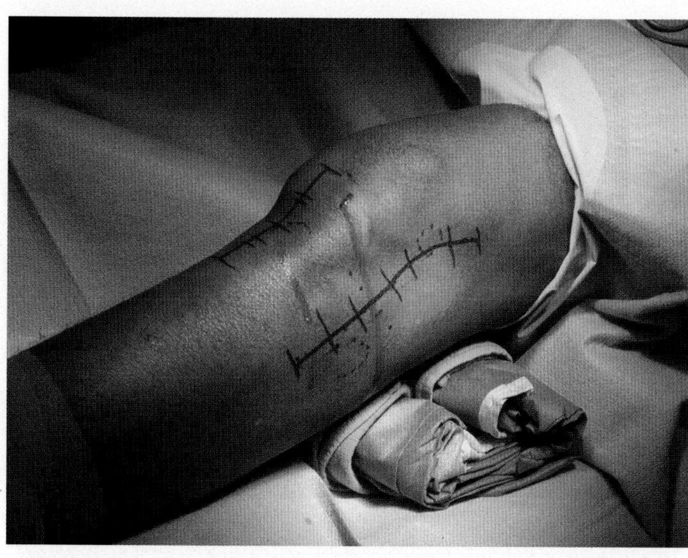

FIGURE 26-3
Incision markings. (Copyright JHJ Choi.)

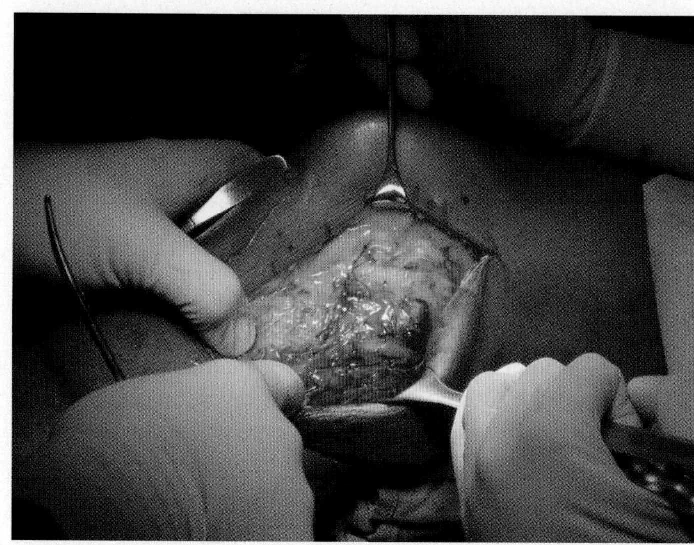

FIGURE 26-4
Superficial approach. (Copyright JHJ Choi.)

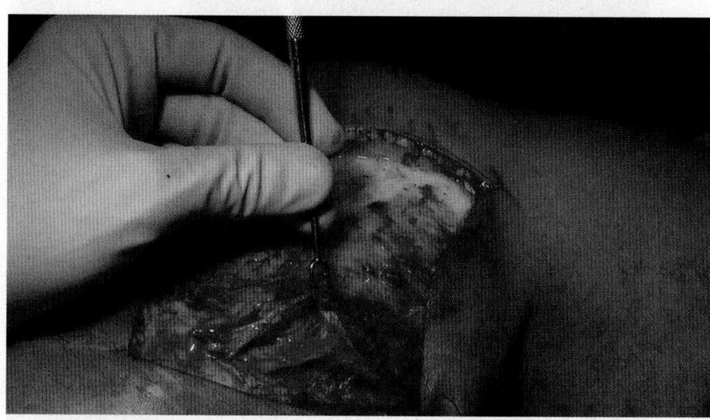

FIGURE 26-5
Identification of peroneal nerve. (Copyright JHJ Choi.)

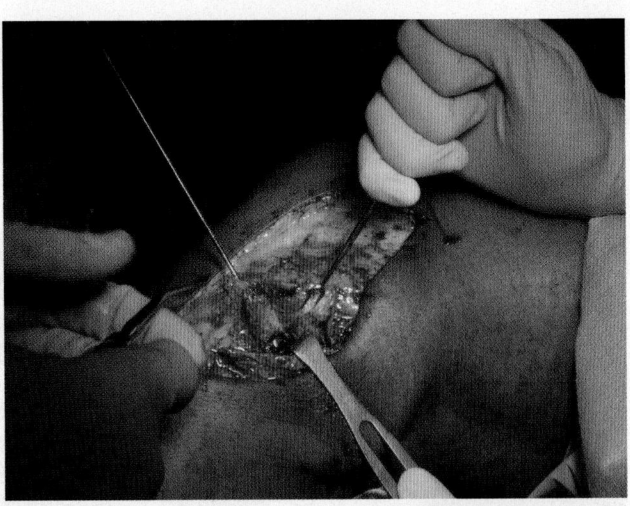

FIGURE 26-6
Fibular tunnel. (Copyright JHJ Choi.)

identifiable, it is recommended to tag these PLC structures for primary repair after completion of reconstruction. Primary repair of PLC structures may be accomplished after reconstruction with direct sutures to bone, suture anchors, or soft tissue screws and washers at the surgeon's discretion.

The IT band is longitudinally split centrally starting at Gerdy tubercle and extending proximally to expose the LCL origin on the femur and popliteus insertion on the femur as well as the biceps femoris insertion onto the fibular head. This is described by Terry and Laprade as their first window. The fibular head is then exposed using Hohmann retractors and the peroneal nerve again identified as it courses past the fibular head and protected. A guide wire is placed in the expected track of the tunnel approximately 1 to 1.5 cm distal to the superior tip of the fibular head, orienting slightly anterolateral to posteromedial, then the tunnel created with a 6- or 7-mm reamer, illustrated by Figure 26-6. This tunnel location provides an adequate bony bridge proximal to the tunnel. Next, a passing portal is created in the interval between the IT band and the biceps femoris midway from the fibular head to the lateral epicondyle. The graft is passed through the fibular head and up through the newly created passing portal seen in Figures 26-7 to 26-9.

Attention is then directed to the lateral epicondyle of the femur where the LCL origin and popliteus insertion are exposed and identified. A point equidistant to these two landmarks is marked, tapped, and a 6.5-mm screw with 18-mm washer placed leaving it elevated off the bone to facilitate graft passage as demonstrated in Figure 26-10. The anterior limb of the graft is passed posterior to the screw and docked under the femoral post screw, while the posterior portion of the graft is passed anteriorly in a figure-of-eight fashion. The graft limb ends are then brought back toward the fibular head via the passing portal, and the sutures for the strand that is located posterior to the screw (the strand originally exiting the fibular tunnel posteriorly) are passed through the tunnel as

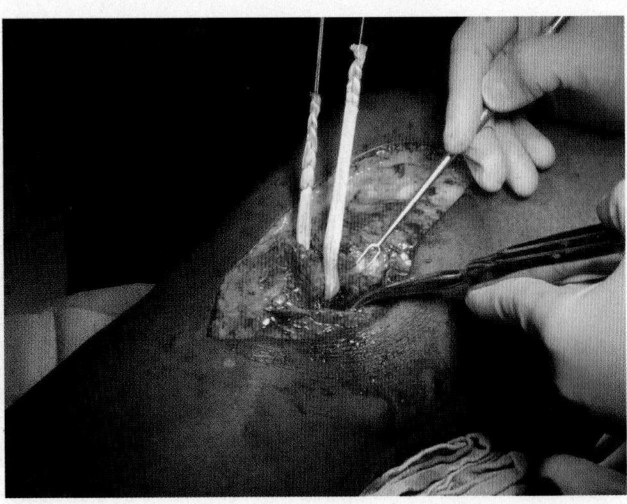

FIGURE 26-7
Graft passage though fibular tunnel. (Copyright JHJ Choi.)

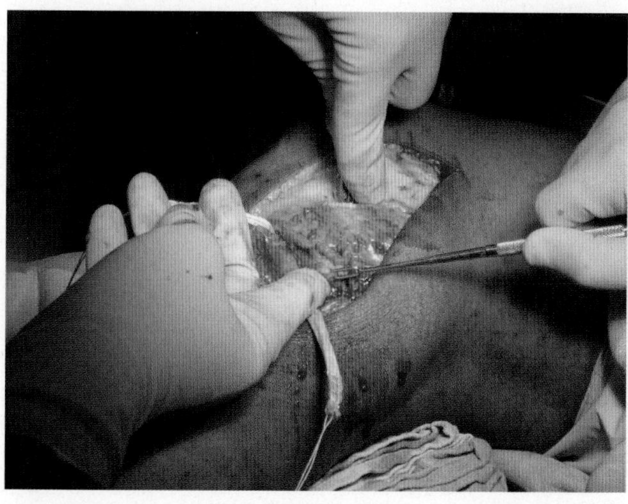

FIGURE 26-8

Passing graft through passing portal. (Copyright JHJ Choi.)

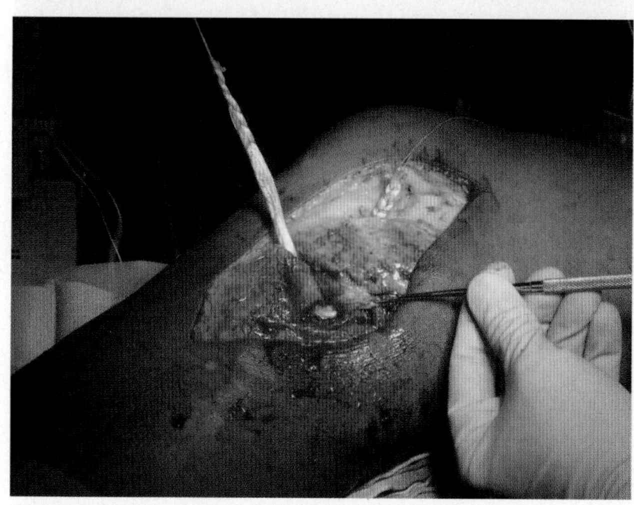

FIGURE 26-9

Passing graft through passing portal. (Copyright JHJ Choi.)

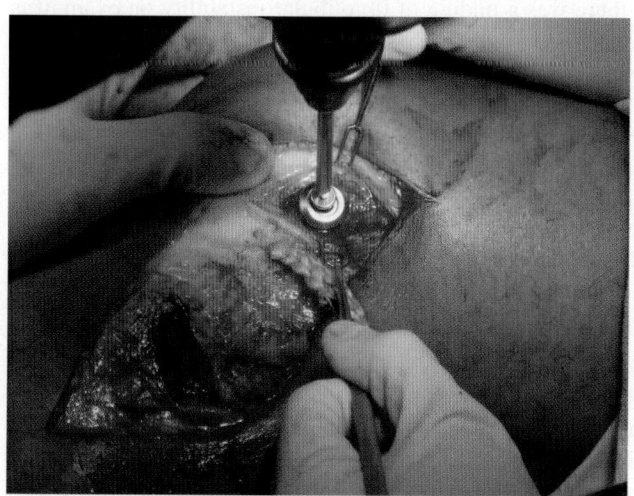

FIGURE 26-10

Femoral postscrew placement. (Copyright JHJ Choi.)

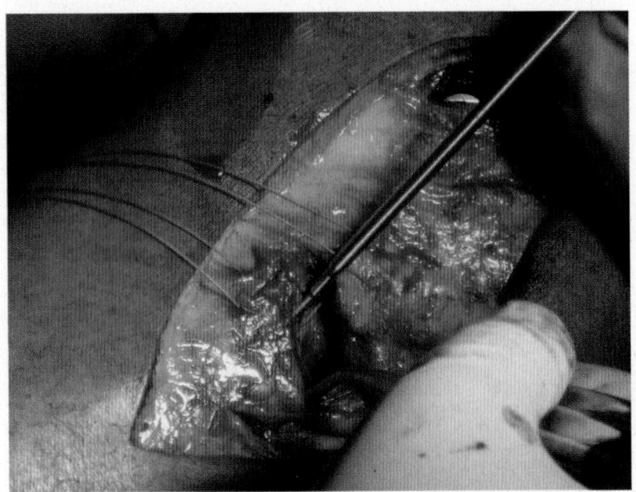

FIGURE 26-12

Primary repair in acute injury. (Copyright JHJ Choi.)

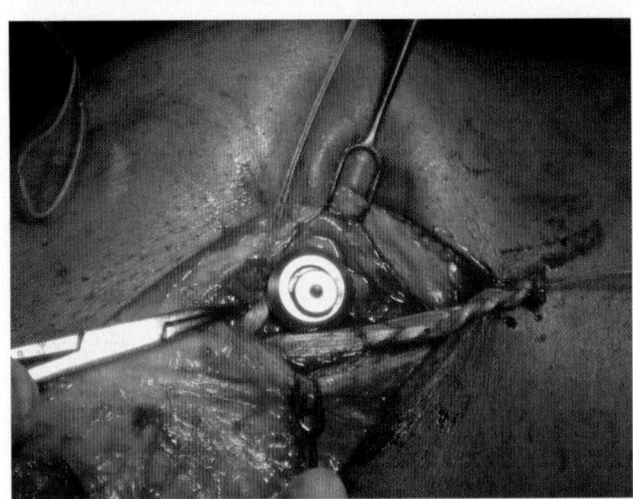

FIGURE 26-11

Graft passage around the post. (Copyright JHJ Choi.)

seen in Figure 26-11. Tensioning of the reconstruction is completed with the knee in 30 degrees of flexion, valgus, and internal rotation, and the knees examined for stability before the sutures securing the ends of the graft are tied together. The femoral postscrew is then tightened as the final step to secure the graft. Primary repair of any acutely injured PLC structures is completed at this time as shown in Figure 26-12. If there was a finding of tibiofibular instability on exam, it is recommended to complete the PLC reconstruction first then utilize two tight ropes for tibiofibular stabilization as it provides more normal micromotion—this avoids the risks of damaging the tight ropes when reaming the tunnels for PLC reconstruction. The wound is copiously irrigated then incisions in the joint capsule and IT band are closed with absorbable, braided 0 suture, the skin closed with 2-0 absorbable, braided suture and 3-0 monofilament running suture. The incisions are then dressed with Steri-Strips, Xeroform, and sterile dressing before Polar Care and hinged knee brace are applied (5,12).

PEARLS AND PITFALLS

Ensuring that the soft tissues in the zone of injury are ready for surgical intervention and that the patient has regained as much knee range of motion as possible are major considerations for preventing postoperative surgical complications. Patient with vascular repair at the time of their injury should have clearance from their vascular surgeon before proceeding with PLC reconstruction—typically, patients are able to proceed with ligament reconstruction 6 weeks following vascular repair. Intraoperatively, careful dissection and exposure of the soft tissues and identification of the common peroneal nerve can reduce the chances of iatrogenic nerve injury and improve the

TABLE 26-2 Technique Pearls and Pitfalls
1. Ensure soft tissues in the zone of injury are ready for surgical intervention
2. Maximize knee range of motion preoperatively
3. Patients with vascular repair should have clearance from their vascular surgeon before proceeding with PLC reconstruction
4. Careful dissection and exposure of the soft tissues and identification of the common peroneal nerve can reduce the chances of iatrogenic nerve injury and improve the possibility of identifying critical structures in the case that they can be repaired
5. Identifying appropriate tunnel placement first and drilling the tunnel on single pass will reduce the risk of fibular head fracture or weakening of the bone
6. Appropriate tensioning of the graft in 30 degrees of flexion, valgus, and internal rotation

possibility of identifying critical structures in the case that they can be repaired. Identifying appropriate tunnel placement first and drilling the tunnel on single pass will reduce the risk of fibular head fracture or weakening of the bone. Appropriate tensioning of the graft is a critical step to ensuring success of the reconstruction—tensioning in 30 degrees of flexion, valgus, and internal rotation of the knee provides the appropriate alignment and stability and maximizes the patient's potential for a satisfactory outcome (Table 26-2).

POSTOPERATIVE MANAGEMENT

Postoperative management for PLC reconstruction patients remains a balance in permitting the reconstruction to heal and incorporate versus the risks of knee stiffness with prolonged immobilization and also must accommodate the rehabilitation program for other associated reconstructions. Physical therapy is usually twice to three times weekly over the first 2 months. For PCL reconstruction purposes, postoperative patients are kept in a hinged knee brace locked in extension with touchdown weight bearing for the first 4 weeks. The patient begins passive knee range of motion and quadriceps exercises under the supervision of a physical therapist at their first postoperative visit a few days following surgery. No active hamstring contracture/resistance is permitted for the first 6 weeks. Weight bearing is advanced, and initiation of active range of motion starting with extension in an unlocked knee brace starts at 4 weeks postoperatively then includes flexion (hamstring activation) at 6 weeks. The brace is worn until 8 to 10 weeks postoperatively, and crutches are used until the patient is able to ambulate without a limp. Patients are usually able to initiate running 4 to 6 months postoperatively with a return to play anywhere from 6 to 12 months postoperatively.

COMPLICATIONS

The most site-specific complication for PLC reconstruction is development of common peroneal nerve palsy, other complications shared with other knee and ligament reconstruction surgeries are arthrofibrosis, failure of reconstruction, persistent pain, and infection (1,2). Common peroneal nerve palsy is of concern due to its proximity to the zone of injury and surgical field during reconstruction. Injury to the nerve at the time of index event must be considered, especially in the high-energy, acute injury. Nerve function should be documented from time of injury and followed serially (7). Intraoperatively, great care is taken to identify and decompress the peroneal nerve as it courses through the zone of injury and also to identify it proximally and distally to this area. Postoperative nerve function changes are most likely due to compression, either externally by dressings or internally by soft tissue edema or hematoma formation. Intraoperative transection of the nerve requires immediate repair by a microsurgeon. Patient postoperatively with new onset of neuropraxia without known intraoperative injury or overt compression of the nerve from external or internal causes are monitored in close serial follow-up with placement of ankle-foot-orthosis to prevent equinus contracture and consideration of electrodiagnostic studies at approximately the 6-week point to evaluate nerve function if there has been no or limited improvement. Arthrofibrosis is a rare sequela of PLC reconstruction but as with other knee surgeries can occur postoperatively. For patients found to have limited knee range of motion, a review of their postoperative rehabilitation protocol with the therapist and patient is warranted, and if necessary, reinforcement or adjustments to the program undertaken may be necessary. If patients have persistent stiffness despite appropriate physical therapy, a manipulation under anesthesia may be indicated but no earlier than 6 weeks postoperatively. Failure of the PLC reconstruction also is rare and may be due to either graft failure or fixation hardware failure due to improperly tensioned or sized graft, a graft that is too short for appropriate fixation, improperly or multiply drilled holes for screw placement, and reinjury—particularly in the near postoperative period. Infection in the present day of perioperative antibiotic coverage is a rare complication but does occur. First-generation cephalosporins remain the most effective prophylactic antibiotic for coverage of the majority of skin flora responsible for surgical site infections. Allografts do present a very small risk to transmit infectious disease, and patients should be informed preoperatively of the use of allograft material and the associated risks.

RESULTS

PLC injury is becoming increasingly recognized as a cause of knee derangement and failure for other knee ligament reconstructions. Reconstruction of the PLC has been shown to improve knee stability through cadaveric biomechanical studies; however, long-term and large population–based outcome studies have not revealed consensus, in large part due to the low incidence of this injury (13,14). Fibular-based reconstruction of the PLC provides surgeons with a straightforward, easily reproducible, and functional solution for their patients with this potentially disabling injury pattern.

REFERENCES

1. Piasecki DP, Bach BR. Posterolateral corner reconstruction. *Tech Knee Surg.* 2010;9(3):181–187.
2. Cooper JM, McAndrews PT, LaPrade RF. Posterolateral corner injuries of the knee: anatomy, diagnosis, and treatment. *Sports Med Arthrosc.* 2006;14(4):213–220.
3. Andrews JR, Baker C, Curl W, et al. Surgical repair of acute and chronic lesions of the lateral capsular ligamentous complex of the knee. In: Feagin JA, ed. *The crucial ligaments: diagnosis and treatment.* New York: Churchill Livingston; 1988:425–438.
4. LaPrade RF, Resig S, Wentorf F, et al. The effects of grade III posterolateral knee complex injuries on anterior cruciate ligament graft force. A biomechanical analysis. *Am J Sports Med.* 1999;27:469–475.
5. Larsen MW, Moinfar, AR, Moorman CT. Posterolateral corner reconstruction, fibular-based technique. *J Knee Surg.* 2005;18(2):163–166.
6. Rauh PB, Clancy WG, Jasper LE, et al. Biomechanical evaluation of two reconstruction techniques for posterolateral instability of the knee. *J Bone Joint Surg Br.* 2010;92-B:1460–1465.
7. Fanelli GC, Stannard JP, Stuart MJ, et al. Management of complex knee ligament injuries. *J Bone Joint Surg.* 2010;92:2235–2246.
8. Cooper DE. Tests for posterolateral instability of the knee in normal subjects. *J Bone Joint Surg.* 1991;73A:30–36.
9. Jakob RP, Hassler H, Staubli HU. Observations on rotatory instability of the lateral compartment of the knee. Experimental studies of the functional anatomy and pathomechanism of the true and reverse pivot shift sign. *Acta Orthop.* 1981;52:1–32.
10. Fanelli GC. Treatment of combined anterior cruciate ligament posterior cruciate ligament-lateral side injuries of the knee. *Clin Sports Med.* 2000;19:493–501.
11. LaPrade RF. Arthroscopic evaluation of the lateral compartment of knees with grade 3 posterolateral complex knee injuries. *Am J Sports Med.* 1997;25:596–602.
12. Terry GC, LaPrade RF. The posterolateral aspect of the knee. Anatomy and surgical approach. *Am J Sports Med.* 1996;24:732–739.
13. Levy BA, Dajani KA, Morgan JA, et al. Repair versus reconstruction of the fibular collateral ligament and posterolateral corner in the multiligament-injured knee. *Am J Sports Med.* 2010;38(4):804–809.
14. Camarda L, Condello V, Madonna V, et al. Results of isolated posterolateral corner reconstruction. *J Orthop Traumatol.* 2010;11:73–79.

27 PLC Reconstruction with Tibial/Fibular-Based Tunnels: Anatomic Reconstruction

Robert F. LaPrade, Samuel G. Moulton, Tyler R. Cram, and Nicholas I. Kennedy

INDICATIONS/CONTRAINDICATIONS

The posterolateral side of the knee used to be known as "the dark side of the knee," in part due to the complexity of the soft tissue structures and the inherent bony instability of the relatively convex lateral femoral condyle and lateral tibial plateau (1). Instability occurs due to increased lateral compartment gapping along with posterolateral subluxation of the lateral tibial plateau relative to the lateral femoral condyle (2). While posterolateral corner (PLC) injuries are reported to range from 5% to 9% of all knee ligament injuries (3), up to 70% of PLC injuries are misdiagnosed at initial presentation (4). Additionally, unmanaged injuries or improper treatment can lead to failure of anterior cruciate ligament (ACL) reconstructions and posterior cruciate ligament (PCL) reconstructions (5,6). Physical examination is a key part of the diagnosis of PLC injuries; specific maneuvers include the external rotation recurvatum test, varus stress test, dial test, posterolateral drawer test, and reverse pivot shift. Increased anterior or posterior translation on the Lachman test and posterior drawer test may also indicate a PLC injury.

Recent biomechanical research has advanced our understanding of PLC injuries. The PLC includes an interdependent series of musculotendinous structures, ligaments, and neurovasculature. The three main static stabilizers of the PLC are the fibular collateral ligament (FCL), the popliteus tendon, and the popliteofibular ligament (7). Quantitative studies describing the anatomic footprints of the tendons and ligaments led to the advent of anatomically based surgical repairs and reconstructions (8–10). Biomechanical studies have validated the anatomic reconstruction technique with tibial and fibular tunnels.

Understanding the anatomy and function is the basis for performing an anatomic reconstruction of the posterolateral structures of the knee. The FCL originates proximally at its femoral attachment 1.4 mm proximal and 3.1 mm posterior to the lateral epicondyle (11). The fibers course distally inserting on the lateral aspect of the fibular head. Additional fibers extend further distally with the peroneus longus fascia. The FCL measures on average 70 mm in its entirety (11). The FCL is the primary stabilizer against unwanted varus motion. Sectioning the FCL has been shown to result in an additional 2.7 mm of lateral compartment gapping (12). Between 0 and 60 degrees of flexion, the FCL has a constant varus load response, which decreases beginning at 90 degrees of flexion. Between 0 and 30 degrees of knee flexion, the FCL provides stability against external rotatory forces (7).

The popliteus tendon originates on the lateral femoral condyle and courses distally in a posterior medial direction toward its insertion on the posteromedial tibia (10). The femoral insertion attaches along the anterior fifth of the popliteal sulcus and is located 18.5 mm anterior and distal to the FCL insertion (11). The popliteofibular ligament consists of two divisions coursing distally and laterally toward the fibula (11). The two divisions originate at the popliteus musculotendinous junction. The anterior division inserts 2.8 mm distal to the fibular styloid process on the anteromedial downslope, while the posterior division inserts 1.6 mm distal to the fibular styloid process on the posteromedial downslope (11). Sectioning the popliteus tendon has been reported to lead to an additional 5.9 degrees of external rotation at 90 degrees of knee flexion compared to a native knee and 1.7 degrees of varus angulation at 60 degrees of knee flexion (10). Additionally, the popliteofibular ligament has been reported to be a stabilizer against pathologic external rotation (7,10).

Additionally, reported clinical outcomes have confirmed the benefit of an anatomic reconstruction of grade III PLC injuries for patients (9,13–15). As a result, patients have improved posterolateral stability and preservation of their ACL and PCL ligaments, resulting in improved objective and subjective outcomes.

A grade I or II PLC injury should be managed nonoperatively and typically does not warrant surgery. For the first 3 weeks, the patient's injured leg should be immobilized in full extension. At 3 weeks, the patient can start working on increasing his or her range of motion with the supervision of a physical therapist. At 6 weeks, the physical therapist should initiate a functional rehabilitation program involving a stationary bike, light leg presses to a maximum of 70 degrees of flexion, and a functional walking program. At 2 to 3 months, the physical therapist should increase the exercise program based on the patient's increased strength levels. It is important to assess for residual posterolateral pain or instability after completion of the nonoperative program. Surgery may be indicated if any residual pain or instability persists.

Anatomic reconstruction is indicated for acute and chronic grade III PLC injuries or for a combined grade II PLC injury with a cruciate injury. Popliteus tendon or FCL avulsions can be managed using an anatomic repair within the first 2 weeks (14,16). However, for midsubstance tears or complex tears, anatomic reconstruction provides superior outcomes compared to repair (17,18). A chronic (>2 to 3 months) PLC injury presenting with genu varus malalignment needs to first be worked up for a first-stage proximal tibial osteotomy to correct the malalignment, or the PLC reconstruction has a high risk of failure. The osteotomy will correct the mechanical axis and by itself improve knee stability (19,20). One study found that 38% of patients had sufficient knee stability following a proximal tibial osteotomy and did not require a follow-up PLC reconstruction (19).

PREOPERATIVE PLANNING

Timing is imperative in treating patients with PLC injuries. Early diagnosis and surgical treatment has been shown to improve patient outcomes (14). Surgery is best performed 1 to 2 weeks after injury. Beginning at 3 weeks postinjury, scarring sets in, which can significantly affect patients' long-term outcomes (21).

Proper management requires the use of all resources available. Patient history, physical examination, and diagnostic imaging, including magnetic resonance imaging (MRI) and stress radiographs, help form an accurate diagnosis of the extent of injury to the knee, including damage to the PLC, cruciate ligaments, menisci, and medial-sided knee structures. PLC injuries are generally classified into three grades (1). Although there is no standardized classification, grading can be accomplished based on physical examination findings (Table 27-1) and stress radiographs (Table 27-2).

TABLE 27-1 Examination of PLC Injuries

Examination	Grade of Injury
Varus opening	Grade I—minimal increase in varus opening Grade II—< 1 cm of opening at 30 degrees of knee flexion Grade III—≥ 1 cm of opening at 30 degrees of knee flexion
External rotation	Grade I—minimal increase in external rotation Grade II—< 10 degrees increase compared to contralateral knee at 30 degrees of knee flexion Grade III—≥ 10 degrees increase compared to contralateral knee at 30 degrees of knee flexion
Posterolateral translation	Grade I—minimal increase in posterolateral translation Grade II—no more than a 1 grade increase compared to contralateral knee at 90 degrees of knee flexion Grade III—1–2 grade increase compared to contralateral knee at 90 degrees of knee flexion

TABLE 27-2 Significance of Varus Stress Radiographs (12)

Extent of injury	Side to Side Difference in Varus Gapping (mm)
No injury	<2.7 mm
Isolated FCL injury	2.7 mm– < 4.0 mm
Grade III PLC injury	≥4.0 mm

It is also important to keep in mind the differential diagnosis for a PLC injury. Patients with advanced medial compartment arthritis and genu varus alignment may present with a history and clinical findings similar to chronic PLC injuries. Varus and valgus stress radiographs can aid in differentiating medial versus lateral joint pathology (12), and Rosenberg view plain radiographs can further determine the extent of medial or lateral joint space narrowing. Additionally, patients with anteromedial rotatory instability due to superficial medial collateral ligament and posterior oblique ligament tears may present with clinical findings that can be confused with a PLC injury. Once again, varus and valgus stress radiographs can objectively determine whether the patient has a medial- or lateral-sided knee injury.

Assessment of the patient starts with taking a thorough patient history. It is important to ask the patient about the mechanism of injury, potential instability and pain, history of knee injuries and prior surgeries, as well as any associated lower extremity numbness or weakness.

Prior to performing specific physical examination maneuvers, it is important to inspect both knees of the patient. The examination should start with the uninjured leg in order to form a baseline of the patient's normal range of motion and laxity. Each knee should be evaluated for swelling, ecchymosis, or tenderness over the posterolateral structures of the knee.

A variety of physical examination maneuvers are used to evaluate PLC injuries. The external rotation recurvatum test compares the amount of recurvatum by measuring heel height and varus position of the knee compared to the contralateral knee (Fig. 27-1). The test is considered positive if there is a notable increase in recurvatum and varus positioning compared to the unaffected knee. A positive test is often indicative of a combined PLC injury and an ACL tear (22).

The varus stress test is also important in the evaluation of PLC injuries (Fig. 27-2). Varus gapping is compared between the two legs at 0 and 30 degrees of flexion. The dial test is an additional test that assesses the amount of external rotation compared to the uninjured leg (Fig. 27-3). A significant increase in external rotation at 30 degrees of flexion and little to no difference at 90 degrees suggests an isolated PLC injury, while an increase in external rotation at 30 and 90 degrees suggests a combined PCL and PLC injury (23). Other tests include the posterolateral drawer test (Fig. 27-4), where the amount of posterolateral rotation is compared to the contralateral knee with the knee externally rotated 15 degrees and in 90 degrees of flexion. The reverse pivot shift test is used to assess for reduction of a subluxated tibia relative to the femur as the knee is passively moved from 70 degrees of flexion to full extension (Fig. 27-5). In addition to assessing for ligamentous laxity, it is imperative to ensure that patient is neurovascularly intact. Both motor and sensory function of the common

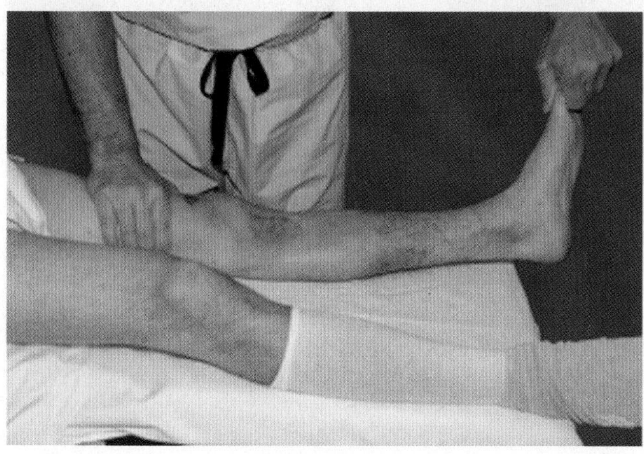

FIGURE 27-1
The external rotation recurvatum test.

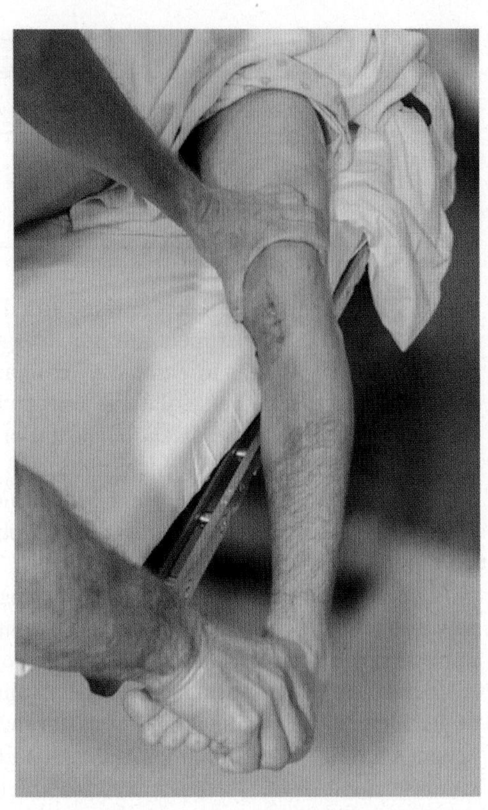

FIGURE 27-2
Varus stress test at 30 degrees.

peroneal nerve should be evaluated (1), as patients with PLC laxity may incur nerve damage during an acute traumatic injury.

Both radiographs and MRI are important components in the preoperative workup of a PLC injury. Standing posterior-anterior (PA) flexion radiographs should be performed to assess for medial joint line narrowing, which may contribute to medial compartment pseudolaxity

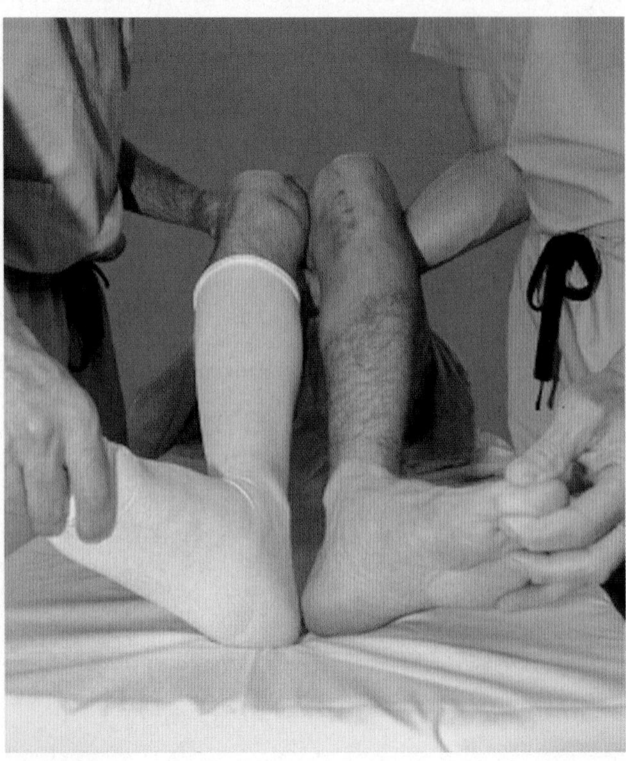

FIGURE 27-3
Dial test at 90 degrees.

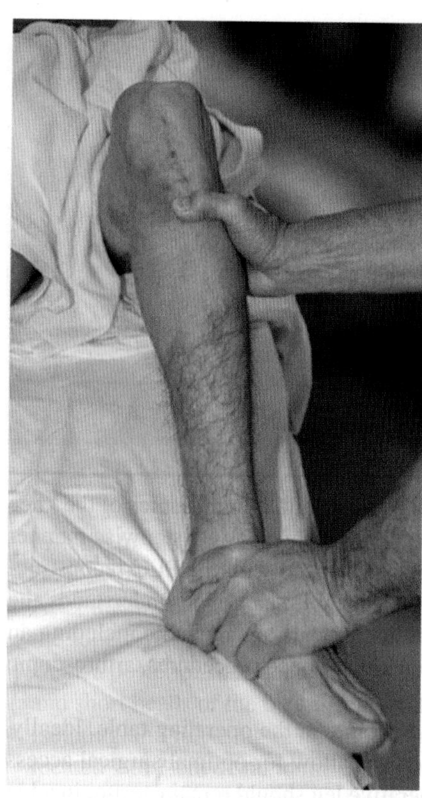

FIGURE 27-4
The posterolateral drawer test.

on clinical examination. Varus stress radiographs are also important diagnostically to evaluate lateral compartment gapping and differentiate an isolated FCL tear and a grade III posterolateral knee injury (Table 27-2). Bilateral varus stress radiographs should be performed at 20 degrees of flexion to appropriately assess lateral compartment opening (12,24). It is important that the clinician performing the radiographs applies the same varus load to both legs to observe any true pathologic lateral laxity. Valgus stress radiographs can also be performed to assess for any possible medial compartment laxity. Fibular head avulsion fractures, Segond fractures, and osteoarthritis need to be ruled out through AP, lateral, sunrise, and tunnel radiographs. Bilateral long-leg radiographs should be obtained to assess for genu malalignment (25). Additionally, MRI studies should be performed in conjunction with radiographic imaging to confirm the extent of injury to the PLC (26). A nerve conduction study may be necessary in cases of patients with residual posterolateral knee pain with no laxity or complain of pain to palpation of the common peroneal nerve (27). During surgical management, arthroscopic evaluation of the lateral compartment is beneficial to assess articular and cartilage damage and increases in lateral compartment gapping, also known as the drive-through sign (1).

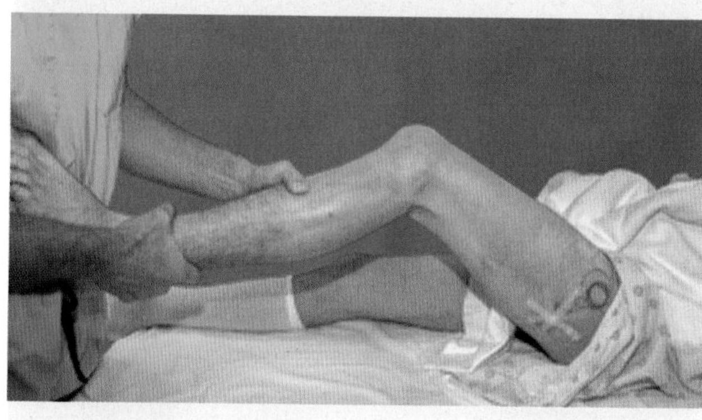

FIGURE 27-5
The reverse pivot shift test.

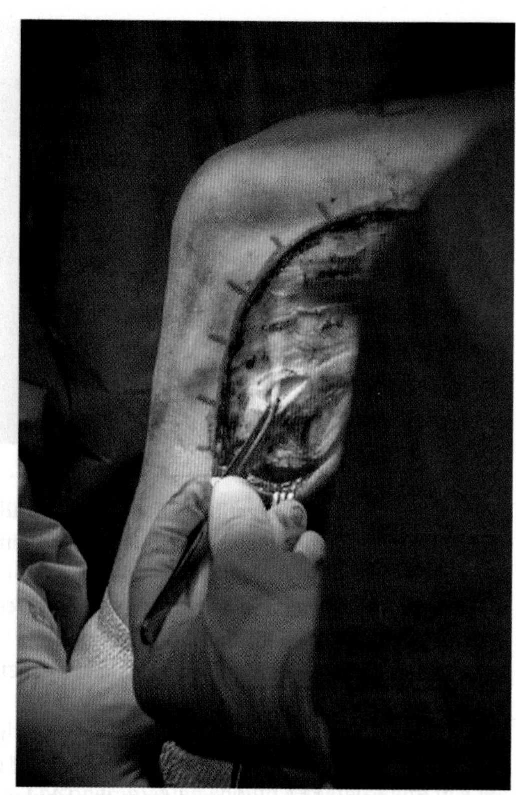

FIGURE 27-9
Identification of the FCL.

surrounding soft tissue structures. Identify the posteromedial aspect of the fibular head where the popliteofibular ligament inserts, and palpate the musculotendinous junction of the popliteus muscle.

- A horizontal incision should be made through the anterior arm of the long head of biceps femoris proximal to the fibular head, extending through the biceps bursa. The incision should allow direct visualization of the midsubstance of the FCL down to its fibular attachment (Fig. 27-9). A traction stitch should be inserted into the midportion of the FCL to allow for identification of the proximal FCL attachment on the femur.
- The fibular attachment of the FCL should be dissected down to the bone and the saddle where the popliteofibular ligament attaches on the posteromedial aspect of the fibular head should be identified.
- After identification of the main structures on the fibula and posterolateral tibia, the next step is to drill the fibular and tibial reconstruction tunnels. Start by drilling the fibular head tunnel. The direction of the tunnel is from the FCL attachment on the lateral aspect of the fibular head to the posteromedial downslope of the fibular styloid at the popliteofibular ligament attachment.
- Use a cruciate aiming device with a retractor placed behind the posteromedial aspect of the fibular head to protect the neurovasculature while drilling in a guide pin.
- Once the guide pin is in the proper orientation (Fig. 27-10), use a 7-mm reamer to ream the fibular head tunnel and place a passing suture into the fibular tunnel to help pass the graft at the end of the case.
- After forming the fibular head tunnel, attention should be turned to the tibial tunnel. Start by exposing the location of the anterior aperture of the tibial tunnel, located at the flat portion on the proximal tibia, distal and medial to Gerdy's tubercle. This area is just lateral to the lateral aspect of the patellar tendon and the tibial tubercle.
- Once the anterior site for the tibial tunnel is located, dissect down to the tibial bone using a rongeur to free the area of soft tissue.
- The posterior aperture of the tibial tunnel should then be formed. Identify the musculotendinous junction of the popliteus tendon between the gastrocnemius and soleus musculature. The posterior aperture will be 1 cm medial and 1 cm proximal to the fibular tunnel at the level of the musculotendinous junction of the popliteus.

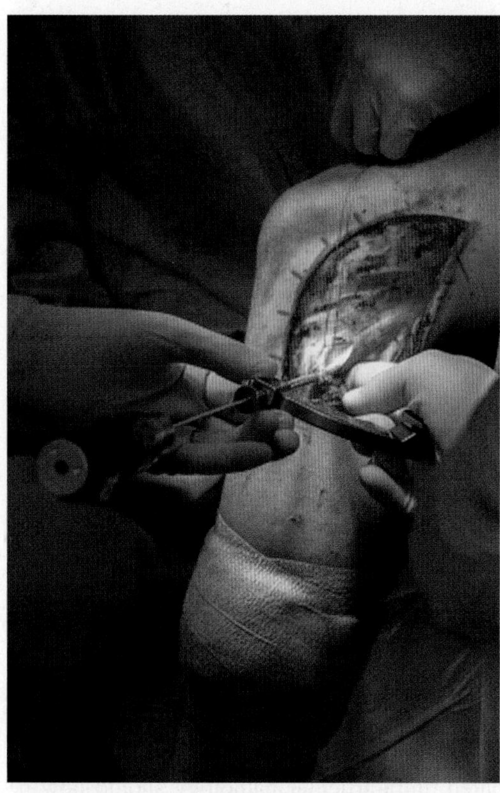

FIGURE 27-10

Drilling a guide pin anterolateral to posteromedial into the fibular head.

- Use an ACL aiming device to direct a guide pin anterior to posterior to form the tibial tunnel. A retractor should be placed behind the location of the posterior aperture of the tibial tunnel to protect the neurovasculature.
- With the retractor still in place, use a 9-mm reamer to create the tibial tunnel and insert a passing stitch (Fig. 27-11).
- Attention is turned to the femur. Place traction on the FCL by pulling the suture to help locate and palpate the femoral FCL attachment site.
- Once the femoral site is located, split the superficial fibers of the iliotibial band in parallel to the muscle fibers to help visualize the femoral FCL attachment.
- The proximal femoral attachment of the popliteus tendon should be located 18.5 mm anterior to the FCL insertion, in the anterior fifth of the popliteus hiatus (1).
- A vertical incision should be formed in the lateral capsule to directly visualize the proximal popliteus tendon attachment.
- Next, the FCL and popliteal femoral tunnels should be reamed. First, start by creating the FCL reconstruction tunnel. Pass a guide pin in the FCL attachment site in an anteromedial orientation

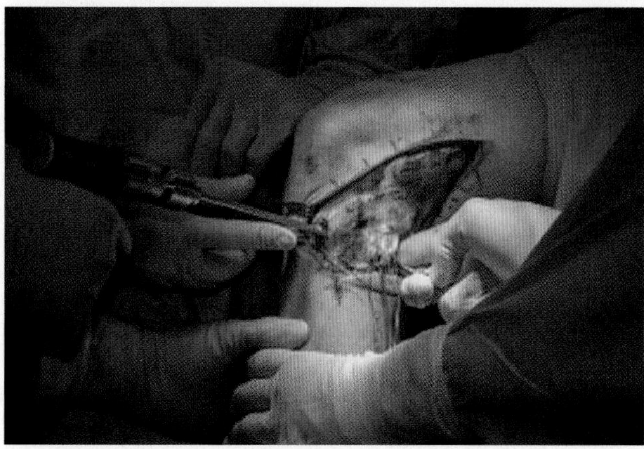

FIGURE 27-11

Reaming the tibial tunnel anterior to posterior with a 9-mm reamer.

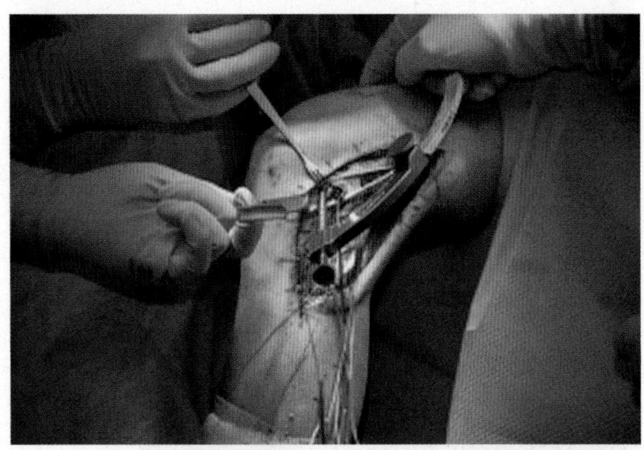

FIGURE 27-12

Drilling guide pins into femoral attachments of the popliteus tendon and the FCL.

across the distal thigh. The guide pin needs to be directed anterior enough to avoid the saphenous nerve, intercondylar notch, and cruciate femoral tunnels.

- Next, a guide pin should be passed through the popliteus tendon femoral attachment site. The FCL guide pin can be used as reference to ensure that the two guide pins are parallel with one another and the tunnels do not converge (Fig. 27-12).
- Prior to reaming the femoral tunnels, the distance of the pins should be checked. For proper anatomic placement, this distance should measure 18.5 mm. With the guide pins in position, the tunnels can be reamed. Using a 9-mm reamer, closed socket tunnels should be drilled to a depth of 25 mm followed by the placement of a passing stitch.
- Once the reconstruction tunnels have been prepared, intra-articular pathology should now be addressed. Secure any concurrent ACL and PCL grafts into the femur; perform any meniscectomy, meniscal repair, or articular cartilage treatment as needed.
- Grafts for the posterolateral reconstruction can be prepared while intra-articular pathologies are addressed. The senior author prefers a split Achilles tendon allograft because it can withstand the native forces of the PLC of the knee.
- Split the calcaneal portion of the Achilles graft down the middle to form two 9 × 25 mm bone plugs (Fig. 27-13).
- Tubularize the distal aspects of the Achilles tendon grafts to fit through a 9-mm tunnel.
- It is important that the initial 70 mm length of the FCL graft, and the initial 60 mm of the popliteus graft remain relatively thick to replicate the strength of the FCL and popliteus tendon. Place passing sutures into the soft tissue and bone plug ends of the grafts.
- The femoral ends of the FCL and popliteus tendon grafts should be fixed into their respective femoral reconstruction tunnels. Place the femoral bone plug end of the graft into the tunnel and use the passing suture to pull the bone plug completely into the femoral tunnel. Confirm that the graft and bone plug fit securely into the tunnel. Repeat the previous steps for the other graft.
- Secure each graft into its femoral tunnel with a 7 × 20 mm cannulated titanium screw with a handheld drill chuck and a 3-cm guide pin. Place the guide pin in the margin between the bone plug

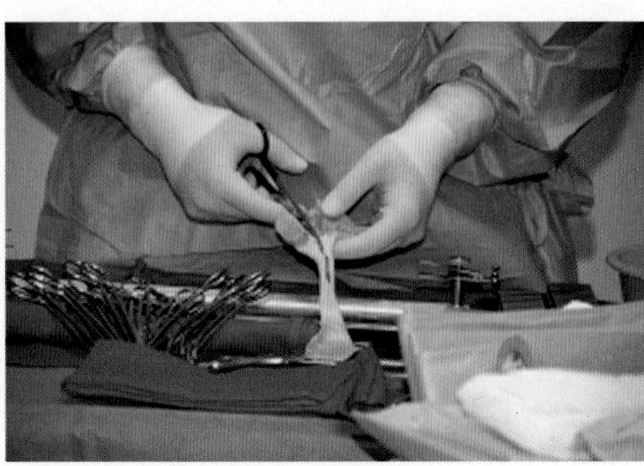

FIGURE 27-13

Preparing the grafts by splitting the Achilles allograft.

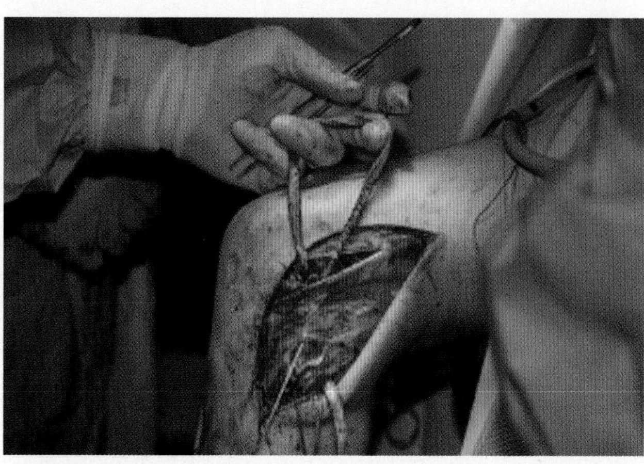

FIGURE 27-14

Passing the FCL graft deep to the iliotibial band.

and the rim of the femoral tunnel and fix the screw in place. Verify the graft is secure by checking for laxity with a firm lateral pull.

- The popliteus tendon should now be passed distally along the popliteal hiatus and ensure that the graft exits the knee between the lateral gastrocnemius and the soleus muscles.
- Next, take the FCL graft and pass it deep (medial) to the superficial iliotibial band and the lateral head of the biceps femoris (Fig. 27-14). With the FCL graft in the proper orientation, pass it through the fibular head tunnel.
- Now is the time to secure the tibial fixation of a concurrent PCL graft.
- The FCL graft can then be secured into the fibular tunnel. With the graft under tension, apply a valgus force to the knee at 20 degrees of flexion with the foot in neutral rotation. Fix the graft into the tunnel with a 7-mm bioabsorbable screw.
- With the grafts secured, the knee should be tested to ensure resolution of varus instability.
- The two PLC grafts are then ready to be passed posterior to anterior through the tibial tunnel to reconstruct the popliteus tendon and the popliteofibular ligament (Fig. 27-15).
- While placing tension on the grafts, the knee should be cycled through a full range of motion to ensure that there is no residual laxity.
- Prior to tibial fixation, palpate the posterior tibial aperture to verify that the grafts are not bunched together.

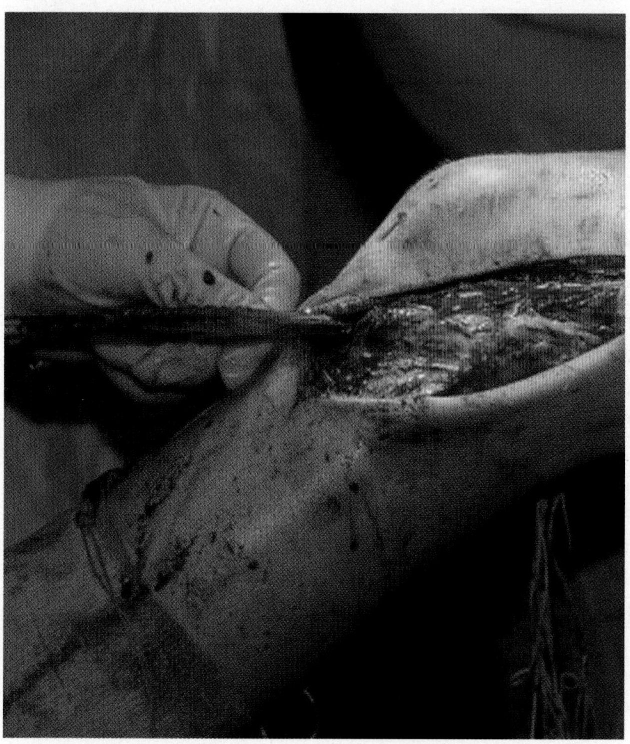

FIGURE 27-15

Passing both grafts through the tibial tunnel posterior to anterior.

- With the knee at 60 degrees of flexion, in neutral rotation, and under tension, fix the grafts with a 9-mm bioabsorbable screw into the anterior aperture of the tibial tunnel.
- Assess posterolateral rotatory stability by performing a dial test and a posterolateral drawer test.
- Now fix the tibial attachment of any concurrent ACL graft and finish treating other concomitant knee pathologies

PEARLS AND PITFALLS

- If the common peroneal nerve is difficult to identify, the nerve can be palpated 2 cm distal to the fibular head.
- A blunt obturator from an arthroscopy set can be placed in the reamed fibular head tunnel to help locate the site of the posterior tibial tunnel aperture.
- By placing the injured leg in 70 degrees of flexion, the femoral attachment of the popliteus can be identified by following the direction of the fibular shaft across the knee. The FCL will run parallel to the fibular shaft, and the popliteus tendon insertion will be approximately 1 cm anterior to the FCL attachment.
- For cruciate ligament reconstructions, fix the femoral end of the grafts while leaving the tibial end of the grafts free to prevent any external rotation deformities.
- A suture passer can help pass the FCL graft through the fibular head if it is difficult to pass the graft through the tunnel.
- If the fibular head tunnel is too proximal, the tunnel will minimize the cortical rim of the bone at the superior fibular head and increase the risk of fracture.
- The fibular head tunnel should be formed first to ensure that the tibial tunnel is located 8 to 10 mm proximally. If the tibial tunnel is formed prior to the fibular head tunnel, there is an increased risk of a horizontal popliteofibular ligament graft.
- If the femoral guide pins are placed too horizontal, there is an increased risk of convergence with the ACL femoral tunnel or crossing the intercondylar notch.
- If the grafts are insufficiently tubularized, the grafts may bunch and not be able to be passed in the tibial or fibular tunnels.
- For osteopenic bone, the grafts should be fixed on the tibia with a staple for secure fixation.

POSTOPERATIVE MANAGEMENT

Anatomic placement of the newly reconstructed PLC allows for early rehabilitation without putting excess stress on the grafts while minimizing the risk for arthrofibrosis and significant quadriceps atrophy. Passive range of motion is ideally initiated on day 1 postoperatively and is limited to 90 degrees until 2 weeks following surgery. The patient should also remain non–weight bearing for 6 weeks. Isolated hamstring activation as well as excess external rotation should be avoided until 4 months. Progression into frontal plane activities can be begin between 5 to 6 months postoperatively but only after the healing of the grafts are assessed by physical exam and varus stress radiographs. A sample rehabilitation protocol is presented below.

- *The first 2 weeks*: Quadriceps activation is maintained with quadriceps activation sets and straight leg raises in an immobilizer. Passive range of motion is allowed from 0 to 90 degrees and patella mobilizations should be performed daily. Focus should also be placed on maintaining full extension during the entire non–weight-bearing period.
- *At week 2*: If the patient is able to perform a straight leg raise without an extension lag, he or she can discontinue the use of the immobilizer during these exercises. The patient should also continue to perform their quad contraction sets. Passive range of motion can gradually be increased past 90 degrees as tolerated.
- *6 weeks*: The patient will transition to a functional ligament brace and can initiate weight bearing with crutches. Once the patient is able to walk without a limp, he or she is able to discontinue the use of the crutches. At this time, the patient can also begin using an indoor stationary bike without resistance.
- *12 weeks*: At this time point, the focus turns to single plane strengthening exercises as well as increasing the resistance on the stationary bike.

- *6 months*: In order to transition to frontal plane exercises, healing of the grafts should be confirmed on physical exam and varus stress radiographs.
- *7 to 9 months*: The patient can progress to multiplanar and plyometric exercises. Higher-level sport-specific drills and activities should be included at this time. Prior to full safe return to sport, a functional sports test should be administered to include strength, agility, and endurance.

COMPLICATIONS

While the surgical procedure generally benefits patients, complications do exist. Physicians need to understand the potential pitfalls in order to avoid complications. Like any procedure, there is always the risk of infection or wound dehiscence. Patients should be given prophylactic antibiotics prior to surgery. In addition, proper sterile technique will help minimize the risk of infection.

Deep venous thrombosis is another potential complication. A 6-week course of enteric-coated aspirin prophylaxis and the use of compression socks will help minimize the formation of deep venous thrombi. For patients with a history of hypercoagulability, consult with a hematologist to create a proper anticoagulation protocol.

Laceration of the common peroneal nerve or neurapraxia can occur due to the proximity of the nerve to the site of injury. Damage to the common peroneal nerve can lead to postoperative footdrop or sensory loss in the distal leg. Performing a proper peroneal neurolysis, including releasing the nerve from the peroneus longus fascia, allows the nerve to be secured away from the site of injury, limiting the opportunity for damage.

Improper placement of the two guide pins will lead to a nonanatomic reconstruction, which can lead to increased risk of graft failure and laxity. Placing both guide pins first and then measuring between them helps to avoid improper tunnel placement.

Graft failure is another potential pitfall. Postoperative follow-up with the patient is essential to assess for graft integrity. Additionally, the patient may have residual posterolateral instability. Follow-up physical examination and varus stress radiographs can assess for potential instability.

The patient may also have postoperative arthrofibrosis. Arthrofibrosis is a known complication following any intra-articular knee surgery, with a reported incidence of 4% to 35% (28). Early ROM and rehabilitation aid in minimizing arthrofibrosis; however, in the case of significant stiffness, the patient will need to return for manipulation or debridement postoperatively.

RESULTS

There have been few studies reporting clinical outcomes following anatomic PLC reconstruction surgery. However, the few reports published have shown promising results. Geeslin and LaPrade reported the outcomes of 29 patients who had PLC reconstruction or repair with a mean follow-up of 2.4 years. They found that the postoperative objective and subjective scores significantly increased following surgery (13).

Similarly, LaPrade et al. (15) found both subjective and objective scores to be significantly improved at a mean follow-up of 4.3 years. This study followed 64 patients who had grade III chronic posterolateral instability who were treated with anatomic reconstruction at a mean of 4.4 years postinjury. The total modified Cincinnati follow-up scores averaged 65.7, and objective IKDC scores for varus opening at 20 degrees, external rotation at 30 degrees, reverse pivot shift, and single-leg hop all significantly improved.

Levy et al. (29) compared postoperative Lysholm scores, IKDC scores, and failure rates following PLC reconstruction, at a mean follow-up of 28 months, and PLC repair, at a mean follow-up of 34 months. Both the repair and reconstruction groups had improved IKDC scores, average 77 for reconstruction and 79 for repair, and Lysholm scores, average 85 for repair and 88 for reconstruction. However, they found the repair group had a significantly higher failure rate (4 failures in 10 repairs) compared to the reconstruction group (1 failure in 18 reconstructions).

All studies mentioned also found that range of motion was largely maintained or improved following reconstruction. While these preliminary follow-up studies only report short-term outcomes, they show promise for long-term outcomes following anatomic PLC reconstruction.

ACKNOWLEDGMENT

The authors would like to acknowledge Angelica Wedell for her expertise in acquiring photos of the surgical technique.

REFERENCES

1. LaPrade RF. *Posterolateral knee injuries: anatomy, evaluation, and treatment*. New York: Thieme; 2006:1–226.
2. DeLee JC, Riley MB, Rockwood CA Jr. Acute posterolateral rotatory instability of the knee. *Am J Sports Med.* 1983;11:199–207.
3. LaPrade RF, Wentorf FA, Fritts H, et al. A prospective magnetic resonance imaging study of the incidence of posterolateral and multiple ligament injuries in acute knee injuries presenting with a hemarthrosis. *Arthroscopy.* 2007;23:1341–1347.
4. Ranawat A, Baker CL III, Henry S, et al. Posterolateral corner injury of the knee: evaluation and management. *J Am Acad Orthop Surg*. 2008;16:506–518.
5. LaPrade RF, Muench C, Wentorf F, et al. The effect of injury to the posterolateral structures of the knee on force in a posterior cruciate ligament graft: a biomechanical study. *Am J Sports Med*. 2002;30:233–238.
6. LaPrade RF, Resig S, Wentorf F, et al. The effects of grade III posterolateral knee complex injuries on anterior cruciate ligament graft force. A biomechanical analysis. *Am J Sports Med.* 1999;27:469–475.
7. LaPrade RF, Tso A, Wentorf FA. Force measurements on the fibular collateral ligament, popliteofibular ligament, and popliteus tendon to applied loads. *Am J Sports Med*. 2004;32:1695–1701.
8. Crum JA, LaPrade RF, Wentorf FA. The anatomy of the posterolateral aspect of the rabbit knee. *J Orthop Res*. 2003;21:723–729.
9. LaPrade RF, Johansen S, Wentorf FA, et al. An analysis of an anatomical posterolateral knee reconstruction: an in vitro biomechanical study and development of a surgical technique. *Am J Sports Med*. 2004;32:1405–1414.
10. LaPrade RF, Wozniczka JK, Stellmaker MP, et al. Analysis of the static function of the popliteus tendon and evaluation of an anatomic reconstruction: the "fifth ligament" of the knee. *Am J Sports Med*. 2010;38:543–549.
11. LaPrade RF, Ly TV, Wentorf FA, et al. The posterolateral attachments of the knee: a qualitative and quantitative morphologic analysis of the fibular collateral ligament, popliteus tendon, popliteofibular ligament, and lateral gastrocnemius tendon. *Am J Sports Med*. 2003;31:854–860.
12. LaPrade RF, Heikes C, Bakker AJ, et al. The reproducibility and repeatability of varus stress radiographs in the assessment of isolated fibular collateral ligament and grade-III posterolateral knee injuries. An in vitro biomechanical study. *J Bone Joint Surg Am*. 2008;90:2069–2076.
13. Geeslin AG, LaPrade RF. Outcomes of treatment of acute grade-III isolated and combined posterolateral knee injuries: a prospective case series and surgical technique. *J Bone Joint Surg Am*. 2011;93:1672–1683.
14. LaPrade RF, Griffith CJ, Coobs BR, et al. Improving Outcomes for Posterolateral Knee Injuries. *J Orthop Res*. 2014;32:485–491.
15. LaPrade RF, Johansen S, Agel J, et al. Outcomes of an anatomic posterolateral knee reconstruction. *J Bone Joint Surg Am*. 2010;92:16–22.
16. Fanelli GC, Feldmann DD. Management of combined anterior cruciate ligament/posterior cruciate ligament/posterolateral complex injuries of the knee. *Oper Tech Sports Med*. 1999;7:143–149.
17. Lunden JB, Bzdusek PJ, Monson JK, et al. Current concepts in the recognition and treatment of posterolateral corner injuries of the knee. *J Orthop Sports Phys Ther*. 2010;40:502–516.
18. Terry GC, LaPrade RF. The posterolateral aspect of the knee. Anatomy and surgical approach. *Am J Sports Med*. 1996;24:732–739.
19. Arthur A, LaPrade RF, Agel J. Proximal tibial opening wedge osteotomy as the initial treatment for chronic posterolateral corner deficiency in the varus knee: a prospective clinical study. *Am J Sports Med*. 2007;35:1844–1850.
20. Noyes FR, Barber-Westin SD, Albright JC. An analysis of the causes of failure in 57 consecutive posterolateral operative procedures. *Am J Sports Med*. 2006;34(9):1419–1430.
21. LaPrade RF, Wentorf F. Diagnosis and treatment of posterolateral knee injuries. *Clin Orthop Rel Res*. 2002;402:110–121.
22. LaPrade RF, Ly TV, Griffith C. The external rotation recurvatum test revisited: reevaluation of the sagittal plane tibiofemoral relationship. *Am J Sports Med.* 2008;36:709–712.
23. Kim JG, Lee YS, Shim JC, et al. Correlation between the rotational degrees of the dial test and arthroscopic and physical findings in posterolateral rotatory instability. *Knee Surg Sports Traumatol Arthrosc*. 2010;18:123–129.
24. Gwathmey FW Jr, Tompkins MA, Gaskin CM, et al. Can stress radiography of the knee help characterize posterolateral corner injury? *Clin Orthop Relat Res*. 2012;470:768–773.
25. Babazadeh S, Dowsey MM, Bingham RJ, et al. The long leg radiograph is a reliable method of assessing alignment when compared to computer-assisted navigation and computer tomography. *Knee*. 2013;20:242–249.
26. LaPrade RF, Gilbert TJ, Bollom TS, et al. The magnetic resonance imaging appearance of individual structures of the posterolateral knee. A prospective study of normal knees and knees with surgically verified grade III injuries. *Am J Sports Med.* 2000;38:191–199.
27. Roy PC. Electrodiagnostic evaluation of lower extremity neurogenic problems. *Foot Ankle Clin*. 2011;6:225–242.
28. Biggs-Kinzer A, Murphy B, Shelbourne KD, et al. Perioperative rehabilitation using a knee extension device and arthroscopic debridement in the treatment of arthrofibrosis. *Sports Health*. 2010;2:417–423.
29. Levy BA, Dajani KA, Morgan JA, et al. Repair versus reconstruction of the fibular collateral ligament and posterolateral corner in the multiligament injured knee. *Am J Sports Med*. 2010;38:804–809.

RECOMMENDED READINGS

Coobs BR, LaPrade RF, Griffith CJ, et al. Biomechanical analysis of an isolated fibular (lateral) collateral ligament reconstruction using an autogenous semitendinosus graft. *Am J Sports Med*. 2007;35:1521–1527.

Geeslin AG, LaPrade RF. Outcomes of treatment of acute grade-III isolated and combined posterolateral knee injuries: a prospective case series and surgical technique. *J Bone Joint Surg Am*. 2011;93:1672–1683.

Harner CD, Vogrin TM, Hoher J, et al. Biomechanical analysis of a posterior cruciate ligament reconstruction. Deficiency of the posterolateral structures as a cause of graft failure. *Am J Sports Med.* 2000;28:32–39.

LaPrade RF. Posterolateral knee injuries: anatomy, evaluation, and treatment. New York: Thieme; 2006:1–226.

LaPrade RF, Johansen S, Wentorf FA, et al. An analysis of an anatomical posterolateral knee reconstruction: an in vitro biomechanical study and development of a surgical technique. *Am J Sports Med.* 2004;32:1405–1414.

LaPrade RF, Ly TV, Wentorf FA, et al. The posterolateral attachments of the knee: a qualitative and quantitative morphologic analysis of the fibular collateral ligament, popliteus tendon, popliteofibular ligament, and lateral gastrocnemius tendon. *Am J Sports Med.* 2003;31:854–860.

LaPrade RF, Muench C, Wentorf F, et al. The effect of injury to the posterolateral structures of the knee on force in a posterior cruciate ligament graft: a biomechanical study. *Am J Sports Med.* 2002;30:233–238.

LaPrade RF, Resig S, Wentorf F, et al. The effects of grade III posterolateral knee complex injuries on anterior cruciate ligament graft force. A biomechanical analysis. *Am J Sports Med.* 1999;27:469–475.

LaPrade RF, Wozniczka JK, Stellmaker MP, et al. Analysis of the static function of the popliteus tendon and evaluation of an anatomic reconstruction: the "fifth ligament" of the knee. *Am J Sports Med.* 2010;38:543–549.

Levy BA, Dajani KA, Morgan JA, et al. Repair versus reconstruction of the fibular collateral ligament and posterolateral corner in the multiligament injured knee. *Am J Sports Med.* 2010;38:804–809.

28 Surgical Technique for Knee Dislocation

John Jasko, G. Keith Gill, Gehron Treme, and Robert C. Schenck Jr

DIAGNOSIS

Classically, a knee dislocation (KD) is defined as greater than 100% displacement of the tibiofemoral articulation evidenced on radiographs. Since the 1990s, the existence of spontaneously reduced knee dislocations has been well recognized. With an incidence as high as 50% of all KDs, these knees present reduced but have multiple injured ligaments (usually including both cruciates), instability on stress testing in extension, and significant swelling. A study from our institution showed that the incidence of vascular injury in reduced dislocations was equal to that of knees that presented dislocated. Therefore, any patient with a swollen knee and associated multitrauma must be evaluated for multiligamentous knee pathology and potential vascular injury. We utilize a KD protocol that documents initial ankle-brachial indices (ABIs) and involves serial vascular assessments of all knee dislocation patients with normal ABIs. Vascular surgery is consulted at the time of admission for all patients in order to involve this specialist early in the process and to obtain any additional recommendations on further workup/treatment. Computerized tomographic angiography (CTA) is commonly used in the patient with a dislocated knee and/or multitrauma to also insure a normal vascular tree.

The patient's knee should be evaluated using the standard and accepted physical exam tests for each ligament of the knee. First, we measure range of motion of the knee then examine the ligaments: posterior drawer for the PCL, varus, and valgus stress at 0 and 30 degrees for the collaterals; dial test at 30 and 90 and posterolateral drawer for the PLC; and Lachman and pivot shift for the ACL. The pivot shift test may be affected by severe medial injury giving a false-negative result. Use of a stabilized Lachman can be useful to help with both collateral and cruciate ligamentous examination.

Although most knee dislocations involve tears of both the PCL and anterior cruciate ligament (ACL), case reports of cruciate-intact knee dislocations do exist. A PCL-intact knee dislocation was first described in 1975. Several authors have described patients with a radiographically documented knee dislocation that, upon reduction, demonstrated an intact, functional cruciate ligament on physical examination. In most PCL-intact knee dislocations, the tibia is perched anterior on the distal femur, and in addition to an ACL tear, there is often complete rupture of either the medial collateral ligament (MCL) or posterolateral corner (PLC). Similarly, ACL-intact knee dislocations have also been reported. These are also extremely rare injuries. The tibia is perched posterior on the femur, and there is a complete tear of the PCL associated with a complete collateral ligament injury. Again, the presence of a functional ACL provides increased stability in the knee and changes the management of these injuries. A classification system for knee dislocations must take into account the presence of both reduced and cruciate-intact knee dislocations (Fig. 28-1A,B).

CLASSIFICATION

Several different classification systems for knee dislocations have been proposed and used over the years. All systems have their strength and weaknesses. However, like all orthopedic classifications, the most useful systems are easy to apply, are applicable to all patients, and serve as a guide to communication about and treatment for an injury. The most common classifications for knee dislocations are based on position, injury velocity, and anatomy.

In 1963, Kennedy was the first to classify knee dislocations proposing a classification system based on the tibial position with respect to the femur. He identified five types of dislocations: anterior, posterior, lateral, medial, and rotatory. Rotatory dislocations were further subdivided into four groups:

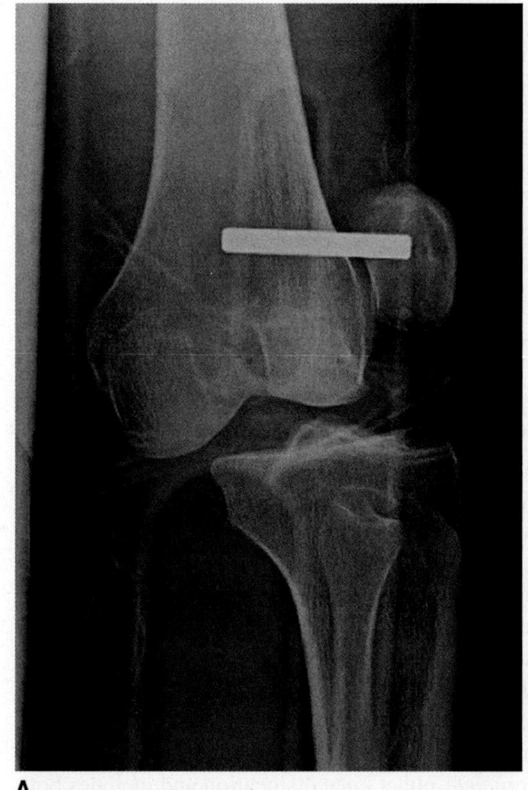

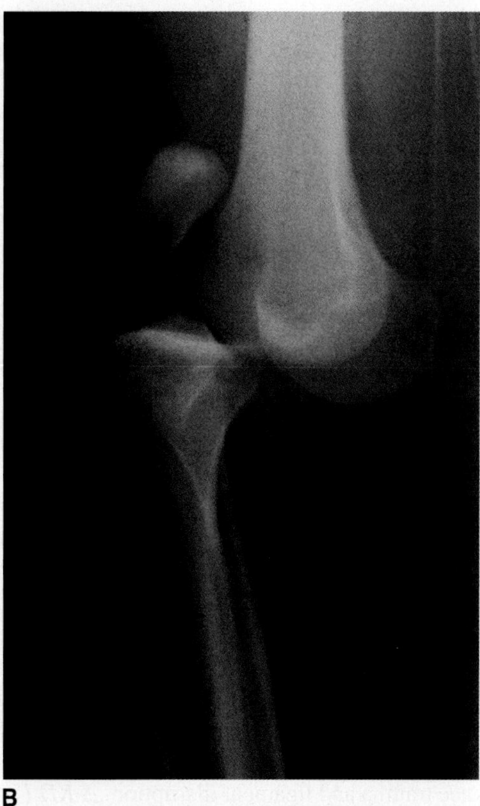

A B

FIGURE 28-1

A: Obvious multiligamentous knee injury that is not classifiable by position. **B:** KD I with an intact PCL with tearing of the ACL and PLC. (Image courtesy of and copyrighted by R.C. Schenck, Jr MD.)

anteromedial, anterolateral, posteromedial, and posterolateral. This classification system provides the treating physician with a guide to reduction and includes the posterolateral knee dislocation pattern that may require urgent operative reduction. This pattern frequently involves invagination of the medial sleeve into the joint, may present with skin furrowing along the joint line, and can result in tissue necrosis if left malreduced. Unfortunately, this system does not apply to all KDs as 50% present reduced. Additionally, with the exception noted above, this classification provides little guidance to treatment for the physician as there is no note of which ligaments are disrupted and need surgical intervention.

KDs have also been classified by the degree of energy imparted to the knee joint resulting in ligamentous injury. Most commonly, knee dislocations result from high-energy mechanisms such as motor vehicle collisions, industrial accidents, and falls from height. The injury mechanisms in high-energy knee dislocations often cause significant multisystem injuries as well as soft tissue injury about the affected knee. Many of these associated injuries can be life threatening, and their management takes precedence over treatment of the knee ligaments. KDs can also occur from low-energy trauma such as that seen in sports activities or in minor falls from low heights. These injuries tend to be more isolated with less multisystem involvement. Recently, Azar and colleagues proposed a third group of patients presenting to emergency departments with increasing frequency. These are morbidly obese individuals who present with a dislocated knee from a fall from standing height or from stepping awkwardly. They termed this group *ultra-low-velocity (ULV) knee dislocation*. These patients tend to have a body mass index (BMI) greater than 48 kg/m^2 and are more commonly female. They have a high rate of popliteal artery and nerve injury, are challenging to image, and have difficulty with rehabilitation after treatment. This patient group can be considered for early external fixation to mitigate some of these issues.

Finally, a classification system that is based on the ligamentous structures injured has been described by the senior author of this chapter (RCS) and has become universally accepted. This system applies to all patients once the knee is evaluated, guides treatment for the surgeon, aids in communication, and is easily applied and reproducible. Furthermore, this system has been correlated with patient outcomes after treatment with worsening functional scores found as the anatomic severity of the knee injury increases. The ligament anatomy of the knee is complex, with many injury patterns possible

TABLE 28-1 Anatomic Classification of Knee Dislocations

Class[a]	Injury
KD I	PCL- or ACL-intact KD, variable collateral involvement
KD II	Both cruciates torn, collaterals intact
KD III	Both cruciates torn, one collateral torn, subset M or L
KD IV	All four ligaments torn
KD V	Periarticular fracture-dislocation

[a]Subtypes: C, arterial injury; N, nerve injury.
ACL, anterior cruciate ligament; KD, knee dislocation; L, lateral; M, medial; PCL, posterior cruciate ligament.

when a knee dislocation occurs. The knee can be separated into four simply identifiable structures: the ACL, the PCL, the medial ligamentous structures, and the PLC. This simplistic representation of knee anatomy can be useful to the clinician in planning treatment of a dislocated knee.

In order to classify a KD by the injured anatomy, it is important to obtain a complete assessment of the injured knee using modern ligamentous exam maneuvers in order to determine which structures are functionally compromised. Magnetic resonance imaging (MRI) is critical in the evaluation and treatment of the dislocated knee, but functional evaluation of the ligaments ultimately determines the specific class of injury. Because of pain and limited motion, an exam under anesthesia (EUA) may be required to determine whether a ligament is completely and functionally torn. Stress radiographs are often valuable when there question of an involved collateral ligament in diagnosing a KD III versus a KD IV.

With the anatomic classification of a KD, five major injury patterns may occur (Table 28-1). Injuries are classified by roman numerals with higher-numbered injuries having sustained greater knee trauma and ligament disruption. A *KD I* is a cruciate-intact knee dislocation and includes both PCL-intact and ACL-intact injuries. A *KD II* is a bicruciate injury with functionally intact collateral ligaments. *KD III*, the most common injury pattern, involves tears of both cruciate ligaments and one of the collateral ligaments (M or L). *KD IV* involves complete disruption of all four major knee ligaments. Finally, the *KD V* group (as modified by Wascher and Schenck) is a KD with the presence of a major periarticular fracture and is described by other authors as a fracture-dislocation of the knee. Fracture-dislocations of the knee involve a ligamentous injury to the knee in association with a major fracture of the tibial plateau or femoral condyles that further destabilize the knee joint. Although avulsion injuries are frequently seen in purely ligamentous knee dislocations (arcuate avulsion fractures, tibial spine avulsions, or Segond fractures), they should be classified as a ligamentous injury in one of the first four categories, despite the small fracture present.

The final component of the anatomic classification is the use of additional labels to identify associated neurovascular injuries. A subtype C indicates a significant arterial injury and alerts the clinician to the need for revascularization of the limb. A subtype N indicates a peripheral nerve injury, either the tibial nerve or, more commonly, the peroneal nerve. This N subtype is used for any neurological deficit (neurapraxia, neurotmesis, or axonotmesis). For example, a dislocated knee with complete tears of the ACL, PCL, and PLC with an associated popliteal artery injury and a peroneal nerve palsy would be classified as a KD III-L-CN.

INDICATIONS/CONTRAINDICATIONS

Treatment of the dislocated knee involves several factors that must be weighed when choosing surgery and timing of surgery. In several series, nonoperative treatment has produced inferior results to surgical treatment of KDs regardless of energy or anatomical class. However, the patient presentation including vascular status, soft tissue integrity, closed head trauma, ability to participate in rehabilitation, neurologic status, and treatment of other long bone fractures will affect the treatment and timing of the KD. In some circumstances, the treating surgeon will be forced to treat KD patients nonoperatively (permanently or for a time) despite the knowledge of surgical treatment's superior outcomes.

In one study by Taylor et al., the authors found that immobilization for 4 to 6 weeks provided enough scarring to allow functional stability. The senior authors at our institution utilize this time period when nonoperative treatment is unavoidable due to patient traumatic comorbidities. In these situations, external fixation may be used to allow for "controlled arthrofibrosis" with a plan for delayed reconstruction or for this to be the definitive treatment depending on the patient's condition. Figure 28-2A to E highlights a patient that nonoperative management of the ligaments was necessitated by patient presentation.

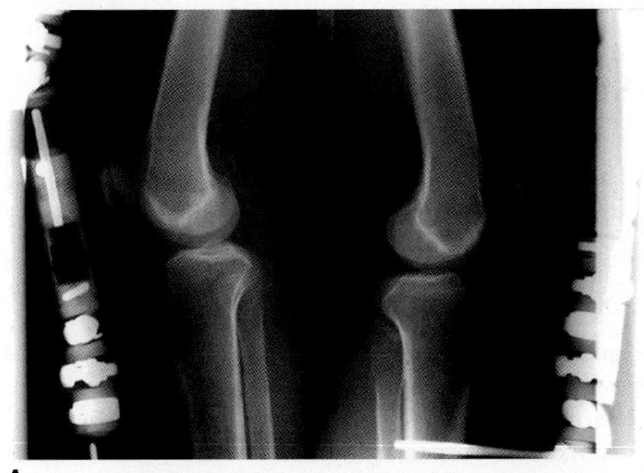

A

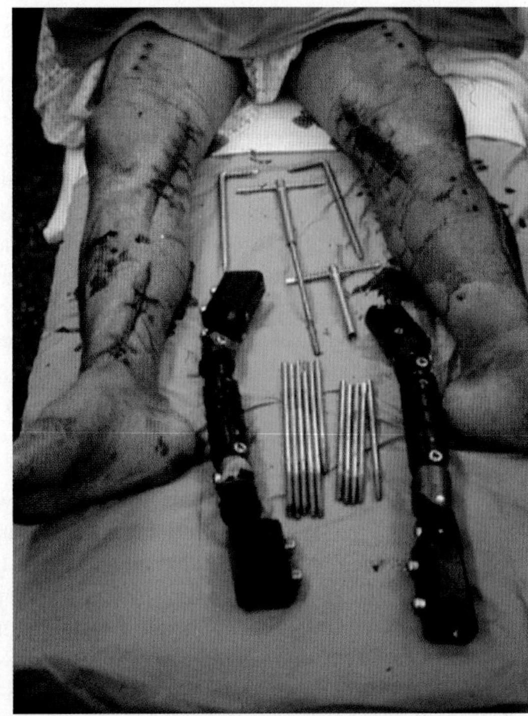

B

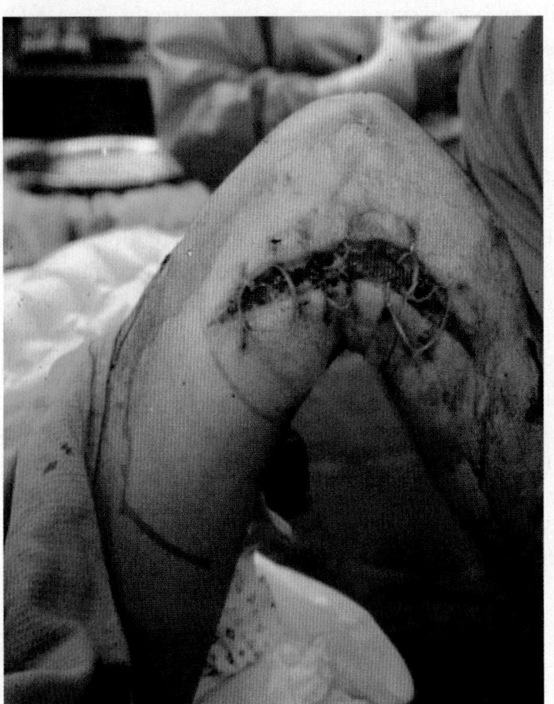

C

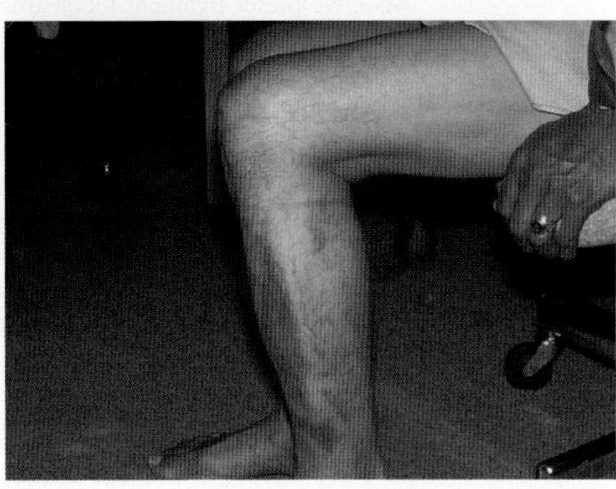

D

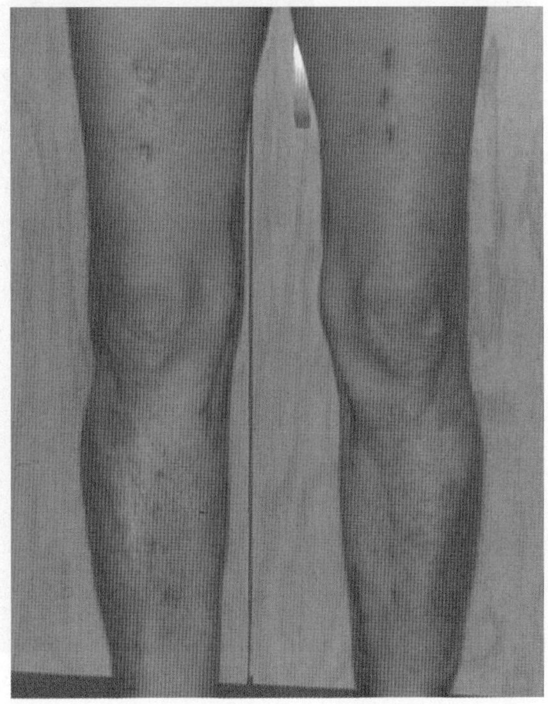

E

FIGURE 28-2

A–E: A 37-year-old male hit by a train with bilateral KDs with bilateral arterial injuries requiring bilateral reverse saphenous vein grafting and bilateral four compartment fasciotomies for bilateral compartment syndromes. External fixation utilized for 6 weeks followed by removal and manipulation under anesthesia. Note on lateral normalized tibiofemoral position on manipulation photograph. Wounds at this point would not allow safe arthroscopy or ligamentous reconstruction, and at long-term follow-up, patient did not require ligamentous surgery. (Images courtesy of and copyrighted by R.C. Schenck, Jr MD.)

PREOPERATIVE PLANNING

The surgical treatment of KDs requires surgical efficiency during the procedure. However, preoperative planning is essential to allow this efficiency to take place the day of surgery. Planning should include arrangement of implants and surgical sets with which the surgeon is familiar, ordering of allograft tissue of proper dimension as needed for the reconstruction, admission of the patient overnight for monitoring, decisions regarding anticoagulation strategy and rehabilitation, and setting patient expectations appropriately.

When evaluating the KD for surgical treatment, a variety of approaches exist. Orthopedic traumatologists often rely upon external fixation versus early operative repair. Orthopedic sports medicine surgeons frequently rely upon early or late repair versus reconstruction or staged or simultaneous reconstructions and often avoid external fixation. Despite an aversion to external fixation, this approach is sometimes required for extremely unstable KDs particularly if other injuries require that the joint be stabilized quickly without addressing the soft tissues directly. Most KDs can be externally fixed with a uniplanar frame spanning the knee joint with pins placed anterolaterally in the femur and anteromedially in the tibia. However, some KDs are so unstable that a hybrid fixator with a ring on the tibia just below the joint line and half pins in the femur is required to gain adequate stability and alignment. If the surgeon must use external fixation, anatomic reduction without joint distraction should be obtained and weekly radiographs taken to ensure that interval subluxation or dislocation has not occurred (Fig. 28-3).

In most cases, we plan to address all ligament injuries at one time once motion is reestablished. Also, we prefer ligament reconstructions rather than repairs in most cases. Exceptional situations that preclude waiting for motion restoration include irreducible posterolateral dislocation, extensor tendon and bony ligamentous avulsions, a Stener-type lesion of the MCL, and locked meniscal tears among others. See Figures 28-4A,B, 28-5A,B, and 28-6, for examples, of exceptions requiring early repair. Early repair of the collaterals has received great attention by investigators at separate institutions. Both Stannard and Levy have shown PLC repair failure rates of approximately 40% when done along with staged reconstruction of the cruciate ligaments. Despite some advantages to this approach, treating both the collaterals and cruciates with reconstruction in a single operation may avoid this high failure rate. Nonetheless, when applicable, a Krackow suture technique is useful with a screw and washer or bone tunnel technique (Schenck, 1994) as seen in Figure 28-7.

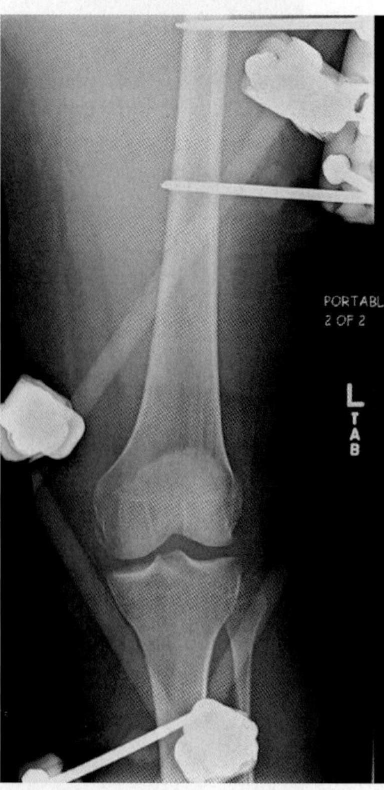

FIGURE 28-3

Use of external fixation in patient with a closed head injury, multitrauma, and an inability to maintain reduction of a KD IV injury film shown in Figure 28-1A. Joint distraction was re-reduced. (Image courtesy of and copyrighted by R.C. Schenck, Jr MD.)

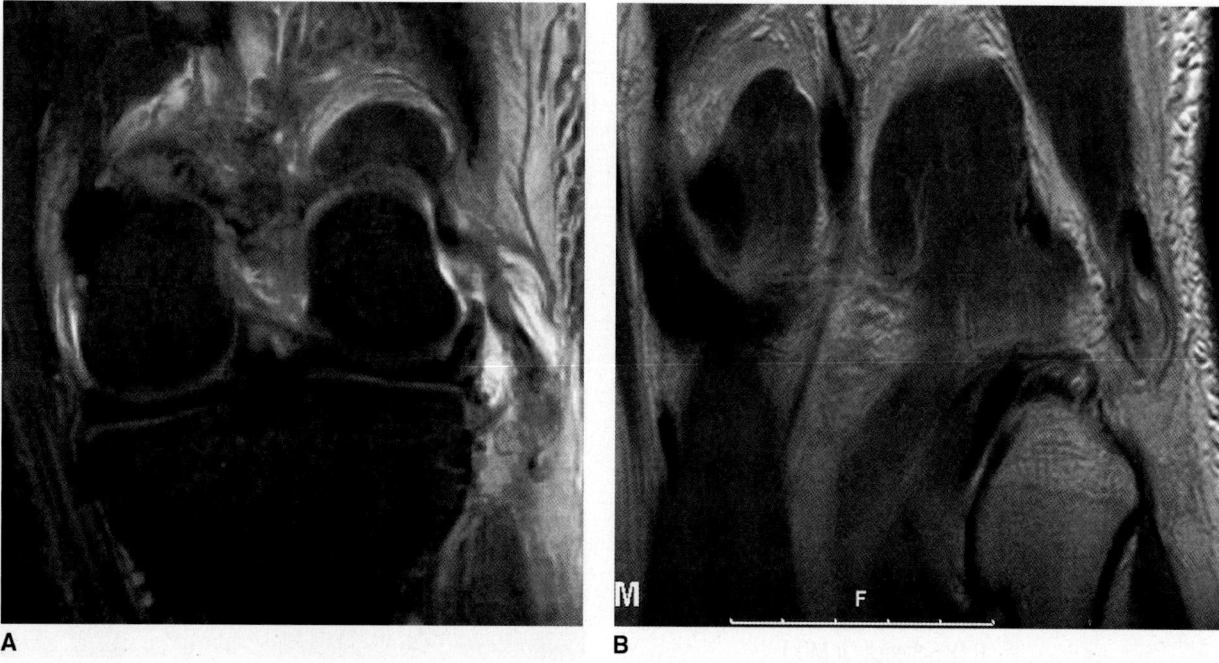

FIGURE 28-4

A, B: Avulsions of the lateral ligamentous structures and biceps femoris in a KD I in a collegiate athlete necessitating early repair. (Images courtesy of and copyrighted by R.C. Schenck, Jr MD.)

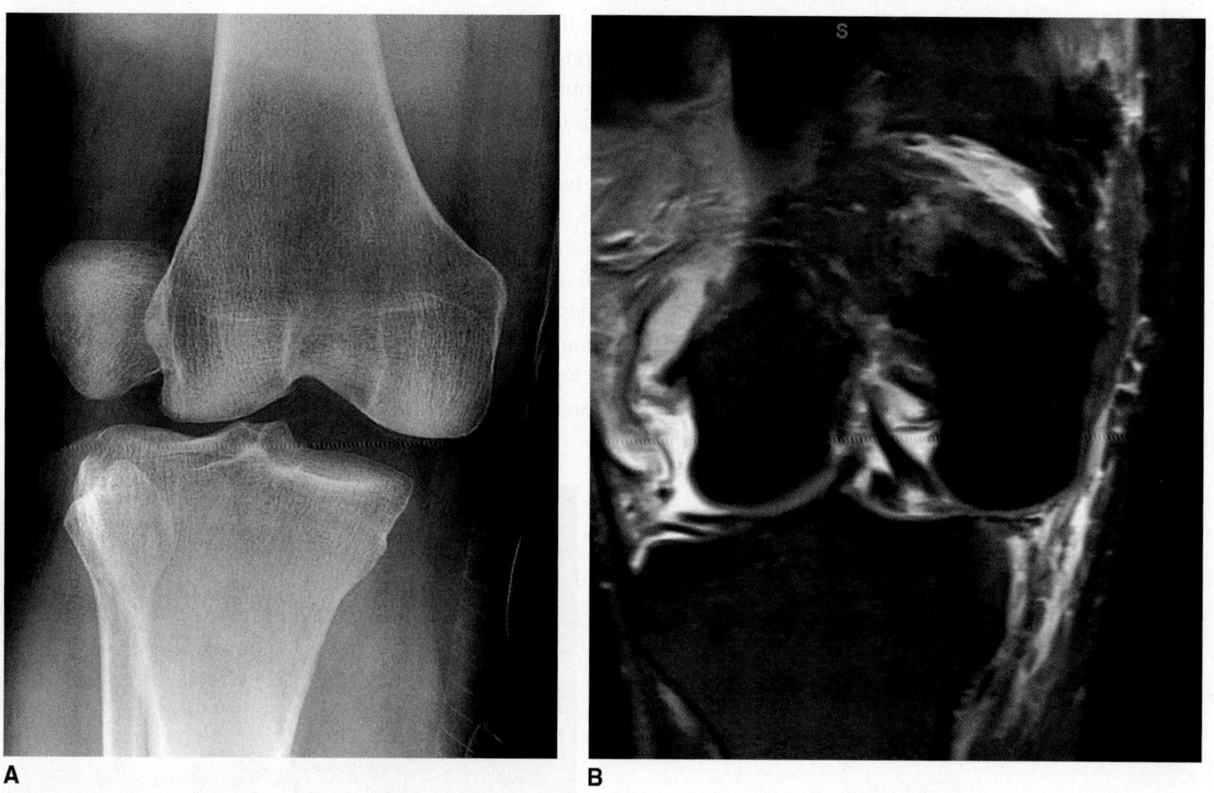

FIGURE 28-5

A, B: A 40-year-old injured in snowboarding accident with an isolated irreducible KD IV (variant of a PL dislocation) with plain film and corresponding MR coronal T2-weighted image. Early repair required 2 days after injury. (Images courtesy of and copyrighted by R.C. Schenck, Jr MD.)

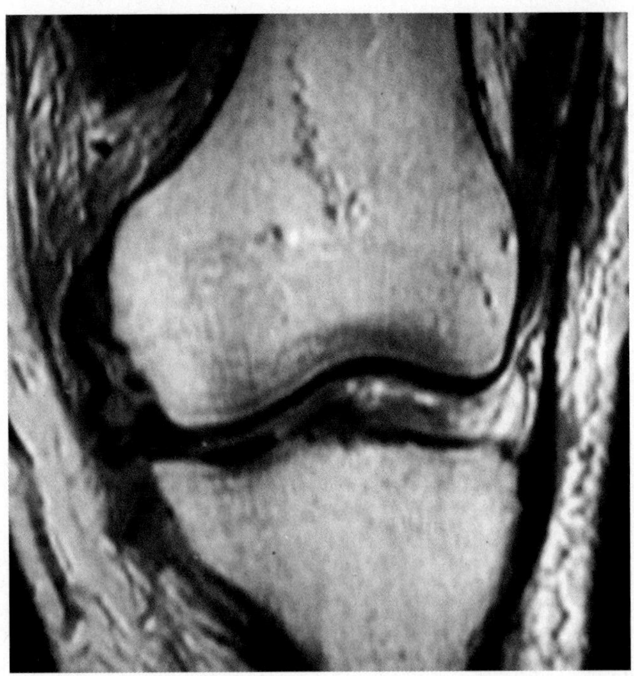

FIGURE 28-6

Avulsion of the tibial collateral ligament, flipped outside the pes anserinus and creating a Stener lesion of the knee. (Images courtesy of and copyrighted by R.C. Schenck, Jr MD.)

Surgical treatment of knee dislocations follows similar concepts as in isolated knee ligament surgery. However, because of the complexity and relative rarity for most surgeons, extra time for preoperative planning and the procedure is always required. We recommend that extra experienced assistants be available to help the case run smoothly and to divide the multiple tasks. Additionally, ample time should be allowed in the surgeon's day for these cases and overscheduling should be avoided. Allograft preparation prior to the start of the case can allow for more efficiency once the case starts and decrease the overall surgical time for the patient.

Proper equipment and implants should be arranged far in advance. Predetermine the need for implants such as suspensory devices, interference screws, and suture anchors and check your center's supply. Spiked soft tissue washers, small and large fragment screws, and staples are particularly helpful with repairs and are useful for backup fixation if needed. Specialized sets such as PCL and collateral ligament reconstruction trays are available from various vendors, but may need to be special ordered for the operation if they are not routinely used.

A final important factor in preoperative planning involves consideration of bone tunnel placement for the ligament reconstructions in order to avoid convergence. This is especially important on the femoral condyles with respect to ACL and PLC reconstructions and with PCL and MCL combination reconstructions. Creating bony sockets of minimal required depth can help prevent such convergence as can understanding the 3-dimensional orientation of each tunnel.

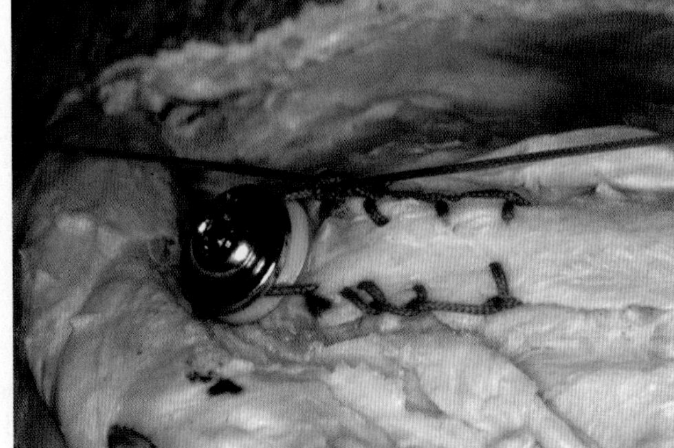

FIGURE 28-7

Use of a Krackow suture technique in performing repair of obvious ligament or tendon avulsions. (Image courtesy of and copyrighted by R.C. Schenck, Jr MD.)

OPERATIVE TREATMENT

The patient is positioned supine on the operative bed with the knee joint placed at the bend in the table. Variable degrees of knee flexion can be achieved by hanging the operative leg off the side of the bed or by adjusting the bend in the foot of the bed. The nonoperative leg is padded well under the thigh, fibular head, calf, and heel and may be gently secured to the bed with wide tape, especially if movement of the foot of the bed is anticipated. A foot or calf pump is placed to provide mechanical DVT prophylaxis during the case. A lateral post is secured to the bed to allow for valgus stressing during surgery. We prefer a modular post that can be flipped or swung out of the way when needed. A padded thigh tourniquet is placed as high as possible to allow maximum access to the extremity. The arthroscopy tower with monitor and surgical tables are positioned to allow maximum efficiency and provide access for c-arm imaging as needed during the case. The procedure is performed under general anesthesia and combined with preoperative femoral regional nerve blockade. Muscular relaxation, which is especially important when repairing avulsions or harvesting autografts, may also be useful and should be administered prior to tourniquet inflation.

As noted earlier, an EUA with comparison to the uninjured knee is critical to determine the integrity of ligaments and verifies the anatomic classification made prior to surgery. EUA is especially important in cases where the degree of collateral injury is not clear based on imaging or the in-office exam and includes the same tests described in the diagnosis section. Preoperative or intraoperative stress radiographs comparing both knees at full extension and 25-degree knee flexion can be extremely valuable. Arthroscopic EUA is very useful if questions remain regarding ligament integrity or for verification of the preoperative plan. The amount of medial compartment opening with valgus stress is an important indicator of the degree of medial-sided injury. Likewise, the presence of a drive-through sign and any injury to the intra-articular portion of the popliteus tendon provides valuable information regarding PLC integrity.

Arthroscopic portals should be planned with all intra-articular procedures considered. Similarly, the incisions for the open portions of the surgery should be positioned to maximize interval skin bridges. We prefer to perform the initial arthroscopy without tourniquet inflation in order to save tourniquet time for the open portion of the procedure. Frequently, once the joint is cleared of residual bloody effusion, visualization is adequate without need for the tourniquet. However, during procedures when visualization is not sufficient and the tourniquet needs to be used, we limit its use to 2 hours total time. If the procedure occurs 2 to 3 weeks after injury, the knee capsule has usually healed sufficiently to allow arthroscopically assisted procedures using a fluid pump system with the inflow pressure kept at or below 35 mm Hg. In those patients undergoing early repair, gravity flow is used as the capsule has had little time to heal. In all cases, frequent monitoring of potential extracapsular extravasation and calf compartment swelling is important, and one of the team members other than the primary surgeon is assigned the task of monitoring. In the presence of significant calf swelling, arthroscopy should be discontinued, and open reconstruction or suspension of the procedure altogether should be considered.

As this text contains chapters on individual reconstruction techniques for each ligament and structure potentially involved in a knee dislocation, we will not recapitulate each procedure here but will focus on surgical strategy and provide our most common choices for reconstruction of each ligament. The PCL is reconstructed with an Achilles or quadriceps tendon allograft with bone plug attached. These grafts can be used for either transtibial or inlay techniques. We most commonly utilize a transtibial approach, reserving inlay reconstruction for revision settings. Inlay is also used in some primary KD cases requiring medial reconstruction as described by the senior author (RCS). The ACL is addressed with autograft or allograft hamstring tissue using suspensory fixation on the femur and interference screw fixation on the tibia. MCL injuries are reconstructed using a hamstring allograft for the superficial MCL and imbrication of the posteromedial capsule. Lastly, the PLC is addressed with the technique described by LaPrade using an Achilles allograft. As some patients request the use of all autograft tissue for reconstruction, the surgeons may need to access the contralateral knee to provide adequate tissue. Hamstrings, quadriceps tendon, and patella tendon are all available in this situation. Meniscus tears are addressed as needed with particular attention paid to repairable tears in order to preserve as much of the secondary stabilizer affect as possible.

We prefer to perform arthroscopic procedures first prior to opening the corners for reconstruction in order to maximize arthroscopic fluid containment. The arthroscopic portion of the case includes meniscal debridement, meniscal repair, cruciate debridement, and cruciate ligament tunnel creation as well as any cartilage work that may be required. The order of ligament reconstruction is complex and cruciate ligament grafts are passed and secured on one end during this portion of the procedure. However, final fixation and tensioning is done in sequence as the procedure progresses. Our preferred order of final graft fixation is PCL, MCL, PLC, and ACL when performing a KD IV with this order adjusted as needed in the setting of other anatomic patterns.

Once the other arthroscopic procedures are completed, we begin the intra-articular portion of cruciate reconstruction. The notch is debrided of its contents to allow full visualization of the cruciate femoral footprints. Proposed insertion sites for the grafts are marked on the femur. The PCL tibial tunnel is then prepared, and pin placement is accomplished through the use of an accessory posteromedial portal. We utilize a safety incision, as described by Fanelli and others, to assist in safely creating the tibial tunnel. Care must be taken with the PM portal to avoid a large arthrotomy as soft tissue swelling can occur with a poor capsular seal around a cannula. The tibial tunnel for the PCL must be created carefully with intraoperative radiographs taken if there is question that the pin is not in optimal position. Careful controlled drilling of this tunnel should be performed first such that visualization of this critical part is optimized. The PCL femoral tunnel is then created by using an endoscopic inside out placement of a drill tip guide pin followed by overreaming with an acorn bit of appropriate diameter. The two PCL tunnels should create only minimal fluid extravasation and do not typically affect visualization. The femoral tunnel of the ACL is then created in the footprint of the old ACL using standard anatomic landmarks through an accessory anteromedial portal. Finally, the tibial tunnel of the ACL is created and the grafts are passed and fixed on the femoral side.

Our approach to final graft fixation allows a stepwise progression for reestablishing knee stability with anatomic reduction while moving efficiently through each ligament reconstruction. Femoral cruciate fixation is straightforward during the arthroscopic portion of the case whether utilizing interference screw or suspensory fixation. The PCL is tensioned with the knee at ninety degrees flexion, holding the knee in the anatomic neutral position such that the tibia is not subluxated anteriorly. We then move to the medial side with the hip externally rotated and complete the MCL reconstruction. Next, the leg is brought over the side of the table allowing for exposure of the lateral side of the knee along with dissection and protection of the common peroneal nerve. Tunnels for the PLC reconstruction can then be created and graft passage and fixation completed. Given the concern for potential tunnel convergence and disruption of the ACL femoral fixation, the tibial side of the ACL graft is tensioned after the PLC reconstruction is completed. This step allows for assessment of the femoral side integrity of the ACL. Once all grafts are passed and secured, intraoperative radiographs are obtained, incisions are closed with standard technique and a sterile, soft bandage is placed along with a long hinged knee brace locked in extension.

POSTOPERATIVE MANAGEMENT

If not already an inpatient, patients undergoing surgical reconstruction of the dislocated knee are admitted to the hospital for close observation of the neurovascular status of the leg and for supplemental pain control. Pedal pulses, microcirculatory appearance of the foot, and distal sensorimotor function are assessed every 4 hours for the first 24 hours postop. Any concern should prompt repeat ABI measurement followed by angiography and vascular surgery consultation if indicated. The high-energy nature of most knee dislocations required immobilization after injury, and subsequent surgical treatment renders each individual who sustains a multiligamentous knee injury at risk for developing a venous thromboembolic event (VTE). Therefore, we use mechanical prophylaxis during the hospital stay and start chemoprophylaxis 24 hours postoperatively. Our typical routine is to use low molecular weight heparin for 3 weeks followed by enteric-coated aspirin for 3 weeks, thus fulfilling the recommendations for "major orthopedic surgery" as outlined in the ACCP Antithrombotic Guidelines.

As with all ligamentous surgery of the knee, postoperative rehab must balance the protection of the soft tissue and grafts with the prevention of long-term stiffness, which portends a poor result. Recent studies have shown less ROM deficits and no significant increased laxity in patients allowed earlier ROM exercises. Our current regimen is to place the knee in a long-leg hinged brace locked in extension prior to leaving the operating room. Quad isometrics and assisted straight leg raises in brace are begun immediately. Patients are instructed to be NWB for the first 6 weeks with the brace locked in extension to protect the collateral ligament repairs. Range of motion is begun gently and progressively once sutures are removed. Full extension is emphasized but not hyperextension. To minimize the hamstring-mediated shear forces across the PCL, flexion past 30 degrees is performed in the side-lying or prone position until 6 weeks postop. New antishear device such as the PCL Jack Brace (Albrecht, Germany) can aid in resisting gravitational posterior forces while allowing ROM. Starting week 7, the patient begins progressive WB with crutches with the brace unlocked from 0 to 90. Once 105 degrees of flexion is achieved, work with an exercise bike is started. Transition off of crutches and into a hinged brace typically occurs at 9 to 10 weeks. Resisted hamstring activity and closed kinetic chain exercises past 70 degrees of flexion is restricted until 4 months postop. Patients are counseled that maximal improvement and return to sporting exercise takes 9 to 12 months.

Complications

Neurovascular injuries are the most difficult problems to manage with knee dislocations and their treatment. A high level of suspicion is required for rapid recognition, and if ischemia is present, immediate revascularization with a reverse saphenous vein graft is needed. As noted previously with external fixation, joint stabilization is a critical component in assisting the trauma team in their efforts on revascularization. For that reason, use of the posteromedial approach for revascularization is recommended as a posterior approach has significant disadvantages (see Fig. 28-8). The posterior approach is not extensile; requires a prone position, which adds risk to the multitrauma patient; and requires careful patient turning to the supine position to then apply external fixation. With the posteromedial approach, the patient is kept supine, and once revascularization is successful, the orthopedic team can apply an external fixator. In many scenarios, with good teamwork, the orthopedic surgeons can efficiently apply an ex-fix rapidly just prior to the vascular surgeon making their PM approach.

Of the neurologic complications, injury to the peroneal nerve is very debilitating and significantly limits patient return to function. In such scenarios, the nerve usually undergoes a significant stretch injury but is rarely torn. Early exploration and neurolysis has produced inconsistent results but in one study showed return of motor function in one in four patients. Because the PLC (KD IIIL or KD IV) is often involved with the peroneal nerve, treatment of the PLC always involves release of the peroneal nerve aiding in the potential recovery of neural deficits there. Nonetheless, treatment of a chronic foot drop is often as significant of a problem for patients as knee instability. Small patient series have utilized sural nerve grafts for peroneal nerve reconstruction, but results are often unpredictable with a success rate of less than 50% and usually only recommended in ideal candidates. Alternatively, use of a posterior tibial tendon transfer to the lateral cuneiform through the interosseous membrane accompanied by a percutaneous Achilles tendon release is predictable and leads to great improvement in the patient's function.

Ligament failure is an unfortunate complication with multiligamentous reconstructions and may involve an unrecognized involvement of a corner or cruciate, loss of fixation after reconstruction, or allograft tissue mediated failure. It is critical that the surgeon makes an accurate ligamentous diagnosis using a combination of EUA, stress radiographs, and arthroscopic EUA. Abnormal joint line opening must be recognized and treated with an appropriate corner reconstruction along with

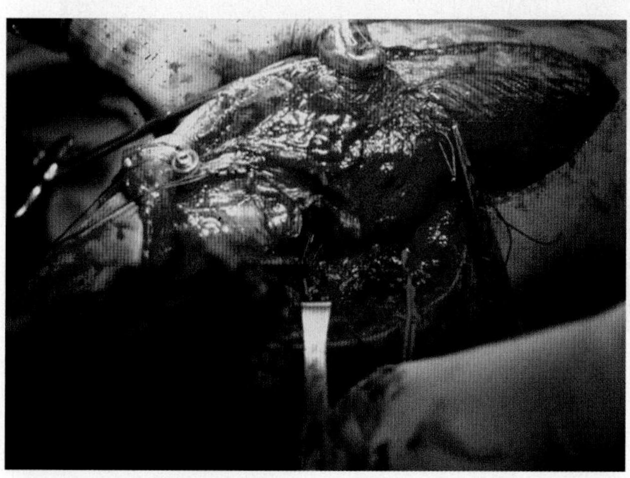

FIGURE 28-8

Posteromedial approach when performing a reverse saphenous vein graft reconstruction of the popliteal artery. Patient underwent simultaneous ligamentous repairs of the PCL and MCL (KD IIIMC) with delayed reconstruction of the ACL at 3 months postinjury. (Image courtesy of and copyrighted by R.C. Schenck, Jr MD.)

the involved cruciates. In the chronic multiligament-deficient knee, presence of a varus thrust must be managed with joint realignment procedures prior to ligamentous reconstructions.

As noted decades ago with knee dislocation outcomes by Marshall and Warren, "a stiff knee is worse than a loose knee." Arthrofibrosis is commonly seen in postreconstructed KDs, and virtually one in four patients will need arthroscopic lysis of adhesions and/or manipulation (see Fig. 28-9A,B). Careful observation for full extension and flexion past 90 degrees at 8 weeks is an important marker for the surgeon in the postoperative phase. Preoperative range of motion, avoidance of surgery on a knee that is inflamed, and involvement of a vigilant physical therapist pre- and postoperatively are extremely important.

Postoperative evaluation at 2, 4, 8, and 12 weeks is valuable in managing patient goals and in avoidance of arthrofibrosis. Presence of a flexion contracture at 2 to 3 weeks must be aggressively managed with prone leg hangs and manual stretching and, in recalcitrant cases, with the use of nighttime and passive stretch bracing. It is extremely useful to educate patients on goals such as obtaining 90 degrees of flexion by 6 to 8 weeks in avoiding a second surgery. Nonetheless, if by 10 weeks 90 degrees hasn't been reached, arthroscopic evaluation with lysis of adhesions and gentle manipulation are very useful and will result in improved outcomes. If the patient has both a flexion contracture and limited flexion, then the treatment should include admission with CPM and epidural anesthesia for 72 hours. In contrast, if the patient has full extension and just limited flexion near 90 degrees, then LOA and manipulation as an outpatient followed by immediate return to physical therapy is often successful.

Infection is the most difficult complication as it adds significant complexity to an already difficult clinical problem. Quick recognition and aggressive management with surgical washouts and intravenous antibiotics can often salvage the grafts and avoid repeat reconstruction. Ligamentous reconstruction after external fixation carries increased infection risk, and the surgeon must carefully judge the timing of knee surgery after external fixation removal.

In summary, avoidance of complications is always the surgeon's goal. Unfortunately with knee dislocations, complications are frequent and need to be managed aggressively when encountered. Initial careful examination for adequate vascularity, detection of any neurologic abnormality, vigilance for deep venous thrombosis, preoperative range of motion, waiting for inflammation to resolve before surgery, wound management/infection management, and prompt aggressive treatment of arthrofibrosis when observed are all part of managing the patient with a knee dislocation.

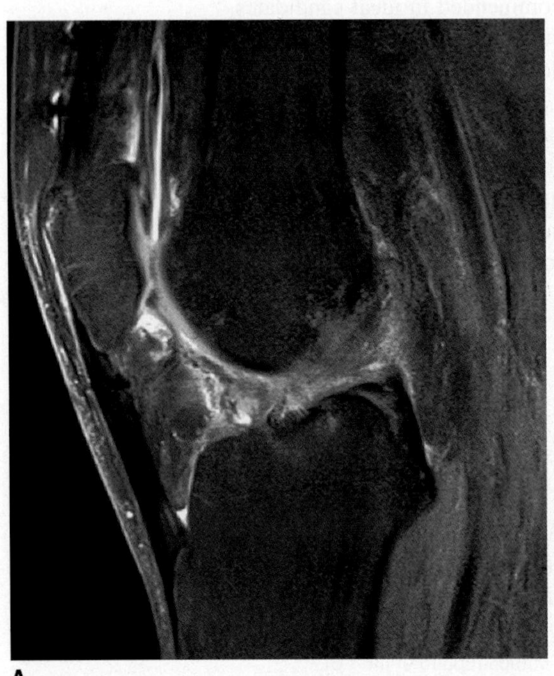
A

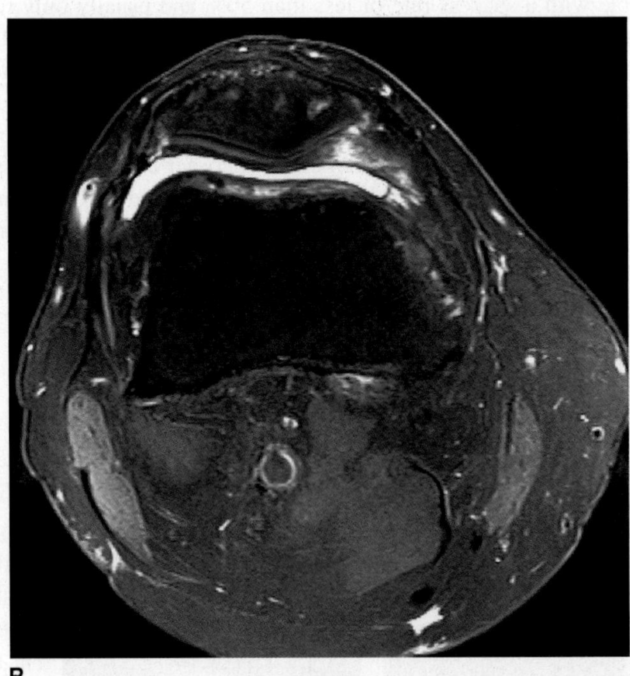
B

FIGURE 28-9

A, B: Extensive scarring in a multiligamentous knee injury requiring arthroscopic lysis of adhesions and gentle manipulation. (Image courtesy of and copyrighted by R.C. Schenck, Jr MD.)

PEARLS AND PITFALLS

Pearls

- KD treatment must be individualized depending upon patient presentation. Multitrauma, closed head injury, vascular injury, and soft tissue status must be included in any treatment decision.
- KDs should be classified by what is torn, anatomically.
- Operative treatment of ligament injuries is more successful and reliable than nonoperative management.
- Closed treatment with external fixation is often needed in the presence of limb-threatening associated injuries.
- Reconstructions are preferred over repairs, but surgeon experience and preference often dictate an approach. Collateral ligament repairs without an associated cruciate reconstruction carry a 40% failure rate.
- When performing repairs, the surgeon should consider simultaneous cruciate reconstructions.

Pitfalls

- Have a high degree of suspicion for a spontaneously reduced knee dislocation and associated vascular injury with any swollen knee in a multitrauma patient.
- When using external fixation, careful plain radiographs with weekly repeat films are critical to avoid subluxation.
- When using arthroscopy in a dislocated knee, soft tissue swelling is a signal to end the arthroscopy and either delay surgery or proceed to open procedures.
- When performing bicruciate reconstructions alongside corner reconstructions, the surgeon must be cautious with tunnel convergence to avoid damaging a well-placed graft.
- A stiff knee is routinely a worse outcome than a loose or unstable knee.

RECOMMENDED READINGS

Azar FM, Brandt JC, Miller RH, et al. Ultra-low-velocity knee dislocations. *Am J Sports Med.* 2011;39:2170–2174.

Hill JA, Rana NA. Complications of posterolateral dislocation of the knee: case report and literature review. *Clin Orthop Relat Res.* 1981;154:212–215.

Kennedy JC. Complete dislocation of the knee joint. *J Bone Joint Surg Am.* 1963;45:889–904.

LaPrade RF, Johansen S, Wentorf FA, et al. An analysis of an anatomical posterolateral knee reconstruction: an in vitro biomechanical study and development of a surgical technique. *Am J Sports Med.* 2004;32:1405–1414.

Medina O, Arom GA, Yeranosian MG, et al. Vascular and nerve injury after knee dislocation: a systematic review. *Clin Orthop Relat Res.* 2014;472(9):2621–2629.

Mook WR, Miller MD, Diduch DR, et al. Multiple-ligament knee injuries: a systematic review of the timing of operative intervention and postoperative rehabilitation. *J Bone Joint Surg Am.* 2009;91:2946–2957.

Muscat JO, Rogers W, Cruz AB, et al. Arterial injuries in orthopaedics: the posteromedial approach for vascular control about the knee. *J Orthop Trauma.* 1996;10:476–480.

Richter D, Wascher CD, Schenck RC. A novel posteromedial approach for tibial inlay PCL reconstruction in KDIIIM injuries: avoiding prone patient positioning. *Clin Orthop Relat Res.* 2014;472(9):2680–2690.

Schenck RC. The dislocated knee. *Instr Course Lect.* 1994;43:127–136.

Shuler MS, Jasper LE, Rauh PB, et al. Tunnel convergence in combined anterior cruciate ligament and posterolateral corner reconstruction. *Arthroscopy.* 2006;22(2):193–198.

Stannard JP, Sheils TM, Lopez-Ben RR, et al. Vascular injuries in knee dislocations: the role of physical examination in determining the need for arteriography. *J Bone Joint Surg Am.* 2004;86-A:910–915.

Taylor AR, Arden GP, Rainey HA. Traumatic dislocation of the knee. A report of forty-three cases with special reference to conservative treatment. *J Bone Joint Surg Br.* 1972;54:96–102.

Wascher DC, Dvirnak PC, DeCoster TA. Knee dislocation: initial assessment and implications for treatment. *J Orthop Trauma.* 1997;11:525–529.

29 Surgical Management of Malalignment in the Cruciate-Deficient Knee—Proximal Tibia and Distal Femur

Benjamin V. Herman and Robert Litchfield

INDICATIONS AND CONTRAINDICATIONS

Knees with a chronic anterior cruciate ligament (ACL) or posterior cruciate ligament (PCL) injury are susceptible to further meniscal or chondral injury, particularly on the medial side of the knee. Malalignment of the lower limb can put a cruciate-deficient patient at risk for further damage. Traditionally, osteotomies around the knee have been used in the setting of unicompartmental osteoarthritis in an effort to unload the affected compartment. High tibial osteotomy (HTO) is most commonly used for varus malalignment while distal femoral osteotomy (DFO) is reserved for valgus malalignment. The role of osteotomy in the setting of ACL or PCL deficiency has expanded over the years and can be used with or without a ligament reconstruction to address cruciate-deficient knees with or without gonarthrosis.

How Does an Osteotomy Help with Malalignment and Cruciate Deficiency?

The purpose of an osteotomy is to realign the weight-bearing axis of the lower extremity. Even with normal alignment, the knee experiences a varus/adduction moment during the gait cycle due to the adducted orientation of the femoral and tibial anatomical axes. This increases the compression in the medial compartment and tension on the lateral structures and is exacerbated with varus alignment. Conversely, with valgus alignment, there is a valgus/abduction moment at the knee, resulting in increased compression in the lateral compartment and tension on the medial soft tissue structures. These adduction/abduction moments at the knee can create forces that a cruciate-deficient knee may have trouble resisting, thus resulting in episodes of instability. Reorienting the weight-bearing axis can alter and decrease these forces at the knee.

Patients who are chronically ACL or PCL deficient tend to increase the contact pressures and accelerate wear in the medial compartment, thus causing further varus deformity. Noyes et al. have coined the terms "primary," "double," and "triple" varus to describe such knees. Primary varus is due to tibiofemoral bony alignment as well as any additional varus that results from medial compartment meniscectomy or chondral injury. Double varus knees are a result of this bony alignment and lateral compartment widening due to a posterolateral corner injury or lateral soft tissue deficiency. Triple varus knees have the same issues as do double varus knees in addition to increased external tibial rotation, hyperextension, and abnormal varus recurvatum.

Genu valgum is an issue that is seen less with cruciate injuries. However, ACL ruptures have a high association with lateral meniscal injuries. In the presence of a lateral meniscectomy, the lateral compartment is at an increased risk for accelerated wear due to the convex shape of the tibial articular surface. Articular contact pressures can become significantly greater than when a functioning meniscus is present to improve the lateral compartment congruity. Giffin et al. has described a classification for valgus knees that is similar to Noyes' for varus knees. Primary valgus is described as occurring for lateral compartment wear. Double valgus is due to lateral compartment wear and a valgus thrust secondary to medial femoral condylar liftoff from elongated medial soft tissues. Triple valgus is due to lateral compartment wear, valgus thrust, and failure of the posteromedial structures resulting in a rotational deformity.

The importance of sagittal alignment (posterior tibial slope) and its association with sagittal stability (anterior/posterior tibial translation) has become increasingly acknowledged. The resting position of the femur on the tibia is dependent on the tibial slope. When the slope is increased, the femur slides posteriorly in relation to the tibia (or the tibia translates anteriorly). When the cruciate ligaments are intact, there is a greater stress on the ACL and less on the PCL. When the ACL is injured, further anterior translation occurs. However, when the PCL is injured, the relatively anterior resting position of the tibia is advantageous to the posterior stability of the knee. Conversely, with decreased (flatter) tibial slope, the femur slides anteriorly in relation to the tibia. In the uninjured knee, the stress is greater on the PCL and less on the ACL. The ACL-deficient knee is aided by the relatively posterior resting position of the tibia while the PCL-deficient knee incurs further posterior translation and instability.

When Does Alignment Become "Malalignment?"

Normal alignment of the lower limb is considered anything between 3 degrees of varus and 3 degrees of valgus. There are patients who have normal inherent varus alignment—defined either as greater than 3 degrees of varus or a weight-bearing line falling medial to the medial tibial spine—or normal inherent valgus alignment—defined as greater than 3 degrees of valgus or a weight-bearing line falling lateral to the lateral tibial spine. Malalignment indicates a patient has had a change in his or her normal anatomy or that a patient's knee is now symptomatic with pain or instability that is exacerbated by the patient's varus/valgus alignment. The authors tend to define malalignment based on where the weight-bearing axis falls in relation to the tibial spine in a symptomatic patient.

Does the Patient Need an Osteotomy?

Symptoms of a chronically cruciate-deficient knee include instability and pain. A full history will reveal the severity of the symptoms and other pertinent information (see *Preoperative Planning*). Before considering any operative intervention, an appropriate course of nonoperative management should be trialed. Judicious use of analgesics, anti-inflammatories, injections, physical therapy, and braces should be employed. Once it has been determined that nonoperative management is not useful or has failed, the surgical options can be considered, including osteotomy.

In the presence of malalignment, there are four general parameters (Table 29-1) that must be addressed with the cruciate-deficient patient. First, it must be determined if this is an acute injury or a chronic issue. The more acute an injury, the less likely subtle malalignment issues will need to be addressed. Only in the rare case of severe coronal or sagittal malalignment should an osteotomy be considered. Second, the presence or absence of degenerative changes or cartilaginous injury must be determined and, if present, which compartment(s) of the knee is/are affected. An ideal outcome requires a situation in which the weight-bearing axis will fall within a relatively pristine compartment. Third, in the setting of revision cruciate ligament reconstruction, the factors contributing to the failure must be established. There is an extensive body of literature showing that varus malalignment and increased posterior tibial slope are risk factors for ACL injury and graft failure due to increased stress on the ligament. Last, the physiologic age, activity level, and expectations of the

TABLE 29-1 Four Parameters to Assess in Cruciate Patients with Malalignment

1. Acute versus chronic injury
2. Presence of chondral injury or arthritic changes
3. Possible revision surgery and factors leading to failure
4. Physiologic age, activity level, and expectations of the patient

TABLE 29-2 Most Common Clinical Scenarios and Surgical Procedures Required

Ligament Deficiency	Coronal Malalignment	Clinical Scenario/Symptoms	Surgical Procedure
ACL	Varus	Chronic with arthrosis	MOW HTO[a] + decrease slope
ACL	Varus	Instability +/− arthrosis	MOW HTO[a] +/− decrease slope + ACL reconstruction
ACL	Normal	Chronic with arthrosis	MOW HTO[a] + decrease slope +/− ACL reconstruction
ACL	Valgus	Instability	MCW DFO + ACL reconstruction
PCL	Varus	Chronic with arthrosis, failed PCL reconstruction	MOW HTO[a] + increase slope

[a]A tibial tubercle osteotomy may be required as part of an HTO, depending on preoperative templating.
ACL, anterior cruciate ligament; PCL, posterior cruciate ligament; MOW, medial opening wedge; HTO, high tibial osteotomy; MCW, medial closing wedge; DFO, distal femoral osteotomy.

patient must be elucidated. Osteotomy without ligament reconstruction is a good surgical option in the older patient who is involved in noncompetitive athletics or wants improvement in his or her activities of daily living.

What Type of Osteotomy Should the Patient Receive?

Several surgical options exist to achieve lower limb realignment. Combinations of opening wedge, closing wedge, laterally based, medially based, high tibial, and distal femoral osteotomies can be used to realign the weight-bearing axis. Each has its own advantages and disadvantages (Table 29-2).

Opening wedge osteotomies allow for an easier correction of both coronal and sagittal alignment. Only one cut is required, and it is easier to titrate the wedge size than two parallel cuts. The opening wedge preserves the patient's bone stock and may help tighten soft tissues around the knee. The main disadvantage is the resultant void space and need for bone graft—either autograft or allograft. There is also a risk of delayed union or nonunion and potential for delayed weight bearing without a solid construct (i.e., locking plate).

Closing wedge osteotomies require two parallel cuts to remove a wedge of bone. This can make it difficult to obtain the exact correction needed. However, once the wedge has been closed, there is cortical contact, meaning no need for bone grafting, and weight bearing can begin earlier.

Lateral-based osteotomies of the tibia violate the anterior compartment leading to increased risk of compartment syndrome. The common peroneal nerve and proximal tibiofibular joint is in close proximity and at risk for iatrogenic injury. When used on the femur, the lateral osteotomy may be easier to perform as the contralateral limb is not impeding access to the surgical field. However, prominent hardware can irritate the iliotibial band.

Medial-based osteotomies of the tibia avoid neurovascular and compartment violation issues of the lateral side. However, prominent hardware can irritate the pes tendons. The superficial medial collateral ligament must be addressed and protected postoperatively. On the femoral side, the medial osteotomy avoids the IT band irritation, but further proximal exposure may be limited.

Osteotomy of the tibia can affect symptoms through the entire range of motion. Femoral osteotomy has a more profound effect of symptoms in stance phase rather than flexion. HTO is typically used for varus deformity to realign a patient in slight valgus while a DFO is used for valgus deformity to create more varus. However, exceptions to these rules exist on a patient-by-patient basis.

Should the Patient Have an Associated Ligament Reconstruction and, If So, When Should it be Staged?

In the acute or subacute setting, the majority of patients with an ACL injury or high-grade PCL injury (most low-grade PCL injuries are successfully treated nonoperatively) will be candidates for a ligamentous reconstruction without an osteotomy. Older or less active patients may be treated nonoperatively. There are two situations in the patient with a first-time cruciate injury where osteotomy should be strongly considered. First, a primary osteotomy procedure should take place in patients with severe malalignment where the weight-bearing axis falls outside (medial or lateral to) the tibial plateau surface. The osteotomy should be healed prior to proceeding with the

TABLE 29-3 Indications for Osteotomy in the Setting of Cruciate Deficiency

Setting	Indications
Acute setting	• Severe malalignment • Associated chondral injury
Failed previous reconstruction	• Any varus malalignment with weight-bearing axis medial to medial tibial spine • Tibial slope > 10–12 degrees
Chronic	• Unstable knee in older and less active patients • Painful knee with unicompartmental degenerative changes • Double and triple varus knees

reconstruction. This may take 4 to 6 months. Second, young patients with significant malalignment who suffer severe chondral injuries that require a cartilage restoration procedure may be considered for an osteotomy with a chondral procedure concurrently or prior to a ligamentous reconstruction.

In the setting of a failed ACL reconstruction, a lower threshold should be held to address malalignment and slope, particularly with a noncontact mechanism of injury. The size of correction, status of the bone tunnels (need for bone graft), and associated meniscal or chondral injuries are all considerations when deciding on whether to stage or perform the osteotomy concurrently.

The chronic setting may be more challenging to determine the need for a ligamentous procedure as patients may have been functioning well with the cruciate deficiency. Typically, a young or highly active patient with symptomatic instability and progressive degenerative changes in the medial compartment secondary to varus malalignment and ACL deficiency are candidates for a combined osteotomy and ligament reconstruction. The size of correction can help guide the decision on whether or not to stage the procedures. Older or less active patients complaining of instability with or without pain, patients with pain only, and patients with severe chronic deformity (i.e., double and triple varus) can be first addressed with a realignment osteotomy. The decision to proceed with a ligamentous procedure can be made on a later date after adequate rehabilitation from the osteotomy (Table 29-3).

CONTRAINDICATIONS

Absolute contraindications to osteotomy in the setting of cruciate deficiency include the presence of an active infection and a poor ambulatory status for reasons other than the knee injury. Other strong contraindications include severe tricompartment osteoarthritis and contralateral compartment total meniscectomy or chondral injury. Reorienting the weight-bearing axis through an injured compartment will not result in a more functional or pain-free knee. Inflammatory arthritis is similar in that the disease is present throughout the entire the joint and reorienting the weight-bearing axis still puts it through a compromised compartment. A lack of functional range of motion cannot be improved through an osteotomy, and patients with such should be steered away from such an operation.

Relative contraindications include moderate to severe obesity and advanced age, though such patients may be considered after carefully exploring their expectations and activity levels. Diabetics and smokers should also be approached with caution as these patients have been shown to suffer from increased complication rates (Table 29-4).

TABLE 29-4 Contraindications to Osteotomy

- Severe tricompartmental osteoarthritis
- Contralateral compartment meniscectomy, articular cartilage defect
- Inflammatory arthritis
- Flexion contracture > 10 degrees
- Inability to flex > 100 degrees
- Moderate to severe obesity
- Advanced age
- Smoker
- Diabetic

PREOPERATIVE PLANNING

Patient Assessment

A full history should be taken first, and the patient's concerns should be elucidated. As mentioned previously, instability and pain are the typical presenting complaints. It should be determined when instability occurs—whether it is present during sporting or everyday activities. Pain is more worrisome and can indicate further injury to the knee, particularly meniscal injury and/or chondral injury. In the setting of a chronic cruciate injury, there may be posttraumatic osteoarthritic changes. Pain associated with weight bearing or at night is correlative with such degenerative changes.

A focused physical exam should follow. One should assess the standing coronal alignment for genu varum or valgum. Observing the patient's gait will detect the presence of a varus (with or without hyperextension) or valgus thrust. Assess the range of motion—both actively and passively—for any hyperextension, varus recurvatum, blocks to movement, or crepitus. Laxity of the cruciate and collateral ligaments as well as the posterolateral and posteromedial corners should all be assessed. Determining if there are additional ligamentous injuries to the cruciate injury is paramount to a successful outcome as missed collateral or corner injuries can lead to failure of cruciate reconstructions or further instability. In the chronic setting, it can sometimes be difficult to assess the normal reduced position of the knee as it "teeter-totters" about the tibial spines. Varus and valgus stress radiographs (see later) will help in this situation. Lastly, a neurovascular exam should be completed as multiligamentous injuries can have associated peroneal nerve or popliteal artery injuries.

Imaging for preoperative planning will include both radiographs and magnetic resonance imaging (MRI). Standard radiographs include bilateral weight-bearing anteroposterior (AP) views of the knee in full extension and in 30 to 45 degrees of flexion (Rosenberg view), lateral, skyline, and weight-bearing hip-to-ankle AP views. AP views will allow assessment of degenerative changes in the knee, with the tunnel views being more sensitive to assess loss of joint space. The lateral view is used to measure posterior tibial slope and patellar height as well as assess the patellofemoral joint for degenerative changes. The full-length standing films are used to assess the deformity and mechanical/anatomical axes and template an osteotomy.

Alignment (or malalignment) can be determined on the full-length standing films in one of two ways. First, the weight-bearing axis can be drawn from the center of the femoral head to the center of the talus. Assessing the position of this axis within the knee dictates the severity of deformity. Normal alignment is defined as the weight-bearing axis falling between the tibial spines whereas an axis that falls outside the knee would be considered severe genu varum or valgum. The second method is to draw mechanical axes of the femur and tibia intersecting at the center of the knee. The resultant angle is the degree of deformity.

Stress radiographs can be used in complex knee cases when there is difficulty in assessing the ligamentous injury on physical exam. A PCL stress radiograph can be taken with the patient kneeling and assessing the side-to-side difference of posterior tibial translation. Other methods exist to perform a stress radiograph, including using gravity, hamstring contraction, or a Telos device, but the authors find kneeling to be the fastest and easiest way for the patient. Collateral stress radiographs are simply obtained by performing a varus or valgus stress test using protective gloves at the time of imaging. Side-to-side differences are used to determine the severity of the injury. These are indicated in the setting of double and triple varus/valgus knees. The reader is directed to the recommended readings of LaPrade.

The authors do not routinely order MRIs for isolated ACL injuries but will for isolated PCL injuries to rule out additional ligamentous injuries (i.e., posterolateral corner). MRI should be employed on all patients with multiple ligamentous injuries to help determine all soft tissue injuries and corroborate the physical exam. As mentioned previously, a full understanding of the ligamentous deficiencies is important as missed collateral, posterolateral, or posteromedial corner injuries can lead to a failed outcome. MRI can help with planning graft options and additional surgical instruments (i.e., meniscal repair).

Preoperative Templating

First, confirm that there is no obvious anatomical abnormality of the tibia or femur accounting for the malalignment. The osteotomy is best performed on the abnormal bone if one exists. If both bones are essentially normal, proceed as follows. The mechanical axes must be templated to the position where the new weight-bearing axis will be (the correction point). When instability is the indication for surgery, the center of the knee is used as the correction point. In the presence of varus malalignment and medial compartment pathology, the downslope of the lateral tibial spine is sufficient. Conversely, the downslope of the medial tibial spine can be used in cases of valgus malalignment and lateral compartment pathology. Once the correction point is established, the remainder of the templating is the same (Fig. 29-1A–C).

1. Draw the femoral mechanical axis from the center of the femoral head through the correction point in the knee.
2. Draw the tibial mechanical axis from the center of talus through the correction point.
3. Draw the proposed osteotomy, and measure the length of this line
   a. In the tibia, this starts on the proximal medial cortex and extends proximally toward the lateral metaphyseal flare, such that the osteotomy ends approximately 20 mm from the joint line. Stop the osteotomy approximately 5 to 10 mm from the lateral cortex.
   b. In the femur, this starts on the supracondylar medial cortex and extends distally toward the proximal aspect of the lateral femoral condyle. Stop the osteotomy approximately 5 to 10 mm from the lateral cortex.
4. Starting at the correction point, superimpose the proposed osteotomy line over one of the mechanical axes lines.
5. Determine the proposed osteotomy wedge size by measuring the distance between the two mechanical axes at the end of the superimposed osteotomy line.

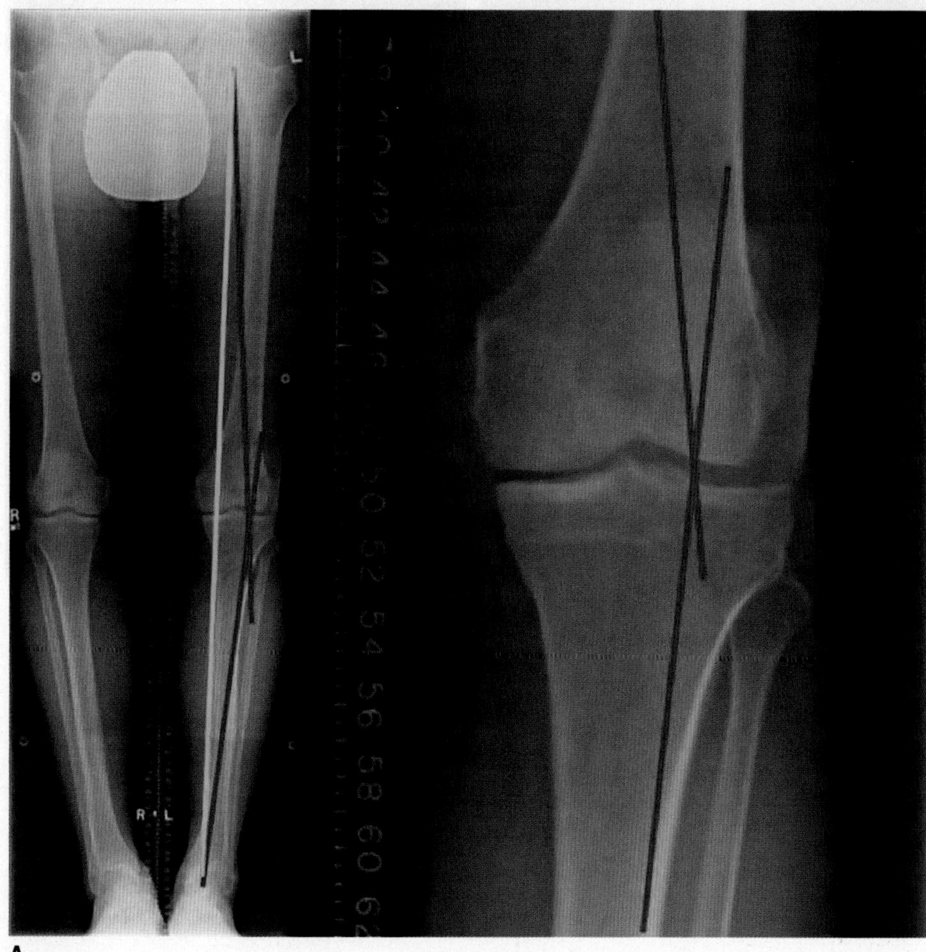

A

FIGURE 29-1

A–C: The templating process. The downslope of the lateral tibial spine has been used as the correction point, which would indicate the patient has medial pain in addition to his or her instability. The *green line* is the patient's current weight-bearing axis. The *red lines* are the templated mechanical axes. The *yellow lines* indicate the proposed osteotomy site and the same length overlaying the mechanical axis. The *blue line* indicates the size of the wedge.

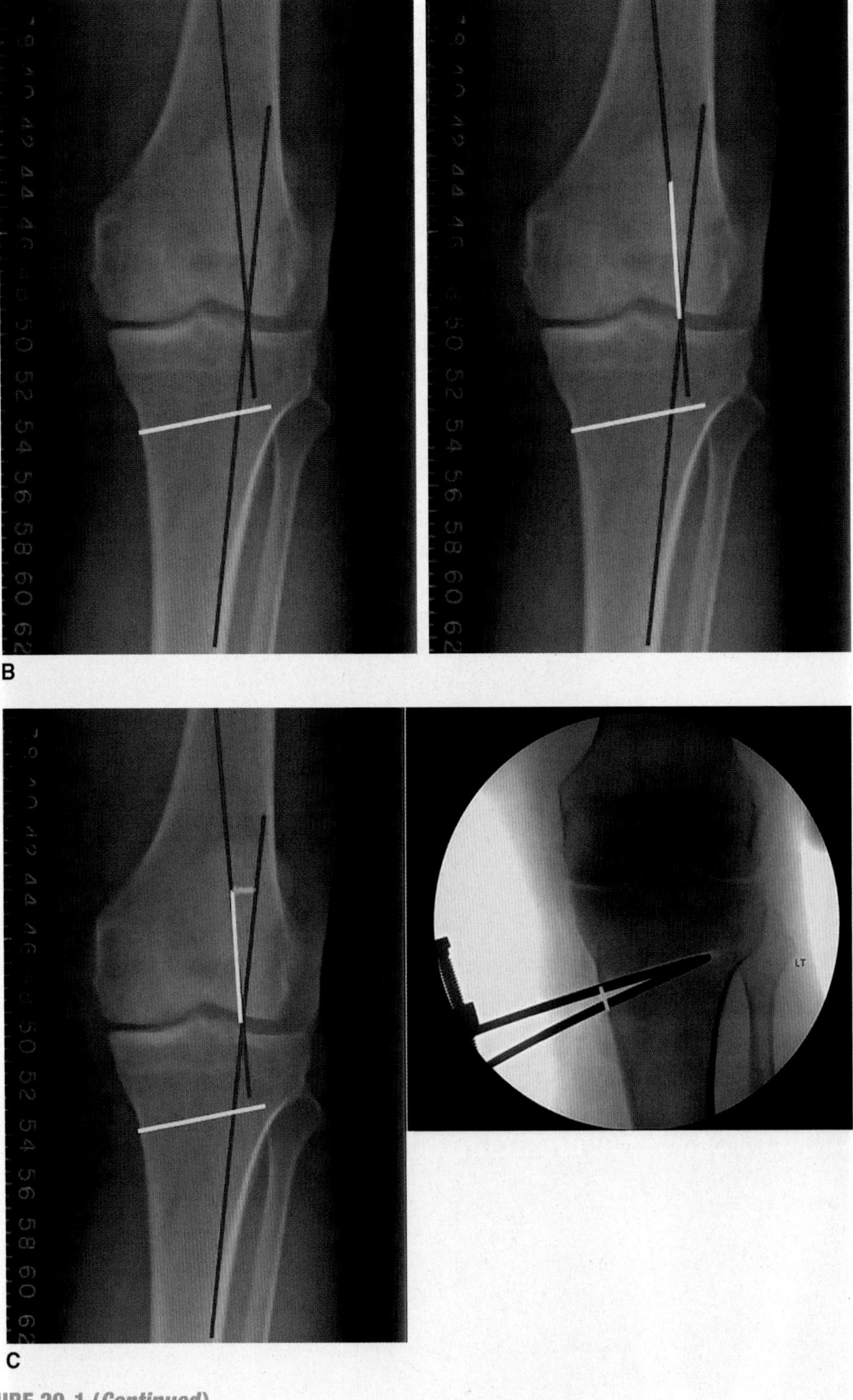

FIGURE 29-1 (*Continued*)

Lastly, the lateral radiograph should be assessed for patellar height, posterior tibial slope (Fig. 29-2), and any degenerative changes of the patellofemoral joint. The patellar height can be determined by a number of different ratios (Insall-Salvati, Blackburne-Peel, Caton-Deschamps). If a medial opening wedge HTO is being used and a patient has patellar baja or patellofemoral arthritis, or if a large correction is being made (i.e., 15 degrees or greater), plans for a biplanar osteotomy with a tibial tubercle osteotomy (TTO) should be made. The posterior tibial slope is determined by

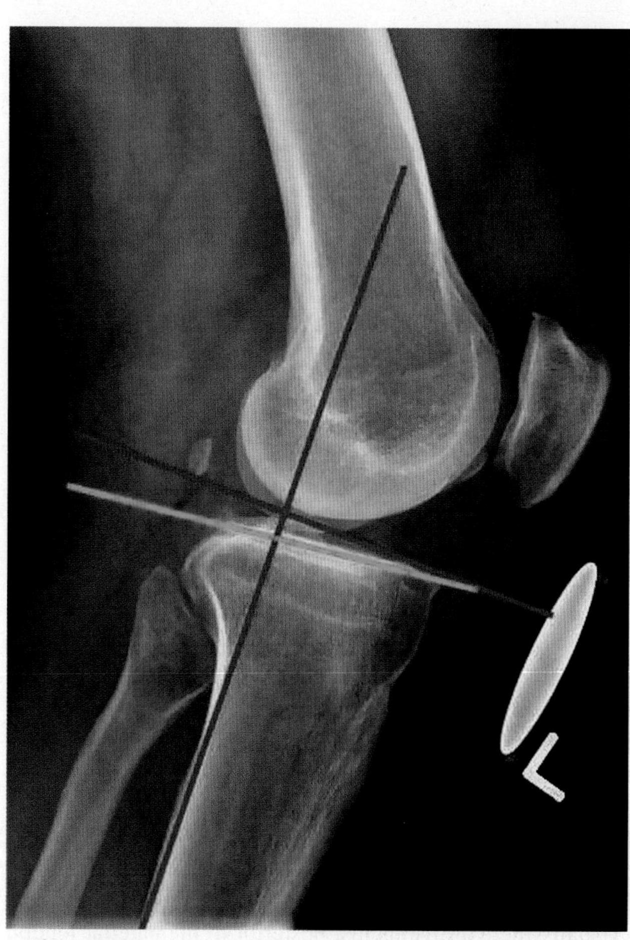

FIGURE 29-2

Determining posterior tibial slope with a lateral radiograph.

drawing a line along the posterior cortex of the tibial shaft and a line perpendicular to it at the level of the knee joint. A line is then drawn along the medial tibial joint line, and the angle between this and the perpendicular line is the slope. The particular cruciate deficiency and size of the slope will help determine the intraoperative management of the proposed HTO.

SURGICAL PROCEDURE AND TECHNIQUE

Patient Setup

Preoperative templating is confirmed, and a surgical checklist is conducted. The patient is placed in the supine position on a radiolucent operating table with all bony prominences well padded and a tourniquet applied to the upper thigh. A general anesthetic is administered, and the patient is intubated. Supplementary regional nerve blocks have been described for these procedures; however, we would discourage their use, particularly in laterally based tibial osteotomies or biplanar medially based osteotomies due to the risk of masking symptoms of a possible compartment syndrome. Appropriate preoperative antibiotics should be administered prior to the incision. A padded bump can be placed beneath the ipsilateral hip to prevent excessive external rotation of the hip, particularly if a laterally based procedure is being done. A lateral post at the thigh and a foot post can be added if a concurrent arthroscopic exam or ACL reconstruction is being planned.

After appropriate prepping and draping of the limb, C-arm fluoroscopy should be draped and easily accessible. When doing a medially based procedure, the C-arm should come in from the ipsilateral side and the surgeon should stand on the contralateral side and vice versa for a laterally based procedure. A sterile positioning bundle can be used to elevate the operative limb. This helps with obtaining intraoperative fluoroscopic images without interference from the contralateral limb. After elevating the leg and inflating the tourniquet, the surgical procedure can proceed. If a diagnostic arthroscopy is required, this should be done prior to the osteotomy.

TABLE 29-5 A "La Carte" Surgical Options for Osteotomies

Surgical Approach Options	Coronal Osteotomy Options	Sagittal Osteotomy Options[a]
Medial HTO	Opening wedge	Increase tibial slope[a]
Lateral HTO	Closing wedge	Decrease tibial slope[a]
Medial DFO	Tibial tubercle[a]	
Lateral DFO		

[a]With HTO only.

Surgical Technique

As mentioned previously, there are certain clinical scenarios that are more common, and these will be the focus of this section. The reader should be aware that there are options for more rare cases and can use an "a la carte" approach when the clinical scenario dictates it (Table 29-5).

ACL Deficiency with Varus Gonarthrosis

A MOW HTO is used, and the tibial slope is decreased through the osteotomy. The medial incision can be oriented either vertically midway between the tibial tubercle and posteromedial border of the tibia or obliquely just superior to the pes tendons. Blunt dissection is used to expose the first layer of fascia. This sartorial fascia can then be incised superior to and in line with the gracilis tendon. The pes attachments (gracilis and semitendinosis) are then released off the tibia distally for 1 cm. It is important to stay superficial to the superficial MCL when performing this release. Electrocautery is then used to open to the fascia posterior to the MCL along the tibial metaphyseal flare for a length of approximately 5 cm. A Cobb or periosteal elevator is slid along the posterior cortex to bluntly release the soft tissues to aid in placing a blunt-tipped retractor to protect neurovascular structures. Anteriorly, the tibial tubercle and medial border of the patellar tendon are identified and the fascia is opened longitudinally using cautery. Usually there are veins just posterior to the patellar tendon at the superior edge of the tubercle, and hemostasis should be obtained to aid visualization. A blunt retractor is placed beneath the tendon to protect it. If a TTO has been planned, it should be performed at this point (see below).

A break-away guide pin is drilled under fluoroscopic guidance at the upper margin of the proposed osteotomy site. The authors aim for the lateral metaphyseal flare with a gentle superior angle from the medial side and plan the osteotomy to finish 5 to 10 mm short of the lateral cortex. The tibial width is measured off the guide pin and should be similar to the templated distance. A wide osteotome helps visualize the proposed osteotomy angle pass just superior to the tibial tubercle. The sagittal plane cut angle should generally follow the normal tibial slope, which provides more proximal bone for screw fixation. Cautery is used to mark the proposed cut. At this point, the authors release the MCL in line with the proposed cut with the cautery. Others may choose to elevate the MCL distally and allow it to fall back over the osteotomy at the conclusion.

Retractors are appropriately positioned to be in line with the cut once ready. A small oscillating saw blade is used to perform the initial cut on the distal side of the guide pin. Fluoroscopy helps to ensure the saw blade does not drift off-line. A thin osteotome is then used to continue making the bony cut. Once the osteotomy has been completed along the anterior and posterior cortices and is lateral enough using the thin osteotomes, a wide, rigid osteotome can be inserted. The mobility of the site is assessed, and, if adequate, the proposed opening wedge can be created using stacked osteotomies, wedges, or laminar spreaders. Measure off the posteromedial cortex to determine the absolute size of the correction.

Adjustments to the tibial slope adjustments can now be assessed and made. In the ACL-deficient knee, the posterior cortex must be opened more than the anterior cortex to flatten the slope and thus change the resting position of the femur on the tibia. Because of the triangular nature of the tibia, an increased tibial slope will result if the anterior and posterior cortices are opened to the same the degree. When trying to flatten the slope, it is best to keep a laminar spreader or wedge in the posterior aspect of the osteotomy site while the knee is placed in extension with a positioning bundle under the foot. The osteotomy site is essentially placed in an extended position to help close the anterior cortex while the hardware is positioned and secured. The amount of correction needed to improve the resting position of the femur on the tibia is only 3 to 4 degrees. Once the surgeon is happy with the clinical and fluoroscopic appearance of the slope in comparison to the preoperative films, final fixation can be placed. The authors prefer a locking plate construct to maintain stability during the consolidation period (i.e., Synthes Tomofix), but several options exist. The plate is positioned on the fascial layer and using fluoroscopic guidance to ensure it is below the joint line. The distal aspect of the plate is assessed clinically to ensure it is not prominent anteriorly. Screws can be placed with fluoroscopic guidance.

After the hardware is placed, the defect may be filled with bone graft (autograft or allograft) or a substitute. To avoid donor site morbidity, the authors prefer cancellous bone chip allograft combined with 1 g of vancomycin for any opening wedge correction greater than 8 mm. The routine postoperative management is outlined below.

Considerations When Performing ACL Reconstruction with a Concurrent MOW HTO

The initial surgical steps are similar to any ACL reconstruction. The arthroscopic assessment can confirm the patient has a relatively intact lateral compartment to tolerate a valgus-producing osteotomy. Graft selection, preparation, and sizing follow. The authors recommend autograft and most commonly use ipsilateral hamstrings in a primary reconstruction, but other graft options exist. The femoral tunnel is then prepared in the typical fashion. At this point, the osteotomy is completed as previously described. The major concern is to ensure the proximal screws do not interfere with the tibial tunnel. Placing the plate as posterior as possible can help avoid this. The situation may dictate that a shorter screw be used or even left out of the most anterior screw hole. If that is the case, the surgeon must ensure a plate system is used that allows for adequate fixation in the proximal fragment. The authors' preference in such cases is a locking plate (Synthes Tomofix). Once the plate is affixed to the bone, the tibial tunnel can be drilled. The authors' experience is that the tunnel tends to exit the anterior aspect of the tibia at the proximal aspect of the osteotomy site. The graft can then be passed and secured. Tibial fixation is left to the surgeon's discretion.

ACL Deficiency with Valgus Malalignment

A varus-producing osteotomy is required, which is best accomplished in the distal femur. Typically, valgus is a product of an anatomical abnormality of the distal femur (i.e., hypoplastic lateral femoral condyle) and, as mentioned previously, it is best to address the "abnormal" bone. The authors prefer to use a medial-sided approach, for reasons stated above, with a closing wedge osteotomy. A femoral-based osteotomy does not address tibial slope and thus, the realignment procedure must be done in conjunction with an ACL reconstruction to restore stability. Fewer considerations are made with a concurrent ACL reconstruction because the medial DFO hardware should not interfere with tunnel placement. The osteotomy can be performed followed by the ACL reconstruction in the typical fashion.

The medial closing DFO uses a subvastus approach and begins with a longitudinal incision starting distally at the medial epicondyle and extending proximally for 5 cm. Blunt dissection is employed to avoid iatrogenic saphenous nerve injury until the fascia of the vastus medialis obliques (VMO) is reached. Fascia is incised in line with the incision, and the muscle compartment is followed posteriorly by bluntly sweeping away the muscle fibers off the posterior fascia. Once the femur has been reached, a blunt retractor is placed over the top of the bone to protect the VMO and extensor mechanism. A Cobb elevator is used to bluntly dissect across the posterior aspect of the femur to place a retractor.

The guide pin is drilled under fluoroscopic guidance starting on the supracondylar medial cortex and aiming lateral and distal toward the proximal aspect of the lateral femoral condyle. It should stop approximately 5 to 10 mm from the lateral cortex. This guides the distal cut of the closing wedge osteotomy. A second pin is then placed proximal to guide the second cut. It should be directed towards and converge with the first pin. The oscillating saw is used to create the first cut under fluoroscopic guidance on the proximal side of the most distal pin. Thin osteotomes are used to reach the desired width. The second cut is made on the distal side of the proximal pin. This cut should gradually converge to meet the first cut at the lateral margin of the osteotomy. It is important to remain parallel as the cut is initiated at the medial cortex to ensure better cortical contact once the osteotomy is closed. A variation that the authors prefer is to perform a biplanar cut anteriorly to aid in stability of the osteotomy prior to application of hardware. It also avoids rotational deformity

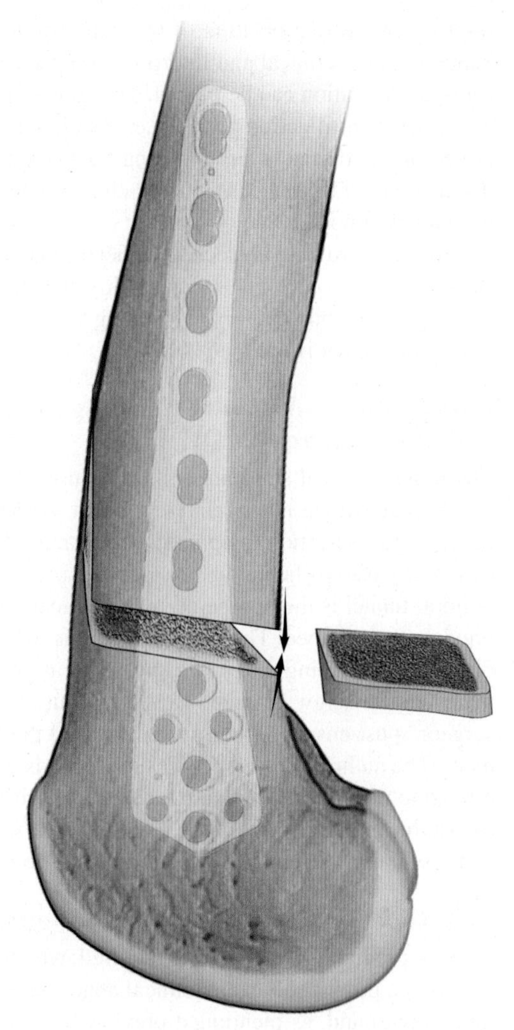

FIGURE 29-3

The biplanar closing wedge distal femoral osteotomy has added stability and surface area for osteotomy site healing.

through the osteotomy in the event of lateral cortical breach. The biplanar cut is made by stopping short of the anterior cortex with the first cut and then making a cut parallel to the axis of the femur (perpendicular to the first cut) for a length of 2 to 3 cm (Fig. 29-3).

Once the osteotomy is completed and the mobility is adequate, the site is held closed and hardware is applied. The plate is placed directly on the bone, and the proximal position must be assessed to ensure it is not prominent anteriorly. Once all hardware is inserted, final fluoroscopic images are taken to confirm position. Bone graft is not needed while wound closure and postoperative management are similar to those in an HTO.

In the atypical setting of tibial valgus deformity, a lateral opening wedge HTO can be used. This has the advantages of allowing adjustments in the tibial slope and can have an effect on flexion athletes (i.e., skiers). However, hardware interference with the tibial tunnel of the ACL reconstruction is a challenge. The approach uses an anterolateral longitudinal incision extending distally from Gerdy tubercle. Full-thickness soft tissue flaps are created, and the fascia of the anterior compartment is incised in line. Muscles of the anterior compartment are bluntly elevated from the anterolateral tibia using a Cobb elevator and retracted posteriorly. The proximal tibiofibular joint capsule is incised anteriorly to allow the joint to be mobile when the osteotomy is opened. The lateral edge of the patellar tendon is exposed to aid in placing a retractor under the tendon. A retractor is also placed posterior to the tibia to protect the neurovascular structures. The osteotomy is then created in the same fashion as a MOW HTO.

PCL Deficiency with Varus Gonarthrosis

An MOW HTO is used and to increase tibial slope, and the approach is used as previously described. The tibial slope is then increased through the osteotomy site, or the osteotomy is placed into a slightly flexed position. The osteotomy is made parallel to that of the patient's natural tibial

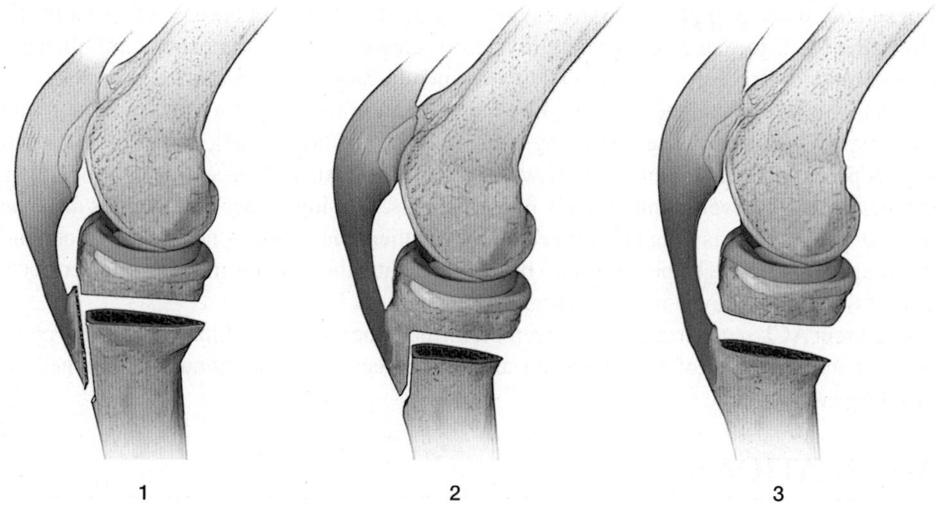

FIGURE 29-4

There are two techniques to perform the tibial tubercle osteotomy. No. 1 shows a separate tubercle fragment, which allows the surgeon to place the tubercle at the desired height but requires more fixation. No. 2 shows the tubercle attached to the proximal tibia with a biplanar cut. While technically more difficult, it can give slightly increased osteotomy stability, healing surface area while avoiding patella baja.

slope, and the anterior cortex can be opened as much (or even a few more millimeters if needed) as the posterior cortex. This will alter the resting position of the femur on the tibia to a more anterior position. Usually, it is easier to increase slope than decrease it. However, if required, laminar spreaders can be placed more anteriorly within the osteotomy site, provided they do not interfere with the placement of hardware. Once the surgeon is satisfied with the fluoroscopic appearance of the slope, hardware can be applied. The use of bone graft, closure, and postoperative management is the same as above.

Tibial Tubercle Osteotomy

When an HTO is planned and the patient has preexisting patella baja or significant patellofemoral arthritis or a large correction is templated (>15 degrees), a concurrent biplanar tibial tubercle should be performed. Three techniques exist (Fig. 29-4), but the authors' preferred method will be explained here. After the appropriate surgical exposure of the tibial tubercle and distal patellar tendon is complete, electrocautery is used to mark out the proposed osteotomy line, which begins at the superior aspect of the tibial tubercle and extends distal for 6 cm. An oscillating saw is used to create a wafer of bone approximately 5 to 10 mm thick across the anterior tibia. The fascia of the anterior compartment must be released on the lateral side to allow the tibial tubercle to be mobilized.

If a separate tubercle fragment has been created, it can be reduced after the wedge osteotomy is complete and fixation is in place. The superior aspect of the tubercle is aligned with the physeal scar, which tends to be at the distal aspect of the proximal fragment of the osteotomy. Once reduced, two bicortical lag screws are placed in an anterior-to-posterior direction under fluoroscopy to get compression. If the tubercle has remained attached to the proximal fragment, one bicortical screw is usually sufficient. Care should be taken not to plunge through the posterior cortex. If necessary, a washer can be used with the screw for better fixation of the tubercle fragment.

POSTOPERATIVE MANAGEMENT

The wound is closed in layers over a drain, which is removed on postoperative day 1. The drain is used to avoid wound complications from the accumulation of a hematoma. When a medial opening wedge HTO is used, the anterior compartment is not violated; thus the risk of compartment syndrome is low and the use of a drain does not have a bearing on this concern. Patients will receive one dose of postoperative antibiotics while thromboprophylaxis is given to higher-risk patients (i.e., previous deep vein thrombosis/pulmonary embolism, history of cancer).

A hinged knee brace is applied prior to leaving the operating room. In the case of an MOW HTO, this allows the MCL to scar in after being divided or elevated during the exposure. Full range of motion is permitted. Brace use is continued in a weaned fashion for approximately 6 weeks.

Weight-bearing status is dependent on the type of fixation used (locking plate versus nonlocking plate), type of osteotomy used (opening wedge versus closing wedge), and size of correction. The authors permit patients to immediately weight bear as tolerated in the setting of a locking plate (see Synthes Tomofix), even in moderately obese patients. Closing wedge osteotomies also can be permitted to weight bear as tolerated immediately. If patients have had a nonlocking plate and an opening wedge HTO, weight bearing may be delayed until the 4-week mark. Larger corrections (>15 degrees) are also delayed in weight bearing.

If a concurrent ACL reconstruction has been performed, the ACL rehabilitation protocol prevails, and range of motion goals of full extension and 90 degrees of flexion should be reached at the 6-week postoperative mark.

COMPLICATIONS

The incidence of complications following an osteotomy around the knee is multifactorial. Patient factors such as body mass index, systemic illness (diabetes), and smoking status in addition to surgical factors such as the type and location of osteotomy used, size of correction, and hardware system used all play a significant role in the possibility for postoperative complications. Moreover, reported complication rates will be affected by how and when the surgeon defines a delayed union or nonunion. The authors define delayed union as greater than 6 months without radiographic evidence of union (bridging is best seen on the posterior cortex in a MOW HTO) and 12 months for a nonunion.

Historically, the list of complications following an osteotomy includes infection, thromboembolic disease, nonunion/delayed union, neurovascular injury, arthrofibrosis, patella baja, tibial plateau fracture, loss of correction, fibular nonunion, and compartment syndrome.

The senior author has published an article that investigates the complication rate in the most common osteotomy performed in our center—the MOW HTO. Complications were classified as Classes 1, 2, or 3. Class 1 complications are minor ones that do not require any treatment such as delayed wound healing, lateral cortical fracture, or undisplaced tibial plateau fracture. Class 2 complications are those that require short-term nonoperative treatment such as a deep vein thrombosis, superficial infection, or delayed union. Class 3 complications require additional surgery or long-term nonoperative treatment such as hardware failure, deep infection, or nonunion.

Of the 323 procedures that were reviewed, 17% were done in conjunction with a ligament reconstruction, 26% were done in conjunction with a TTO, and cancellous allograft was used to fill the osteotomy site in 94% of cases. Nonlocking plates were used in 83% of cases. The results found that severe class 3 adverse events occurred 7% of the time with nonunions occurring 3.2% of the time. The most common complication requiring an extended course of nonoperative treatment was delayed union (12%). In the subgroup analysis, it was found that the class 3 adverse event rate was only 3% with careful patient selection (avoid dependant diabetic patients), precise technique, and use of a locking plate. With that said, one adverse event that may be unreported in the literature is prominent bothersome hardware. The need for hardware removal may be as high as 30% to 40%, in the author's experience. This should be delayed until the osteotomy site is fully healed (typically 1 year).

ILLUSTRATIVE CASES

Case 1—An otherwise healthy 55-year-old mechanic suffered an ACL rupture and failed 2 years of nonoperative management with an ACL brace. He complained of instability during daily activities and led a very active lifestyle. Physical examination revealed genu varum and a varus thrust. There was a grade 2 Lachman test and grade 2 pivot shift test. Standing radiographs revealed varus malalignment with significant decreased joint space of the medial compartment. The other compartments were relatively well-preserved. Because of his healthy active lifestyle, failure of nonoperative management, and varus gonarthrosis with ACL deficiency, the decision was made to perform a concurrent MOW HTO and ACL reconstruction with hamstring autograft. He was allowed to toe touch weight bear and range his knee as tolerated immediately post-op. He went on to return to activities as tolerated at 1 year postoperative (Fig. 29-5A–C).

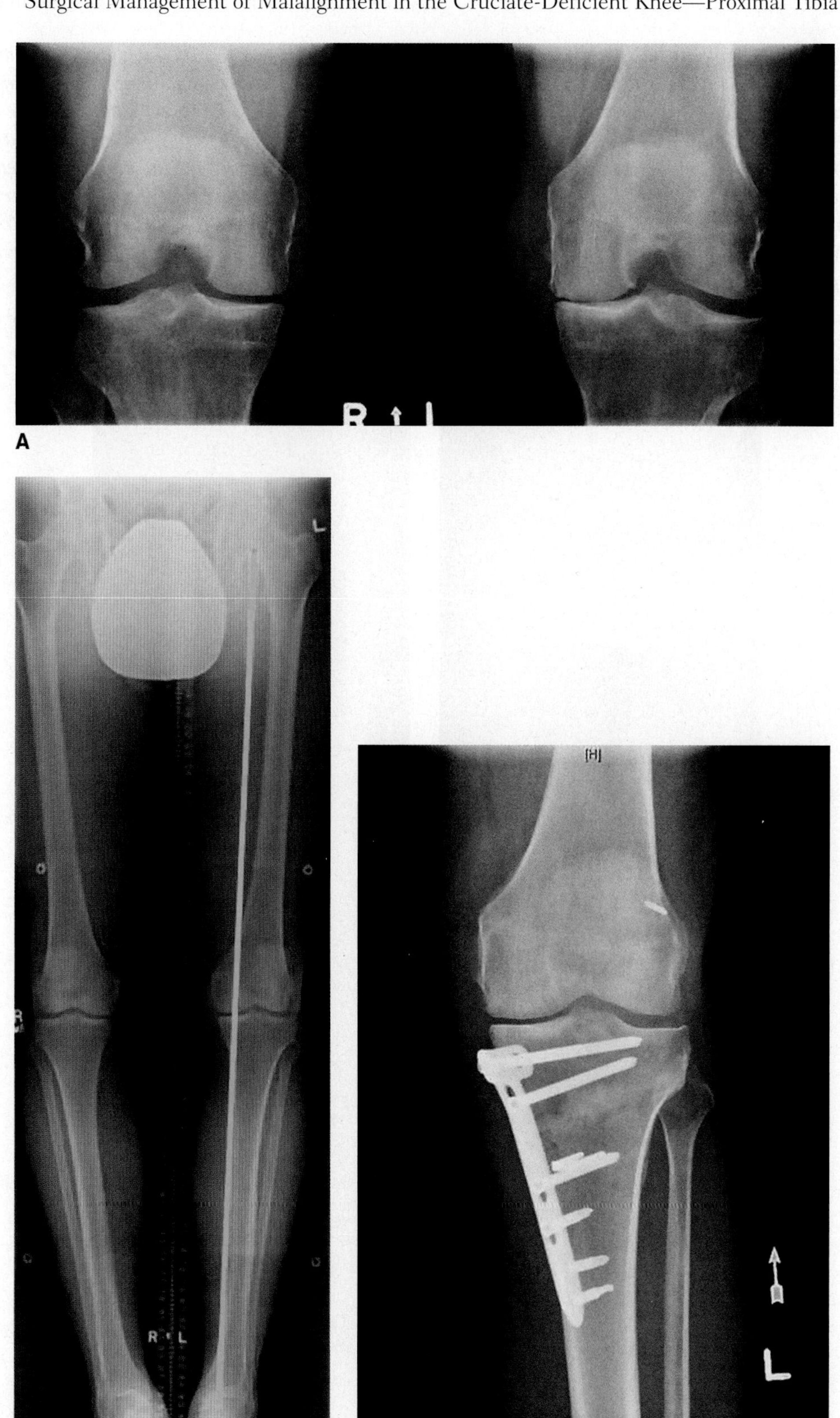

FIGURE 29-5

A–C: A patient with a chronic left ACL deficient knee. Radiographs show decreased joint space in the medial compartment with a weight-bearing line falling within the medial compartment. An MOW HTO with ACL reconstruction using femoral Endobutton fixation and staple tibial fixation was performed.

Case 2—A 33-year-old professional hockey player sustained a PCL injury and was initially treated nonoperatively. After several months of rehabilitation, brace wear, and corticosteroid injections, he complained of instability, pain, and swelling after activity. Physical exam confirmed a low-grade PCL injury with an endpoint on posterior drawer testing. Imaging showed mild varus alignment and a normal posterior slope. A diagnostic arthroscopy confirmed the PCL insufficiency but also found a large medial femoral chondral defect on the weight-bearing surface. The lateral compartment was pristine. After a discussion with the patient, the decision was made to perform an MOW HTO to unload the medial compartment while increasing the tibial slope to improve the symptoms from his PCL insufficiency (Fig. 29-6A, B).

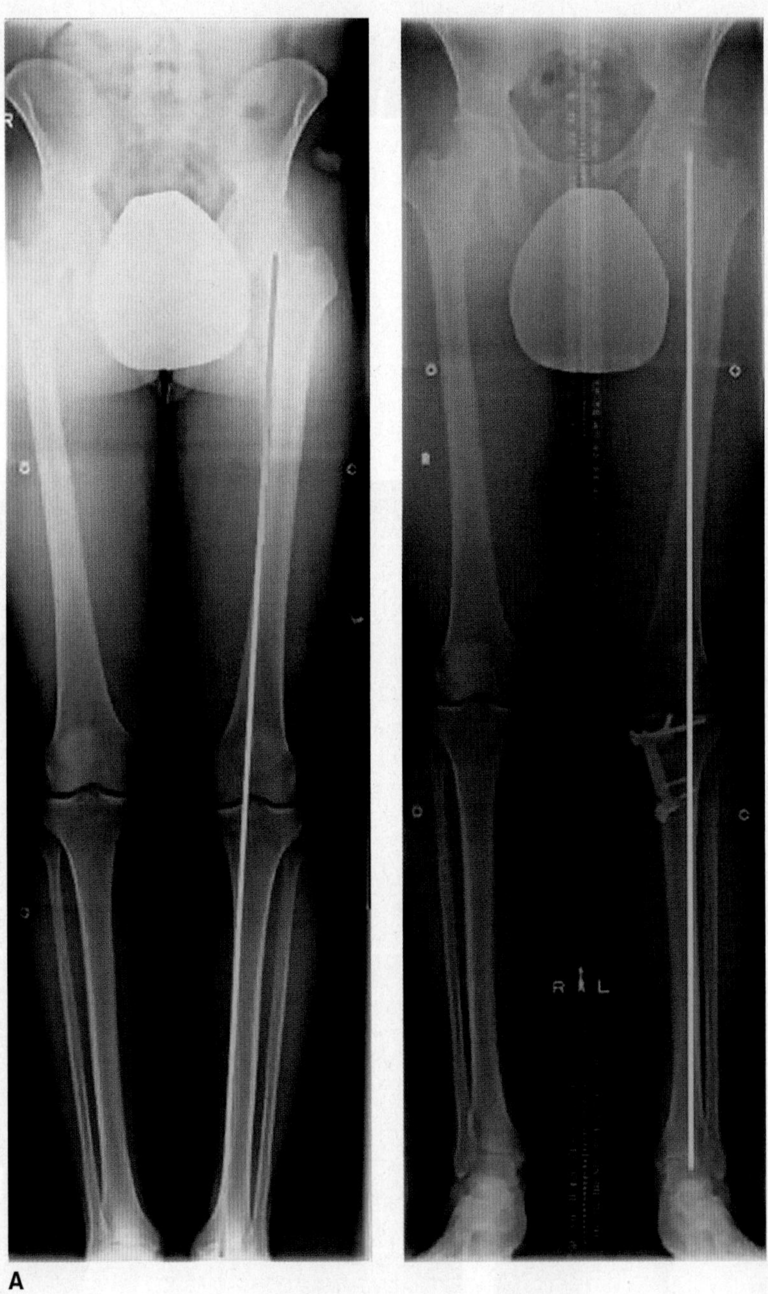

FIGURE 29-6

A, B: Before and after radiographs of a patient with PCL deficiency and a large chondral defect in the medial compartment with mild varus alignment. An MOW HTO with an increase in the tibial slope was performed to help with his symptoms of instability and medial-sided knee pain.

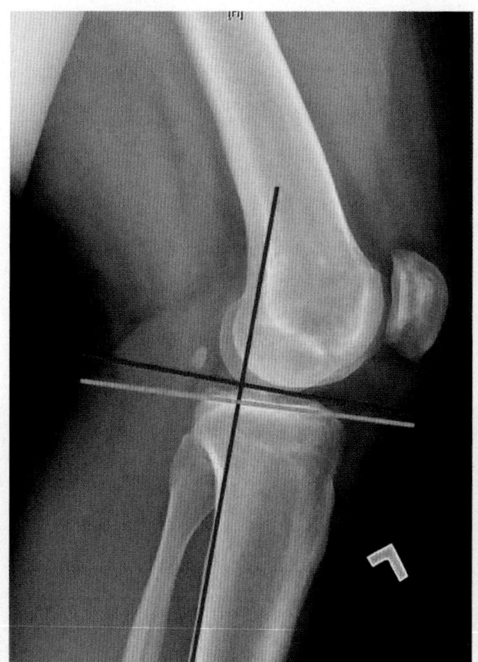

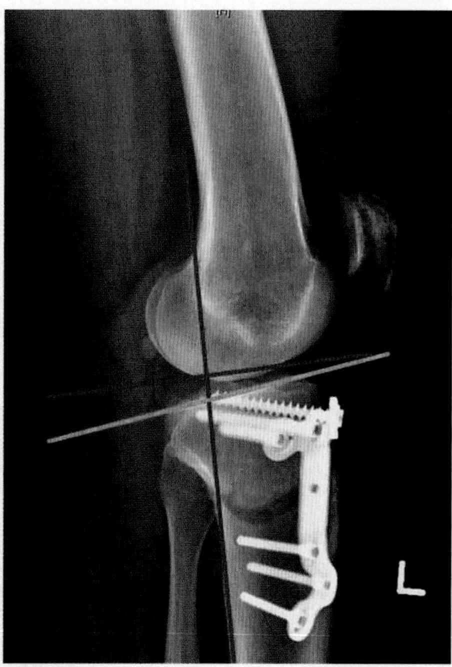

B

FIGURE 29-6 ***(Continued)***

Case 3—A 26-year-old professional motocross racer failed two previous ACL reconstructions with autograft. He complained of both instability and pain upon referral to clinic. Clinical examination was consistent with ACL insufficiency. Standing films revealed valgus malalignment and decreased joint space in the lateral compartment. The patient was consented for a revision ACL reconstruction with allograft and a concurrent MCW DFO. He followed the regular ACL reconstruction post-op protocol (Fig. 29-7A–C).

PEARLS AND PITFALLS

- Malalignment is defined as a weight-bearing axis that falls medial or lateral to the tibial spine in a symptomatic patient.
- Symptoms of pain and/or instability need to be elucidated prior to determining a surgical plan.
- Plan to stage the osteotomy and ligament reconstruction for patients requiring large corrections (>15 degrees), revision ligament reconstruction with bone tunnels larger than 16 mm, and older patients with triple varus knees.
- Opening wedge osteotomies are easier to titrate with a single cut while closing wedge osteotomies may be more theoretically more stable.
- When templating, correct to the center of the knee for symptoms of isolated instability. Correct to the downslope of the lateral tibial spine for varus patients with pain and instability and to the medial tibial spine for valgus patients with pain and instability.
- When performing an HTO, assess patellar height and be prepared to perform TTO for preexisting patella baja, patellofemoral arthritis, and correction greater than 15 degrees.
- Measure the correction size off the posteromedial cortex in an HTO.
- When trying to maintain a neutral slope or decrease the tibial slope, place the wedge or laminar spreader in the posterior aspect of the osteotomy and keep the leg extended to help close the anterior cortex.
- When performing a concurrent ACL reconstruction with HTO, place the plate slightly posterior or avoid placing a screw through the anterior screw hole in the plate proximally so as not to interfere with the tibial tunnel.
- Early weight bearing can be allowed, particularly in the setting of a locking plate.
- Be wary of complications in the smoker or diabetic patient.

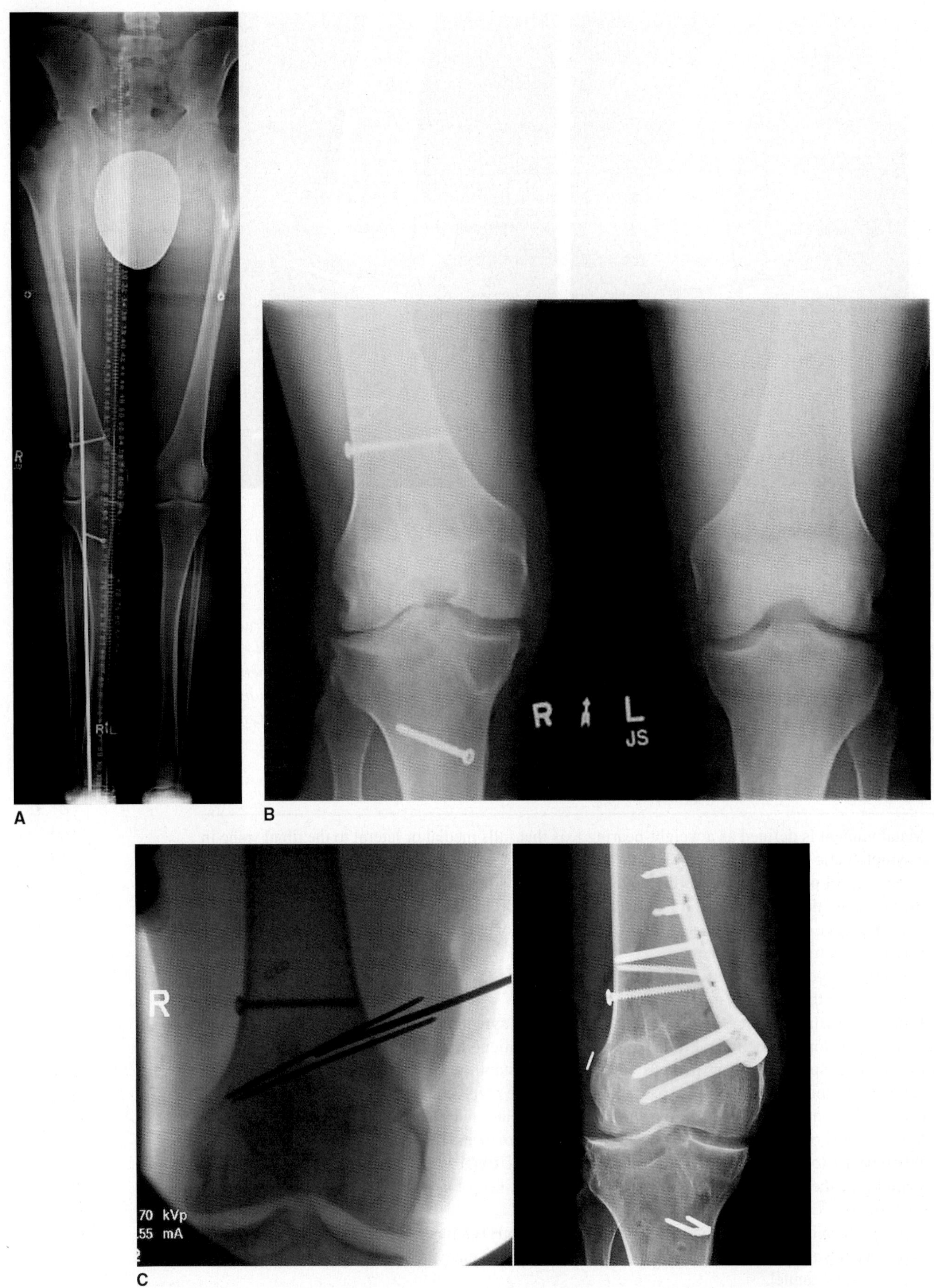

FIGURE 29-7

A–C: A patient who failed two previous right ACL reconstructions has decreased lateral joint space and stands with valgus malalignment. An MCW DFO was performed in conjunction with a revision ACL reconstruction using Endobutton femoral fixation and staple tibial fixation.

RECOMMENDED READINGS

Dugdale TW, Noyes FR, Styer D. Preoperative planning for high tibial osteotomy. The effect of lateral tibiofemoral separation and tibiofemoral length. *Clin Orthop Relat Res.* 1992;274:248–264.

Giffin JR, Vogrin TM, Zantop T, et al. Effects of increasing tibial slope on the biomechanics of the knee. *Am J Sports Med.* 2004;32(2):376–382.

Giffin JR, Shannon FJ. The role of the high tibial osteotomy in the unstable knee. *Sports Med Arthrosc.* 2007;15(1):23–31.

Hulet C, Sebilo A, Collon S. Results of combined high tibial osteotomy (HTO) and ACL reconstruction. In: Siebold R, ed. *Anterior cruciate ligament reconstruction: A practical surgical guide.* Heidelberg: Springer; 2014:441–446.

LaPrade RF, Bernhardson AS, Griffith CJ, et al. Correlation of valgus stress radiographs with medial knee ligament injuries: an in vitro biomechanical study. *Am J Sports Med.* 2010;38(2):330–338.

LaPrade RF, Heikes C, Bakker AJ, et al. The reproducibility and repeatability of varus stress radiographs in the assessment of isolated fibular collateral ligament and grade-III posterolateral knee injuries. An in vitro biomechanical study. *J Bone Joint Surg Am.* 2008;90(10):2069–2076.

Martin R, Birmingham TB, Willits K, et al. Adverse event rates and classifications in medial opening wedge high tibial osteotomy. *Am J Sports Med.* 2014;42(5):1118–1126.

Noyes FR, Barber-Westin SD, Hewett TE. High tibial osteotomy and ligament reconstruction for varus angulated anterior cruciate ligament-deficient knees. *Am J Sports Med.* 2000;28(3):282–296.

Noyes FR, Simon R. The role of high tibial osteotomy in the anterior cruciate ligament-deficient knee with varus alignment. In: DeLee JC, Drez D, eds. *Orthopaedic sports medicine: principles and practice.* Philadelphia: WB Saunders; 1994:1401–1443.

Savarese E, Bisicchia S, Romeo R, et al. Role of high tibial osteotomy in chronic injuries of posterior cruciate ligament and posterolateral corner. *J Orthop Traumatol.* 2011;12:1–17.

PART IV ARTICULAR CARTILAGE AND SYNOVIUM

30 Chondroplasty and Synovectomy

Kushal V. Patel and Eric McCarty

INDICATIONS/CONTRAINDICATIONS

Chondroplasty

Chondroplasty is performed as part of a diagnostic arthroscopy and debridement. Chondroplasty, defined as surgical shaping of the articular cartilage, is a technique that involves debridement of unstable, degenerative cartilage segments and flaps to ultimately improve the articular surface contour and establish stable cartilage edges. Thus, the mechanical symptoms from the unstable fragments are alleviated. On many occasions, pain rather than mechanical symptoms from chondromalacia is the primary complaint. Chondroplasty can also be very beneficial in these situations. Furthermore, the inflammatory cascade resulting from the devitalized articular fragments is mitigated by a chondroplasty as well as by the joint irrigation itself. The lavage removes particulate debris and proteins present that are involved in inflammation.

As a result, patients who have symptomatic, unstable articular cartilage lesions generally do quite well because of the twofold intervention. The mechanical symptoms are generally alleviated; however, the degree and length of pain/inflammatory improvement are variable, particularly when chondromalacia pain is primary presentation. Chondroplasty likely does not alter the natural history of articular cartilage degeneration. The surrounding cartilage of unstable, degenerative segments experiences altered forces before and after a chondroplasty. The altered mechanical environment in combination with other multifactorial influences contributes to further degradation of the articular cartilage. Despite continued articular cartilage degeneration, symptoms can be highly variable.

Generally, mechanical symptoms resulting from the articular cartilage fragmentation, loosening, or impingement are an indication for chondroplasty. Symptoms can include localized pain with range of motion, catching or locking, and recurrent effusions. The pathologic articular cartilage can commonly detach and become loose bodies and present with similar symptoms. Discussion with the patient regarding the severity of symptoms is important.

Symptoms, either mechanical or pain as described above, should be interfering with activities of daily living and impacting the quality of life. Attempt at conservative treatment is an option for patients with minimal symptoms. These include viscosupplementation, activity modification, bracing, physical therapy, corticosteroid injection, oral anti-inflammatories, assistive devices such as a cane, and weight loss. However, in our experience, when mechanical symptoms are present, arthroscopic evaluation and chondroplasty are generally recommended. The procedure for mechanical symptoms has excellent prognosis, and in many patients, conservative treatment

TABLE 30-1 Two Classifications of Chondromalacia

Grade	Outerbridge Classification	International Cartilage Repair Society (ICRS) Classification
0	Normal cartilage	Normal cartilage
1	Cartilage softening/swelling	A. Cartilage softening/fibrillations B. Superficial cartilage fissuring
2	Cartilage fissuring not to subchondral bone or <1.5 cm in diameter	Cartilage lesions <½ depth
3	Cartilage fissuring to subchondral bone and >1.5 cm in diameter	Cartilage lesions >½ depth
4	Exposed subchondral bone	Cartilage lesions violating the subchondral plate

does not alleviate mechanical symptoms. In addition, as our aging population continues to be more active, arthroscopic debridement and chondroplasty can be an important tool in patients with early chondromalacia void of mechanical symptoms. These patients usually present more with pain from either chondromalacia or concomitant degenerative meniscal tears or a combination of the two. Therefore, when arthroscopic evaluation is performed, a chondroplasty is performed when unstable cartilage fragments are encountered. As a result, another relative indication for chondroplasty is for grade 3 or 4 (Table 30-1) chondromalacia that is encountered at time of diagnostic/debridement arthroscopy for pain secondary to degenerative wear. Importantly, counseling patients for chondroplasty in the presence of degenerative wear is different than in patients with mechanical symptoms. Patients with mechanical symptoms can anticipate good to excellent outcomes. Contrary, results in patients with primarily pain are highly variable as to degree and length of symptom relief. Variables such as subchondral edema, degenerative involvement of multiple compartments, and severity of degeneration can influence prognosis. Establishing realistic patient expectations is critical.

Synovectomy

Synovectomy, defined as the excision of the synovium, was first described by Volkmann for the treatment of tuberculosis arthritis. Since its initial open description, advances in arthroscopic technique and application to other disease processes, arthroscopic synovectomy has become an important treatment option for certain patients. Synovitis is defined as the inflammation of the synovial tissue, a specialized mesenchymal lining of joints that supplies nutrients to the articular cartilage and produces lubricant for joints. Synovitis can be either local or diffuse depending on the etiology. In a majority of cases, patients have had long-standing symptoms prior to surgical intervention. Therefore, the synovium typically has undergone hyperplasia, vascular angiogenesis, and increased cellularity with lymphocytes and macrophages at the time of arthroscopic synovectomy. The goals of an arthroscopic synovectomy are to not only alleviate the patient's symptoms but also prevent the potential articular cartilage destruction that accompanies prolonged synovitis.

Generally, failure of conservative treatment is an indication for arthroscopic synovectomy with continued pain, swelling, or mechanical symptoms. Conservative treatment includes activity modification, use of assistive devices, bracing or orthotics, corticosteroids or viscosupplementation injections, weight loss, oral anti-inflammatories, disease modifying antirheumatic drugs, and physical therapy. Patient symptoms ideally limit or interfere with activities of daily living and function. Common etiologies of synovitis are listed in Table 30-2. Symptoms from systemic/autoimmune etiologies of synovitis generally improve as medical management of the disease is maximized. In these patients, we prefer treatment via a comprehensive team approach with involvement from an internist or rheumatologist.

Recurrent synovitis is a possibility after synovectomy, and therefore, the patient should be counseled regarding this. This is particularly more common in patients with systemic disease. In a majority of cases, patients respond well to surgical intervention, but the degree and length of relief can be variable. The condition of the articular cartilage and meniscus are variables potentially impacting outcomes. In general, our two contraindications for arthroscopic synovectomy are advanced joint destruction and active infection.

TABLE 30-2 Common Etiologies of Synovitis

Rheumatoid Arthritis	Synovial Chondromatosis	Persistent Synovitis Following Infection
PVNS	Seronegative arthropathy	Posttraumatic synovitis
Crystalline synovitis	Nonspecific synovitis	Hemophilic synovitis

PREOPERATIVE PLANNING

Patient evaluation begins with a thorough history of symptoms (including recurrent pain, swelling, warmth, stiffness, and mechanical symptoms), functional impact of symptoms, and trails of conservative treatment. Particularly important in patients with synovitis is questioning, in addition to the above, medical and family history of any autoimmune or hematologic disorders, potential involvement of other joints, sexual history, and previous joint or systemic infections. Patients with rheumatoid arthritis will also have involvement of the small joints of the hand, whereas pigmented villonodular synovitis (PVNS) is monoarticular involvement. Patients with chondromalacia commonly present with joint line pain similar to meniscal symptoms. Symptomatic medial compartment chondromalacia is more common than lateral. Patients will typically report deep ache and burning at night and with activities. This may be compounded by mechanical symptoms if an unstable cartilage fragment is present. Reports of stiffness and swelling are present in patients with more advanced wear. Stiffness is common after prolonged rest or at the end of the day in patients with advanced degenerative changes, whereas patients with autoimmune-related synovitis will report morning stiffness that improves with activity. A majority of the time, there is absence of trauma and gradual onset of symptoms. However, younger patients more commonly report a trauma damaging an isolated area of cartilage with or without subchondral bone edema. Patients with synovitis present differently. No focal area of pain is identified. Rather, the entire joint is inflamed and symptomatic. Typically, joint swelling does not correlate with amount of activities.

Physical exam can be vital in facilitating the differential diagnosis and should document:

- Presence and degree of joint infusion
- Signs of infection/local inflammation including warmth, tenderness, and erythema
- Presence of any masses
- Pain with range of motion; active and passive arcs of motion to evaluate for arthrofibrosis, flexion contracture, mechanical block, or limited range of motion secondary to pain
- Ligament competency of the anterior cruciate, posterior cruciate, medial collateral, lateral collateral, and posterolateral corner ligaments
- Thorough skin examination for any rheumatoid nodules, malar rash, psoriasis, nail pitting
- Cervical spine evaluation specifically in patients with confirmed or suspected rheumatoid arthritis
- Limb malalignment indicative of advanced joint destruction
- Hip range of motion to rule out any referred pathology
- Examination of noninvolved knee to provide baseline physical findings

Radiographs are important to evaluate the severity of joint destruction and can aid in differential diagnosis. Radiographs should include weight-bearing AP, lateral, merchant, and PA flexion/Rosenberg views. In our clinic, we obtain bilateral views as to compare both the alignment and degree of joint degeneration. Rosenberg views provide a better understanding of the degree of osteoarthritis. The posterior femoral condyle is typically involved in osteoarthritis; therefore, joint space narrowing not present on the AP view may be present on the Rosenberg views (Fig. 30-1). Other clues of osteoarthritis along with joint space narrowing are subchondral sclerosis, osteophytes, pointed tibial spines, squaring of the femoral condyles, and cyst formation. Most commonly, the medial compartment will be involved. Autoimmune and inflammatory arthritis have symmetric joint space narrowing, osteopenia, and periarticular erosions. Calcifications can also be visualized indicating synovial chondromatosis or pseudogout/chondrocalcinosis (Fig. 30-2).

If there is concern of malalignment, then hip-to-ankle radiograph may be warranted to fully assess the mechanical alignment. Typically, we obtain large cassette weight-bearing films, and they can

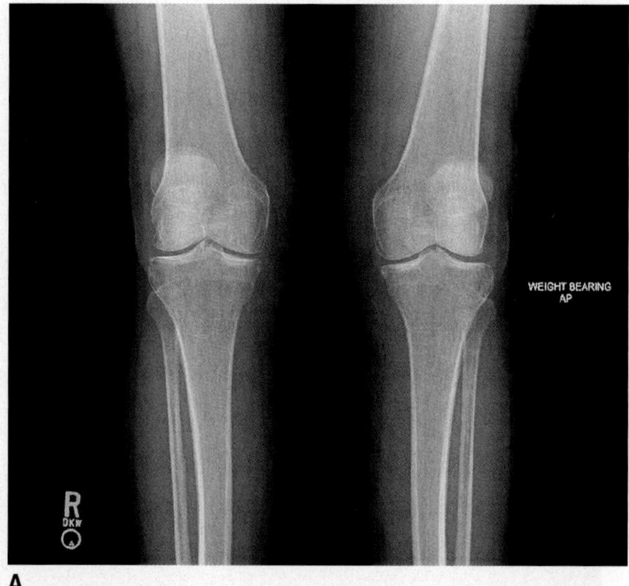

A

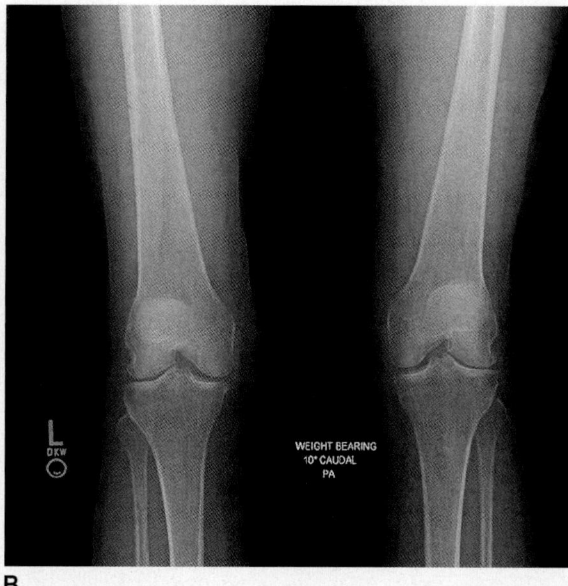

B

FIGURE 30-1

A, B: Weight-bearing large cassette radiographs of patient with right knee pain. **A:** AP view illustrates mild joint space narrowing with no significant signs of arthritis and comparison to the contralateral knee. **B:** PA flexion view demonstrates decreased joint space of the lateral compartment on both knees with greater change present in the right knee.

suggest any mechanical alignment. In patients with well-preserved joint and minimal degenerative findings, hip-to-ankle radiographs are obtained to help with surgical planning if necessary. Genu varus is encountered more commonly than genu valgus. Advanced imaging such as magnetic resonance imaging (MRI) can be very helpful to assess one, the condition of the joint and articular cartilage especially if radiographs are normal (Fig. 30-3). The MRI is thoroughly evaluated for chondromalacia, subchondral edema, and meniscal tears. Asymptomatic patellofemoral compartment involvement can be encountered in patients who present primarily with medial or lateral joint line pain. The MRI

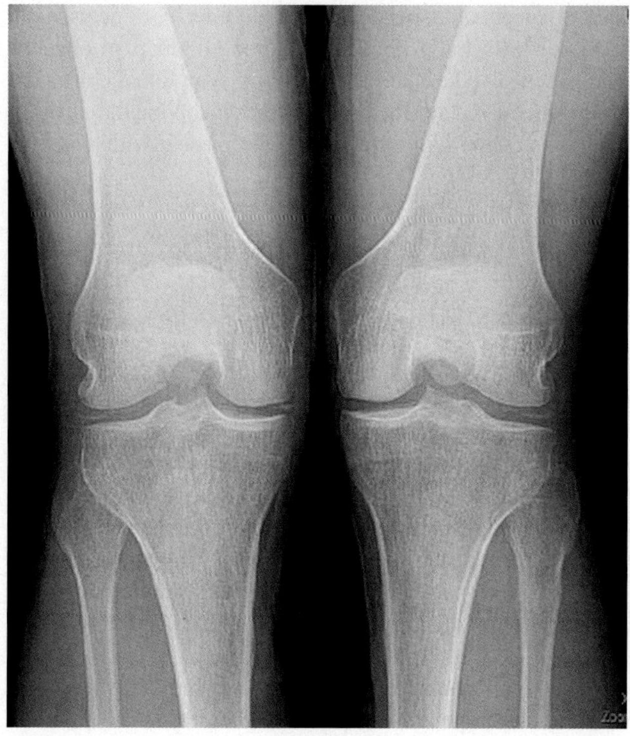

FIGURE 30-2

Flexion PA films demonstrating bilateral chondrocalcinosis. The calcification within the meniscus is classically seen in chondrocalcinosis.

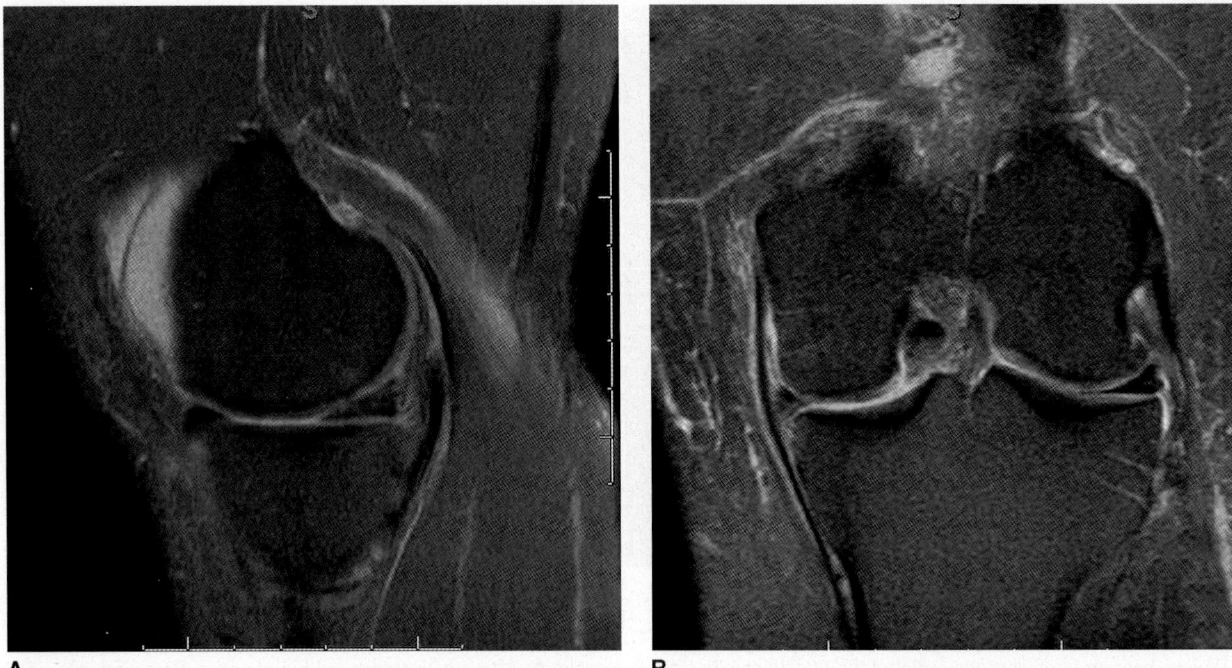

FIGURE 30-3

A, B: MRI images of the knee. **A:** Sagittal image illustrating cartilage thinning along the posterior medial femoral condyle with mild subchondral edema. **B:** Coronal image demonstrating heterogeneity and thinning of the articular cartilage of the medial femoral condyle. Particularly, a linear signal located at the lateral edge of the condyle.

images should be reviewed with the patient. This will help guide patient treatment and more importantly postoperative expectations. In some instances, the cartilage may be well preserved by MRI; however, during arthroscopic evaluation, there may be softening and fissuring not appreciated by MRI. The MRI is also helpful in documenting any subchondral edema and status of the meniscus. In particular, the fat suppressed proton density (FSPD) and T2-weighted images are most helpful in evaluating the cartilage. A majority of the articular cartilage pathology will be found in the medial compartment on the femoral side. Advanced chondromalacia is associated with a degenerative meniscus in the involved compartment. Thorough discussion with the patient regarding the findings of physical exam, imaging, and history is critical. The patient is educated on potentially symptomatic articular cartilage and the implications on prognosis of generalized degenerative changes involving the cartilage and meniscus. MRI can also facilitate evaluation of the joint in patients who present with synovitis (Fig. 30-4). The MRI findings of synovitis included:

- Thickened synovium
- Joint effusion
- Articular cartilage changes with erosions
- Hypointense signal on T1 and T2 images secondary to hemosiderin deposition if present
- Postcontrast enhancement of synovium

The MRI can also demonstrate the extent of synovial proliferation particularly when involvement in the popliteal fossa is present. Understanding the extent of synovial proliferation is critical to surgical planning. Furthermore, in patients with rheumatoid arthritis, cervical spine x-rays including AP, open mouth odontoid, and lateral views are ordered. A radionucleotide bone scan is seldom utilized and, however, can be beneficial in patients who have pain out of proportion to objective findings or those patients who cannot undergo a MRI. Particularly, we utilize bone scans to evaluate any increased hypermetabolic regions that can attribute to patient symptoms. This commonly occurs in the presence of malalignment with abnormal forces on the joint surface. Generalized uptake is more indicative of advanced degenerative changes.

Further evaluation of a patient who presents with an inflamed, painful knee should involve joint aspiration. Joint aspiration can be diagnostic and therapeutic. Simply removal of synovial fluid and

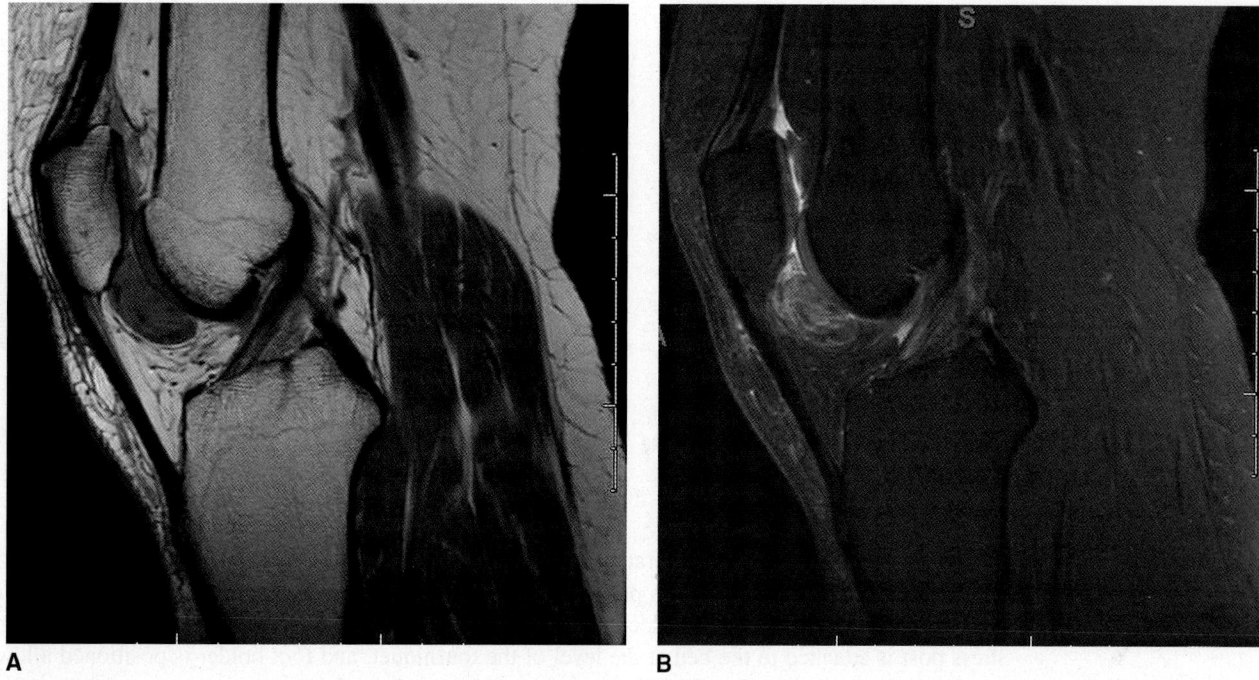

FIGURE 30-4

A, B: Sagittal MRI images of the knee. TI and T2 images demonstrate a well-circumscribed mass anterior to the lateral femoral condyle with hemosiderin deposition consistent with PVNS.

decreasing the tension upon the joint capsule can lead to improved pain. It is imperative to note that once a needle has been introduced into the joint, the removal of as much synovial fluid as possible is attempted. Angling the needle in different directions and milking the joint concurrently may be helpful especially in the presence of synovial proliferation or hematoma that can potentially block the needle lumen. In our practice, we perform aspirations with a 60-mL syringe and an 18-gauge needle. We feel that the 18-gauge needle provides the largest lumen diameter allowing aspiration of large volume more feasibly and efficiently. In addition, the synovial fluid should be sent off for fluid analysis including examination of crystals, rheumatoid factor, compliment levels, cell count, gram stain, and cultures. Gross hematoma can be indicative of PVNS or a blood disorder.

The expected length of symptom improvement can be variable from either a chondroplasty or synovectomy. The procedure may not be the final one. Medical history such as obesity and autoimmune/inflammatory conditions that can impact the postoperative improvement is also discussed. In some instances, there is none to minimal relief or even worsening symptoms after surgery especially if mechanical symptoms are not present. We have found this to be very uncommon, but the patient should be notified of the possibility. Again, patient expectations should be guided by collectively examining history, physical, and radiographic findings.

SURGICAL TECHNIQUE

Informed consent is obtained prior to surgical intervention and encompasses discussion on risks, benefits, postoperative course and rehabilitation, and prognosis. Again, the patient should understand potential recurrence of symptoms and variable relief. In the preoperative area, patient questions are answered again and clarified. We confirm that a physical therapy appointment has been scheduled within a week of surgery and educate the patient on the prescribed postoperative medications. The operative limb is marked next to the knee to ensure that the mark is visible after the limb is draped and prepped.

Once in the operating room and after appropriate anesthesia has been provided, the operative knee is examined focusing on the range of motion and ligamentous exam. On occasion, passive range of motion can be affected in cases of diffuse synovial hypertrophy and commonly in the presence of advanced degenerative changes. Visual inspection and palpation may demonstrate presence of an

FIGURE 30-5

Setup of knee arthroscopy. Image demonstrates the operative knee exposed with support from a lateral thigh post and foot holder. The monitor is positioned on the opposite side of the operative.

effusion. The contralateral nonoperative knee is examined to provide a baseline of normalcy. Next, a nonsterile tourniquet is placed as proximal as possible on the thigh. Commonly, the tourniquet is not inflated unless intracapsular bleeding is unable to be controlled (Figs. 30-5 and 30-6). A thigh stress post is attached to the bed at the level of the tourniquet, and foot holder is positioned allowing the knee to stay flexed at 90 degrees. A foot pedal for the arthroscopic resector is placed on the side of surgery to prevent searching for it under the operative table once the patient is draped. The monitor for the arthroscope is positioned at eye level at the head of the bed on the contralateral side. We utilize gravity-flow irrigation with four three-liter bags positioned as high as possible to distend the joint and minimize intracapsular bleeding. We also place 1 mL of epinephrine (1 mg/mL) into the each three-liter saline bag to aid in hemostasis.

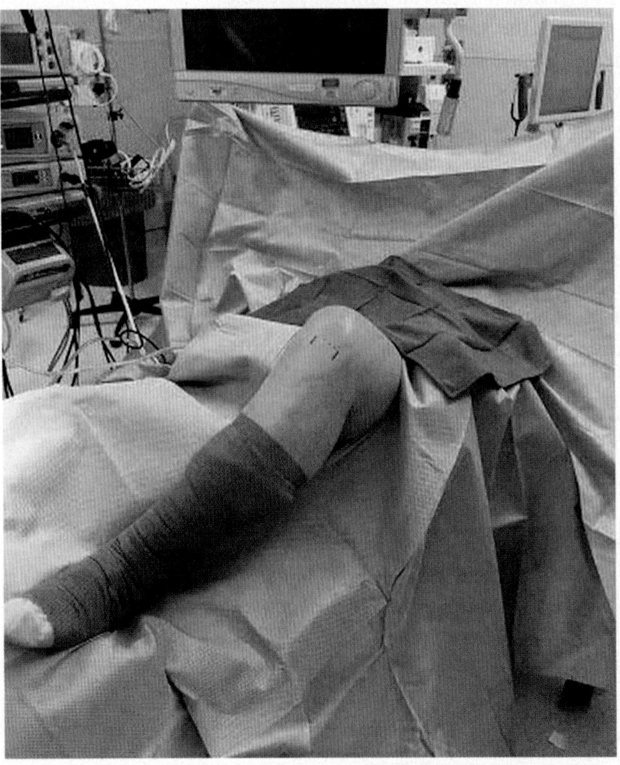

A

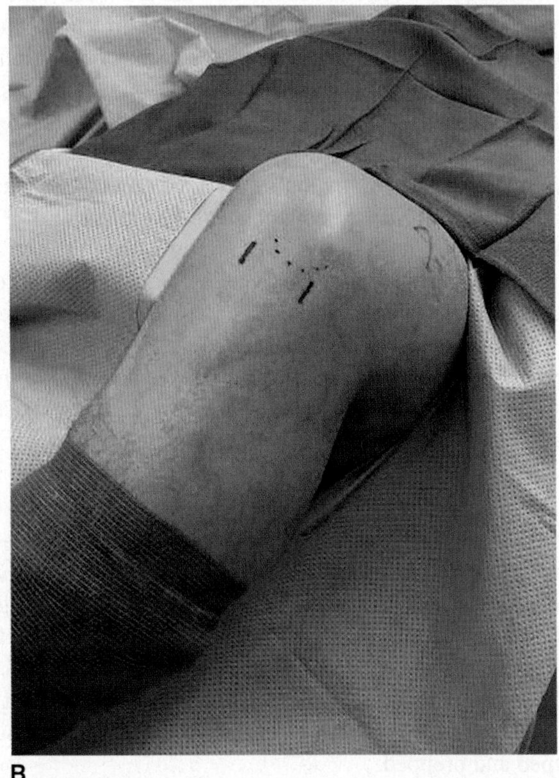

B

FIGURE 30-6

A, B: The inferior pole of the patella has been marked out with a *dotted line*. The anteromedial and anterolateral portal sites have been marked. Also note the visualized marked initials on the lateral thigh indicating correct operative site.

Diagnostic Arthroscopy

After sterile prep and draping of the operative limb, the anticipated vertical anteromedial and anterolateral portal sites and landmarks are marked with the knee in 90 degrees of flexion. The anterolateral portal is usually marked just lateral to the patella tendon starting at the level of the inferior pole of the patella and measuring 1 cm in length. The anteromedial portal is marked in a similar fashion; however, the site is usually one fingerbreadth medial to the medial border of the patellar tendon. We utilize a scope trocar with both inflow and outflow vents and therefore do not utilize any other portals. A mixture of 5 mL 1% lidocaine with epinephrine and 5 mL 0.5% Marcaine is injected subcutaneously at the portal sites to minimize bleeding and help with postoperative pain. Next, a spinal needle is placed intra-articular superolaterally with the knee in full extension, and 60 mL of solution containing 30 mL of saline and 15 mL of both 0.5% Marcaine and 1% Lidocaine without epinephrine is injected.

The marked anterolateral portal is incised with the knee in 90 degrees of flexion. The incision is made with the scalpel angled and directed toward the intercondylar notch. Next, a blunt trocar placed in an arthroscope cannula is inserted using a similar angle. On many occasions, once through the skin, with slow maintained progression, the trocar abutting the capsule is appreciated. The trocar can then be pumped as to bounce upon the capsule and then penetrate the capsule with an appreciable loss of resistance. Once through the capsule, the knee is brought into extension, and the trocar is positioned into the suprapatellar pouch. The blunt trocar is removed and a 30-degree (4-mm) arthroscope is placed into cannula. The irrigation inflow value is opened to distend the capsule. We then sequentially close and open the inflow and outflow valves to help remove any debris and blood in the joint. Next, the lens focus is adjusted, and the arthroscope is white balanced. In patients who have hypertrophied or inflamed synovitis in the suprapatellar pouch, we do not proceed to resect the synovium as to avoid any bleeding that may hinder the diagnostic evaluation (Figs. 30-7 to 30-11).

Joint Evaluation

Our diagnostic evaluation follows a very methodical process every time as to prevent overlooking any pathology. The suprapatellar pouch is evaluated for any debris, loose bodies, and potentially symptomatic plicas. We then proceed to evaluate the patella and its respective facets as well as the trochlea. The lateral gutter is examined for any loose bodies followed by the medial gutter. The leg is then placed on the hip, and a valgus force is applied with aid from the stress post. The medial compartment is visualized with the arthroscope. A spinal needle is inserted into the medial

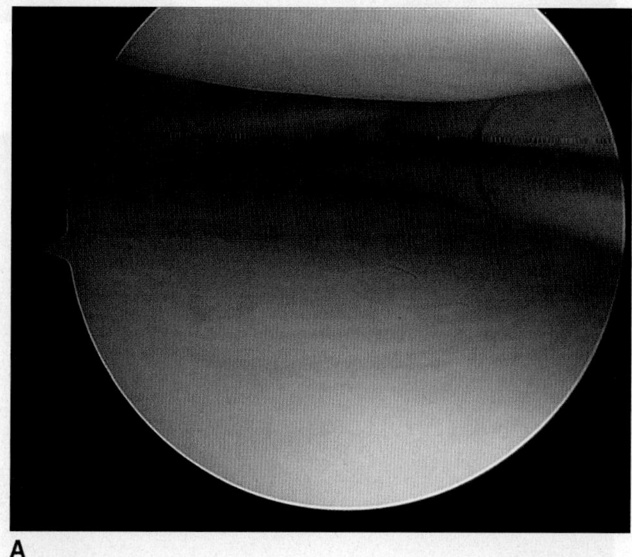
A

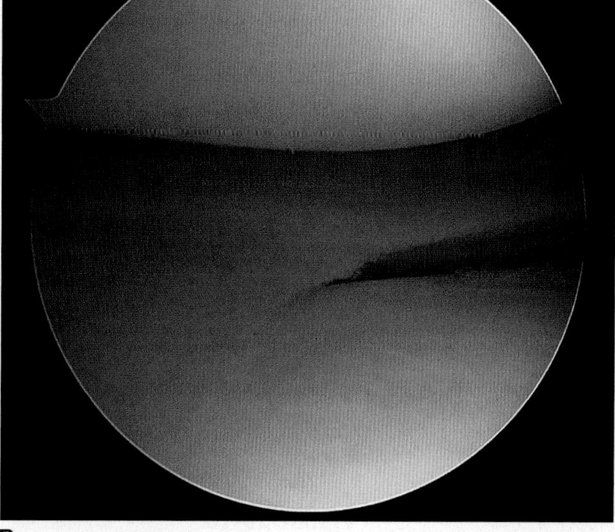
B

FIGURE 30-7

A, B: Arthroscopic images of normal articular cartilage.

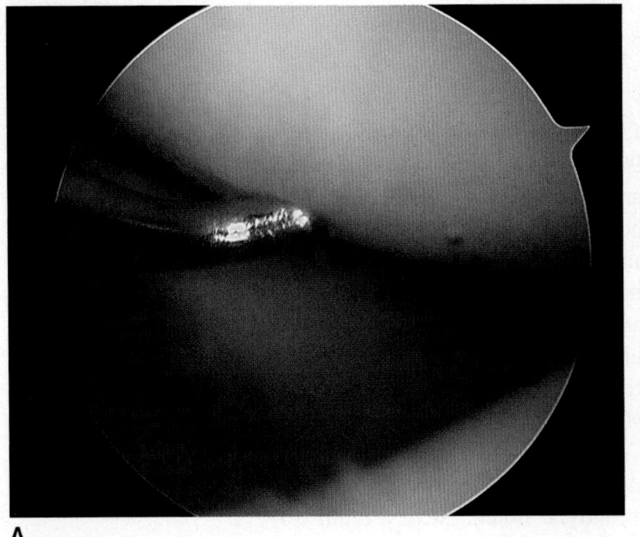
A

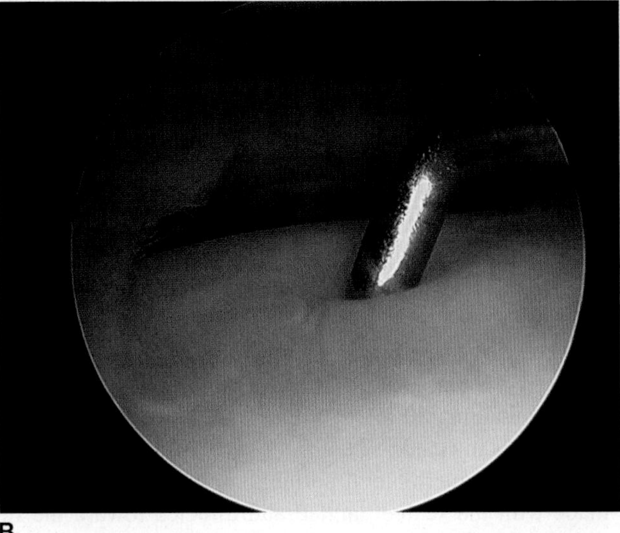
B

FIGURE 30-8

A, B: Arthroscopic images of grade 1 articular cartilage softening. The soft articular cartilage is noted as the surface indents while probed.

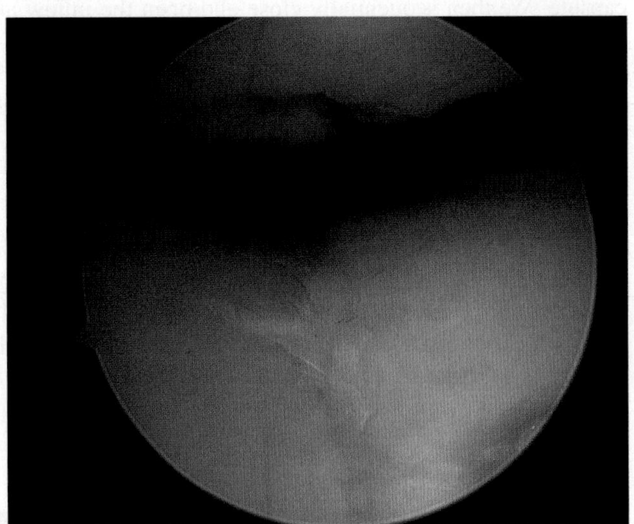

FIGURE 30-9

Arthroscopic image of grade 2 articular cartilage degeneration of the femoral trochlea.

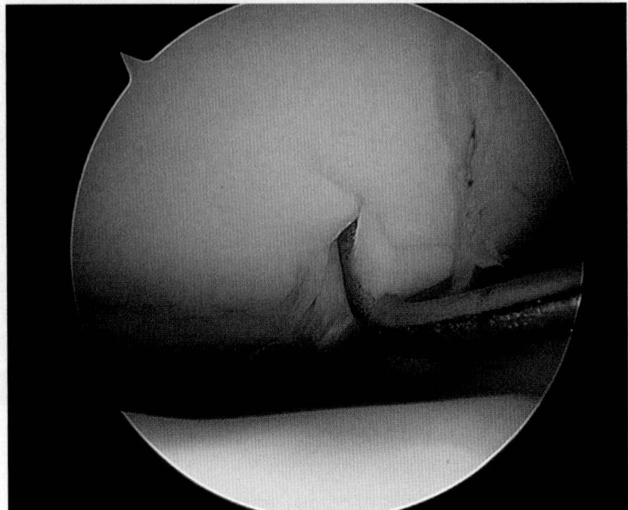

FIGURE 30-10

Arthroscopic image of grade 3 articular cartilage lesion involving the medial facet of the patella.

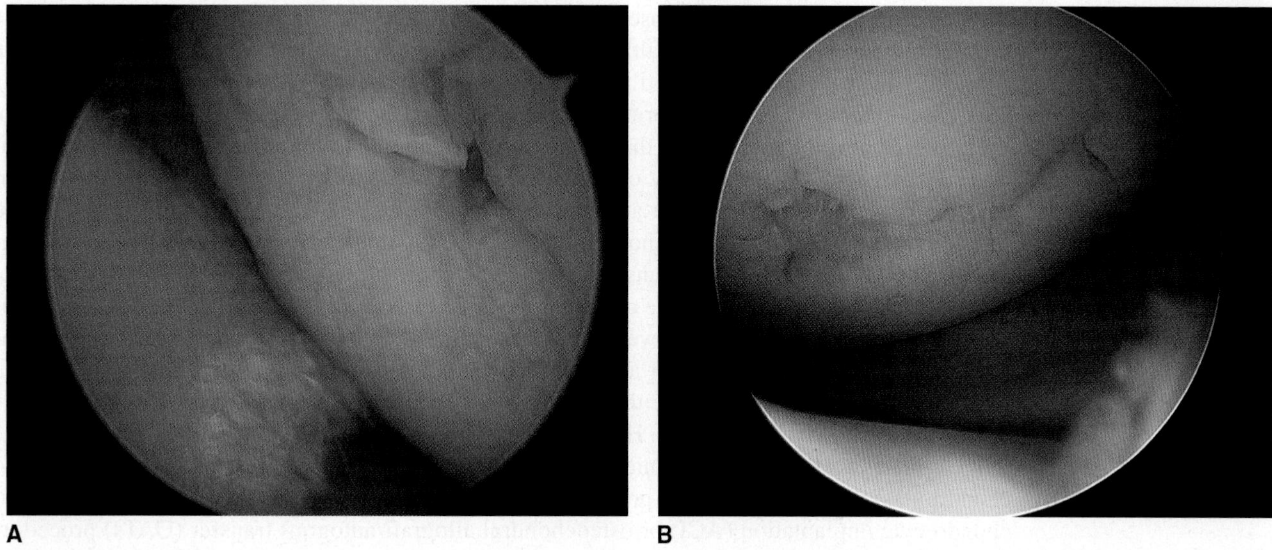

FIGURE 30-11
A, B: Arthroscopic images of grade 4 articular cartilage lesions. The subchondral bone is exposed.

compartment through the marked anteromedial portal to ensure appropriate placement. Changing the arthroscope view from the 9 o'clock view in a right knee to 3 o'clock helps visualize the spinal needle preventing iatrogenic injury to the articular surface. After appropriate portal site is confirmed, skin and capsule are incised. Again, the knife tip entering the joint can be directly visualized as stated above. The blunt trocar is placed to expand the capsule followed immediately by a right-angled probe. The arthroscope view can now be placed back to the 9 o'clock view. The meniscus is probed for tears and posterior root attachment. While the posterior horn is being examined, outflow suction is opened, and the popliteal fossa is palpated by the assistant as to suction any loose bodies. Adjusting the amount of valgus force and knee flexion helps maximize the visualization of the posterior horn of the medial meniscus. To visualize the anterior horn, the arthroscope view is positioned between 4 and 6 o'clock for a right knee. The articular cartilage is visualized entirely by flexing and extending the knee. The arthroscope is then placed in the intercondylar notch, and anterior cruciate ligament (ACL) and posterior cruciate ligament (PCL) are probed and evaluated with the knee at 90 degrees of flexion. The lateral compartment is next evaluated with the knee in a figure-of-four position. The foot is placed on nonoperative limb at 90 degrees of flexion or less and supported by an assistant. By doing so, the hip is externally rotated and abducted, and a varus force is placed on the knee. In cases of a very tight lateral compartment, downward pressure on the distal thigh while the limb is a figure-of-four position can further help open the lateral compartment. The lateral compartment is evaluated in a similar manner as the medial. In a majority of cases involving synovitis, the meniscus is spared, whereas the cartilage may demonstrate fraying and fissuring. The arthroscope is then placed in the suprapatellar pouch along with an arthroscopic resector. The joint is thoroughly irrigated via suction on the resector as the assistant lightly taps the popliteal fossa. This is to help remove any remaining debris within the joint.

Chondroplasty

The joint is evaluated during the diagnostic arthroscopy as stated above. More advanced chondromalacia is clearly evident. Early pathologic articular cartilage swelling and softening can be appreciated with a probe. The cartilage will have a bungee affect. For cartilage softening, fraying, and superficial fissuring, a chondroplasty is not performed. This is reserved for higher-grade lesions. Nevertheless, these lesions should be documented. Commonly, palpation with a probe will demonstrate unstable fragments that warrant a chondroplasty. With the probe, any delaminated cartilage from the subchondral bone should be noted. The goal is remove these fragments. An arthroscopic shaver is utilized to smoothen the edges and obtain a stable edge.

We prefer to use a mechanical oscillating resector rather than an aggressive teethed edge to prevent unwanted removal of healthy cartilage and iatrogenic injury when entering the joint. A radiofrequency ablator is not utilized for chondroplasty. The thermal energy transmitted can have deleterious effects on the normal cartilage, matrix, and exposed bone. The shaver resector tip is angled at right angles with the cartilage, and gentle motion void of excessive pressure is used. The suction is opened fully on the shaver while resecting. This allows the unstable cartilage to be drawn into the shaver and preserve the healthy cartilage, which generally will not. Intermittent re-evaluation of the chondroplasty and remaining cartilage is done to appreciate the progress. Generally, there is a transition between abnormal and normal cartilage in degenerative knees, and therefore, the edge can be sloped off. In younger patients, this transition can be abrupt, and a curette can help develop stable edges. When exposure of the subchondral bone is encountered unexpectedly after a chondroplasty, we generally follow two pathways. One, if degenerative changes are diffuse either involving the compartment or multiple compartments, no additional treatment is performed. However, if the lesion is isolated with relative well-preserved joint, a marrow stimulation technique is performed. We prefer a microfracture technique. A chondroplasty is also performed prior to a cartilage restoration procedure such as autologous chondrocyte implantation (ACI) or osteochondral allograft/autograft transfer (OATs) procedure to prepare the site. This can be performed either via an open or arthroscopic technique. When performed open, similar principles are applied of eliminating the abnormal cartilage to a normal rim (see Figs. 30-14 to 30-19).

Synovectomy

Once the diagnostic evaluation is completed as above, focus can be turned to the synovitis. We begin our synovial resection in the suprapatellar pouch. An arthroscopic ablator should be available. In many cases, a sequential combination of the resector and ablator is utilized to prevent excessive bleeding and disruption of visualization. Occasionally, the bleeding is difficult to stop, and the tourniquet is inflated. If the tourniquet is inflated, prior to completion of the procedure, the tourniquet is deflated, and any excessive bleeding is ablated to prevent a postoperative hematoma. The synovectomy is performed sequentially by focusing on each compartment individually, starting in the suprapatellar pouch, followed by the retropatellar space, lateral gutter, medial gutter, medial compartment, intercondylar notch, lateral compartment, and finally the posterior compartment. Essentially, the synovectomy starts in the suprapatellar pouch and then progresses distally, medially, and laterally. The arthroscope can be placed in the anteromedial portal as needed for improved visualization and aid in synovectomy by using the anterolateral portal as a working portal. Synovitis spanning from the intercondylar notch or present in the retropatellar space can initially be resected with the knee in extension. The arthroscope view is angled between the 3 and 6 o'clock position for a right knee. Resection in near full extension can minimize iatrogenic injury to the intermeniscal ligament and ACL. The synovectomy starts at the superior aspect of the trochlea and progresses distally. When resecting with the knee in 90 degrees of flexion, the resector face is always visualized to prevent iatrogenic injury especially when synovitis prevents adequate visualization. In certain circumstances where retropatellar or intercondylar synovitis is extensive, a 70-degree arthroscope can be placed through an accessory superolateral portal. By doing so, one is enabled to visualize directly upon the retropatellar region. This technique is done with the knee in extension. If synovitis is present in the posterior aspect of the joint, an accessory posteromedial portal used primarily as working portal may be necessary as well as a 70-degree arthroscope. We create a posteromedial portal utilizing an inside-out technique as follows. First, visualization of the posterior joint and capsule is obtained. This is done by placing the arthroscope between the lateral wall of the medial femoral condyle and the PCL. Without moving the cannula, the arthroscope is switched out for a blunt trocar. Next, lateral force is placed on the PCL to create space between the PCL and medial femoral condyle. This is performed by bringing the hand toward the patellar tendon. The blunt trocar is then advanced gently under control into the posterior joint. The blunt trocar is replaced by a 30-degree arthroscope and position confirmed. While visualizing the posteromedial capsule, a spinal needle is placed into the joint. The trajectory of the spinal needle is evaluated ensuring access to the majority of the posterior joint. Once confirmed, a longitudinal skin incision is made at the entry point approximately 1 to 2 cm. On many occasions, we leave the spinal needle in place and slide a switching stick adjacent and parallel to the spinal needle to help with placement. Once through the capsule, the spinal needle is removed, and a cannulated portal dilator is placed over the switching stick. A 6.5-mm cannula can then be placed, ensuring several threads placed through the capsule to prevent the cannula from backing up. The switching stick is removed. The working portal is now ready for a resector or ablator. Similar technique is used for a posterolateral portal when necessary. We try to avoid using the posterolateral portal secondary to concerns of iatrogenic common peroneal nerve injury. If necessary, the portal should be anterior to the biceps femoris tendon. Initially, we use a 30-degree arthroscope but commonly transition a 70-degree for optimal visualization. When utilizing the resector or ablator, we ensure that the face of the instrument is never directly on the posterior capsule. The instrument is either facing 90 or 180 degrees from the capsule to prevent unwarranted arthrotomy and potential injury to the popliteal fossa neurovascular bundle.

The incisions are closed with a nonabsorbable suture. Five milliliters of plain local anesthetic is injected intra-articularly through the superolateral puncture site from the start of the case. Sterile dressing is applied including a nonadhesive, two 4 × 4 gauze folded in half, and medium Tegaderms followed by a compressive wrap. For patients who underwent a synovectomy, an abdominal pad is added without a Tegaderm. Again, a gentle compressive wrap is placed to help with postoperative swelling and hematoma. Thigh-high antiembolism compressive sleeves are placed bilaterally for all patients. A cooling device is placed on the knee before the patient leaves the operating room (Figs. 30-12 to 30-19).

Arthroscopic images are taken throughout the procedure to document the pathology encountered for medical record and, perhaps most importantly, to provide a visual guide for the patient. At the first postoperative visit, the images are reviewed with the patient. The patient is educated and provided with an understanding of his or her joint. This can be especially critical when degenerative changes are present and patient expectations are unrealistic or to establish patient expectations. We print two copies, one for the patient and one for our medical records. All pictures are labeled. The set for the patient is labeled in nontechnical or medical terms.

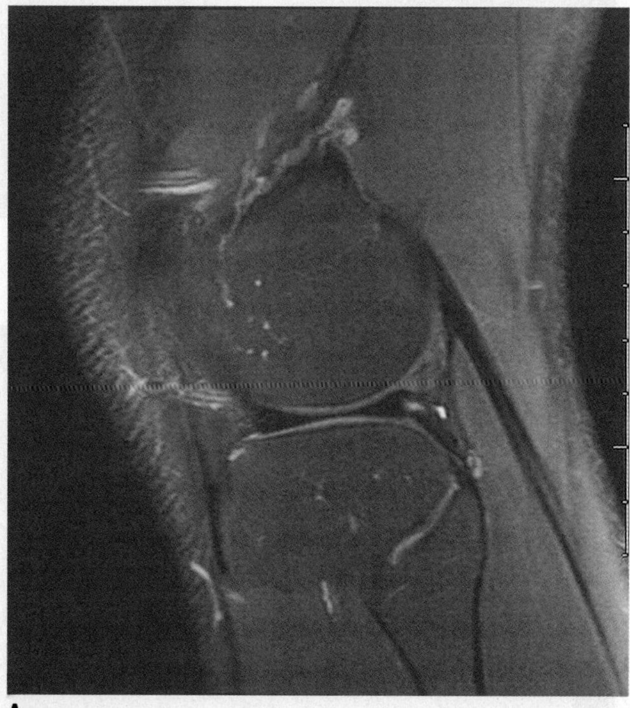
A

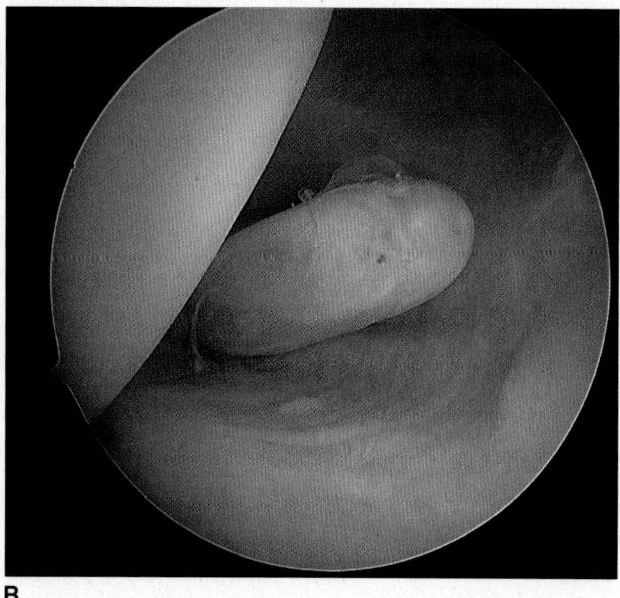
B

FIGURE 30-12

A: MRI sagittal image demonstrating localized PVNS in the posterolateral knee joint. Note the heterogeneity of the mass with hypointense areas corresponding to hemosiderin deposition. **B:** A notch view with a 70-degree arthroscope illustrating the PVNS.

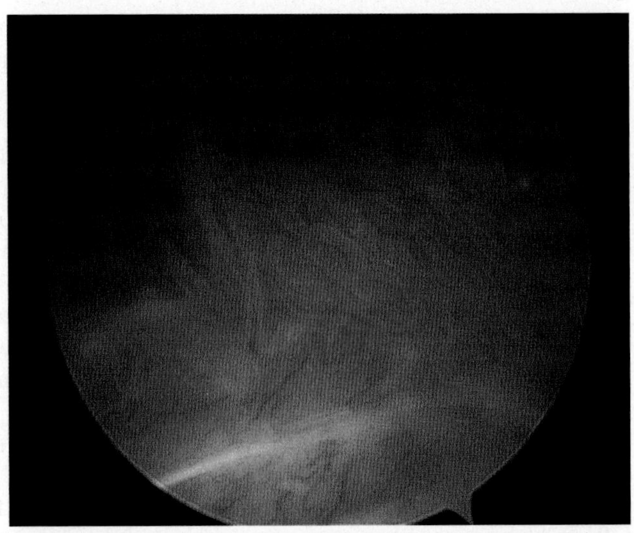

FIGURE 30-13
Arthroscopic image of inflamed synovium in the suprapatellar pouch.

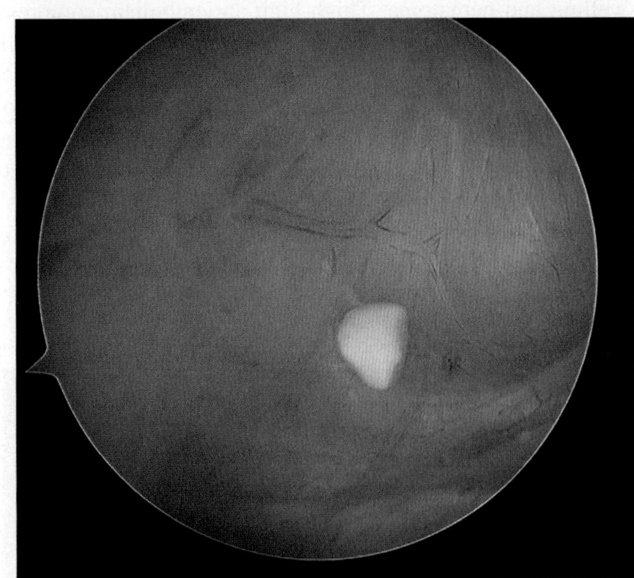

FIGURE 30-14
Arthroscopic image of a loose articular cartilage fragment. Documenting findings as such is important for patient education and expectations.

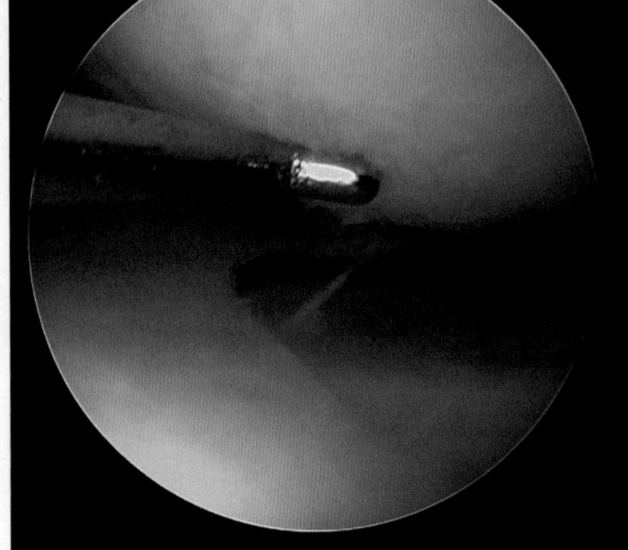

FIGURE 30-15
Arthroscopic image illustrating evaluation of the articular surface with a probe. The probe can also facilitate sizing lesions. The inner length of the probe is 3 mm from the bend, and the outer length is 5 mm.

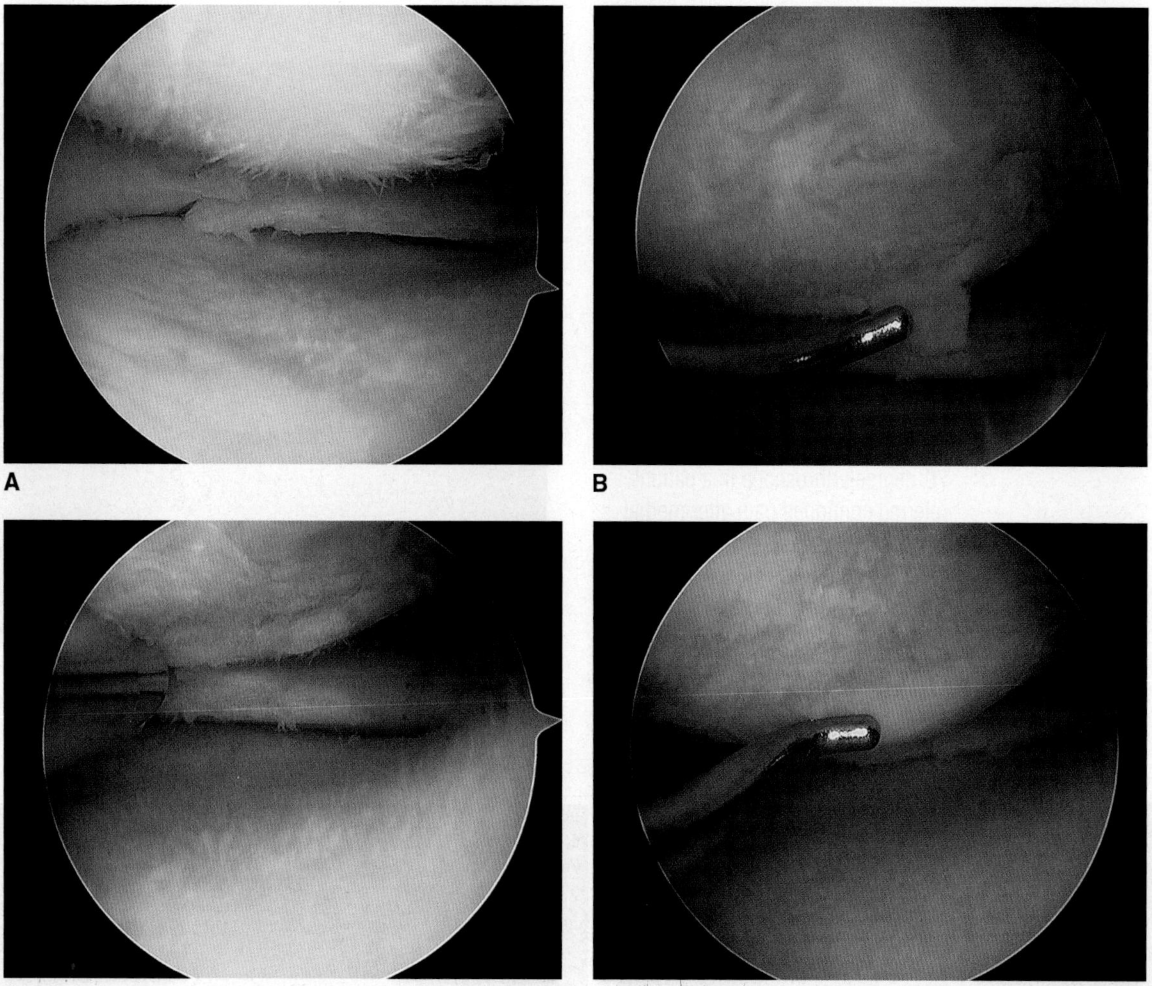

A

B

C

D

FIGURE 30-16

A–D: Arthroscopic images of the medial compartment. **A:** There are diffuse grade 3 articular cartilage changes on the medial femoral condyle with an associated degenerative posterior horn medial meniscus tear. **B:** Increased knee flexion exposes an unstable articular cartilage segment. The probe helps identify these lesions. **C:** An arthroscopic resector is utilized to perform a chondroplasty removing the frayed and unstable articular cartilage. **D:** Postchondroplasty image demonstrating stable articular cartilage edge and removed fraying.

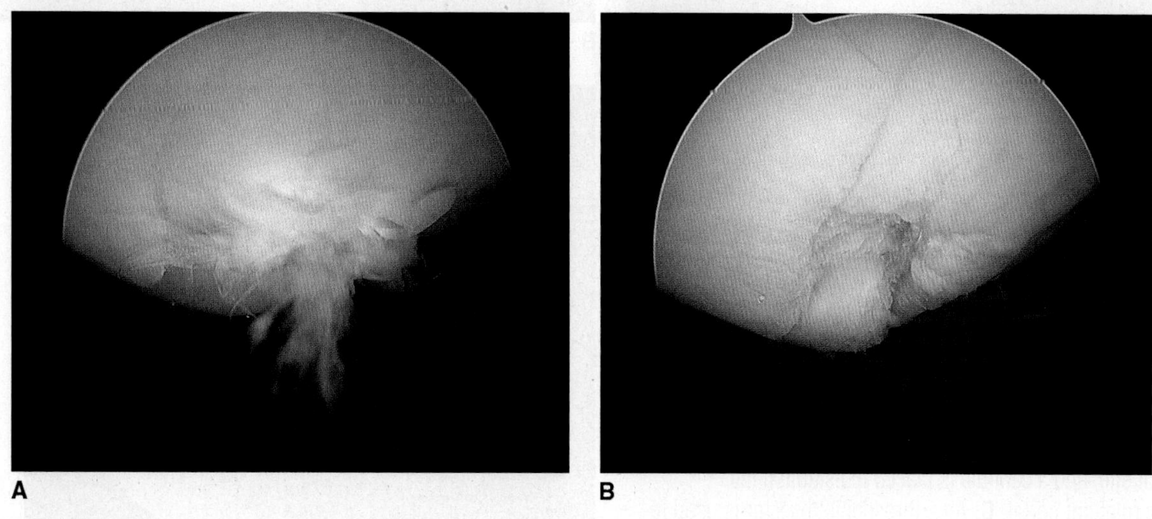

A

B

FIGURE 30-17

A, B: Arthroscopic images of pre- and postchondroplasty of grade 3 chondromalacia involving the patella.

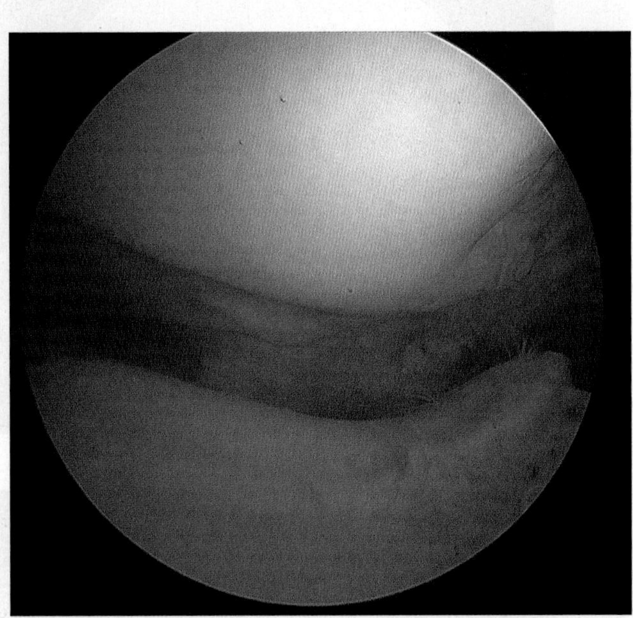

FIGURE 30-18

Arthroscopic image of the patellofemoral joint from the superolateral portal utilizing a 70-degree arthroscope in a patient referred continued pain after medial patellofemoral ligament reconstruction. This view allows great evaluation of the patella position within the trochlea as well as the retropatellar space.

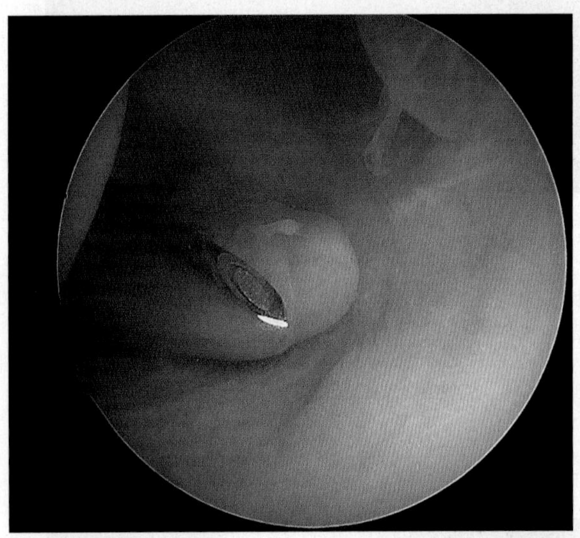

A

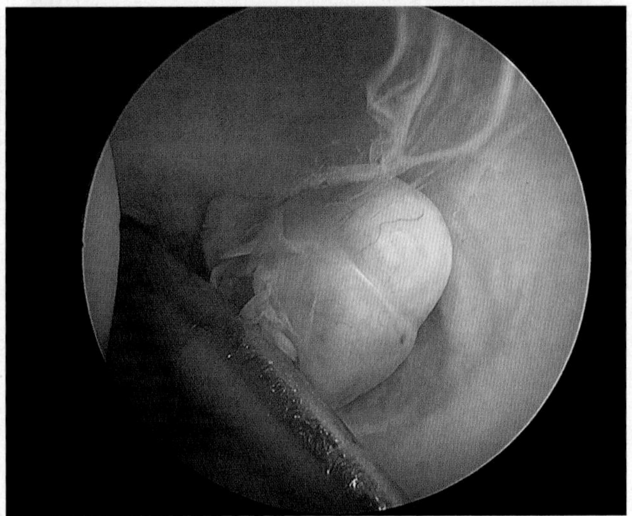

B

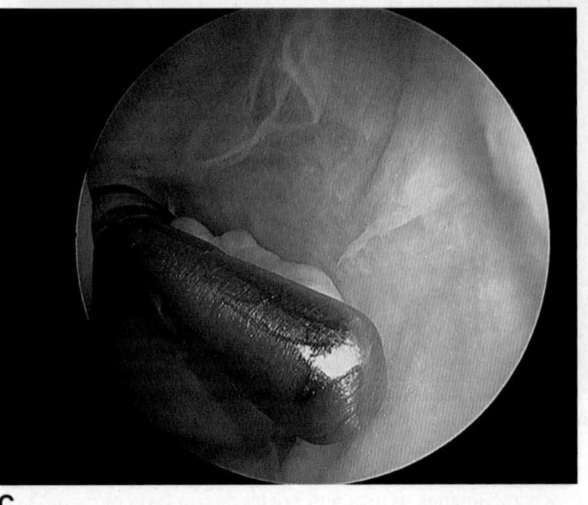

C

FIGURE 30-19

A–D: Removal of PVNS lesion in the posterolateral knee joint. **A:** Needle localization to establish an appropriate posterolateral portal via a notch view with a 70-degree arthroscope. **B:** Blunt trocar is placed through the anticipated portal site, and a cannula is placed to establish the posterolateral portal. **C:** An arthroscopic resector is used to amputate the mass at its base and avoiding resection of the mass itself.

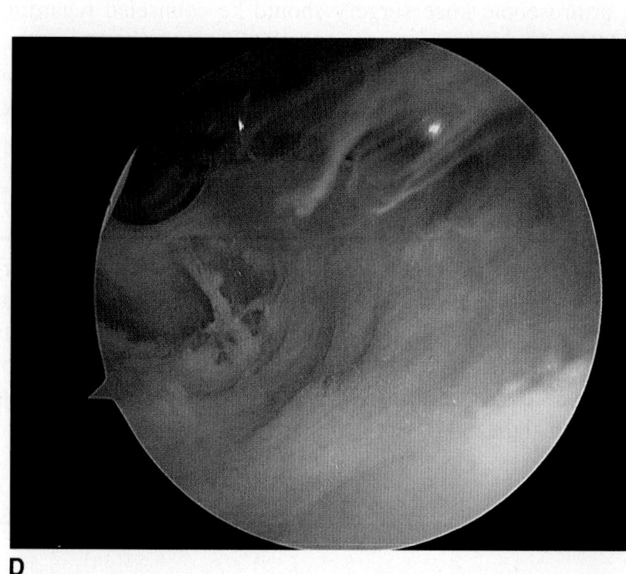

D

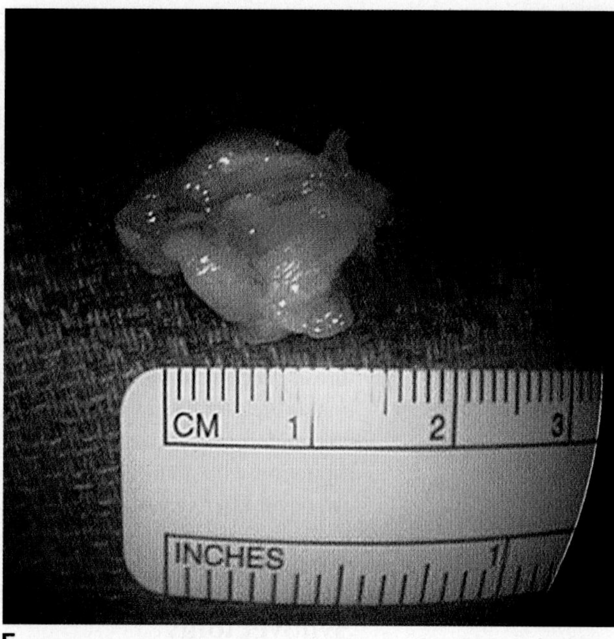

E

FIGURE 30-19 (*Continued*)

D: The lesion has been excised, and any remaining PVNS has been removed. **E:** The mass is measured and sent for pathology.

POSTOPERATIVE MANAGEMENT

Generally, all patients undergo outpatient surgery. In the postoperative area, the cooling device is continued and the limb is elevated. We recommended keeping the antiembolism compressive sleeve on for 2 to 3 days postoperation or until ambulatory. Crutches are provided during the same time frame. Physical therapy is initiated within a week of surgery to regain range of motion, minimize swelling, and to focus on quadriceps activation. Patients are typically weight bearing as tolerated with crutches. Once the general anesthesia has worn off, we discuss the operative findings and procedures performed. Intraoperative arthroscopic pictures are utilized for visual confirmation. All patients receive a folder that contains a copy of the arthroscopic pictures, their diagnosis, the operation performed, surgical findings, physical therapy recommendations, and therapy goals for the first 2 weeks. We also have postoperative instructions on the dressing, emphasizing limb elevation and cryotherapy use, concerning signs and symptoms, and explanations on common postoperative experiences such as nausea and swelling. Patients usually discontinue crutch use in 1 week. They follow up also within a week for evaluation, wound examination, answer questions, and again discuss surgical findings with arthroscopic pictures as well as expected postoperative course/outcomes. As pain and inflammation from surgery improve, cycling and quadriceps strengthening are initiated. In our practice, we encourage formal physical therapy within a week of surgery. The guidance and support provided by the therapist facilitate not only physical but also mental recovery. The therapist can also provide feedback and apply modalities as needed.

PEARLS AND PITFALLS

- Have a 70-degree arthroscope available when performing a synovectomy.
- Turbulent flow should be limited with small capsular incisions preventing fluid leak during the surgery.
- Use 1 mg/mL epinephrine solution in saline irrigation bags to assist in hemostasis during arthroscopy.
- For chondroplasty, in reviewing the MRI with the patient, and there being a change of microfracture, it should be discussed on its implications of nonweight bearing.
- Aggressive chondroplasty of articular cartilage lesions in the femoral trochlea can lead to mechanical symptoms with range of motion as the patella tracks. These lesions are often of minimal symptoms or an incidental finding and should be addressed with care.

- Patients with bone marrow edema generally do not improve from arthroscopic chondroplasty.
- Preoperative MRI images demonstrating subchondral edema may be the initial presentation of osteonecrosis. Patients undergoing arthroscopic knee surgery should be counseled regarding spontaneous osteonecrosis if clinical presentation indicates such possibility and thus preventing any confusion postoperatively if pain does not resolve or MRI images demonstrate progression of disease. Postarthroscopic osteonecrosis is also a complication of arthroscopic knee surgery; however, much less common.

COMPLICATIONS

The morbidity of arthroscopic knee surgery is low. Complications include septic arthritis, hemarthrosis, deep vein thrombosis, pulmonary embolism, and cutaneous nerve injury. Sinus tract formation at the portal sites and neurovascular injury of the popliteal fossa are very uncommon. Patients who undergo a synovectomy are at higher risk of hemarthrosis. If a hemarthrosis does develop, joint aspiration with a large-bore needle may be necessary and arthroscopic washout if needed. Stiffness can occur after synovectomy and early physical therapy.

RESULTS

Synovectomy

Arthroscopic synovectomy has promising results. Goetz et al. evaluated arthroscopic and radiation synovectomy for rheumatoid arthritis in 32 knees with 14-year follow-up. They noted a reoperation rate of 56% at 10 years and improved function for at least 5 years. In rheumatoid patients, arthroscopic synovectomy has a survival rate of 88.5% at 5 years, 53.9% at 10 years, and 39.6% at 14 years with an endpoint of a total knee replacement (1). Another study demonstrated similar improvements in function at 28 months postsynovectomy. In patients with hemophilia, arthroscopic synovectomy can help improve range of motion, function, and decrease incidence of recurrent hemarthrosis; however, it does not alter the natural history of joint degeneration (2). A main predictor of outcomes is the degree of joint degeneration on preoperative radiographs (3).

Auregan et al. retrospectively evaluated the functional outcome in patients with PVNS treated with arthroscopic synovectomy. At an average of 7 years, in 21 patients with both local and diffuse forms, there was significant improvement in function (4). Recurrence-free survival at 2 years was 62% and 48% at 5 years in patients who underwent arthroscopic synovectomy with local and diffuse PVNS (5).

Chondroplasty

Unlike arthroscopic synovectomy, arthroscopic chondroplasty lacks studies that provide insight on outcomes. If mechanical symptoms are present from unstable cartilage, the anticipated improvement is good to excellent. However, when pain and degenerative changes are the primary presentation, the situation is vastly different. The numerous compounding variables present make it difficult to develop high-power studies that can ultimately guide our profession and treatment of these patients. Arron et al. concluded that the severity of degenerative changes present ultimately correlated with outcomes. Generally, this reflects our experience. The severity of pain preoperatively also translates to postoperative pain. Educating patients that the degree and length of symptom improvement are highly variable is critical. Arthroscopic chondroplasty is a temporizing procedure available for the middle-aged patient with symptomatic mild to moderate articular degeneration.

REFERENCES

1. Goetz M, Klug S, Gelse K, et al. Combined arthroscopic and radiation synovectomy of the knee joint in rheumatoid arthritis: 14-year follow-up. *Arthroscopy.* 2011;27(1):52–59.
2. Wiedel JD. Arthroscopic synovectomy of the knee in hemophilia: 10-to-15 year follow up. *Clin Orthop Relat Res.* 1996;328:46–53.
3. Verma N, Valentino LA, Chawla A. Arthroscopic synovectomy in haemophilia: indications, technique and results. *Haemophilia.* 2007;13(suppl 3):38–44.
4. Auregan JC, Bohu Y, Lefevre N, et al. Primary arthroscopic synovectomy for pigmented villo-nodular synovitis of the knee: recurrence rate and functional outcomes after a mean follow-up of seven years. *Orthop Traumatol Surg Res.* 2013;99(8):937–943.
5. Sharma V, Cheng EY. Outcomes after excision of pigmented villonodular synovitis of the knee. *Clin Orthop Relat Res.* 2009;467(11):2852–2858.

RECOMMENDED READINGS

Browne JE, Branch TP. Surgical alternatives for the treatment of articular cartilage lesions. *J Am Acad Othrop Surg.* 2000;8:180–189.

Ewing JW. Arthroscopic treatment of degenerative meniscal lesions and early degenerative arthritis of the knee. In: Ewing JW, ed. *Articular cartilage and knee joint function: basic science and the arthroscope*. New York: Raven Press; 1990:137–145.

Hanssen AD, Stuart MJ, Scott RD, et al. Surgical options for the middle-aged patient with osteoarthritis of the knee joint. *J Bone Joint Surg.* 2000;82-A:1768–1781.

Harwin SF. Arthroscopic debridement for osteoarthritis of the knee: predictors of patient satisfaction. *Arthroscopy.* 1999;15:142–146.

Jackson DW, Simon TM, Aberman HA. Symptomatic articular cartilage degeneration: the impact in the new millennium. *Clin Orthop Relat Res.* 2001;391S:S14–S25.

Jackson RW, Dieterichs C. The results of arthroscopic lavage and debridement of osteoarthritic knees based on the severity of degeneration: a 4- to 6-year follow-up. *Arthroscopy.* 2003;19:13–20.

McCauley TR, Disler DG. Magnetic resonance imaging of articular cartilage of the knee. *J Am Acad Orthop Surg.* 2001;9:2–8.

Mosely JB, O'Malley K, Petersen NJ, et al. A controlled trial arthroscopic surgery for osteoarthritis of the knee. *N Engl J Med.* 2002;347:81–88.

Simon TS, Jackson DW. Articular cartilage: injury pathways and treatment options. *Sports Med Arthrosc Rev.* 2006;14(3):146–154.

31 Microfracture Technique: Treatment of Full-Thickness Chondral Lesions

Ian D. Hutchinson, Arielle J. Hall, and Scott A. Rodeo

INTRODUCTION

The "microfracture" technique was developed by JR Steadman, MD over 20 years ago to enhance chondral resurfacing by directly accessing the regenerative cellular and biological elements of subchondral bone and bone marrow. Due to its minimally invasive approach, limited surgical morbidity, and cost effectiveness, microfracture is considered a first-line treatment for symptomatic chondral lesions in the knee and other joints. Following adequate debridement of a chondral lesion, purposely designed awls are used to make multiple perforations, or "microfractures," in the subchondral bone plate producing a regenerative mesenchymal clot and initiating fibrocartilage formation. Patient-reported outcomes have shown significant improvement in the short term with a progressive decline in the performance of the repair tissue from the medium to long term. In the clinical and preclinical setting, microfracture is considered the gold standard for comparison of emerging cartilage repair technologies. Concurrently, due to the relative ease of translation, strategies to augment microfracture using matrices, cells, growth factors, and other biologic agents targeting the repair site and the whole joint homeostasis are also under investigation.

INDICATIONS/CONTRAINDICATIONS

Indications

Microfracture is primarily indicated for symptomatic, full-thickness articular lesions in the weight-bearing regions of the femur, tibia, and in the patellofemoral joint (Table 31-1). A review of the current literature suggests that the following preoperative characteristics are associated with more successful outcomes following microfracture:

- *Patient-related characteristics:* age less than 40 years; body mass index (BMI) less than 30 kg/m^2
- *Defect characteristics:* minimal symptom duration; defect size less than 4 cm^2; location on the femoral condyle; primary surgery on the presenting defect

While discrete lesions may be appreciated preoperatively on magnetic resonance imaging (MRI), areas of intact cartilage that are unstable to probing at the time of arthroscopy are also indicated. Patients with acute chondral injuries are ideally treated as soon as possible after the diagnosis is made, especially if the knee is being treated concurrently for meniscal or anterior cruciate ligament (ACL) pathology.

Microfracture is also performed for focal degenerative defects in knees with appropriate axial alignment and ligamentous stability. It is worth noting that while many lesions may be practically amenable to the microfracture procedure, the biological potential of the mesenchymal clot to fill the repair site with robust cartilaginous tissue, particularly in the setting of early joint degeneration in a patient aged greater than 45 years may be limited. In addition, it may be difficult to distinguish

TABLE 31-1 Indications and Contraindications for Microfracture

Indications	Contraindications
Full-thickness chondral defect	Partial-thickness defects
Unstable full-thickness cartilage segment	Uncorrected axial malalignment
Isolated, contained degenerative chondral lesions	Global degenerative osteoarthrosis
Patient capable of rehabilitation protocol	Poor patient compliance or questionable commitment to prolonged rehabilitation

symptoms attributed to isolated lesions from general prodromal symptoms of osteoarthritis in the older patient population (e.g., pain predicated by certain movements or prolonged standing, etc.). Therefore, microfracture in the setting of early degenerative changes warrants careful discussion with the patient regarding realistic goals and expectations of the procedure. It is generally recommended that patients with chronic or degenerative chondral lesions are initially treated conservatively (activity modification, physical therapy, nonsteroidal anti-inflammatory drugs, viscosupplementation, etc.) and that microfracture should only be considered in refractory cases.

Contraindications

Contraindications of microfracture consist of patient-related, knee and defect characteristics that make successful generation of an in situ clot, tissue regeneration, and successful rehabilitation unlikely. Specifically, these include:

- *Patient-related characteristics:* poor compliance and motivation, inability to use the opposite leg for weightbearing during protected weightbearing or nonweightbearing, autoimmune disorders, tumor, infection, inflammatory arthropathy, and intrinsic diseases of articular cartilage
- *Knee characteristics:* uncorrected axial malalignment, high-grade ligamentous instability, patellar maltracking or instability, and global degenerative osteoarthritis
- *Defect characteristics:* lack of an intact peripheral rim of cartilage tissue that is necessary to contain the mesenchymal clot

Relative contraindications include patients older than 65 years because of expected limited biologic potential difficulties with crutch walking and the extended rigorous rehabilitation (Table 31-1).

PREOPERATIVE PLANNING

Patients with symptomatic chondral defects present with knee joint pain and should be assessed accordingly at the initial consultation. A careful patient history may provide important information about the chronicity of symptomatic lesions and the presence of concomitant soft tissue pathology. In addition, patient-related factors that may affect the generation of a successful mesenchymal clot (e.g., age, medical comorbidities, medications) are noted. During examination of the knee, definitive clinical diagnosis of chondral lesions may be challenging; identification of point tenderness on the femur/tibia or compression of patellofemoral joint is useful, but not diagnostic.

Standard radiographs are acquired to observe for angular deformity and joint space narrowing, often suggestive of articular cartilage loss. Specifically, anteroposterior and lateral radiographs of both knees as well as weight-bearing views with the knees in 30 to 45 degrees of flexion are acquired. The patellofemoral joint is assessed for patellar (height and tilt) and trochlear morphology with axial "sunrise" views (e.g., axial Merchant view). MRI has become standard in the assessment of soft tissue defects. Standard fast spin-echo pulse sequences are useful in locating pathology, including use of both T1-weighted and T2-weighted sequences. Important information about tissue composition is provided by quantitative sequences (qMRI), including T1rho (proteoglycan content) and T2 relaxation time mapping (collagen organization).

Uncorrected malalignment is a relative contraindication to microfracture, and realignment procedures may be planned prior to or in conjunction with cartilage restoration. In each microfracture patient, long leg standing radiographs are used to evaluate limb alignment. The mechanical axis should fall between the central quarters of the medial and lateral compartments or between the tibial spines. The authors have a relatively low threshold for consideration of osteotomy to correct malalignment in the setting of cartilage repair.

Preoperative planning concludes with a discussion of patient-related considerations, the rationale for the procedure, the expected postoperative rehabilitation, and a careful discussion of alternative options between the operating surgeon and the patient. The factors that predict successful outcome are discussed with the patient. This helps to provide realistic expectations for the patient. The patient should understand that the results of cartilage repair surgery could be somewhat variable and unpredictable. The possibility of progressive degenerative changes in the future and the need for further surgical treatment should be discussed. Finally, it is important to keep in mind that violation of the subchondral plate with microfracture may potentially diminish future cartilage restoration attempts.

TECHNIQUE

Patient Positioning and Preparation

The patient is placed in the supine position, general or regional anesthesia (spinal or epidural) is administered, and routine skin preparation and draping for knee arthroscopy are initiated. Positioning of the operated knee must allow for motion, without restriction. A tourniquet is placed on the proximal aspect of the thigh but not routinely utilized; in the setting of microfracture, arthroscopic fluid pump pressure is used to control bleeding. The leg is covered with impermeable stockinet and conformed to the leg using an adhesive bandage. Standard arthroscopic portals may be used for microfracture: anterolateral and anteromedial portals access lesions on the central femoral condyles; superolateral portals may be used for patellar and trochlear lesions; and accessory further medial or lateral portals may be added to access peripheral defects, as required.

Diagnostic Knee Arthroscopy

A diagnostic arthroscopic examination of the knee should always precede a microfracture procedure. All anatomic areas of the knee joint are systematically assessed: suprapatellar pouch, medial and lateral gutters, patellofemoral joint, intercondylar notch, and both the medial and lateral compartments (including the posterior horns of both menisci). It is important to carefully evaluate for plicae and lateral retinacular tightness leading to lateral patellar tilt when treating patellofemoral lesions.

Concomitant Procedures

All pathology present should be addressed surgically. Careful preoperative planning, with consideration of symptoms, physical examination, and imaging studies, will identify all pathology that needs to be addressed. Concurrent management of malalignment, meniscal lesions, ligament disruption, multiple chondral defects, or patellar maltracking is encouraged in a single-stage approach to minimize repetitive operative morbidity and extended rehabilitation. We generally address concomitant procedures prior to microfracture given the potential for attenuation of visibility caused by fat droplets and blood within the knee from microfracture holes. Addressing the other soft tissues before microfracture also minimizes the potential of pumping fluid into the subchondral bone and marrow from raised intra-articular fluid pressures.

Chondral Lesion Preparation

After inspecting and probing the periphery of the full-thickness articular cartilage defect, existing cartilage flaps are debrided back to a stable peripheral margin using an arthroscopic shaver or ring curette. A stable full-thickness border of cartilage is necessary to contain the clot and regenerating tissue and provides a more robust tissue-clot interface during early loading. It is also important to note that if a stable rim of cartilage cannot be achieved, microfracture should not be undertaken since the clot will not be contained. The prepared defect is measured with a calibrated probe and correlated to the arc of motion of the joint; these details are recorded for the operative note and have important implications for postoperative rehabilitation (Fig. 31-1). It is critical to remove the calcified cartilage layer while taking care to preserve the underlying subchondral bone plate. Underresection of the calcified cartilage layer has been shown to compromise binding of the clot and regenerated tissue at the repair site. Conversely, violation of the subchondral plate has been associated with osseous overgrowth within the defect, compromising the repair and rendering the articular cartilage surface vulnerable to progressive degeneration. Removal of the calcified cartilage

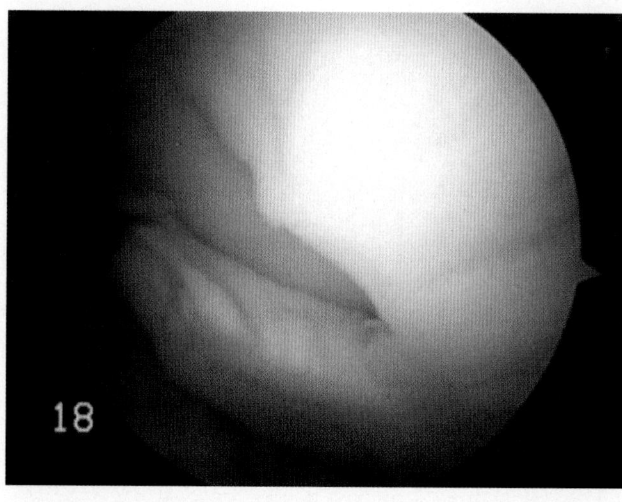

FIGURE 31-1
Loose, marginally attached cartilage is removed from the surrounding rim of the lesion.

layer is facilitated by manual tactile feedback using a curette, which allows the surgeon to differentiate the calcified cartilage layer from the harder subchondral bone (Fig. 31-2).

Microfracturing the Defect

After careful preparation of the lesion, an arthroscopic awl (e.g., Linvatec, Largo, FL) is used to make multiple holes, or "microfractures," in the exposed subchondral bone plate at the base of the defect. Arthroscopic awl tips with conical shape and angulations of 30, 45, and 90 degrees are favored over the drilling technique (Pridie drilling) in order to avoid thermal injury (Fig. 31-3). The tip of the awl is placed perpendicular to the subchondral bone, and the plate is penetrated to a depth of 2 to 3 mm. To achieve this, the 30 and 45 degrees awls are gently toed (to reduce the risk of skiving) and impacted directly using a mallet. It can be difficult to achieve a perpendicular orientation to the patellar surface. The patella can be manually tilted to improve access, and counterpressure on the patella is required when impacting the awl. Consideration can be made for retrograde drilling from the superficial aspect of the patella to access the patellar surface. It is critically important to avoid horizontal slippage of the awl ("skiving") on the subchondral plate, as this can compromise the integrity of the subchondral bone.

The microfracture holes are developed from the periphery of the lesion toward the center in a spiral pattern allowing homogenous distribution of the holes within the defect (Fig. 31-4). A four-millimeter bone bridge is maintained between each hole, thus maintaining the integrity of the subchondral plate. The release of fatty droplets from the marrow cavity via the microfracture holes indicates that the requisite depth of penetration has been achieved (Fig. 31-5). Osseous debris is

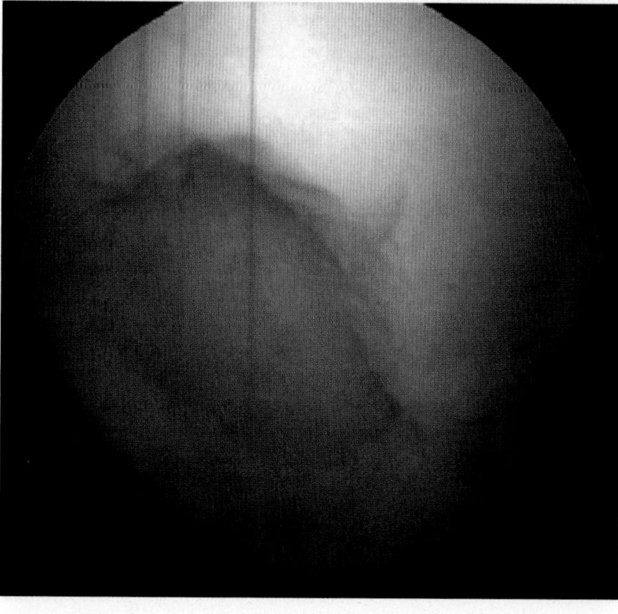

FIGURE 31-2
The calcified cartilage layer must be removed carefully using a curette.

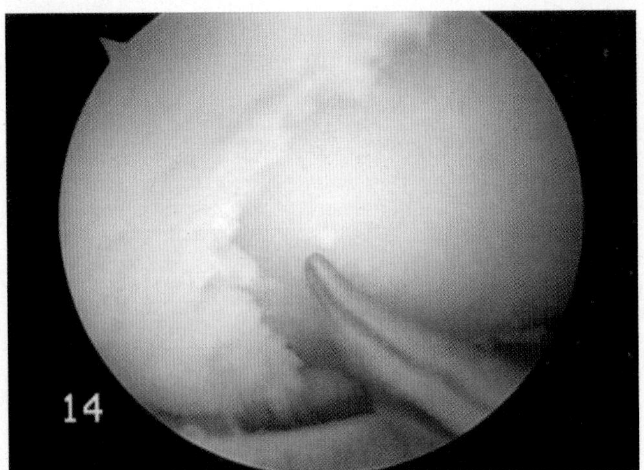

FIGURE 31-3

Awls with angulated tips allow the microfracture technique to remain perpendicular to bone throughout the lesion.

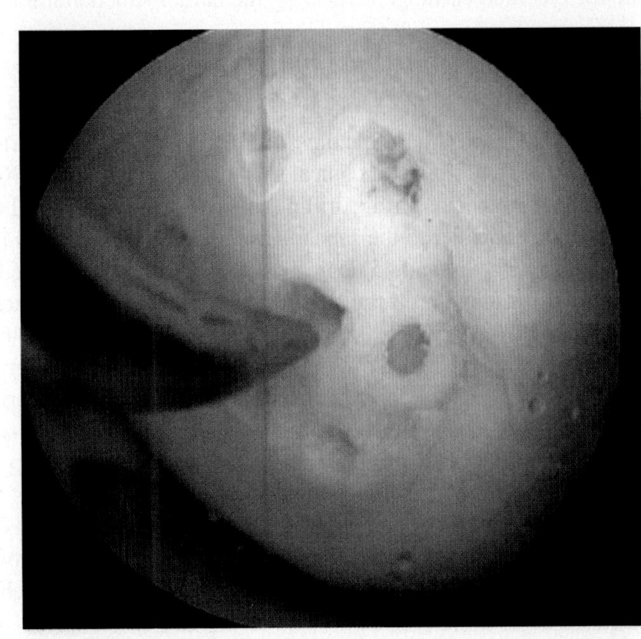

FIGURE 31-4

The appropriate depth has been reached when fat droplets are seen coming from the marrow cavity (~3 to 4 mm).

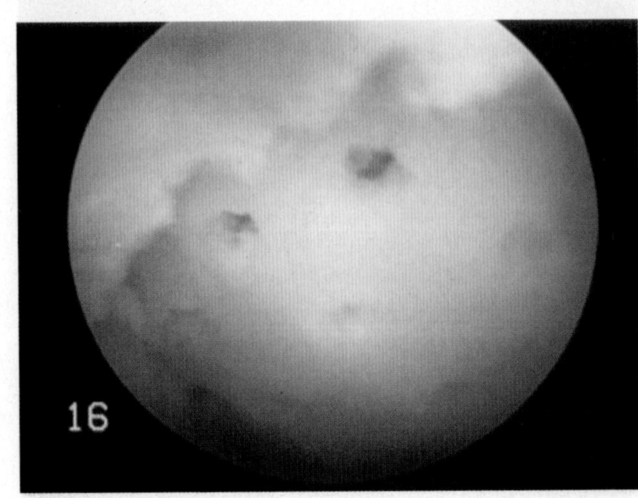

FIGURE 31-5

Microfracture holes are created around the periphery of the defect first, working concentrically toward the center of the defect.

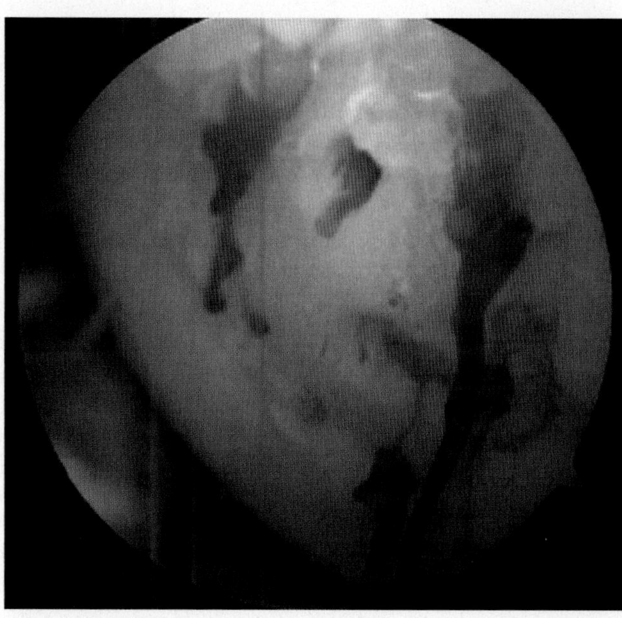

FIGURE 31-6

Reducing the arthroscopic irrigation fluid pump pressure facilitates direct visualization of marrow fat droplets and blood flowing from the microfracture holes into the prepared lesion.

removed from the defect using a curette or shaver, and the lesion is again inspected to ensure a sufficient number of holes have been made before reducing the arthroscopic irrigation fluid flow to verify bleeding from the holes.

Maintaining the Microfracture Mesenchymal Clot

After the arthroscopic irrigation fluid pump pressure is reduced, the flow of marrow fat droplets and blood from the microfracture holes into the prepared lesion is visualized and judged to be adequate when marrow elements are seen to flow from each hole (Fig. 31-6). Since the clinical success of microfracture has been correlated to the degree of fill of the defect, we feel that robust bleeding from each hole will optimize initial coverage of the defect with a fibrin clot (Fig. 31-7). The arthroscopic instruments are removed, the joint is evacuated, and the incisions are closed without the use of a drain. Intra-articular drains should not be used because they may allow for drainage of the clot (rich in marrow elements) required to form and stabilize over the lesion and may physically disrupt any clot during postoperative transferring and joint mobilization. A pressure dressing is applied to the knee, and cryotherapy is initiated to decrease pain and swelling. Cryotherapy is typically continued for approximately 7 to 10 days postoperatively and is associated with decreased pain and swelling.

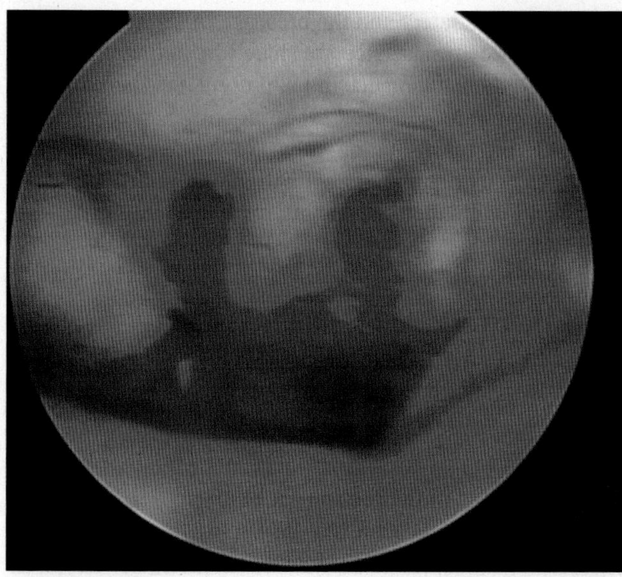

FIGURE 31-7

The quantity of marrow contents flowing into the joint is judged to be adequate when marrow elements are seen to flow from all the microfracture holes, filling the entire defect.

Additional Considerations: Chronic Lesions

In chronic degenerative-type chondral lesions, eburnated bone and bony sclerosis cause a thickening of the effective subchondral plate making adequate access to the underlying bone marrow elements more difficult. In such instances, it may be necessary to use a motorized burr to remove excess sclerotic bone until punctate bleeding is evident. Sclerotic bone is removed uniformly over the surface of the lesion, taking care to maintain the radius of curvature of the articular surface; the microfracture procedure can now be performed on the new base of the lesion as previously described.

PEARLS AND PITFALLS

- Complete a diagnostic arthroscopic diagnostic examination before microfracture and treat all pathology in a single-stage approach, where possible.
- Perform all other intra-articular procedures before completing microfracture, as this aids arthroscopic visualization.
- Debride all loose or marginally attached cartilage down to exposed bone in the prepared chondral defect—aids clot attachment.
- Remove the calcified cartilage layer to the tidemark with a handheld curette without penetrating the subchondral bone using tactile feedback.
- Microfracture the periphery of the lesion before spiraling toward the center utilizing the appropriate angulated awls.
- Maintain 3 to 4 mm between the holes to preserve the subchondral plate; 3- to 4-mm penetration is usually adequate to access the marrow elements.
- Successful microfracture results from meticulous technique; a miniarthrotomy may be used if necessary, particularly in inexperienced hands.
- Observation of defect filling is achieved by reducing the irrigation pump pressure (and/or tourniquet).
- Postoperative drain in the joint should not be used.
- The importance of postoperative continuous passive range of motion (CPM) and protected weightbearing should be emphasized.
- A carefully designed postoperative rehabilitation program is critical and may be affected by other concomitant procedures performed. Close correspondence with the treating physical therapist on an individualized basis is advised.

POSTOPERATIVE MANAGEMENT

The rehabilitation program following microfracture strives to maintain the integrity of the clot and regenerating tissue at the repair site. Therefore, postoperative management is individualized to a degree depending on both the location and size of the defect and the presence of concomitant procedures. Common principles of postoperative joint convalescence are shared including graduation of weightbearing on the operated surfaces, CPM, and maintenance of the musculature in the kinetic chain. It is imperative that the patient is clearly aware of the need for strict compliance and long-term engagement with physical therapy goals during rehabilitation to ensure the best possible outcome for the procedure. A recent systematic review by Schmitt et al. highlighted significant deficits in quadriceps strength, gait deviations, and functional deficits persisting for 5 to 7 years following microfracture.

REHABILITATION PROTOCOL FOR PATIENTS WITH LESIONS ON THE FEMORAL CONDYLE OR TIBIAL PLATEAU

Continuous Passive Motion

Following microfracture of a chondral lesion on the weight-bearing surfaces of the femoral condyles or tibial plateau, continuous passive motion is initiated in the recovery room from 0 to 60 degrees and gradually increased until full passive range of motion is achieved. Regaining full passive ROM of the injured knee as soon as possible after surgery is critical to maintain cartilage metabolism (exchange of nutrition and waste products) and direct mesenchymal stem cell differentiation within the defect, while protecting the integrity of the regenerating tissue from excessive compressive and shear forces. CPM is prescribed for a minimum of 3 to 4 hours per day for 6 weeks (typically divided into several sessions over the course of the day). The rate of the machine is usually one cycle per minute initially, but this can be customized based on patient preference and comfort. For those patients unable to use the CPM machine, instructions are given for passive flexion and extension of the knee with up to 300 repetitions 3 times per day.

Weightbearing

Protected weightbearing is recommended for 6 weeks, beginning with toe touch weightbearing for the first 2 to 3 weeks with gradual progression to partial weightbearing after 3 to 4 weeks. After the 6 week postoperative point, the patient is progressed to weightbearing as tolerated, typically weaning off crutches within 1 week. Initial weightbearing is done with the knee in a double metal upright, hinged brace locked in full extension. Once the patient can perform a straight-leg raise with minimal quadriceps inhibition and no extensor lag, indicating good quadriceps function, the hinges on the brace are opened. The range of flexion allowed may be determined by the location of the lesion, which determines the flexion angle where the lesion would be loaded with weightbearing. Factors directing the return to full weightbearing include patient symptoms (pain, effusion) and specific characteristics of the defect (size and shape), and for most patients, 6 to 8 weeks is adequate time to limit weightbearing.

Knee Joint Rehabilitation

The patient begins physical therapy immediately following surgery with an emphasis on control of the effusion, restoration of quadriceps contraction, and reversal of pain–induced quadriceps inhibition, patellar mobility, and range of motion. Patients are instructed to perform medial to lateral and superior to inferior movement of the patella as well as medial to lateral movement of the quadriceps and patellar tendons. Mobilization is essential to prevent patellar tendon fibrous adhesions and resultant increases in patellofemoral joint reaction forces.

Range-of-motion exercises (without range-of-motion limitations), quadriceps sets, straight-leg raises, hamstring stretching, and ankle pumps are also initiated immediately postoperatively. Stationary biking without resistance is initiated when full passive range of motion is achieved at 1 to 2 weeks postoperatively.

Restoration of normal muscular function through the use of low-impact exercises is emphasized during weeks 9 through 16. Core strengthening is an important part of the rehabilitation process. Stationary biking with increasing resistance, treadmill walking on a 7% incline, and elliptical training are all initiated during this phase. Closed-chain double knee bends and elastic cord exercise are added to the regimen at about 12 weeks. The ability to achieve predetermined goals for sets and repetitions of elastic resistance cord exercises is a useful indicator for progressing to weight training. Free or machine weights are allowed when the patient has achieved the early goals of the rehabilitation program, but not before 16 weeks.

A progressive run-to-walk program and initial agility drills are commenced between 16 to 24 weeks postoperatively. Initial running is completed on a forgiving surface, using a ratio of 1 minute running followed by 4 minutes walking. Once the patient can perform 20 minutes at a 1:4 ratio, the ratio is gradually progressed to 4 minutes running and 1 minute walking before the patient is allowed to run continuously. Initial agility drills include single-plane activities completed at 25% speed with increases in duration made before increases in intensity.

Return to Regular Activities/Return to Sport

Return to regular activities is generally achieved 6 to 8 months postoperatively when strength and neuromuscular control are achieved. Return-to-sport criteria require serial clinical and functional performance examinations and are individualized based on achievement of functional criteria, the size of the patient, the sports and lesion characteristics (location and the size). In general, patients are not cleared to return to sports that involve pivoting, cutting, and jumping for at least 6 to 8 months following successful completion of physical therapy protocols.

REHABILITATION PROTOCOL FOR PATIENTS WITH PATELLOFEMORAL LESIONS

Patients treated using microfracture for patellofemoral lesions are placed in a hinged knee brace locked in full extension when full weightbearing is initiated. Thereafter, the knee brace is locked at 0 to 20 degrees for the first 6 weeks postoperatively. This brace position limits compression and shearing of the regenerating surfaces of the patellofemoral joint. CPM is undertaken from 0 to 80 degrees for 6 weeks postoperatively with the same parameters as for tibiofemoral lesions.

Rehabilitation protocols following microfracture in the patellofemoral joint should incorporate the location of the lesion and joint angles observed at the time of arthroscopy to determine where the defect comes into contact with the patellar facet or the trochlear groove during strength training. It is preferable to avoid operated areas during strength training for up to 4 months.

Patients are allowed to weightbear as tolerated in their brace in full extension at 2 weeks following surgery. After 6 to 8 weeks, range of motion in the knee brace is gradually increased before the brace is discontinued. Stationary biking without resistance is allowed 2 weeks postoperatively; resistance is gradually added at 6 to 8 weeks after microfracture coincident with the removal of the brace. After the 12 week postoperative point, progression of the rehabilitation program is the same as for those on the femoral condyle or tibial plateau, as described above.

COMPLICATIONS

Most patients tolerate the postoperative period and rehabilitation without significant issues. Mild transient pain is most frequently encountered following microfracture of the patellofemoral joint. Alterations of the articular surface topography of the patellofemoral joint may produce a grating sensation (crepitus) within the joint; this sensation typically manifests on restoration of full weightbearing through the range of motion, is painless, and usually resolves spontaneously over a period of weeks to months. Additionally, if a steep perpendicular rim was created in the trochlear groove, patients may perceive a “catching” or “locking” as the apex of the patella rides over this lesion during joint motion. These symptoms usually gradually dissipate within 3 months with progressive fill of the defect and maturation of the reparative tissue. When locking is painful, weightbearing is protected at the symptomatic joint angle, and cryotherapy is initiated. Joint swelling and effusion are expected to resolve within 6 to 8 weeks after microfracture. In patients with femoral condyle microfracture, recurrent effusions are occasionally encountered on a return to weightbearing and are usually painless, responding to conservative treatment.

Regarding the repair tissue, bony overgrowth within the microfractured chondral defect can occur in 20% to 70% of patients. Although the factors contributing to bony overgrowth are unclear, extensive resection of subchondral bone and calcified cartilage during defect preparation have been implicated. Bony overgrowth within the defect may have negative biomechanical implications for the repair and the articulating cartilage surface, although this finding has not been associated with inferior clinical outcome. In fact, a longitudinal MRI study of bony overgrowth in 72 microfracture-based treatments by Shive et al. demonstrated less than expected bony overgrowth; in 80% of patients who developed some bony overgrowth, the volume was less than 10% of the original defect. Interestingly, bony overgrowth tended to recur in defects where it had been debrided at the time of surgery, and at 12 months follow-up, there was no correlation between bony overgrowth and patient symptoms.

RESULTS

When interpreting the clinical results of microfracture, it is important to recognize the distinct patient populations, defect characteristics, surgical technique, and rehabilitation protocols that are critical to interpreting the data accurately and applying the principles to surgical practice. In addition, optimal results can only be expected for the patient by adhering to specific indications, recommended techniques, and addressing existing comorbidities.

As a regenerative surgical technique, microfracture is ultimately dependent on the biological potential of the stem cells contained within the mesenchymal clot, and it is not surprising that patient age is emerging as an important prognostic factor. It is well documented that aging tissues that exhibit diminished regenerative capabilities and degenerative changes of tissue-specific stem cells, niches, and homeostatic mechanisms that direct their activity are directly implicated. Kreuz et al. focused on the effect of age in their prospective study and divided their patient population into those greater and less than 40 years of age (mean age = 39 years). Their findings in 85 patients at 3 years demonstrated that while both groups experienced significant clinical improvement at 18 months, only the younger group had sustained improvement and defect fill on MRI at 36 months. In addition, de Windt et al. demonstrated prospectively that the Knee injury and Osteoarthritis Outcome Score (KOOS) improvement was significantly better for patients less than 30 years compared with older patients at 3 years. In a prospective cohort study, Mithoefer et al. observed that a lower BMI and short duration of preoperative symptoms correlated with higher scores for the activities of daily living and SF-36 in a prospective study of 48 symptomatic patients with isolated full-thickness articular defects who underwent microfracture. The worst results were seen in those patients with a BMI greater than 30 kg/m^2.

Regarding the defect characteristics, Gudas et al. demonstrated in a prospective, randomized clinical study that superior outcomes (International Knee Documentation Committee—IKDC score) in young athletes (mean age = 24.3 years) were associated with a lesion size less than 2 cm^2. Another prospective, randomized clinical study by Knutsen et al. (comparing microfracture to ACI) demonstrated significantly higher short form 36 (SF-36) scores in microfracture patients associated with lesions under 4 cm^2; again the best results were seen in younger and more active patients.

The effect of defect location was assessed by de Windt et al. in a prospective cohort study of microfracture and ACI, where chondral defects in the medial compartment were associated with a significantly better KOOS than those in the lateral compartment at 3 years. Kreuz et al. investigated the anatomic location of the defect prospectively and observed early clinical outcome scores that were significantly improved at 18 months for all lesions of the femoral condyles, tibiae, trochlea, and retropatellar surface. However, there was deterioration in clinical gains for each location except the femoral condyle in the subsequent 18 months; femoral condyle lesions also maintained the best fill on MRI.

Refinements in the degree and precise technique of marrow stimulation (including microfracture and drilling) may have the potential to improve outcome by impacting both the quality of the cartilage repair tissue and the restorative capacity of the subchondral bone plate. Chen et al. (1) used the rabbit model to compare the effect of 2-mm microfracture holes created with an awl to drill holes of 2- and 6-mm depth using cooled irrigation drilling on early subchondral bone morphology. At day 1 postoperatively, there was increased osteocyte necrosis evidenced by empty lacunae around the microfracture holes versus the drilling group. It appeared that the drilling technique provided sustained access to marrow stroma; in contrast, microfracture produced fractured and compacted bone around holes. Deeper drilling (to 6 mm) was sufficient to penetrate the epiphyseal scar in the rabbit model and resulted in a greater degree of subchondral hematoma. As part of a larger study, Marchand et al. (2) compared smaller 0.5- and 0.9-mm diameter drill holes in the rabbit model and did not see any difference in cartilage tissue repair or subchondral bone metrics at 6.5 months. Eldracher et al. (3) performed a similar study using the sheep model and reported improved cartilage repair for 1.0-mm diameter drilling versus 1.8 mm at 6 months. There was no difference in cartilage degeneration surrounding the defect between groups. The microstructures of the subchondral bone plate (higher bone volume and reduced thickening) and the subarticular spongiosa (higher bone volume and more and thinner trabeculae) were both better restored after 1.0-mm compared to 1.8-mm drilling. Bone mineral density of the subchondral bone in the 1.8-mm drill holes was reduced; for the 1.0-mm drill holes, it remained similar to the adjacent subchondral bone. No subchondral bone cysts were seen in any group while there was an upward migration of the subchondral bone plate in both groups. Finally, there were no significant correlations between cartilage repair and subchondral bone restoration at 6 months for these trochlear lesions.

Recently, the same group compared the efficacy of microfracture using 1.0-mm awls versus 1.2-mm awls for a 4 × 8-mm full-thickness chondral defect in the medial femoral condyle of the sheep model (4). Interestingly, histological repair tissue quality was significantly better for the smaller 1.0-mm awl with particular gains relating to surface regularity and integration with the surrounding cartilage. The smaller awl decreased the relative bone volume of the subarticular spongiosa; however, subchondral bone cysts and intralesional osteophytes were observed with similar frequency. In addition, the biochemical analysis of the repair tissues and evidence of degeneration in the surrounding cartilage were similar in both awl groups. These data contrasted with an existing study by Kok et al. (5) who found no difference in outcome comparing 0.45- and 1.1-mm diameter awls a talar osteochondral defects using a goat model; however, the significant mechanical and biological differences between the knee and ankle joints make both findings difficult to compare directly.

Focusing on reoperation, Salzmann et al. presented a retrospective study of 560 microfracture patients with a minimum follow-up of 2 years. In their study, one quarter of patients underwent reoperation at an average of 18 months following clinical failure; the reoperated lesions were smaller and had undergone more previous surgeries. Patients with a higher probability of reoperation had presented with lower preoperative numeric analogue scales of pain and function, where smokers had patellofemoral lesions.

Goyal et al. presented a systematic review of level I and II studies on microfracture and concluded that while short-term symptomatic improvement is seen in smaller lesions and lower postoperative demands, treatment failures are to be expected after 5 years. In addition, they identified heterogeneity of patient selection, defect description, outcome scoring, surgical technique, and rehabilitation; such variations may contribute to disparity among individual studies and centers. Critically, clinical interpretation of the long-term utility of microfracture remains hampered by the lack of appropriate control groups (chondral defect with no surgical intervention/conservative treatment).

In particular, arthroscopic treatment of the degenerative knee lesions remains controversial. The goals of microfracture in this setting are to alleviate pain, maximize function, and prevent further degenerative changes. This surgical strategy is generally conserved for patients who fail conservative measures, often temporizing the patient to a definitive arthroplasty solution. Bae et al. reported the survival analysis of microfractured defects in the osteoarthritic knee with greater than 10 years follow-up (11.2 years) with failure defined as total knee arthroplasty. In 134 knees (mean age 61 ± 6.8 years; BMI 25.8 ± 3.4), they observed a survival rate of 88.8% at 5 years and 67.9% at 10 years. Increased survival was associated with smaller defect size on the femoral condyle (<2 cm^2) and better axial alignment of the operated knee. The success of microfracture undertaken in combination with high tibial osteotomy (HTO) for medial compartment lesions and malalignment is also well documented.

Finally, the emergence of augmented microfracture techniques, potentially subjected to fewer regulatory hurdles, has demonstrated enhanced efficacy in many clinical studies. Augmentation of the microfracture technique aims to increase defect fill volume and produce more hyaline-like cartilage tissue, often focusing clinically at the medium term where benefits will be more easily distinguished. There have been three general approaches: clot containment using hydrogels or matrices, the use of cell and/or biological augments at the repair site, and the intra-articular delivery of a drug or biologic targeting joint homeostasis. Shive et al. recently tested the repair benefits of the BST-CarGel scaffold as an adjuvant to microfracture, with patients showing improvements in function, pain, and stiffness at 5 years postoperatively. Results showed greater quality and quantity of the repair tissue at 5-year follow-up. Power et al. used an rhFGF-18 intra-articular injection in an ovine model to augment healing following microfracture, with improved formation of hyaline-like cartilage repair tissue. Xing et al. used an osteochondral paste implantation in a rabbit model, and Xu et al. used a kartogenin intra-articular injection, both with positive results. Karakaplan et al. added autologous conditioned plasma (ACP) to a preclinical rabbit model of microfracture; regenerated cartilage in the ACP group demonstrated enhanced filling of the defect with a cartilage matrix that histologically demonstrated a more hyaline-like character.

ACKNOWLEDGMENTS

The authors would like to acknowledge the contributions of J. Richard Steadman, MD, and William G. Rodkey, DVM, MS, to this chapter in the previous editions.

REFERENCES

1. Chen H, Sun J, Hoemann CD, et al. Drilling and microfracture lead to different bone structure and necrosis during bone-marrow stimulation for cartilage repair. *J Orthop Res.* 2009;27(11):1432–1438.
2. Marchand C, Chen G, Tran-Khanh N, et al. Microdrilled cartilage defects treated with thrombin-solidified chitosan/blood implant regenerate a more hyaline, stable, and structurally integrated osteochondral unit compared to drilled controls. *Tissue Eng Part A.* 2012;18(5–6):508–519.
3. Eldracher M, Orth P, Cucchiarini M, et al. Small subchondral drill holes improve marrow stimulation of articular cartilage defects. *Am J Sports Med.* 2014;42(11):2741–2750.
4. Orth P, Duffner J, Zurakowski D, et al. Small-diameter awls improve articular cartilage repair after microfracture treatment in a translational animal model. *Am J Sports Med.* 2016;44(1):209–219.
5. Kok AC, Tuijthof GJ, den Dunnen S, et al. No effect of hole geometry in microfracture for talar osteochondral defects. *Clin Orthop Relat Res.* 2013;471(11):3653–3662.

RECOMMENDED READINGS

Asik M, Ciftci F, Sen C, et al. The microfracture technique for the treatment of full-thickness articular cartilage lesions of the knee: midterm results. *Arthroscopy.* 2008;24(11):1214–1220.

Bae DK, Song SJ, Yoon KH, et al. Survival analysis of microfracture in the osteoarthritic knee-minimum 10-year follow-up. *Arthroscopy.* 2013;29(2):244–250.

Frisbie DD, Morisset S, Ho CP, et al. Effects of calcified cartilage on healing of chondral defects treated with microfracture in horses. *Am J Sports Med.* 2006;34:1824–1831.

Frisbie DD, Oxford JT, Southwood L, et al. Early events in cartilage repair after subchondral bone microfracture. *Clin Orthop.* 2003;407:215–227.

Gudas R, Gudaite A, Pocius A, et al. Ten-year follow-up of a prospective, randomized clinical study of mosaic osteochondral autologous transplantation versus microfracture for the treatment of osteochondral defects in the knee joint of athletes. *Am J Sports Med.* 2012;40(11):2499–2508.

Knutsen G, Engebretsen L, Ludvigsen TC, et al. Autologous chondrocyte implantation compared with microfracture in the knee. A randomized trial. *J Bone Joint Surg Am.* 2004;86-A(3):455–464.

Salzmann GM, Sah B, Sudkamp NP, et al. Reoperative characteristics after microfracture of knee cartilage lesions in 454 patients. *KSSTA.* 2013;21(2):365–371.

Kocher MS, Steadman JR, Briggs KK, et al. Reliability, validity, and responsiveness of the Lysholm knee scale for various chondral disorders of the knee. *J Bone Joint Surg Am.* 2004;86A:1139–1145.

Kreuz PC, Erggelet C, Steinwachs MR, et al. Is microfracture of chondral defects in the knee associated with different results in patients aged 40 years or younger? *Arthroscopy.* 2006;22(11):1180–1186.

Krych AJ, Harnly HW, Rodeo SA, et al. Activity levels are higher after osteochondral autograft transfer mosaicplasty than after microfracture for articular cartilage defects of the knee: a retrospective comparative study. *J Bone Joint Surg Am.* 2012;94(11):971–978.

Miller DJ, Smith MV, Matava MJ, et al. Microfracture and osteochondral autograft transplantation are cost-effective treatments for articular cartilage lesions of the distal femur. *Am J Sports Med.* [Epub ahead of print] 2015.

Miller BS, Steadman JR, Briggs KK, et al. Patient satisfaction and outcome after microfracture of the degenerative knee. *J Knee Surg.* 2004;17:13–17.

Mithoefer K, Williams RJ III, Warren RF, et al. The microfracture technique for the treatment of articular cartilage lesions in the knee. A prospective cohort study. *J Bone Joint Surg Am.* 2005;87(9):1911–1920.

Orth P, Duffner J, Zurakowski D, et al. Small-diameter awls improve articular cartilage repair after microfracture treatment in a translational animal model. *Am J Sports Med.* 2016;44(1):209–219.

Steadman JR, Briggs KK, Rodrigo JJ, et al. Outcomes of microfracture for traumatic chondral defects of the knee: average 11-year follow-up. *Arthroscopy.* 2003;19:477–484.

Steadman JR, Miller BS, Karas SG, et al. The microfracture technique in the treatment of full-thickness chondral lesions of the knee in National Football League players. *J Knee Surg.* 2003;16:83–86.

Steadman JR, Rodkey WG, Briggs KK. Microfracture chondroplasty: indications, techniques, and outcomes. *Sports Med Arthrosc Rev.* 2003;11:236–244.

Sterett WI, Steadman JR. Chondral resurfacing and high tibial osteotomy in the varus knee. *Am J Sports Med.* 2004;32:1243–1249.

32 Osteochondral Autograft Transplantation (OAT)

Megan Gleason and Mark D. Miller

INTRODUCTION

Articular cartilage injuries pose a significant challenge to the treating orthopedic surgeon. Lesions, whether traumatic, degenerative, or spontaneous (e.g., osteochondritis dissecans), have compromised healing due to a lack of a direct blood supply and a subsequent reliance on synovial and interstitial fluid for nutrient diffusion. Furthermore, articular cartilage chondrocytes have low mitotic activity and slow turnover, making spontaneous healing unlikely.

Investigations into cartilage healing suggest vital nutrients are available beneath the calcified cartilage layer. Cartilage injuries that breach the tidemark or restorative techniques that penetrate this layer are thought to show improved healing. Marrow stimulation or microfracture leads to the formation of fibrocartilage (type I collagen). While this tissue replaces the void left by cartilage damage, it does not function in the same manner as does native hyaline cartilage. Fibrocartilage tends to be less stiff and has poor wear characteristics, thus failing to replicate the biomechanical properties of articular cartilage (Fig. 32-1).

Interest in restoring hyaline cartilage to articular defects has led to the development of various surgical techniques. Osteochondral plug transplantation, autologous chondrocyte implantation (ACI), and osteochondral allografts aim to restore the articular cartilage surface with hyaline cartilage or a hybrid of hyaline and fibrocartilage. The goals of these procedures are symptom relief, improved function, and stabilization to prevent further progression of cartilage damage.

Osteochondral autograft transplantation (OAT) or mosaicplasty is a technique used to restore the hyaline cartilage to cartilage lesions. Donor grafts of articular hyaline cartilage and the underlying subchondral bone are harvested from low-contact regions of the knee and transplanted to the site of the lesion. The goal is incorporation of the bone plug with reconstitution of the articular surface. Depending on the size of the lesion, small areas of fibrocartilage may heal around the transplanted grafts.

Donor plugs are usually less than 10 mm in diameter, and several small grafts can be used on one area. The plugs are traditionally taken from the medial or lateral aspect of the femoral condyle or the intercondylar notch. The most common recipient areas are the weight-bearing portions of the medial femoral condyle, the patella, and the lateral femoral condyle (1).

SUMMARY

Options for cartilage restoration

1. Microfracture is best for small defects (<2.5 cm^2 diameter). The end result is fibrocartilage (type I collagen). This procedure is minimally invasive and not technically difficult. Microfracture involves removing the zone of calcified cartilage and penetrating the subchondral bone with awl to cause bleeding and clot formation.
2. Osteochondral allograft/autograft plug transfer is used for medium-sized lesions (2 to 5 cm^2). It is more technically demanding than microfracture. The goal of this technique is restore hyaline cartilage to the defect (see details below).
3. Autologous chondrocyte implantation (ACI): This technique may be used on a variety of sized lesions (ranging from 2 to 12 cm^2). The drawbacks to ACI are the high cost and requirement for two surgical procedures. Autologous chondrocytes are harvested from the knee via biopsy, cultured in the laboratory, and then reimplanted in the cartilage defect and secured with a periosteal patch. The end result is both hyaline cartilage and fibrocartilage.

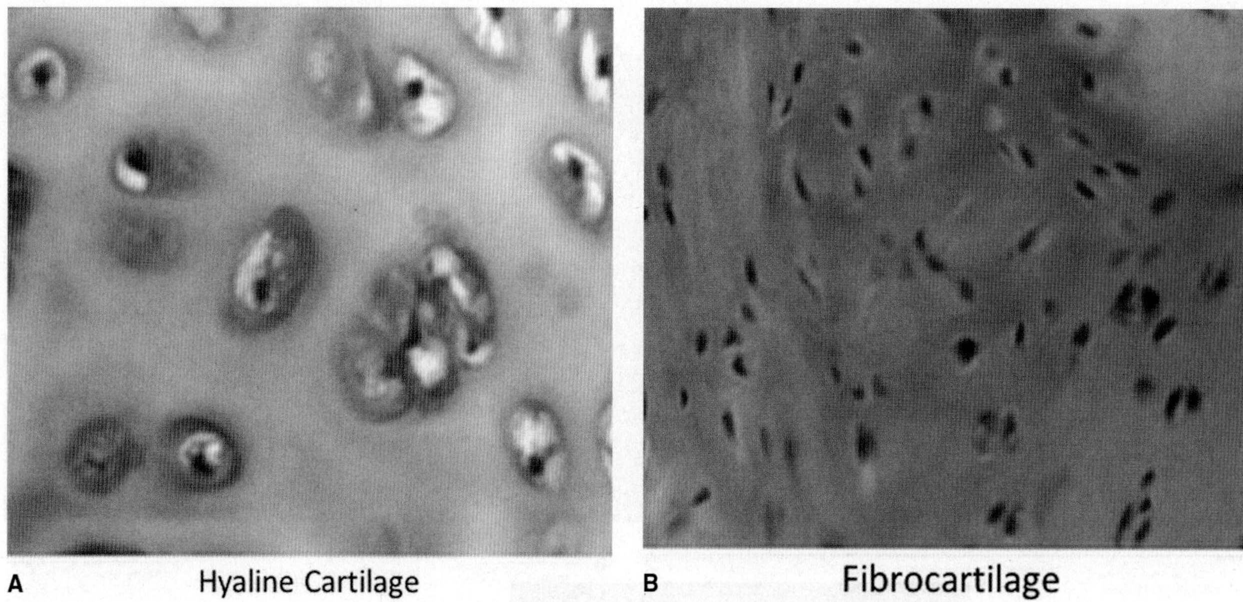

FIGURE 32-1
Microscopic comparison of (**A**) hyaline cartilage and (**B**) fibrocartilage (mcgraw hill, mhhe.com).

OSTEOCHONDRAL AUTOGRAFT TRANSPLANTATION

A plug of cartilage and subchondral bone is transferred from a non–weight-bearing/low-contact pressure region of knee to the weight-bearing region with the focal chondral defect. This is analogous to changing the pin on a putting green (Fig. 32-2)!

Indications/Contraindications

The goals of an OAT procedure include symptom relief, improved function, stabilization to prevent further progression of cartilage damage, and restoration of hyaline cartilage when possible

OATs are best suited for focal, full-thickness cartilage defects on the weight-bearing surfaces of the knee. The ideal patient is physiologically young and active; therefore, there is no specific age range for this procedure. The area of the lesion should fall within 2 to 5 cm^2. The defects may be accessed by either an open or arthroscopic approach.

Contraindications to OATs include diffuse chondrosis/osteoarthritis and/or kissing lesions ("bipolar lesions"). It is important to assess the patient's overall limb alignment prior to proceeding with OATs, as lesions will tend to recur or fail to heal if malalignment is present. In addition, any ligamentous instability, such as ACL deficiency, must also be addressed to ensure cartilage damage does not recur or worsen with recurrent instability episodes. Obesity is a relative contraindication to the OAT procedure. Finally, the location of the lesion must be considered as it must be accessible by arthroscopic or open means.

Preoperative Planning

Patients with focal cartilage defects often present with knee pain, swelling, and mechanical symptoms including locking and catching. A good history is key to understanding the cause of the cartilage lesion, whether traumatic or idiopathic (e.g., osteochondritis dissecans).

The physical exam should document the presence or absence of an effusion, a ligamentous exam, areas of focal tenderness, and other finding that may support chondral defects in the differential diagnosis, such as mechanical symptoms or crepitus.

Initial imaging should include weight-bearing x-rays of the affected knee and long alignment films, if indicated. While lesions may be seen on plain films, they are better characterized with advanced imaging. A noncontrast, nonarthrogram MRI of the knee is valuable in assessing the location and size of cartilage lesions. If the lesion is not seen on x-ray, the provider must have a high level of suspicion for a cartilage injury given the patient's presentation and physical examination (Fig. 32-3).

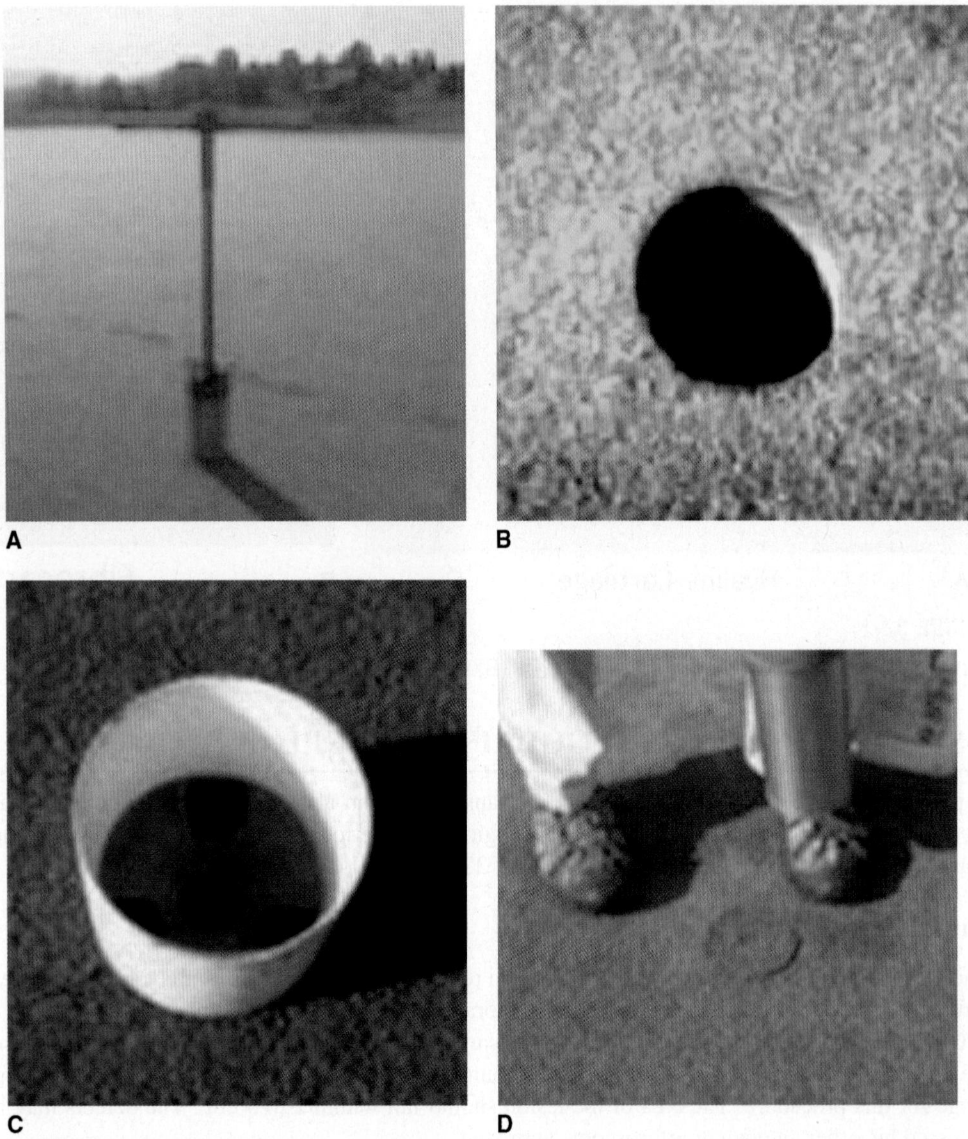

FIGURE 32-2

A–D: OAT can be compared to replacing the hole on a putting green. **A:** A cup cutter with a standard diameter is used to remove a plug of grass and underlying soil, (**B**) a new hole is created, (**C**) the new hole becomes the new cup, and (**D**) the plug is placed in the old hole and gently stamped into place, where grass resumes growth. (Images courtesy of Dr. M.D. Miller.)

Once the osteochondral lesion is identified and the decision to proceed with autograft transfer is made, a transplantation system should be selected. There are several commercially available systems, including Arthrex Osteoarticular Transfer System (OATS), Smith & Nephew Mosaicplasty, and DePuy Mitek COR. Each system allows for harvesting and transplantation of various graft sizes. The diameter and number of autograft plugs may be estimated by measuring the lesion on MRI; however, the final decision should be made after arthroscopic evaluation of the lesion following debridement.

SURGICAL PROCEDURE/TECHNIQUE

1. *Diagnostic knee arthroscopy* is performed to evaluate the cartilage lesion as well as any other intra-articular pathology. This is performed under anesthesia with the patient supine, commonly with a thigh tourniquet on operative extremity. The standard anterolateral and anteromedial portals are used, and additional portals may be created as needed. Localize the portal trajectory with a spinal needle prior to skin incision for ideal portal placement.

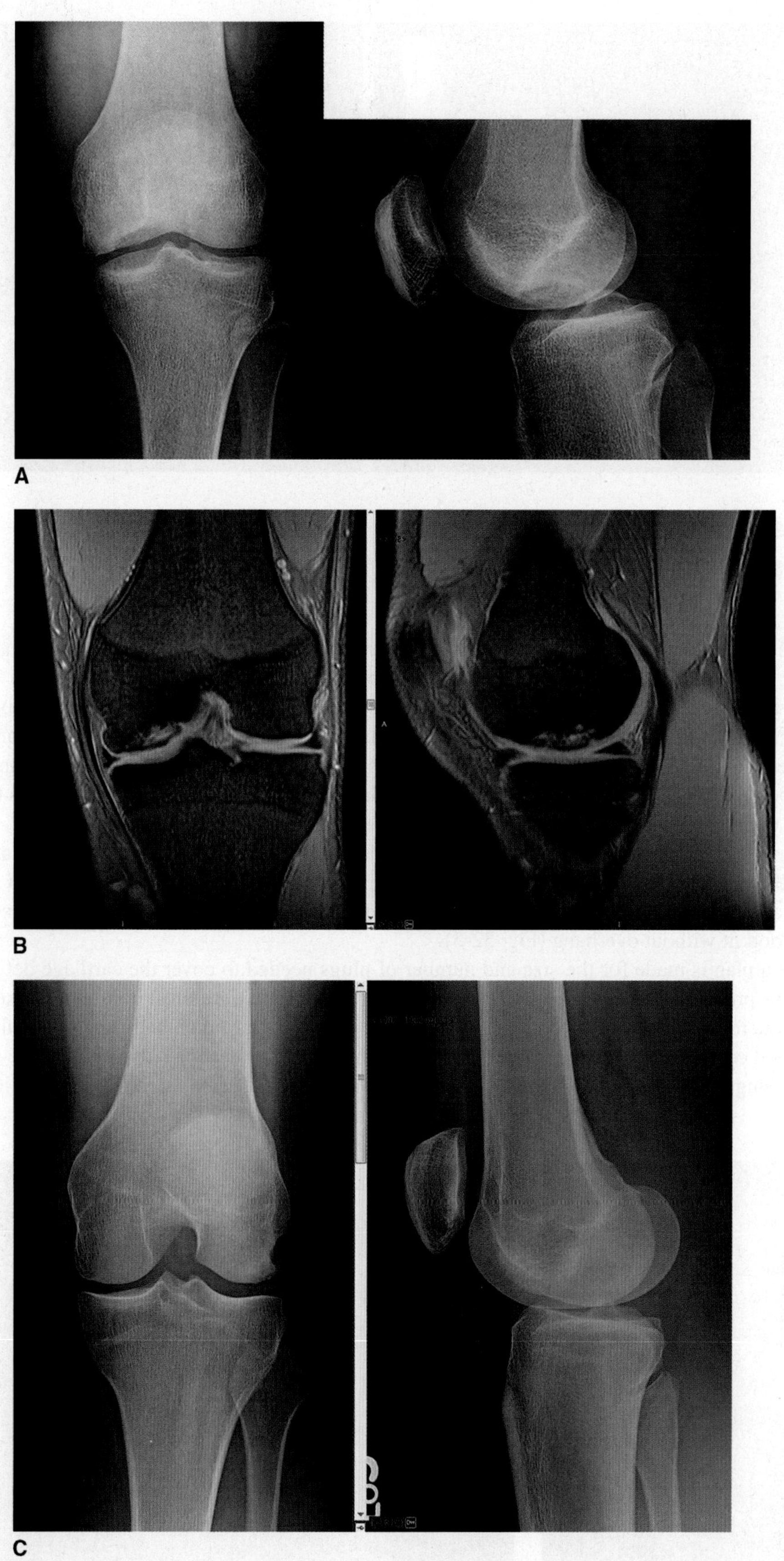

FIGURE 32-3

A: X-ray imaging of the knee shows abnormality of the medial femoral condyle. **B:** The corresponding MRI of the knee in figure A better delineates the lesion. **C:** X-ray imaging may show subtle changes on x-ray that may be missed on initial review; however, a follow-up MRI

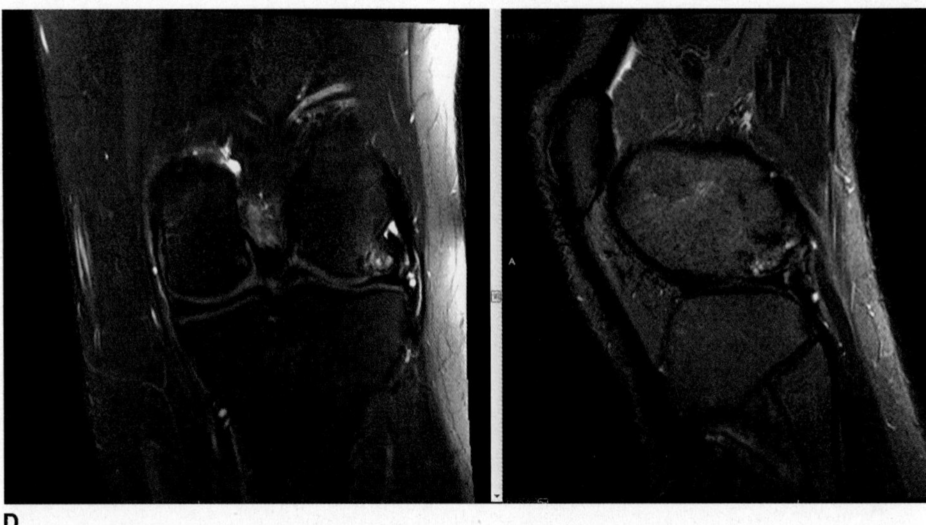

D

FIGURE 32-3 (*Continued*)

(**D**) shows the defect.

2. Once the lesion is identified, *sharp debridement* of lesion edges is performed to remove any flaps and establish a stable border. This may be done with a beaver blade or small curette. Debridement of the base of the lesion should be taken down to calcified cartilage. This is also the time to evaluate access to lesion. A small bump, triangle, or Alvarado knee positioner may be needed to maintain the position of the leg in optimal knee flexion to access the lesion. If it is not possible to obtain a perpendicular path to the lesion via arthroscopic means, this is the best time to proceed with an open approach to the knee (Fig. 32-4).
3. The next step is to measure the lesion and *determine the "best fit"* for autograft transplantation, namely, the size and number of plugs (e.g., one 10-mm plug vs. two 6-mm plugs). A sizer is available with the autograft system and should be used to determine the size of the plugs needed for good fit without overhang (Fig. 32-5).
4. Once a plan is made for the size and number of plugs needed to cover the cartilage defect, it is best to proceed with *harvesting of autograft plugs*. The plugs are most commonly taken from the superolateral lateral femoral condyle, but the intercondylar notch and superomedial medial femoral condyle may also be used. If necessary, the opposite knee may also be a source of autograft plugs; however, this is avoided when possible due to increased morbidity (Fig. 32-6).

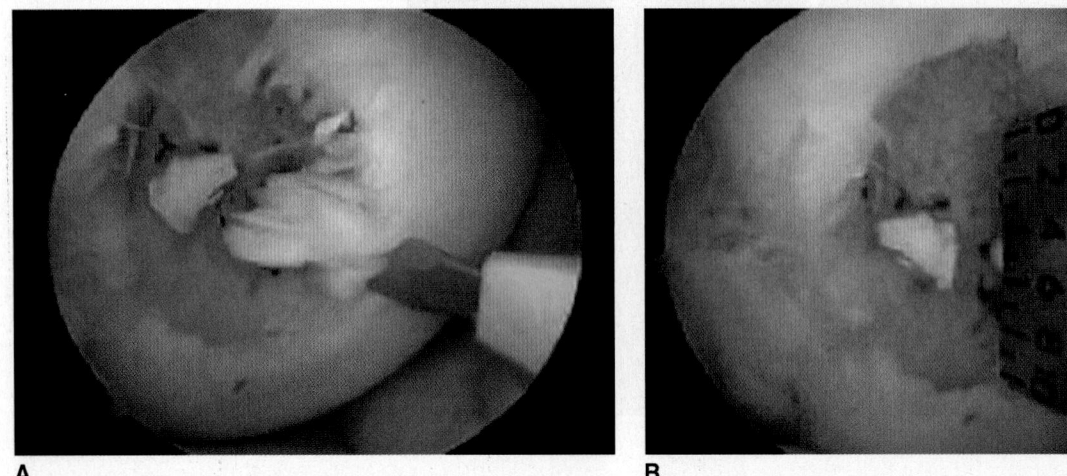

A B

FIGURE 32-4

A: Sharp debridement of the lesion using a beaver blade. **B:** Accurate measurement of the lesion following debridement.

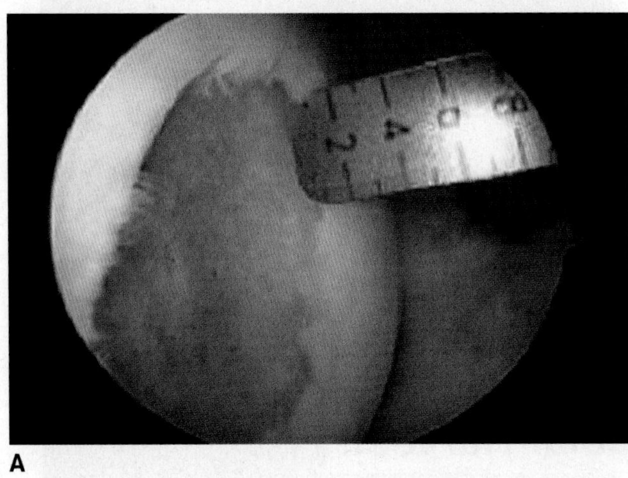
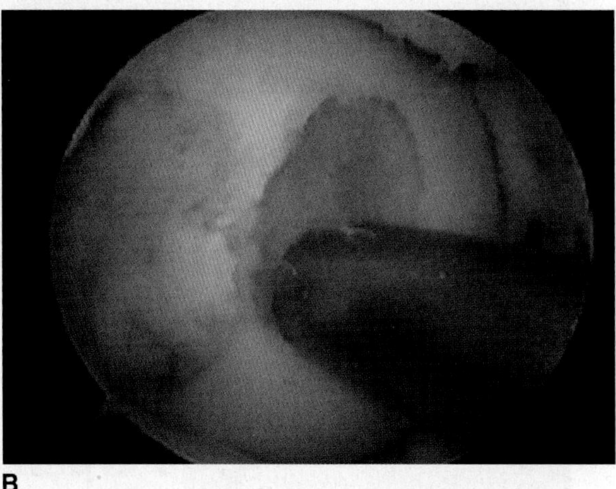

A B

FIGURE 32-5

A: An arthroscopic ruler is used to determine the length and width of the lesion prior to graft harvesting. **B:** A sizer with a standard diameter is placed in the lesion to assess best fit.

5. To harvest from the lateral femoral condyle, a lateral parapatellar incision is made from the superior pole of the patella to the lateral joint line. An arthrotomy is made in the lateral capsule approximately 5 mm from the lateral edge of the patella, extending from the vastus lateralis to the lateral tibial plateau. Care should be taken to protect the underlying structures during the arthrotomy. All plugs should be taken from the region proximal to the sulcus terminalis and approximately 2 mm apart to avoid convergence. The patella and surrounding soft tissues are gently retracted for access to the superolateral lateral femoral condyle. The autograft harvest system is then used to remove the plug. Whether autograft plugs are harvested open or arthroscopically, the surgeon must use great care to ensure the graft harvest system is perpendicular to articular surface. The depth of the autograft is usually 10 to 15 mm, with a relative goal of the length of graft 2 mm greater than the diameter. Once the autograft plug is removed, it should be taken in the back table and assessed. If the graft harvester was perpendicular to the articular cartilage, the plug will have uniform circumferential cartilage thickness (Figs. 32-7 and 32-8).
6. After the appropriate size autograft plug has been obtained, the *recipient site should be prepared for transplantation*. This is often done arthroscopically if the lesion is accessible. First, drill the recipient lesion with the appropriate diameter drill to the same depth as the plug harvest. For example, if an 8-mm plug was harvested to a depth of 12 mm, the lesion should be drilled with an 8-mm reamer to the depth of 12 mm. A drill guide is used to protect the surrounding tissues and keep the drill perpendicular to articular surface. Next, the graft is guided into the knee via the delivery tube. The edges of the delivery tube should rest on normal cartilage. The autograft

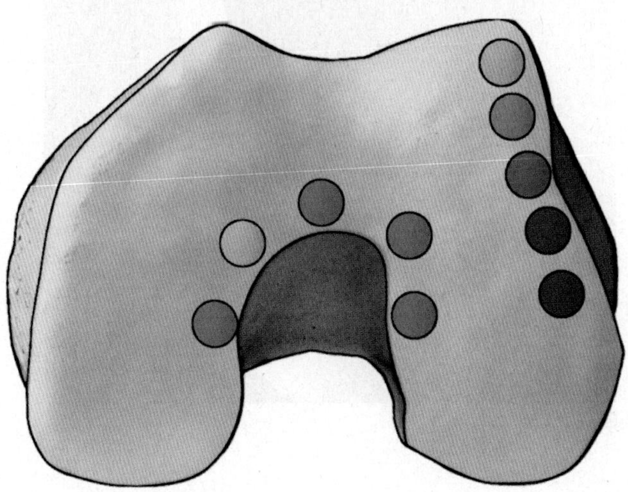

FIGURE 32-6

A gray-scale drawing of the relative mean color density measurements at each of the donor sites; the darker the color, the greater the pressure. * significantly different from sites of greatest pressure. (Redrawn from Simonian PT, Sussmann PS, Wickiewicz TL, et al. Contact pressures at osteochondral donor sites in the knee. *Am J Sports Med.* 1998;26(4):491–494.)

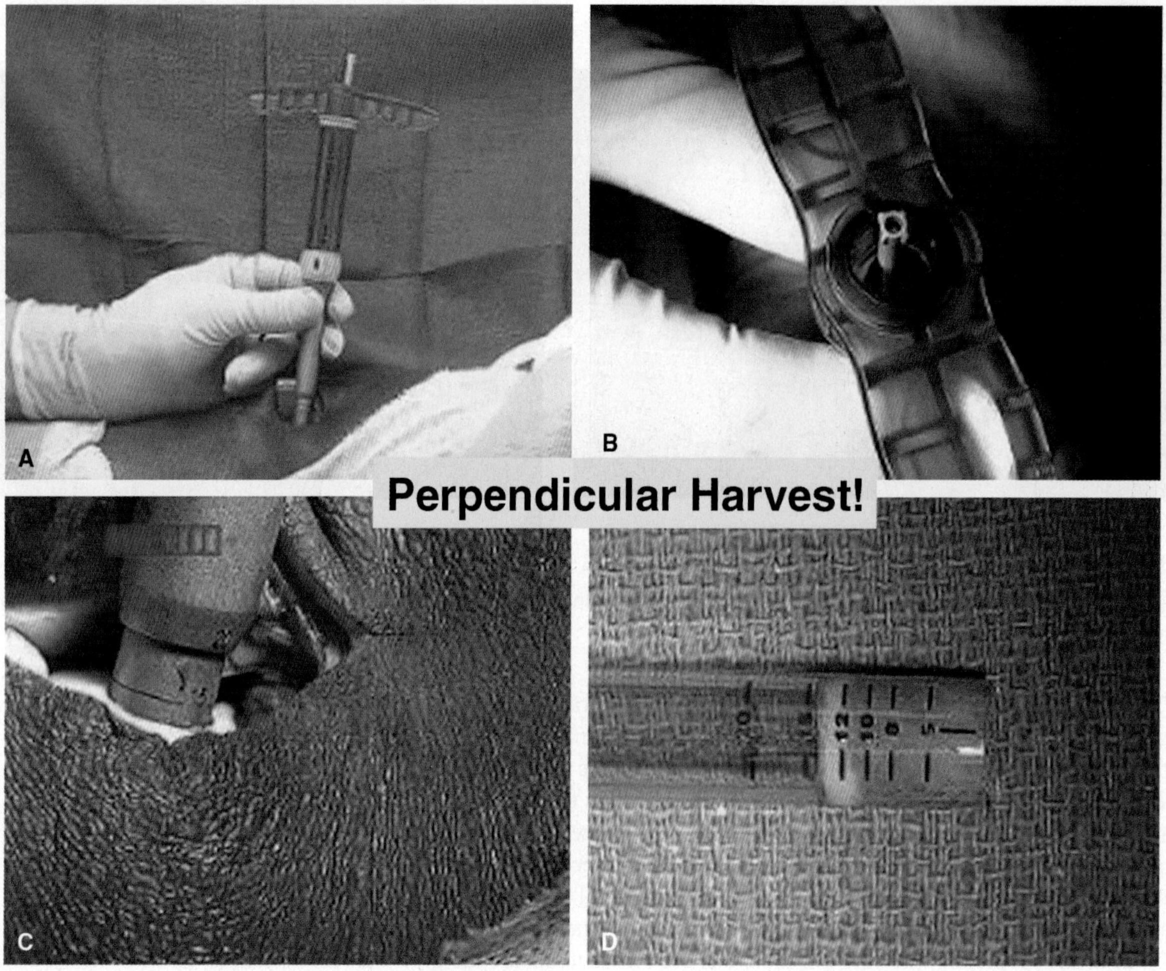

Perpendicular Harvest!

FIGURE 32-7

Osteochondral autograft harvest. **A:** A superolateral arthrotomy is made and the Harvester is positioned. **B:** Centering the guide will help insure perpendicular harvesting. **C:** The laser lines on the harvester are used as a secondary check for alignment. The lines should be parallel to the articular surface. **D:** After the plug is harvested, it is checked for perpendicularity. Note that the articular surface, not the bone cartilage junction, is the important feature.

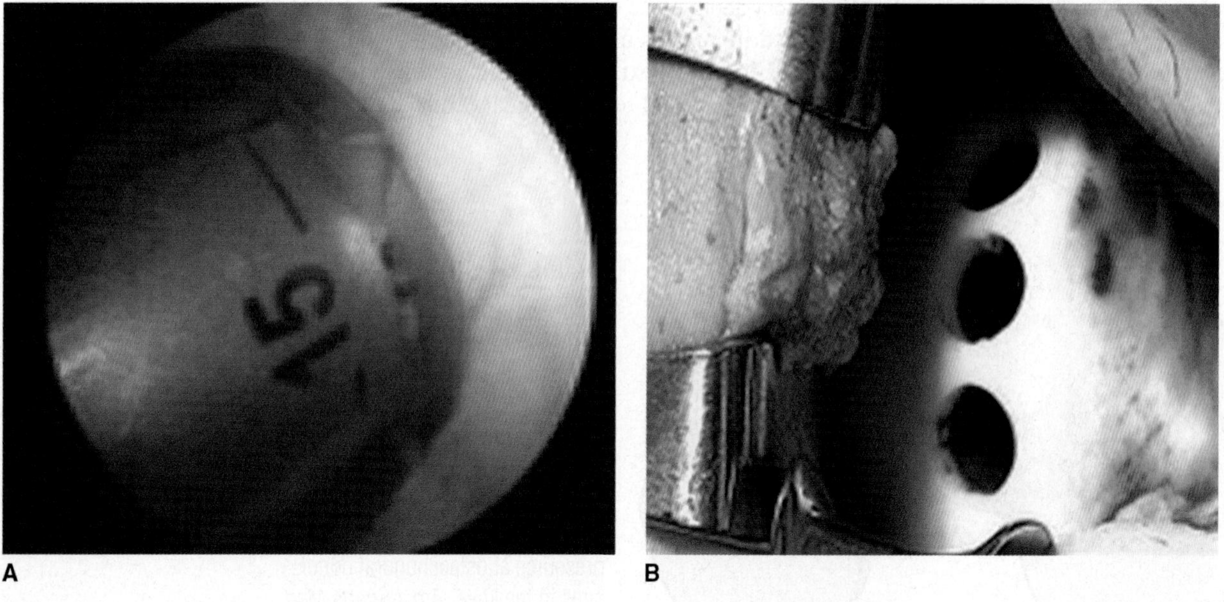

FIGURE 32-8

A: Monitor the depth of the plug circumferentially while harvesting. **B:** Maintain a minimum of 2 mm between plugs to prevent convergence of the donor sites and minimize the risk of collapse or fracture.

plug is gently tapped in place, perpendicular to the intact articular cartilage. A tamp is used to carefully position the plug to the appropriate depth. If additional plugs are needed, reassess the size of the defect and then harvest. Place one graft at a time. If possible, consider overlapping plugs to best fill the cartilage lesion (Fig. 32-9).

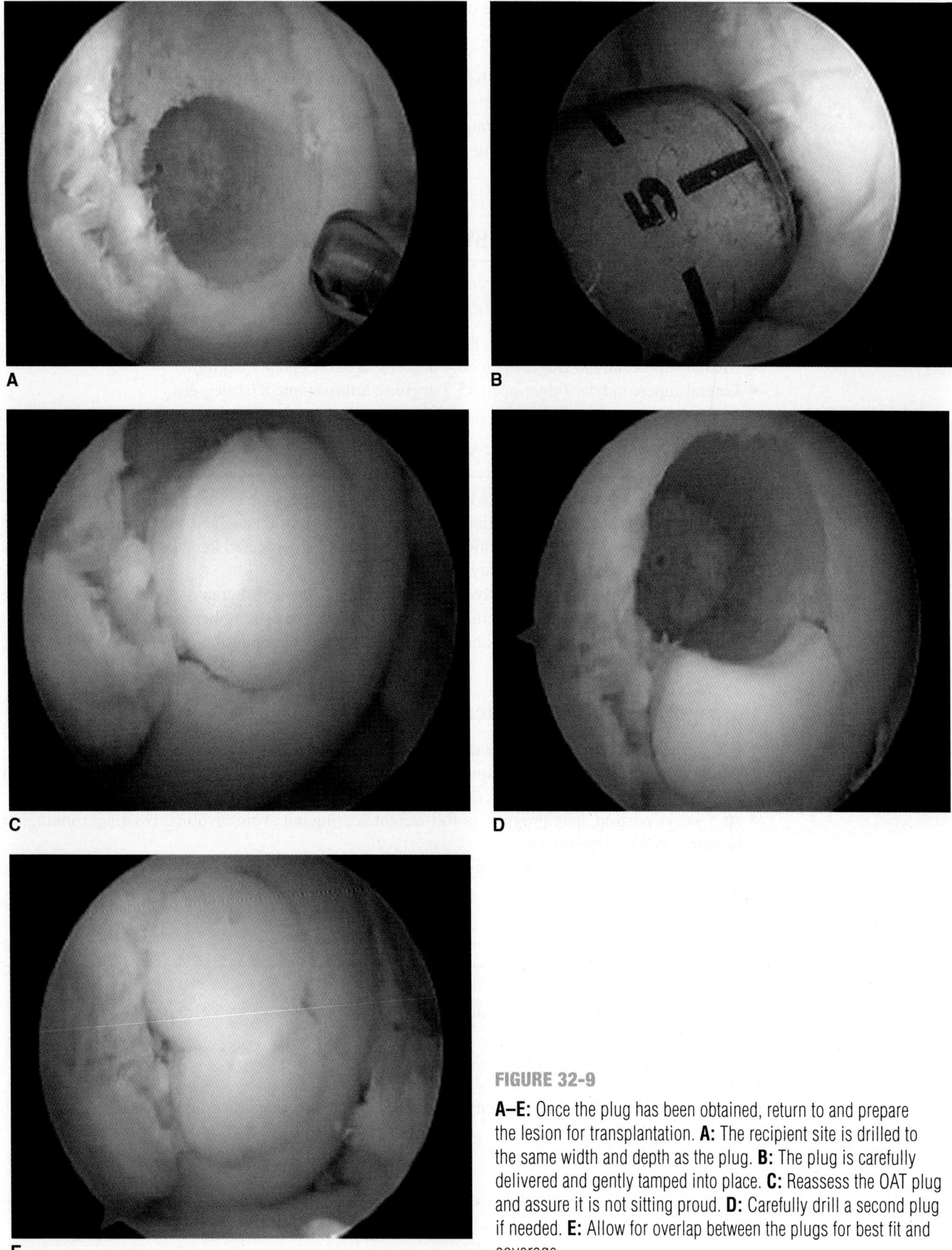

FIGURE 32-9

A–E: Once the plug has been obtained, return to and prepare the lesion for transplantation. **A:** The recipient site is drilled to the same width and depth as the plug. **B:** The plug is carefully delivered and gently tamped into place. **C:** Reassess the OAT plug and assure it is not sitting proud. **D:** Carefully drill a second plug if needed. **E:** Allow for overlap between the plugs for best fit and coverage.

7. After placement of the osteochondral plugs, *reassess the grafts*. Proud plugs may be gently tapped into place with a tamp. Recessed plugs may be carefully removed using a threaded K-wire. Bone graft can be added to the recipient site and the plug carefully replaced and tamped into place. If the plug is altogether too loose, it can be stabilized with headless screws or pins. At the conclusion of the procedure, take the knee through a full range of motion to ensure smooth articulation of the plugs with the corresponding articular surface.

Things to consider:

Why must the graft harvester be perpendicular to the articular surface when harvested and transplanted?
Perpendicular plugs allow for congruence between donor and recipient; better congruence leads to better healing of graft. As little as 1 mm of step-off can lead to poor incorporation and poor healing (2).

ARTHROSCOPIC VERSUS OPEN HARVESTING?

Epstein et al. (3) performed a cadaver study looking at mini-open versus arthroscopic harvesting of plugs to determine which allowed for more perpendicular grafts.

- Lateral intercondylar notch: open 84.1 degrees, arthroscopic 84.2 degrees
- Medial supracondylar ridge: open 88.4 degrees, arthroscopic 81 degrees*
- Lateral supercondylar ridge: open 85.7 degrees, arthroscopic 87.1 degrees

POST-OP MANAGEMENT

After OAT, patients should be 50% weight bearing on the operative extremity for 5 weeks. No post-operative bracing is needed. The patient should maintain full extension and work on range of motion with either a continuous passive motion (CPM) machine or dedicated knee flexion exercises (goal: flexion greater than 200 times per day).

Care is taken to treat postoperative pain and edema. Physical therapy should be started in the week following surgery with a specific protocol for quadriceps strengthening and range of motion, progressing to full weight bearing and strengthening. One example of a therapy protocol is listed below.

Postoperative physical therapy protocol:

- 0 to 2 weeks post-op, focus on quad recruitment, straight leg raises, and heel slides
- At 2 weeks post-op, may begin aquatic therapy, stationary bike with elevated seat, leg press with 50% body weight, leg extension/curls with low weight, and high repetition
- At 5 weeks post-op, may progress to full weight bearing but avoid pivoting, twisting, running, or jumping. Work on proprioception.
- At 10 weeks post-op, may begin plyometrics with both legs and gradually progress to single leg; begin jogging

COMPLICATIONS

- Donor site morbidity
- Bone necrosis/failure of incorporation
- Graft mismatch
- Progression of chondral injury
- Donor site overgrowth
- Donor site giant cell reaction when backfilled with a synthetic bone graft material

*A significant difference was found in the perpendicularity in the medial supracondylar ridge between open and arthroscopic harvesting.

PEARLS AND PITFALLS

Pearls:

- Careful preparation: sharp debridement and estimation of size/number of plugs before harvesting.
- Harvest plugs first—graft harvest perpendicular to surface.
- Graft delivery perpendicular to surface.
- Plug tamped until flush with surface; slightly recessed better than slightly proud. If proud, tamp into place. If remains proud, remove and trim plug.

Pitfalls:

- Evaluate axial alignment prior to surgery—mechanical axis issues in the affected compartment must be addressed for optimal healing.
- Cyst beneath articular lesion? Fill with bone graft prior to placing plug.
- Convergence of grafts may lead to subsidence.

OUTCOMES

Several studies looking at subjective outcomes following OAT have shown good to excellent results in 76.7% to 92% of patients, including high-level athletes (4–6) Hyaline cartilage restoration tends to have better outcomes than do other restoration techniques at 3 to 5 years' follow-up (7).

OAT and microfracture have been compared in several studies. OATs does well in the short term, with good to excellent results in 96% of patient (vs. 52% who underwent microfracture); better subjective scores at 1, 2, and 3 years; and faster return to sport, with 93% of patients returning to

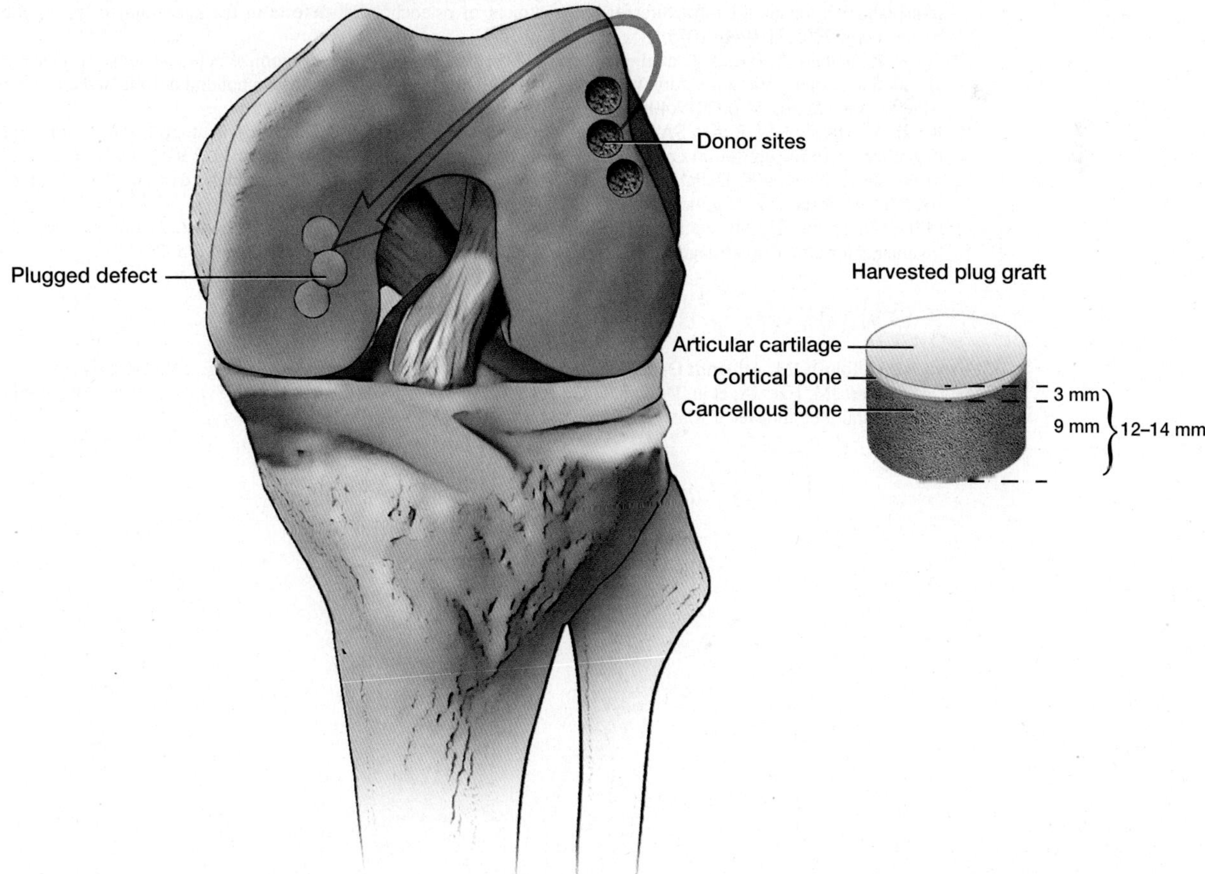

FIGURE 32-10

Composite figure demonstrating the technique for osteochondral autograft harvesting from the superolateral femur and delivery into the defect (in this case in the medial femoral condyle). Image modified from www.cartilagerestoration.org.

sport at 6 months versus 52% in the microfracture group (8). Intermediate- and long-term subjective outcomes, however, show a similarity between the two groups but osteochondral autografts tend to maintain a higher level of athletic activity (9,10). Approximately 91% of patients who undergo OATs procedure return to sport on average 7 months after surgery (11). The reoperation rate was noted to be 28.6% following microfracture versus 12.5% after OATs, and the net cost and cost-effectiveness of the two procedures are comparable (12).

OAT offers a reliable solution to full-thickness cartilage defects in the weight-bearing regions of the knee. While it can be technically challenging, a familiarity with the autograft transplant systems and good preoperative and perioperative planning allows for restoration of areas of the knee with devastating cartilage damage. With good short- and long-term clinical outcomes, this technique stands to be an important tool for restoration of articular cartilage lesions and may have similar future application to other regions, including the elbow and talus (Fig. 32-10).

REFERENCES

1. Safran MR, Seiber KS. The evidence for surgical repair of articular cartilage in the knee. *J Am Acad Orthop Surg.* 2010;18(5):259–266.
2. Pearce SG, Hurtig MB, Clarnette R, et al. An investigation of 2 techniques for optimizing joint surface congruency using multiple cylindrical osteochondral autografts. *Arthroscopy.* 2001;17:50–55.
3. Epstein DM, Choung E, Ashraf I, et al. Comparison of mini-open versus arthroscopic harvesting of osteochondral autografts in the knee: a cadaveric study. *Arthroscopy.* 2012;28:1867–1872.
4. Maracci M, Kon E, Delcogliano M, et al. Arthroscopic autologous osteochondral grafting for cartilage defects of the knee: prospective study results at a minimus 7-year follow up. *Am J Sports Med.* 2007;35(12):2014–2021.
5. Panics G, Hangody LR, Balo E, et al. Osteochondral autograft and mosaicplasty in the football athlete. *Cartilage.* 2012;3(1 suppl):25S–30S.
6. Hangody L, Fules P. Autologous osteochondral mosaicplasty for the treatment of full-thickness defects of weight-bearing joints: ten years of experimental and clinical experience. *J Bone Joint Surg Am.* 2003;85(suppl 2):25–32.
7. Hangody L, Kish G, Karpati Z. Arthroscopic autogenous osteochondral mosaicplasty: a multicentric, comparative, prospective study. *Index Traumat Sport.* 1998;5:3–9.
8. Gudas R, Kalesinskas RJ, Kimtys V, et al. A prospective randomized clinical study of mosaic osteochondral autologous transplantation versus microfracture for the treatment of osteochondral defects in the knee joint in young athletes. *Arthroscopy.* 2005;21:1066–1075.
9. Gudas R, Gudaite A, Pocius A, et al. Ten-year follow-up of a prospective, randomized clinical study of mosaic osteochondral autologous transplantation versus microfracture for the treatment of osteochondral defects in the knee joint of athletes. *Am J Sports Med.* 2012;40(11):2499–508.
10. Krych AJ, Harnly HW, Rodeo SA, et al. Activity levels are higher after osteochondral autograft transfer mosaicplasty than after microfracture for articular cartilage defects of the knee. *J Bone Joint Surg.* 2012;94(11):971–978.
11. Mithoefer K, Hambly K, Della Villa S, et al. Return to sports participation after articular cartilage repair in the knee: scientific evidence. *Am J Sports Med.* 2009;37(S1):2051–2063.
12. Miller DJ, Smith MV, Matava MJ, et al. Microfracture and osteochondral autograft transplantation are cost-effective treatments for articular cartilage lesions of the distal femur. *Am J Sports Med.* 2015;43:2175–2181.

RECOMMENDED READINGS

Fitzpatrick K, Tokish JM. Allograft OATS: decision-making and operative steps. *J Knee Surg.* 2011;24:101–108.

Fowler DE, Hart JM, Hart JA, et al. Donor site Giant Cell reaction following backfill with Synthetic Bone Material During osteochondral plug transfer. *J Knee Surg.* 2009;22:371–374.

33 Autologous Chondrocyte Implantation

Christian Lattermann and Michael P. Elliott

INDICATIONS/CONTRAINDICATIONS

Autologous chondrocyte implantation (ACI) is an effective two-stage, cell-based treatment option for symptomatic, full-thickness chondral and osteochondral defects (OCD) of the knee that have failed to improve with nonoperative management. The first procedure involves arthroscopic harvest of chondrocytes from a non–weight-bearing portion of the knee. The cells then undergo aseptic processing, viability and potency testing, and culture expansion (4 to 6 weeks). Implantation of the chondrocytes on a prepared defect occurs in a second procedure. The ideal candidate is a young, active patient presenting with pain, swelling, recurring effusions, catching or locking with activity, and a full-thickness chondral defect between 2 and 10 cm^2 that is surrounded by a healthy cartilage rim in a mechanically stable knee joint with normal axial alignment.

Chondral lesions that can be considered for treatment with ACI should be Outerbridge grade III or IV (International Cartilage Repair Society [ICRS] grade 3 or 4; Fig. 33-1) defects between 2 and 12 cm^2 in size. Ideally, the opposing articular surface should be undamaged or have minor cartilage wear (Outerbridge grade I or II, ICRS grade 1 or 2).

ACI can be used to treat lesions on the femoral condyles, trochlea, and patella. Tibial plateau defects and bipolar ("kissing") lesions may also be considered for ACI, as newer techniques have emerged and more studies have shown improved results over time (1). Multiple lesions (two or more lesions in one joint) have also shown satisfactory mid- to long-term results after undergoing ACI.

Absolute contraindications to performing ACI are documented presence of inflammatory arthritis or established high-grade osteoarthritis with radiographic joint space narrowing over 50%, significant loss of motion or arthrofibrosis, inability to comply with postoperative restrictions and rehabilitation, and history of a gentamicin allergy. Relative contraindications, if uncorrected, are ligamentous instability, meniscus deficiency, axial malalignment, and habitual factors such as smoking, age greater than 50, and body mass index (BMI) greater than 35; studies have shown these factors negatively influence the overall outcomes of patients undergoing cartilage procedures (2). In many cases, ligament reconstruction, corrective osteotomies, and meniscal transplants to correct some of the relative contraindications may be required in combination with ACI in either a staged or simultaneous procedure to provide an optimal environment for successful outcomes.

PREOPERATIVE PLANNING

A thorough preoperative assessment of patients undergoing ACI is critically important. A careful history should be obtained, which includes mechanism of injury, onset and timing of symptoms, and prior treatment and the response to treatments.

Examination and Evaluation

A detailed physical exam will help to reveal the relative contribution of coexisting abnormalities such as ligamentous instability, meniscal pathology, and mechanical malalignment of the lower extremity. Point tenderness, crepitance, locking, catching, or an effusion may indicate underlying cartilage pathology. When evaluating lesions of the patella, careful attention should be paid to patellofemoral instability or malalignment.

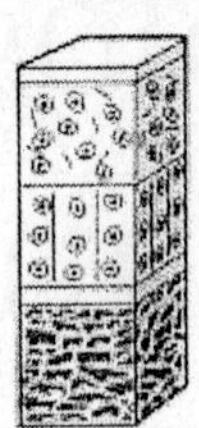

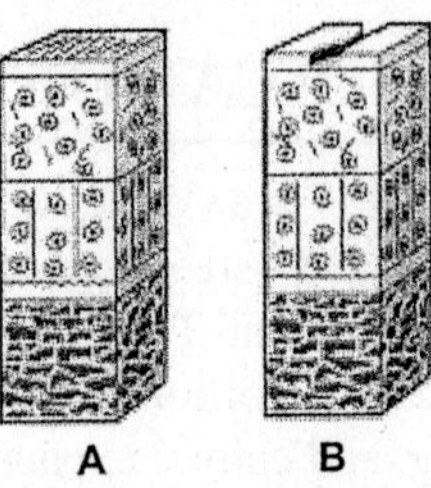

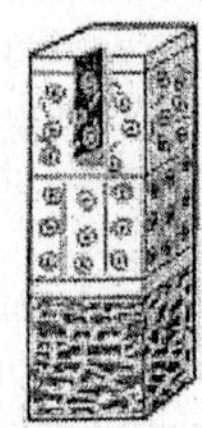

ICRS Grade 3—Severely Abnormal
Cartilage defects extending down >50% of cartilage depth (A) as well as down to calcified layer (B) and down to but not through the subchondral bone (C). Blisters are included in this Grade (D)

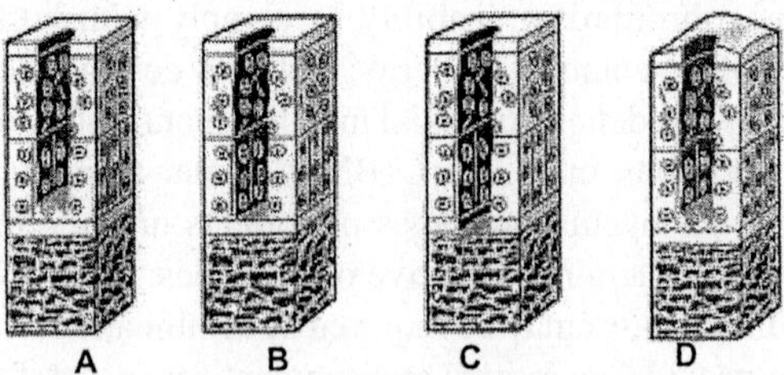

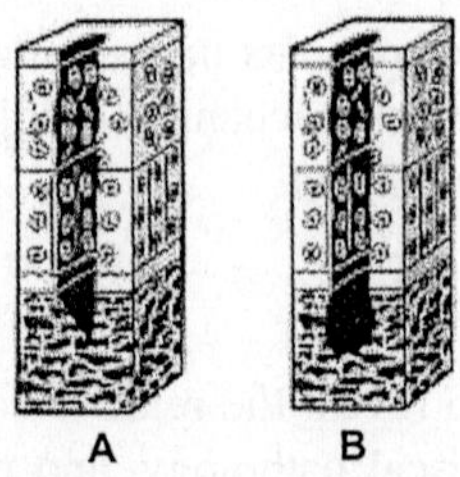

FIGURE 33-1

ICRS classification of cartilage lesions. (Reprinted with permission from the International Cartilage Repair Society, ICRS Cartilage Injury Evaluation Page, 2000.)

Imaging

Radiographic evaluation should include standing AP, lateral, Merchant, and 45 degrees of flexion PA weight-bearing views, as well as bilateral long-leg alignment films. Computerized tomography (CT) scans may be helpful when evaluating for patellofemoral dysplasia and instability or in the case of adolescent OCD lesions where a CT scan with intra-articular contrast may be helpful to assess the stability of the lesion. Magnetic resonance imaging (MRI) is useful to identify location, size, and depth of the lesions as well as underlying subchondral bone abnormalities such as edema or cysts. The biochemical homeostasis of articular cartilage can be analyzed using MRI T1rho or T2 sequencing; however, this is only available in few centers and has to be considered experimental at this time.

Arthroscopic Evaluation

Thorough arthroscopic evaluation is an important step, which allows the opportunity to assess and verify the location, topical geography, surface area, and depth of the lesion, and potential bone loss. It also allows for the evaluation of comorbidities such as status of the meniscus and cruciate ligaments, as well as opposing articular surfaces and other unsuspected cartilage defects. The examination should proceed as follows:

- General or regional anesthesia is administered.
- Exam under anesthesia is performed to assess ligamentous stability.
- Thorough arthroscopic examination is performed of the articular surfaces, menisci, synovial lining, and cruciate ligaments with an arthroscopic probe.
- If present, debris and loose bodies should be removed using an arthroscopic grasper or shaver.
- Evaluate the location, size, depth, and containment of the cartilage lesion.
- Measure the defect size with a mechanical tool, such as a metal ruler or flexible ruler (Fig. 33-2).
- Document the lesion characteristics carefully in the OR report as this information is later needed for insurance approval!
- If the lesion is suitable for ACI, proceed with cartilage biopsy.
- A biopsy of normal hyaline cartilage can be taken from either the superomedial edge of the trochlea or the lateral/medial edge of the intercondylar notch (our preferred site) using an open-ring curette or gouge.
- The biopsy should be taken down through subchondral bone to ensure bleeding and eventual healing with fibrocartilage. Care should be taken to minimize capture of synovial tissue.

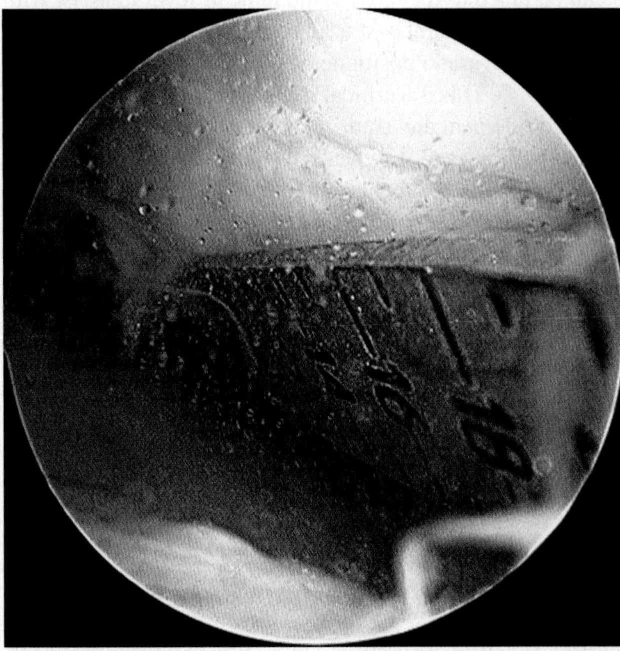

FIGURE 33-2

Arthroscopic picture of measuring full-thickness cartilage defect with ruler.

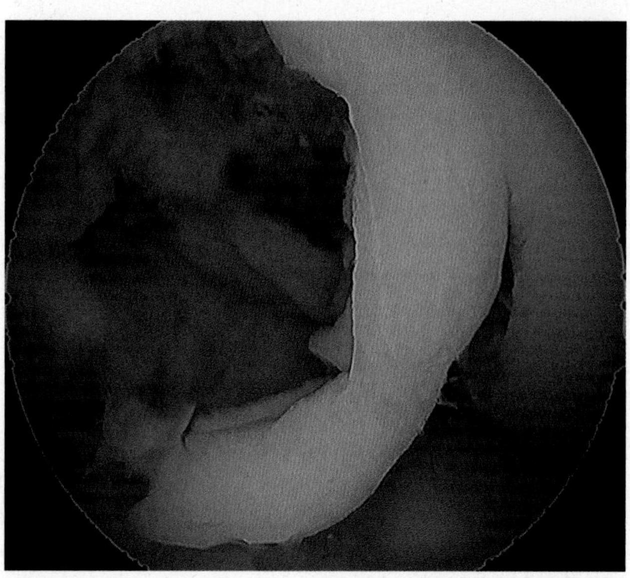

FIGURE 33-3

Arthroscopic picture of cartilage biopsy after harvesting with ringed curette (notice that the superior portion of the biopsy is left attached, to facilitate removal).

- Leaving one end of the biopsy attached will allow for easier removal of the specimen using a grasper (Fig. 33-3).
- The volume of the biopsy should be approximately 200 to 300 mg, or a 5 × 10 mm surface area (two or three "Tic Tacs").
- The specimen is placed in a sterile collection vial and sent to Vericel Inc. (Cambridge, MA) for processing and cellular expansion, which takes approximately 4 to 6 weeks. Chondrocytes can be cryopreserved for up to 2 years.
- Meniscal pathology should be treated at the time of the cartilage biopsy.
- The second procedure for implantation of the expanded chondrocytes is performed at a minimum 4 weeks following the index procedure to allow for in vitro expansion of harvested chondrocytes.

SURGICAL PROCEDURE

Chondral Lesions

Positioning and Approach

General or regional anesthesia is administered. The patient is positioned supine on a standard operating table. A 3-L saline bag or sandbag can be taped to the table at the midcalf level to assist with keeping the leg flexed to approximately 90 degrees. A lateral post is also used to keep the knee vertically positioned. We prefer to use a De Mayo or Alvarado positioner, as this allows us to fine-tune the knee position to assist with exposure (Fig. 33-4). This is a critical step in the set up; it will ensure stable positioning during the open chondral debridement and suturing process.

A nonsterile tourniquet is placed on the thigh; however, it typically is not inflated until after the defect is prepared in order to allow for the assessment of subchondral bleeding. Exposure depends upon defect location; for patellofemoral lesions, we prefer to perform a tibial tubercle osteotomy. In most cases, patellofemoral chondral defects will undergo a tubercle anteriorization or medialization in our practice. This offers an atraumatic approach to the patellofemoral joint. Alternatively, a midline skin incision with medial or lateral parapatellar arthrotomy can be performed, and the patella can be pushed aside or everted if access to multiple lesions is needed. Femoral condyle lesions can be accessed through limited parapatellar arthrotomies (Fig. 33-5). A mid- or subvastus approach can be used to gain increased exposure if needed.

Preparation of Defect and Collagen Membrane Patch

- Excise all fibrocartilage covering the lesion as well as damaged or loose articular flaps.
- The perimeter of the lesion should be demarcated with a fresh no. 15 blade, cutting perpendicular to the articular surface down to subchondral bone.
- It is helpful to score the articular cartilage in a grid shape with a no. 15 blade as it facilitates removal of the articular cartilage with a curette.

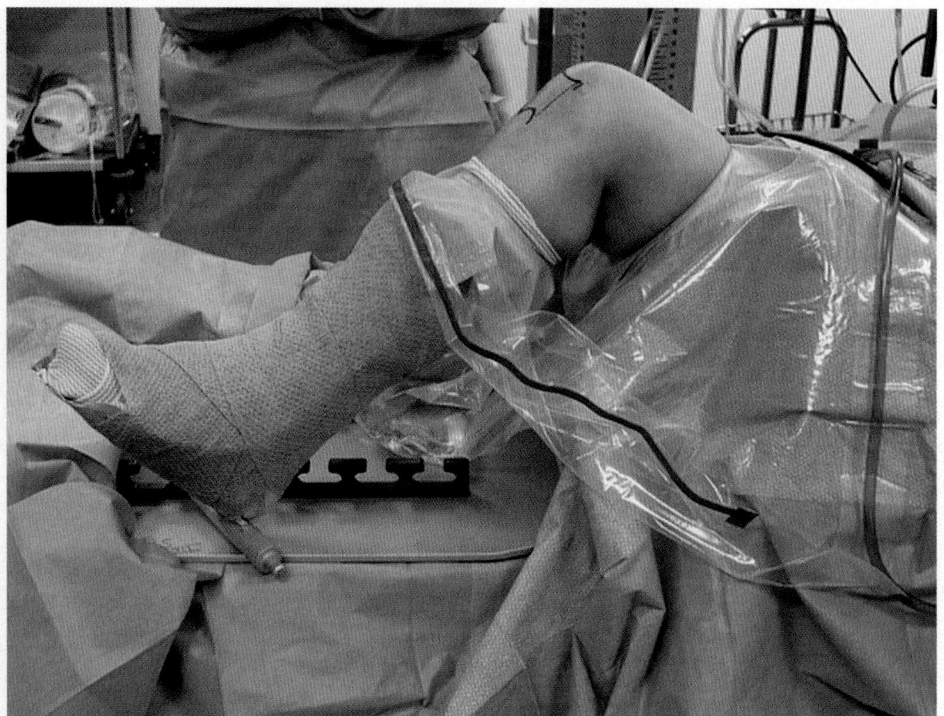

FIGURE 33-4
Proper position of the knee with the assistance of an Alvarado knee holder.

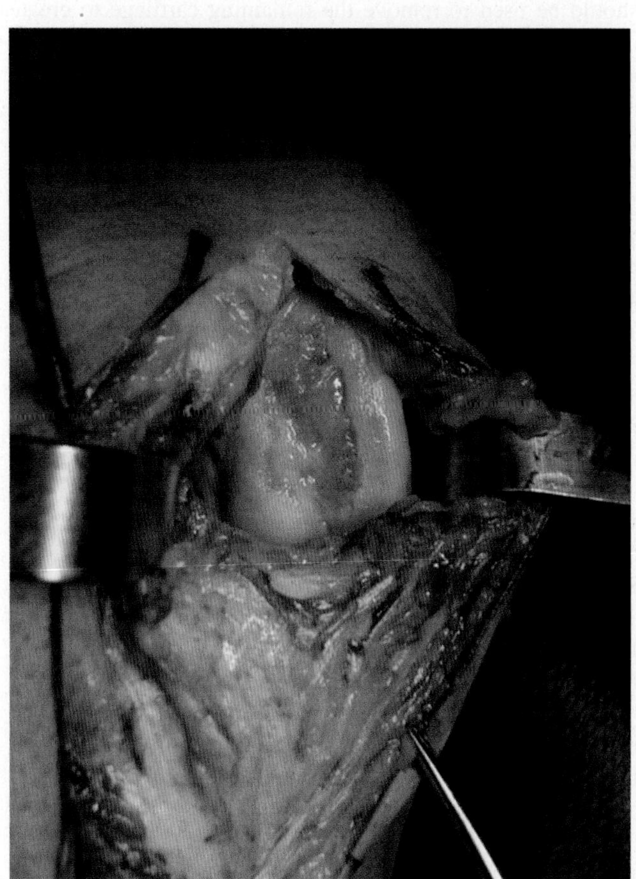

FIGURE 33-5
Exposure of a femoral condyle defect through a parapatellar arthrotomy, prior to debridement of the cartilage.

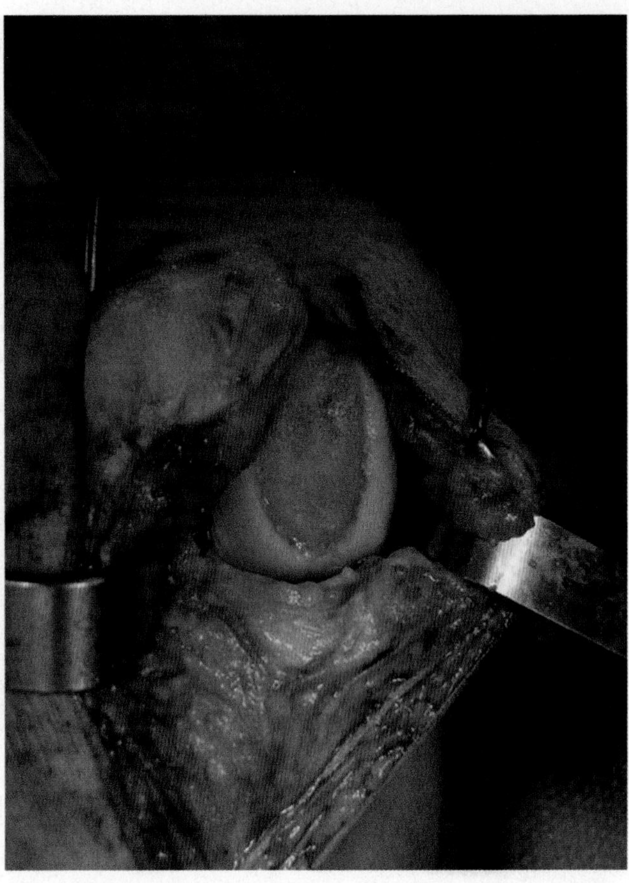

FIGURE 33-6

Femoral condyle defect after excision and debridement of all damaged, unhealthy cartilage.

- Straight, angled, and ring curettes should be used to remove the remaining cartilage to create stable, vertical walls of healthy cartilage shouldering the lesion (Fig. 33-6).
- A circular or oval-shaped defect should be prepared.
- All efforts should be made to keep the lesion "contained" by cartilage as well as avoid violating the subchondral bone causing bleeding into the defect.
- If bleeding occurs, hemostasis can be achieved most easily using commercially available fibrin glue (Tisseel, Baxter Healthcare Corp, Glendale, CA). A small amount should be deposited in the base of the lesion, and a gloved finger is used to press the glue into the subchondral bone. Usually, all bleeding will stop after holding pressure for a minute. Older techniques such as application of neuropatties soaked with a dilute 1:1,000 epinephrine solution can be tried but are often ineffective.
- The defect is then measured to determine the proper size of the bilayer collagen membrane patch (Bio-Gide, Geistlich Pharma North America). Sterile paper (glove paper) or a small piece of aluminum foil from the scalpel blade is placed over the lesion and marked with a surgical marking pen to create a template that is a negative of the defect.
- The template is then positioned upside down onto the collagen membrane. This is important if the shape is asymmetric.
- The bilayer collagen membrane should be cut along the template using a fresh no. 15 blade scalpel or tenotomy scissors and should be handled with jeweler's forceps.
- It is important to understand that periosteum and the newer bilayer membranes (Bioguide) behave differently. While periosteum would shrink and had to be slightly oversized, the bilayer membrane actually stretches and therefore should be exactly sized or even slightly undersized.
- A commonly used modification of the traditional cell application technique (ACI-collagen membrane seeding) is to place one vial of cells onto the rough surface of the membrane at the beginning of the preparation. After approximately 10 minutes, the cells have adhered to the membrane and form a firmly attached layer. This so-called poor man's membrane-associated chondrocyte implantation (MACI) has become the standard in most cartilage centers in the United States (3).
- Once the patch is prepared, keep it in a moist chamber until utilized.

Collagen Membrane Patch Suturing

- Inspect the defect again for any bleeding and address accordingly.
- Cover the defect with the membrane patch.
- Anchor the membrane patch with one suture in each corner using a cutting needle with 6-0 Vicryl (Ethicon, Somerville, NJ) sutures, soaked in glycerin or mineral oil, anchoring the patch flush with the surrounding articular cartilage (we prefer a colored suture for better visibility).
- Place the first four sutures at the 12, 6, 3, and 9 o'clock positions.
- Sutures should be placed at 3 to 5 mm intervals around the periphery of the lesion (Fig. 33-7).
- Suture is passed first through the patch 2 mm from the edge and then articular cartilage exiting approximately 4 mm from the edge, tying knots over the patch.
- If the surrounding cartilage is unable to hold suture, microanchors with absorbable suture may be used. For uncontained areas, bone tunnels may be created with 0.45-mm Kirschner wires or a 1-mm drill, and 6-0 sutures may be passed through the transosseous tunnels.
- Tension the flap like the skin over a drum with interrupted sutures in a Z pattern. This can also be done using a running suture technique; however, if the initial or last knot unravels, the risk of losing the patch is high.
- Leave an opening in the most superior portion for the injection of the chondrocytes.
- Fibrin glue should be used to seal the distances between sutures.
- Stable fixation and a good fit of the patch are crucial to the surgical outcome.

Watertightness Testing

- A nonantibiotic saline–filled tuberculin syringe and 18-gauge 2-in Angiocath can be used to test if the patch is watertight. Gently insert the Angiocath through the superior opening and slowly inject the saline. The "chamber" should contain the fluid without leaks, and one should be able to see the level of saline steadily rise toward the top. Once satisfied with the seal, aspirate the saline completely to avoid diluting the cells.

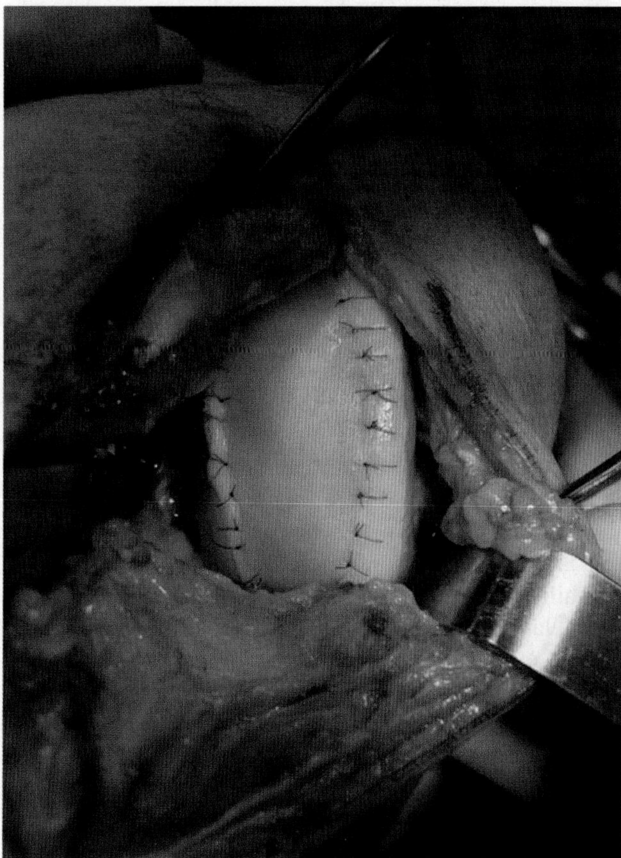

FIGURE 33-7

Final appearance of the membrane after interrupted sutures are placed every 3 to 5 mm along the periphery, securing the membrane.

- If there is a leak, additional sutures can be placed at leakage locations; the edges surrounding the patch are then gently dried and sealed with fibrin glue. Retest if the patch is watertight as described above.

Implantation of Cells

- Aspirate the chondrocytes into the tuberculin syringe using an 18-gauge 2-in Angiocath.
- Fill the defect by advancing the Angiocath into the most distal aspect of the defect and gently inject the chondrocytes.
- Slowly withdraw the Angiocath as you inject the chondrocytes, evenly distributing the cells throughout the defect.
- Close the superior opening with additional sutures and fibrin glue.
- If the defect is large, an upper and lower opening may be necessary for proper filling of the defect. Inject cells into the lower part of the defect first, close the injection window in the membrane, and then start filling through the upper opening.
- Intra-articular drains should not be used, as they can harm the patch and suck out transplanted chondrocytes. If a drain must be used, ensure it is without suction.
- Close the wound in layers and apply a sterile dressing.

POSTOPERATIVE MANAGEMENT

The rehabilitation protocol following ACI in the knee is slow process with gradual progression that extends up to 9 to 18 months, based on the three phases of the natural maturation process of chondrocytes. Initially after surgery, the patient may be immobilized in a total range-of-motion brace (TROM, DonJoy International, Guildford, England) and made nonweight bearing for 4 to 6 weeks. Use of continuous passive motion (CPM) begins postoperative day 1, for 6 to 8 hours per day, starting at 30 degrees and advancing by 5 to 10 degrees per day with a goal of 90 degrees by 4 weeks and 120 degrees by 6 weeks. The brace is discontinued at 4 to 6 weeks when weight bearing begins, advancing to full weight bearing by 6 to 12 weeks. Early in the rehabilitation, closed chain exercises are recommended, and by 6 to 12 weeks, patients will begin open chain exercises and balancing activities. Quadriceps and hamstring strengthening is focused on throughout the rehabilitation. Gradual reintroduction to low-impact exercises such as exercise bike or elliptical begins around the 12-week mark, with advancement to greater impact loading exercises and eventual return to sporting activity around 4 to 6 months. During the rehabilitation process if the patient develops swelling and a persistent, significant effusion, a Medrol Dosepak can be useful to help assist with inflammation control and resolution of the effusion.

CONCOMITANT SURGERY

Creating an optimal environment to allow for tissue healing is an important aspect of cartilage surgery, and concomitant pathology should also be addressed at the time of cell harvest or at the time of implantation. The mantra "the knee of the patient lead to the cartilage lesion in normal articular cartilage" should be respected. Any articular cartilage repair will not succeed if the same uncorrected abnormal environment persists. Therefore, any abnormal alignment or biomechanical challenge for the involved compartment should be optimized. In order to achieve neutral tibial-femoral joint alignment, a high tibial osteotomy may be performed (Fig. 33-8A–D) most commonly for varus malalignment and a distal femoral osteotomy most commonly for valgus malalignment. Patellofemoral instability may need to be addressed with procedures such as anteromedialization of the tibial tubercle, lateral retinacular lengthening, and/or medial patellofemoral ligament reconstruction. Unstable meniscus tears should be repaired or resected; in the setting of meniscal insufficiency, a meniscus transplant may need to be performed. Cruciate ligaments should be intact and competent; therefore, a deficient ACL or PCL should be reconstructed, restoring mechanical stability. In most cases, concomitant pathology should be addressed at the time of implantation, once the cartilage lesion is debrided but before the chondrocytes are injected. In some cases, adjunct procedures may be performed separately or at the time the biopsy is taken.

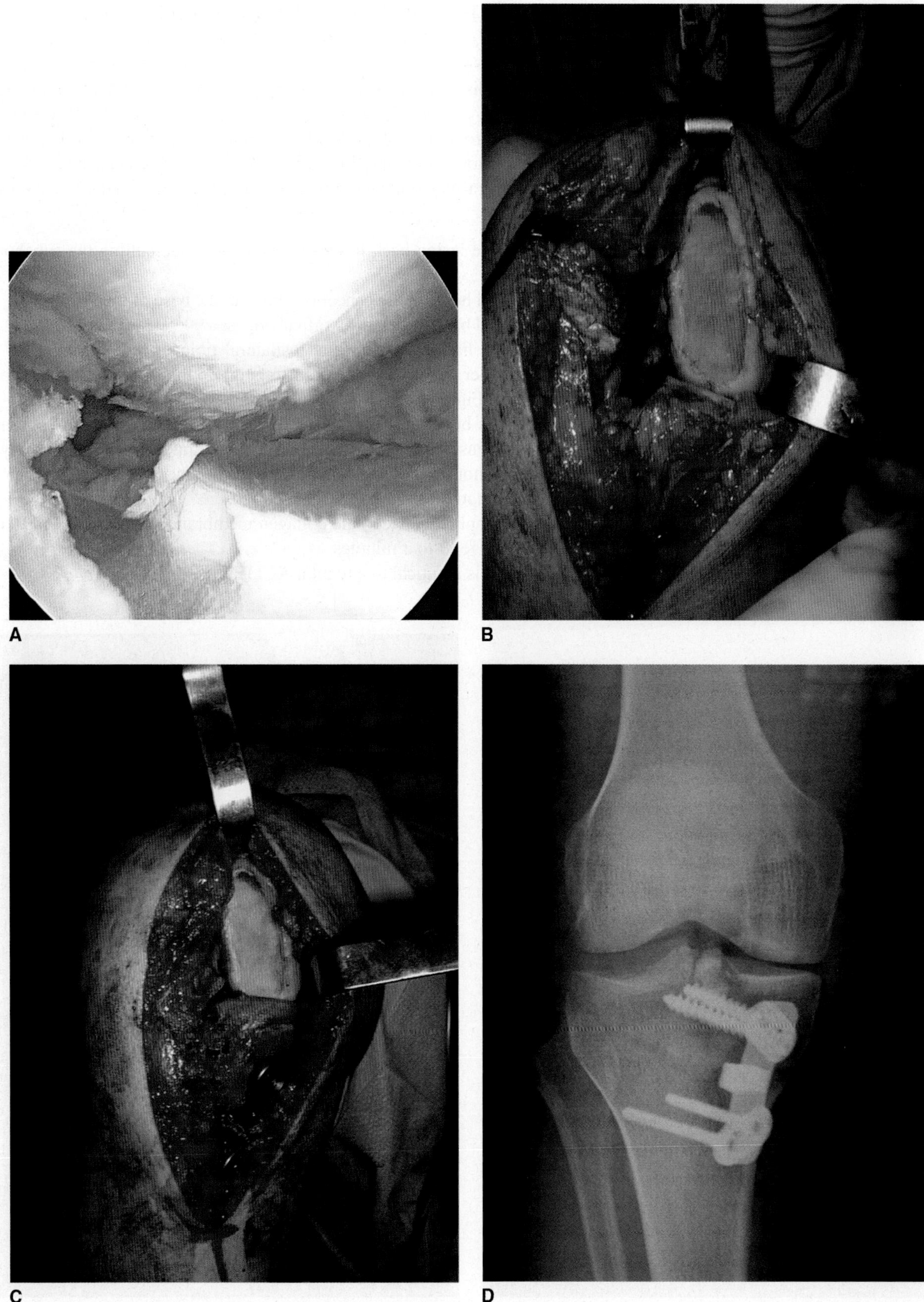

FIGURE 33-8

Arthroscopic picture **(A)** of full-thickness femoral condyle lesion along with meniscal insufficiency. Femoral condyle defect **(B)** prior to debridement. High tibial osteotomy and meniscus transplant **(C)** performed to correct underlying concomitant pathology. Postoperative x-rays **(D)** demonstrating correction of tibiofemoral alignment with high tibial osteotomy.

OSTEOCHONDRAL LESIONS (OSTEOCHONDRITIS DISSECANS)

When addressing osteochondritis dissecans with ACI, it is important to note the depth of the defect. Bony defects less than 6 to 8 mm can be treated in the same manner as a chondral lesion. Care should be taken to debride the sclerotic base of the lesion; bleeding occurs frequently and has to be carefully managed and stopped prior to implantation. If the bony defect is greater than 6 to 8 mm (Fig. 33-9A,B), autologous bone grafting along with ACI should be performed. This so-called sandwich ACI is done as follows:

- Debride the sclerotic base of the lesion back to cancellous bone, undercutting the subchondral bone.
- A 2-mm drill can be used to drill holes in the cancellous bone at the base of the lesion.
- The cartilage should be debrided back to healthy, vertical edges.
- Autologous bone graft may be harvested from the ipsilateral tibia or femoral condyle. This amount will almost always render sufficient bone graft to build up the defect to the level of the surrounding subchondral bone (Fig. 33-9C).
- Pack the defect with autologous bone graft starting at the bottom of the defect and contour the cancellous bone over the defect just below the level of the subchondral bone. Typically, only corner sutures are necessary to anchor the membrane in place. Fibrin glue may be placed under the membrane to assist with fixation to the bone graft (Fig. 33-9D).
- Once the fibrin glue has been applied between the collagen membrane and the bone graft, compress the area with a dry sponge for 2 to 3 minutes.
- The remainder of the procedure is identical to a regular ACI (Fig. 33-9E).

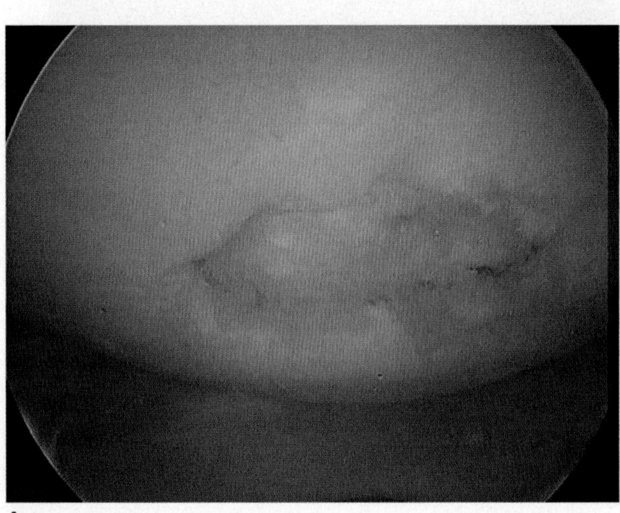

A

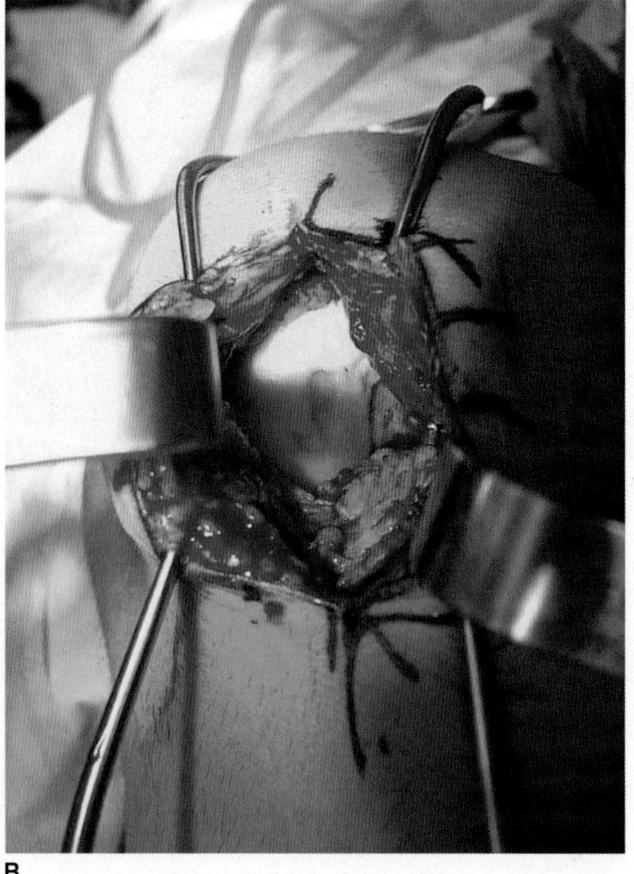

B

FIGURE 33-9

Arthroscopic photo of osteochondritis dissecans involving femoral condyle **(A)**. The defect prior to debridement **(B)** and after debridement and filling of the bony defect with cancellous bone graft **(C)**.

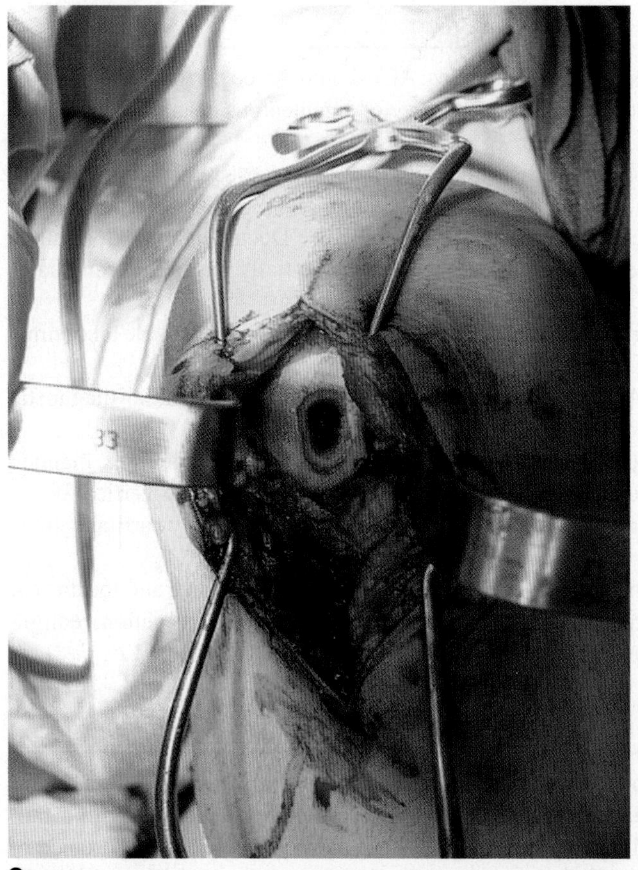

C

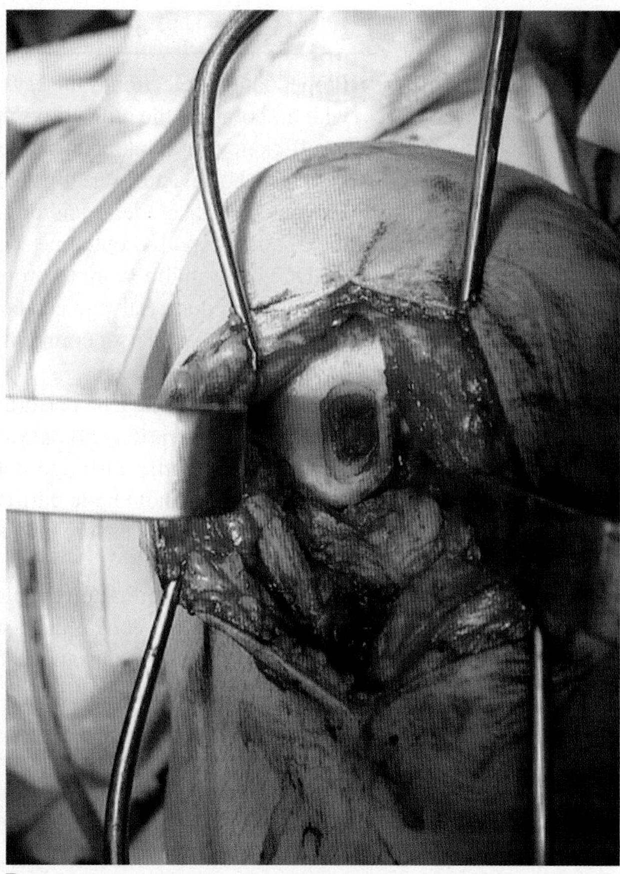

D

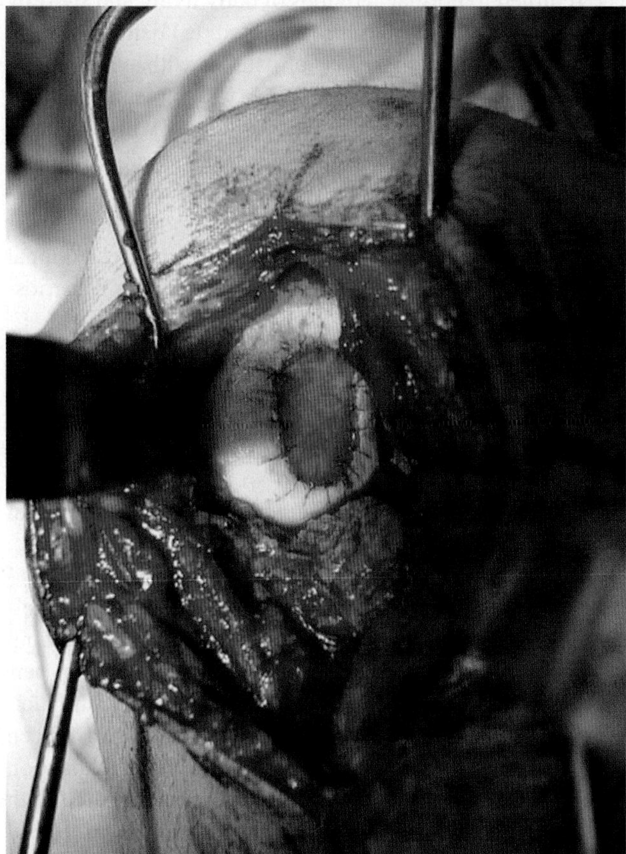

E

FIGURE 33-9 (*Continued*)

The defect is then covered with a membrane **(D)**, followed by second membrane overlying defect under which the chondrocytes are injected **(E)**. Arthroscopic photo of the transplanted area 3 years after the transplantation was completed.

PEARLS AND PITFALLS

- Proper patient selection is the *key* to successful outcomes. ACI should not be performed in patients who do not meet the indications described or have uncorrected ligamentous instability, meniscus insufficiency, or axial malalignment.
- Patients who have fully established osteoarthritis with radiographic changes greater than Kellgren-Lawrence (KL) grade II and/or are complaining of excessive amounts of pain that may cause their patient reported outcome scores such as the International Knee Documentation Committee (IKDC) or Lysholm score to drop below approximately 35 are potentially unsuitable candidates for this procedure. Salvage can be expected in these patients at best.
- Consider all possible concomitant procedures that may be required in order to provide an optimal environment for success.
- The surgeon planning to perform ACI should be the one who performs the initial diagnostic arthroscopy and cartilage biopsy.
- Debridement of the cartilage defect should be done with care and in a meticulous manner, ensuring that all nonviable cartilage is removed and only healthy cartilage with vertical edges remains. One way to ensure this is to incorporate a 1- to 2-mm margin of healthy cartilage in the debridement.
- Postoperative rehabilitation should be individualized for the patient based on size and location of the lesion as well as concomitant surgical procedures such as ligamentous reconstruction, realignment osteotomy, or meniscus treatment.

RESULTS

Long-term studies have shown good to excellent results reported in 86% of patients at 5 to 11 years after undergoing ACI using a periosteal graft for femoral and patellofemoral lesions, with a failure rate of approximately 16% (4). More importantly, this study demonstrated the importance of patient status at 2 years as an indicator of future outcome. In most cases of graft failure, the grafts failed within the first 2 years. Patients who returned to normal activities of daily living and sport by 2 years after ACI were able to continue these activities long term. Minas et al. (5) demonstrated a survivorship of 71% at 10 to 15 years and improved function in 75% of patients with symptomatic cartilage defects of the knee at a minimum of 10-year follow-up after surgery. Of note, a prior history of marrow stimulation as well as very large defects (>15 cm^2) was associated with increased risk of graft failure. Rate of reoperation for graft-related issues was 51%. Zaslav et al. (6) looked at the effectiveness of ACI in 154 patients with a mean follow-up of 4 years who failed prior treatments for articular cartilage defects in the knee. Seventy-six percent of patients reported significant improvement in both symptoms and function, including activities of daily living and recreational activities. However, 49% required subsequent surgical procedures, most commonly for graft/periosteal hypertrophy or arthrofibrosis.

Historically, ACI procedures performed for patellofemoral lesions have shown fewer good to excellent results as well as higher failure rates when compared with femoral condyle lesions. However, Gomoll et al. (7), in a recent multicenter study involving 110 patients followed for a minimum of 4 years, showed 92% of patients would choose to undergo ACI again, with 86% rating their knees as good or excellent at the time of final follow-up, and an 8% failure rate. They stressed the importance of attention to biomechanics when performing ACI for patellofemoral lesions.

Comparisons of ACI with other cartilage treatment methods, such as microfracture, osteochondral allograft, and mosaicplasty, have showed equivalent or superior outcomes when treating patellofemoral and femoral condyle lesions. ACI is associated with potential complications including arthrofibrosis, periosteal graft hypertrophy, delamination, and graft failure. Periosteal graft hypertrophy requiring subsequent surgical procedures is common, and in an effort to decrease the incidence of periosteal autograft hypertrophy and donor site morbidity, advanced techniques have been developed such as collagen-covered ACI (CACI) and matrix-induced chondrocyte implantation (MACI). Both of these techniques have demonstrated improved clinical outcomes compared with microfracture. At our institution, we no longer use periosteal grafts due to the issues with graft hypertrophy and donor site morbidity and have transitioned to CACI exclusively. This has markedly reduced the need for reoperation.

REFERENCES

1. Ossendorf C, Steinwachs M, Kreuz P, et al. Autologous chondrocyte implantation (ACI) for the treatment of large and complex cartilage lesions of the knee. *Sports Med Arthrosc Rehabil Ther Technol.* 2011;3:11.
2. Lattermann C, Luckett MR. Staging and comorbidities. *J Knee Surg.* 2011;24(4):217–224.
3. Steinwachs M. A new technique for cell-seeded collagen matrix-supported autologous chondrocyte transplantation. *Arthroscopy.* 2009;25(2):208–211.
4. Peterson L, Brittberg M, Kiviranta I, et al. Autologous chondrocyte transplantation: biomechanics and long-term durability. *A J Sports Med.* 2002;30(1):2–12.
5. Minas T, Von Keudell A, Bryant T, et al. A minimum 10-year outcome study of autologous chondrocyte implantation. *Clin Orthop Relat Res.* 2014;472(1):41–51.
6. Zaslav K, Cole B, Brewster R, et al. A prospective study of autologous chondrocyte implantation in patients with failed prior treatment for articular cartilage defect of the knee. *Am J Sports Med.* 2009;37(1):42–55.
7. Gomoll A, Gillogy S, Cole B, et al. Autologous chondrocyte implantation in the patella: a multicenter experience. *Am J Sports Med.* 2014;42(5):1074–1081.

RECOMMENDED READINGS

Aldrian S, Zak L, Wondrasch B, et al. Clinical and radiological long-term outcomes after matrix induced autologous chondrocyte transplantation: a prospective follow-up at a minimum of 10 years. *Am J Sports Med.* 2014;42(11):2680–2688.

Bentley G, Biant LC, Carrington RW, et al. A prospective, randomized comparison of autologous chondrocyte implantation versus mosaicplasty for osteochondral defects of the knee. *J Bone Joint Surg Br.* 2003;85:223–230.

Cole BJ, Cole BJ, DeBerardino T, et al. Outcomes of chondrocyte implantation in study of the treatment of articular repair (STAR) patients with osteochondritis dissecans. *Am J Sports Med.* 2012;40(9):2015–2022.

Ebert JR, Fallon M, Ackland TR, et al. Arthroscopic matrix-induced autologous chondrocyte implantation: 2-year outcomes. *Arthroscopy.* 2012;28(7):952–964.

Horas U, Pelinkovic D, Herr G, et al. Autologous chondrocyte implantation and osteochondral cylinder transplantation in cartilage repair of the knee joint: a prospective, comparative trial. *J Bone Joint Surg Am.* 2003;85:185–192.

Knutsen G, Drogset JO, Engebretson L, et al. A randomized trial comparing autologous chondrocyte implantation with microfracture: findings at five years. *J Bone Joint Surg Am.* 2007;89:2105–2112.

Schneider U, Rackwitz L, Andereya S, et al. A prospective multicenter study on the outcome of type I collagen hydrogen-based autologous chondrocyte implantation (CaReS) for the repair of articular cartilage defects in the knee. *A J Sports Med.* 2011;39(1):2558–2565.

34 Allograft Osteochondral Plugs

William Bugbee

Fresh osteochondral allografts (OCAs) are now a well-established option in the cartilage restoration algorithm and are increasingly popular because of their versatility and favorable clinical outcomes. The ability to restore diseased or damaged cartilage with mature hyaline cartilage tissue is attractive, and the surgical technique for implanting plugs or dowel-type grafts in simple femoral condyle lesions is fairly straightforward. A large body of basic science and clinical outcome data support the use of fresh OCAs in clinical practice (1,2).

INDICATIONS/CONTRAINDICATIONS

Fresh OCAs possess the ability to restore a wide spectrum of articular and osteoarticular pathology. The clinical indications for allografts include a broad range of pathology. As is true for other restorative procedures, in addition to evaluating the particular articular lesion, the careful assessment of the entire joint, as well as the individual, is important. Many proposed treatment algorithms suggest the use of allografts for large lesions (>2 or 3 cm) or for salvage in difficult reconstructive situations where bone loss is also present. In our experience, allografts can be considered as a primary treatment option for osteochondral lesions greater than 2 cm (approximately) in diameter, as is typically seen in osteochondritis dissecans (OCD) and osteonecrosis. Fresh allografts are also useful as a salvage procedure when other cartilage-restorative procedures, such as microfracture, osteoarticular transfer system (OATS), and autologous chondrocyte implantation, have been unsuccessful (3). The increasingly recognized relationship between articular cartilage and underlying subchondral bone (the so-called osteochondral unit), particularly with respect to cartilage injury and disease, makes OCA an attractive option due to its ability to restore diseased cartilage and subchondral bone.

Additionally, allografts often are used for salvage reconstruction of posttraumatic defects of the tibial plateau or the femoral condyle. Other indications for allografting in the knee include treatment of patellofemoral chondrosis or arthrosis and in very select cases of unicompartmental tibiofemoral arthrosis (Table 34-1).

Relative contraindications to the allografting procedure include uncorrected joint instability or uncorrected malalignment of the limb. An allograft may be considered in combination or as part of a staged procedure in these settings. Allografting should not be considered an alternative to prosthetic arthroplasty in an individual with symptoms and acceptable age and activity level for prosthetic replacement. In the younger individual, bipolar and multicompartmental allografting have been modestly successful and probably should be considered an interim procedure. The use of fresh OCAs in individuals with altered bone metabolism, such as is seen in chronic steroid use, smoking, or even nonsteroidal anti-inflammatory agents, has not been studied extensively. Unlike other cartilage procedures, relative size of the lesion (large or small) is not considered a contraindication to allografting.

PREOPERATIVE PLANNING

Common to all fresh allografting procedures is matching the donor with recipient, which is done on the basis of size. In the knee, an anteroposterior radiograph with a magnification marker is used, and a measurement of the medial-lateral dimension of the tibia, just below the joint surface, is made (Fig. 34-1). Alternatively, measurements from magnetic resonance imaging (MRI) or CT scans can be used. The image-based measurement is corrected for magnification, and the

TABLE 34-1 Major Indications for Fresh Osteochondral Allografting of the Femoral Condyle

1. Chondral lesions: traumatic or degenerative
2. Osteochondritis dissecans
3. Postfracture reconstruction
4. Osteonecrosis
5. Salvage of previous cartilage procedure (microfracture, OATS, autologous chondrocyte implantation)

tissue bank makes a direct measurement on the donor tibial plateau. Alternatively, a measurement of the affected femoral condyle can be performed. A match is generally considered acceptable at ±2 mm; however, it should be noted that there is a significant variability in anatomy that is not reflected in size measurements. In particular, in treating OCD, the pathologic condyle typically is larger, wider, and flatter; therefore, a larger donor generally should be used. When using allograft plugs or dowels, one is generally safe with a larger donor. Small donor condyles lead to problems with matching radius of curvature, particularly for grafts over 20 mm in diameter. Recently, we have shown that it may be acceptable to use a contralateral lateral femoral condyle for many medial condyle lesions particularly if the lesion is 20 mm or less (i.e., a left lateral femoral condyle can be used for a right medial femoral condyle lesion) (4). This is important as the higher demand for medial condyles leads to relative scarcity and lateral femoral condyles are more readily available.

Most femoral condyle lesions can be treated using dowel-type grafts. Commercially available instruments (Arthrex, Naples, FL; Joint Restoration Foundation, Denver, CO) simplify the preparation, harvesting, and insertion of these grafts, which may be up to 35 mm in size (Fig. 34-2). Perhaps the most important step in preoperative planning is understanding that one is using living human tissue and performing a transplantation procedure. Respecting the donation process and understanding the recovery, processing, and safety issues are minimum requirements necessary for the surgeon wishing to use fresh allograft tissue.

SURGERY

For most femoral condyle lesions, allografting can be performed through a miniarthrotomy. In most situations, a diagnostic arthroscopy has been performed recently and is not a necessary component of the allografting procedure. However, if there are any unanswered questions regarding meniscal status, or the status of the other compartments, a diagnostic arthroscopy can be performed prior to the allografting procedure. Examination under anesthesia is done in the standard fashion, as is the diagnostic arthroscopy when the surgeon feels this is indicated. Only rarely do we perform arthroscopy, as adequate data have typically been collected to properly indicate the patient for the OCA procedure prior to beginning the process of graft acquisition.

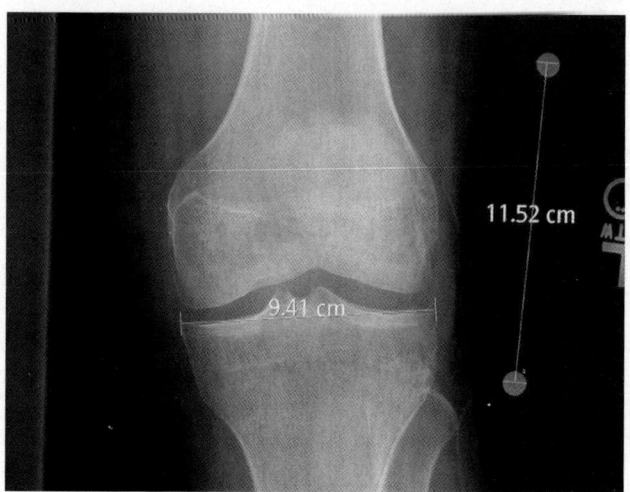

FIGURE 34-1

Radiographic technique for graft sizing. In this example, the corrected tibial width is 81 mm (9.41 × 10/11.52).

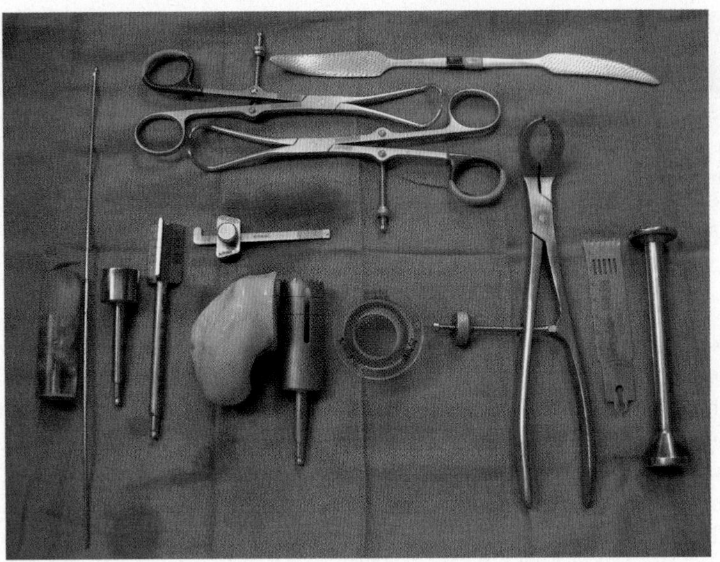

FIGURE 34-2
Commonly used instruments for allograft plug technique.

Patient Positioning

The patient is positioned supine with a tourniquet on the thigh. A leg holder is valuable in this procedure to position the leg in between 40 and 120 degrees of flexion and to access the lesion (Fig. 34-3). Trochlea and patellar lesions are best accessed with the knee in low flexion angles, medial femoral condyle lesions with the knee in 70 to 100 degrees of flexion, and lateral femoral condyle lesions with the knee between 90 and 120 degrees or more of knee flexion. At least one surgical assistant is necessary to provide adequate retraction and leg position for working through the mobile window of the small arthrotomy.

Technique

The fresh graft is inspected to confirm the adequacy of the size match and quality of the tissue prior to opening the knee joint. It is important to keep the graft moist during the procedure; generally, it is left in the packaging media when not being instrumented.

A midline incision is made with the knee in flexion from the center of the patella to the tip of the tibial tubercle. This incision is preferred in anticipation of further surgery in the patient's lifetime. This incision is elevated subcutaneously, either medially or laterally to the patellar tendon, depending on the location of the lesion (either medial or lateral). A retinacular incision is then made from the superior aspect of the patella inferiorly. Great care is taken to enter the joint

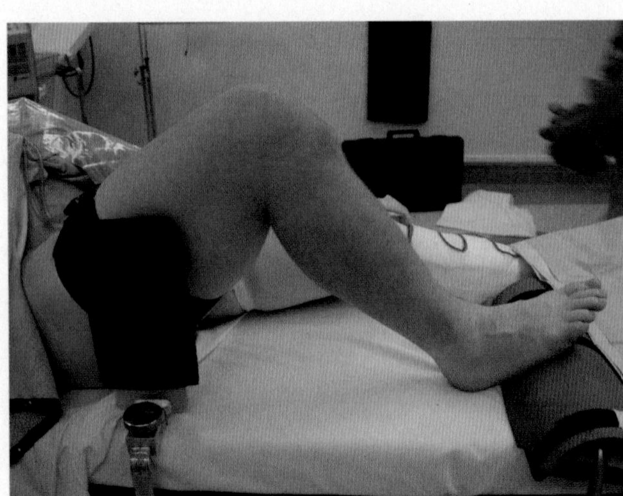

FIGURE 34-3
Position of the leg for access to a typical medial femoral condyle lesion.

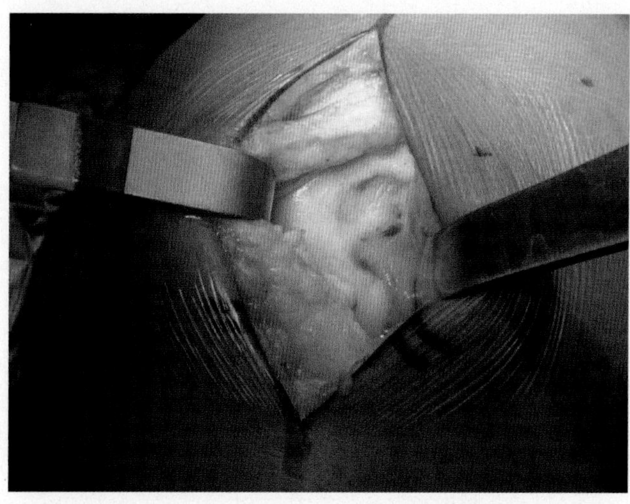

FIGURE 34-4

Miniarthrotomy with Z retractor and bent Hohmann in notch, exposing the OCD lesion of the medial femoral condyle.

and to incise the fat pad without disrupting the anterior horn of the meniscus. In some cases in which the lesion is posterior or very large, the meniscus must be detached and reflected; generally, this can be done safely, leaving a small cuff of tissue adjacent to the anterior attachment of the meniscus for later repair. This is most common for large OCD lesions of the lateral femoral condyle.

Once the joint capsule and synovium have been incised and the joint has been entered, retractors are placed medially and laterally. Care is taken in the positioning of the retractor within the notch to protect the cruciate ligaments and the articular cartilage. This notch retractor is essential to adequately mobilize the patella. The knee is then flexed and/or extended until the proper degree of flexion is noted that presents the lesion into the arthrotomy site (Fig. 34-4). Excessive degrees of flexion limit the ability to mobilize the patella. If access is difficult, extending the arthrotomy proximal is warranted. The lesion then is inspected and palpated with a probe to determine the extent, margins, and maximum size. After a size determination is made, a guidewire is driven into the center of the lesion, perpendicular to the curvature of the articular surface. It is critical to place the guidewire perpendicular to the joint surface. The size of the proposed graft is determined using sizing dowels (Fig. 34-5), the remaining articular cartilage is scored, and a coring drill is used to remove the remaining articular cartilage and 3 to 4 mm of subchondral bone (Figs. 34-6 and 34-7). In deeper lesions, the pathologic bone is removed until there is healthy, bleeding bone. In cases of very deep lesions, we believe the depth of this coring should not exceed 10 mm, and bone grafting should be performed to fill any deeper or more extensive osseous defects. Our experience suggests that the minimal amount of allograft bone should be transplanted, and our grafts are rarely more than 5 to 8 mm in total thickness. The guide pin then is removed, depth measurements are made in the four quadrants of the prepared recipient site, and a simple map is created (Fig. 34-8). The corresponding anatomic location

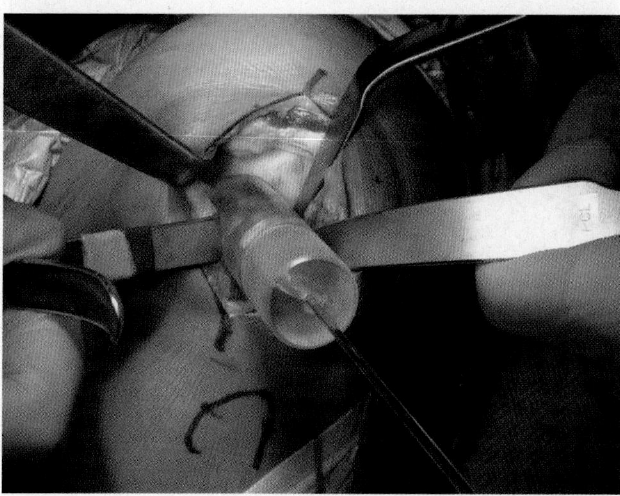

FIGURE 34-5

Guidewire in place and sizing dowel measuring lesion diameter.

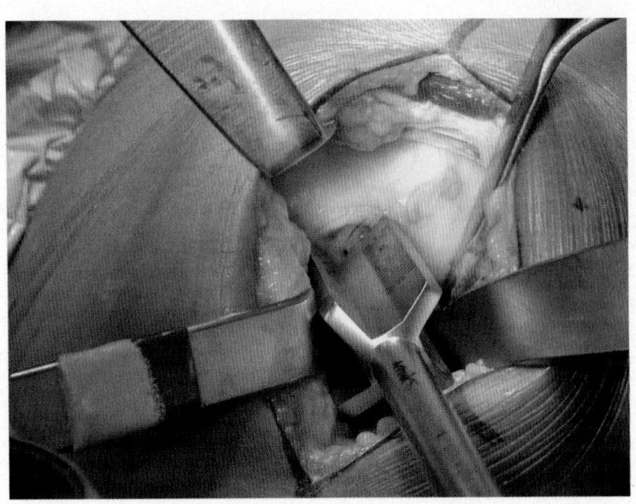

FIGURE 34-6

The cutting reamer placed over the guidewire with soft tissues well protected.

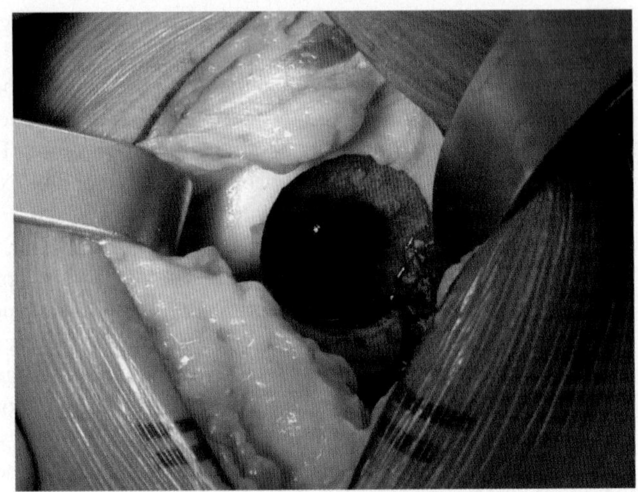

FIGURE 34-7

Recipient socket after preparation. Note the minimal depth.

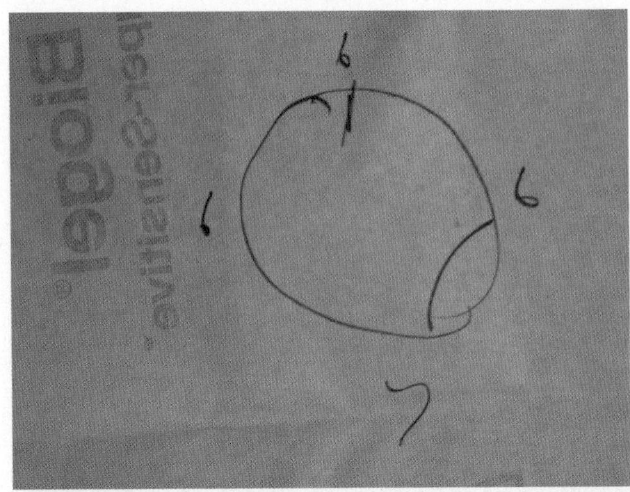

FIGURE 34-8

Depth map of recipient site. The position of the free edge is marked.

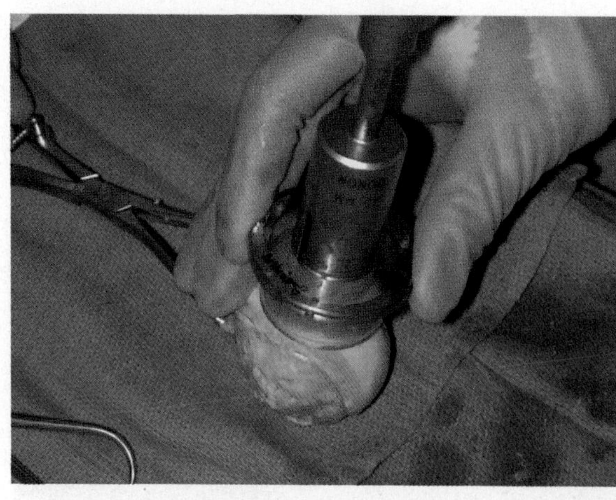

FIGURE 34-9

Harvesting of the plug from the allograft condyle. The graft and guide are held as one unit.

of the recipient site then is identified on the graft. In cases of size or shape mismatch between the recipient and graft condyles, it is appropriate to harvest a graft anywhere on the condyle that provides the best contour match. The graft is placed into a graft holder (or alternately, held with bone-holding forceps). A saw guide then is placed in the appropriate position, again perpendicular to the articular surface; and an appropriate-sized graft harvesting reamer is used to core out the graft (Figs. 34-9 and 34-10). Prior to removing the graft from the condyle, an identifying mark is made to ensure proper orientation. Once the graft is removed, depth measurements, which were taken from the recipient, are transferred to the graft; this graft then is cut with an oscillating saw and then is trimmed with a rasp to the appropriate thickness in all four quadrants (Figs. 34-11 and 34-12). Often, this must be done multiple times to ensure precise thickness and to match the prepared defect in the patient.

The graft now is irrigated copiously with a high-pressure lavage to remove all marrow elements, and the recipient site is dilated to ease the insertion of the graft and to prevent excessive impact loading of the articular surface when the graft is inserted. At this point, any remaining osseous defects are grafted.

The graft is then inserted by hand in the appropriate rotation and is gently tamped in place until it is flush (Figs. 34-13 and 34-14). Recent studies have shown that impact loading during insertion of osteochondral grafts causes chondrocyte death (1). Thus, gentle manual pressure followed by joint range of motion may be a more reasonable method of graft insertion. If the graft does not fit, refashioning of either the recipient site (deepening or dilating) or the graft itself (tapering or thinning) is performed carefully. An excessively tight fit is not necessary. We accept mismatches of no more than 1 mm from flush with the surrounding joint surfaces and avoid countersinking of the graft. Retaining bone from the defect preparation process is valuable, and this can be used for autografting cysts or building up the recipient site if the graft is inadvertently too thin for the recipient site depth.

Once the graft is seated, a determination is made whether additional fixation is required. If the graft is captured and not rocking with direct pressure, then no further fixation is generally required. Absorbable polydioxanone pins or chondral darts can be used, particularly if the graft is large or

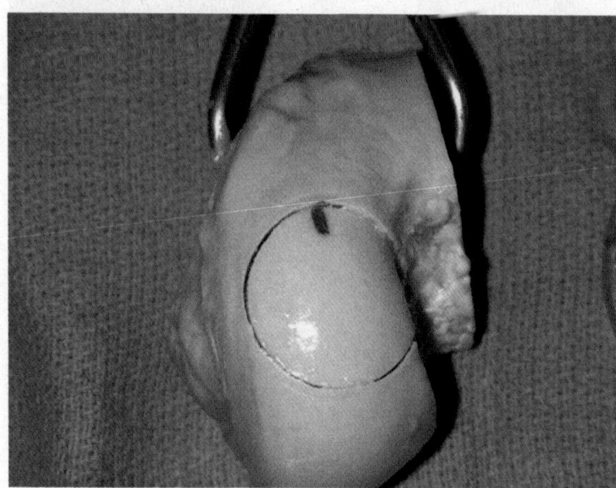

FIGURE 34-10

Allograft plug is marked and ready for removal from condyle.

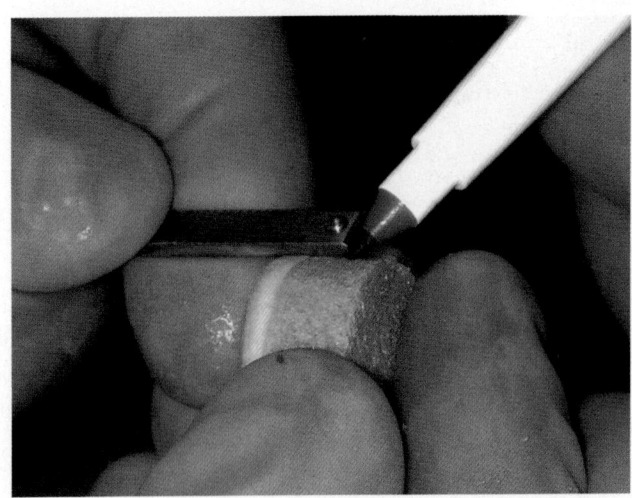

FIGURE 34-11

Depth measurements from the recipient socket are transferred to the plug.

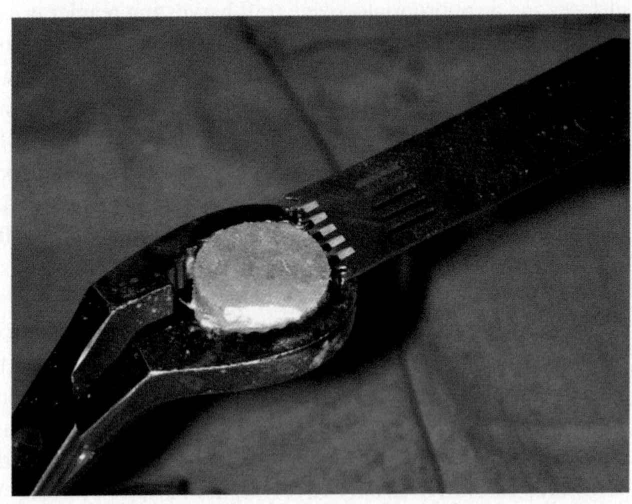

FIGURE 34-12

Allograft plug is trimmed carefully to the appropriate thickness.

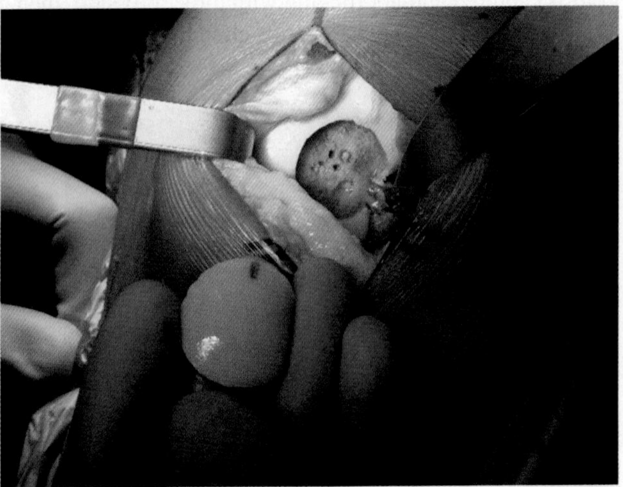

FIGURE 34-13

After lavage, the graft is ready for implantation. Correct rotation is determined.

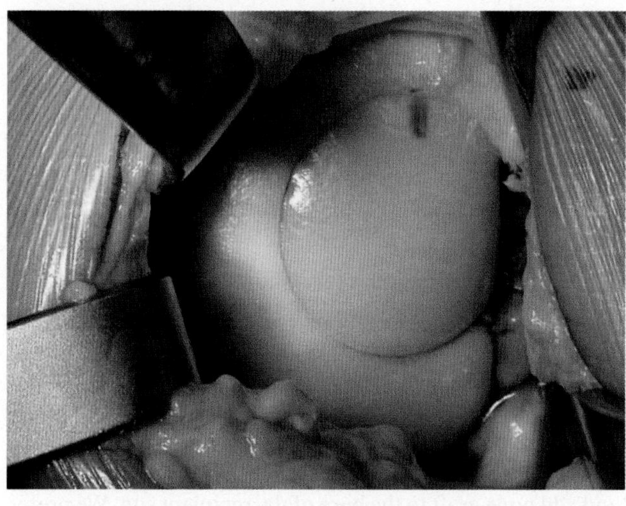

FIGURE 34-14

The graft is seated, and rotation, step-off, and stability are checked. At this time, the joint is carried through a range of motion to completely seat the graft.

has an exposed edge within the notch (Fig. 34-15). We have used small diameter absorbable pins through the graft surface for years without any deleterious effect; however, we currently rarely use any additional fixation for typical plug grafts. Occasionally, the graft needs to be trimmed in the notch region to prevent impingement. The knee is then brought through a complete range of motion to confirm that the graft is stable and no catching or soft-tissue obstruction is noted. At this point, the wound is irrigated copiously, and routine closure is performed. We typically use a small drain for 24 hours to prevent painful hemarthrosis from developing.

Lesions of the trochlea and patella are approached in a similar manner; however, these are much more technically challenging, as the anatomy of the patellofemoral joint is much more complex, leading to technical issues in creating symmetric matching recipient sites and donor grafts. In this setting, extensive care must be taken to match the anatomic location and the angle of approach.

PEARLS AND PITFALLS

- Preoperative assessment of the biological and mechanical environment of the joint are critical. Be sure of the necessity of concomitant procedures, such as finding and removing loose bodies, meniscectomy or repair, anterior cruciate ligament reconstruction, and osteotomy.
- Adequate confirmation of appropriateness of the lesion for fresh osteochondral allografting is necessary. Don't be surprised by new or enlarging lesions.
- A careful, informed consent process, including risks of infection and disease transmission, should be in place.
- Confirm graft recipient match in both size and side. Do this before induction of anesthesia.

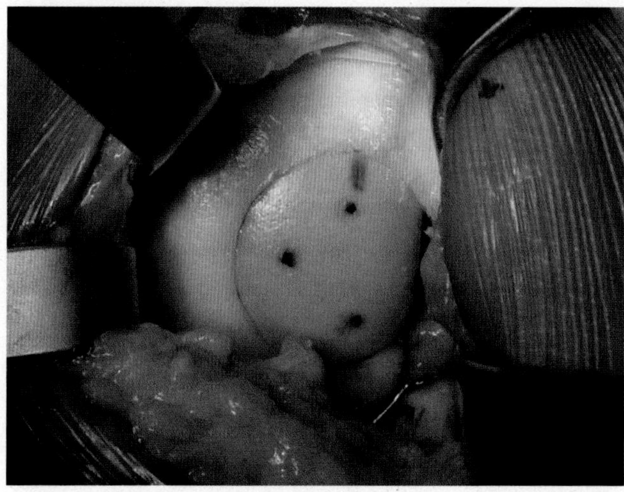

FIGURE 34-15

Three PDS pins have been placed through the graft for additional fixation.

- Inspect the allograft before making an incision. If it is a small graft, don't try to make a big plug (30 mm) from it. The curvature will not match the recipient condyle.
- All cutting instruments should contact the condyle (recipient and graft) perpendicular to the articular surface.
- Use reamers rather than drills for all cutting and irrigate copiously.
- Save reamings for possible bone grafting.
- For in-between sizes, always start preparing for the smaller graft. One can always enlarge the recipient site. Avoid removing too much normal cartilage.
- Two or more plug grafts can be placed overlapping for large lesions (snowman technique).
- Be prepared to use a freehand (shell graft) technique, if necessary, for large or posterior lesions.
- Minimize the osseous portion of the allograft at 3 to 6 mm. Use bone graft from the recipient site reaming (or the allograft) to fill any deeper defects.
- Always remove all soft tissue and perform pressurized lavage of graft prior to insertion.
- Avoid excessive impacting of the graft during insertion. Loose fitting grafts can be pinned.
- Use adjunctive fixation, including absorbable pins, chondral darts, or even screws.
- If the graft ends up too thin, remove it and add bone graft to the base of the recipient site. We prefer the graft flush, but 1 mm proud is better than 1 mm countersunk.
- Adequate and prolonged quadriceps rehabilitation is essential. Often, these patients are multiply operated and have had a long period of disability prior to allografting.
- Nonunion of the graft is very rare. Late fragmentation is a more common event.

POSTOPERATIVE MANAGEMENT AND REHABILITATION

The rehabilitation of the knee allograft patient in the early postoperative period includes management of pain, swelling, restoration of limb control, and range of motion. Assuming rigid graft fixation, patients are limited to 25% weight bearing for 4 to 8 weeks postoperatively, or until bony union is determined by radiographs. We are currently allowing accelerated weight bearing for small contained lesions. For femoral condyle allografts, no bracing is needed; but if an osteotomy is performed, a hinged range-of-motion brace is used for protection until healing is apparent. Weight bearing is progressed slowly between the second and fourth month, with full weight bearing using a cane or crutch. Continuous passive motion is not used, but we encourage early use of cycling in the rehabilitation process. The main objective is restoration of range of motion and strengthening of the quadriceps/hamstrings using isometric exercises and avoidance of open chain exercises. We believe one of the great advantages of OCA is the simple and relatively rapid recovery. Since the grafts are fully mature hyaline cartilage with stable fixation, requiring only bone healing for healing, there is little need for complex and extended rehabilitation protocols such as those used for microfracture or autologous chondrocyte implantation.

Clinical follow-up includes radiographs at 4 to 6 weeks, 3 months, 6 months, and yearly thereafter. Careful radiographic assessment of the graft-host interface is important. Any concern of delayed healing or incomplete functional recovery should lead to a more cautious approach to weight bearing and other high-stress activities. We generally see radiographic evidence of osseous union by 8 to 16 weeks.

Patients will typically experience continued improvement over the first postoperative year and often continue to demonstrate functional improvement between years 1 and 2. This often depends on patient motivation, desired activity level, and adherence to a rehabilitation program. Return to sports and recreational activities is individualized in the period between 3 and 6 months year (Table 34-2).

TABLE 34-2 Postoperative Management of Femoral Condyle Allografts

1. Partial weight bearing, 4–8 wk
2. Range-of-motion restoration
3. Quadriceps contraction exercises
4. Stationary bicycle at 2–4 wk
5. Progressive weight bearing beginning at 4–8 wk
6. Sports/recreation at 3–6 mo

COMPLICATIONS

Early complications unique to the allografting procedure are few. There does not appear to be any increased risk of surgical site infection with the use of allografts as compared with other procedures. The most unique issue regarding possible postoperative complications with fresh allografts relates to transmission of disease from the graft itself. In our series of over 1,000 allografts, we have yet to record a graft-associated bacterial or viral infection.

The use of a miniarthrotomy in the knee theoretically increases the risk of postoperative stiffness. Occasionally, one sees a persistent effusion, which is typically a sign of over use, but which may indicate an inflammatory synovitis. Delayed union or nonunion of the fresh allograft is the most common early finding. This is evidenced by persistent discomfort and/or visible graft-host interface on serial radiographic evaluation. Delayed or nonunion is more common in larger grafts or in the setting of compromised bone, such as in the treatment of osteonecrosis. In this setting, patience is essential, as complete healing or recovery may take an extended period. Decreasing activities and prolonging weight-bearing precautions are appropriate interventions. In this setting, careful evaluation of serial radiographs can provide insight into the healing process. MRI scans are rarely helpful, particularly before 6 months postoperatively, as they typically show extensive signal abnormality that is difficult to interpret. CT scans can be useful as they provide more information about the bone interface and healing of the graft. It should be noted that with adequate attention to postoperative weight-bearing restrictions and adequate graft fixation, delayed or nonunion requiring repeat surgical intervention within the first year is extremely uncommon. The natural history of the graft that fails to osseointegrate is unpredictable. Clinical symptoms may be minimal, or there may be progressive clinical deterioration and radiographic evidence of fragmentation, fracture, or collapse. Typical symptoms of this type of graft failure include increased pain or sudden onset, often associated with minor trauma. Effusion, crepitus, or focal, localized pain is commonly seen. Careful evaluation of serial radiographs typically will demonstrate collapse, subsidence, fracture, or fragmentation. Fresh OCAs rarely fail due to the cartilage portion of the graft; most failures originate within the osseous portion. It is important to note that the allografted joint may suffer from the same pathology that is present in any other joint, such as meniscus or ligamentous injury or even another cartilage injury. It should also be noted that radiographic and magnetic resonance abnormalities are commonly noted, even in well-functioning allografts, and great care must be taken in interpreting and correlating the imaging studies with clinical findings.

Treatment options for failed allografts include observation, if the patient is minimally symptomatic and the joint is thought to be at low risk for further progression of disease. Arthroscopic evaluation and debridement also may be used. In many cases, revision allografting is performed and generally has led to a success rate equivalent to primary allografting. This appears to be one of the particular advantages to fresh osteochondral allografting, in that fresh allografting does not preclude a revision allograft as a salvage procedure for failure of the initial allograft.

RESULTS

In general, OCA has demonstrated good to excellent outcomes for the treatment of idiopathic focal chondral or osteochondral lesions of the femoral condyles. This technique has shown a 5-year survival rate of 77.5% to 100%, a 10-year survival rate of 71% to 85%, and survival of 74% at up to 15 years. Worse results are seen with bipolar lesions, larger lesions, increasing patient age, chronic lesions, uncorrected malalignment, and worker's compensation. Results are also favorable for the diagnoses of OCD and steroid-associated osteonecrosis, with each demonstrating graft survival rates of 89% to 91% at up to 5 years (Table 34-3).

SUMMARY

Fresh OCA plugs are useful for a wide variety of chondral and osteochondral lesions of the femoral condyle of the knee. The surgical technique is straightforward but does require special instruments and careful attention to detail. Postoperative management is not complex and complications are uncommon.

TABLE 34-3 Clinical Outcomes of Osteochondral Allografting in the Knee

Author/Year	Number of Patients	Knee Location	Follow-up Time (Mean and Range) Years	Age (Mean and Range/SD) Years	Main Outcome: Type Outcome	Main Outcome: Preoperative Score (Mean or Range)	Main Outcome: Postoperative Score (Mean and Range)	Failure (*n* [%])	Comments
Gracitelli et al./2014 (5)	27 (28 knees)	PF	9.7 (1.8–30.1)	33.6 (14–64)	IKDC	36.5	66.5[a]	8 (28.5%)	45% required further surgeries (not failures)
Meric et al./2014 (6)	46 (48 knees)	TF, PF	7 (2–19.7)	40 (15–66)	IKDC pain IKDC function	7.5 ± 2.2 3.4 ± 1.5	4.7 ± 3.1[a] 7.0 ± 2.0[a]	22 (46%)	Bipolar lesions
Murphy et al./2014 (7)	39 patients/43 knees	MFC, LFC, plateau, patella, trochlea	8.4 (1.7–27.1)	16.4 (11.0–17.9)	IKDC	42.0 ± 16.6	75.2 ± 20.2[a]	5 (11.6%)	88% good/excellent results
Shaha et al/2013 (8)	38	MFC, LFC	4.1 (1–9)	29.83 ± 5.3	KOOS	N/A	249.51 ± 51.26	0	Disappointing results in an active-duty population
Horton et al./2013 (9)	33	MFC, LFC, plateau, patella, trochlea	10 (2.4–26)	33 (16–64)	IKDC	NA	70.5 (25–95)	13 (39%)	Only revised allografts
Giorgini et al./2013 (10)	11	MFC, LFC, plateau, "kissing lesion"	2.2 (1–4.5)	34 (18–66)	IKDC	27.4 ± 14.9	47.4 ± 15.7	1 (9%)	Short follow-up time
Raz et al./2014 (11)	58	MFC, LFC	21.8 (15–32)	28 (11–48)	HSS	NA	86 at 15 y	13 (22.4%)	62% of concomitant realignment procedure
Krych et al./2012 (12)	43	MFC, LFC, trochlea	2.5 (1–11)	33 (18–49)	IKDC	46.3 ± 14.9	79.3 ± 15.5[a]	No failure	NA
Levy et al./2012 (13)	122 (129 knees)	MFC, LFC	13.5 (2.4–27.5)	32.8 (15–68)	IKDC pain IKDC function	7.0 ± 1.9 3.4 ± 1.3	3.8 ± 2.9 7.2 ± 2.0[a]	31 (24%)	Largest cohort
Scully et al./2011 (14)	18	MFC, LFC	3.4	27 (30–35)	Return to duty	NA	9 of 16 completed MEB; 1 of 12 soldiers returned to combat duty; 1 retired; 1 was considered noncombatant	0	Short follow-up time
Gortz et al./2010 (15)	22 (28 knees)	MFC, LFC, bicondylar	5.6 (2–19.5)	24.3 (16–44)	IKDC pain IKDC function	7.1 3.5	2.0[a] 8.3[a]	5 (18%)	Steroid-associated osteonecrosis
La Prade et al./2009 (16)	23	MFC, LFC, multiple	3 (1.9–4)	31 (18–47)	IKDC	52	68.5[a]	0	
Rue et al./2008 (17)	30 (31 knees)	MFC, LFC	2.9 (1.9–5)	37 (20–48)	IKDC	31.4 ± 12.8	57.1 ± 17.8[a]	2 (6.4%)	Combined meniscal allograft transplantation and cartilage restoration procedures

Pearsall et al./2008 (18)	48	MFC, LFC, trochlea, patella	3.08 (2–5.2)	46 (16–71)	KSS	112.8	154.2[a]	9 (19%)	Mixed population (autograft, allograft fresh, and frozen)
Davidson et al./2007 (19)	67	MFC, trochlea, MFC + trochlea	3.3 (1.6–5)	33 (21–48)	IKDC	27 (9–55)	79 (56–99)[a]	NA	Also included histological study
McCulloch et al./2007 (20)	25	MFC, LFC, multiple	2.9 (2–5.6)	35 (17–49)	IKDC	29	58	2 (8%)	Meniscal transplant included
Williams et al./2007 (21)	19	MFC, LFC	2.9 (2–5.6)	34 (19–49)	ADLS	56 ± 24 (20–100)	70 ± 22 (30–98)[a]	4 (21%)	NA
Emmerson et al./2007 (22)	64 (66 knees)	MFC, LFC	7.7 (2–22)	29 (15–54)	Merle D'Aubigné-Postel	3.0 ± 1.7	16.4 ± 2.0[a]	5 (7.5%)	70% good or excellent results
Gross et al./2005 (23)	60	MFC, LFC, plateau	MFC/LFC, 10 (4.8–21.5); plateau, 11.8 (2–24)	FC, 27 (15–47); TP, 43 (26–69)	HSS	NA	FC, 83; plateau, 85.3 ± 11	FC, 12 (60%), Plateau 21 (65%)	Survival analysis revealed 95% survival at 5 y, 80% at 10 y, and 65% at 15 y
Jamali et al./2005	18 (20 knees)	Patella, trochlea	7.8 (2–17.8)	42 (19–64)	Merle D'Aubigné-Postel	11.7 (7–15)	16.3 (12–18)[a]	5 (20%)	8 patients were extremely satisfied and 6 were satisfied

REFERENCES

1. Sherman SL, Garrity J, Bauer KL, et al. Fresh osteochondral allograft transplantation for the knee: current concepts review. *J Am Acad Orthop Surg.* 2014;22(2):121–133.
2. Bugbee WB, Pallante-Kichura AL, Gortz S, et al. Osteochondral allograft transplantation in cartilage repair: graft storage paradigm, translational models and clinical applications. *J Orthop Res.* 2016;34(1):31–38.
3. Gracitelli GC, Meric GM, Briggs D, et al. Fresh osteochondral allografts in the knee: comparison of primary transplantation versus transplantation after failure of previous subchondral marrow stimulation. *Am J Sports Med.* 2015;43(4):885–891.
4. Mologne TS, Cory E, Hansen BC, et al. Osteochondral allograft transplant to the medial femoral condyle using a medial or lateral femoral condyle allograft: is there a difference in graft sources? *Am J Sports Med.* 2014;42(9):2205–2213.
5. Gracitelli GC, Meric GM, Pulido PA, et al. Fresh osteochondral allograft transplantation for isolated patellar cartilage injury. *Am J Sports Med.* 2015;43(4):879–884.
6. Meric GM, Gracitelli GC, Pulido PA, et al. Fresh osteochondral allograft transplantation for bipolar reciprocal osteochondral lesions of the knee. *Am J Sports Med.* 2015;43(3):709–714.
7. Murphy RT, Pennock AT, Bugbee WD. Osteochondral allograft transplantation of the knee in the pediatric and adolescent population. *Am J Sports Med.* 2014;42(3):635–640.
8. Shaha JS, Cook JB, Rowles DJ, et al. Return to an athletic lifestyle after osteochondral allograft transplantation of the knee. *Am J Sports Med.* 2013;41:2083–2089.
9. Horton MT, Pulido PA, McCauley JC, et al. Revision osteochondral allograft transplantations: do they work? *Am J Sports Med.* 2013;41(11):2507–2511.
10. Giorgini A, Donati D, Cevolani L, et al. Fresh osteochondral allograft is a suitable alternative for wide cartilage defect in the knee. *Injury.* 2013;44(suppl 1):S16–S20.
11. Raz G, Safir OA, Backstein DJ, et al. Distal femoral fresh osteochondral allografts: follow-up at a mean of twenty-two years. *J Bone Joint Surg Am.* 2014;96(13):1101–1107.
12. Krych AJ, Robertson CM, Williams RJ III, et al. Return to athletic activity after osteochondral allograft transplantation in the knee. *Am J Sports Med.* 2012;40(5):1053–1059.
13. Levy YD, Gortz S, Pulido PA, et al. Do fresh osteochondral allografts successfully treat femoral condyle lesions? *Clin Orthop Relat Res.* 2013;471(1):231–237.
14. Scully WF, Parada SA, Arrington ED. Allograft osteochondral transplantation in the knee in the active duty population. *Mil Med.* 2011;176(10):1196–1201.
15. Gortz S, De Young AJ, Bugbee WD. Fresh osteochondral allografting for steroid-associated osteonecrosis of the femoral condyles. *Clin Orthop Relat Res.* 2010;468(5):1269–1278.
16. LaPrade RF, Botker J, Herzog M, et al. Refrigerated osteoarticular allografts to treat articular cartilage defects of the femoral condyles. A prospective outcomes study. *J Bone Joint Surg Am.* 2009;91(4):805–811.
17. Rue JP, Kilcoyne K, Dickens J. Complex knee problems in a young, active duty military population. Part I: ACL reconstruction, allograft OATS, and treatment of meniscal injuries. *J Knee Surg.* 2011;24(2):71.
18. Pearsall AW, Madanagopal SG, Hughey JT. Osteoarticular autograft and allograft transplantation of the knee: 3 year follow-up. *Orthopedics.* 2008;31(1):73.
19. Davidson PA, Rivenburgh DW, Dawson PE, et al. Clinical, histologic, and radiographic outcomes of distal femoral resurfacing with hypothermically stored osteoarticular allografts. *Am J Sports Med.* 2007;35(7):1082–1090.
20. McCulloch PC, Kang RW, Sobhy MH, et al. Prospective evaluation of prolonged fresh osteochondral allograft transplantation of the femoral condyle: minimum 2-year follow-up. *Am J Sports Med.* 2007;35(3):411–420.
21. Williams RJ III, Ranawat AS, Potter HG, et al. Fresh stored allografts for the treatment of osteochondral defects of the knee. *J Bone Joint Surg Am.* 2007;89(4):718–726.
22. Emmerson BC, Gortz S, Jamali AA, et al. Fresh osteochondral allografting in the treatment of osteochondritis dissecans of the femoral condyle. *Am J Sports Med.* 2007;35(6):907–914.
23. Gross AE, Shasha N, Aubin P. Long-term followup of the use of fresh osteochondral allografts for posttraumatic knee defects. *Clin Orthop Relat Res.* 2005;435:79–87.
24. Jamali AA, Emmerson BC, Chung C, et al. Fresh osteochondral allografts: results in the patellofemoral joint. *Clin Orthop Relat Res.* 2005;437:176–185.

35 Surgical Techniques for Osteochondritis Dissecans in the Skeletally Immature

James L. Carey, Zachary B. Domont, and Theodore J. Ganley

Osteochondritis dissecans (OCD) is an important condition involving the focal alteration of subchondral bone with a risk for instability of a bony progeny fragment and the adjacent articular cartilage from the surrounding parent bone. This chapter considers the treatment of OCD in the setting of open physes about the knee.

The surgeon should ask the child about the presence and frequency of pain and mechanical symptoms (catching and locking). Physical examination of the knee should assess for range of motion, effusion, point tenderness, and palpable crepitus. X-rays and an MRI provide meaningful information about the status of the physis and specific features of the OCD lesion.

With respect to stability, the following features on MRI are associated with instability: high-intensity signal between the progeny fragment and the parent bone, cysts and edema in the adjacent parent bone, and radially oriented low-intensity signal within the articular cartilage at the margins of the lesion.

For a stable-appearing OCD lesion in a skeletally immature patient, Wall et al. developed a nomogram for predicting probability of healing following nonoperative treatment, using normalized lesion length, normalized lesion width, and symptoms (1). This estimated probability of healing can inform the shared decision-making process. Ultimately, the surgeon, the patient, and the patient's family discuss this value in the context of all other factors and decide if this probability is acceptable or not.

INDICATIONS FOR SURGERY

- An OCD lesion that appears unstable
- An OCD lesion that appears stable but there is an unacceptable probability of healing
- An OCD lesion that appears stable and there was initially an acceptable probability of healing, but the lesion failed to demonstrate any appreciable healing following at least 3 months of nonsurgical treatment

CONTRAINDICATIONS FOR SURGERY

- Active infection
- Advanced arthritis (very rare in children)
- Inadequate trial of nonoperative treatment measures, when appropriate

PREOPERATIVE PLANNING

In these cases, it is important that the patient and the family understand that the final treatment decisions are often made at the time of surgery.

Specifically, arthroscopy inspection and probing will reveal whether the progeny fragment is immobile or mobile with respect to the surrounding parent bone and cartilage.

Further, a fragment can be classified as salvageable or nonsalvageable. A salvageable fragment can be saved by definition. A fragment is typically considered salvageable when it has sufficient bone underlying the articular cartilage, has essentially intact overlying articular cartilage, and consists of one major fragment.

SCENARIO 1: IMMOBILE, SALVAGEABLE PROGENY

Surgical Procedure—Drilling

- Arthroscopically confirm that the OCD lesion is not mobile. The margin may be subtly demarcated.
- For transarticular drilling (Fig. 35-1)
  - Place a drill sleeve or a cannula through the portal to protect the soft tissue.
  - Advance a 0.062-in (1.6-mm) diameter drill into the center of the OCD lesion to a sufficient depth to facilitate healing, without threatening the growth plate—typically about 15 mm or so.
  - Repeat with drill holes approximately 3 to 5 mm apart, covering the entire lesion.
  - Use a motorized shaver attached to suction to ensure that the articular surface is smooth and that all particles are removed.
- For retroarticular drilling
  - Bring fluoroscopy machine in position.
  - Make a small longitudinal incision and insert a 0.062-in (1.6-mm) diameter Kirschner wire, starting just distal to the growth plate and ending within the center of the OCD lesion. Do not advance through the articular cartilage.
  - Confirm placement into the center of the OCD lesion on AP and lateral imaging. Leave this wire in place as a guide for further wire placement.
  - Use a parallel wire guide to repeat with holes approximately 3 to 5 mm apart, covering the entire lesion.
- Arthroscopically confirm again that the OCD lesion is not mobile.

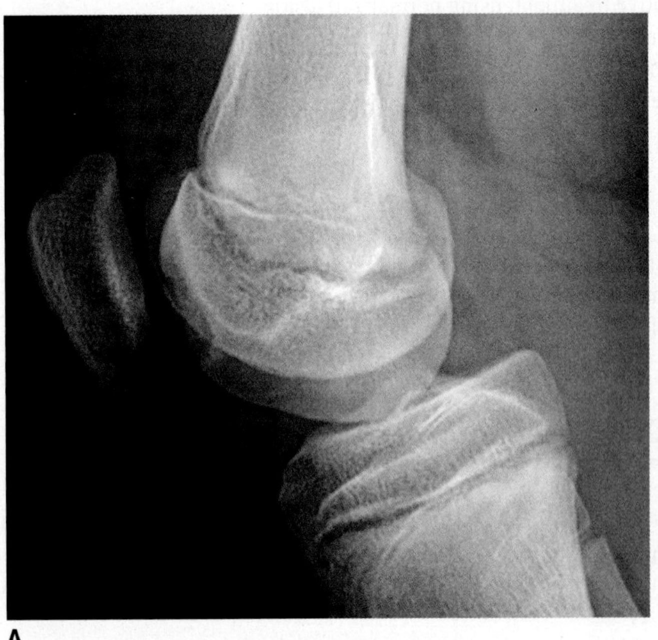

A

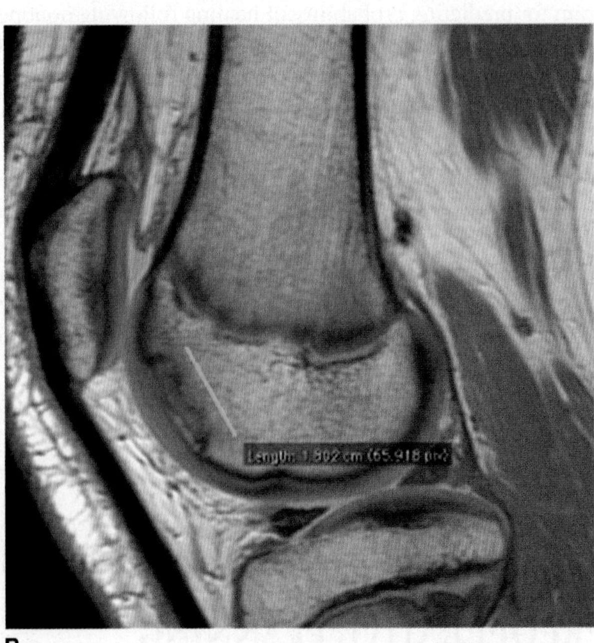

B

FIGURE 35-1

OCD of the trochlea in a 14-year-old boy. **A:** Lateral x-rays demonstrating the radiolucent region of the trochlea. **B:** MRI revealing no appreciable abnormality of the overlying articular cartilage.

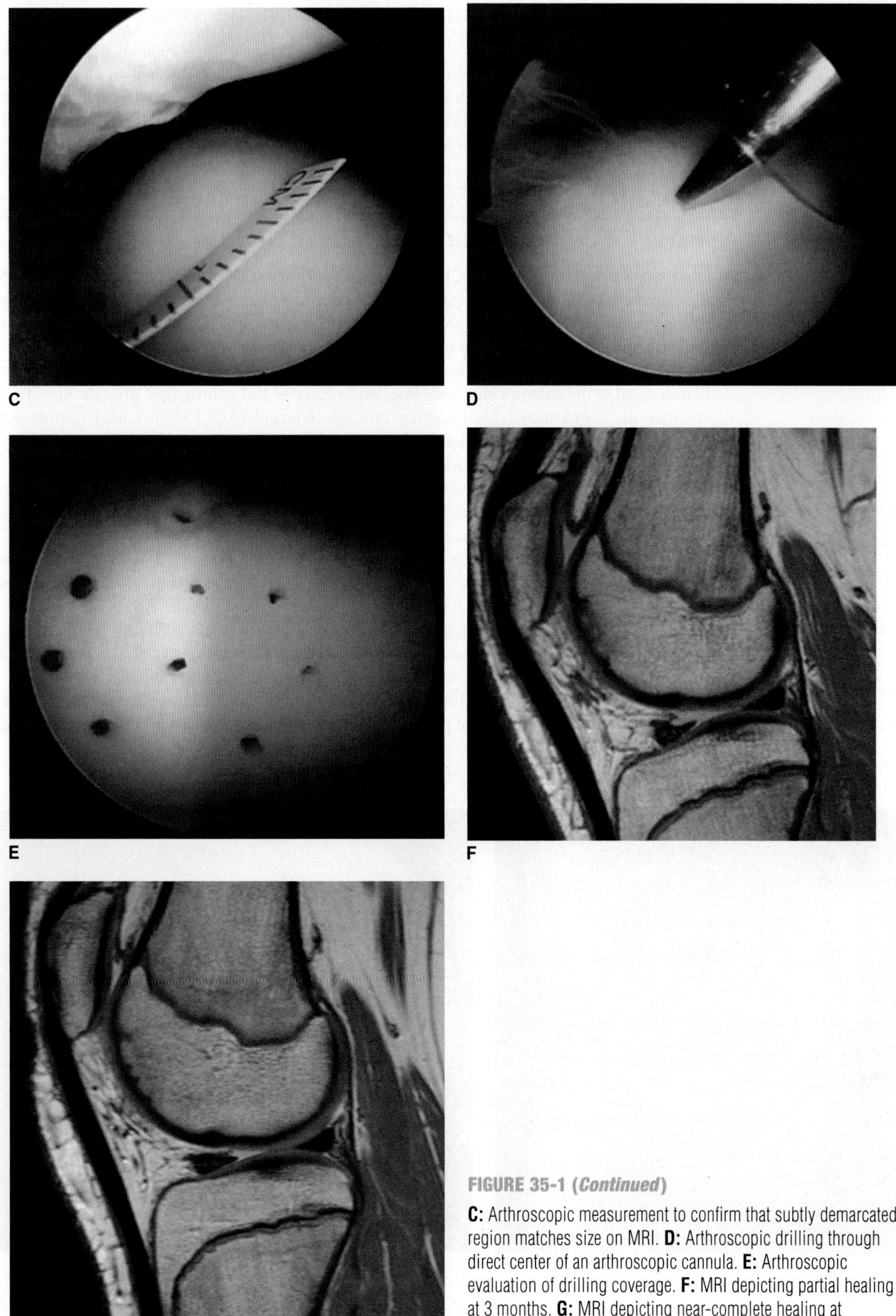

FIGURE 35-1 (*Continued*)

C: Arthroscopic measurement to confirm that subtly demarcated region matches size on MRI. **D:** Arthroscopic drilling through direct center of an arthroscopic cannula. **E:** Arthroscopic evaluation of drilling coverage. **F:** MRI depicting partial healing at 3 months. **G:** MRI depicting near-complete healing at 6 months.

Postoperative Management

Following drilling, the patient typically has protected weight bearing—touchdown (~25%) weight bearing—for 6 weeks. Motion is unlimited. After 6 weeks, an unloader brace is often used in order to minimize weight bearing through the affected compartment. Impact activities may be resumed after 12 weeks. After radiographic healing is confirmed and return-to-play criteria are met, contact and collision sports may be resumed after 18 weeks.

SCENARIO 2: MOBILE, SALVAGEABLE PROGENY

Surgical Procedure—Fixation with Bone Grafting

- Arthroscopically confirm that the OCD lesion is mobile. The archetypal OCD lesion of the medial femoral condyle can open like a trap door, hinging on some soft tissue about the posterior cruciate ligament.
- Through a parapatellar arthrotomy, carefully remove sclerotic and necrotic bone as well as fibrous tissue interposed between the parent bone and progeny fragment.
- Harvest autogenous cancellous bone from the ipsilateral proximal tibia from a region about 25 mm distal to the anteromedial joint line, using curettes and arthroscopic grasper. Specifically, penetrate the cortex near typical anterior cruciate ligament (ACL) tibial tunnel starting point, using a small curette. Serially dilate with larger curettes until the arthroscopic grasper can pass through. Place bone graft into sterile cup for later use.
- Drill periphery of the parent bone with a 0.062-in (1.6-mm) drill to facilitate the efflux of marrow elements to augment healing. Place bone graft into defect to fill void and facilitate healing without limiting ability for door to close completely.
- In the setting of adequate bone on the progeny fragment (i.e., bone >3 mm thick), fix fragment with variable pitch metallic screws (Herbert/Whipple Bone Screw, Zimmer, Warsaw, IN), which do not require subsequent removal (Fig. 35-2).
- In the setting of inadequate bone on the progeny fragment (i.e., bone <3 mm thick), fix fragment with 1.5-mm solid screws (Titanium Modular Hand System, Synthes, Paoli, PA), which do require removal about 8 weeks postoperatively. Of note, removal can most often be performed arthroscopically.
- Perform formal "approach and withdraw" with fluoroscopy machine to ensure no prominence of variable pitch screws and minimal prominence of regular screws, with respect to the subchondral bone.

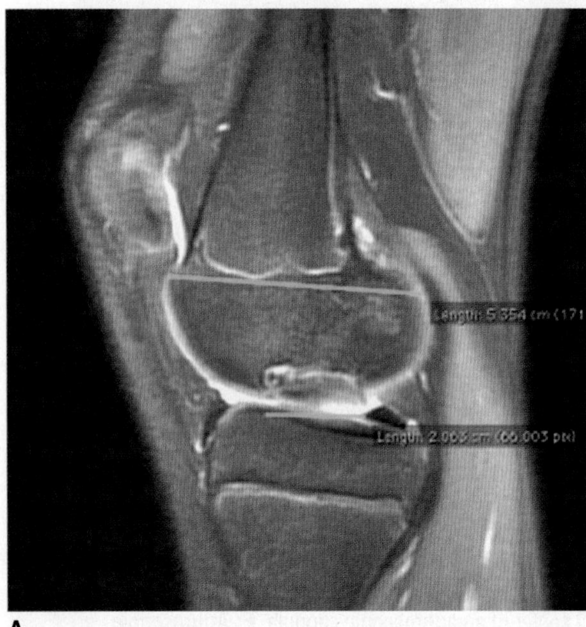

A

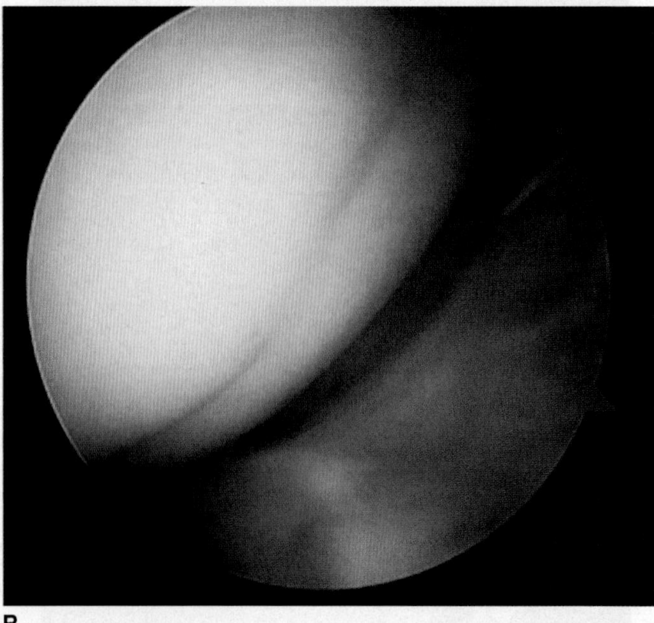

B

FIGURE 35-2

OCD of the medial femoral condyle in a 14-year-old girl. **A:** MRI depicting high-intensity signal between progeny fragment and parent bone. **B:** Arthroscopic evaluation of distinct margin.

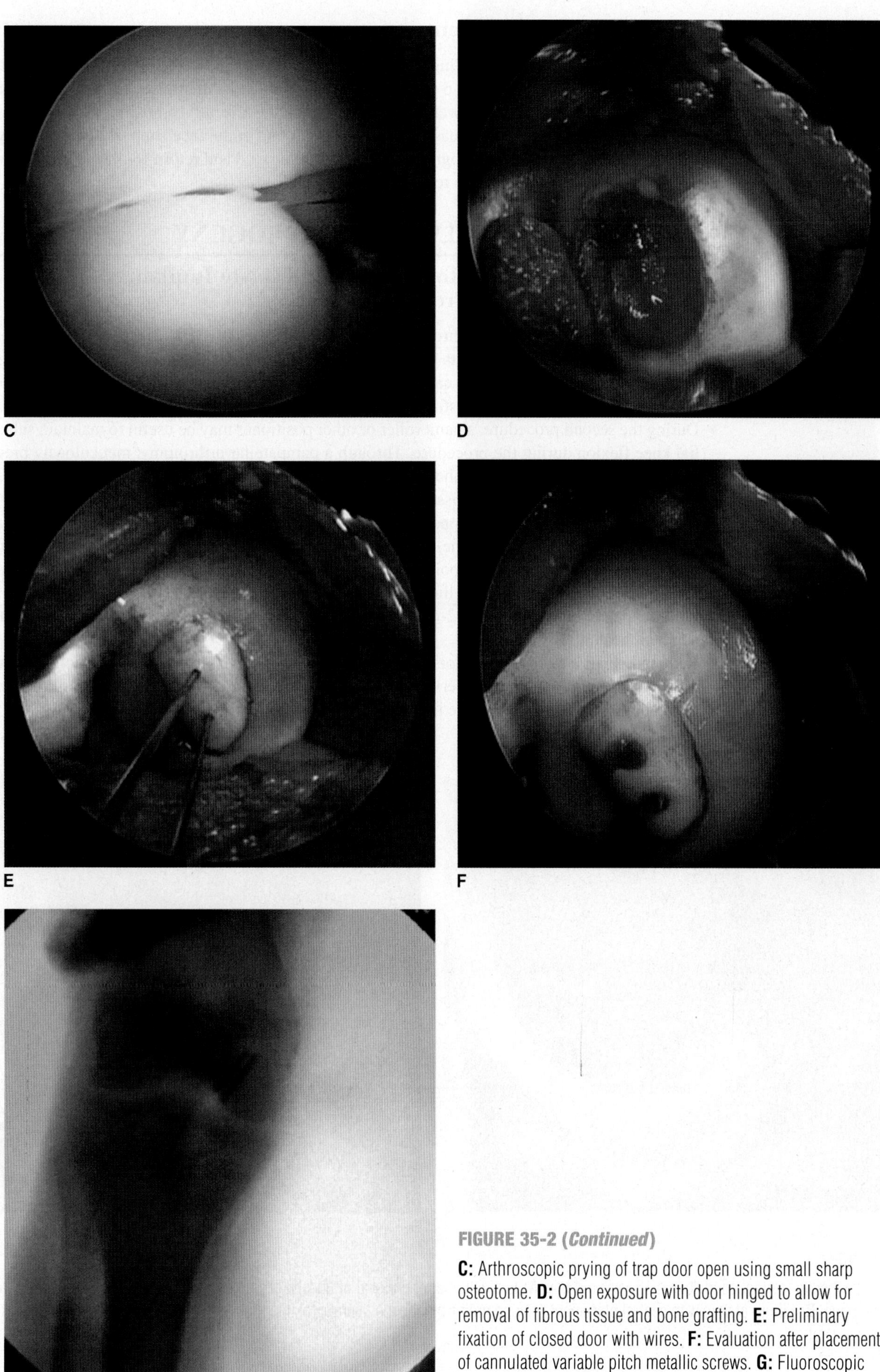

FIGURE 35-2 (*Continued*)

C: Arthroscopic prying of trap door open using small sharp osteotome. **D:** Open exposure with door hinged to allow for removal of fibrous tissue and bone grafting. **E:** Preliminary fixation of closed door with wires. **F:** Evaluation after placement of cannulated variable pitch metallic screws. **G:** Fluoroscopic view after dynamic approach and withdraw.

Postoperative Management

Following fixation with bone grafting, the patient typically has protected weight bearing—touch-down (~25%) weight bearing—for 6 weeks. Motion is unlimited. After 6 weeks, an unloader brace is often used in order to minimize weight bearing through the affected compartment.

After 3 months, the patient increases muscle strength and endurance. Impact activities may be resumed after 18 weeks. After radiographic healing is confirmed and return-to-play criteria are met, contact and collision sports may be resumed after 24 weeks.

SCENARIO 3: NONSALVAGEABLE PROGENY

Surgical Procedure—Autologous Chondrocyte Implantation with Bone Grafting (Staged Procedure)

- During the first procedure, arthroscopically confirm that the OCD lesion is unsalvageable. Remove any prominent fragments and smooth edges of defect with motorized shaved. Harvest a full-thickness biopsy of articular cartilage from the margin of the trochlea or intercondylar notch. Send the biopsy to the proper destination.
- During the second procedure, a paint roller or other positioner may be useful to maintain substantial knee flexion during the procedure. Through a parapatellar arthrotomy, meticulously prepare the OCD lesion removing all unhealthy articular cartilage, all sclerotic-appearing and necrotic-appearing bone, and all fibrous tissue from the deep and peripheral aspects (Fig. 35-3).
- Harvest autogenous cancellous bone from the ipsilateral proximal tibia from a region about 25 mm distal to the anteromedial joint line, using curettes and arthroscopic grasper. Specifically, penetrate the cortex near ACL tibial tunnel point, using a small curette. Serially dilate with larger curettes until the arthroscopic grasper can pass through. Place bone graft into sterile cup for later use.
- Drill the parent bone with a 0.062-in (1.6-mm) drill to facilitate the efflux of marrow elements to augment healing.
- Rethread small absorbable anchors (MICROFIX Anchors, DePuy Mitek, Raynham, MA) with 5-0 Vicryl suture (Ethicon, Somerville, NJ). Place these anchors circumferentially in the parent bone about 1 to 2 mm deep to the interface of the cartilage and subchondral bone.

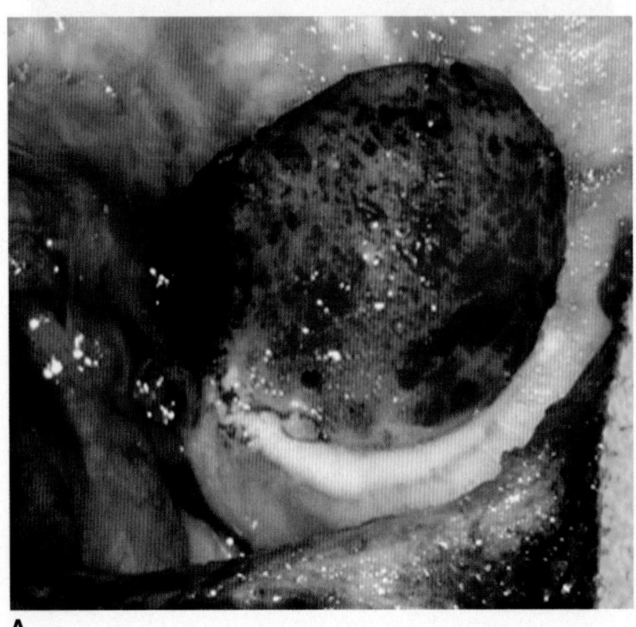
A

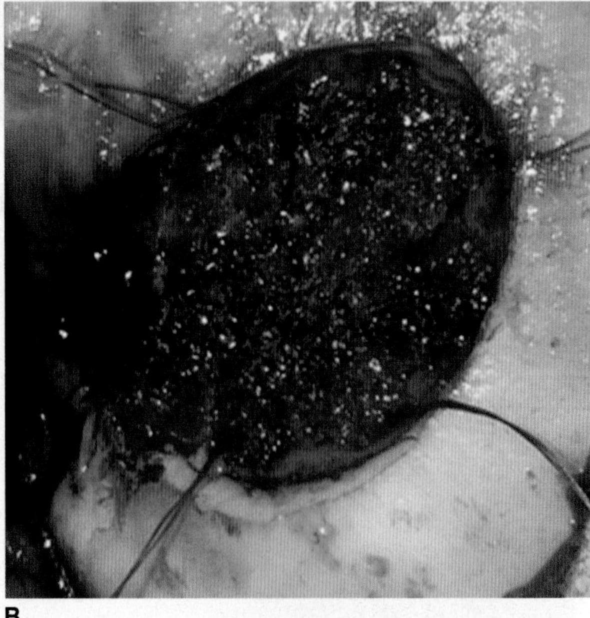
B

FIGURE 35-3

OCD of the medial femoral condyle in a 16-year-old boy. **A:** Evaluation after removal of unsalvageable progeny fragment, fibrous tissue, and sclerotic bone. **B:** Filling of void with central placement of bone graft from the ipsilateral proximal tibia and peripheral placement of four anchors with suture.

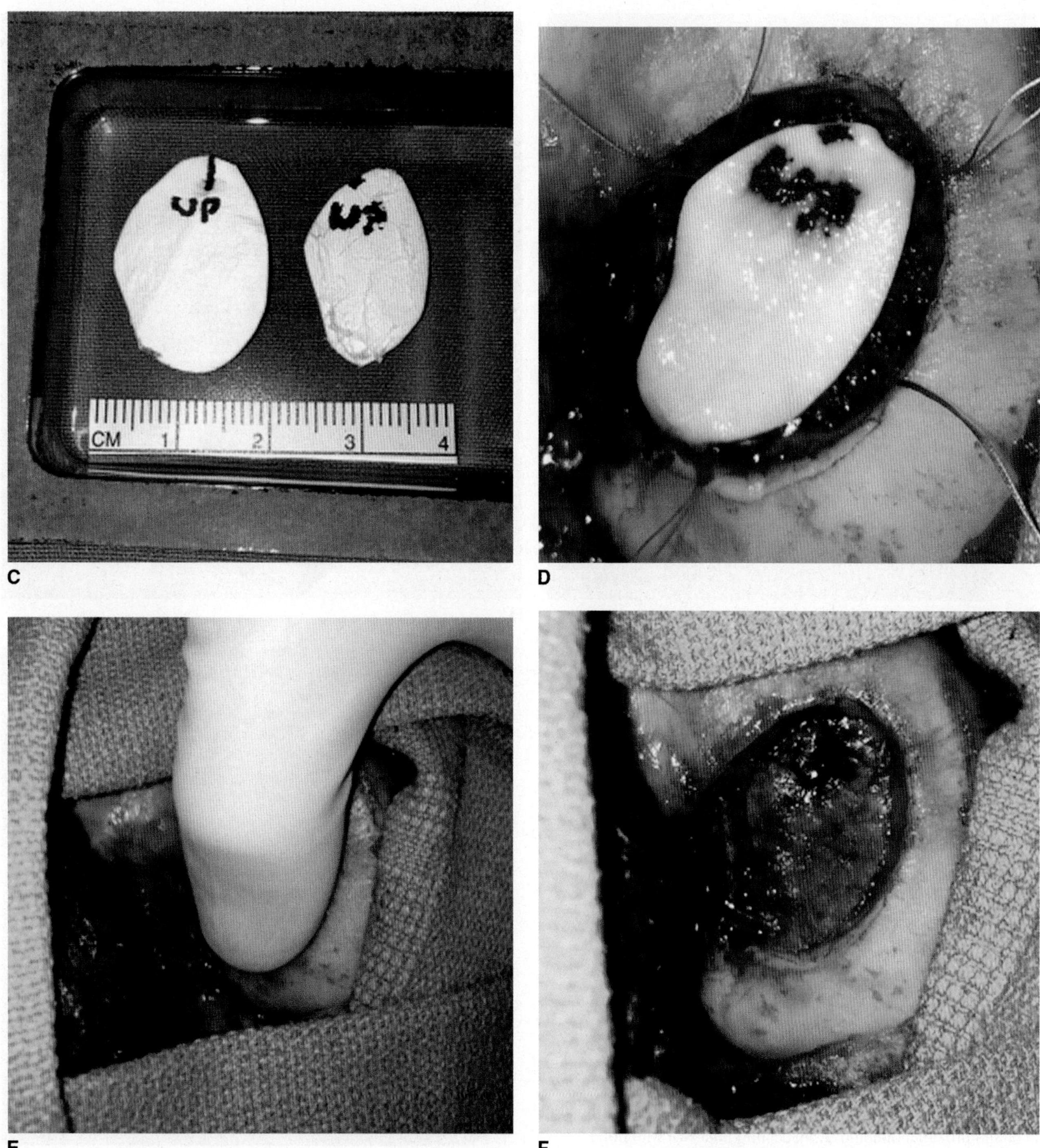

FIGURE 35-3 (*Continued*)

C: Superficial (**left**) and deep (**right**) collagen membranes with care taken to maintain orientation so that rough surfaces are adjacent to cells. **D:** Positioning of deep membrane over bone graft. **E:** Holding pressure for 30 seconds with the thumb after administration of fibrin sealant about periphery and deep surface of membrane. **F:** View after completion of bone grafting.

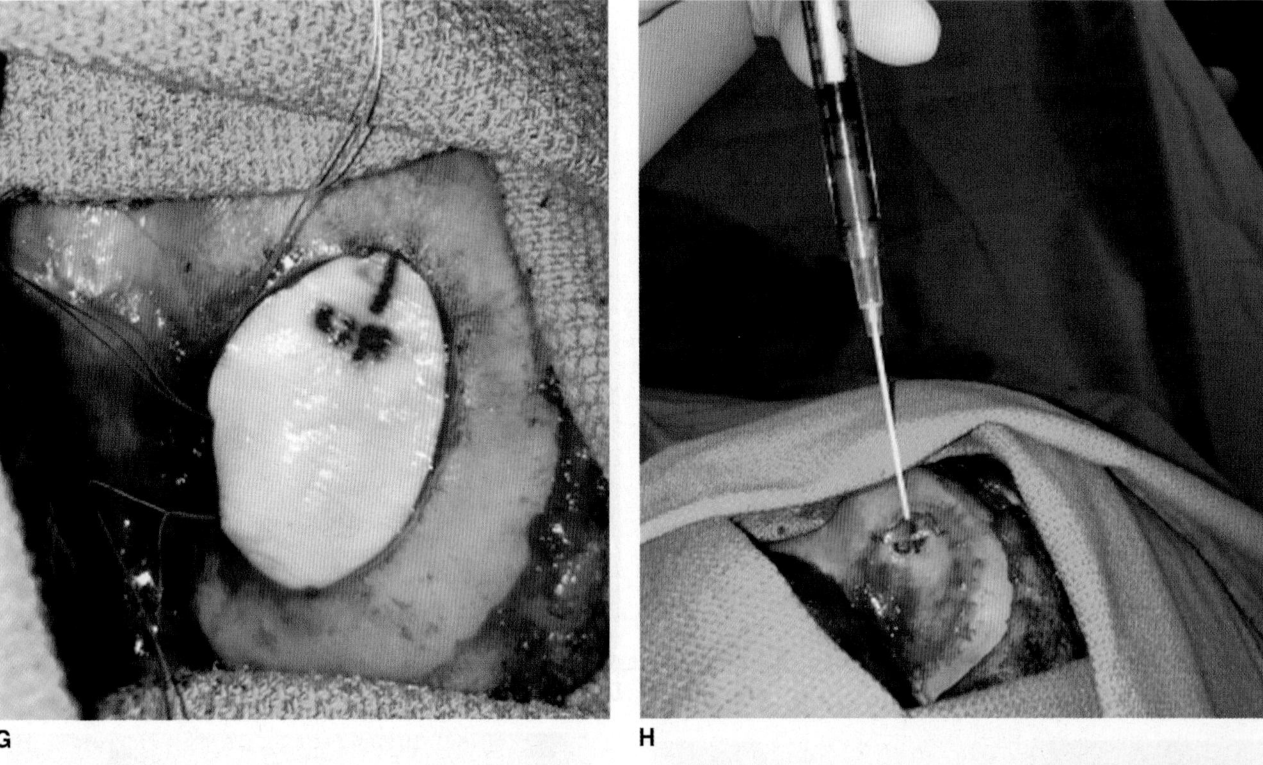

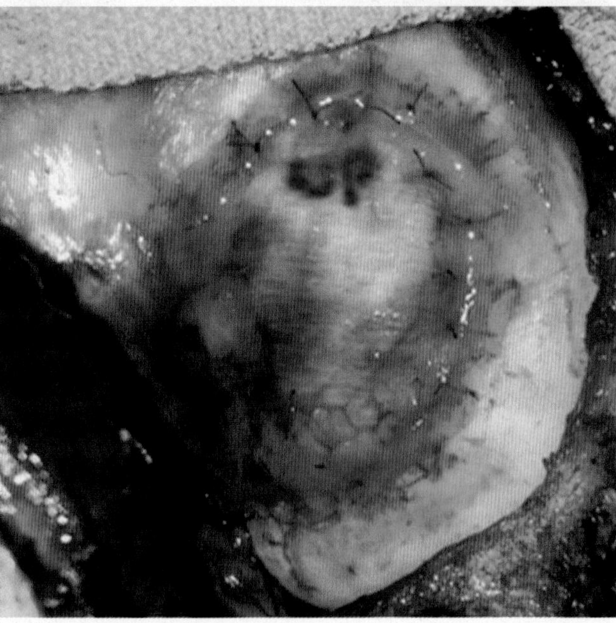

FIGURE 35-3 (*Continued*)

G: Positioning of superficial membrane and three anchors with suture in uncontained region about intercondylar notch. **H:** Injecting of cells in proximal opening. **I:** Inspecting final ACI with bone grafting.

- Place the bone graft into the defect. Impact with a tamp and mallet.
- Cut porcine-derived collagen cover (Bio-Gide, Geistlich Pharma, Princeton, NJ) before wetting since it is much easier to work with when dry. Plan for slight expansion when the membrane becomes wet. Secure over bone graft with the suture in the anchors.
- Place fibrin sealant (Tisseel, Baxter, Westlake Village, CA) deep to the membrane along the periphery to ensure separation of marrow elements and bleeding from implanted chondrocytes.
- Subsequently, autologous chondrocyte implantation (ACI) is performed in the usual manner as described in Chapter 33 by Dr. Lattermann. These OCD lesions are often uncontained in the region adjacent to the intercondylar notch, requiring the preparation a few other anchors in a manner as described in step 5. These anchors are placed at the edge of the intercondylar notch.

(Of note, a large unsalvageable OCD lesion may also be treated by osteochondral allograft transplantation, as described in Chapter 34 by Dr. Bugbee.)

Postoperative Management

Following ACI with bone grafting, the patient typically has protected weight bearing—touchdown (~25%) weight bearing for the first 6 weeks. The patient wears a brace that is locked in extension while ambulating. Range of motion is often facilitated by a continuous passive motion (CPM) machine during this time period.

In general, after these first 6 weeks, the patient may progress weight bearing as tolerated. The original knee brace that was locked in extension is discontinued. An unloader brace is commonly ordered at this point in order to minimize weight bearing through the affected compartment. The patient gradually increases functional activities like standing and walking.

After 3 months, the patient increases muscle strength and endurance. Bicycling is an important component of rehabilitation. Emphasis should be placed on a gradual advancement of activities, progressing to light jogging and running by 9 months, and eventually jumping by 12 months. Contact and collision sports are resumed after 12 months.

PEARLS AND PITFALLS

- When surgery is indicated, the key for success when treating OCD lesions is to do the last procedure first. Do not perform procedures with low success rates just because they are technically easier or less invasive.
- When fixing an OCD lesion, treat the interface between the progeny fragment and parent bone like a nonunion—with removal of fibrous tissue and bone grafting.
- When treating an unsalvageable OCD lesion with ACI, remember to bone graft when the bony involvement is more than 5 mm or so. Otherwise, you may be building a house on a bad foundation.

COMPLICATIONS

Avoid infection by keeping salvageable fragments in the body (and off the floor) whenever possible. Specifically, for the unstable OCD lesion of the medial femoral condyle, leave the progeny fragment attached to the soft tissue about the posterior cruciate ligament. The lesion opens like a trap door and allows access for all work without difficulty.

Avoid harmful radiation exposure for the patient by placing lead under and over the patient.

Avoid damage to opposing articular surface by ensuring that all permanent hardware (like a headless screw) is entirely within subchondral bone, all temporary hardware (like a regular screw) is removed prior to weight bearing, and all progeny cartilage is perfectly flush or gently recessed. Nothing should be proud with respect to the surrounding parent bone and cartilage.

REFERENCE

1. Wall EJ, Vourazeris J, Myer GD, et al. The healing potential of stable juvenile osteochondritis dissecans knee lesions. *J Bone Joint Surg Am.* 2008;90:2655–2664.

RECOMMENDED READINGS

Carey JL, Ganley TJ, Grimm NL. Osteochondritis dissecans in the knee: treatment algorithms. In: Carey JL, ed. *Osteochondritis dissecans.* Rosemont, IL: American Academy of Orthopaedic Surgeons; 2015:1–7.

Chambers HG, Shea KG, Anderson AF, et al. AAOS clinical practice guideline summary: diagnosis and treatment of osteochondritis dissecans. *J Am Acad Orthop Surg.* 2011;19:297–306.

Edmonds EW, Polousky J. A review of knowledge in osteochondritis dissecans: 123 years of minimal evolution from Konig to the ROCK study group. *Clin Orthop Rel Res.* 2013;471:1118–1126.

Gunton MJ, Carey JL, Shaw CR, et al. Drilling juvenile osteochondritis dissecans: retro- or trans-articular? *Clin Orthop Relat Res.* 2013;471:1144–1151.

Konig F. Ueber freie korper in den gelenken [On loose bodies in the joint]. *Dtsch Z Chir.* 1887;27:90–109.

36 Proximal Tibial/Distal Femoral Osteotomy for Management of Unicompartmental Arthritis

Annunziato Amendola and Davide E. Bonasia

INTRODUCTION

High tibial osteotomy (HTO) and distal femoral osteotomy (DFO) are widely performed procedures. HTO and DFO achieved good results with appropriate patient selection and a precise surgical technique. Clinical indications include malalignment of the knee associated with (a) medial or lateral unicompartmental arthrosis, (b) knee instability, (c) medial or lateral compartment overload in postmeniscectomized knees, and (d) osteochondral defects requiring resurfacing procedures. Both coronal (varus or valgus) and sagittal (tibial slope) alignment should be thoroughly evaluated. Many techniques have been described for HTO and DFO, with or without combined procedures. In this chapter, the indications, preoperative workup, preoperative planning, surgical techniques, and complications are outlined.

HIGH TIBIAL OSTEOTOMY

Indications

HTO is a widely performed procedure, and clinical indications include varus alignment of the knee associated with

1. Medial compartment arthrosis/overload
2. Chronic knee instability (i.e., varus thrust)
3. Medial compartment overload in postmeniscectomized knees
4. Osteochondral lesions (OCL) requiring resurfacing procedures

Negative prognostic factors:

- Severe joint destruction (≥Ahlback grade III)
- Age greater than or equal to 65 years
- Range of motion (ROM) less than 90 degrees
- Flexion contracture greater than or equal to 15 degrees
- Rheumatoid arthritis
- Advanced patellofemoral arthritis
- Inadequate postoperative physical therapy

Positive prognostic factors:

- Young age (<60 years)
- Isolated unicompartmental osteoarthritis

- Good ROM
- Adequate postoperative physical therapy

The influence of body mass index (BMI) remains a controversial factor. Although originally instability was considered as a contraindication for osteotomy, recently HTO, with or without combined ligamentous reconstruction, has raised in popularity for the treatment of malalignment and (a) chronic knee instability, (b) ligament reconstruction failure, and (c) combined medial arthrosis and knee instability.

Many techniques have been described for HTO (with or without combined procedures) including the following:

- Lateral closing wedge HTO
- Medial opening wedge HTO
- Dome HTO
- Progressive callus distraction HTO with external fixator
- Chevron HTO

In the past, lateral closing wedge HTO was considered the gold standard. However, this technique presents some drawbacks: (a) fibular osteotomy or proximal tibiofibular joint disruption, (b) risk of peroneal nerve injury, (c) bone stock loss, and (d) more demanding subsequent total knee replacement (TKR). For these reasons, medial opening wedge HTO has replaced lateral closing as the primary means of HTO. However, also this technique has some disadvantages, and these include the necessity of bone graft and possible collapse or loss of correction. Currently, there is no evidence regarding the superiority of one procedure over the other, and the choice of the technique remains a matter of preference of the surgeon. The authors commonly prefer opening wedge HTO, reserving the closing wedge technique to heavy smokers, who are not amenable to other procedures. Cigarette smoke has been proven to increase the risk of nonunion. Leg length discrepancy may be a consideration with larger corrections. In selected cases, when tibial tubercle osteotomy is not planned, preoperative patellar height abnormality can guide the choice of the procedure. Closing wedge HTO has been proven to increase patellar height, whereas opening wedge HTO has shown the opposite effect and therefore care should be taken to avoid this alteration. In the young patient with concomitant early patellofemoral arthritis, a combined HTO and tibial tubercle osteotomy could be considered.

Planning

Preoperative radiographic evaluation for HTO includes bilateral weight-bearing anteroposterior (AP) views in full extension as well as tunnel views at 30 degrees of flexion or Rosenberg views at 45 degrees of flexion. Lateral and skyline views are also obtained. A weight-bearing hip-to-ankle AP view is obtained to measure the lower extremity alignment. The MRI can help identify any other bony or soft tissue pathologies (meniscal tears, ligamentous lesions, osteochondral defects, osteonecrosis, etc.) and the subchondral edema, typical in case of the overload. The degree of degeneration in the medial compartment is evaluated on the x-rays. The patellar height is evaluated on the lateral view of the knee with the Insall-Salvati, Blackburne-Peel, or Caton Deschamps index. Severe patellar height abnormalities can dictate the need for a combined tibial tubercle osteotomy or guide the choice between closing versus opening wedge HTO.

The planning for opening wedge and closing wedge HTO is as described in Figures 36-1 and 36-2, respectively. In HTO for medial compartment arthrosis, the planning on the sagittal plane is not as important as for knee instability. Nevertheless, attention should be paid not to alter the anatomical tibial slope (Video 36-1).

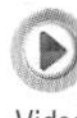
Video 36-1

Patient Preparation and Positioning

- Spinal or general anesthesia.
- Patient supine on a radiolucent operating table.
- Appropriate preoperative i.v. antibiotic prophylaxis.
- Tourniquet at the proximal thigh.
- Lateral post at the level of the thigh, if arthroscopy is planned.

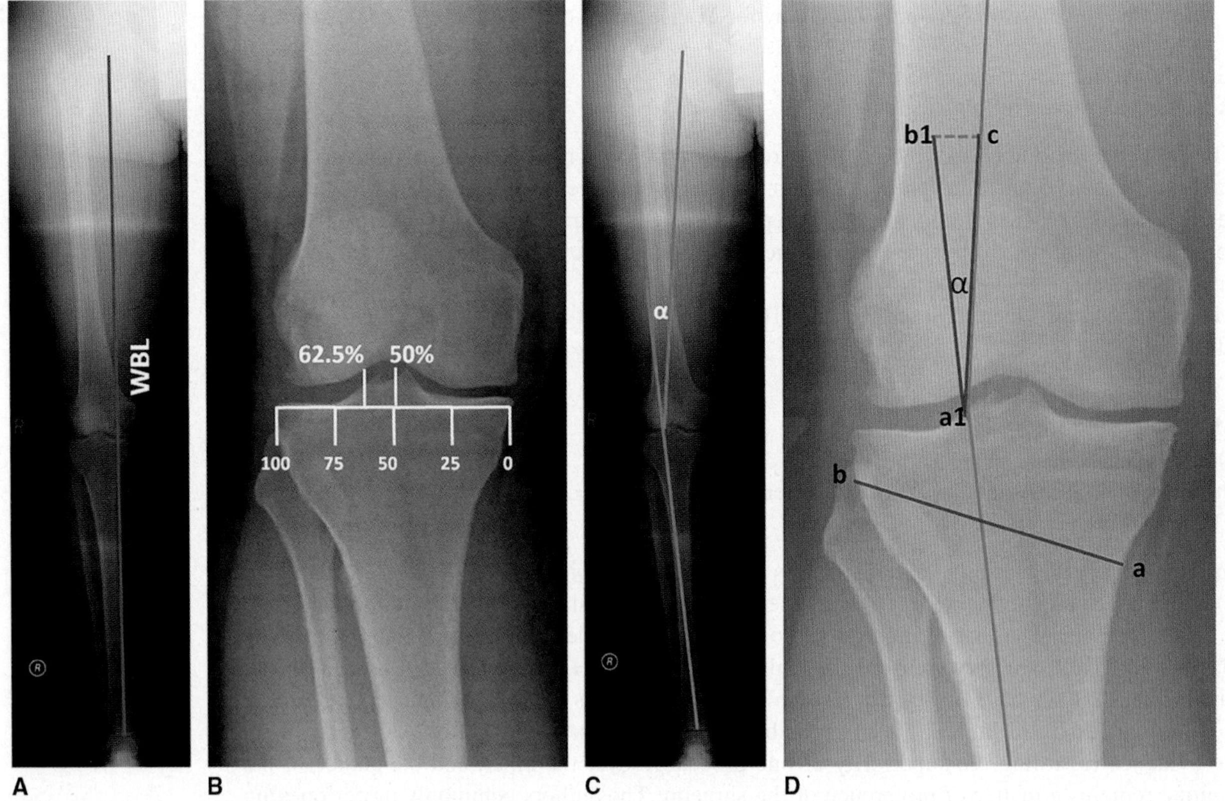

FIGURE 36-1

Planning for opening wedge HTO. **A:** The alignment is evaluated drawing the weight-bearing line (connecting the center of the hip to the center of the ankle). **B:** The osteotomy is commonly planned in order to have a WBL passing through a point at 62.5% of the tibial width. A neutral alignment (50% of the tibial width) is planned in younger patients. **C:** Then, the angle of correction is determined (α). **D:** Then, the osteotomy line is defined from medial (≈4 cm below the joint line) to lateral (tip of the fibular head) and measured (line ab). This measure is transferred to both rays of the α angle from the vertex (lines a1b1 and a1c). In this fashion, the α angle is defined by two identical segments (equal to the osteotomy length), and these are connected by another line (b1c). b1c corresponds to the size of the toothed plate and to the opening that should be achieved at the osteotomy site.

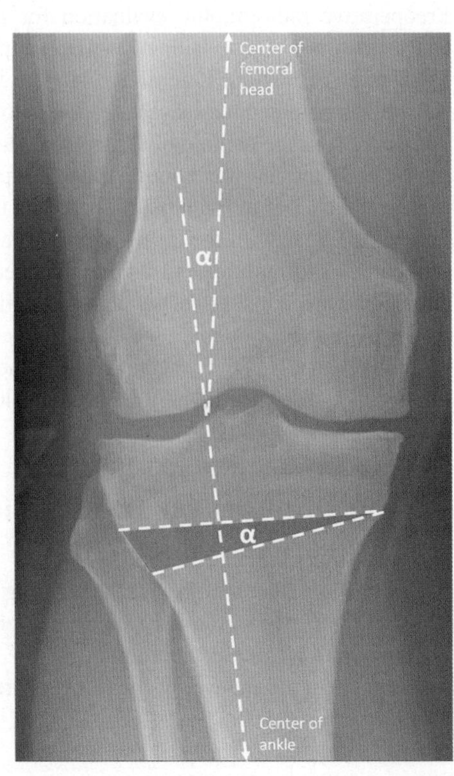

FIGURE 36-2

Planning for closing wedge HTO. The planning is similar to opening wedge HTO. The α angle is calculated as previously described, but the osteotomy is different and entails two cuts. The proximal osteotomy line is usually horizontal and placed 2 to 2.5 cm distal to the joint line. The proximal and distal osteotomy should define the angle of correction (α).

- In case of opening wedge HTO, the C-arm of the image intensifier enters from the side of the affected limb, while surgery is performed from the side of the contralateral limb (for easier approach to the medial tibia). Opposite position in case of closing wedge HTO.
- If arthroscopy is planned, the screen is usually positioned opposite to the C-arm.

SURGICAL TECHNIQUE FOR OPENING WEDGE HTO

- If necessary, arthroscopy can be performed through standard anteromedial and anterolateral portals (possible additional superomedial portal for outflow) (Video 36-1).
- A 5- to 7-cm longitudinal incision on the anteromedial aspect of the proximal tibia. The incision is started proximally 1 cm below the medial joint line, midway between the medial border of the tubercle and the posteromedial border of the tibia (Fig. 36-3A).
- The medial border of the patellar tendon is identified, retracted laterally, and protected with a hook or a Hohmann retractor (Fig. 36-3B).
- The sartorial fascia is exposed by sharp dissection (Fig. 36-3C) and the pes anserinus is then retracted distally with a blunt retractor, exposing the superficial medial collateral ligament (sMCL).
- The sMCL is partially detached at the distal tibial insertion with a Cobb elevator. A blunt retractor is then positioned on the posteromedial border of the tibia in order to protect the posterior neurovascular structures (Fig. 36-3D).
- A guidewire is then positioned (Fig. 36-4). The guidewire should enter the anteromedial tibia at the level of the superior border of the tibial tubercle (about 4 cm distal from the joint line) (Fig. 36-4A). The wire must be inserted aiming to the tip of the fibular head (1 cm below the lateral articular surface). The guidewire positioning is assessed by image intensifier (Fig. 36-4B).

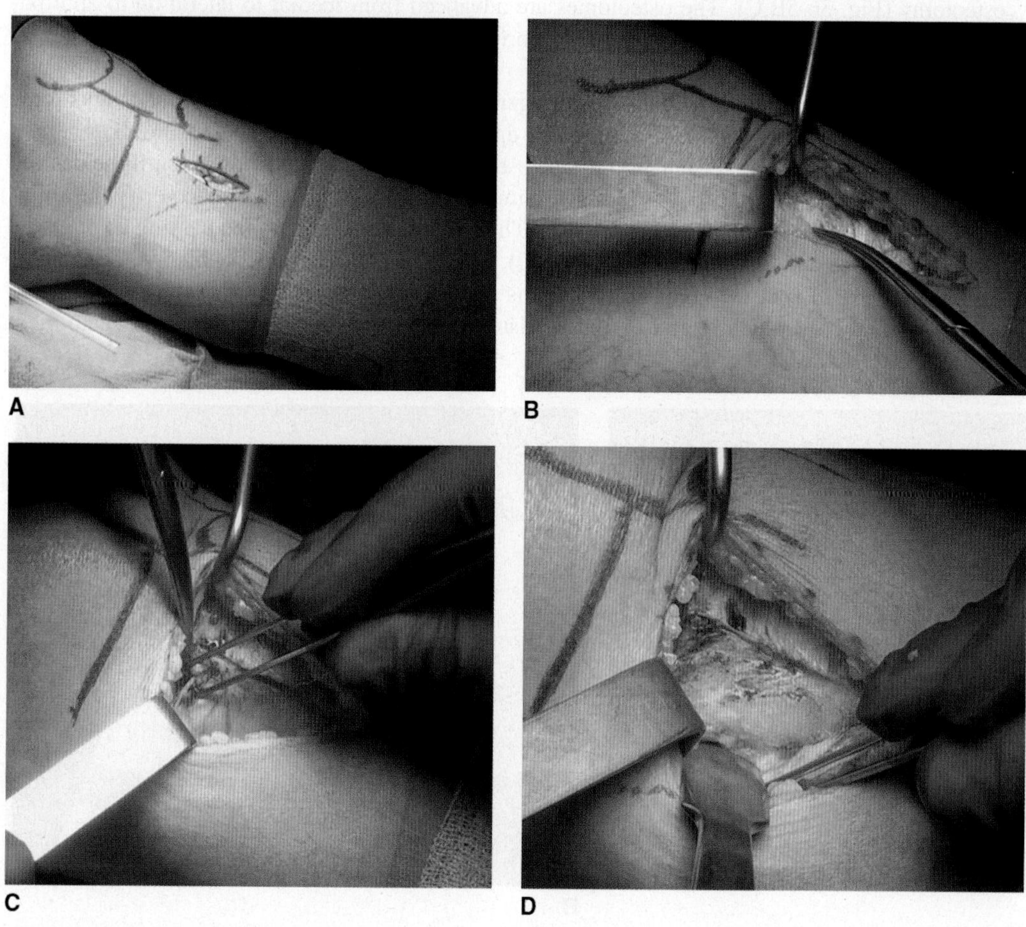

FIGURE 36-3

Opening wedge HTO. Surgical approach (see text).

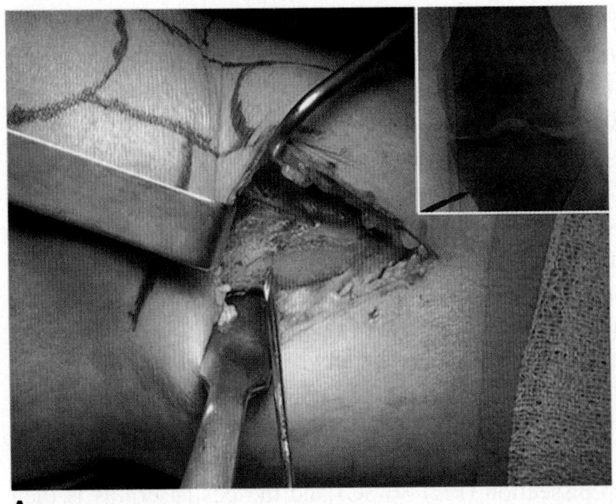
A

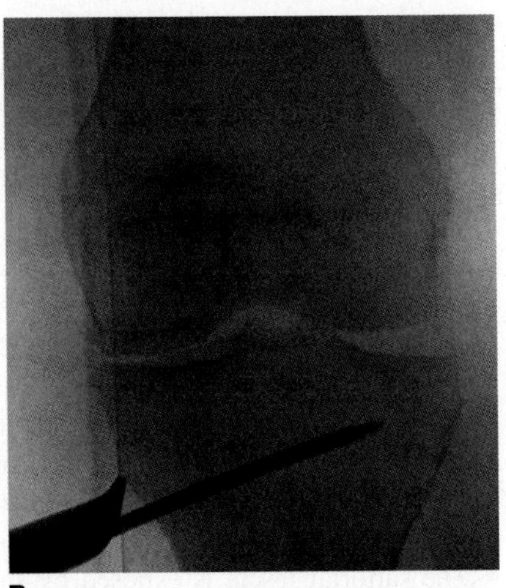
B

FIGURE 36-4

Opening wedge HTO. Guidewire position (see text).

- The tibial osteotomy is performed distal to the guide pin in order to avoid proximal migration of the osteotomy into the joint. The slope of the osteotomy in the sagittal plane is critical and should mimic the proximal tibial joint slope (around 10 degrees from anterior to posterior). A small oscillating saw is used to cut the tibial cortex from the tibial tubercle around to the posteromedial corner under direct vision (Fig. 36-5A). Thin, flexible osteotomes are then used to advance the osteotomy (Fig. 36-5B,C). The osteotomes are advanced from medial to lateral up to approximately 1 cm of distance from the lateral tibial cortex. This is achieved using graduated osteotomes under image intensifier control (Fig. 36-5D).
- The mobility of the osteotomy is checked by gentle manipulation of the leg with a valgus force (Fig. 36-6A) and encouraged, if needed, piling up two or three osteotomes (Fig. 36-6B).
- Calibrated wedges are then engaged into the osteotomy and advanced slowly, until the desired opening is achieved (Fig. 36-7A). A long alignment rod (Fig. 36-7B) is used to verify the alignment with the image intensifier (Fig. 36-7C). The rod should be positioned passing through the center of the hip and ankle joints (Fig. 36-7C). The position of the rod (which is the weight-bearing line [WBL]) at the level of the knee is then evaluated. The sagittal plane should also be assessed fluoroscopically and by direct visualization: in order to preserve the anatomical

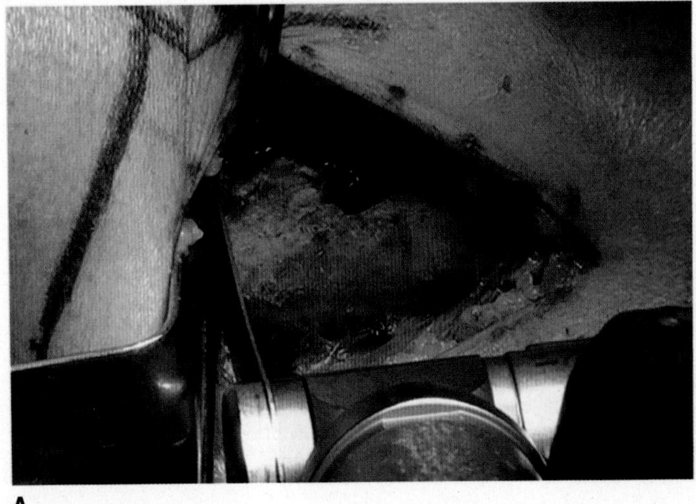
A

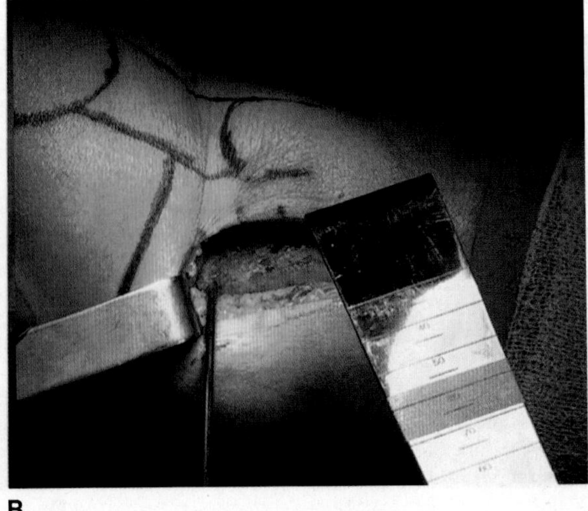
B

FIGURE 36-5

Opening wedge HTO. Osteotomy (see text).

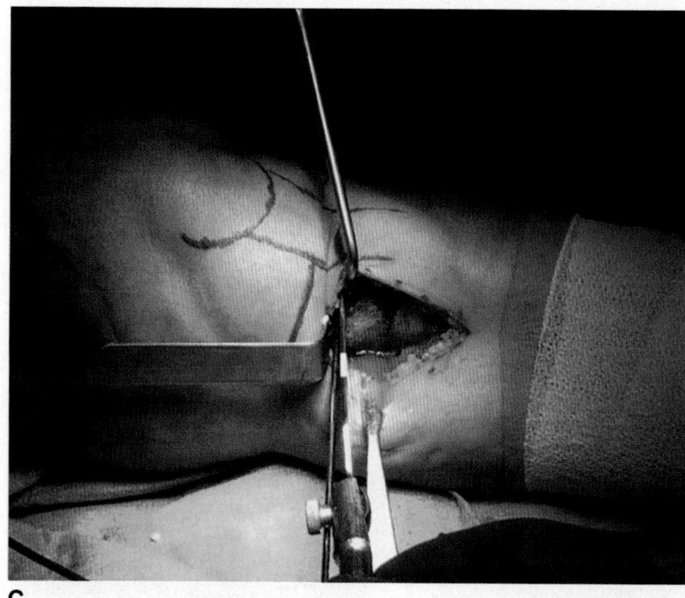
C

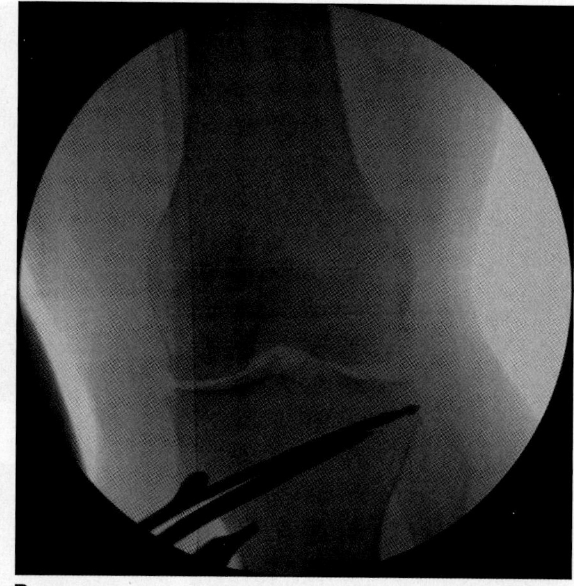
D

FIGURE 36-5 (*Continued*)

slope, the anterior opening should be less than the posteromedial, because of the triangular shape of the tibia.

- Once the desired correction is achieved, plating is performed and the wedges are removed (Fig. 36-8A,B). Fluoroscopic control is used to assess positioning of the screws (Fig. 36-8C). Various plates are available for opening wedge HTO fixation, and these include (a) short or long, (b) locked or nonlocked, and (c) with rectangular (or tapered) spacer or without spacer. Locking spacer plates and long locking plates are the most commonly used devices for HTO fixation. Recently, PEEK osteotomy plates and PEEK wedged implants have been introduced in the market. These implants use specific instrumentation.
- The defect is then grafted using the preferred bone graft (iliac crest autograft, allograft, bone substitutes). Corticocancellous auto- or allograft, or synthetic calcium phosphate wedges may be used. Grafting is recommended for more than 10 mm opening. For smaller corrections, bone grafting is not mandatory.

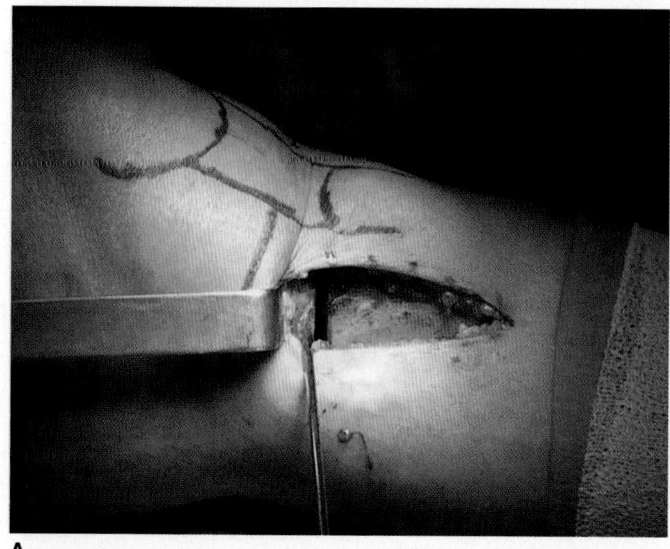
A

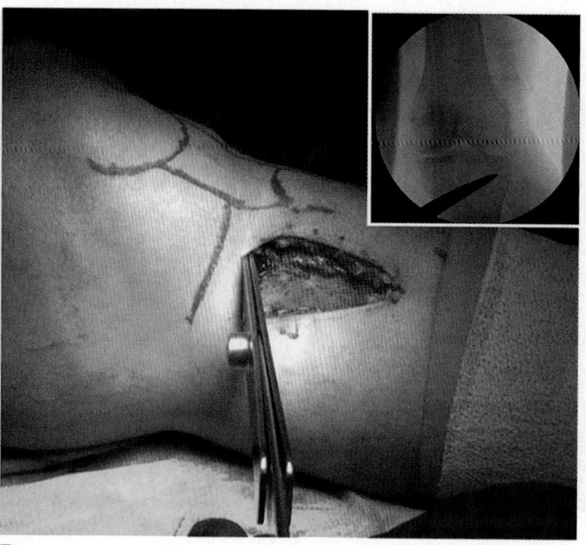
B

FIGURE 36-6

Opening wedge HTO. Checking the completeness and mobility of the osteotomy (see text).

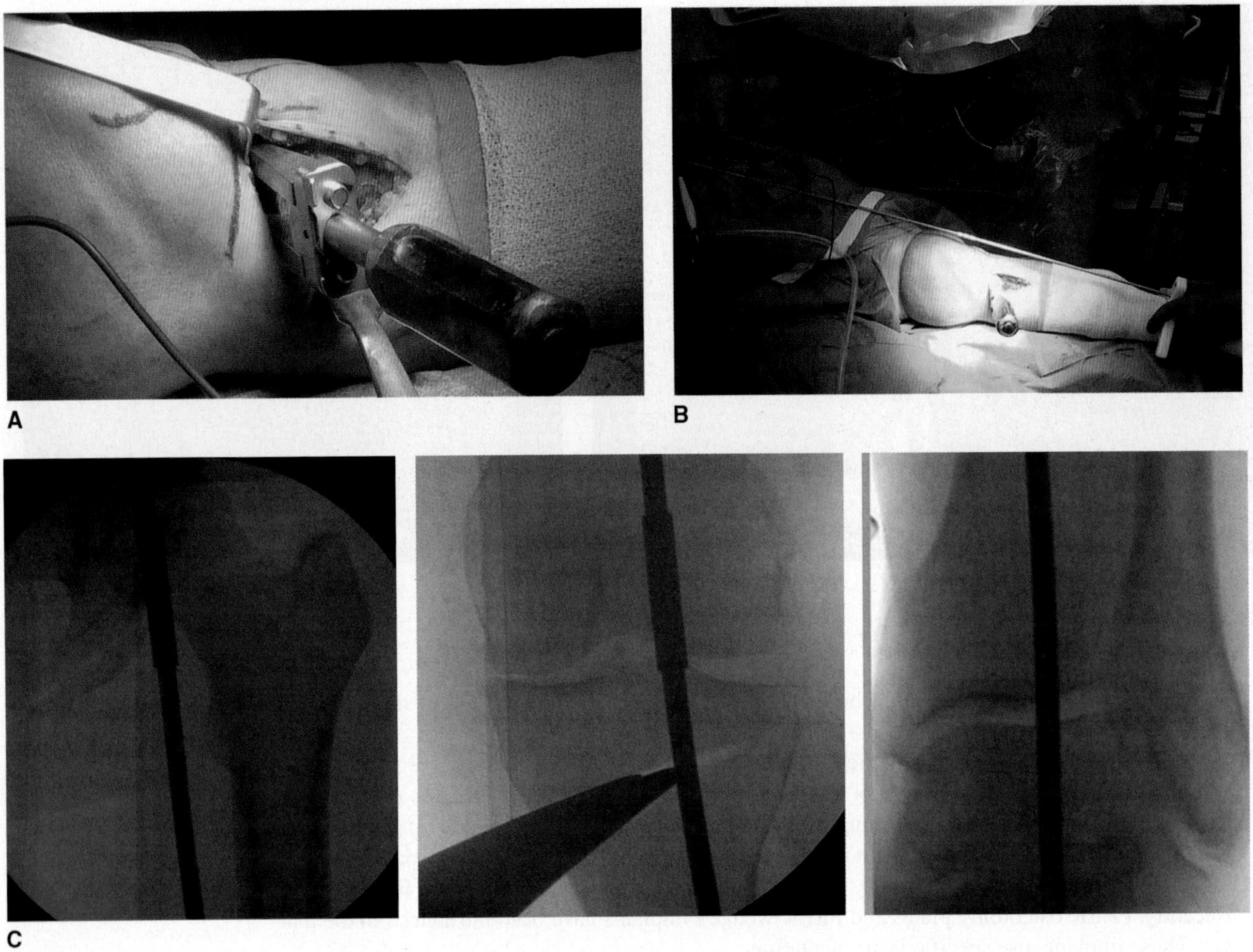

A B

C

FIGURE 36-7

Opening wedge HTO. Opening of the osteotomy and fluoroscopic control of the alignment (see text).

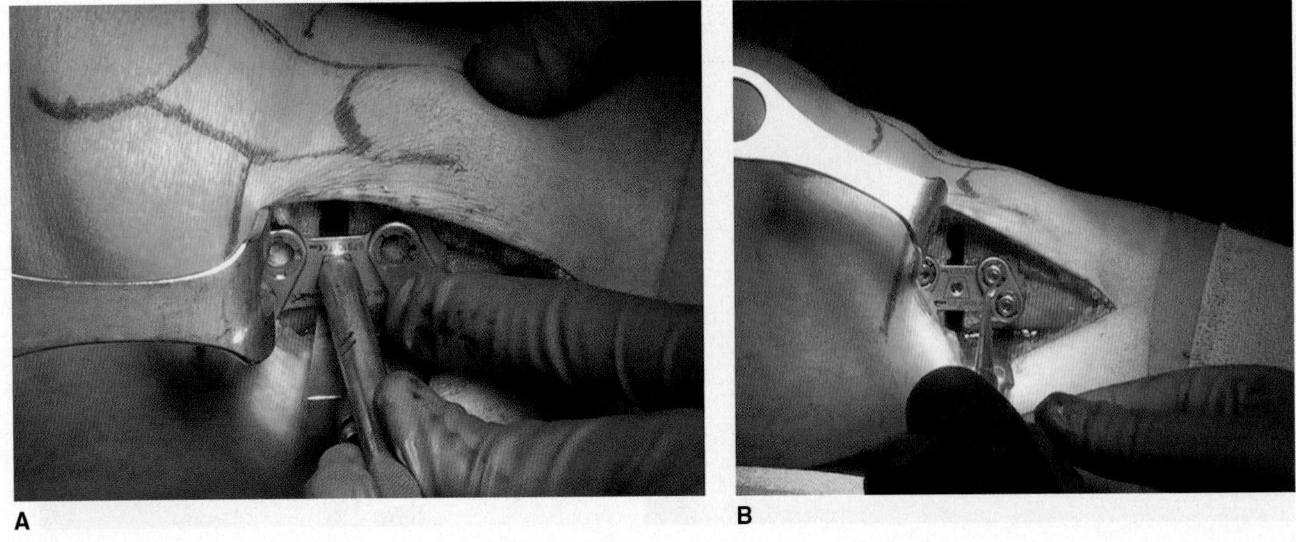

A B

FIGURE 36-8

Opening wedge HTO. Plating (see text).

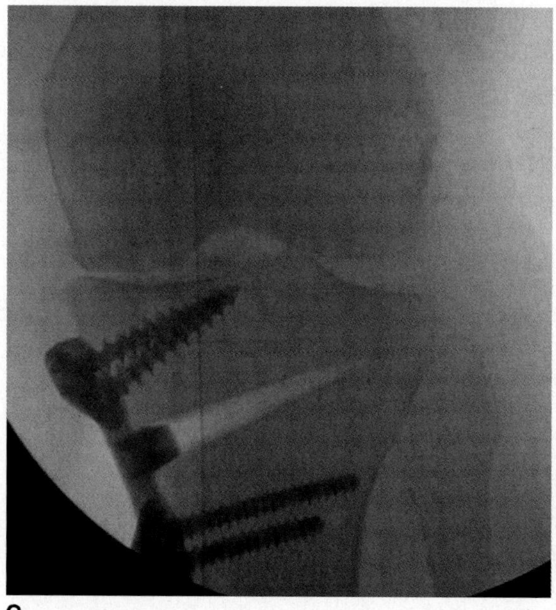
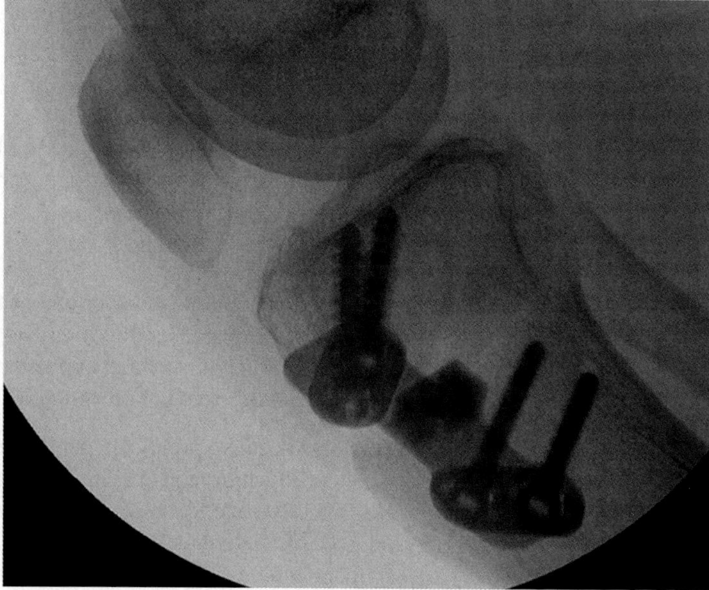

C

FIGURE 36-8 (*Continued*)

SURGICAL TECHNIQUE FOR CLOSING WEDGE HTO

- An anterolateral L-shaped incision, with the vertical portion of the incision running along the lateral edge of the tibial tubercle and the horizontal portion running parallel to the lateral joint line (1 cm distal).
- The fascia of the anterior compartment is incised along the anterolateral crest of the tibia. A Cobb elevator is used to elevate the tibialis anterior muscle and the inferior portion of the iliotibial band from Gerdy tubercle proximally.
- It is not necessary to dissect or protect the common peroneal nerve throughout the procedure since we are proximal to it, but certainly can be exposed if the surgeon prefers.
- Many techniques have been described for addressing the proximal tibiofibular joint, including (a) joint excision or disruption, (b) fibular osteotomy (10 cm distal from the fibular head), and (c) excision of the fibular head.
- The lateral edge of the patellar tendon is identified and protected with a retractor. A second retractor is positioned on the posterolateral tibial edge to protect the neurovascular structures.
- A laterally based wedge is removed with an angular cutting guide. The base of the wedge should be 2 to 3 mm smaller than the planned osteotomy. During closure of the osteotomy, this will allow the distal cortex of the proximal fragment to overlap the proximal cortex of the distal fragment, without the risk of overcorrection.
- To reduce the risk of intra-articular fracture, the outer cortex and a large portion of the wedge, along with the medial half, can be removed with saw cuts, using a combination of curettes, rongeurs, and osteotomes, to within 1 cm of the medial cortex.
- The completeness of wedge removal is assessed fluoroscopically. The osteotomy is closed, and alignment is checked under fluoroscopy.
- Fixation can be achieved with step staples driven from lateral to medial just anterior to the fibula. More rigid fixation can be achieved with a laterally applied contoured T-plate or a locking plate.

Postoperative Management

- ROM brace set at 0 to 90 degrees.
- Touch weight bearing for 6 weeks.
- From weeks 6 to 12, the brace is discontinued and weight bearing is gradually progressed

The postoperative management may vary according to the fixation device used. Earlier weight bearing can be allowed when using long locking plates. Short radiographs are taken at 6 and 12 weeks, and long leg alignment films are obtained at 6 months.

DISTAL FEMORAL OSTEOTOMY

Indications

DFO is indicated in case of valgus malalignment and

1. Unicompartmental arthritis/overload of the lateral compartment
2. Chronic valgus knee instability (i.e., valgus thrust)
3. Lateral compartment overload in postmeniscectomized knees
4. OCL requiring resurfacing procedures

Positive and negative prognostic factors are as described for HTO.

Both lateral opening and medial closing DFO have been described. No superior results have been described for one technique over the other. The authors' technique of choice is lateral opening wedge DFO. Medial closing wedge DFO preferred in case of heavy smokers and when massive osteochondral allografts are used to treat malunited lateral tibial plateau fractures.

Planning

The planning is similar to HTO, with a different osteotomy line (Video 36-1). The osteotomy line for opening wedge DFO has craniocaudal inclination of 20 degrees, from lateral (6 to 7 cm above the joint line) to medial (4 to 5 cm above the joint line). Generally, no varus overcorrection should be planned in these cases. Correction to a neutral alignment is advisable in order to obtain durable results (Fig. 36-9A,B).

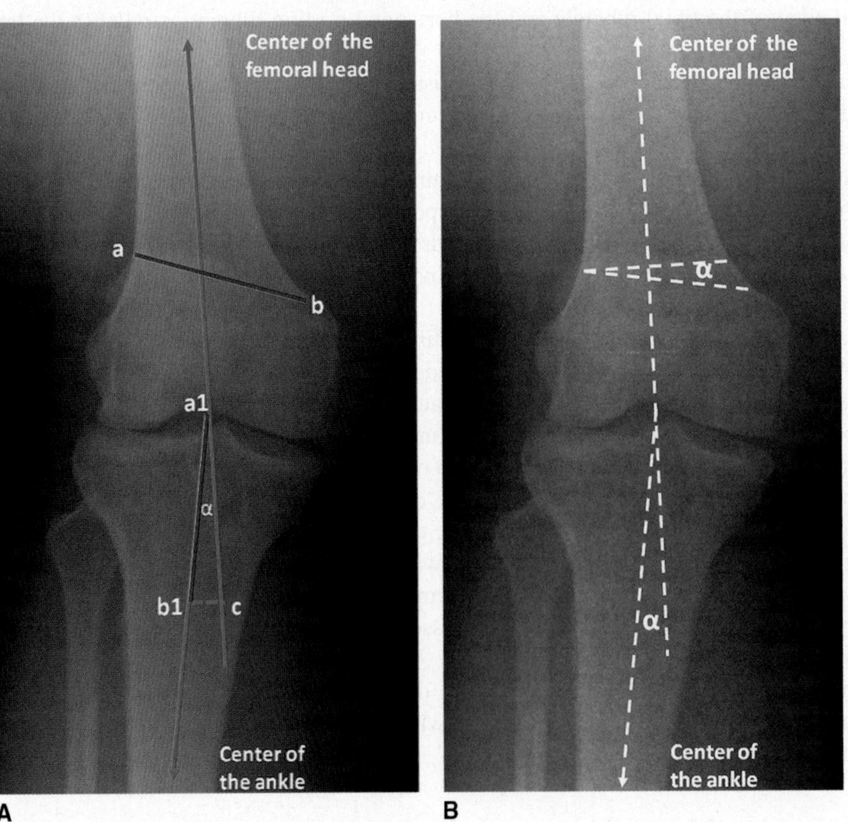

FIGURE 36-9

Planning for opening wedge DFO (**A**) and closing wedge DFO (**B**). The planning is similar to HTO except for the osteotomy line direction and the degree of correction. The osteotomy line for opening wedge DFO has craniocaudal inclination of 20 degrees, from lateral (6 to 7 cm above the joint line) to medial (4 to 5 cm above the joint line). Correction to a neutral alignment (no overcorrection) is recommended.

Patient Preparation and Positioning

As described for HTO, except for the position of the C-arm. In case of opening wedge DFO, the C-arm of the image intensifier enters from the side of the unaffected limb, while surgery is performed from the side of the affected limb (for easier approach to the lateral femur). Opposite position in case of closing wedge DFO.

SURGICAL TECHNIQUE FOR OPENING WEDGE DFO

- A 10- to 15-cm longitudinal lateral distal femoral incision is performed starting 2 cm distal to the femoral condyle and prolonging it proximally (Video 36-1). The iliotibial band is split to the level of the joint line, and the vastus lateralis is retracted from the intermuscular septum using a curve blunt retractor placed ventrally (Fig. 36-10A). The bone plane is better exposed with a slight knee flexion.
- Under fluoroscopic control, a guidewire is inserted in the middle of the lateral femur, with a craniocaudal inclination of 20 degrees, from lateral (6 to 7 cm above the joint line) to medial (4 to 5 cm above the joint line) (Fig. 36-10A).
- The exposed cortex is cut with a small oscillating saw above the guidewire. Sharp and thin AO osteotomes are then used to complete the osteotomy to within 1 cm from the medial cortex, under fluoroscopic guidance (Fig. 36-10B).
- The site of osteotomy at this point is opened with a wedge opener to the desired correction (Fig. 36-11A). Fluoroscopy and alignment rod are used to assess the limb correction, as previously described (Fig. 36-11B).
- A DFO plate (regular or locked) is then used for fixation (Fig. 36-12A) under image intensifier (Fig. 36-12B). Bone grafting or bone substitutes are used to fill the gap (Fig. 36-12C).

SURGICAL TECHNIQUE FOR CLOSING WEDGE DFO

- A longitudinal 10- to 15-cm anteromedial incision is performed on the distal femur (Fig. 36-13A). The fascia over the vastus medialis muscle is incised, and the muscle is separated from the intermuscular septum and retracted superiorly.
- A guidewire is inserted parallel to the joint line. A slot for a blade plate is then prepared parallel to the guidewire and, an osteotomy is made about 2 to 3 cm proximal to the slot (Fig. 36-13B).
- The medial cortex and large portion of the wedge can be removed with saw cuts, along with the medial half using a combination of curettes, rongeurs, and osteotomes, to within 1 cm of the lateral cortex (Fig. 36-13C).

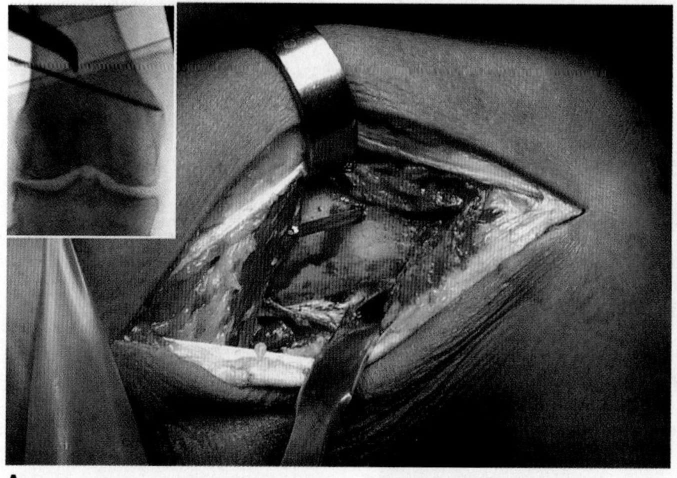
A

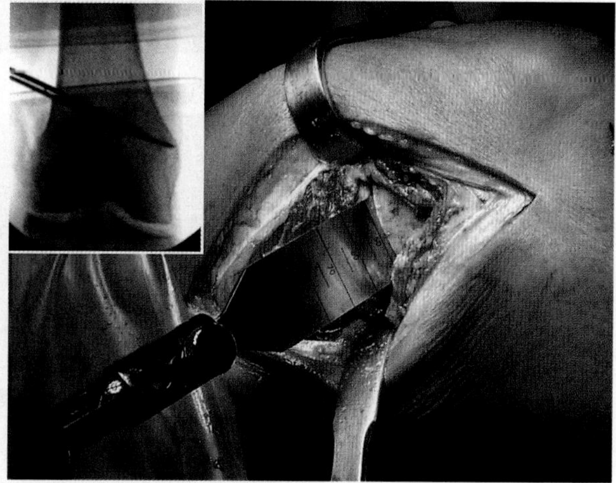
B

FIGURE 36-10

Opening wedge DFO. Guide wire position and osteotomy creation (see text).

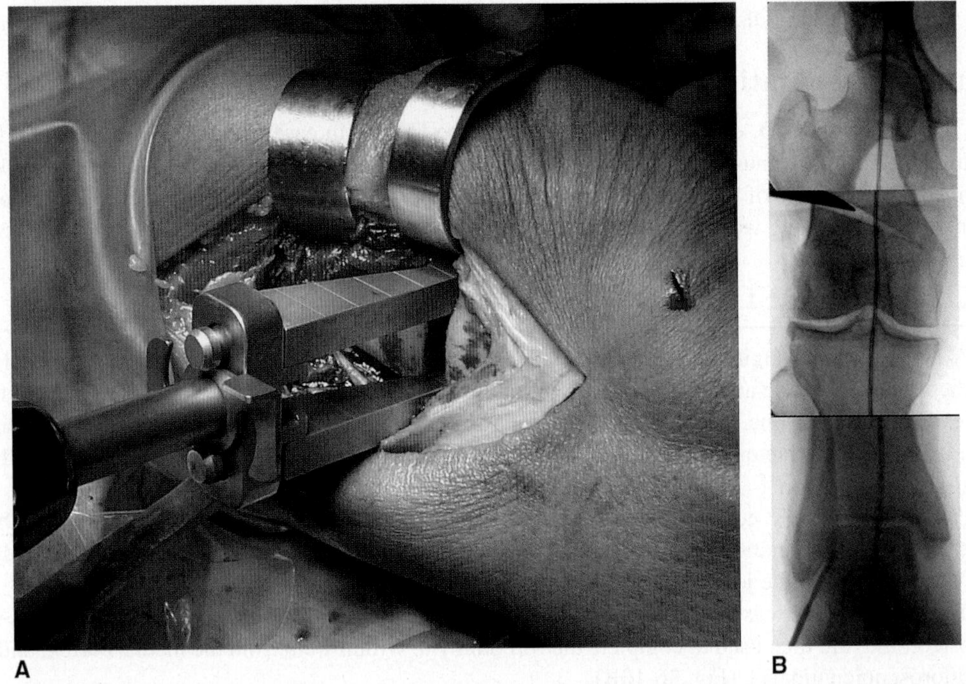

FIGURE 36-11

Opening wedge DFO. Opening of the osteotomy with wedges and alignment control with image intensifier (see text).

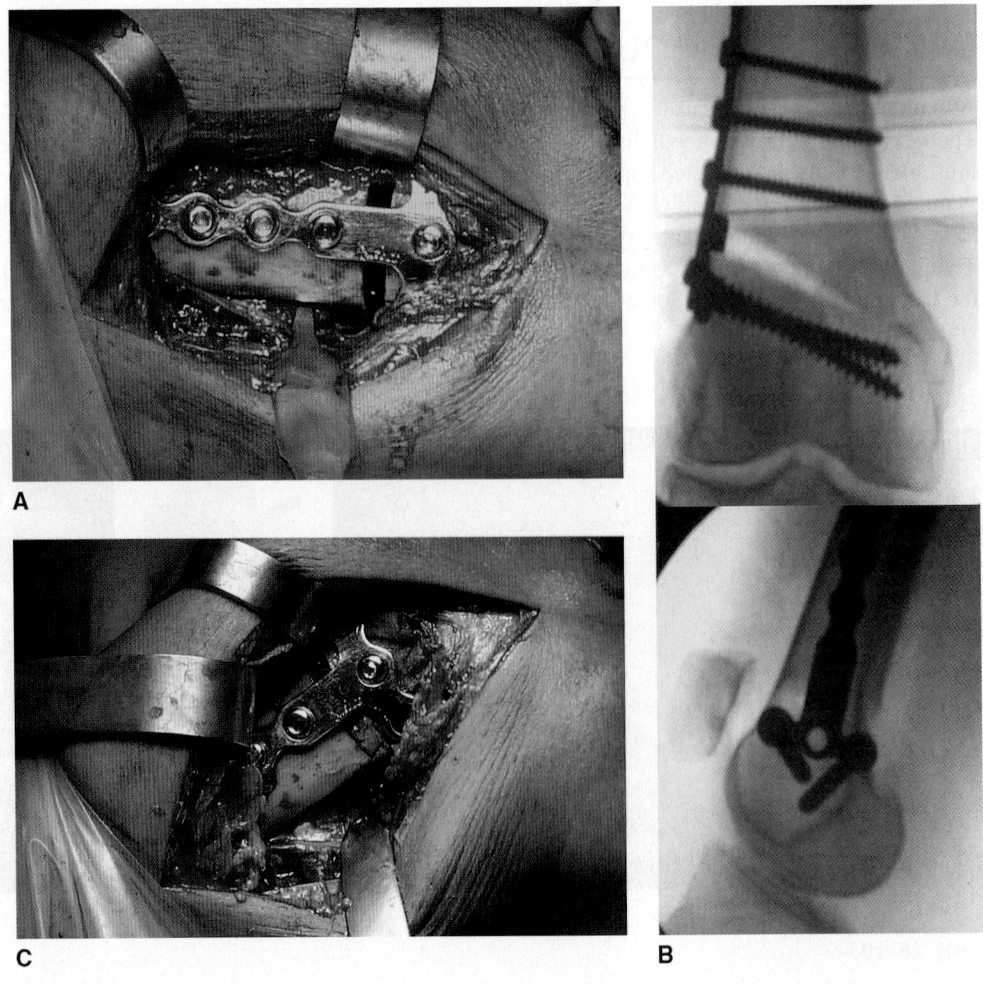

FIGURE 36-12

Opening wedge DFO. Plating, final control with image intensifier, and bone grafting (see text).

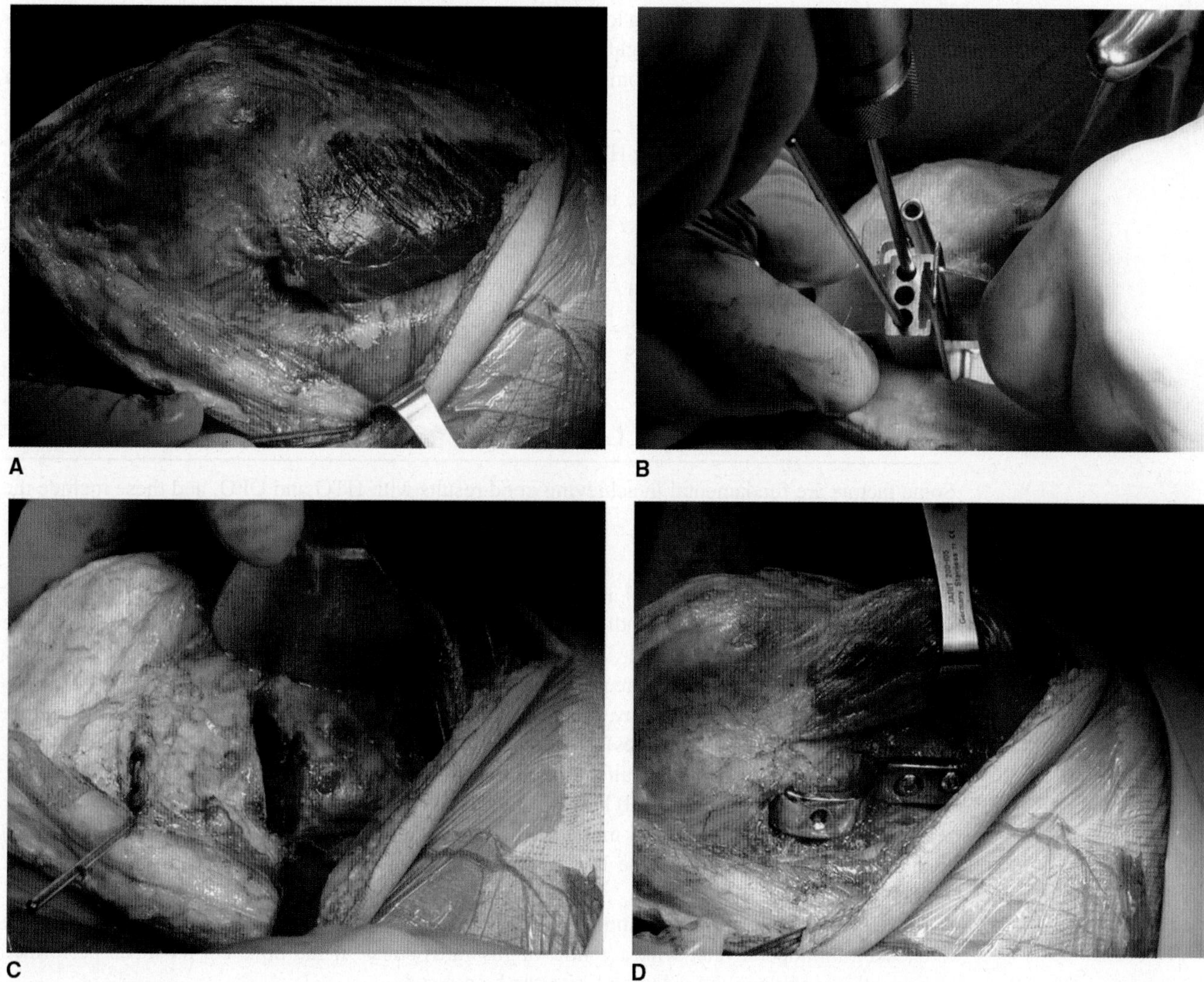

FIGURE 36-13
Closing wedge DFO (see text).

- A 90-degree angle blade plate is inserted in the prepared slot. Manual varus reduction is performed, allowing the medial spike of the proximal part to dig into the distal cancellous bone (Fig. 36-13D). The rigid fixation is achieved with the anatomic knee axis of 0 degree, after fluoroscopic assessment of the correction.

Postoperative Regimen

The postoperative regimen of DFO is generally slightly more cautious than HTO.

- ROM brace set at 0 to 90 degrees.
- Touch weight bearing for 6 weeks.
- From weeks 6 to 12, full ROM is allowed in the brace and weight bearing is gradually progressed to 50% of the body weight.
- At 12 weeks, after short knee radiographs are taken to confirm maintenance of correction and healing of the osteotomy, full weight bearing is allowed.

COMPLICATIONS

Intraoperative Complications of HTO and DFO Include the following:

- Disruption of the medial/lateral hinge: when using short nonlocking plates, this complication needs to be addressed intraoperatively, with additional hardware (cannulated screws opposite to the plate or staples). When using locking plates, no further treatment is needed, except for cautious postoperative regimen (nonweight bearing for 6 weeks).

- Intra-articular fractures: this complication needs to be addressed intraoperatively, usually with cannulated screws.

Postoperative Complications of HTO and DFO Include the following:

- General complications, that is, infection, deep venous thrombosis, bleeding, surgical wound problems, etc.
- Nonunion
- Malunion and loss of correction
- Persistent pain
- Pain at the level of the hardware

PEARLS AND PITFALLS

Some factors are fundamental in achieving good results with HTO and DFO, and these include the following:

- Correct indications.
- Precise planning on both frontal and sagittal planes.
- Correct patient position of the radiolucent table (make sure that the hip, knee, and ankle are visible with image intensifier).
- Correct position of the guidewire.
- When performing the osteotomy, the guidewire must be between the joint line and the cutting instruments (saw and osteotomes) in order to avoid intra-articular migration of the osteotomy.
- Make sure the osteotomy is parallel to the tibial slope.
- Make sure the lateral (or medial) hinge is preserved in opening wedge HTO (or DFO).
- Make sure not to preserve too much of the lateral cortex in opening wedge HTO. As shown in Figure 36-14, "b" should be longer than "a" in order to reduce the risk of intra-articular fractures.
- Make sure the osteotomy is complete at the level of anterior and posterior cortexes. This can be checked intraoperatively, with a gentle valgus/varus stress. If the bone cut has been performed correctly, opening of the osteotomy site can be noticed.
- Postoperative regimen based on stability of the osteotomy.

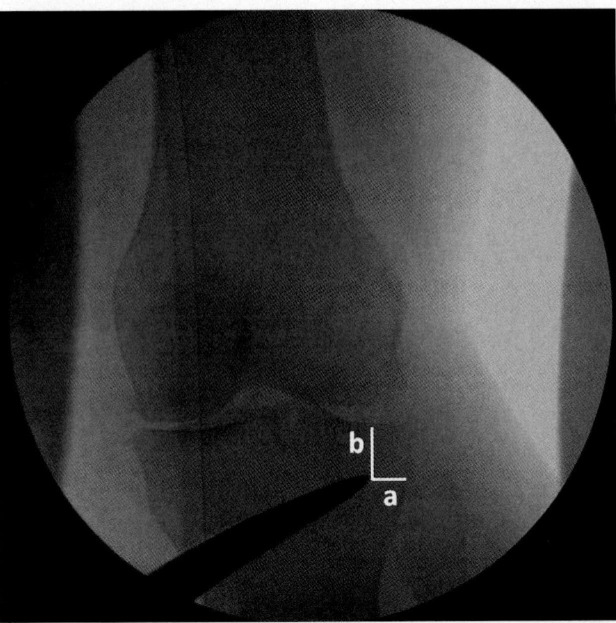

FIGURE 36-14

When performing an osteotomy make sure that b is greater than a in order to avoid intra-articular migration of the osteotomy line (see text).

RECOMMENDED READINGS

Amendola A, Bonasia DE. Results of high tibial osteotomy: review of the literature. *Int Orthop.* 2010;34(2):155–160. doi:10.1007/s00264-009-0889-8. Epub 2009 Oct 17. Review. PubMed PMID: 19838706; PubMed Central PMCID: PMC2899364.

Amendola A. Unicompartmental osteoarthritis in the active patient: the role of high tibial osteotomy. *Arthroscopy.* 2003;19(suppl 1):109–116.

Bonasia DE, Dettoni F, Sito G, et al. Medial opening wedge high tibial osteotomy for medial compartment overload/arthritis in the varus knee: prognostic factors. *Am J Sports Med.* 2014;42(3):690–698. doi:10.1177/0363546513516577. Epub 2014 Jan 21. PubMed PMID: 24449807.

Bonasia DE, Governale G, Spolaore S, et al. High tibial osteotomy. *Curr Rev Musculoskelet Med.* 2014;7(4):292–301. doi:10.1007/s12178-014-9234-y. PubMed PMID: 25129702.

Brouwer RW, Bierma-Zeinstra SMA, Raaij TM, et al. Osteotomy for medial compartment arthritis of the knee using a closing wedge or an opening wedge controlled by a Puddu plate. *J Bone Joint Surg Br.* 2006;88:1454–1459.

Phisitkul P, Wolf BR, Amendola A. Role of high tibial and distal femoral osteotomies in the treatment of lateral-posterolateral and medial instabilities of the knee. *Sport Med Arthrosc Rev.* 2006;14:96–104.

Puddu G, Cipolla M, Cerullo G, et al. Osteotomies: the surgical treatment of the valgus knee. *Sports Med Arthrosc.* 2007;15(1):15–22.

Rossi R, Bonasia DE, Amendola A. The role of high tibial osteotomy in the varus knee. *J Am Acad Orthop Surg.* 2011;19(10):590–599. Review. PubMed PMID: 21980024.

Rosso F, Margheritini F. Distal femoral osteotomy. *Curr Rev Musculoskelet Med.* 2014;7(4):302–311. doi:10.1007/s12178-014-9233-z. PubMed PMID: 25142271.

Vena G, D'Adamio S, Amendola A. Complications of osteotomies about the knee. *Sports Med Arthrosc.* 2013;21(2):113–120. doi:10.1097/JSA.0b013e3182900720.

37 Unicompartmental Knee Arthroplasty in the Athletically Active

David P. Lustenberger, Jourdan M. Cancienne, and David R. Diduch

INTRODUCTION

With the continuing trend toward less invasive surgery, combined with encouraging clinical outcomes, unicompartmental knee arthroplasty (UKA) has seen a significant increase in popularity in recent years. The procedure itself has evolved, and the indications for the procedure have expanded to the younger and more active population. Candidacy for the procedure involves unicompartmental degeneration with pain isolated to the degenerative compartment, with intact cruciate ligaments and near-normal motion. The benefits of this unique procedure versus total knee arthroplasty (TKA) include more rapid rehabilitation, better maintenance of normal knee kinematics, and less blood loss. Appropriate surgical technique is the keystone to success, and with technically sound technique, patients can have an accelerated recovery and ultimately return to recreation and sport with reduced pain.

INDICATIONS

Classically, the indications for a UKA included unicompartmental degeneration (medial or lateral compartment), age over 60 years, low demand, range of motion greater than 90 degrees with less than a 5-degree flexion contracture, weight less than 82 kg, and an angular deformity less than 15 degrees correctable to neutral mechanical alignment (1). These guidelines, if followed, have been shown to have positive results (2). While these indications provide a reasonable early set of guidelines, the indications for UKA have expanded recently.

The indications for UKA now are (3) as follows:

- Unicompartmental degeneration (medial or lateral compartment)
- Symptoms confined to the compartment with degeneration
- No clinical patellofemoral symptoms
- Degeneration from primary osteoarthritis
- No inflammatory arthropathy
- A maximum of 10 degrees of varus or 5 degrees of valgus deformity
- No flexion contracture greater than 10 degrees
- Intact anterior cruciate ligament
- No joint subluxation in the coronal plane

Although symptomatic patellofemoral degeneration is a contraindication to UKA, radiographic findings of patellofemoral degeneration do not necessitate exclusion from consideration for UKA (4,5). Although the presence of an intact ACL as a prerequisite for UKA has been debated (4,6,7), we do not recommend lateral UKA in the ACL-deficient knee. In addition, recent studies have shown success in the younger patient population, obviating the need to limit the procedure to only those over 60 years of age (8,9).

PREOPERATIVE PLANNING

A thorough history is taken that includes assessment of current symptoms and functional limitations. Particular attention should be pain to the location of the patient's symptoms, as pain limited

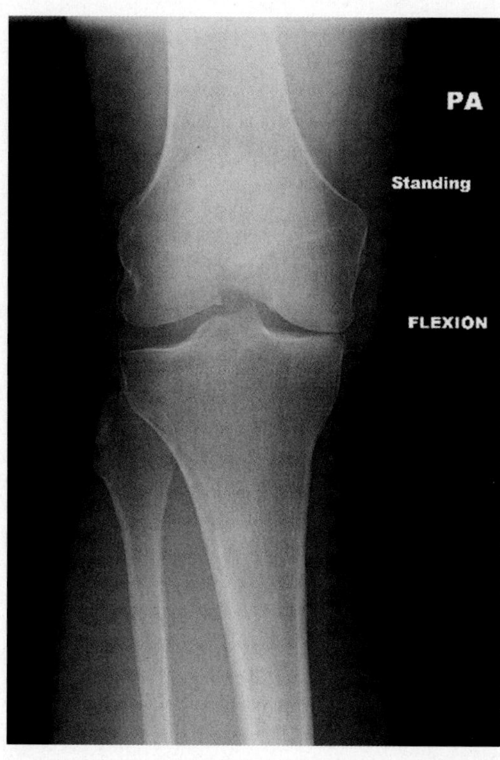

FIGURE 37-1

PA flexion radiograph of the left knee of a 61-year-old active male with isolated medial compartment pain. Medial compartment joint space narrowing with relative preservation of lateral compartment.

to the degenerative compartment to be replaced is a key to successful UKA. A physical exam should include evaluation of range of motion, joint line pain on palpation and during joint motion, and any pain in the patellofemoral joint. All knee ligaments should be assessed, and the patient's gait should be observed as well. Any flexion contracture or instability should be carefully assessed.

Of particular importance in the preoperative assessment is the localization of pain by the patient. The pain should be limited to the compartment in question, and the patient should have minimal to no pain in the opposite compartment, in addition to an asymptomatic patellofemoral compartment (4).

Diagnostic imaging includes an AP radiograph of the knee in full extension, a flexed knee weight-bearing PA radiograph, a sunrise view of the patella, and a lateral radiograph (see Figs. 37-1 to 37-3).

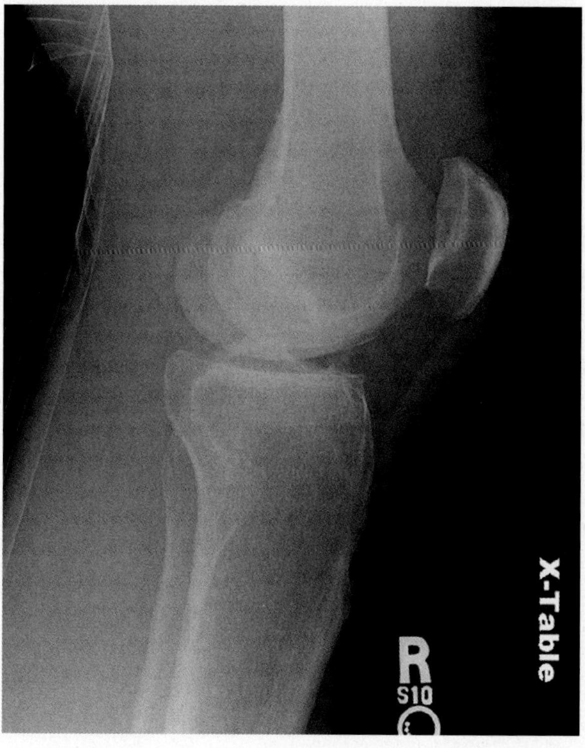

FIGURE 37-2

Lateral radiograph of the left knee of a 61-year-old active male with isolated medial compartment pain.

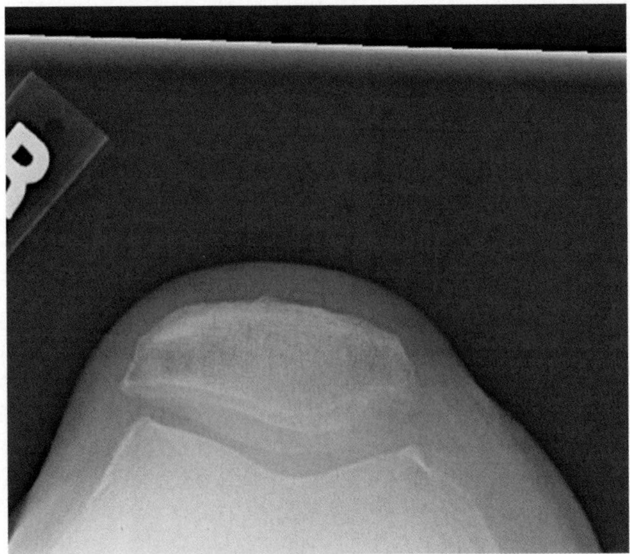

FIGURE 37-3
Sunrise radiograph of the left knee of a 61-year-old active male with isolated medial compartment pain.

SURGICAL TECHNIQUE

The goals of UKA are to restore neutral or near-neutral mechanical alignment of the knee in order to improve limb function and to reduce pain. As opposed to an osteotomy where overcorrection is often sought to displace the weight-bearing forces away from the affected compartment, in a unicompartmental arthroplasty, it is essential to avoid overcorrection of the limb as this may increase the stress in the contralateral compartment and cause advanced cartilage breakdown and subsequent arthrosis. Once appropriate preoperative evaluation is complete, surgery can be undertaken. We routinely use an extramedullary alignment technique, but both this and the intramedullary options are outlined here.

The patient is positioned in the supine position on the operating room table with a tourniquet applied, and the knee is ranged under anesthesia. If the knee is unable to flex 120 degrees, a larger incision may be necessary to create adequate exposure. The patient is then prepped and draped in standard sterile fashion. It is important to avoid bulky dressings on the distal tibia, ankle, and foot as this can displace the tibial resector guide leading to inaccurate cuts. The incision can be made in either flexion or extension, and several different locations can be used depending on the compartment being replaced. If a lateral incision is used, the surgeon must be mindful of future incisions such as those needed for TKA.

An abbreviated medial parapatellar approach is used for a medial UKA. With the knee flexed to 90 degrees, an incision is made from the medial margin of the patella to a point approximately 3 cm distal to the joint line (Fig. 37-4). The capsular incision is then extended obliquely and medially for 1 to 2 cm into the vastus medialis (Fig. 37-5). A portion of the retropatellar fat pad can then be excised for further exposure, and the ACL is inspected. All osteophytes are then removed from the medial aspect of the medial femoral condyle and from the intercondylar notch.

For a lateral parapatellar incision for lateral UKA, the incision runs from just lateral to the superior pole of the patella to 2 to 4 cm below the joint line and slightly lateral to the tibial tubercle. The lateral margin of the patellar tendon is then marked and a lateral parapatellar arthrotomy is made. If necessary, the distal 1 to 2 cm of vastus lateralis muscle can be released to help mobilize the patella. The fat pad can then be excised with special attention to avoid the anterior horn of the medial meniscus. Soft tissue is then subperiosteally resected from the tibia along the joint line laterally toward the LCL, protecting the popliteus tendon. The anterior third of the lateral meniscus is then excised to expose the tibial plateau to facilitate position of the tibial cutting guide. Alternatively, a standard medial parapatellar arthrotomy can be performed as needed for exposure.

Without everting the patella, the knee is then flexed to approximately 30 degrees, and a retractor is used to displace the patella medially or laterally depending on the exposure. The tibial saw guide

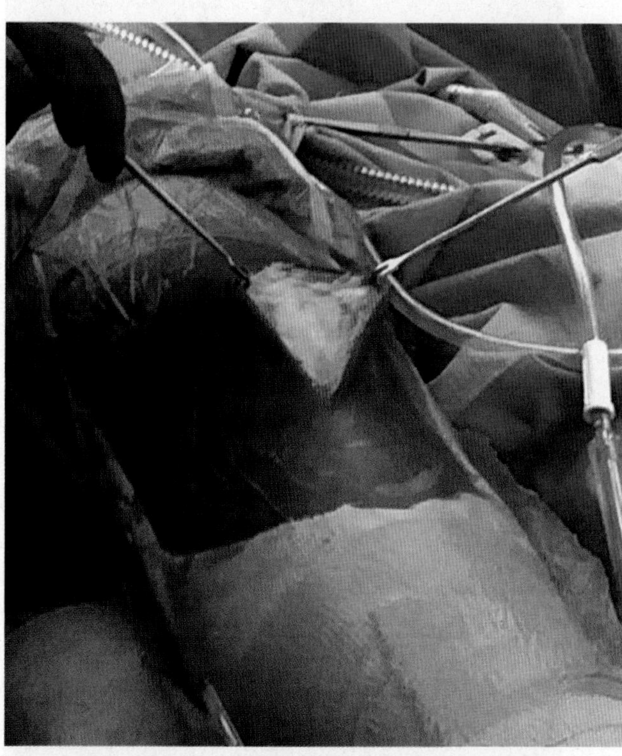

FIGURE 37-4

Initial incision from the medial margin of the patella to a point approximately 3 cm distal to the joint line.

is then applied with its shaft parallel with the long axis of the tibia in both planes (Fig. 37-6). The level of resection is estimated based on both preoperative templating and intraoperative findings. It is recommended that the saw cut pass 1 to 2 mm below the deepest part of the wear within the compartment. A cut that passes too deeply into the cancellous bone of the tibia can result in component subsidence and early loosening. Therefore, sclerotic bone should be preserved to support the tibial component. In general, it is better to start with a conservative first cut, as the tibia can easily be recut if needed. A reciprocating saw is then used to make the vertical cut, taking care to protect the cruciate ligaments (Fig. 37-7). Then, with a retractor inserted to protect the collateral ligament, the horizontal cut is made (Fig. 37-8). When the plateau is loose, it is levered up with an osteotome and removed, completing the tibial cut (Fig. 37-9). The posterior horn of the meniscus is then removed, and the excised plateau is taken to the back table as a guide in selecting the appropriate size of the tibial implant.

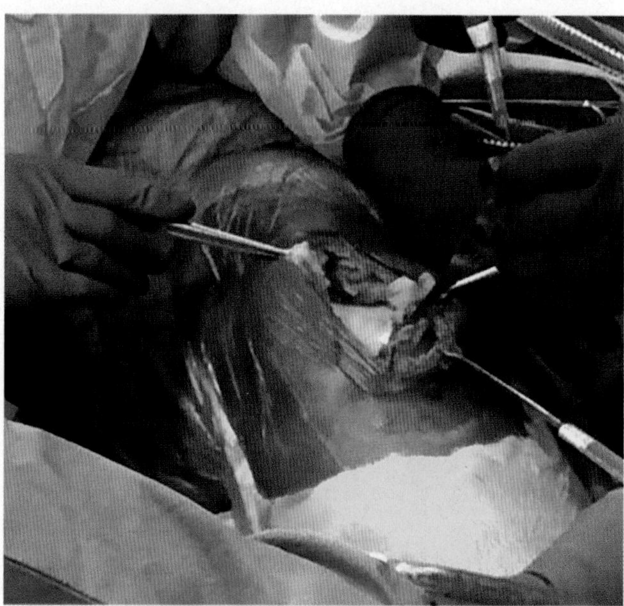

FIGURE 37-5

Deep extension of dissection through the capsule.

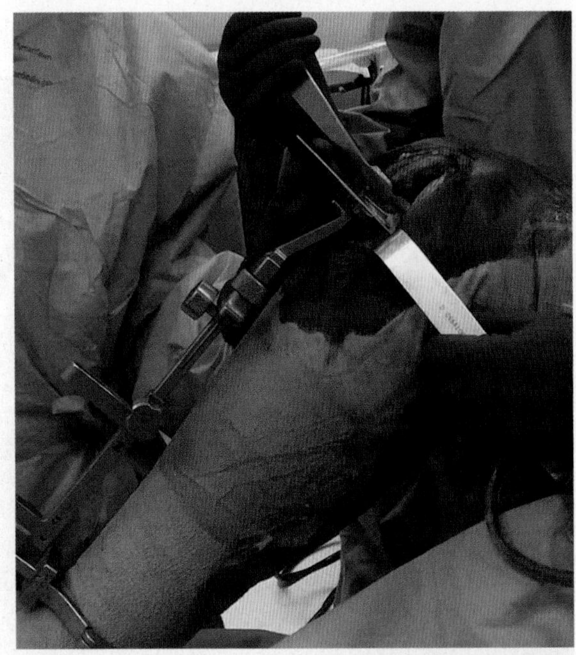

FIGURE 37-6

Tibial saw guide application. Ensure guide is parallel to the tibia in coronal and sagittal planes.

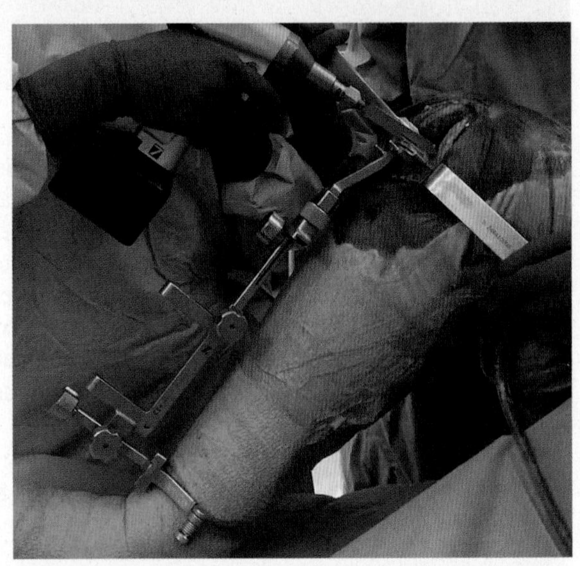

FIGURE 37-7

Making the vertical cut with cruciates well protected.

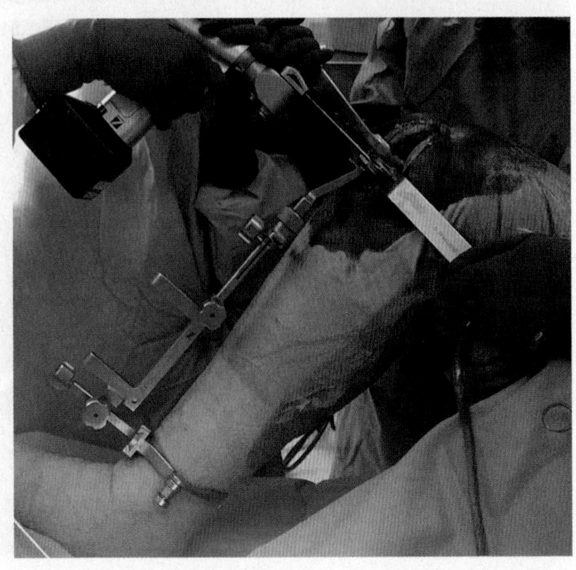

FIGURE 37-8

Horizontal cut passing 1 to 2 mm below the deepest part of the wear within the compartment.

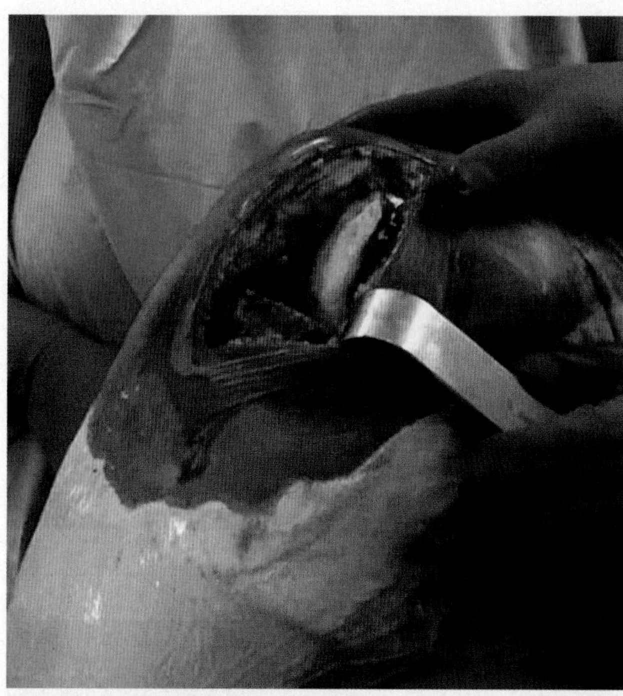

FIGURE 37-9
Completed tibial cuts.

Once sufficient bone has been removed from the tibia to accommodate the tibial template, attention is turned to cutting and sizing the femoral component. A spacer block with parallel cutting guide is placed within the joint space and the knee taken to full extension (Fig. 37-10). With the long alignment rod positioned along the mechanical axis of the lower extremity (from a point 2 finger breadths medial to the anterior superior iliac spine, through the knee, and then along the crest of the tibial shaft), the distal femoral cut is made parallel to the previous tibial cut and perpendicular to the mechanical axis (Fig. 37-11). Using this cut, a femoral finishing guide is selected that is 1 to 2 mm smaller than the outer margin of the cut bone, taking care to avoid patellar impingement. This is pinned in place and the femoral chamfer cuts performed (Fig. 37-12), thus completing the femoral cuts (Fig. 37-13).

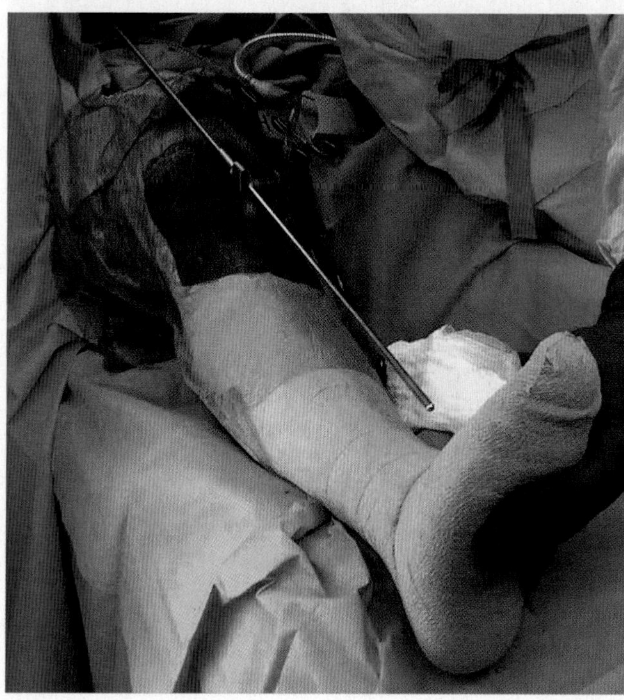

FIGURE 37-10
Positioning of the long alignment rod.

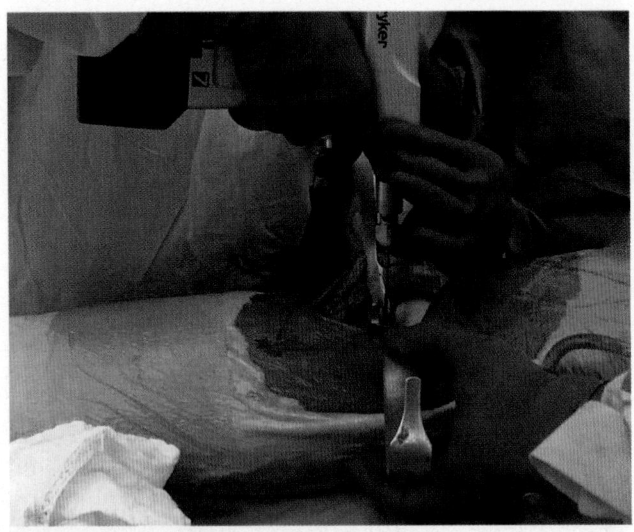

FIGURE 37-11
Distal femoral cut made parallel to the previous tibial cut and perpendicular to the mechanical axis.

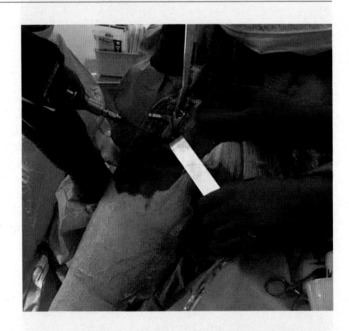

FIGURE 37-12
Completing the femoral chamfer cuts.

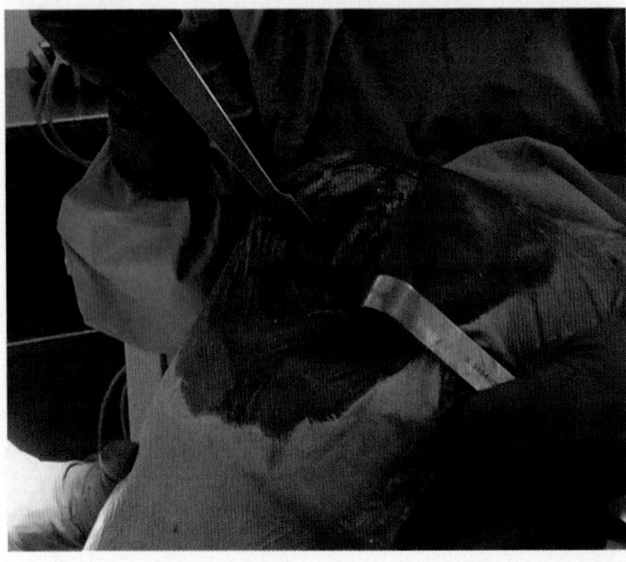

FIGURE 37-13
Both tibial and femoral cuts completed.

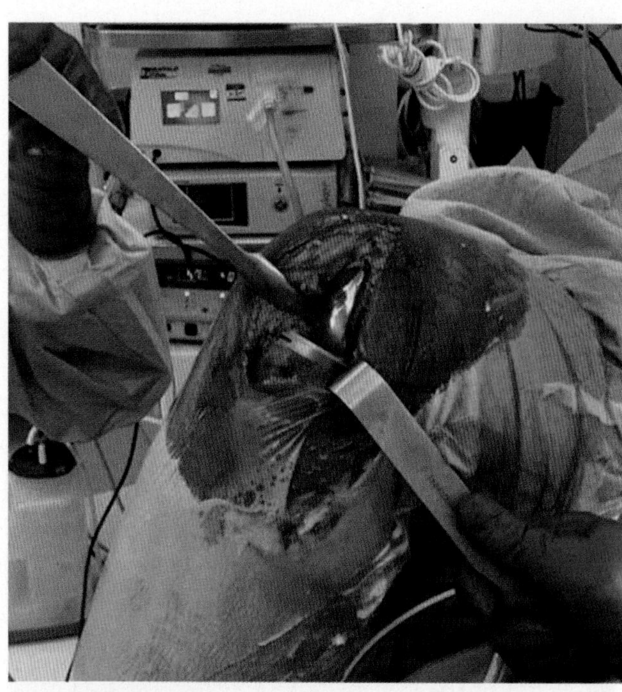

FIGURE 37-14
Final components in place.

Alternatively, for an intramedullary alignment system, the knee is flexed approximately 45 degrees, and a hole is made into the intramedullary canal of the femur with an awl or drill. The correct starting point for intramedullary insertion is approximately 1 cm anterior to the anteromedial corner of the intercondylar notch above the PCL insertion. The femoral drill guide is then inserted and positioned such that it lies in the middle of the condyle and is parallel with the long axis of the tibia. Flexion and extension, in addition to internal and external rotation of the tibia, are used to ensure drill guide position. The drill is then passed and the femoral saw block placed into the drilled holes. The posterior facet of the femoral condyle and distal femur cuts are then made.

After completion of tibial and femoral cuts and final lug hole drilling for the components, flexion and extension gaps are then measured and balanced, and appropriate trial components are selected. Trial components must be flushed to bone, and then a trial meniscal bearing of chosen thickness is inserted. With the bearing in place, the knee is taken through a full range of motion to test stability of the joint and bearing, ensuring the absence of impingement. The thickness of the bearing should be such that the ligaments are at their natural state of tension at both 90 degrees of flexion and full extension. Once the knee has been appropriately balanced in extension and flexion, components are selected, and the femoral and tibial surfaces are power irrigated to prepare for cementing. The tibial component is inserted first from posterior to anterior so that excess cement can be removed anteriorly with a small curette. The femoral component is then applied to the condyle and impacted with excess cement removed in a similar fashion, thus completing component insertion (Fig. 37-14). Following cement hardening, the trial bearing is replaced with the final bearing, although we typically place the final bearing surface prior to tibial component insertion. A final examination of the knee is performed, testing range of motion and stability. Visual inspection for appropriate component positioning and articulation is then performed (Figs. 37-14 and 37-15). The knee is then thoroughly irrigated and closed in layers in standard fashion.

POSTOPERATIVE MANAGEMENT

Early mobilization and range of motion are the primary goal of the postoperative rehabilitation program. Knee range-of-motion exercises with progressively increasing flexion are key. Patients are allowed to be immediately weight bearing as tolerated. Early discharge from the hospital is typical. Many patients are now managed as outpatients. Formal physical therapy can be initiated soon postoperatively, although is not necessary for a successful outcome (10). Knee range of motion is examined in postoperative visits, and emphasis is placed on continued range-of-motion

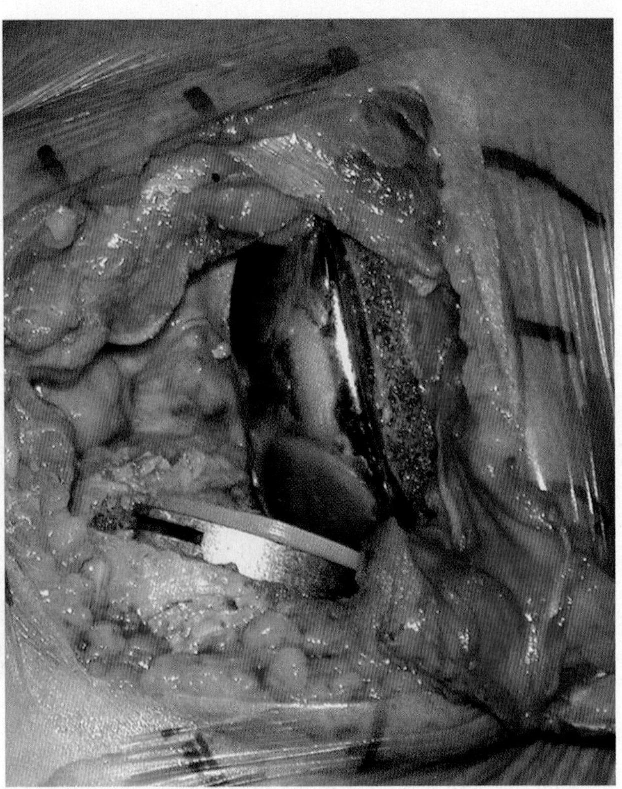

FIGURE 37-15

Intraoperative photograph of a medial unicompartmental knee arthroplasty, with final components in place.

gains (Fig. 37-16). Return to light recreational activities can be initiated in a matter of weeks postoperatively, although patients are advised to avoid repetitive high-impact activity and particularly strenuous athletics in the interest of component longevity. Low-impact activities or lateral movement sports are preferred, such as swimming, cycling, golf, tennis, and skiing.

Each patient should have clinical follow-up to assess appropriate progression in muscular conditioning and restoration. If patients lack the appropriate muscle tone or control, particularly quadriceps and hamstring function, then return to sport is delayed until appropriate muscular function can be assured.

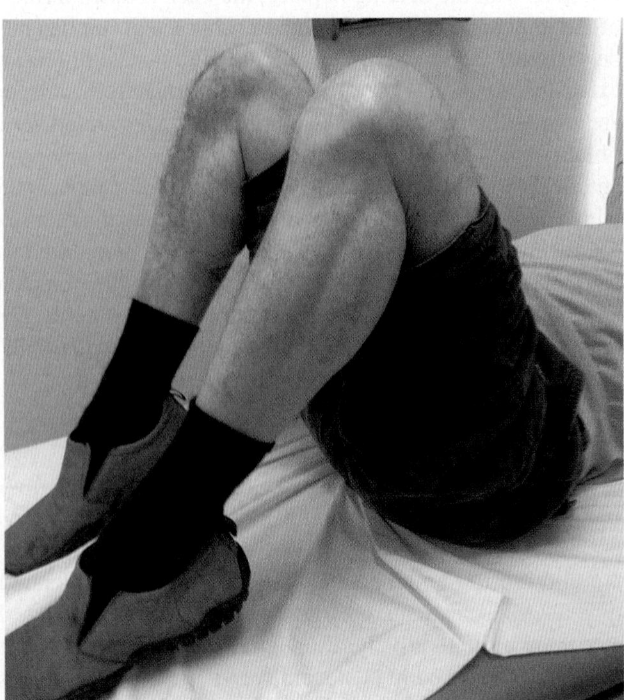

FIGURE 37-16

Clinical photograph of a 61-year-old active male 6 weeks status postmedial UKA, demonstrating successful return to symmetric knee flexion.

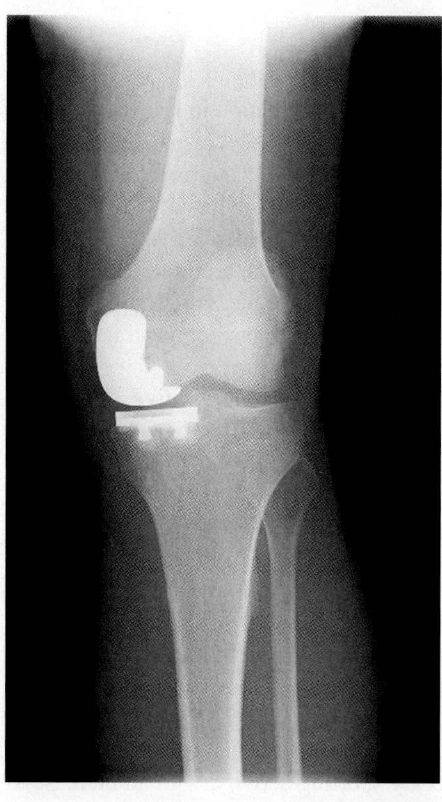

FIGURE 37-17

AP radiograph of the left knee of a 61-year-old active male, 6 weeks status postmedial UKA.

Radiographic follow-up is also important to closely screen for component loosening, change in position, or imminent failure (3) (Figs. 37-17 and 37-18).

RESULTS

Numerous studies have shown favorable outcomes in UKA, particularly in return to activity. With UKAs being performed in younger patients with significant return to sporting activity postoperatively, concern regarding implant longevity may be elicited. However, studies have demonstrated excellent implant survivorship, showing UKA provides early and high levels of return to sports without sacrificing longevity.

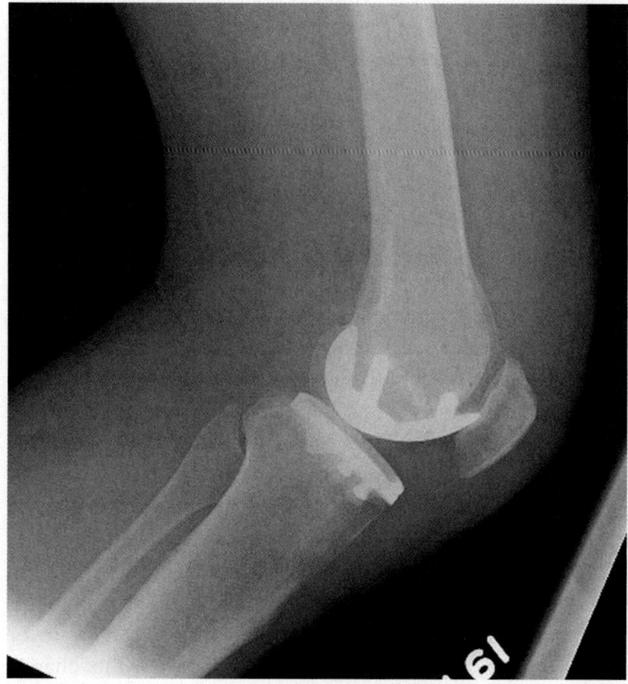

FIGURE 37-18

Lateral radiograph of the left knee of a 61-year-old active male, 6 weeks status postmedial UKA.

Activity

Remarkable return to activity was shown by Naal et al. in a group of 83 patients having undergone UKA. The return to activity rate, as measured by patient-reported participation in sporting endeavors before and after surgery, was noted to be 95%. The vast majority (90%) of patients reported that UKA had maintained or improved their ability to participate in sport and recreation. These authors did note a decrease in the variety of activities performed, which likely resulted from a shift by the patients away from high-impact activities (3). Fisher et al. also demonstrated a superior level of return to sports with a metal backed mobile bearing UKA in 76 patients, at a rate of 93% (11). Similarly, Pietschmann et al. found that 80% of 131 patients studied after medial UKA returned to preoperative level of sports at a mean follow-up of 4 years, and the patients demonstrated a shift from away from high-impact sports postoperatively.

Further evidence demonstrating excellent return to activity for the athletically active after lateral UKA was noted by Walker et al. (12). In a group of 45 patients at mean follow-up of 3 years, 98% of patients returned to recreational activity after lateral UKA, and two-thirds of the patients reached a high activity level postoperatively based on the University of California, Los Angeles (UCLA), activity scale. Similar to the trend seen in medial UKA, patients returned to low- and medium-impact recreational activities at the greatest levels, with high-impact activity avoided (12).

The younger and athletically active patient was also shown to do very well after UKA by Biswas et al. (8). Seventy-five patients underwent medial UKA at a mean age of 49 years and were evaluated prospectively. At a mean of 4 years, the Knee Society score improved from a mean of 49 points preoperatively to a mean of 95.1 points postoperatively, and the mean UCLA activity score was 7.5 (range 5 to 9). The estimated survivorship for the group was 96.5% at 10 years (8).

Jahnke et al. (13) recently demonstrated increased levels of sport participation after UKA. Preoperatively, 100 out of 135 patients participated in weekly sporting activity, with an increase to 114 patients participating in sports weekly at an average of 2 years after surgery. Low- to medium-impact activities such as hiking, cycling, and swimming saw the greatest increase in participation postoperatively. Interestingly, the greatest increase in sport participation postoperatively was seen in those patients with higher body mass index, although the authors note this is likely due to much lower preoperative activity level in this population (13). Overall, this study supports the use of UKA for the athletically active patient, with evidence that sport participation can actually be increased by the procedure.

Survivorship

A combination of excellent return to activity and implant longevity after UKA was demonstrated by Felts et al. (14). Sixty-five UKAs were performed in 62 patients younger than 60. At a mean follow-up of 11.2 years, the average functional and activity scores increased, 83% of the patients returned to their previous sport activities, and 90% reported no or slight limitation during sporting endeavors. In addition, the 12-year Kaplan-Meier survivorship was 94%. A similar study by Pennington et al. (9) also demonstrated excellent survivorship in younger patients, expanding the indications for UKA. Forty-five knees, which had undergone UKA at an age younger than 60 years, were followed for a mean duration of 11 years. Thirty-nine of the 45 knees (93%) had excellent outcome scores, and Kaplan-Meier analysis showed 11-year survivorship at 92% (9).

Excellent long-term results were reported by Berger et al. in a series of 49 cemented modular unicompartmental knees followed for a minimum of 10 years, with 45/49 (92%) of knees having a good or excellent result. Only two knees with well-fixed components were revised to TKA because of progression of patellofemoral arthritis, making overall survival 96% (2).

Longer-term data are also encouraging. Nineteen cemented fixed bearing UKA knees in 16 patients were noted to have 15-year survivorship of 93%, with no patients presenting with aseptic loosening or osteolysis, similar to that reported for TKA (15).

A recent comprehensive meta-analysis of randomized controlled trials of UKA versus TKA (16) showed that in three studies, the UKA group had function scores better than the TKA group, but to a degree that did not reach statistical significance. Two studies compared the mean values of maximum knee flexion between UKA and TKA with no significant difference found.

Of note, the risk of complications was lower in the UKA group with an RR of 0.39 when compared to the TKA group. Thus, the likelihood of having a postoperative complication was 60% lower after a UKA than a TKA. The risk of revision surgery was higher in the UKA group, with a chance of requiring revision approximately 5.4 times higher in the UKA group versus the TKA group. However, this noted that high risk of revision data comes from two of the three articles reviewed regarding this outcome. In the trial by Sun and Jia, all the revisions of the UKAs were within the first 2 years of the procedure being performed by the authors, and in the article itself, the need for the UKA revisions was attributed to technical failures and a steep learning curve (17). In the article by Costa et al., all of the prostheses that failed had an all-polyethylene tibial component, a very specific type of UKA and one whose survivorship data may not be generalizable to other UKA prosthesis designs (18). Therefore, the quoted risk of revision from the meta-analysis stems from one study in which the revisions were attributed to user error, and another in which one particular component design showed a high early failure rate.

The third article included in the meta-analysis regarding revision rates, by Newman et al., showed only a 1.04 RR of revision in UKA versus TKA, an article in which UKA patients were shown to have less perioperative morbidity, regain knee movement more rapidly, and have earlier hospital discharge, with the overall finding that UKA has better results than TKA through at least 5 years (19). Additionally, in a follow-up study of that same cohort, the better early results with UKA were upheld at 15 years, with a 15-year survivorship rate of 89.8% for UKA versus 78.7% for TKA (20).

CONCLUSIONS

Unicompartmental arthroplasty is a procedure that can produce excellent results in patients with symptoms and degeneration in the knee confined to a single compartment. The procedure has seen a recent increase in interest due to expanding indications with successful outcomes, particularly for younger, active patients.

Despite the broadening indications, several key prerequisites exist for UKA, including pain isolated to the compartment in question and noninflammatory arthropathy. Careful patient selection and meticulous surgical technique are key factors in optimizing patient outcome.

The less invasive nature of the surgery and the accelerated return to activity are beneficial for all patients, with particular appeal for the younger, active patient who desires rapid return to activity. The procedure provides a shorter hospital stay and recovery period and has been shown to have an overall excellent rate of return to activity. We perform the procedure routinely now as an outpatient in the absence of serious medical comorbidities. As the procedure continues to evolve and indications expand for younger patients, it will continue to benefit the athletically active patient and provide pain relief and rapid return to activity.

REFERENCES

1. Kozinn SC, Scott R. Unicondylar knee arthroplasty. *J Bone Joint Surg Am.* 1989;71(1):145–150.
2. Berger RA, Meneghini RM, Jacobs JJ, et al. Results of unicompartmental knee arthroplasty at a minimum of ten years of follow-up. *J Bone Joint Surg Am.* 2005;87(5):999–1006.
3. Naal FD, Fischer M, Preuss A, et al. Return to sports and recreational activity after unicompartmental knee arthroplasty. *Am J Sports Med.* 2007;35(10):1688–1695.
4. Borus T, Thornhill T. Unicompartmental knee arthroplasty. *J Am Acad Orthop Surg.* 2008;16(1):9–18.
5. Price AJ, Waite JC, Svard U. Long-term clinical results of the medial oxford unicompartmental knee arthroplasty. *Clin Orthop Relat Res.* 2005;435:171–180.
6. Engh GA, Ammeen DJ. Unicondylar arthroplasty in knees with deficient anterior cruciate ligaments. *Clin Orthop Relat Res.* 2014;472(1):73–77. doi:10.1007/s11999-013-2982-y.
7. Hernigou P, Deschamps G. Posterior slope of the tibial implant and the outcome of unicompartmental knee arthroplasty. *J Bone Joint Surg Am.* 2004;86-A(3):506–511.
8. Biswas D, Van Thiel GS, Wetters NG, et al. Medial unicompartmental knee arthroplasty in patients less than 55 years old: minimum of two years of follow-up. *J Arthroplasty.* 2014;29(1):101–105. doi:10.1016/j.arth.2013.04.046.
9. Pennington DW, Swienckowski JJ, Lutes WB, et al. Unicompartmental knee arthroplasty in patients sixty years of age or younger. *J Bone Joint Surg Am.* 2003;85-A(10):1968–1973.
10. Munk S, Dalsgaard J, Bjerggaard K, et al. Early recovery after fast-track oxford unicompartmental knee arthroplasty. 35 patients with minimal invasive surgery. *Acta Orthop.* 2012;83(1):41–45. doi:10.3109/17453674.2012.657578.
11. Fisher N, Agarwal M, Reuben SF, et al. Sporting and physical activity following oxford medial unicompartmental knee arthroplasty. *Knee.* 2006;13(4):296–300.
12. Walker T, Gotterbarm T, Bruckner T, et al. Return to sports, recreational activity and patient-reported outcomes after lateral unicompartmental knee arthroplasty. *Knee Surg Sports Traumatol Arthrosc.* 2015;23(11):3281–3287. doi:10.1007/s00167-014-3111-5.
13. Jahnke A, Mende JK, Maier GS, et al. Sports activities before and after medial unicompartmental knee arthroplasty using the new Heidelberg sports activity score. *Int Orthop.* 2015;39(3):449–454. doi:10.1007/s00264-014-2524-6.
14. Felts E, Parratte S, Pauly V, et al. Function and quality of life following medial unicompartmental knee arthroplasty in patients 60 years of age or younger. *Orthop Traumatol Surg Res.* 2010;96(8):861–867. doi:10.1016/j.otsr.2010.05.012.

15. Foran JR, Brown NM, Della Valle CJ, et al. Long-term survivorship and failure modes of unicompartmental knee arthroplasty. *Clin Orthop Relat Res.* 2013;471(1):102–108. doi:10.1007/s11999-012-2517-y.
16. Arirachakaran A, Choowit P, Putananon C, et al. Is unicompartmental knee arthroplasty (UKA) superior to total knee arthroplasty (TKA)? A systematic review and meta-analysis of randomized controlled trial. *Eur J Orthop Surg Traumatol.* 2015;25(5):799–806. doi:10.1007/s00590-015-1610-9.
17. Sun PF, Jia YH. Mobile bearing UKA compared to fixed bearing TKA: a randomized prospective study. *Knee.* 2012;19(2):103–106. doi:10.1016/j.knee.2011.01.006.
18. Costa CR, Johnson AJ, Mont MA, et al. Unicompartmental and total knee arthroplasty in the same patient. *J Knee Surg.* 2011;24(4):273–278.
19. Newman JH, Ackroyd CE, Shah NA. Unicompartmental or total knee replacement? Five-year results of a prospective, randomised trial of 102 osteoarthritic knees with unicompartmental arthritis. *J Bone Joint Surg Br.* 1998;80(5):862–865.
20. Newman J, Pydisetty RV, Ackroyd C. Unicompartmental or total knee replacement: the 15-year results of a prospective randomised controlled trial. *J Bone Joint Surg Br.* 2009;91(1):52–57. doi:10.1302/0301-620X.91B1.20899.

Index

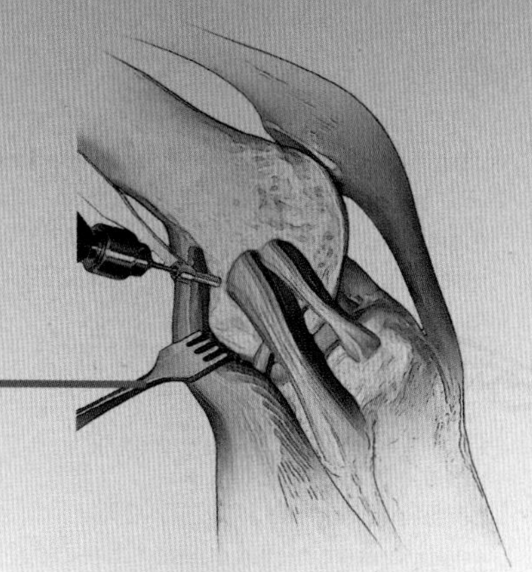

Note: Page numbers in italics denote figures; those followed by "t" denote tables.

B

C